WHO Classification of Tumours

Central Nervous System Tumours

WHO Classification of Tumours Editorial Board

International Agency for Research on Cancer

 World Health Organization

Suggested citation

WHO Classification of Tumours Editorial Board. Central nervous system tumours.
Lyon (France): International Agency for Research on Cancer; 2021.
(WHO classification of tumours series, 5th ed.; vol. 6).
https://publications.iarc.fr/601.

Sales, rights, and permissions

Print copies are distributed by WHO Press, World Health Organization, 20 Avenue Appia, 1211 Geneva 27, Switzerland
Tel.: +41 22 791 3264; Fax: +41 22 791 4857; email: bookorders@who.int; website: https://whobluebooks.iarc.fr

To purchase IARC publications in electronic format, see the IARC Publications website (https://publications.iarc.fr).

Requests for permission to reproduce or translate IARC publications – whether for sale or for non-commercial distribution – should be submitted
through the IARC Publications website (https://publications.iarc.fr/Rights-And-Permissions).

Third-party materials

If you wish to reuse material from this work that is attributed to a third party, such as figures, tables, or boxes, it is your responsibility to determine
whether permission is needed for that reuse and to obtain permission from the copyright holder. See *Sources*, pages 493–499. The risk of claims
resulting from infringement of any third-party-owned component in the work rests solely with the user.

General disclaimers

The designations employed and the presentation of the material in this publication do not imply the expression of any opinion whatsoever on the
part of WHO or contributing agencies concerning the legal status of any country, territory, city, or area, or of its authorities, or concerning the
delimitation of its frontiers or boundaries. Dotted and dashed lines on maps represent approximate border lines for which there may not yet be full
agreement.

The mention of specific companies or of certain manufacturers' products does not imply that they are endorsed or recommended by WHO or
contributing agencies in preference to others of a similar nature that are not mentioned. Errors and omissions excepted, the names of proprietary
products are distinguished by initial capital letters.

All reasonable precautions have been taken by WHO to verify the information contained in this publication. However, the published material is
being distributed without warranty of any kind, either expressed or implied. The responsibility for the interpretation and use of the material lies with
the reader. In no event shall WHO or contributing agencies be liable for damages arising from its use.

First print run (7500 copies)

Updated corrigenda can be found at https://publications.iarc.fr

IARC Library Cataloguing-in-Publication Data

Names: WHO Classification of Tumours Editorial Board.
Title: Central nervous system tumours / edited by WHO Classification of Tumours Editorial Board.
Description: Fifth edition. | Lyon: International Agency for Research on Cancer, 2021. | Series: World Health Organization classification of tumours.
  | Includes bibliographical references and index.
Identifiers: ISBN 9789283245087 (pbk.) | ISBN 9789283245094 (ebook)
Subjects: MESH: Central Nervous System Neoplasms.
Classification: NLM WL 15

This volume was produced in collaboration with

The Consortium to Inform Molecular and Practical Approaches to
CNS Tumor Taxonomy (cIMPACT)

The WHO classification of central nervous system tumours presented in this book reflects
the views of the WHO Classification of Tumours Editorial Board that convened
via video conference 24–26 August 2020.

For the complete list of all contributors and their affiliations, see pages 483–488.

The WHO Classification of Tumours Editorial Board (continued)

For the complete list of all contributors and their affiliations, see pages 483–488.

WHO Classification of Tumours
Central Nervous System Tumours

Edited by	The WHO Classification of Tumours Editorial Board
IARC Editors	Ian A. Cree
	Dilani Lokuhetty
	Laura A.N. Peferoen
	Valerie A. White
Epidemiology	Ariana Znaor
Project Assistant	Asiedua Asante
Assistants	Anne-Sophie Hameau
	Laura Brispot
Technical Editing	Jessica Cox
	Julia Slone-Murphy
Principal Information Assistant	Alberto Machado
Information Assistant	Catarina Marques
Layout	Meaghan Fortune
Radiology Advisor	Sona A. Pungavkar, Global Hospitals, Mumbai, India
Printed by	Maestro Gestion D'Edition
	69100 Villeurbanne, France
	Printed in Italy
Publisher	International Agency for Research on Cancer (IARC)
	150 Cours Albert Thomas
	69372 Lyon Cedex 08, France

Contents

List of abbreviations

AIDS	acquired immunodeficiency syndrome
AMT PET	α-[11C]methyl-L-tryptophan positron emission tomography
ATP	adenosine triphosphate
bp	base pair(s)
cAMP	cyclic adenosine monophosphate
CBTRUS	Central Brain Tumor Registry of the United States
cIMPACT	Consortium to Inform Molecular and Practical Approaches to CNS Tumor Taxonomy
CMV	cytomegalovirus
CNS	central nervous system
COG	Children's Oncology Group
CSF	cerebrospinal fluid
CT	computed tomography
DNA	deoxyribonucleic acid
EBV	Epstein–Barr virus
ER	estrogen receptor
EU-RHAB	European Rhabdoid Registry
FDG PET	18F-fluorodeoxyglucose positron emission tomography
FET PET	18F-fluoroethyltyrosine positron emission tomography
FISH	fluorescence in situ hybridization
FLAIR	fluid-attenuated inversion recovery
FNA	fine-needle aspiration
G-CIMP	glioma CpG island methylator phenotype
H&E	haematoxylin and eosin
HBV	hepatitis B virus
HGVS	Human Genome Variation Society
HHV6	human herpesvirus 6
HIV	human immunodeficiency virus
HPF	high-power field(s)
HPV	human papillomavirus
HTLV	human T-lymphotropic virus
IARC	International Agency for Research on Cancer
ICD-11	International Classification of Diseases, 11th revision
ICD-O	International Classification of Diseases for Oncology
ICD-O-3	International Classification of Diseases for Oncology, 3rd edition
Ig	immunoglobulin
ITD	internal tandem duplication
M:F ratio	male-to-female ratio
MALT	mucosa-associated lymphoid tissue
MALT lymphoma	extranodal marginal zone lymphoma of mucosa-associated lymphoid tissue
MIM number	Mendelian Inheritance in Man number
MITF	melanogenesis-associated transcription factor
MRI	magnetic resonance imaging
mRNA	messenger ribonucleic acid
N:C ratio	nuclear-to-cytoplasmic ratio
NCCN	National Comprehensive Cancer Network
NEC	not elsewhere classified
NOS	not otherwise specified
NSE	neuron-specific enolase
OS	overall survival
PAS	periodic acid–Schiff
PCR	polymerase chain reaction
PCV	procarbazine, lomustine, and vincristine
PET	positron emission tomography
PET-CT	positron emission tomography–computed tomography
PFA	posterior fossa group A
PFB	posterior fossa group B
PFS	progression-free survival
PR	progesterone receptor
RNA	ribonucleic acid
RT-PCR	reverse transcriptase polymerase chain reaction
SEER Program	Surveillance, Epidemiology, and End Results Program
SNP	single-nucleotide polymorphism
SSTR PET	somatostatin receptor positron emission tomography
TAM	tumour-associated macrophage
TKD	tyrosine kinase domain
TNM	tumour, node, metastasis
Treg cell	T regulatory cell
tRNA	transfer ribonucleic acid
t-SNE	t-distributed stochastic neighbour embedding
VATER/VACTERL association	vertebral defects, anal atresia, cardiac malformations, tracheo-oesophageal fistula with oesophageal atresia, radial or renal dysplasia, and limb abnormalities

Foreword

The WHO Classification of Tumours, published as a series of books (also known as the WHO Blue Books) and now as a website (https://tumourclassification.iarc.who.int), is an essential tool for standardizing diagnostic practice worldwide. It also serves as a vehicle for the translation of cancer research into practice. The diagnostic criteria and standards that make up the classification are underpinned by evidence evaluated and debated by experts in the field. About 200 authors and editors participate in the production of each book, and they give their time freely to this task. I am very grateful for their help; it is a remarkable team effort.

This sixth volume of the fifth edition of the WHO Blue Books has, like the preceding five, been led by the WHO Classification of Tumours Editorial Board, composed of standing and expert members. The standing members, who have been nominated by pathology organizations, are the equivalent of the series editors of previous editions. The expert members for each volume, equivalent to the volume editors of previous editions, are selected on the basis of informed bibliometric analysis and advice from the standing members. The diagnostic process is increasingly multidisciplinary, and we are delighted that several radiology and clinical experts have joined us to address specific needs.

The most conspicuous change to the format of the books in the fifth edition is that tumour types common to multiple systems are dealt with together – so there are separate chapters on mesenchymal (non-meningothelial) tumours, melanocytic tumours, haematolymphoid tumours, and germ cell tumours. There is also a chapter on genetic tumour syndromes. Genetic disorders are of increasing importance to diagnosis in individual patients, and the study of these disorders has undoubtedly informed our understanding of tumour biology and behaviour over the past decade.

We have attempted to take a more systematic approach to the multifaceted nature of tumour classification; each tumour type is described on the basis of its localization, clinical features, epidemiology, etiology, pathogenesis, histopathology, diagnostic molecular pathology, staging, and prognosis and prediction. We have also included information on macroscopic appearance and cytology, as well as essential and desirable diagnostic criteria. This standardized, modular approach makes it easier for the books to be accessible online, but it also enables us to call attention to areas in which there is little information, and where serious gaps in our knowledge remain to be addressed.

The organization of the WHO Blue Books content now follows the normal progression from benign to malignant – a break with the fourth edition, but one we hope will be welcome.

The volumes are still organized by anatomical site (digestive system, breast, soft tissue and bone, etc.), and each tumour type is listed within a hierarchical taxonomic classification that follows the format below, which helps to structure the books in a systematic manner:

Site: e.g. CNS embryonal tumours

    Category: e.g. medulloblastoma

        Family (class): e.g. molecularly defined medulloblastomas

            Type: e.g. SHH-activated and *TP53*-wildtype medulloblastoma

                Subtype: e.g. provisional molecular subgroup SHH-1

The issue of whether a given tumour type represents a distinct entity rather than a subtype continues to exercise pathologists, and it is the topic of many publications in the literature. We continue to deal with this issue on a case-by-case basis, but we believe there are inherent rules that can be applied. For example, tumours in which multiple histological patterns contain shared truncal mutations are clearly of the same type, despite the differences in their appearance. Equally, genetic heterogeneity within the same tumour type may have implications for treatment. A small shift in terminology in the fifth edition is that the term "variant" in reference to a specific kind of tumour has been wholly superseded by "subtype", in an effort to more clearly differentiate this meaning from that of "variant" in reference to a genetic alteration.

Another important change in this edition of the WHO Classification of Tumours series is the conversion of mitotic count from the traditional denominator of 10 HPF to a defined area expressed in mm^2. This serves to standardize the true area over which mitoses are enumerated, because different microscopes have high-power fields of different sizes. This change will also be helpful for anyone reporting using digital systems.

We are continually working to improve the consistency and standards within the classification. In addition to having moved to the International System of Units (SI) for all mitotic counts, we have standardized genomic nomenclature by using Human Genome Variation Society (HGVS) notation. For CNS tumours, mutation of histone genes is of particular importance, and we have incorporated the latest nomenclature to ensure that histone sequence variants have an unambiguous description in the classification. We have also further standardized our use of units of length, adopting the convention used by the International Collaboration on

Cancer Reporting (http://www.iccr-cancer.org) and the UK Royal College of Pathologists (https://www.rcpath.org/), so that the size of tumours is now given exclusively in millimetres (mm) rather than centimetres (cm). This is clearer, in our view, and avoids the use of decimal points – a common source of medical errors.

The WHO Blue Books are much appreciated by pathologists and of increasing importance to practitioners of other clinical disciplines involved in cancer management, as well as to researchers. The editorial board and I certainly hope that the series will continue to meet the need for standards in diagnosis and to facilitate the translation of diagnostic research into practice worldwide. It is particularly important that cancers continue to be classified and diagnosed according to the same standards internationally so that patients can benefit from multicentre clinical trials, as well as from the results of local trials conducted on different continents.

Dr Ian A. Cree

Head, WHO Classification of Tumours Programme
International Agency for Research on Cancer
November 2021

ICD-O topographical coding of central nervous system tumours

The ICD-O topography codes for the main anatomical sites covered in this volume are as follows {990}:

C70 Meninges
    C70.0 Cerebral meninges
    C70.1 Spinal meninges
    C70.9 Meninges, NOS

C71 Brain
    C71.0 Cerebrum
    C71.1 Frontal lobe
    C71.2 Temporal lobe
    C71.3 Parietal lobe
    C71.4 Occipital lobe
    C71.5 Ventricle, NOS
    C71.6 Cerebellum, NOS
    C71.7 Brain stem
    C71.8 Overlapping lesion of brain
    C71.9 Brain, NOS

C72 Spinal cord, cranial nerves, and other parts of central nervous system
    C72.0 Spinal cord
    C72.1 Cauda equina
    C72.2 Olfactory nerve
    C72.3 Optic nerve
    C72.4 Acoustic nerve
    C72.5 Cranial nerve, NOS
    C72.8 Overlapping lesion of brain and central nervous system
    C72.9 Nervous system, NOS

C75 Other endocrine glands and related structures
    C75.1 Pituitary gland
    C75.2 Craniopharyngeal duct
    C75.3 Pineal gland

ICD-O morphological coding: Introduction

The ICD-O coding system uses a topography (T) code and a morphology (M) code together, but these are presented in separate lists for ease of use. Behaviour is coded /0 for benign tumours; /1 for unspecified, borderline, or uncertain behaviour; /2 for carcinoma in situ and grade III intraepithelial neoplasia; /3 for malignant tumours, primary site; and /6 for malignant tumours, metastatic site. Behaviour code /6 is not generally used by cancer registries. For various reasons, the ICD-O morphology terms may not always be identical to the entity names used in the WHO classification, but they should be sufficiently similar to avoid confusion. The designation "NOS" ("not otherwise specified") is provided to make coding possible when subtypes exist but exact classification may not be possible in small biopsies or certain other scenarios. Therefore, it is usual to have "NOS" even when a more specific alternative term is listed in ICD-O.

ICD-O coding of central nervous system tumours

ICD-O-3.2   ICD-O label (subtypes are indicated in grey text, with the label indented);
Please note that the WHO classification of tumour types is more readily reflected in the table of contents

Gliomas, glioneuronal tumours, and neuronal tumours
Adult-type diffuse gliomas

	Astrocytoma, IDH-mutant
9400/3	Astrocytoma, IDH-mutant, grade 2
9401/3	Astrocytoma, IDH-mutant, grade 3
9445/3	Astrocytoma, IDH-mutant, grade 4
	Oligodendroglioma, IDH-mutant and 1p/19q-codeleted
9450/3	Oligodendroglioma, IDH-mutant and 1p/19q-codeleted, grade 2
9451/3	Oligodendroglioma, IDH-mutant and 1p/19q-codeleted, grade 3
9440/3	Glioblastoma, IDH-wildtype

Paediatric-type diffuse low-grade gliomas

9421/1	Diffuse astrocytoma, *MYB-* or *MYBL1*-altered[†]
9431/1	Angiocentric glioma
9413/0	Polymorphous low-grade neuroepithelial tumour of the young[†]
9421/1	Diffuse low-grade glioma, MAPK pathway–altered[†]

Paediatric-type diffuse high-grade gliomas

9385/3	Diffuse midline glioma, H3 K27–altered[†]
9385/3	Diffuse hemispheric glioma, H3 G34–mutant[†]
9385/3	Diffuse paediatric-type high-grade glioma, H3-wildtype and IDH-wildtype[†]
9385/3	Infant-type hemispheric glioma[†]

Circumscribed astrocytic gliomas

9421/1	Pilocytic astrocytoma
9421/3*	High-grade astrocytoma with piloid features
9424/3	Pleomorphic xanthoastrocytoma
9384/1	Subependymal giant cell astrocytoma
9444/1	Chordoid glioma
9430/3	Astroblastoma, *MN1*-altered[†]

Glioneuronal and neuronal tumours

9505/1	Ganglioglioma
9492/0	Gangliocytoma
9412/1	Desmoplastic infantile ganglioglioma
9412/1	Desmoplastic infantile astrocytoma
9413/0	Dysembryoplastic neuroepithelial tumour
n/a	Diffuse glioneuronal tumour with oligodendroglioma-like features and nuclear clusters (provisional entity)
9509/1	Papillary glioneuronal tumour
9509/1	Rosette-forming glioneuronal tumour
9509/1	Myxoid glioneuronal tumour[†]
9509/3*	Diffuse leptomeningeal glioneuronal tumour
9509/0*	Multinodular and vacuolating neuronal tumour
9493/0	Dysplastic cerebellar gangliocytoma (Lhermitte–Duclos disease)
9506/1	Central neurocytoma
9506/1	Extraventricular neurocytoma
9506/1	Cerebellar liponeurocytoma

Ependymal tumours

9391/3	Supratentorial ependymoma, NOS[†]
9396/3	Supratentorial ependymoma, *ZFTA* fusion–positive[†]
9396/3	Supratentorial ependymoma, *YAP1* fusion–positive[†]
9391/3	Posterior fossa ependymoma, NOS[†]
9396/3	Posterior fossa group A (PFA) ependymoma[†]
9396/3	Posterior fossa group B (PFB) ependymoma[†]
9391/3	Spinal ependymoma, NOS[†]
9396/3	Spinal ependymoma, *MYCN*-amplified[†]
9394/1	Myxopapillary ependymoma
9383/1	Subependymoma

Choroid plexus tumours

9390/0	Choroid plexus papilloma
9390/1	Atypical choroid plexus papilloma
9390/3	Choroid plexus carcinoma

Embryonal tumours

Medulloblastomas, molecularly defined

9475/3	Medulloblastoma, WNT-activated
9471/3	Medulloblastoma, SHH-activated and *TP53*-wildtype
9476/3	Medulloblastoma, SHH-activated and *TP53*-mutant
9477/3	Medulloblastoma, non-WNT/non-SHH

Medulloblastomas, histologically defined

9470/3	Medulloblastoma, histologically defined
9471/3	Desmoplastic nodular medulloblastoma
9471/3	Medulloblastoma with extensive nodularity
9474/3	Large cell medulloblastoma
9474/3	Anaplastic medulloblastoma

Other CNS embryonal tumours

9508/3	Atypical teratoid/rhabdoid tumour
n/a	Cribriform neuroepithelial tumour (provisional entity)
9478/3	Embryonal tumour with multilayered rosettes
9500/3	CNS neuroblastoma, *FOXR2*-activated[†]
9500/3	CNS tumour with *BCOR* internal tandem duplication[†]
9473/3	CNS embryonal tumour, NEC/NOS

Pineal tumours

9361/1	Pineocytoma
9362/3	Pineal parenchymal tumour of intermediate differentiation
9362/3	Pineoblastoma
9395/3	Papillary tumour of the pineal region
n/a	Desmoplastic myxoid tumour of the pineal region, *SMARCB1*-mutant (provisional entity)

Cranial and paraspinal nerve tumours

9560/0	Schwannoma
9540/0	Neurofibroma
9550/0	Plexiform neurofibroma
9571/0	Perineurioma
9563/0	Hybrid nerve sheath tumour
9540/3	Malignant melanotic nerve sheath tumour
9540/3	Malignant peripheral nerve sheath tumour
8693/3	Cauda equina neuroendocrine tumour (previously paraganglioma)

Meningioma

9530/0	Meningioma

Mesenchymal, non-meningothelial tumours involving the CNS

Fibroblastic and myofibroblastic tumours

8815/1	Solitary fibrous tumour

Vascular tumours

9121/0	Cavernous haemangioma
9131/0	Capillary haemangioma
9123/0	Arteriovenous malformation
9161/1	Haemangioblastoma

Skeletal muscle tumours

8910/3	Embryonal rhabdomyosarcoma
8920/3	Alveolar rhabdomyosarcoma
8901/3	Rhabdomyosarcoma, pleomorphic-type
8912/3	Spindle cell rhabdomyosarcoma

Tumours of uncertain differentiation

n/a	Intracranial mesenchymal tumour, FET::CREB fusion–positive (provisional entity)
9367/3	*CIC*-rearranged sarcoma
9480/3	Primary intracranial sarcoma, *DICER1*-mutant[†]
9364/3	Ewing sarcoma

Chondrogenic tumours

9240/3	Mesenchymal chondrosarcoma
9220/3	Chondrosarcoma
9243/3	Dedifferentiated chondrosarcoma

Notochordal tumours

9370/3	Chordoma

Melanocytic tumours

Diffuse meningeal melanocytic neoplasms

8728/0	Meningeal melanocytosis
8728/3	Meningeal melanomatosis

Circumscribed meningeal melanocytic neoplasms

8728/1	Meningeal melanocytoma
8720/3	Meningeal melanoma

Haematolymphoid tumours involving the CNS

CNS lymphomas

9680/3	Primary diffuse large B-cell lymphoma of the CNS
9766/1	Lymphomatoid granulomatosis
9766/1	Lymphomatoid granulomatosis, grade 1
9766/1	Lymphomatoid granulomatosis, grade 2
9766/3	Lymphomatoid granulomatosis, grade 3
9712/3	Intravascular large B-cell lymphoma

Miscellaneous rare lymphomas in the CNS

9699/3	MALT lymphoma of the dura
9671/3	Lymphoplasmacytic lymphoma
9690/3	Follicular lymphoma
9714/3	Anaplastic large cell lymphoma (ALK+/ALK−)
9702/3	T-cell lymphoma
9719/3	NK/T-cell lymphoma

Histiocytic tumours

9749/3	Erdheim–Chester disease
9749/3	Rosai–Dorfman disease[†]
9749/1	Juvenile xanthogranuloma[†]
9751/1	Langerhans cell histiocytosis
9755/3	Histiocytic sarcoma

ICD-O label (subtypes are indicated in grey text, with the label indented);
Please note that the WHO classification of tumour types is more readily reflected in the table of contents

Germ cell tumours

9080/0	Mature teratoma
9080/3	Immature teratoma
9084/3	Teratoma with somatic-type malignancy
9064/3	Germinoma
9070/3	Embryonal carcinoma
9071/3	Yolk sac tumour
9100/3	Choriocarcinoma
9085/3	Mixed germ cell tumour

Tumours of the sellar region

9351/1	Adamantinomatous craniopharyngioma
9352/1	Papillary craniopharyngioma
9432/1	Pituicytoma
9582/0	Granular cell tumour of the sellar region
8290/0	Spindle cell oncocytoma
8272/3	Pituitary adenoma / pituitary neuroendocrine tumour (PitNET)[†]
8273/3	Pituitary blastoma

These morphology codes are from the International Classification of Diseases for Oncology, third edition, second revision (ICD-O-3.2) {1414}. Behaviour is coded /0 for benign tumours; /1 for unspecified, borderline, or uncertain behaviour; /2 for carcinoma in situ and grade III intraepithelial neoplasia; /3 for malignant tumours, primary site; and /6 for malignant tumours, metastatic site. Behaviour code /6 is not generally used by cancer registries.

This classification is modified from the previous WHO classification, taking into account changes in our understanding of these lesions.

n/a, not available (provisional entity).

* Codes marked with an asterisk were approved by the IARC/WHO Committee for ICD-O at its meeting in May 2021.

† Labels marked with a dagger have undergone a change in terminology of a previous code.

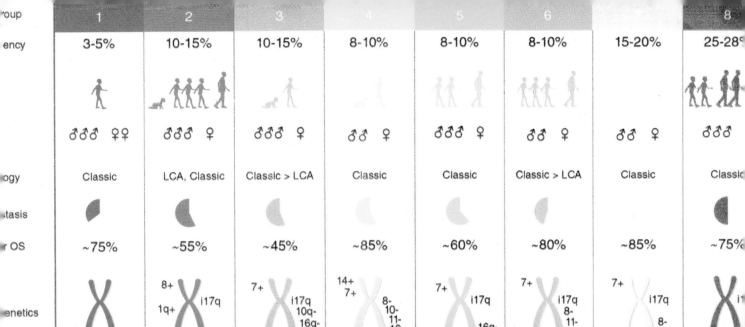

roup	1	2	3	4	5	6		8
ency	3-5%	10-15%	10-15%	8-10%	8-10%	8-10%	15-20%	25-28%
ogy	Classic	LCA, Classic	Classic > LCA	Classic	Classic	Classic > LCA	Classic	Classic
tasis								
OS	~75%	~55%	~45%	~85%	~60%	~80%	~85%	~75%
enetics		8+ 1q+ i17q	7+ i17q 10q- 16q-	14+ 7+ 8- 10- 11- 16-	7+ i17q 16q-	7+ i17q 8- 11-	7+ i17q 8-	i1 8-

1

Introduction to CNS tumours

Introduction to CNS tumours

Louis DN
Ellison DW
Perry A
Wesseling P

The fifth-edition *Central nervous system tumours* volume of the WHO Classification of Tumours series (also known as the WHO Blue Books) is based on the revised fourth-edition volume published in 2016, on the many developments in the field that followed the 2016 classification, and on the recommendations of the Consortium to Inform Molecular and Practical Approaches to CNS Tumor Taxonomy (cIMPACT) {1933,1932,1935,838, 356,1946,1934,1944,357,836}. The fifth-edition classification is presented in the table of contents of this volume. The fifth edition moves further in advancing the role of molecular diagnostics in CNS tumour classification but remains rooted in other established approaches to tumour characterization, including histology and immunohistochemistry. The increasing impact of molecular approaches has necessitated a series of changes, which are summarized in this introductory chapter.

CNS tumour taxonomy
CNS tumour classification has long been based on histological findings supported by ancillary tissue-based tests (e.g. immunohistochemical, ultrastructural). The 2016 classification introduced molecular markers as key aspects of classification for a relatively small set of entities. Given the large increase in knowledge of the molecular basis of these tumours, the current fifth edition refers to numerous molecular changes that are important for the most accurate classification of CNS neoplasms. A summary of the most salient molecular alterations for each CNS tumour type is listed in Table 1.01.

As the molecular underpinnings of brain and spinal cord tumours have been further elucidated, challenges have arisen in how to organize the classification of these lesions. Some tumour types are readily and consistently characterized by molecular features; some are only sometimes able to be classified by molecular parameters; and others are rarely or never diagnosed using such approaches. The resulting nosological organization is therefore also mixed. For some tumour families, the fifth edition has grouped tumours according to the genetic changes that effect a complete diagnosis (e.g. IDH and H3 status); for some, by looser, oncogenic associations (e.g. MAPK pathway alterations); for others, by histological and histogenetic similarities even though molecular signatures vary (e.g. see neoplasms discussed in Chapter 2: *Gliomas, glioneuronal tumours, and neuronal tumours*); and for many (e.g. medulloblastoma), by using molecular features to define new subtypes. This hybrid taxonomy represents the current state of the field, maturing from what was possible for the 2016 WHO classification but probably only an intermediate stage on the way to an even more molecular future classification. Examples where the transitional state of the current classification is especially apparent include the family of paediatric-type diffuse low-grade gliomas (p. 56), in which some entities have been lumped and others split, with such consensus decisions being based on the state of the field at the time of final editorial discussions.

In this fifth-edition volume, for consistency with the other fifth-edition WHO Blue Books, the term "type" is used instead of "entity", and "subtype" is used instead of "variant". Only types are listed in the classification, with the subtypes listed in the *Subtype(s)* subsections and then described in the *Histopathology* or *Diagnostic molecular pathology* subsections of individual sections. As a result of this change and because grading is being applied within types (see below), meningioma is treated as a single type with only one entry in the classification, with its many histological subtypes and different grades described within that entry.

CNS tumour nomenclature
For CNS tumour nomenclature, the fifth edition follows the recommendations of the cIMPACT-Utrecht meeting to make nomenclature more consistent and simple {1944}. In the past, some tumour names included anatomical site modifiers (e.g. "chordoid glioma of the third ventricle") whereas others did not, despite occurring in specific locations (e.g. "medulloblastoma"), and some included genetic modifiers (e.g. "glioblastoma, IDH-wildtype") whereas others did not, despite having specific genotypes (e.g. "atypical teratoid/rhabdoid tumour"). Names have therefore been simplified as much as possible, and only location, age, or genetic modifiers with remaining clinical utility have been used (e.g. "extraventricular neurocytoma" vs "central neurocytoma"). Importantly, for tumours with features that are highly characteristic (e.g. the stereotypical location of chordoid gliomas in the third ventricle), these specific features are included in the tumour definitions and descriptions even if they are not part of the tumour name. Moreover, tumour names sometimes reflect characteristic features that are not found in all such lesions. For example, some myxopapillary ependymomas are not myxoid, some are not papillary, and some are neither myxoid nor papillary in substantial ways; and xanthomatous change is found in a relatively small percentage of pleomorphic xanthoastrocytomas. Nonetheless, such names represent characteristic, if not universal, features. The terms may also reflect historical associations that have become embedded in common usage; for instance, although a medulloblast has not been identified in developmental studies, the term "medulloblastoma" is deeply ingrained in tumour terminology, and changing the name could be quite disruptive to clinical care, scientific experiments that rely on prior data, and epidemiological studies. Lastly, with the change to grading within tumour types (see below), modifier terms like "anaplastic" are not routinely included; familiar names like "anaplastic astrocytoma" and "anaplastic oligodendroglioma" do not, therefore, appear in this classification.

Gene and protein nomenclature for CNS tumour classification
The fifth edition of the WHO Classification of Tumours follows the Human Genome Organisation (HUGO) Gene Nomenclature Committee (HGNC) system for gene symbols and gene names

(https://www.genenames.org/) {390}, the Human Genome Variation Society (HGVS) recommendations for sequence variants (https://varnomen.hgvs.org/) {735}, and the International System for Human Cytogenetic Nomenclature (ISCN) 2020 reporting guidelines for chromosomal alterations {2053}. Gene symbols are presented in italics, but proteins and gene groups (e.g. the family of IDH genes) are not italicized.

A sequence alteration relative to a transcript reference sequence is reported using the prefix "c." for the coding DNA sequence, followed by the nucleotide number and the nucleotide change. The predicted protein sequence change then follows the prefix "p.", specifying the reference amino acid, the amino acid number, and the variant amino acid resulting from the mutation. For example, the most common BRAF variant is

Table 1.01 The most common diagnostic molecular alterations in major primary CNS tumours (continued on the next page)

Tumour type	Characteristically altered genes / molecular profiles[a]
Adult-type diffuse gliomas	
Astrocytoma, IDH-mutant	IDH1, IDH2
Oligodendroglioma, IDH-mutant and 1p/19q-codeleted	IDH1, IDH2, 1p/19q
Glioblastoma, IDH-wildtype	IDH-wildtype, chromosomes 7 and 10, TERT, EGFR, others
Paediatric-type diffuse low-grade gliomas	
Diffuse astrocytoma, MYB- or MYBL1-altered	MYB, MYBL1
Angiocentric glioma	MYB
Polymorphous low-grade neuroepithelial tumour of the young	BRAF, FGFR genes
Diffuse low-grade glioma, MAPK pathway–altered	MAPK pathway genes
Paediatric-type diffuse high-grade gliomas	
Diffuse midline glioma, H3 K27–altered	H3 p.K28 (K27), EGFR, EZHIP
Diffuse hemispheric glioma, H3 G34–mutant	H3 p.G35 (G34)
Diffuse paediatric-type high-grade glioma, H3-wildtype and IDH-wildtype	IDH-wildtype, H3-wildtype, methylome
Infant-type hemispheric glioma	RTK genes
Circumscribed astrocytic gliomas	
Pilocytic astrocytoma	KIAA1549::BRAF, BRAF
High-grade astrocytoma with piloid features	Methylome
Pleomorphic xanthoastrocytoma	BRAF, CDKN2A
Subependymal giant cell astrocytoma	TSC1, TSC2
Chordoid glioma	PRKCA
Astroblastoma, MN1-altered	MN1, BEND2
Glioneuronal and neuronal tumours	
Ganglion cell tumours	BRAF
Dysembryoplastic neuroepithelial tumour	FGFR1
Diffuse glioneuronal tumour with oligodendroglioma-like features and nuclear clusters	Methylome
Papillary glioneuronal tumour	PRKCA
Rosette-forming glioneuronal tumour	FGFR1, PIK3CA, NF1
Myxoid glioneuronal tumour	PDGFRA
Diffuse leptomeningeal glioneuronal tumour	KIAA1549::BRAF, 1p, methylome
Multinodular and vacuolating neuronal tumour	MAPK pathway genes
Dysplastic cerebellar gangliocytoma (Lhermitte–Duclos disease)	PTEN
Extraventricular neurocytoma	FGFR genes (FGFR1::TACC1), IDH-wildtype
Ependymal tumours	
Supratentorial ependymomas	ZFTA (C11orf95), YAP1
Posterior fossa ependymomas	PFA molecular profile, PFB molecular profile
Spinal ependymomas	NF2, MYCN

C19MC, chromosome 19 microRNA cluster; PFA, posterior fossa group A; PFB, posterior fossa group B; RTK, receptor tyrosine kinase; SHH, sonic hedgehog.
[a]Details of molecular alterations are found in the respective sections.

Tumour type	Characteristically altered genes / molecular profiles[a]
Embryonal tumours	
Medulloblastoma, WNT-activated	WNT pathway genes
Medulloblastoma, SHH-activated	SHH pathway genes, *TP53*
Medulloblastoma, non-WNT/non-SHH	Methylome
Atypical teratoid/rhabdoid tumour	*SMARCB1, SMARCA4*
Embryonal tumour with multilayered rosettes	C19MC, *DICER1*
CNS neuroblastoma, *FOXR2*-activated	*FOXR2*
CNS tumour with *BCOR* internal tandem duplication	*BCOR*
Desmoplastic myxoid tumour of the pineal region, *SMARCB1*-mutant	*SMARCB1*
Meningioma	*NF2, AKT1, TRAF7, SMO, PIK3CA*; and in subtypes *KLF4, SMARCE1, BAP1*
Solitary fibrous tumour	*NAB2::STAT6*
Meningeal melanocytic tumours	*NRAS* (diffuse); *GNAQ, GNA11, PLCB4, CYSLTR2* (circumscribed)
Tumours of the sellar region	
Adamantinomatous craniopharyngioma	*CTNNB1*
Papillary craniopharyngioma	*BRAF*

C19MC, chromosome 19 microRNA cluster; PFA, posterior fossa group A; PFB, posterior fossa group B; RTK, receptor tyrosine kinase; SHH, sonic hedgehog.
[a]Details of molecular alterations are found in the respective sections.

BRAF:c.1799T>A p.Val600Glu (or *BRAF*:c.1799T>A p.V600E if single-letter amino acid codes are preferred, as have been used throughout this volume). Notably, however, this example assumes that a particular *BRAF* transcript reference sequence accession and version have previously been defined (e.g. NM_004333.5).

For some genes, such as those in the H3 histone group, which are sometimes altered in CNS tumours, there is the potential for confusion with amino acid numbering. Histone amino acid positions are typically described in the context of the protein sequence lacking the initiating methionine, resulting in a single amino acid difference in numbering compared with the predicted sequence derived from the corresponding gene transcript. Therefore, the description of histone sequence alterations in many cancers has, to date, differed from the HGVS numbering by omitting the first amino acid. Next-generation sequencing reports, however, follow HGVS guidelines. The coexistence of these two nomenclatures may lead to confusion for pathologists, oncologists, and researchers. To address this issue, the fifth edition uses the legacy protein numbering system in parentheses after the protein-level variant description, for example "*H3-3A*:c.103G>A p.G35R (G34R)" or "*H3-3A*:c.83A>T p.K28M (K27M)". In these examples, as noted above, prior definition of the accession and version of the reference transcript is required.

CNS tumour grading

CNS tumour grading has for many decades differed from the grading of other (non-CNS) neoplasms, since brain and spinal cord tumours have had grades applied across different entities {1943}. As discussed below, the fifth edition has moved CNS tumour grading closer to how grading is done for non-CNS neoplasms, but it has retained some key aspects of traditional CNS tumour grading because of how embedded such grading is in neuro-oncology practice. Two specific aspects of CNS tumour

grading have changed for the fifth edition: neoplasms are graded within tumour types (rather than across different types), and Arabic numerals are used (rather than Roman numerals). Nonetheless, because CNS tumour grading still differs from other tumour grading, the fifth edition endorses the use of the term "CNS WHO grade" when assigning grade.

Grading within types

As mentioned, CNS tumours have traditionally had a grade assigned to each entity, and grades were applied across different entities {1943}. For example, in recent prior editions of the WHO classification, if a tumour had been classified as an anaplastic astrocytoma, it was automatically assigned a CNS WHO grade of III; there was no option to grade an anaplastic astrocytoma as grade I, II, or IV. Notably, anaplastic (malignant) meningiomas were also assigned a CNS WHO grade of III. Even though tumours like meningiomas and astrocytomas are biologically unrelated, grade III tumours in these different categories had somewhat similar survival times. But these were only roughly similar, with the behaviour of an anaplastic astrocytoma often being quite different from that of an anaplastic (malignant) meningioma. This approach thus correlated grade to an idealized clinical–biological behaviour: at one end of the spectrum, grade I tumours were curable if they could be surgically removed; at the other, grade IV tumours were highly malignant, leading to death in a relatively short period of time.

This entity-specific and clinical approach to CNS tumour grading was different from the approach used for other (non-CNS) tumour types {1943}. Most tumours in other organ systems are graded *within* tumour types; for example, a malignant peripheral nerve sheath tumour can be grade 1, 2, or 3. In the 2016 WHO classification of CNS tumours, solitary fibrous tumour / haemangiopericytoma was graded in the latter manner, using a single name but with the option of three grades. In this fifth-edition volume, the shift to within-type grading has been extended to all categories. This change was made for a few major reasons: (1) to provide more flexibility in using grade relative to the tumour type, (2) to emphasize biological similarities within tumour types (rather than to approximate clinical behaviour), and (3) to conform with WHO grading of non-CNS tumour types.

Clinicopathological grading

Nonetheless, because CNS tumour grading has for decades been linked to overall expected clinical–biological behaviours (see above), the fifth-edition WHO classification of CNS tumours has generally retained the ranges of grades used for tumour types in prior editions. In this context, for example, IDH-mutant astrocytomas extend from grade 2 to grade 4, and meningiomas from grade 1 to grade 3; in other words, at least at the present time, there is neither a grade 1 IDH-mutant astrocytoma nor a grade 4 meningioma. Moreover, given that tumours are graded on the basis of their expected natural history, highly malignant tumours for which there are treatments that may greatly modulate their behaviour (e.g. medulloblastoma, germinoma) are still assigned a grade 4 designation in the fifth edition.

The above approach to grading is a compromise, since the original underlying prognostic correlations were based on natural history, at a time when few effective therapies were available. Today, however, estimating natural history is nearly impossible, since practically all patients receive therapies that can affect overall survival {3346}. In the current context of modern therapies that markedly affect patient survival, the necessity of grading every tumour type is questionable. In fact,

in editorial discussions for the fifth edition, it was argued that grades should not be assigned if designation of a grade could confuse clinical care. For instance, WNT-activated medulloblastoma is an embryonal tumour with an aggressive behaviour if left untreated, but it is responsive to current therapeutic regimens such that nearly all patients have long-term survival. Designating this tumour as grade 4 (equivalent to many untreatable paediatric brain tumours with a dismal outcome) could give an incorrect impression of the prognosis when therapeutic options are discussed in the clinic. Likewise, designating this tumour as grade 1, as one might do with neoplasms having a similar prognosis on the basis of surgery alone, could give a false sense that the tumour is biologically benign. Examples of how this might apply in other settings are given in Box 1.01.

Combined histological and molecular grading

CNS tumour grading has traditionally been based exclusively on histological parameters, but many molecular markers can now provide powerful prognostic information. For this reason, molecular parameters have now been added for grading and estimating prognosis in multiple tumour types. Examples in the fifth edition include *CDKN2A* and/or *CDKN2B* homozygous deletion in IDH-mutant astrocytomas, as well as *TERT* promoter mutation, *EGFR* amplification, and +7/–10 copy-number changes in IDH-wildtype glioblastoma. In these situations, a molecular parameter often overrides histological findings in assigning a grade. Specific instances are discussed with the relevant tumour types.

Box 1.01 Layered report structure, with two examples

Information to be included:

Tumour site

Integrated diagnosis (combined tissue-based histological and molecular diagnosis)

Histopathological classification

CNS WHO grade

Molecular information (listed)

Example A

This layered report illustrates (1) use of site in the diagnosis, (2) use of a histological diagnosis that does not designate "anaplasia" but the report still assigns a grade, and (3) use of the NOS designation (in this instance because the case cannot be worked up adequately at a molecular level).

Cerebrum:

Integrated diagnosis:	Supratentorial ependymoma NOS
Histopathological classification:	Ependymoma
CNS WHO grade:	3
Molecular information:	Derivatives extracted from FFPE tissue were of insufficient quality for sequencing, and insufficient tissue remained for FISH studies.

Example B

This layered report illustrates (1) a tumour type with a subtype, (2) lack of a definite grade, and (3) that the integrated diagnosis does not necessarily include the histological designation.

Cerebrum:

Integrated diagnosis:	Diffuse low-grade glioma, MAPK pathway–altered *Subtype:* diffuse low-grade glioma, *FGFR1* TKD–duplicated
Histopathological classification:	Oligodendroglioma
CNS WHO grade:	Not assigned
Molecular information:	Duplication of the *FGFR1* TKD (next-generation sequencing)

FFPE, formalin-fixed, paraffin-embedded; TKD, tyrosine kinase domain.

Table 1.02 Approximate number of fields per 1 mm² based on the field diameter and its corresponding area

Field diameter (mm)	Field area (mm²)	Approximate number of fields per 1 mm²
0.40	0.126	8
0.41	0.132	8
0.42	0.138	7
0.43	0.145	7
0.44	0.152	7
0.45	0.159	6
0.46	0.166	6
0.47	0.173	6
0.48	0.181	6
0.49	0.188	5
0.50	0.196	5
0.51	0.204	5
0.52	0.212	5
0.53	0.221	5
0.54	0.229	4
0.55	0.237	4
0.56	0.246	4
0.57	0.255	4
0.58	0.264	4
0.59	0.273	4
0.60	0.283	4
0.61	0.292	3
0.62	0.302	3
0.63	0.312	3
0.64	0.322	3
0.65	0.332	3
0.66	0.342	3
0.67	0.352	3
0.68	0.363	3
0.69	0.374	3

Arabic versus Roman numerals

Traditionally, CNS WHO tumour grades were given as Roman numerals. However, a danger of using Roman numerals in a within-type grading system is that a "II" and a "III" or a "III" and a "IV" can quite easily be mistaken for one another, and an uncaught typographical error could have clinical consequences (this was less likely when each tumour type had a different name, e.g. when "anaplastic" was present in addition to "grade III"). Moreover, the fifth-edition WHO Blue Books emphasize a more uniform approach to tumour classification and grading across organ systems, and they favour the use of Arabic numerals. Given these considerations, particularly to decrease the possibility of errors, all CNS WHO grades have been changed to Arabic numerals in the fifth edition (in this

volume, Roman numerals have been used only in discussions referring to studies that used the older designations).

NOS and NEC diagnoses

As detailed elsewhere {1946,1934}, the designations "not otherwise specified (NOS)" and "not elsewhere classified (NEC)" allow the ready separation of standard, well-characterized WHO diagnoses from those diagnoses that result from either (1) a lack of necessary diagnostic (e.g. molecular) information or (2) non-diagnostic (i.e. for a WHO diagnosis) or negative results. The "NOS" designation indicates that the diagnostic information (histological or molecular) necessary to assign a specific WHO diagnosis is not available, alerting the oncologist that a full molecular workup has not been undertaken or was not successful. In contrast, the "NEC" designation indicates that the necessary diagnostic testing has been successfully performed but that the results do not readily allow for a WHO diagnosis – for example, if there is a mismatch between clinical, histological, immunohistochemical, and/or genetic features. NEC diagnoses are similar to what pathologists have termed "descriptive diagnoses", in which the pathologist uses a non-WHO term to describe the tumour. In this regard, the "NEC" designation alerts the oncologist that the tumour does not conform to a standard WHO diagnosis, despite the case having received an adequate pathological workup. NOS and NEC diagnoses are facilitated by the use of layered integrated reports (see below and Box 1.01, p. 11).

Novel diagnostic technologies

Over the past century, many novel technologies have impacted tumour classification, including light microscopy, tissue stains, electron microscopy, immunohistochemistry, molecular genetics, and most recently a variety of broad molecular profiling approaches. Each new method burst onto the scene promising to revolutionize classification, and each then eventually found a specific niche alongside the existing methods, rather than replacing them. In the past couple of decades, nucleic acid–based approaches (e.g. DNA and RNA sequencing, DNA FISH, RNA expression profiling) have clearly shown their abilities to contribute to tumour diagnosis and classification, as evidenced by the changes in the revised fourth-edition WHO classification of CNS tumours (2016) and in this fifth-edition volume. The global availability of such technologies was already increasing as the 2016 volume was being prepared {62,112}, and the past few years have witnessed a further expansion of their use, as well as the emergence of skilful ways to adapt histological to molecular classification recommendations {2808,2994}. This fifth-edition WHO Blue Book thus incorporates more molecular approaches for the classification of CNS tumours.

Over the past decade, methylome profiling – the use of arrays to determine DNA methylation patterns across the genome – has also emerged as a powerful approach to CNS tumour classification {460,463,1458}. Most CNS tumour types and subtypes can be reliably identified by their methylome profile, although caveats remain in that the optimal methodological approaches for methylome profiling have not yet been determined, regulatory issues have yet to be resolved, and the technology is currently not widely available {1944}. Copy-number profiles can also be derived from methylation or other data (e.g. 1p/19q codeletion, +7/–10 signature, amplifications, homozygous deletions, and indications of fusion events). At this time, methylome profiling can be recommended as an effective method for brain and spinal cord tumour classification when used alongside standard technologies, including histology. Indeed, most tumour types and subtypes can also be reliably identified by other techniques (e.g. by a combination of histology and a defining genetic alteration). However, methylome profiling may be the most effective way to characterize some diagnostically challenging neoplasms, and it may be the only way (currently) to identify some rare tumour types and subtypes. The method also has utility when small biopsy samples are limiting for standard technologies. Methylome profiling may also be used as a surrogate marker for genetic events, for instance when a methylome signature is characteristic of an IDH-wildtype glioblastoma in the absence of IDH mutation testing; but methylome profiling cannot serve as a surrogate when the demonstration of specific mutations prior to patient treatment is required for targeted therapies or clinical trial participation. Moreover, in the interpretation of methylome profiling results, careful attention must be paid to the common calibrated score threshold. As discussed in detail elsewhere {463}, thresholds may be set at 0.84 or 0.90; pathologists should be wary about endorsing suggested diagnoses with scores < 0.84 and should probably discard recommendations if scores are < 0.50. As with other diagnostic tests, the pathologist must take into account histological features (e.g. tumour cell amount and purity) in interpreting results. For the fifth-edition WHO classification of CNS tumours, therefore, it is assumed that most tumour types have a distinct methylation signature {460}, and this is not specified in each definition; however, information about diagnostic methylation profiling is included in the *Definition* and *Essential and desirable diagnostic criteria* subsections of the tumour types for which such information can provide more critical guidance for diagnosis.

Quantification of mitotic counts

The fifth-edition WHO Blue Books aim to standardize mitotic counting across tumour types. In this CNS volume, therefore, where possible, mitotic counts have been expressed as the number of mitoses per a defined area in mm², as well as per the commonly used denominator of 10 HPF. Given that individual microscopes have high-power fields of different sizes, this change should standardize the true area over which mitoses are enumerated. The approximate number of fields per 1 mm² based on field diameter and corresponding area is presented in Table 1.02. As an example, the discussion on diagnosis of atypical meningiomas specifies "≥ 2.5 mitoses per mm² (4 mitoses per 10 consecutive 0.16 mm² fields)". Therefore, a diagnosis of atypical meningioma based on mitotic count requires the finding of ≥ 4 mitoses within a 1.6 mm² area. If, for instance, one's ocular or digital field dimensions are > 0.16 mm², then the conversion could come out to only 7 or 8 consecutive high-power fields rather than 10.

It is recognized, however, that such a conversion introduces a number of practical challenges, including that mitotic counting has been reported in many older studies without specifically quantifying high-power field size. In the future, ideally, cut-off values using measured high-power fields should be established via new and/or repeated studies. And as pathologists adopt digital approaches to counting mitoses, the use of defined field sizes will prove helpful, such as for assessing variability

Box 1.02 Newly recognized tumour types

Diffuse astrocytoma, *MYB-* or *MYBL1*-altered

Polymorphous low-grade neuroepithelial tumour of the young

Diffuse low-grade glioma, MAPK pathway–altered

Diffuse hemispheric glioma, H3 G34–mutant

Diffuse paediatric-type high-grade glioma, H3-wildtype and IDH-wildtype

Infant-type hemispheric glioma

High-grade astrocytoma with piloid features

Diffuse glioneuronal tumour with oligodendroglioma-like features and nuclear clusters (provisional entity)

Myxoid glioneuronal tumour

Multinodular and vacuolating neuronal tumour

Supratentorial ependymoma, *YAP1* fusion–positive

Posterior fossa group A ependymoma

Posterior fossa group B ependymoma

Spinal ependymoma, *MYCN*-amplified

Cribriform neuroepithelial tumour (provisional entity)

CNS neuroblastoma, *FOXR2*-activated

CNS tumour with *BCOR* internal tandem duplication

Desmoplastic myxoid tumour of the pineal region, *SMARCB1*-mutant

Intracranial mesenchymal tumour, FET::CREB fusion–positive (provisional entity)

CIC-rearranged sarcoma

Primary intracranial sarcoma, *DICER1*-mutant

Pituitary blastoma

in counts across specimens. In practice, most quantification of proliferation (mitotic counting, Ki-67/MIB1 labelling) has prioritized hotspots (e.g. in meningiomas), but it can be useful to include background proliferation estimates in such assessments as well (e.g. focally elevated labelling in a diffuse glioma). Digital assessments based on defined-area fields will facilitate this.

Integrated and layered diagnoses

Because of the growing importance of molecular information in CNS tumour classification, diagnoses and diagnostic reports need to combine different data types into a single integrated diagnosis. Such integrated diagnoses form the backbone of the fifth-edition WHO classification of CNS tumours. Even diagnostic terms that do not incorporate a molecular term may require a molecular characteristic for diagnosis (e.g. atypical teratoid/rhabdoid tumour). Thus, to display the full amount of diagnostic information available, the use of layered (or tiered) diagnostic reports is strongly encouraged, as endorsed by the International Society of Neuropathology – Haarlem consensus guidelines {1939} and the International Collaboration on Cancer Reporting {1945}. Such reports feature an integrated diagnosis at the top, followed by layers that display histological, molecular, and other key types of information (see Box 1.01, p. 11).

For some tumour types in this fifth-edition volume, the listed diagnostic terms are general ones (e.g. "diffuse high-grade paediatric-type glioma, H3-wildtype", "diffuse low-grade glioma, MAPK pathway–altered"), and mix-and-match approaches, using a matrix of histological and molecular features, are necessary to arrive at a specific integrated diagnosis. These approaches are described for each of these tumour groups and are similar to how the 2016 volume classified medulloblastomas

Astrocytoma, IDH-mutant

Diffuse midline glioma, H3 K27–altered

Chordoid glioma

Astroblastoma, *MN1*-altered

Supratentorial ependymoma, *ZFTA* fusion–positive

Embryonal tumour with multilayered rosettes

Malignant melanotic nerve sheath tumour

Solitary fibrous tumour

Mesenchymal chondrosarcoma (formerly a subtype)

Adamantinomatous craniopharyngioma (formerly a subtype)

Papillary craniopharyngioma (formerly a subtype)

Pituicytoma, granular cell tumour of the sellar region, and spindle cell oncocytoma (now grouped rather than separate)

Pituitary adenoma / pituitary neuroendocrine tumour

{1939} and to what cIMPACT update 4 recommended for paediatric low-grade diffuse gliomas {838}: an integrated diagnosis optimally combines a term from a histologically defined list of tumours and a term from a genetically defined list of tumours (e.g. see *Example B* in Box 1.01, p. 11). Even though each list may contain many items, some combinations are more common than others, such that the resulting number of routinely used integrated diagnoses is typically manageable.

In this fifth-edition volume, the essential and desirable diagnostic criteria for each tumour type are presented in systematically structured text boxes, in the hope that such a format will make it easier for the user to evaluate whether key diagnostic criteria are present and to discern what combinations of such criteria are sufficient for diagnosis. The essential diagnostic criteria are considered must-have features, but there may be different combinations that can confirm a diagnosis (i.e. not all criteria are necessarily required for the diagnosis to be rendered). For the tumour types for which this is the case, the user should pay close attention to the "OR" designations under the "Essential" heading within the *Essential and desirable diagnostic criteria* boxes. The desirable diagnostic criteria are nice-to-have features (i.e. they support a diagnosis but are not mandatory).

Newly recognized entities and revised nomenclature

The major changes to the classification are discussed in the introduction sections relating to the families of tumours (e.g. see *Gliomas, glioneuronal tumours, and neuronal tumours: Introduction*) and are only briefly mentioned here.

A number of newly recognized types (see Box 1.02, p. 13) have been accepted into the fifth-edition WHO classification of CNS tumours. In addition, changes have been made to the nomenclature of some entities, both to clarify molecular alterations and to follow the nomenclature guidelines in cIMPACT update 6 {1944} (see Box 1.03). Other nomenclature changes were made to standardize type names with those in other WHO Blue Books, such as for peripheral nerve and other soft tissue tumours.

Some proposed tumour types were discussed and provisionally accepted as types because they appeared to be distinct clinicopathological entities, but additional published studies are needed for full acceptance; these provisional entities are designated as such in Box 1.02 (p. 13). Others were also discussed, but it was decided that the published literature left too many unanswered questions about the nature of the proposed type for it to be added as a provisional entity at this time. An example of this is neuroepithelial tumour, *PATZ1* fusion–positive, few cases of which are described in the literature {2928,3037,410}. Although unpublished data suggest that these lesions have distinct molecular alterations, there is marked heterogeneity in their histopathological appearances and clinical courses, and therefore more published data are needed to evaluate whether neuroepithelial tumour, *PATZ1* fusion–positive, is truly a distinct tumour type.

Prior editions of the WHO classification of CNS tumours included more comprehensive lists of "non-brain" tumours. But because some of these neoplasms are only rarely encountered in the CNS and their diagnostic information is more comprehensively covered in other WHO Blue Books, this fifth-edition CNS volume lists fewer tumours in some sections, such as those on mesenchymal, non-meningothelial tumours and haematolymphoid tumours. The reader is referred to the corresponding WHO Blue Books for information on those types.

Conclusion

All classifications are imperfect representations, reflecting the state of understanding in a field at a particular time as well as how that information is interpreted by a handful of experts. The fifth-edition *Central nervous system* volume of the WHO Classification of Tumours series, like its predecessors, should therefore be seen as a work in progress, as a stage in evolution. We have attempted to introduce new knowledge into the classification as carefully but progressively as possible, by introducing newly recognized entities, phasing out ostensibly obsolete tumour types, and adjusting the taxonomic structure. It is hoped that such changes and their explanations provide practical guidance to pathologists and specialists in neuro-oncology around the world and that such progress benefits the patients who are affected by CNS tumours.

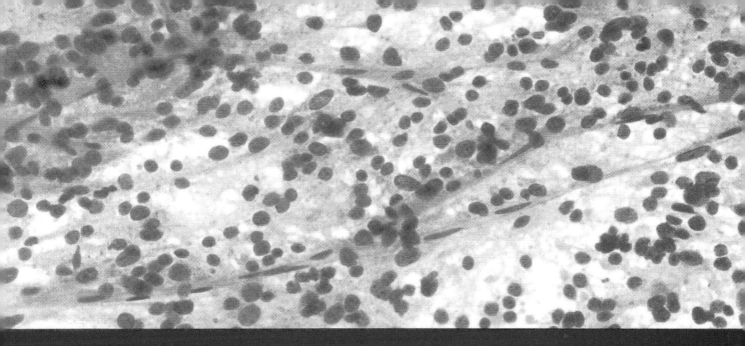

2

Gliomas, glioneuronal tumours, and neuronal tumours

Edited by: Brat DJ, Ellison DW, Figarella-Branger D, Hawkins CE, Louis DN, Perry A, Pfister SM, Reifenberger G, von Deimling A

Gliomas, glioneuronal tumours, and neuronal tumours: Introduction

Louis DN Perry A
Brat DJ Pfister SM
Ellison DW Reifenberger G
Figarella-Branger D von Deimling A
Hawkins CE

Gliomas, glioneuronal tumours, and neuronal tumours are the most common and most varied tumours affecting the parenchyma of the CNS. This fifth edition of the WHO classification of CNS tumours divides them into six different groups: (1) adult-type diffuse gliomas (the brain tumours that often constitute the bulk of adult neuro-oncology practice, e.g. glioblastoma, IDH-wildtype), (2) paediatric-type diffuse low-grade gliomas (typically associated with a favourable outcome), (3) paediatric-type diffuse high-grade gliomas (generally aggressive tumours), (4) circumscribed astrocytic gliomas ("circumscribed" referring to their more contained growth pattern, as opposed to the inherently "diffuse" tumours in groups 1, 2, and 3), (5) glioneuronal and neuronal tumours (a diverse group of tumours, commonly featuring neuronal differentiation), and (6) ependymal tumours (ependymomas; now classified by site as well as histological and molecular features). Notably, choroid plexus tumours, with their marked epithelial characteristics, are now separated from the category of gliomas, glioneuronal tumours, and neuronal tumours. To illustrate some biological relationships among these groups, they are compared in a series of t-distributed stochastic neighbour embedding (t-SNE) plots based on DNA methylome data: Fig. 2.01 shows an overall plot of gliomas, glioneuronal tumours, and neuronal tumours, and the rest of the figures in this introduction show individual plots of adult-type diffuse gliomas, paediatric-type diffuse low-grade gliomas, paediatric-type diffuse high-grade gliomas, circumscribed astrocytic gliomas, and glioneuronal and neuronal tumours.

A number of newly recognized types have been added to the classification of the gliomas as well as the glioneuronal and neuronal tumours: diffuse astrocytoma, *MYB*- or *MYBL1*-altered; polymorphous low-grade neuroepithelial tumour of the young; diffuse low-grade glioma, MAPK pathway–altered; diffuse hemispheric glioma, H3 G34–mutant; diffuse paediatric-type high-grade glioma, H3-wildtype and IDH-wildtype; infant-type hemispheric glioma; high-grade astrocytoma with piloid features; diffuse glioneuronal tumour with oligodendroglioma-like features and nuclear clusters (provisional); myxoid glioneuronal tumour; and multinodular and vacuolating neuronal tumour.

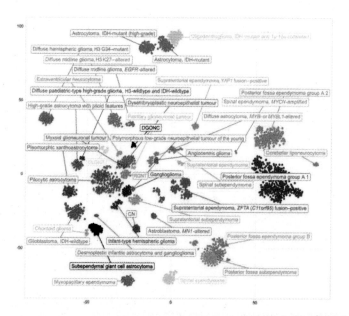

Fig. 2.01 Gliomas, glioneuronal tumours, and neuronal tumours: molecular groups. Unsupervised, non-linear t-distributed stochastic neighbour embedding (t-SNE) projection of methylation array profiles from 2632 tumours. Samples were selected from a large database of > 50 000 brain tumour datasets to serve as reference profiles for training a supervised classification model based on strict criteria: all these samples showed a high calibrated classification score (> 0.9) when applying the brain tumour classifier available at https://www.molecularneuropathology.org. CN, central neurocytoma; DGONC, diffuse glioneuronal tumour with oligodendroglioma-like features and nuclear clusters; DLGNT, diffuse leptomeningeal glioneuronal tumour; RGNT, rosette-forming glioneuronal tumour.

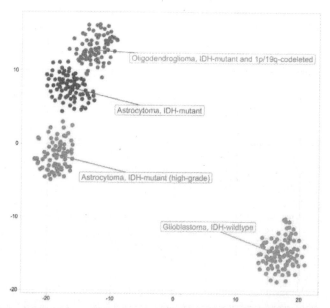

Fig. 2.02 Adult-type diffuse gliomas: molecular groups. Unsupervised, non-linear t-distributed stochastic neighbour embedding (t-SNE) projection of methylation array profiles from 343 tumours. Samples were selected from a large database of > 50 000 brain tumour datasets to serve as reference profiles for training a supervised classification model based on strict criteria: all these samples showed a high calibrated classification score (> 0.9) when applying the brain tumour classifier available at https://www.molecularneuropathology.org. "Astrocytoma, IDH-mutant" and "Astrocytoma, IDH-mutant (high-grade)" comprise two distinct methylation groups that were strongly associated with survival in several different patient cohorts {2916}. Further molecular heterogeneity of the "Glioblastoma, IDH-wildtype" group can also be assessed by methylation analysis, which has revealed several stable molecular subgroups (not shown here) that appear to be associated with distinct prognosis and/or response to therapy {3427}.

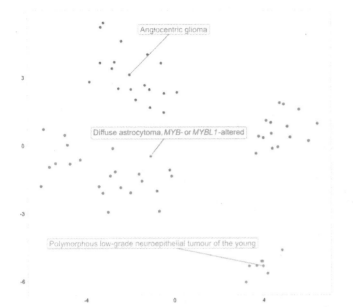

Fig. 2.03 Paediatric-type diffuse low-grade gliomas: molecular groups. Unsupervised, non-linear t-distributed stochastic neighbour embedding (t-SNE) projection of methylation array profiles from 66 tumours. Samples were selected from a large database of > 50 000 brain tumour datasets to serve as reference profiles for training a supervised classification model based on strict criteria: all these samples showed a high calibrated classification score (> 0.9) when applying the brain tumour classifier available at https://www.molecularneuropathology.org.

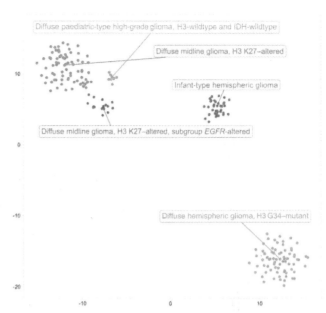

Fig. 2.04 Paediatric-type diffuse high-grade gliomas: molecular groups. Unsupervised, non-linear t-distributed stochastic neighbour embedding (t-SNE) projection of methylation array profiles from 218 tumours. Samples were selected from a large database of > 50 000 brain tumour datasets to serve as reference profiles for training a supervised classification model based on strict criteria: all these samples showed a high calibrated classification score (> 0.9) when applying the brain tumour classifier available at https://www.molecularneuropathology.org.

The ependymomas have been reclassified in two ways: (1) by anatomical site and (2) by the addition of genetic or epigenetic types: supratentorial ependymoma, *YAP1* fusion–positive; posterior fossa group A (PFA) ependymoma; posterior fossa group B (PFB) ependymoma; and spinal ependymoma, *MYCN*-amplified. The approach to classifying ependymal tumours by anatomical site is discussed in *Ependymal tumours: Introduction* (p. 159).

For some of these entities (most notably for diffuse paediatric-type high-grade glioma, H3-wildtype and IDH-wildtype, and for diffuse low-grade glioma, MAPK pathway–altered), histological appearance and defined molecular features must be combined to arrive at an integrated diagnosis. Such data are most effectively displayed as layered diagnoses. These approaches are discussed for the relevant types and subtypes.

There have also been some nomenclature changes to existing entities. For example, the diffuse midline glioma is now designated as "H3 K27–altered" rather than "H3 K27M–mutant" in order to recognize the various manners in which the pathogenic pathway can be altered in these tumours. Astroblastoma has been specified as "*MN1*-altered" to improve diagnostic focus for this entity. For other tumour types, changes in nomenclature relating to the inclusion of genetic and anatomical site modifiers have followed the recommendations of the Consortium to Inform Molecular and Practical Approaches to CNS Tumor Taxonomy (cIMPACT) update 6 {1944}.

As discussed in more detail below, three sets of major changes have affected classification and grading of the diffuse gliomas. The paediatric-type diffuse gliomas have been separated from the adult-type diffuse gliomas. And for the adult-type diffuse gliomas, their classification has been simplified to three

major types; in addition, their nomenclature and grading have been changed.

Division of diffuse gliomas into adult-type and paediatric-type

The fifth edition recognizes the clinical and molecular distinctions between diffuse gliomas that occur primarily in adults (termed "adult-type") and those that occur primarily in children (termed "paediatric-type"). Note the use of the word "primarily" here; paediatric-type tumours may sometimes occur in adults, particularly younger adults, and adult-type tumours may (more rarely) occur in children. Nonetheless, the division of the classification into adult-type and paediatric-type diffuse gliomas is hoped to be a major step forward in clearly separating these clinically and biologically distinct groups of tumours. The need to do so has been considered for a long time, but the elucidation of molecular differences has now made this possible. It is specifically hoped that this distinction will enable better care of children with brain tumours.

Simplification of the classification of common adult-type diffuse gliomas

In the 2016 WHO classification of CNS tumours, the common diffuse gliomas of adults were divided into 15 entities, largely because different grades were assigned to different entities (e.g. anaplastic oligodendroglioma was considered a different type from oligodendroglioma) and because NOS designations were assigned to distinct entities (e.g. diffuse astrocytoma NOS). In contrast, this fifth edition includes only three types: astrocytoma, IDH-mutant; oligodendroglioma, IDH-mutant and 1p/19q-codeleted; and glioblastoma, IDH-wildtype.

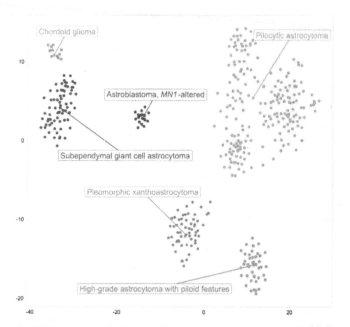

Fig. 2.05 Circumscribed astrocytic gliomas: molecular groups. Unsupervised, non-linear t-distributed stochastic neighbour embedding (t-SNE) projection of methylation array profiles from 420 tumours. Samples were selected from a large database of > 50 000 brain tumour datasets to serve as reference profiles for training a supervised classification model based on strict criteria: all these samples showed a high calibrated classification score (> 0.9) when applying the brain tumour classifier available at https://www.molecularneuropathology.org.

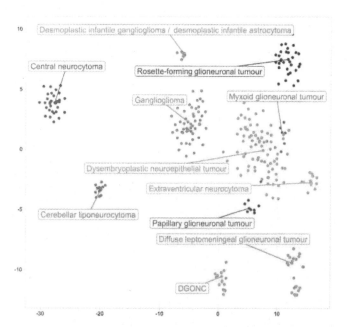

Fig. 2.06 Glioneuronal and neuronal tumours: molecular groups. Unsupervised, non-linear t-distributed stochastic neighbour embedding (t-SNE) projection of methylation array profiles from 297 tumours. Samples were selected from a large database of > 50 000 brain tumour datasets to serve as reference profiles for training a supervised classification model based on strict criteria: all these samples showed a high calibrated classification score (> 0.9) when applying the brain tumour classifier available at https://www.molecularneuropathology.org. DGONC, diffuse glioneuronal tumour with oligodendroglioma-like features and nuclear clusters.

This focusing of the classification has resulted from (1) more ecumenical use of the designations "not otherwise specified (NOS)" and "not elsewhere classified (NEC)", as discussed in the general introduction to this volume and in cIMPACT update 1 {1946}; (2) recognition of the value of molecular diagnostics to assign older entities (e.g. oligoastrocytoma or IDH-wildtype diffuse astrocytoma) to more objectively defined types; and (3) use of grades *within* types {357,1944} rather than requiring each grade to have a different name (see Chapter 1: *Introduction to CNS tumours*).

Nomenclature and grading of common adult-type diffuse astrocytic gliomas

In the 2016 classification, IDH-mutant diffuse astrocytic tumours were assigned to three different tumour types (diffuse astrocytoma, anaplastic astrocytoma, and glioblastoma) depending on histological parameters. In the current classification, however, all IDH-mutant diffuse astrocytic tumours are considered a single type (astrocytoma, IDH-mutant) and are then graded as CNS WHO grade 2, 3, or 4 (see Chapter 1: *Introduction to CNS tumours*). Moreover, grading is no longer entirely histological, because the finding of *CDKN2A* and/or *CDKN2B* homozygous deletion results in a CNS WHO grade of 4 even in the absence of microvascular proliferation or necrosis.

For IDH-wildtype diffuse astrocytic tumours in adults, a number of papers have reported that the presence of at least one of three genetic parameters (*TERT* promoter mutation, *EGFR* gene amplification, and the combination of whole chromosome 7 gain and whole chromosome 10 loss [+7/−10]) appears to be sufficient to assign the highest CNS WHO grade (CNS WHO grade 4) {356,3168}. The fifth edition therefore incorporates these three genetic parameters as criteria for the diagnosis of glioblastoma, IDH-wildtype. As a result, IDH-wildtype glioblastoma can be diagnosed in the setting of an IDH-wildtype diffuse astrocytic glioma if there is microvascular proliferation, necrosis, *TERT* promoter mutation, *EGFR* gene amplification, or +7/−10 chromosome copy-number alteration.

Astrocytoma, IDH-mutant

Brat DJ
Cahill DP
Cimino PJ
Huse JT
Kleinschmidt-DeMasters BK

Komori T
Reuss DE
Šuvà ML
von Deimling A
Weller M

Definition

Astrocytoma, IDH-mutant, is a diffusely infiltrating *IDH1*- or *IDH2*-mutant glioma with frequent *ATRX* and/or *TP53* mutation and absence of 1p/19q codeletion (CNS WHO grade 2, 3, or 4).

ICD-O coding

9400/3 Astrocytoma, IDH-mutant, grade 2
9401/3 Astrocytoma, IDH-mutant, grade 3
9445/3 Astrocytoma, IDH-mutant, grade 4

ICD-11 coding

2A00.0Y & XH6PH6 Other specified gliomas of brain & Astrocytoma, NOS
2A00.0Y & XH2HK4 Other specified gliomas of brain & Diffuse astrocytoma, IDH-mutant

Related terminology

Not recommended: diffuse astrocytoma, IDH-mutant; anaplastic astrocytoma, IDH-mutant; glioblastoma, IDH-mutant; low-grade astrocytoma; lower-grade astrocytoma; high-grade astrocytoma; infiltrating astrocytoma; diffuse glioma.

Subtype(s)

Astrocytoma, IDH-mutant, CNS WHO grade 2; astrocytoma, IDH-mutant, CNS WHO grade 3; astrocytoma, IDH-mutant, CNS WHO grade 4

Localization

Astrocytomas with *IDH1* or *IDH2* mutation can be located in any region of the CNS, including the brainstem and spinal cord, but they most commonly develop in the supratentorial compartment and are usually centred near or within the frontal lobes {1789, 3040,473}. This localization is similar to that of IDH-mutant and 1p/19q-codeleted oligodendroglioma {1790,3617}. A genetically distinct form of IDH-mutant astrocytoma has recently been described in the infratentorial compartment.

Clinical features

Development of signs and symptoms is rarely abrupt unless the diagnosis is revealed by neuroimaging after onset of epileptic seizures. A small subset of tumours are diagnosed incidentally when neuroimaging is performed after trauma or for headache {3417}. Neurocognitive function in patients with IDH-mutant astrocytomas is relatively preserved, compared with that in patients with similar-sized IDH-wildtype tumours {3403}; this may be because of slower growth, which allows for compensatory neuroplasticity. Among IDH-mutant astrocytomas, higher-grade tumours are assumed to be associated with shorter clinical history, but this has not been confirmed in contemporary studies.

Seizures are a common presenting sign; however, subtle neurological abnormalities, such as speech or language

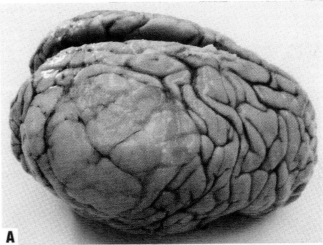

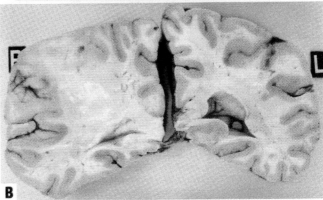

Fig. 2.07 Astrocytoma, IDH-mutant, CNS WHO grade 2. This unsuspected tumour was identified at autopsy in a man in his thirties who had last been known to be alive 2 days prior; he was found dead at home. **A** Note the exophytic right parieto-occipital mass lesion that blurs cortical anatomical features and is associated with cerebral oedema. Herniation was identified at autopsy and histological examination proved IDH-mutant status. **B** Coronal sectioning of the brain (after brief formalin fixation) revealed a non-necrotic, ill-defined gelatinous tumour in the right parieto-occipital lobe, with mass effect. Note the ventricular compression and blurring of the grey matter–white matter junction produced by the tumour compared with the normal left side of the brain.

difficulties, changes in sensory or motor function, or changes in vision, may be pre-existing. With frontal lobe tumours, changes in behaviour or personality may be the initial clinical feature and may have been present for months or even years before diagnosis.

Imaging

Neuroimaging findings of IDH-mutant astrocytomas can vary based on location, extent of disease, and tumour grade. On CT, IDH-mutant astrocytoma, CNS WHO grade 2, is noted as a poorly defined, homogeneous, low-density mass without contrast enhancement. Calcification and cystic change may be present. Midline deviation, extensive oedema, contrast

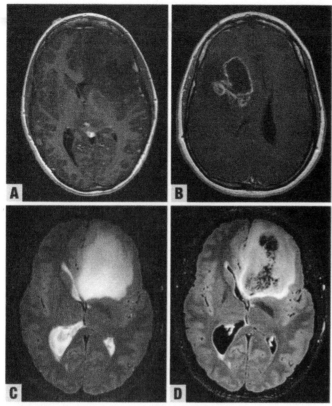

Fig. 2.08 Astrocytoma, IDH-mutant. **A** CNS WHO grade 3 tumour. Postcontrast T1-weighted MRI demonstrating an infiltrative mass involving the left frontal and parietal lobes that is T1-hypointense and without contrast enhancement, a pattern typical of grade 2 and 3 IDH-mutant astrocytomas. **B** CNS WHO grade 4 tumour. Postcontrast T1-weighted MRI showing a mass centred in the right frontoparietal region demonstrating rim enhancement surrounding central necrosis with adjacent T1 hypointensity, typical of a grade 4 IDH-mutant astrocytoma. **C** CNS WHO grade 3 tumour. T2-weighted MRI demonstrating a homogeneously hyperintense mass centred in the left frontal lobe and involving white matter and cortex, with mass effect leading to midline shift. The corresponding FLAIR image (**D**) shows heterogeneous signal across the lesion, and this T2–FLAIR mismatch is characteristic of IDH-mutant astrocytoma. **D** CNS WHO grade 3 tumour from the same patient shown in panel C. FLAIR MRI demonstrating a mass lesion centred in the left frontal lobe involving the white matter and cortex with heterogeneous signal intensity and demonstrating distinct regions of hyperintensity and hypointensity. The corresponding T2-weighted image (**C**) shows homogeneous signal intensity, and this T2–FLAIR mismatch is characteristic of IDH-mutant astrocytoma.

enhancement, and central hypodensity due to necrosis become evident at higher grades. MRI typically shows T1 hypodensity and T2 hyperintensity, with enlargement and distortion of involved areas. T2 hyperintensity is often paired with relative hypointensity on FLAIR sequences (known as the T2–FLAIR mismatch sign), a finding highly suggestive of CNS WHO grade 2 and grade 3 IDH-mutant astrocytomas {2419}. Gadolinium enhancement is uncommon in CNS WHO grade 2 IDH-mutant astrocytomas {3277,3602,1518}, but it is present at increasing frequency in CNS WHO grade 3 and grade 4 tumours. A pattern of rim enhancement around central necrosis is most common in CNS WHO grade 4 tumours. More extensive peritumoural oedema is noted in higher-grade lesions.

Epidemiology

Precise population-based data on the incidence of IDH-mutant astrocytomas are not available. The majority of patients present

in their thirties or forties (median age: 38 years) with CNS WHO grade 2 or 3 tumours {452,2655}. CNS WHO grade 2 and 3 astrocytomas have similar age distributions {2655}, whereas patients with CNS WHO grade 4 tumours tend to be slightly older {2655}. IDH mutations are uncommon in paediatric gliomas; when present, they are usually seen in adolescents {2531, 917}. IDH-mutant astrocytomas are uncommon in patients aged > 55 years {203,2687}. There is a slight male predominance among CNS WHO grade 2 and 3 IDH-mutant astrocytomas {452}. One study of CNS WHO grade 4 tumours found that their M:F ratio is significantly lower than that of IDH-wildtype glioblastomas {2313}. Recent work indicates that most CNS WHO grade 4 IDH-mutant astrocytomas occur de novo, rather than with a history of a lower-grade glioma {1714}.

Etiology

Genetic susceptibility

Most IDH-mutant astrocytomas develop sporadically, in the absence of a familial or hereditary predisposition syndrome. Genome-wide association studies indicate an association between a low-frequency SNP at 8q24.21 and increased risk of IDH-mutant gliomas, including oligodendroglioma and astrocytoma {1466}. Increased IDH-mutant astrocytoma risk is also associated with variants at 8q24.21 (the *CCDC26* locus), as well as with variants at the *PHLDB1*, *AKT3*, *IDH1*, and *D2HGDH* loci {2065,2907,823}. Rare genetic syndromes predispose to IDH-mutant astrocytoma. For example, it is the brain tumour most frequently associated with Li–Fraumeni syndrome, which is characterized by germline *TP53* mutations {1648,2320} (see *Li–Fraumeni syndrome*, p. 446). In patients from three families with Li–Fraumeni syndrome, *IDH1* mutations were observed in five astrocytomas that developed in members with a *TP53* germline mutation. All five contained the *IDH1*:c.394C>T p.R132C mutation {3398}, which in sporadic astrocytic tumours accounts for < 5% of all *IDH1* mutations {186,3397,3514}. This selective occurrence suggests a preference for *IDH1* p.R132C mutations in neural precursor cells that already carry a germline *TP53* mutation. IDH-mutant gliomas (oligodendrogliomas and astrocytomas) have also been diagnosed in patients with inherited Ollier disease, which predisposes to multiple enchondromatosis and chondrosarcoma {980,1332,3123,320}. IDH-mutant astrocytomas have not been associated with other diffuse glioma predisposition syndromes including neurofibromatosis type 1 {675}, *POT1* germline mutation {176,2747}, or melanoma-astrocytoma syndrome {507}.

IDH1-mutant astrocytomas in children and young adults are enriched for germline mutations in mismatch repair genes {766}. For these patients, immunohistochemical staining for mismatch repair proteins is usually an effective screening tool {178}. Importantly, the management of these tumours may be different from that of other *IDH1*-mutant gliomas {3222}.

Other etiological factors

Diffuse gliomas can arise after therapeutic radiation for another CNS malignancy, but these tumours lack IDH mutations {1928}. Although gliomas can be induced experimentally in rats with chemical carcinogens such as ethylnitrosourea and methylnitrosourea, there is no convincing evidence that these substances have an etiological role in human gliomas. Similarly, although polyomavirus (SV40, BK virus, and JC virus) genome sequences and proteins have been reported in gliomas, they were only rarely found in a more recent large series of 225 gliomas {2712}.

Pathogenesis
Cell of origin
Identification of the cell(s) of origin of IDH-mutant astrocytoma remains an area of active investigation (see also *Oligodendroglioma, IDH-mutant and 1p/19q-codeleted*, p. 28). Morphology and single-cell RNA-sequencing analysis of human tumours supports the notion that IDH-mutant astrocytomas are composed of a mixture of malignant cell types that recapitulate astrocytic and oligodendroglial lineages, as well as neural precursor–like cells {3309}. Experimental transformation of immortalized human astrocytes with *IDH1* p.R132H reprogrammes their cellular lineage and favours the emergence of a neural precursor state {3239}. Experiments in transgenic mice indicate that astrocytomas may originate from different CNS cell types, including neural precursor cells, oligodendrocyte precursor cells, and astrocytes {3619}. Neural and oligodendrocyte precursor cells may give rise to either oligodendroglial or astrocytic phenotypes in gliomas, depending on the genes driving transformation {1915,1901,1685}. This suggests an interplay between oncogenic events and the cell(s) of origin, and indicates that both are critical in determining the resulting glioma phenotype. IDH-mutant gliomas and IDH-wildtype glioblastomas may derive from different precursor cells. The differing patient ages, sex distribution, and clinical outcome suggest that IDH-mutant and IDH-wildtype gliomas have distinct cellular pathogenetic mechanisms {2313}. Compared

with IDH-wildtype glioblastomas, IDH-mutant gliomas show a much stronger predilection for involving frontal locations, indicating that they may originate from precursor cells located in (or migrating to) the frontal lobe. Moreover, the preferential frontal lobe localization may be a consequence of the frontally restricted expression of the glutamate dehydrogenase gene *GLUD2*, which encodes GDH2, a hominoid-specific enzyme that facilitates glutamate turnover in human forebrain {540, 3354}. GDH2 activity may partially compensate for IDH mutation–induced metabolic alterations, thereby facilitating the early stages of IDH-mutant astrocytoma growth. Together, these observations support the hypothesis that IDH-mutant astrocytic gliomas develop from a distinct population of precursor cells, although this has not yet been studied carefully across grades {2313,3309}.

Genetic profile
IDH mutations were first reported in 2008 {2405} and are a defining feature for IDH-mutant astrocytoma, CNS WHO grades 2, 3, and 4. IDH mutations are an early event in gliomagenesis and persist during tumour progression in most cases. Analysis of serial biopsies from the same patients have not yet uncovered cases in which an *IDH1* mutation occurred after the acquisition of a *TP53* mutation {3397}. An exception is *IDH1* mutations in patients with Li–Fraumeni syndrome, in which the germline *TP53* mutation is the initial genetic alteration and influences the subsequent acquisition of the *IDH1* mutation (see *Li–Fraumeni syndrome*, p. 446) {3398}. Reported *IDH1* mutations are usually located at the first or second base of codon 132 {186,2405,

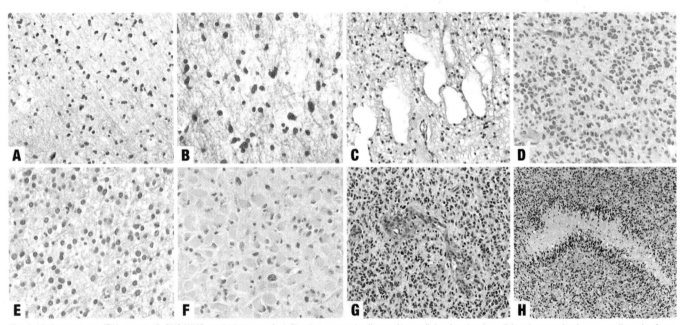

Fig. 2.09 Astrocytoma, IDH-mutant. **A** CNS WHO grade 2 tumour. An infiltrating astrocytic glioma of low cell density, showing mild nuclear atypia of tumour cells and a dense fibrillar background with mild oedema. **B** CNS WHO grade 2 tumour. The nuclei of IDH-mutant astrocytomas are elongate, irregular, and hyperchromatic. **C** CNS WHO grade 2 tumour. Microcystic change / microcyst formation in the tumour stroma is a frequent feature. **D** CNS WHO grade 3 tumour. CNS WHO grade 3 IDH-mutant astrocytomas show greater cellularity and nuclear atypia than do CNS WHO grade 2 tumours, as well as increased mitotic activity. **E** CNS WHO grade 3 tumour. Some IDH-mutant astrocytomas have tumour cells with relatively round nuclei, showing histological overlap with oligodendroglioma cells. The case shown here was IDH-mutant and showed loss of ATRX expression and *TP53* mutation, diagnostic of an IDH-mutant astrocytoma. **F** CNS WHO grade 3 tumour. Gemistocytic differentiation can be seen focally or extensively in IDH-mutant astrocytomas and consists of tumour cells with enlarged, rounded cell bodies containing abundant eosinophilic cytoplasm and an eccentrically located nucleus. **G** CNS WHO grade 4 tumour. Microvascular proliferation, noted as accumulation of hyperplastic endothelial cells and pericytes in the vessel wall, forming budding projections, is a histological feature of CNS WHO grade 4 in IDH-mutant astrocytoma. **H** CNS WHO grade 4 tumour. Palisading cells around a central focus of necrosis are a histological feature of CNS WHO grade 4 in IDH-mutant astrocytoma.

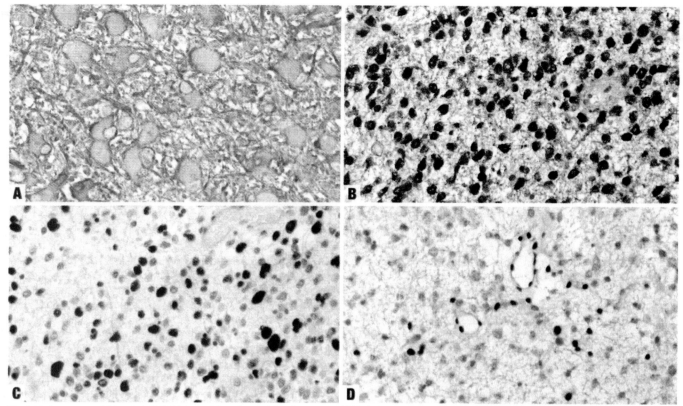

Fig. 2.10 Astrocytoma, IDH-mutant, CNS WHO grade 3. **A** Immunohistochemistry for GFAP shows strong and diffuse immunoreactivity in the tumour cell cytoplasm and glial processes in this IDH-mutant astrocytoma with gemistocytic differentiation. **B** Immunohistochemistry for IDH1 p.R132H demonstrates strong cytoplasmic reactivity in all neoplastic cells, indicating an *IDH1* p.R132H mutation. **C** Immunohistochemistry for p53 shows strong nuclear staining in a large percentage of neoplastic cells, which correlates well with *TP53* mutation in the setting of IDH-mutant astrocytoma. **D** Immunohistochemistry for ATRX reveals loss of nuclear staining in neoplastic cells, but retention of nuclear staining in non-neoplastic endothelial cells and glia, indicating ATRX loss or mutation in this IDH-mutant astrocytoma.

3397}. The most frequent is the *IDH1*:c.395G>A p.R132H muta-tion, found in 83–91% of IDH-mutant gliomas {186,3397,3514}. Other mutations are rare, including *IDH1*:c.394C>T p.R132C (found in 3.6–4.6% of cases), p.R132G (in 0.6–3.8%), p.R132S (in 0.8–2.5%), and p.R132L (in 0.5–4.4%) {186,3397,3514}. The *IDH2* gene encodes the only human protein homologous to IDH1 that also uses NADP+ as an electron acceptor. *IDH2* mutations in gliomas are located at residue p.R172, with the p.R172K mutation being the most frequent {3502,3514}. IDH2 p.R172 is the analogue of the p.R132 residue in IDH1, and it is located in the enzyme's active site, forming hydrogen bonds with the isocitrate substrate. *IDH2* mutations are much less fre-quent than *IDH1* mutations in IDH-mutant astrocytoma.

Glioma-associated *IDH1* and *IDH2* mutations impart a gain-of-function phenotype to the respective metabolic enzymes IDH1 and IDH2, which then overproduce the oncometabolite 2-hydroxyglutarate {674}. The physiological consequences of 2-hydroxyglutarate overproduction are widespread and include profound effects on cellular epigenomic states and gene regu-lation {591,931}. The introduction of mutant *IDH1* into primary human astrocytes alters specific histone markers and induces extensive DNA hypermethylation (termed the "glioma-associ-ated CpG island methylator phenotype [G-CIMP]"), suggesting that the presence of an *IDH1* mutation is sufficient to estab-lish a hypermethylation phenotype {3240}. Widespread hyper-methylation in gene promoter regions is thought to silence the expression of several important cellular differentiation factors

{1948,3240} and to favour the emergence or maintenance of a stem cell–like state prone to self-renewal and tumorigenesis {3239}. IDH mutations may also promote glioma formation by disrupting the binding of the methylation-sensitive insulator protein CTCF, thus affecting chromosomal topology and allow-ing aberrant chromosomal regulatory interactions that induce oncogene expression {945}. *MGMT* promoter methylation is also commonly observed in IDH-mutant gliomas {2204,3240}. *MGMT* encodes a DNA repair protein {598} that removes pro-mutagenic alkyl groups from the O6 position of guanine in DNA, thereby blunting the treatment effects of some alkylating agents {860,1062} (see also *Glioblastoma, IDH-wildtype*, p. 39). How-ever, the predictive role of *MGMT* promoter methylation may be limited to tumours that additionally exhibit loss of one copy of chromosome 10, where *MGMT* is located (e.g. IDH-wildtype glioblastoma).

IDH-mutant astrocytomas also harbour class-defining loss-of-function mutations in *TP53* and *ATRX* {1474,1547,452}. *ATRX* encodes an essential chromatin-binding protein, and its defi-ciency has been associated with epigenomic dysregulation and telomere dysfunction {611}. In particular, *ATRX* mutations induce an abnormal telomere maintenance mechanism known as alter-native lengthening of telomeres {1276}. *ATRX* mutations and alternative lengthening of telomeres are mutually exclusive with activating promoter mutations of the *TERT* gene, which encodes the catalytic component of telomerase. *TERT* promoter muta-tions are rare in IDH-mutant astrocytomas, but they are present

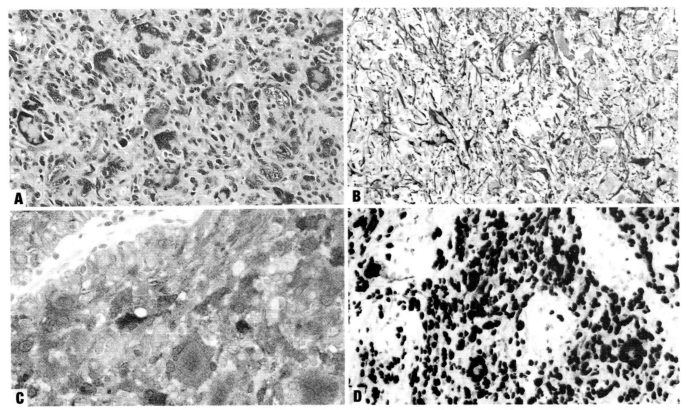

Fig. 2.11 Astrocytoma, IDH-mutant, CNS WHO grade 4 with giant cell features. **A** Giant cell tumours are often IDH-wildtype, but this example was IDH-mutant. Next-generation sequencing revealed biallelic *MLH1* inactivation, as well as hypermutation, including mutations of the *IDH1*, *TP53*, and *ATRX* genes. **B** This tumour with a mismatch repair defect showed GFAP immunoreactivity. **C** Although most giant cell glioblastomas are IDH-wildtype, this one was IDH-mutant, as evidenced by the immunoreactivity for IDH1 p.R132H. **D** This giant cell tumour with a mismatch repair defect showed diffuse p53 positivity, consistent with *TP53* mutation.

in the vast majority of IDH-mutant oligodendrogliomas and IDH-wildtype glioblastomas {452,824,1614}.

ATRX deficiency has also been associated with generalized genomic instability, which can induce p53-dependent cell death in some contexts {628}. Therefore, *TP53* mutations in IDH-mutant astrocytomas may enable tumour cell survival in the setting of ATRX loss. The genomic instability of IDH-mutant astrocytomas is reflected in characteristic DNA copy-number abnormalities, which include low-level amplification events involving the oncogenes *MYC* and *CCND2* in mutually exclusive subsets {452}. Copy-number events typically associated with IDH-wildtype glioblastoma, such as *EGFR* amplification as well as *PTEN* mutation or deletion, are rarely encountered, emphasizing the biological differences between IDH-mutant and IDH-wildtype astrocytomas {452,824,1145}.

Genetic alterations associated with tumour progression
Multiple retrospective studies indicate that homozygous deletion of *CDKN2A* and/or *CDKN2B* is associated with shorter survival in patients with IDH-mutant astrocytomas, corresponding to CNS WHO grade 4 behaviour (see also *Prognosis and prediction*, below) {357}. Alterations in other genes encoding members of the RB1 pathway, including *CDK4* amplification and *RB1* mutation or homozygous deletion, may also be associated with accelerated growth {357}. *PDGFRA* amplification {357}, *MET* alterations {1875,1362}, *MYCN* amplifications, and mutations in *PIK3R1* and *PIK3CA* have been associated with shorter survival and may play a role in tumour progression {357}.

Macroscopic appearance

IDH-mutant astrocytomas of low histological grade are expansile and blur the grey matter–white matter junction. They enlarge and distort invaded anatomical structures and may show large or small cysts. Extensive microcyst formation occasionally produces a gelatinous appearance, or a single large cyst filled with clear fluid. Large, grossly detectable calcifications are not present, but diffuse grittiness is occasionally noted. Higher-grade examples may show similar features, but large coalescent zones of yellowish discolouration due to necrosis and/or haemorrhage may also be present.

Histopathology

IDH-mutant astrocytomas range from well-differentiated, low-cell-density, and slow-growing tumours (CNS WHO grade 2) to highly anaplastic, hypercellular, and rapidly progressive tumours (CNS WHO grade 4).

CNS WHO grade 2 tumours are composed of well-differentiated fibrillary glial cells that diffusely infiltrate the CNS parenchyma individually, usually without cellular cohesion, generating a loosely structured, often microcystic matrix {3303,1398}. Cellularity is mildly to moderately increased compared with that of normal brain, and mild nuclear atypia is characteristic. Tumour cell density and cellular morphology may vary, the latter with respect to cell size, cytoplasmic abundance, and prominence of cellular processes. Histological recognition of neoplastic astrocytes depends mainly on nuclear characteristics. Compared with those in normal astrocytes, the nuclei in IDH-mutant

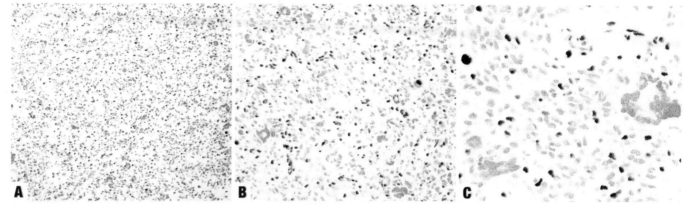

Fig. 2.12 Astrocytoma, IDH-mutant, CNS WHO grade 4 with giant cell features. **A** This tumour with a mismatch repair defect showed loss of ATRX expression by immunohistochemistry. **B** MLH1 expression was lost in tumour nuclei but retained in endothelial cells and other non-neoplastic cells in this tumour with a mismatch repair defect. **C** In addition to loss of MLH1 in tumour cells, secondary PMS2 loss was detected by immunohistochemistry, as expected, given that these two proteins normally form heterodimers.

astrocytomas are enlarged, and they display irregular nuclear contours, an uneven chromatin pattern, and hyperchromasia. Overall, monomorphic nuclei and rounded nuclear contours may be seen, occasionally showing morphological overlap with oligodendroglial tumours. Nucleoli are typically indistinct and are most often not visible. Unlike in cells undergoing reactive astrocytosis, cellular processes in IDH-mutant astrocytomas usually vary from one tumour cell to the next. Mitotic activity is absent or uncommon in CNS WHO grade 2 tumours; a single mitosis within a resection specimen is compatible with a CNS WHO grade 2 designation {357}.

The principal feature distinguishing CNS WHO grade 3 astrocytomas from CNS WHO grade 2 astrocytomas is increased mitotic activity and histological anaplasia (see *Grading*, below). However, the threshold for a CNS WHO grade 3 designation has not been established in IDH-mutant astrocytoma cohorts. One mitotic figure may be sufficient for assigning grade 3 within a very small biopsy, whereas more mitoses are required in larger resection specimens {357}. Grade 3 tumours also often display increased cell density and greater nuclear atypia, including variation in nuclear size and shape, chromatin coarseness, and

dispersion. Multinucleated tumour cells and abnormal mitoses may be seen. By definition, microvascular proliferation (multilayered endothelia within vessels) and necrosis are absent.

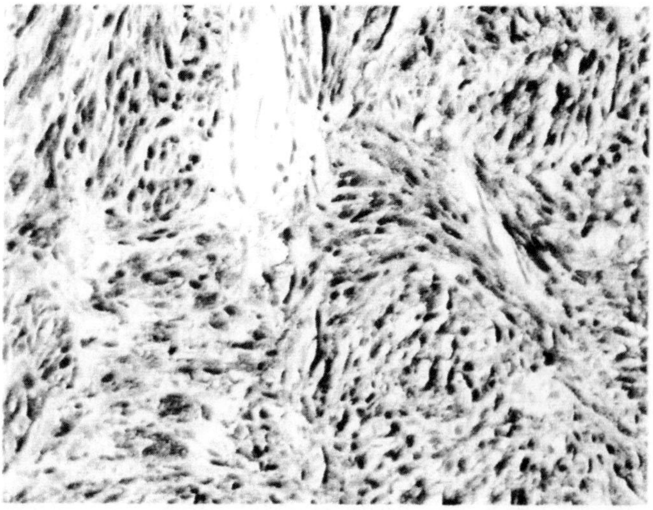

CNS WHO grade 4 tumours must manifest necrosis and/or microvascular proliferation in addition to the features of CNS WHO grade 3 lesions, but the designation of CNS WHO grade 4 IDH-mutant astrocytoma is also warranted if the tumour shows homozygous deletion of *CDKN2A* and/or *CDKN2B*, even in the absence of necrosis or microvascular proliferation (see *Grading* and *Diagnostic molecular pathology*) {357}. For more information about the histopathology of microvascular proliferation, see the *Histopathology* subsection (p. 45) in *Glioblastoma, IDH-wildtype*.

The term "glioblastoma" is no longer applied to CNS WHO grade 4 IDH-mutant astrocytoma. Morphologically, however, the histology of individual cells of CNS WHO grade 4 IDH-mutant astrocytoma has considerable overlap with that of IDH-wildtype glioblastoma, and distinguishing between them requires testing for IDH mutations. Nevertheless, some features differ. Areas of ischaemic zonal and/or palisading necrosis have been observed in 50% of CNS WHO grade 4 IDH-mutant astrocytomas, considerably less frequently than in IDH-wildtype glioblastoma, where they are found in as many as 90% of cases {2269}. Focal oligodendroglioma-like components are more common in CNS WHO grade 4 IDH-mutant astrocytoma than in IDH-wildtype glioblastoma {2269,1789}.

Gemistocytic differentiation can be noted focally, regionally, or nearly uniformly in all grades of IDH-mutant astrocytoma. However, the gemistocytic tissue pattern is not specific to IDH-mutant astrocytomas and can be noted in IDH-wildtype gliomas as well. To be considered a major tissue pattern, gemistocytes should account for (approximately) > 20% of all tumour cells – a somewhat arbitrary, but useful, criterion {3394,1744,3198}. Gemistocytes are characterized by plump, glassy, eosinophilic cell bodies and stout, randomly oriented processes that form a coarse fibrillary network. Nuclei are typically eccentric, with small, distinct nucleoli and densely clumped chromatin. Perivascular lymphocyte cuffing is frequent {417}. This tissue pattern is associated with a focal gain of chromosome 12p encompassing *CCND2* {2780}. No definite associations with clinical behaviour are known.

Fig. 2.13 Astrocytoma, IDH-mutant, CNS WHO grade 4 with gliosarcoma features. Although most gliosarcomas are IDH-wildtype, this example was IDH-mutant, as evidenced by immunoreactivity for IDH1 p.R132H protein.

Proliferation

In older studies, when IDH status was not incorporated into the diagnosis, astrocytomas with ≥ 2 mitoses within the entire specimen were associated with shorter survival than those with < 2 mitoses {633,1091,684}, but several studies of patients with IDH-mutant astrocytoma have not corroborated these thresholds for mitotic activity {3539,2318,809}. However, others have demonstrated that traditional grading schemes based on mitoses can stratify risk among patients with grade 2 and grade 3 IDH-mutant astrocytomas {597,2916,3522}. To date, no studies have established an alternative mitotic count threshold that more reliably stratifies risk among histological CNS WHO grade 2 and grade 3 IDH-mutant astrocytomas.

Similarly, studies of proliferation (e.g. based on the Ki-67 index) have not identified criteria that unequivocally stratify risk among patients with IDH-mutant astrocytomas {809}. The growth fraction as determined by the Ki-67 proliferation index is usually < 4% for CNS WHO grade 2 IDH-mutant astrocytomas. In CNS WHO grade 3 tumours, the Ki-67 proliferation index is usually in the range of 4–10%, but it can overlap with values for CNS WHO grade 2 tumours at one end of the range and CNS WHO grade 4 tumours at the other {632,1457,1557,2601}. Ki-67 proliferation index values in CNS WHO grade 4 IDH-mutant astrocytomas vary considerably and do not appear to be associated with survival {362}.

Grading

Astrocytoma, IDH-mutant, can be designated as CNS WHO grade 2, 3, or 4, according to the criteria in Table 2.01 {357}.

Immunophenotype

Individual tumour cells of IDH-mutant astrocytoma reliably express GFAP, although to varying degrees {1647}. Gemistocytic tumour cells are typically strongly and uniformly positive for GFAP {3395}. OLIG2 is a transcription factor that shows strong nuclear immunoreactivity in most forms of diffuse gliomas, including IDH-mutant astrocytomas. One study concluded that OLIG2 expression was lower in high-grade IDH-mutant astrocytomas than in other IDH-mutant gliomas {1892,2824}. Vimentin is often positive in tumour cells, with a labelling pattern similar to that of GFAP {1296}. Immunohistochemical assays used as surrogates for genetic alterations (e.g. IDH1 p.R132H, p53, ATRX) are discussed below, in the *Diagnostic molecular pathology* subsection.

Differential diagnosis

For CNS WHO grade 2 tumours, the main differential diagnostic considerations are normal brain and reactive astrocytosis. The cytoplasm of normal human astrocytes, in contrast to that of IDH-mutant astrocytoma cells, is not distinct from the background neuropil. Their nuclei are small and regular, displaying delicate and uniform chromatin patterns. Reactive astrocytes are defined by enlarged nuclei (often with a single prominent nucleolus) and clearly distinguished cytoplasm. Reactive gemistocytes are a specific type of astrocytes that are characterized by abundant eosinophilic cytoplasm, eccentric nuclei, and prominent glial processes. Reactive astrocytes are often uniformly distributed throughout tissue and often show similar nuclear and cytoplasmic features, unlike neoplastic cells. Microcystic change strongly favours neoplasia over reactive

Table 2.01 Grading criteria for astrocytoma, IDH-mutant

Grade	Criteria
CNS WHO grade 2	• A diffusely infiltrative astrocytic glioma with an *IDH1* or *IDH2* mutation that is well differentiated and lacks histological features of anaplasia • Mitotic activity is not detected or very low • Microvascular proliferation, necrosis, and homozygous deletions of *CDKN2A* and/or *CDKN2B* are absent
CNS WHO grade 3	• A diffusely infiltrative astrocytic glioma with an *IDH1* or *IDH2* mutation that exhibits focal or dispersed anaplasia and displays significant mitotic activity • Microvascular proliferation, necrosis, and homozygous deletions of *CDKN2A* and/or *CDKN2B* are absent
CNS WHO grade 4	• A diffusely infiltrative astrocytic glioma with an *IDH1* or *IDH2* mutation that exhibits microvascular proliferation or necrosis or homozygous deletion of *CDKN2A* and/or *CDKN2B*, or any combination of these features

astrocytosis. Because most IDH-mutant diffuse astrocytomas have *IDH1* p.R132H mutations, the finding of positive immunostaining for IDH1 p.R132H excludes reactive astrocytosis {445}. Prior freezing of tissue for intraoperative diagnosis, however, may abrogate IDH1 p.R132H immunostaining and can distort nuclear cytological features.

IDH-mutant astrocytoma has a wide differential diagnosis with other diffusely growing brain tumours. The primary considerations are oligodendroglioma, IDH-mutant and 1p/19q-codeleted; glioblastoma, IDH-wildtype; diffuse midline glioma, H3 K27–altered; diffuse hemispheric glioma, H3 G34–mutant; diffuse astrocytoma, *MYB*- or *MYBL1*-altered; diffuse low-grade glioma, MAPK pathway–altered; and high-grade astrocytoma with piloid features.

Cytology

The use of cytological preparations at the time of intraoperative consultation can add value to frozen section evaluation, because certain cellular features (e.g. coarse chromatin, nuclear contour irregularity, fibrillary processes) may be enhanced or accentuated. Individual cells show enlarged, angulated, and hyperchromatic nuclei and may display elongated eosinophilic cellular processes, which often form a loose background of fibrillarity that is helpful in defining glial differentiation. With increasing grade, greater neoplastic cytological pleomorphism and more mitotic figures can be found. In CNS WHO grade 4 IDH-mutant astrocytomas, necrotic debris and/or vessels with endothelial proliferation may also be present in cytological preparations.

Diagnostic molecular pathology

Many of the signature molecular characteristics of IDH-mutant astrocytoma can be demonstrated immunohistochemically. A routine immunohistochemical panel for the initial diagnostic workup of diffuse gliomas in adults involves IDH1 p.R132H, p53, and ATRX {3131,3303}.

Immunohistochemical staining for IDH1 p.R132H is highly sensitive and specific for the *IDH1* p.R132H mutation, and immunopositivity is strong evidence of IDH-mutant glioma {465,351}. IDH1 p.R132H immunohistochemistry has become a critical initial test for the classification of gliomas and also

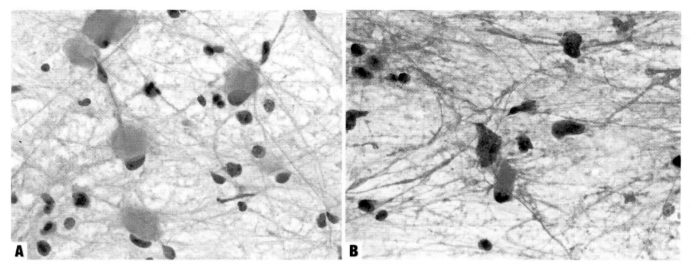

Fig. 2.14 Astrocytoma, IDH-mutant, CNS WHO grade 3. **A** Cytopathological smear preparations highlight the large round eosinophilic cell bodies and delicate glial processes of astrocytoma cells with gemistocytic differentiation. **B** Smear preparation shows IDH-mutant astrocytoma cells with enlarged, hyperchromatic, and irregular nuclei within a background of extensive fibrillarity created by the elongated fibrillar processes emanating from tumour cell bodies.

helps to distinguish true neoplasia from reactive gliosis {445, 464}. The p.R132H variant accounts for approximately 90% of all IDH mutations in supratentorial astrocytomas. Of note, more rarely occurring primary infratentorial IDH-mutant astrocytomas show a distinctively different spectrum of IDH mutations, and about 80% are of the non-p.R132H type {187}. Gene sequencing analysis of *IDH1* codon 132 and *IDH2* codon 172 is recommended in the event of a negative or indeterminate result with the IDH1 p.R132H immunohistochemical stain, in order to rule out the possibility of a non-p.R132H IDH mutation {452,3514}. Given the low frequency of *IDH1* and *IDH2* mutations in CNS WHO grade 4 gliomas arising in patients aged > 55 years, sequencing analysis need not follow a negative IDH1 p.R132H immunostain in this patient population {746,2687,1245}.

In the setting of an IDH-mutant glioma, the detection of strong and diffuse p53 immunopositivity can be used as a surrogate for *TP53* mutations and in support of the diagnosis of IDH-mutant astrocytoma. *TP53* mutation often leads to reduced degradation of the protein, and to its nuclear accumulation; however, not all *TP53* mutations manifest as strong nuclear immunoreactivity, and nonsense mutations in particular can sometimes be associated with a complete absence of staining. Strong nuclear p53 immunohistochemical positivity in > 10% of tumour nuclei correlates well with *TP53* mutations in the setting of an IDH-mutant glioma, but it is best evaluated in the context of morphology and other immunohistochemistry in the diagnostic panel, such as ATRX {3131,1108,3112}. Most IDH-mutant astrocytomas show even more widespread (> 50%) p53 expression {3112}.

Inactivating *ATRX* alterations commonly co-occur with *TP53* mutations in IDH-mutant astrocytomas {821,279,1405}. These often result in a truncated protein and abrogated protein expression, leading to loss of nuclear ATRX immunoreactivity {2657}. ATRX immunopositivity in the nuclei of endothelial cells and neurons serves as an internal positive control {3131} because ATRX protein is prone to rapid degradation in tissue with even minimal hypoxic damage, so areas of tissue showing nuclear ATRX immunopositivity in these cells should be assessed. Loss of nuclear ATRX expression in neoplastic cells strongly

supports the diagnosis of IDH-mutant astrocytoma but is not a surrogate for IDH assessment because loss of nuclear ATRX is also found in H3-altered diffuse gliomas and occasionally in IDH-wildtype gliomas. In addition, although the rate of ATRX loss is > 90% in supratentorial IDH-mutant astrocytomas, the rate in infratentorial IDH-mutant astrocytomas is only about 50% {187}. The combination of mutations in *IDH1* or *IDH2* and *ATRX* in a diffuse glioma (including by immunohistochemistry) is sufficient for the diagnosis of IDH-mutant astrocytoma, obviating the need for 1p/19q testing in order to exclude oligodendroglioma.

Rare cases of dual-genotype IDH-mutant gliomas have been described; distinct regions within these tumours have oligodendroglioma morphology and 1p/19q codeletion, while other regions have astrocytic morphology, ATRX loss, and *TP53* mutations {1382,2587}. A more recent publication documented two dual-genotype IDH-mutant gliomas that displayed uniform tumour morphology throughout, as well as ATRX loss, *TP53* mutations, and 1p/19q codeletion in all tumour regions tested {3588}. These cases, although rare, indicate that the defining molecular alterations of IDH-mutant astrocytomas and oligodendroglioma are not absolutely mutually exclusive. The precise classification for these dual-genotype IDH-mutant gliomas has not been established. However, a layered diagnostic approach that includes morphological findings and molecular alterations, combined with an "NEC" designation, may be appropriate {1946,1939}.

As discussed above, a molecular marker that is strongly associated with unfavourable prognosis in IDH-mutant astrocytoma is homozygous deletion of *CDKN2A* and/or *CDKN2B* {2916}. This has prompted grading of IDH-mutant astrocytoma with homozygous *CDKN2A* and/or *CDKN2B* deletion as CNS WHO grade 4, irrespective of other morphological signs of high-grade malignancy such as necrosis or microvascular proliferation {357}.

Methylation profiling readily identifies IDH-mutant astrocytoma because of the profound influence of IDH mutations on the methylome. Accordingly, the presence of an *IDH1* or *IDH2* mutation can be reliably inferred by this method, although the specific amino acid exchange impacting either *IDH1* or *IDH2* cannot be determined. Methylation profiling can also be used to distinguish between subgroups of IDH-mutant astrocytomas, including those of low and high grade in the supratentorial compartment as well as those in the infratentorial regions {460,187}; see also Fig. 2.02 (p. 16). Copy-number profiles calculated from methylome data can also be useful for determining *CDKN2A* and/or *CDKN2B* and 1p/19q codeletion status.

Essential and desirable diagnostic criteria
See Box 2.01.

Staging
Not clinically relevant

Prognosis and prediction
Clinical prognostic factors
Studies specifically addressing IDH-mutant astrocytomas have confirmed the association of younger age with longer survival {2916,3522}. Similarly, the extent of resection and the presence of postoperative residual tumour have been shown to correlate with overall survival (OS) {1514,3442,234}.

Proliferation
Proliferative activity quantified by mitotic count remains a grading criterion for IDH-mutant astrocytomas, yet several studies of IDH-mutant cohorts have not shown significant risk stratification {3539,2318,809}. Other studies have demonstrated that traditional grading schemes based on mitotic activity can stratify risk among patients with CNS WHO grade 2 and 3 IDH-mutant astrocytomas {597,2916,3522}. In one study of histological grade 2 and 3 diffuse gliomas, investigators were not able to identify a Ki-67 threshold that could reliably stratify risk among IDH-mutant astrocytomas {809}.

Histopathological and genetic factors
The histopathological factors relevant for grading (mitotic activity, microvascular proliferation, and necrosis) are relevant for prognosis (see *Proliferation* and *Grading*, above). Patients with IDH-mutant CNS WHO grade 2 astrocytomas have a median OS of > 10 years {123,2916}. An IDH-mutant astrocytoma that contains considerable mitotic activity and histological anaplasia yet lacks microvascular proliferation, necrosis, and *CDKN2A* and/or *CDKN2B* homozygous deletion currently fits into the designation of CNS WHO grade 3 IDH-mutant astrocytoma, and patients with such tumours have typical median OS in the range of 5–10 years {3346}.

IDH-mutant astrocytomas with microvascular proliferation, necrosis, or *CDKN2A* and/or *CDKN2B* homozygous deletion (or any combination of these features) correspond to CNS WHO

Box 2.01 Diagnostic criteria for astrocytoma, IDH-mutant

Essential:

A diffusely infiltrating glioma

AND

IDH1 codon 132 or *IDH2* codon 172 missense mutation

AND

    Loss of nuclear ATRX expression or *ATRX* mutation

    OR

    Exclusion of combined whole-arm deletions of 1p and 19q

Desirable:

TP53 mutation or strong nuclear expression of p53 in > 10% of tumour cells

Methylation profile of astrocytoma, IDH-mutant

Astrocytic differentiation by morphology

grade 4 {123,2916}, with expected median OS of about 3 years {3346}. The inclusion of *CDKN2A* and/or *CDKN2B* homozygous deletion as a criterion is based on evidence that the occurrence of these deletions in IDH-mutant astrocytomas of histological grade 2 or 3 is associated with worse outcome, corresponding to CNS WHO grade 4. Some studies have further concluded that homozygous deletion of *CDKN2A* and/or *CDKN2B* is associated with worse outcome among patients with histologically defined CNS WHO grade 4 IDH-mutant astrocytomas {1714, 2916}.

In addition to *CDKN2A* and/or *CDKN2B* homozygous deletion, several other molecular alterations in IDH-mutant astrocytoma have been associated with malignant progression. Some of these occur concomitantly in higher-grade tumours, complicating the assessment of the prognostic impact of individual alterations. For example, in some reports, a significantly worse prognosis was associated with homozygous deletion of *RB1* {2916} or amplification of *CDK4* {597,3522,122}, whereas others did not corroborate these associations {596,123}. DNA methylation profiling has identified two grade-related methylation groups that are associated with differences in OS {460,2916}. Amplification of *PDGFRA* was associated with worse prognosis in several studies {2498,2916,3522}. Other copy-number alterations with a reported negative association with prognosis include *MET* amplification {1875}, *MYCN* amplification {2916}, and chromosome 14q loss {3387,596,597}. One study found that activating point mutations in *PIK3R1* were associated with shorter OS in univariate analysis {122}. Evidence suggests that a higher global copy-number variation load also correlates with worse prognosis {122,2122,2123,2741}.

Oligodendroglioma, IDH-mutant and 1p/19q-codeleted

Reifenberger G
Cairncross JG
Figarella-Branger D
Hartmann C
Kros JM
Louis DN
Snuderl M
Suvà ML
Van Den Bent MJ
Yip S
Yokoo H

Definition

Oligodendroglioma, IDH-mutant and 1p/19q-codeleted, is a diffusely infiltrating glioma with *IDH1* or *IDH2* mutation and codeletion of chromosome arms 1p and 19q (CNS WHO grade 2 or 3).

ICD-O coding

9450/3 Oligodendroglioma, IDH-mutant and 1p/19q-codeleted, grade 2
9451/3 Oligodendroglioma, IDH-mutant and 1p/19q-codeleted, grade 3

ICD-11 coding

2A00.0Y & XH7K31 Other specified gliomas of brain & Oligodendroglioma, IDH-mutant and 1p/19q-codeleted

Related terminology

Not recommended: anaplastic oligodendroglioma, IDH-mutant and 1p/19q-codeleted.

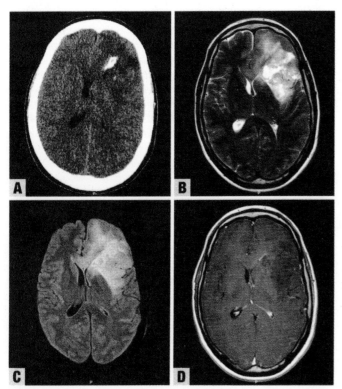

Fig. 2.15 Oligodendroglioma, IDH-mutant and 1p/19q-codeleted, CNS WHO grade 2. A predominantly left frontal low-grade oligodendroglioma. **A** There is involvement of the corpus callosum and mass effect; CT without intravenous contrast shows the presence of a calcification in a hypodense region. **B** Involvement of the corpus callosum and mass effect on T2-weighted MRI. **C** The tumour produces a hyperintense lesion on FLAIR MRI, with cortical involvement, diffuse borders, and signal heterogeneity. **D** There is absence of contrast enhancement after intravenous gadolinium administration on T1-weighted MRI.

Subtype(s)

Oligodendroglioma, IDH-mutant and 1p/19q-codeleted, CNS WHO grade 2; oligodendroglioma, IDH-mutant and 1p/19q-codeleted, CNS WHO grade 3

Localization

Among 5542 histologically defined oligodendrogliomas registered in the Central Brain Tumor Registry of the United States (CBTRUS) database, 59% were located in the frontal lobe, 14% in the temporal lobe, 10% in the parietal lobe, and 1% in the occipital lobe {498}. Among 470 genetically defined CNS WHO grade 3 oligodendrogliomas of the French national POLA network, 62% were frontal tumours, 16% were temporal, 15% were parietal, and 6% were occipital {2542}. Other studies have also shown a clear predilection for the frontal lobes in IDH-mutant and 1p/19q-codeleted oligodendrogliomas {2970,1143,3442}. Less common locations include the posterior fossa, basal ganglia, and brainstem. Exceptional cases of IDH-mutant and 1p/19q-codeleted oligodendroglioma show widespread intracerebral dissemination corresponding to a gliomatosis cerebri pattern {1298}. Leptomeningeal spread is occasionally seen in patients with IDH-mutant and 1p/19q-codeleted oligodendroglioma, in particular at recurrence {106}. Primary leptomeningeal manifestation of IDH-mutant and 1p/19q-codeleted oligodendroglioma has also been reported {183}. Rare cases of intramedullary spinal oligodendroglioma are on record, but data on genotype are usually lacking {970,1264}. Rarely, patients may present with multifocal tumours {1036}. Individual cases of morphologically defined oligodendrogliomas (not genetically characterized) that developed from ovarian teratomas have been reported {3247}.

Clinical features

Seizures are the presenting symptom in approximately two thirds of patients with IDH-mutant and 1p/19q-codeleted oligodendroglioma {3589,401}. Additional common initial symptoms include headache, other signs of increased intracranial pressure, focal neurological deficits, and cognitive changes. These signs and symptoms are nonspecific and depend on the tumour's location and speed of growth. With advanced imaging becoming more widely available for symptom screening, incidental diagnosis is more frequently reported, accounting for 10%′ of cases in one study {3442}.

Imaging

IDH-mutant and 1p/19q-codeleted oligodendrogliomas usually appear on CT as hypodense or isodense mass lesions that are typically located in the cortex and subcortical white matter {2971}. Calcifications are commonly seen, but they are not diagnostic; some tumours show intratumoural haemorrhages and/or areas of cystic degeneration {2971}. MRI typically shows a T1-hypointense and T2-hyperintense mass with indistinct tumour margins. Signal intensities on T1-weighted and T2-weighted MRI are often heterogeneous. Gadolinium contrast enhancement can be detected in < 20% of CNS WHO grade 2 oligodendrogliomas, but it is present in > 70% of CNS WHO grade 3 oligodendrogliomas, where it is associated with microvascular proliferation and less favourable prognosis {1600,3061,1221, 2739}. IDH-mutant and 1p/19q-codeleted oligodendrogliomas showed higher microvascularity (higher rCBV) and higher vascular heterogeneity than IDH-mutant diffuse astrocytomas of corresponding grade {1810}. Magnetic resonance spectroscopy and radiomics can identify differences in certain features between 1p/19q-codeleted and 1p/19q-intact low-grade diffuse gliomas, but these techniques have limited sensitivity and specificity (~80% in validation series) and cannot yet replace molecular diagnostics {387,903,3356,3279}. Demonstration of elevated 2-hydroxyglutarate levels by magnetic resonance spectroscopy is a new means of non-invasively detecting IDH-mutant gliomas (including oligodendrogliomas), but it remains technically challenging {580}. PET imaging may allow the distinction between CNS WHO grade 2 and 3 IDH-mutant gliomas, but reported series tend to be small and unvalidated {2299}.

Spread

IDH-mutant and 1p/19q-codeleted oligodendrogliomas characteristically extend into adjacent brain in a diffuse manner. Like other diffuse gliomas, they occasionally have a gliomatosis cerebri pattern {1298}. In late-stage disease especially, distant leptomeningeal spread may occur in some patients {106}. Rare cases of extracranial metastases of oligodendrogliomas, mostly CNS WHO grade 3, have been reported {2082,2945,420}. At times, patients with progressive tumours without treatment options may show slow clinical deterioration despite the presence of large enhancing lesions.

Epidemiology

The following paragraphs mostly refer to epidemiological data based on histological tumour classification, because population-based data on molecularly defined oligodendrogliomas are not yet available. Thus, the available information must be interpreted with caution as histologically defined oligodendroglial tumours include a considerable subset of gliomas without IDH mutation and 1p/19q codeletion {928,3100,794}.

Incidence

The reported incidence rate (cases per 100 000 person-years) of histologically diagnosed oligodendrogliomas ranges from 0.10 in the Republic of Korea {1826} to 0.50 in France {677}; in the USA, the incidence rate is 0.23 {2344}. For histologically diagnosed CNS WHO grade 3 oligodendrogliomas, the incidence rate is 0.06 in the Republic of Korea {1826}, 0.11 in the USA {2344}, and 0.39 in France {677}. Thus, 0.9% of all brain tumours in the USA are CNS WHO grade 2 oligodendrogliomas and 0.4% are CNS WHO grade 3 oligodendrogliomas {2344}. Approximately one third of all oligodendroglial tumours correspond to CNS WHO grade 3 {2344}. A decrease in the incidence of oligodendrogliomas from 2000 to 2013 has been reported, a finding probably related to changes in diagnostic criteria over time {15}.

Age and sex distribution

Oligodendrogliomas manifest preferentially in adults, with a median age at diagnosis of 43 years reported in the population-based CBTRUS dataset for patients with histologically defined CNS WHO grade 2 oligodendroglioma and 50 years for those with CNS WHO grade 3 oligodendroglioma {2344}. The median ages were comparable for patients with IDH-mutant and 1p/19q-codeleted oligodendrogliomas: 41 years for patients with CNS WHO grade 2 tumours and 47 years for patients with CNS WHO grade 3 tumours {1246}. Overall, histologically defined CNS WHO grade 3 oligodendroglioma shows a slight male predominance, with an M:F ratio of 1.2:1 reported among 5476 patients {2344}. CNS WHO grade 3 oligodendroglioma is more common in White populations than in Black populations, with an incidence ratio of 2.3:1 {2344}. Oligodendrogliomas are rare in children, and few data are available on IDH-mutant and 1p/19q-codeleted oligodendrogliomas in this population. In one study, 3 (14%) of 22 tumours with the typical morphological characteristics of oligodendroglioma demonstrated *IDH1* p.R132H mutation and 1p/19q codeletion {2703}. These 3 patients were aged 16–19 years, indicating that IDH-mutant and 1p/19q-codeleted oligodendrogliomas are rare in children.

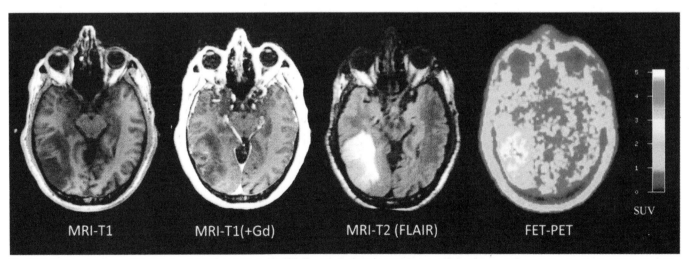

MRI-T1 MRI-T1(+Gd) MRI-T2 (FLAIR) FET-PET

SUV

Fig. 2.16 Oligodendroglioma, IDH-mutant and 1p/19q-codeleted, CNS WHO grade 3. Neuroimaging features. T1-hypointense lesion with focal contrast enhancement after gadolinium administration (+Gd). T2-FLAIR shows the extent of the lesion, and FET PET demonstrates increased metabolic activity.

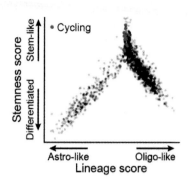

Fig. 2.17 Oligodendroglioma, IDH-mutant and 1p/19q-codeleted. Single-cell RNA-sequencing analysis of human oligodendroglioma. Inferred developmental hierarchy based on genome-wide expression programmes, showing that oligodendroglioma cells can recapitulate stem-like states or more differentiated states along the oligodendroglial or astrocytic lineages. Cycling cells (marked in red) are enriched in stem-like states {3080,3202}.

Etiology

Genetic susceptibility

The etiology of IDH-mutant and 1p/19q-codeleted oligodendroglioma is unclear. Most tumours develop sporadically, in the absence of documented familial clustering or a hereditary cancer predisposition syndrome. However, both familial and sporadic gliomas frequently display shared genomic landscapes, and common core pathways might be targeted by both germline and somatic alterations {1434}. Earlier studies identified SNPs in the *BICRA* (*GLTSCR1*) and *ERCC2* genes as well as the *GSTT1* null genotype with increased risk of oligodendroglioma {3521,1587}. Germline mutations of *POT1*, a shelterin complex gene, have been associated with familial oligodendroglioma {176}. Cases of familial oligodendroglioma with 1p/19q codeletion have been reported {944,2339}. Given that pathological production of 2-hydroxyglutarate, resulting from somatic mutations in *IDH1* or *IDH2*, is found in all oligodendrogliomas and IDH-mutant astrocytomas, it is of interest that variants (particularly rs5839764) in or near the *D2HGDH* gene, which codes for D-2-hydroxyglutarate dehydrogenase, showed genome-wide association with IDH-mutant gliomas {823}. The same study identified rs111976262, located near the *FAM20C* gene, as showing genome-wide association with IDH-mutant, *TERT* promoter–mutant, and 1p/19q-codeleted oligodendrogliomas.

Gliomas have been reported in specific hereditary cancer syndromes including germline *BRCA1* mutations, constitutional mismatch repair deficiency syndrome, Lynch syndrome (also known as hereditary non-polyposis colorectal cancer), and hereditary retinoblastoma, yet oligodendrogliomas are uncommon {1484,3154,2071,1277,22}. Patients with the enchondromatosis syndromes Ollier disease and Maffucci syndrome, which are associated with somatic (or postzygotic) IDH mosaicism, present with multiple benign cartilaginous tumours {95}. A retrospective cohort study showed that those patients may develop gliomas with an anatomical presentation and a grading distribution similar to those of gliomas in non-syndromic patients, but they are typically younger and more often have multicentric lesions {320}. However, none of the gliomas in this enchondromatosis cohort harboured 1p/19q codeletion.

Other etiological factors

The potential role of viral infections in the etiology of IDH-mutant and 1p/19q-codeleted oligodendroglioma has been debated. Several studies have reported the detection of CMV in gliomas including oligodendrogliomas {270,2831}. However, other studies have concluded that CMV is not present in gliomas {222}. Similarly, there have been contradictory findings reported for members of the polyomavirus family (BK virus, JC virus, SV40) {726,2651,2712}. Whole-genome and RNA sequencing, which provided increased sensitivity and specificity for detecting viral genomes and transcripts, revealed only a low-percentage association between HPV and/or HBV and low-grade gliomas including oligodendrogliomas {3054}. It was also determined that previous findings of CMV in gliomas were probably a result of laboratory contamination. Dysregulation of the immune system, including immunodeficiency due to HIV infection, posttransplant immunosuppression therapy, or demyelinating disease, has been associated with rare cases of oligodendroglioma {640, 3041,2835}. However, epidemiological data do not indicate an increased incidence of gliomas in patients with autoimmune disease {1288}. Rat models have shown that nitrosoureas (e.g. ethylnitrosourea and methylnitrosourea) are chemical carcinogens that may induce CNS tumours, including gliomas with an oligodendroglial phenotype {283}. However, cancer studies in humans are not available for these compounds.

Pathogenesis

Cell of origin

The cell (or cells) of origin of IDH-mutant and 1p/19q-codeleted oligodendroglioma remains unknown. Morphology and single-cell RNA-sequencing analysis of human tumours supports the notion that oligodendrogliomas are composed of a mixture of malignant cell types that recapitulate oligodendroglial and astrocytic lineages, as well as neural precursor–like cells {3202}. Experimental transformation of immortalized human glial cells with *IDH1* p.R132H reprogrammes their cellular lineage and favours the emergence of a neural precursor state {3239}. Experiments in transgenic mice indicate that gliomas with oligodendroglial histology may originate from different cell types in the CNS, including neural precursor cells, astrocytes, and oligodendroglial precursor cells {3619}. An oligodendroglioma-like phenotype is commonly found in transgenic brain tumours, despite such tumours showing a variety of targeted cell types and oncogenic events {758,3412}. Studies have suggested that oligodendrogliomas probably originate from oligodendroglial precursor cells {2477,3065}. Oligodendroglial precursor cells have also been suggested as the cell of origin in other classes of gliomas and may give rise to either oligodendroglial or astrocytic phenotypes in gliomas, depending on the genes driving transformation {1915,1901}. Thus, the interplay between oncogenic events and the cell(s) of origin plays a critical role in determining the resulting glioma phenotype.

Genetic profile

The entity-defining alterations in oligodendrogliomas are missense mutations affecting *IDH1* codon 132 or *IDH2* codon 172 combined with whole-arm deletions of 1p and 19q. More than 90% of IDH mutations in oligodendrogliomas correspond to the canonical *IDH1* p.R132H mutation; the remaining tumours carry non-canonical mutations, with a higher proportion of

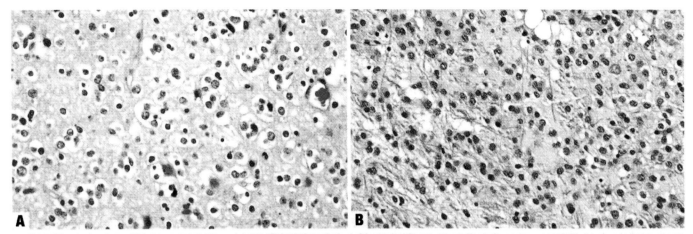

Fig. 2.18 Oligodendroglioma, IDH-mutant and 1p/19q-codeleted, CNS WHO grade 2. **A** Oligodendrogliomas often infiltrate the cortex, and individual tumour cells congregate around neuronal cell bodies. **B** Oligodendroglioma cells are sometimes embedded within a light-blue mucinous matrix.

IDH2 mutations in oligodendrogliomas than in astrocytomas (see also *Astrocytoma, IDH-mutant*, p. 19) {1246,452,824, 126}. The 1p/19q codeletion has been cytogenetically linked to an unbalanced translocation between chromosomes 1 and 19 that results in loss of the der(1;19)(p10;q10) chromosome, causing whole-arm deletions of 1p and 19q, and retention of the der[t(1;19)(q10;p10)] chromosome {1165,1465}. Incomplete/ partial deletions on either chromosome arm are not compatible with the diagnosis of IDH-mutant and 1p/19q-codeleted oligodendroglioma, but they have been detected in a proportion of IDH-wildtype glioblastomas {3339}.

The vast majority of IDH-mutant and 1p/19q-codeleted oligodendrogliomas carry *TERT* promoter hotspot mutations {134, 1614,1678}. However, IDH-mutant and 1p/19q-codeleted oligodendrogliomas arising in teenagers often lack *TERT* promoter mutation {1833}. When present, *TERT* promoter mutation is assumed to be an early (i.e. clonal) event in oligodendroglioma development {3082,881}, which remains stable during tumour progression and at recurrence {44}. Mechanistically, the *TERT* promoter mutations generate de novo ETS transcription factor binding sites {1343}, which results in transcriptional upregulation of TERT expression, thereby driving telomere stabilization, cellular immortalization, and proliferation {1214}.

Mutations of *CIC* (the human orthologue of the *Drosophila melanogaster* capicua gene), located in chromosome band 19q13.2, are also frequent in IDH-mutant and 1p/19q-codeleted oligodendrogliomas {261,3537}, with large-scale sequencing studies reporting *CIC* mutations in as many as 70% of oligodendrogliomas {452,824}. CIC is a constitutive transcriptional repressor of genes essential in development, cellular growth, and metabolism that is relieved by receptor tyrosine kinase signalling {154,3471,38}, and it has been associated with various features of neoplastic behaviour {2940,2317}. *CIC* mutations in oligodendrogliomas are hemizygous and include almost equal proportions of nonsense or truncating mutations and recurrent missense mutations. The latter are preferentially found in the HMG-box DNA-binding domain in exon 5 and the C1 motif in exon 20. They appear to be unique to oligodendroglioma and not present in other *CIC*-mutant tumour types {1823,2317, 2948}. This suggests phenotypic uniqueness of these missense *CIC* mutations in oligodendrogliomas, and that these mutations act cooperatively with IDH mutations to contribute to the pathological upregulation of 2-hydroxyglutarate production {574} and activation of the MAPK signalling pathway {1823,960}. Spatial and temporal profiling of oligodendrogliomas, which have a low mutation burden, has also confirmed the presence of clones bearing unique *CIC* mutations, suggesting the presence of selective pressures to escape normal CIC regulatory control {3082,3202,208}. *CIC* truncating mutations most likely disrupt protein–protein interaction with binding partners including ATXN1L, which appears to result in reciprocal phenotypic alterations {3366,3469,3471}.

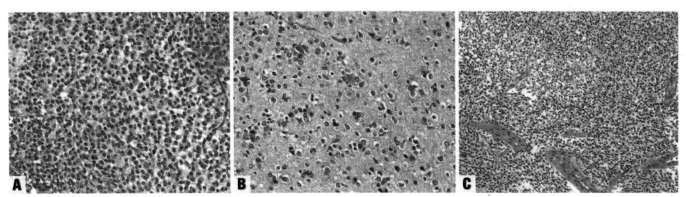

Fig. 2.19 Oligodendroglioma, IDH-mutant and 1p/19q-codeleted, CNS WHO grade 3. **A** Hypercellular region. Many tumour cells retain round to ovoid nuclear morphology. **B** Extensive perineuronal and perivascular satellitosis. **C** Microvascular proliferation.

Approximately 20–30% of IDH-mutant and 1p/19q-codeleted oligodendrogliomas harbour somatic mutations of *FUBP1*, located at chromosome 1p31.1, a region with consistent loss of heterozygosity in these tumours {261,2779}. FUBP1 is a transcriptional regulator essential for normal stem cell self-renewal {2589,1390}. It has recently been identified as a pleiotropic regulator of alternative splicing of tumour suppressor genes and oncogenes {842}. The combined loss of CIC and FUBP1 protein expression, as a surrogate marker of *CIC* and *FUBP1* nonsense or truncating mutations, has been associated with a shorter time to recurrence in patients with 1p/19q-codeleted oligodendroglioma {508}.

Approximately 15% of oligodendrogliomas carry mutations in *NOTCH1*, and less commonly in other NOTCH pathway genes {452,3082}. *NOTCH1* mutation was linked to shorter survival in one study {122}. Other less commonly mutated genes include epigenetic regulator genes such as *SETD2* (and other histone methyltransferase genes), *PIK3CA*, and genes encoding components of the SWI/SNF chromatin remodelling complex {452, 3082}.

Genetic alterations associated with tumour progression
The number of broad copy-number aberrations increases from CNS WHO grade 2 to CNS WHO grade 3 oligodendrogliomas {122}. Deletions on 9p involving the *CDKN2A* and/or *CDKN2B* locus have been associated with CNS WHO grade 3 {2640, 2106}, contrast enhancement on MRI {2658,64}, and shorter

survival {886,64}. In line with these findings, homozygous *CDKN2A* deletion was indicative of short survival in a prospective cohort study of patients with CNS WHO grade 3 IDH-mutant and 1p/19-codeleted oligodendroglioma {123}. Other alterations associated with tumour progression and/or shorter survival include *PIK3CA* mutation {3140,380}, *TCF12* mutation {1778}, and genetic aberrations causing increased MYC signalling {1537}. Whereas IDH mutation, 1p/19q codeletion, and *TERT* promoter mutation are clonal alterations in oligodendrogliomas, mutations in *CIC*, *FUBP1*, *TCF12*, and other genes may be subclonal and thus associated with tumour progression {3082,881}

Epigenetic changes
IDH-mutant and 1p/19q-codeleted oligodendrogliomas show concurrent hypermethylation of multiple CpG islands, corresponding to the glioma CpG island methylator phenotype (G-CIMP){2287}. This phenomenon has been closely linked to IDH mutation causing increased levels of 2-hydroxyglutarate, which functions as a competitive inhibitor of α-ketoglutarate–dependent dioxygenases, including histone demethylases and the TET family of 5-methylcytosine hydroxylases {1948, 3501}. This in turn leads to increased histone methylation and G-CIMP {2287,3240}. DNA methylation profiles of IDH-mutant and 1p/19q-codeleted oligodendrogliomas differ from those of IDH-mutant but 1p/19q-intact astrocytomas, and they can be used for diagnostic purposes {460}. G-CIMP may correlate with epigenetic silencing of multiple genes in oligodendrogliomas,

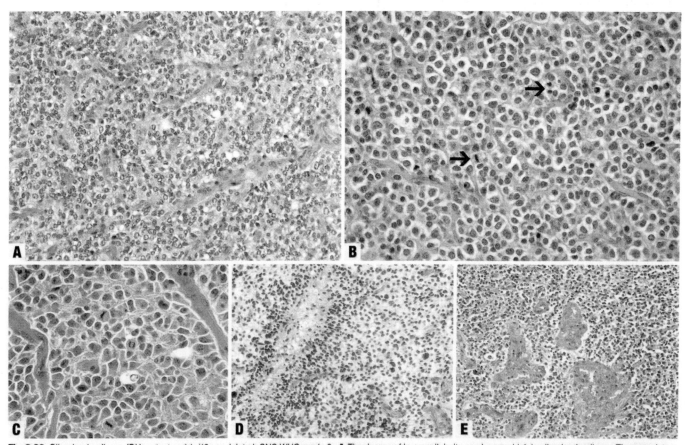

Fig. 2.20 Oligodendroglioma, IDH-mutant and 1p/19q-codeleted, CNS WHO grade 3. **A** The degree of hypercellularity can be very high in oligodendroglioma. The vasculature becomes hypertrophic and proliferative in regions of hypercellularity. **B** Typical image of a cellular glioma with honeycomb cells and mitotic activity (arrows). **C** Marked nuclear atypia and brisk mitotic activity **D** Focal necrosis with palisading tumour cells. **E** Marked microvascular proliferation.

including genes on 1p and 19q, as well as genes on other chromosomes, such as the tumour suppressors *CDKN2A*, *CDKN2B*, and *RB1* {2673}. *MGMT* promoter methylation is detectable in the majority of oligodendrogliomas {2141}. At the mRNA level, IDH-mutant and 1p/19q-codeleted oligodendrogliomas typically show a proneural glioblastoma–like gene-expression signature {798,3418}.

Macroscopic appearance

Oligodendroglioma typically appears macroscopically as a relatively well-defined, soft, greyish-pink mass located in the cortex and white matter, with blurring of the grey matter–white matter boundary. Local invasion into the overlying leptomeninges may be seen. Calcification is frequent and may impart a gritty texture. Occasionally, densely calcified areas may occur as intratumoural stones. Zones of cystic degeneration, as well as intratumoural haemorrhages, are common. Rare cases with extensive mucoid degeneration look gelatinous. Areas of necrosis may be discernible in CNS WHO grade 3 tumours.

Histopathology

Cellular composition

Classic oligodendroglioma cells have uniformly round nuclei that are slightly larger than those of normal oligodendrocytes and show an increase in chromatin density or a delicate salt-and-pepper pattern. A distinct nuclear membrane is often apparent. In formalin-fixed, paraffin-embedded tissue, tumour cells often appear as rounded cells with well-defined cell membranes and clear cytoplasm around the central spherical nucleus. This creates the typical honeycomb or fried-egg appearance, which, although artefactual, is a helpful diagnostic feature. This artefact is not seen in smear preparations or frozen sections, and it may also be absent in rapidly fixed tissue and in formalin-fixed, paraffin-embedded sections made from frozen material. Reactive astrocytes are scattered throughout oligodendrogliomas and are particularly prominent at the tumour borders. Oligodendrogliomas may contain tumour cells that look like small gemistocytes with a rounded belly of eccentric cytoplasm that is positive for GFAP, which are termed "minigemistocytes" or "microgemistocytes". Gliofibrillary oligodendrocytes are typical-looking oligodendroglioma cells with a thin perinuclear rim of positivity for GFAP {1295}. Gliofibrillary oligodendrocytes and minigemistocytes are more commonly seen in CNS WHO grade 3 tumours. GFAP-negative mucocytes or even signet-ring cells are occasionally present, with individual cases reported to consist largely of signet-ring cells {1743}. Eosinophilic granular cells occur in some oligodendrogliomas {3114}. Rare cases with neurocytic or ganglioglioma-like differentiation have also been reported {2466, 2471}. Occasional CNS WHO grade 3 oligodendrogliomas feature multinucleated giant cells {1301}, and rare cases contain sarcomatous areas {1310,2699}. The presence of these various cellular phenotypes does not preclude an oligodendroglioma diagnosis if the tumour is IDH-mutant and 1p/19q-codeleted. Tumour cells with fibrillary or gemistocytic astrocytic morphology are also compatible with this diagnosis when IDH mutation and 1p/19q codeletion are present. Thus, irrespective of oligodendroglial, oligoastrocytic, astrocytic, or ambiguous features on histology, detection of combined IDH mutation and 1p/19q codeletion indicates an IDH-mutant and 1p/19q-codeleted oligodendroglioma {452,3082,3418}.

Mineralization and other degenerative features

Microcalcifications are frequent, found within the tumour itself or in the invaded brain. Calcifications were recorded in 71 (45%) of 157 CNS WHO grade 3 IDH-mutant and 1p/19q-codeleted oligodendrogliomas, {928}. Mineralization along blood vessels typically takes the form of small, punctate calcifications, whereas microcalcifications in the brain (called calcospherites) tend to be larger, with an irregular and sometimes laminated appearance. However, this feature is not specific for oligodendroglioma, and because of incomplete tumour sampling, it is sometimes not found histologically even when clearly demonstrated on CT. Areas characterized by extracellular mucin deposition and/or microcyst formation are frequent. Rare tumours are characterized by marked desmoplasia {1470}.

Vasculature

Oligodendrogliomas typically show a dense network of branching capillaries resembling chicken wire. In some cases, the capillary stroma tends to subdivide the tumour into lobules. In CNS WHO grade 3 tumours, focal or dispersed pathological microvascular proliferation is frequent. Oligodendrogliomas have a tendency to develop intratumoural haemorrhages.

Growth pattern

Oligodendrogliomas grow diffusely in the cortex and white matter; however, some tumours feature distinct nodules of higher cellularity against a background of diffuse infiltration. Occasional tumours show a gliomatosis cerebri–like pattern involving more than two cerebral lobes {1298}. Within the cortex, tumour cells often form secondary structures such as perineuronal satellitosis, perivascular aggregates, and subpial accumulations. Circumscribed leptomeningeal infiltration may induce a desmoplastic reaction. Oligodendrogliomas can have a rare spongioblastic growth pattern consisting of parallel rows of tumour cells with somewhat elongated nuclei forming rhythmic palisades. Occasionally, perivascular pseudorosettes are seen, although some of these are a result of perivascular neuropil formation within foci of neurocytic differentiation {2471}. These patterns are generally present only focally.

Proliferation

Mitotic activity is low or absent in CNS WHO grade 2 oligodendrogliomas, but it is usually prominent in CNS WHO grade 3 tumours. Accordingly, the Ki-67 (MIB1) proliferation index is usually low (< 5%) in CNS WHO grade 2 oligodendrogliomas and elevated in CNS WHO grade 3 oligodendrogliomas, being generally > 10% in the large French national POLA cohort of CNS WHO grade 3 tumours {928,929,2546}. However, a definitive Ki-67 (MIB1) cut-off value has not been established due to marked variability in staining results between institutions and non-uniform counting approaches. One study reported a Ki-67 index of ≥ 15% as an independent marker of shorter survival in patients with IDH-mutant and 1p/19q-codeleted CNS WHO grade 3 oligodendrogliomas {2546}. A mitotic count of ≥ 5 mitoses/mm² was also associated with shorter survival but only on univariate, not multivariate, analysis {2546}. Another study showed that mitotic count was not associated with outcome in patients with IDH-mutant and 1p/19q-codeleted oligodendrogliomas {2318}. Other proliferation markers, such as PCNA {2647}, TOP2A {1717}, MCM2 {3422}, and MCM6 {2546},

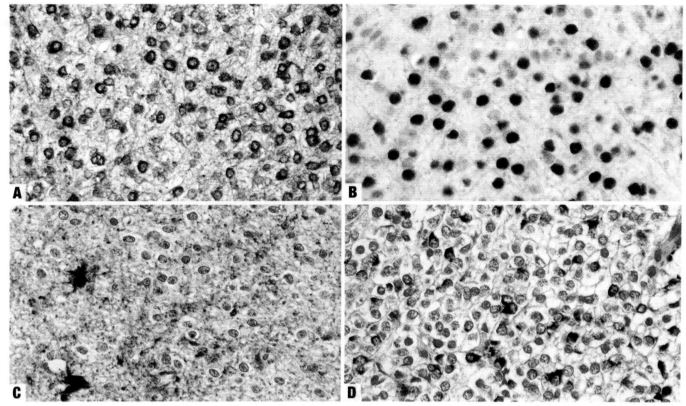

Fig. 2.21 Immunohistochemical features of IDH-mutant and 1p/19q-codeleted oligodendroglioma. **A** MAP2. **B** OLIG2. **C** GFAP. **D** Gliofibrillary oligodendrocytes (GFAP stain).

also correlate with CNS WHO grade and/or survival but do not provide clear advantages over Ki-67 (MIB1).

Grading

Oligodendrogliomas comprise a continuous spectrum of tumours ranging from well-differentiated, slow-growing neoplasms to frankly malignant tumours with rapid growth. In prior editions of the WHO classification of CNS tumours, two grades were distinguished: oligodendroglioma, CNS WHO grade 2, and oligodendroglioma, CNS WHO grade 3. CNS WHO grade retained prognostic significance in patients with IDH-mutant and 1p/19q-codeleted oligodendrogliomas {597}, but the criteria for distinction between grades were not well defined. Histological features that have been linked to higher grade are high cellularity, marked cytological atypia, brisk mitotic activity, pathological microvascular proliferation, and necrosis with or without

palisading. CNS WHO grade 3 oligodendrogliomas usually show several of these features. However, the individual impact of each feature is unclear, in particular because most prognostic studies have not previously been confined to IDH-mutant and 1p/19q-codeleted tumours. Microvascular proliferation and brisk mitotic activity, defined as ≥ 2.5 mitoses/mm² (equating to ≥ 6 mitoses/10 HPF of 0.55 mm in diameter and 0.24 mm² in area) have been reported as indicators of short survival in a study of histologically defined oligodendrogliomas {1096}. Other studies of 1p/19q-codeleted CNS WHO grade 3 oligodendrogliomas suggested that microvascular proliferation and microvascular proliferation with necrosis are linked to shorter survival than is elevated mitotic activity of ≥ 2.5 mitoses/mm² (equating to ≥ 6 mitoses/10 HPF of 0.55 mm in diameter and 0.24 mm² in area) without microvascular proliferation and necrosis {928, 929}. However, data defining a clear cut-off point for a mitotic

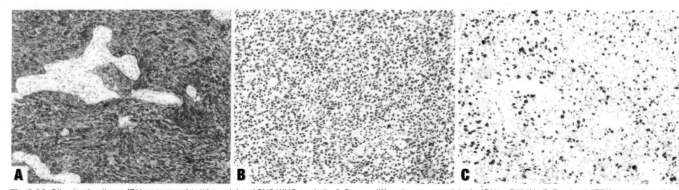

Fig. 2.22 Oligodendroglioma, IDH-mutant and 1p/19q-codeleted CNS WHO grade 3. **A** Strong, diffuse immunoreactivity for IDH1 p.R132H. **B** Retained ATRX immunoreactivity within tumour cell nuclei. **C** An elevated Ki-67 labelling index is typical.

count that distinguishes CNS WHO grade 2 from CNS WHO grade 3 of IDH-mutant and 1p/19q-codeleted oligodendrogliomas are not available. Nevertheless, detection of rare mitoses in a resection specimen is not sufficient for diagnosing CNS WHO grade 3 IDH-mutant and 1p/19q-codeleted oligodendroglioma. In borderline cases, proliferation markers like Ki-67 (MIB1) and attention to clinical and neuroradiological features (e.g. rapid symptomatic growth and contrast enhancement) may provide helpful additional information. Homozygous deletion involving the *CDKN2A* and/or *CDKN2B* locus is found in a small subset (< 10%) of CNS WHO grade 3 oligodendrogliomas but not in CNS WHO grade 2 oligodendrogliomas, and it has been linked to reduced survival, independent of microvascular proliferation with or without necrosis {123}. Therefore, *CDKN2A* homozygous deletion may serve as a molecular marker of CNS WHO grade 3 in IDH-mutant and 1p/19q-codeleted oligodendrogliomas. Although assessment of this marker may not be routinely required in tumours that can histologically be unequivocally assigned to either CNS WHO grade 2 or CNS WHO grade 3, testing for *CDKN2A* homozygous deletion may be helpful, for example in tumour samples with borderline histological features (i.e. when present, a *CDKN2A* homozygous deletion indicates a CNS WHO grade 3 tumour).

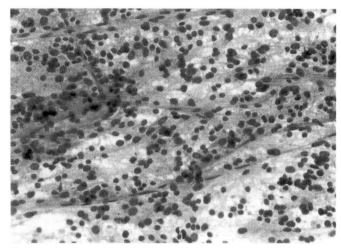

Fig. 2.23 Oligodendroglioma, IDH-mutant and 1p/19q-codeleted, CNS WHO grade 2. Intraoperative smear section of an oligodendroglioma showing tumour cells in a fibrillary background in association with delicate vasculature.

Immunophenotype

Most oligodendrogliomas demonstrate immunoreactivity with the antibody against IDH1 p.R132H {465}, which facilitates the differential diagnosis versus other clear cell tumours as well as non-neoplastic and reactive lesions {461,462}. IDH-mutant and 1p/19q-codeleted oligodendrogliomas retain nuclear expression of ATRX {1916,2657} and typically lack widespread nuclear p53 staining, consistent with the near exclusivity of *ATRX* and *TP53* mutation versus 1p/19q codeletion in IDH-mutant gliomas {452,3082}. Oligodendrogliomas are immunopositive for MAP2, S100, and CD57 (LEU7) {298,2198, 2637}; however, these markers are also positive in astrocytic gliomas. Similarly, the oligodendrocyte lineage transcription factors OLIG1, OLIG2, and SOX10 are expressed in oligodendrogliomas but also in astrocytic gliomas {192,1892}. GFAP is detectable in intermingled reactive astrocytes but may also stain neoplastic cells such as minigemistocytes and gliofibrillary oligodendrocytes {1295,2637}. Antigens expressed by normal oligodendrocytes, including myelin basic protein (MBP), myelin proteolipid protein (PLP), myelin-associated glycoprotein (MAG), galactolipids (e.g. galactocerebroside and galactosulfatide), certain gangliosides, and several enzymes (e.g. CAII [carbonic anhydrase C], CNP, glycerol-3-phosphate dehydrogenase, and LDH) are not diagnostically useful markers for oligodendrogliomas {2198,3073,2199}. Synaptophysin immunoreactivity of residual neuropil between the tumour cells is frequent and should not be mistaken for neuronal or neurocytic differentiation. However, oligodendrogliomas may also contain neoplastic cells that express synaptophysin and/ or NeuN and neurofilaments {2466,2471}. Immunostaining for α-internexin protein is frequent {797} (e.g. in one study it was found in 88.5% of IDH-mutant and 1p/19q-codeleted CNS WHO grade 3 oligodendrogliomas {928}), but it cannot be considered a surrogate marker for 1p/19q codeletion {829}. Similarly, NOGO-A positivity is common but not exclusive {2026}. Reduced nuclear expression of H3 p.K28me3 (K27me3) has

been associated with 1p/19q codeletion in IDH-mutant gliomas {933,904}, but it cannot substitute for 1p/19q testing {2440}.

Differential diagnosis

IDH-mutant and 1p/19q-codeleted oligodendrogliomas may histologically mimic various other lesions. Macrophage-rich lesions such as those characteristic of demyelinating diseases or resulting from cerebral infarction are readily distinguished by immunostaining for macrophage markers and lack of IDH mutation. The relative increase of oligodendrocytes sometimes seen in partial lobectomy specimens performed for intractable seizures also lack IDH mutation. IDH-mutant astrocytomas lack 1p/19q codeletion and show frequent nuclear p53 immunostaining and loss of nuclear ATRX. In fact, loss of nuclear ATRX is sufficient to diagnose an IDH-mutant astrocytoma without additional testing for 1p/19q codeletion {1935}. *TERT* promoter mutations are common in IDH-mutant and 1p/19q-codeleted oligodendrogliomas, although rare cases have been reported to lack *TERT* promoter mutation, and some IDH-mutant but 1p/19q-intact astrocytomas may carry *TERT* promoter mutations {134,1678,1780,3082}. Other morphological mimics, like neurocytoma, liponeurocytoma, and dysembryoplastic neuroepithelial tumour, can be ruled out by their lack of IDH mutation. Ependymomas containing clear cells differ from oligodendrogliomas by their perivascular pseudorosettes and dot-like or ring-shaped EMA immunoreactivity, as well as a lack of IDH mutation and frequent *ZFTA* (*C11orf95*) fusions. Clear cell meningioma can be distinguished by EMA and desmoplakin positivity, IDH-wildtype status, and loss of nuclear SMARCE1 {3148}. Metastatic clear cell carcinomas differ from oligodendrogliomas by their sharp tumour borders, cytokeratin and EMA positivity, and lack of IDH mutation. Pilocytic astrocytomas with oligodendroglial features are IDH-wildtype and carry MAPK pathway gene alterations, in particular *FGFR1* alterations {2932}. However, rare cases of IDH-mutant and 1p/19q-codeleted oligodendrogliomas with *KIAA1549::BRAF* fusions have been reported {171,1628}. In children, diffuse gliomas with *MYB*, *MYBL1*, *FGFR1*, or *BRAF* alterations may have histological features of oligodendroglioma or oligoastrocytoma but are biologically distinct tumours {838}. The differential diagnosis of diffuse

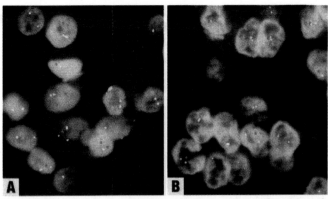

Fig. 2.24 Oligodendroglioma, IDH-mutant and 1p/19q-codeleted, CNS WHO grade 2. FISH demonstrates 1p/19q codeletion (without polysomy). **A** The 1p signal is red and the 1q signal is green. **B** The 19q signal is red and the 19p signal is green.

leptomeningeal glioneuronal tumour is facilitated by the clinical presentation and the combination of MAPK pathway gene alteration (in particular *KIAA1549::BRAF* fusion) and 1p deletion (or 1p/19q codeletion) but absence of IDH mutation {2702}. Malignant small cell astrocytic tumours, including IDH-wildtype glioblastomas and H3 G34–mutant diffuse hemispheric gliomas, must be separated from highly cellular oligodendrogliomas by their IDH-wildtype status and specific alterations, including frequent *EGFR* amplification and chromosome 10 loss {1500, 2464}, or mutations leading to H3 p.G35 (G34) variants.

Oligodendroglioma NOS, oligoastrocytoma NOS, and oligoastrocytoma NEC

Rare cases of diffuse gliomas with classic oligodendroglioma histology in which molecular testing for combined IDH mutation and 1p/19q codeletion failed (e.g. because of limited tissue availability, low tumour cell content, inconclusive test results, or other circumstances impeding molecular testing) or could not be completed can be histologically classified as oligodendroglioma NOS {1946} and designated as CNS WHO grade 2 or 3 depending on the presence or absence of histological features of anaplasia. Immunohistochemical demonstration of IDH mutation and retained nuclear positivity for ATRX may support the oligodendroglioma diagnosis. However, unless successfully tested for 1p/19q codeletion, such tumours cannot be classified as oligodendroglioma, IDH-mutant and 1p/19q-codeleted. Immunohistochemical positivity for oligodendroglioma-associated markers such as α-internexin {797,829} and NOGO-A {2026}, reduced nuclear H3 p.K28me3 (K27me3) immunostaining {933,904}, and immunohistochemical loss of nuclear CIC or FUBP1 expression {221,508} are not sufficient to substitute for 1p/19q codeletion testing.

The diagnosis of oligoastrocytoma NOS is reserved for diffuse gliomas that are composed of a conspicuous mixture of two distinct neoplastic cell types morphologically resembling tumour cells with either oligodendroglial or astrocytic features, and in which testing for IDH mutation, nuclear ATRX expression, and 1p/19q codeletion failed or could not be completed. In such cases, tumour cells with oligodendroglial or astroglial features can be either diffusely intermingled or separated into distinct, biphasic areas. However, the diagnosis of oligoastrocytoma is discouraged because molecular analyses have shown that these tumours carry a genetic profile typical of either

IDH-mutant astrocytoma or IDH-mutant and 1p/19q-codeleted oligodendroglioma {452,2781,3082}. Thus, diffuse gliomas with mixed or ambiguous histological features should be evaluated for IDH mutation and loss of nuclear ATRX expression, as well as for 1p/19q codeletion when nuclear ATRX is retained {1935}.

Rare cases of dual-genotype oligoastrocytomas have been reported. These are characterized by two distinct IDH-mutant tumour cell populations: one showing astrocytoma-associated alterations, such as ATRX loss and *TP53* mutation, and the other showing oligodendroglioma-associated 1p/19q codeletion {2587,204,1382,3444}. The WHO Classification of Tumours does not consider these tumours to be a distinct type or subtype of IDH-mutant diffuse glioma, but they may be tentatively classified as dual-genotype oligoastrocytoma NEC {1946}.

Cytology

In cytological preparations, oligodendroglial tumour cells show uniform round nuclei and well-delineated cytoplasm, with only a modest degree of glial fibrillarity. The perinuclear haloes that are typical of histological preparations are not appreciated in smear specimens. In CNS WHO grade 3 oligodendrogliomas, intensely eosinophilic cytoplasmic granules are occasionally noted. Reactive astrocytes harbouring eosinophilic cytoplasm with multipolar processes may also be present. In some cases, microcalcifications and prominent vasculature can be appreciated.

Diagnostic molecular pathology

Oligodendrogliomas are molecularly defined by *IDH1* or *IDH2* mutations and 1p/19q codeletion. Nearly all tumours have a *TERT* promoter mutation, lack *ATRX* mutation, and show preserved nuclear ATRX expression. *TP53* mutations are uncommon {452,1999,1}. Diagnosis of oligodendrogliomas requires demonstration of IDH mutation by IDH1 p.R132H immunohistochemistry and/or sequencing of the *IDH1* or *IDH2* gene, as well as demonstration of 1p/19q codeletion by FISH, chromogenic in situ hybridization, or molecular genetic testing. In the absence of IDH1 p.R132H-positive immunohistochemistry, sequencing for less common mutations in *IDH1* (codon 132) and *IDH2* (codon 172) should be performed. No particular method for molecular testing for 1p/19q codeletion is required, but it is recommended that 1p/19q assays be able to detect whole-arm chromosomal losses. Only complete losses of both chromosome arms are diagnostic for oligodendroglioma, because partial or isolated loss of 1p or 19q may be present in some IDH-wildtype glioblastomas and IDH-mutant astrocytomas. FISH probes in commonly deleted regions or loss of only a few PCR probes in loss-of-heterozygosity analysis may not reflect whole-arm losses and thus may lead to false positive results {1341}. In addition, any copy-number analysis requires sufficient tumour cell content, preferably > 30%, to avoid false negative results when assessing 1p/19q codeletion. Immunohistochemical detection of IDH1 p.R132H expression and preserved nuclear ATRX expression, without demonstration of 1p/19q codeletion, is not sufficient to diagnose an IDH-mutant and 1p/19q-codeleted oligodendroglioma, even with classic histology. In IDH-mutant gliomas with preserved nuclear ATRX expression by immunohistochemistry, 1p/19q analysis remains critical for accurate molecular diagnosis. Most IDH-mutant and 1p/19q-codeleted oligodendrogliomas carry *TERT* promoter mutations {134}; however, detection of a *TERT* promoter mutation in an IDH-mutant glioma is not sufficient for an oligodendroglioma diagnosis, because rare cases are *TERT*-wildtype, including tumours in teenage patients {1833}. *TERT* promoter mutations are also observed in a subset of 1p/19q-intact IDH-mutant astrocytomas {2442,2277}. DNA methylation array analysis reveals a diagnostic molecular profile by combining the detection of an oligodendroglioma-associated methylation signature and 1p/19q codeletion {460,463}. Copy-number analysis by FISH also provides information on polysomy of 1q and 19p, which has been detected in subsets of 1p/19q-codeleted oligodendrogliomas of CNS WHO grades 2 and 3 and is associated with shorter survival {537,2974,3436}. Homozygous deletion of *CDKN2A* has been detected in a small proportion of CNS WHO grade 3 IDH-mutant and 1p/19q-codeleted oligodendrogliomas, but not in those of CNS WHO grade 2, and it was reported to be an independent marker of shorter survival {123}.

Tumours that cannot be fully analysed for IDH mutation and 1p/19q codeletion but demonstrate classic histological features of oligodendroglioma are classified as oligodendroglioma NOS {1946}. This indicates that the tumour is a histologically classic oligodendroglioma that will probably exhibit clinical behaviour similar to that of an IDH-mutant and 1p/19q-codeleted oligodendroglioma, but that it could not be molecularly analysed or that its test results were inconclusive or uninformative {1946}. Tumours that demonstrate oligodendroglial histology but lack IDH mutation and 1p/19q codeletion should not be classified as oligodendroglioma NOS but must be further evaluated to exclude histological mimics, such as dysembryoplastic neuroepithelial tumour, clear cell ependymoma, neurocytoma, polymorphous low-grade neuroepithelial tumour of the young, and pilocytic astrocytoma, as well as molecularly distinct diffuse gliomas that are characterized by *BRAF, FGFR1, MYB*, or *MYBL1* alterations {838}.

Essential and desirable diagnostic criteria
See Box 2.02.

Staging
Not clinically relevant

Prognosis and prediction
Survival data for histologically diagnosed tumours in older studies and population-based registries are confounded by the inclusion of gliomas without IDH mutation and 1p/19q codeletion. Retrospective molecular stratification of older series confirmed that only subsets (30–80%) of tumours corresponded to IDH-mutant and 1p/19q-codeleted oligodendrogliomas {928,3100, 794}. Overall, IDH-mutant and 1p/19q-codeleted oligodendrogliomas are associated with favourable response to therapy and median survival times of > 10 years. For example, patients with CNS WHO grade 3 IDH-mutant and 1p/19q-codeleted oligodendroglioma who participated in prospective clinical trials and were treated with a combination of radiotherapy and procarbazine, lomustine, and vincristine (PCV) chemotherapy showed a median survival of ≥ 14 years {3276}. Oligodendrogliomas generally recur locally but may show leptomeningeal spread. Malignant progression at recurrence is common, although it usually takes longer in oligodendroglioma than in IDH-mutant astrocytoma {1440}.

Clinical factors
Clinical factors associated with more favourable outcome include younger patient age at diagnosis, frontal lobe location, presentation with seizures, high postoperative Karnofsky score, and macroscopically complete surgical removal {3275}. Many of these factors, including age, are confirmed in studies on molecularly defined oligodendroglioma, but limited follow-up remains an issue {2546,597}.

Imaging
The presence of contrast enhancement on imaging is indicative of worse outcome in IDH-mutant CNS WHO grade 2 and 3 gliomas, including oligodendrogliomas {1221,3061}. An increased growth rate on follow-up MRI has been associated with histological features of anaplasia, including microvascular proliferation and higher mitotic count, with contrast enhancement on neuroimaging, and with shorter progression-free survival (PFS) {2739}.

Surgery
Greater extent of resection has been associated with longer overall survival (OS) and PFS in patients with CNS WHO grade 2 oligodendroglioma, but it did not prolong the time to malignant progression {2977}. Studies using volumetric tumour assessment show that extensive resections are associated with improved outcomes. However, leaving some tumour tissue behind appears to have less impact on the survival of patients with oligodendroglioma than on that of patients with IDH-mutant astrocytoma {3442,2418,759}, perhaps because of the higher sensitivity of oligodendrogliomas to radiotherapy and chemotherapy.

Histological features
Histological features that have been linked to worse prognosis include necrosis, high mitotic activity, increased cellularity, nuclear atypia, cellular pleomorphism, and microvascular proliferation. However, the prognostic significance of each of these requires re-evaluation in patients with molecularly characterized tumours. In IDH-mutant and 1p/19q-codeleted CNS WHO grade 3 oligodendrogliomas, high mitotic count (≥ 2.5 mitoses/mm^2, equating to ≥ 6 mitoses/10 HPF of 0.55 mm in diameter and 0.24 mm^2 in area) was linked to shorter PFS and OS in both univariate and multivariate analyses {929}. The presence of

Box 2.02 Diagnostic criteria for oligodendroglioma, IDH-mutant and 1p/19q-codeleted

Essential:

A diffusely infiltrating glioma

AND

IDH1 codon 132 or *IDH2* codon 172 missense mutation[a]

AND

Combined whole-arm deletions of 1p and 19q

Desirable:

DNA methylome profile of oligodendroglioma, IDH-mutant and 1p/19q-codeleted

Retained nuclear expression of ATRX

TERT promoter mutation

[a]IDH mutation analysis may not be required when DNA methylome profiling is performed and unequivocally assigns the tumour to the methylation class oligodendroglioma, IDH-mutant and 1p/19q-codeleted.

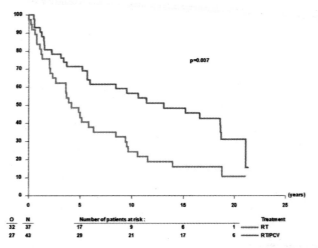

Progression Free Survival

p=0.007

Fig. 2.25 Oligodendroglioma, IDH-mutant and 1p/19q-codeleted. Progression-free survival (PFS) of 80 patients in the prospective randomized European Organisation for Research and Treatment of Cancer (EORTC) 26951 study on adjuvant procarbazine, lomustine, and vincristine (PCV) chemotherapy after 59.4 Gy radiotherapy (RT); the 20-year PFS rate for the patients who received RT plus PCV chemotherapy was 31.3%, versus 10.8% for the patients who received only RT.

microvascular proliferation and/or necrosis was of prognostic significance in cases lacking *CDKN2A* homozygous deletion {123}.

CNS WHO grading

Older studies reported CNS WHO grade as an independent predictor of survival for patients with oligodendroglial tumours {905,1096,1824,2312}. However, these studies antedate the molecular criteria for oligodendroglioma. In one study of patients with gliomas with concurrent IDH mutation and *TERT* promoter mutation, patients with grade 2 tumours had longer survival times than those with grade 3 tumours (median OS: 205.5 months vs 127.3 months, respectively) {1613}. A recent multicentre study observed a median OS of 188 months in patients with grade 2 oligodendrogliomas versus 119 months in patients with grade 3 tumours {974}. This difference remained significant in a multivariate analysis. A study of 176 patients with IDH-mutant and 1p/19q-codeleted oligodendrogliomas (CNS WHO grades 2 and 3) also revealed shorter OS for patients with CNS WHO grade 3 tumours {597}. In contrast, a retrospective analysis of 212 patients with IDH-mutant and 1p/19q-codeleted oligodendrogliomas did not detect CNS WHO grade as a significant predictor of OS {2318}. Similarly, data from a combined cohort from Japan and The Cancer Genome Atlas (TCGA) suggested that grading had a limited prognostic role {3082}. The interpretation of these retrospective studies requires caution because other prognostically relevant factors, such as extent of resection, were not considered, and patients received variable postoperative treatments.

Proliferation

A study of 220 patients with IDH-mutant and 1p/19q-codeleted CNS WHO grade 3 oligodendroglioma revealed that labelling index values of ≥ 50% for MCM6 and ≥ 15% for Ki-67

correlated with shorter OS in univariate and multivariate analyses {2546}. The MCM6 and Ki-67 indices also correlated with OS in 30 patients with CNS WHO grade 2 oligodendrogliomas {2546}. High mitotic count (≥ 2.5 mitoses/mm², equating to ≥ 6 mitoses/10 HPF of 0.55 mm in diameter and 0.24 mm² in area) was associated with an increased growth rate on follow-up MRI and shorter PFS in patients with CNS WHO grade 2 and 3 oligodendrogliomas {2739}.

Genetic alterations

Currently available evidence from retrospective studies suggests that the presence of 1q and 19p co-polysomy detected by FISH concurrent with 1p/19q codeletion is associated with earlier recurrence and shorter survival {537,2974,3436}. Allelic losses on 9p have been detected in about one third of CNS WHO grade 2 IDH-mutant and 1p/19q-codeleted oligodendrogliomas, but they were not associated with shorter survival {3441}. Other studies reported that allelic losses of 9p21.3 (the *CDKN2A* gene locus) were linked to shorter survival in patients with CNS WHO grade 3 oligodendroglioma {886,64}. Homozygous deletion involving the *CDKN2A* gene locus is not observed in CNS WHO grade 2 oligodendrogliomas {3441, 123}, but it is found in a small subset of CNS WHO grade 3 oligodendrogliomas, in which it has been associated with poor outcome {123}. Other alterations that have been linked to less favourable outcome of patients with CNS WHO grade 3 oligodendroglioma include *PIK3CA* mutation {3140,380}, *TCF12* mutation {1778}, and increased MYC signalling {1537}. *PTEN* mutation has been associated with shorter survival of patients with CNS WHO grade 2 oligodendroglioma {3441}. Higher tumour mutation burden was found to predict shorter survival with IDH-mutant gliomas including oligodendrogliomas {73}. *CIC* mutation has been reported as a marker of poor prognosis {1120}, but this finding was not confirmed in other series {794, 3441}. No impact on outcome was observed for *CDK4* amplification or *RB1* homozygous deletion {123}.

Treatment

The optimal postoperative treatment of patients with IDH-mutant and 1p/19q-codeleted oligodendrogliomas of CNS WHO grade 2 is a matter of ongoing discussion. After tumour resection, radiotherapy and chemotherapy are often deferred until tumour progression because therapy-associated neurotoxicity is a major concern {3417}. Patients with symptomatic and progressive tumours, with CNS WHO grade 3 tumours, or with large residual tumours after surgery usually receive immediate further treatment with radiotherapy and/or chemotherapy {3417}. The European Organisation for Research and Treatment of Cancer (EORTC) 22845 trial showed that adjuvant radiotherapy prolonged PFS but not OS in patients with progressive CNS WHO grade 2 gliomas {3272}. Long-term follow-up data from randomized trials showed a major increase in OS after radiotherapy plus PCV chemotherapy in patients with CNS WHO grade 3 oligodendrogliomas {402,3273,438}. Adjuvant chemotherapy with temozolomide or PCV may also be a feasible therapeutic strategy for patients with progressive CNS WHO grade 2 oligodendroglioma {1322,1598,1859,3095}.

Glioblastoma, IDH-wildtype

Louis DN
Aldape KD
Capper D
Giannini C
Horbinski CM
Ng HK

Perry A
Reifenberger G
Sarkar C
Soffietti R
Suvà ML
Wick W

Definition

Glioblastoma, IDH-wildtype, is a diffuse, astrocytic glioma that is IDH-wildtype and H3-wildtype and has one or more of the following histological or genetic features: microvascular proliferation, necrosis, *TERT* promoter mutation, *EGFR* gene amplification, +7/−10 chromosome copy-number changes (CNS WHO grade 4).

ICD-O coding

9440/3 Glioblastoma, IDH-wildtype

ICD-11 coding

2A00.00 & XH5571 Glioblastoma of brain & Glioblastoma, IDH-wildtype

Related terminology

Not recommended: glioblastoma multiforme.

Subtype(s)

Giant cell glioblastoma; gliosarcoma; epithelioid glioblastoma

Localization

Glioblastoma, IDH-wildtype, is most often centred in the subcortical white matter and deeper grey matter of the cerebral hemispheres, affecting all cerebral lobes {2344}. In many cases, tumour infiltration extends into the adjacent cortex and through the corpus callosum into the contralateral hemisphere. Glioblastoma, IDH-wildtype, also affects the brainstem, cerebellum, and spinal cord; however, in midline locations, other diffuse gliomas should also be considered (e.g. diffuse midline glioma, H3 K27–altered).

Clinical features

Symptoms depend largely on tumour location, manifesting as focal neurological deficits (e.g. hemiparesis, aphasia, visual field defects) and/or seizures (in as many as 50% of patients). Symptoms of elevated intracranial pressure, such as headache, nausea, and vomiting, may coexist. Behavioural and neurocognitive changes are common, especially in elderly patients. Neurological symptoms are usually progressive, but in a minority of patients, acute onset may occur due to an intracranial haemorrhage. The time from symptom onset to diagnosis is < 3 months in as many as 68% of patients and < 6 months in as many as 84% {2311}. In general, patients with histological subtypes such as giant cell glioblastoma {2298}, gliosarcoma {975}, and epithelioid glioblastoma {2143,1651,428,3587} present similarly.

Imaging

Glioblastomas are irregularly shaped, often with a ring-enhancing component around a darker central area of necrosis, and surrounding oedema of varying amounts. Less commonly

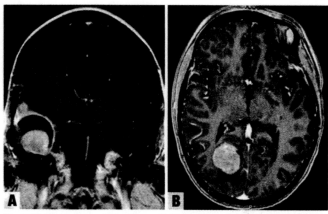

Fig. 2.26 Glioblastoma, IDH-wildtype. **A** Glioblastoma, IDH-wildtype, with sarcomatous component (gliosarcoma). On this postcontrast T1-weighted MRI of a patient with prior history of IDH-wildtype glioblastoma, a solid-appearing component filled the prior resection cavity and was found to be a newly developed sarcomatous component in the recurrent tumour. **B** Epithelioid glioblastoma, IDH-wildtype. Postcontrast T1-weighted MRI showing a solid-appearing enhancing mass.

(e.g. in tumours that meet genetic definitions of IDH-wildtype glioblastoma but lack histological microvascular proliferation and necrosis), tumours show only modest or patchy contrast enhancement or may lack central necrosis. They may extend into adjacent lobes, into the opposite hemisphere through the corpus callosum, and down into the brainstem. In the setting of a ring-enhancing mass, biopsies showing high-grade astrocytoma but without frank histological features of glioblastoma should be suspected to have been inadequately sampled. The morphological subtypes of glioblastoma cannot be distinguished on MRI, although there are some differences: giant cell glioblastomas may be more circumscribed and located subcortically {2298}; gliosarcomas may appear as well-demarcated lesions with a higher risk of cortical involvement and abutting dura {3086,2714,975,3536}; and epithelioid glioblastomas often consist of a well-circumscribed enhancing mass, rarely with a cystic component {384,1370,3587}. Radiomic approaches have been developed to predict gene expression profiles of newly diagnosed glioblastomas based on computational analysis of conventional and advanced MRI images {1978,2209,586,752}, thus increasing diagnostic and prognostic capabilities {141, 3558,1608}.

Spread

A subset (ranging from 0.5% to 35% in different studies) of glioblastomas occur with multiple lesions, termed "multifocal" or "multicentric" glioblastomas {2922,2420,3187,2426,1187,777}. Multifocal glioblastomas demonstrate contiguous pathways of spread between foci, whereas multicentric glioblastomas are widely separated. On careful histological analysis, only 2.4% of glioblastomas are truly multiple independent tumours {216,252,

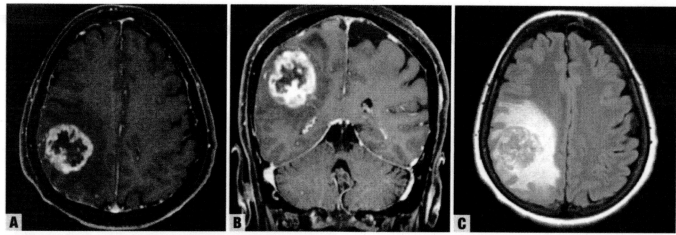

Fig. 2.27 Glioblastoma, IDH-wildtype. Axial (**A**) and coronal (**B**) images of ring-enhancing tumour on postcontrast T1-weighted MRI. **C** FLAIR MRI shows the extent of vasogenic oedema.

2759}. Occasional cases of multifocal epithelioid glioblastoma as well as gliosarcoma have been reported {1046,1688,1758, 2375}. The exact pathogenetic mechanisms of multifocality are unknown, although recent studies have suggested that these tumours have frequent *EGFR* alterations with co-occurrence of *PTEN* and *TERT* promoter mutations {777,12}.

Despite the infiltrative growth of glioblastoma and its ability to seed the cerebrospinal fluid (e.g. along ventricular surfaces or via drop metastases), extension into the dura mater, venous sinuses, and bone is uncommon {136,1159,1081,2534}. Extra-cranial metastasis is rare, occurring in only 0.4–0.5% of cases, mostly at the time of recurrence, with the most common sites being bones, lymph nodes, liver, and lungs {479,658}. Metastasis has also been documented in association with interstitial therapies and ventricular shunts {1224,1958,3355}. Metastases have also occurred in epithelioid glioblastoma and gliosarcoma {384,3253}.

Epidemiology

Glioblastoma is the most frequent malignant brain tumour in adults, accounting for approximately 15% of all intracranial neoplasms and 45–50% of all primary malignant brain tumours. It can manifest in patients of any age but preferentially affects older adults, with peak incidence in patients aged 55–85 years. In children, it accounts for approximately 3% of all CNS tumours {2344}. The M:F ratio for glioblastoma is 1.60:1 in the USA {2345} and 1.28:1 in Switzerland {2310}.

Annual age-adjusted incidence rates for glioblastoma have increased in recent years to 3–6 cases per 100 000 people, as documented in reports from the USA, Canada, England, and Australia {2344,3358,2495,765}. The increase cannot be fully accounted for by improvements in diagnostic techniques and lifestyle changes, and environmental factors might be responsible {2495,692,107,3330,1236,3342}. Glioblastoma may be less common in Asian and African countries, which may be attributable to differences in age distribution and partly to under-ascertainment {747,2003}.

Etiology

The etiology of most glioblastomas remains unknown {2346}. A very small proportion of glioblastomas occur in more than one member of a family or are inherited as part of genetic tumour syndromes {2342}. The latter include Lynch syndrome, constitutional mismatch repair deficiency syndrome, Li–Fraumeni syndrome, and neurofibromatosis type 1. Genome-wide association studies identified genomic variants in *TERT*, *EGFR*, *CCDC26*, *CDKN2B*, *PHLDB1*, *TP53*, and *RTEL1* associated with an increased risk of glioma {2342}; others showed that certain SNPs were associated with increased risk for gliomas, and that these SNPs were different from those in patients with other brain tumours {2065,1634,2346}.

The incidence of glioblastoma seems to be increasing, which suggests that environmental factors have a role in its development {2496}, but although many environmental factors have been studied as potential causes, investigations have been inconclusive or negative for most, including non-ionizing radiation (e.g. from mobile phones) and occupational exposures {3623,2346}. The only validated risk factor is ionizing radiation to the head and neck {3480,2346}. For example, patients who received treatment for acute lymphoblastic leukaemia were more prone to developing glioblastoma {2795,2893,956}, and there is an increased risk of gliomas among survivors of atomic bomb irradiation, but there is no increased risk associated with diagnostic irradiation {2555}. A decreased risk has been observed among individuals with a history of allergies or atopic diseases {2342}.

Pathogenesis

Cell of origin

Mouse modelling experiments suggest that a range of primary CNS cell types can be transformed into malignant cells that recapitulate features of glioblastoma. These include oligodendrocyte precursor cells {1915}, neural precursor cells {1333}, astrocytes {1333}, and neurons {984}, with the susceptibility to transformation declining with lineage restriction {60}. Deep genetic sequencing studies of human glioblastomas suggest that a neural precursor in the subventricular zone is a likely cell of origin {1837}. This interpretation is supported by the coincident anatomical position of neural precursor cells in the subventricular zone and by the identification of stem cell–like cells directly from glioblastomas {2943,2504,1111}. Yet the question of whether stem cell–like cells in glioblastoma are the result of the transformation of a neural precursor in the CNS or are generated by dedifferentiation of a lineage-restricted cell type remains unresolved. Single-cell RNA-sequencing analysis of human tumours supports that glioblastoma is composed of a mixture of cell states that recapitulate neurodevelopmental trajectories (neural progenitor–like, oligodendrocytic progenitor–like, astrocyte-like states) and are influenced by interactions with immune cells (mesenchymal-like state). Genetic events driving glioblastoma may skew the cellular lineages; in addition, the potential for cellular plasticity represents an obstacle in the search for the cell(s) of origin {2226}.

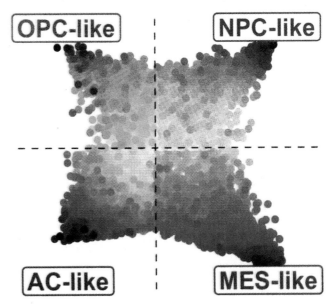

Fig. 2.28 Glioblastoma, IDH-wildtype. Single-cell RNA sequencing of glioblastoma identifies four malignant cellular states and their intermediates. Two-dimensional representation of cellular states, in which each dot represents a malignant cell and each coloured quadrant corresponds to one cellular state. The exact position and colour intensity of each dot reflects the cell's relative score. AC, astrocyte; MES, mesenchymal; NPC, neural progenitor cell; OPC, oligodendrocytic progenitor cell.

Invasion, secondary structures, and metastasis

Infiltrative spread is a defining feature of all diffuse gliomas, but glioblastoma is particularly notorious for its invasion of neighbouring brain structures concurrent with rearrangement of the extracellular matrix {413}. Infiltration occurs most readily along white matter tracts, including the internal capsule, fornix, anterior commissure, and optic radiation, but it can also involve cortical and deep grey matter structures. When infiltration extends through the corpus callosum, with subsequent growth in the contralateral hemisphere, the result can be a bilateral, symmetrical lesion (butterfly glioma).

Other infiltrative patterns (including perineuronal satellitosis, perivascular aggregation, and subpial spread) give rise to secondary structures {3569}. Infiltrative cells are located both inside and outside the contrast-enhancing rim of a glioblastoma and generally create a gradient of decreasing cell density with increasing distance from the tumour centre. Individual infiltrating tumour cells can be histologically identified several centimetres from the tumour epicentre, both in regions that are T2-hyperintense on MRI and in regions that appear uninvolved. These infiltrating cells are the most likely source of local recurrence after initial therapy, because they escape surgical resection, do not receive the highest dose of radiotherapy, and involve regions with an intact blood–brain barrier (which diminishes chemotherapeutic bioavailability) {1101}. In cases where the dominant mass of glioblastoma is effectively controlled by therapy, distant invasion of brainstem structures is recognized as a common cause of death {787}. Interestingly, a pattern of increased infiltration has been observed in a subset of patients with glioblastoma treated with antiangiogenic therapies, presumably due to vascular normalization {702}. Like other diffuse gliomas, glioblastoma can manifest at initial clinical presentation with a gliomatosis cerebri pattern of extensive involvement of the CNS, including multiple cerebral lobes, as well as additional involvement of deep grey matter structures, brainstem, cerebellum, and spinal cord.

Mechanisms that promote invasive properties of glioblastoma cells include those involved in cell motility, cell–matrix and cell–cell interactions, and remodelling of the extracellular matrix, as well as microenvironmental influences {235, 734}. Tumour cells produce migration-enhancing extracellular matrix components and secrete proteolytic enzymes that permit invasion. Gliomas also express a variety of integrin receptors that mediate interactions with molecules in the extracellular space and lead to alterations of the cellular cytoskeleton and activation of intracellular signalling networks such as the AKT, mTOR, and MAPK pathways. Tumour-associated macrophages (TAMs) are also involved in glioma invasion

(see below). Many growth factors expressed in glioblastoma also stimulate migration by activating corresponding receptor tyrosine kinases and downstream mediators that more directly promote migration. In *EGFR*-amplified glioblastomas, cells with amplification are enriched at the infiltrating edges, suggesting that this alteration has a role in peripheral expansion {2975}. The overall mass migration of glioblastoma is radially outwards, away from central necrosis and associated severe hypoxia, with migration rates substantially greater than those of gliomas lacking necrosis {2720,3088}. Hypoxia promotes invasion through the activation of HIF1 and other hypoxia-inducible transcription factors {1574,3571}, and glioma stem-like cells respond to hypoxia by increasing HIF1-dependent expression of alarmin receptors {2386} and additional factors associated with cell motility {358,2720}. Activation of a pro-migration transcriptional programme seems to be associated with a decrease in proliferation, which may have therapeutic consequences {1396,1101,1102}.

Although seeding of the cerebrospinal fluid can occur in the setting of glioblastoma, systemic metastasis is uncommon, and the pathogenesis of glioblastoma metastasis remains largely unknown {2626,2394}. The rarity of metastasis may be attributable to immune mechanisms or inhospitable environments that suppress metastatic implantation and growth, as well as to the relatively short survival of patients with glioblastoma {479,658, 1476,822}. Nonetheless, circulating tumour cells have been identified in the blood of some patients with glioblastoma, and these cells express genes associated with stemness and mesenchymal differentiation {3284,3069}.

Proliferation and apoptosis

Tumour cell proliferation is a hallmark of glioblastoma. In most cases, mitoses are readily visible, but there is often intratumoural

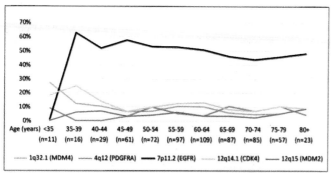

Fig.2.29 Glioblastoma, IDH-wildtype. Rate of recurrent amplifications in 647 molecularly confirmed cases of glioblastoma, IDH-wildtype (methylation groups RTK1, RTK2, and MES) plotted against age at diagnosis. Amplification rates in patients diagnosed after the age of 40 years show little variation. Tumours of the methylation groups RTK1, RTK2, and MES are rare in patients aged < 35 years and possibly do not occur in patients aged < 25 years. Data from {460} combined with institutional cases from Charité Berlin and UZ Leuven. MES, mesenchymal; RTK, receptor tyrosine kinase.

heterogeneity in the density of mitotic figures. Similarly, Ki-67 proliferation index values can vary greatly from region to region within a glioblastoma, sometimes ranging from about 5% to well over 50%. Like other cancers, glioblastomas most commonly overcome RB1-regulated cell-cycle control via molecular events like *CDKN2A* and/or *CDKN2B* deletion, *CDK4* amplification, and *RB1* inactivation {370}. Glioblastoma proliferation is also directly stimulated by neuronal firing via neuron–glioma synapses {3307}. Similar to what has been observed in glial invasion, proliferating glioblastoma cells recapitulate mechanisms found in normal dividing neural/glial progenitor cells {2226}.

Along with mitoses, a common finding in most high-grade CNS tumours (including glioblastoma) is tumour cell apoptosis. Apoptosis is a form of programmed cell death and can be caused by a number of factors, including a hostile microenvironment (e.g. near necrotic areas) and a dysregulated cell cycle. However, glioblastoma cells suppress apoptosis primarily via specific genetic alterations, such as inactivating *TP53* mutations, homozygous *CDKN2A* (*p14ARF*) deletion, and/or *MDM2* or *MDM4* amplification {370}. As a result, although apoptotic cells can be found scattered throughout glioblastomas, they are outnumbered by proliferative cells and have no prognostic value {2110,2836}.

Microvascular proliferation
One of the major histological features of glioblastoma is rapid blood vessel growth, called microvascular proliferation, which manifests as multilayered small-calibre blood vessels. In some glioblastomas, endothelial and smooth muscle cell / pericyte overgrowth is so prominent that the vessels acquire a glomeruloid shape, and can even show mitoses {1211,2194,3421}. Microvascular proliferation is triggered by a number of mechanisms, including perinecrotic hypoxia, which leads to HIF1α-mediated VEGF expression, thereby stimulating new blood vessel growth {361,599}. Despite the prominent role of microvascular proliferation in glioblastoma biology, the anti-VEGF monoclonal antibody bevacizumab does not extend the overall survival (OS) of patients with glioblastoma {1104}.

Necrosis
In addition to microvascular proliferation, the other diagnostic histological feature of glioblastoma is necrosis. There are several postulated mechanisms by which necrosis develops in glioblastoma. One is that rapidly growing blood vessels within the tumour have poorly formed luminal surfaces, which are thrombogenic. This is exacerbated by glioblastoma cells secreting pro-coagulation molecules, such as tissue factor (TF), into the circulation {3256}. Thrombosis leads to infarction of surrounding tissues, creating a microenvironment that is acidic, low in oxygen, and low in glucose. Nearby glioblastoma cells migrate away from such a hostile microenvironment, often creating palisades of HIF1α-expressing, less-proliferative tumour cells {3572, 358,3160,2720,775}. The relationship between thrombosis and necrosis is much stronger in IDH-wildtype glioblastoma than in IDH-mutant CNS WHO grade 4 astrocytomas. In the latter, TF expression is greatly reduced, and when necrosis is present, it is usually less extensive than that in IDH-wildtype glioblastoma and often lacks associated microthrombi {3256,1789}.

Inflammation
Inflammatory infiltrates vary among glioblastomas: the majority (~80%) are myeloid cells, with lymphocytes constituting a smaller proportion {1659}. Myeloid cells are predominantly monocyte-derived macrophages and microglia – collectively referred to as tumour-associated macrophages (TAMs) – whereas neutrophils are less abundant {1659}. CD4+ T cells are the most abundant lymphocytes, followed by CD8+ T cells, NK cells, and B cells {1659}.

TAMs are highly plastic cells that are attracted to and reprogrammed by glioma tumour cells via the secretion of chemokines and other soluble factors to promote invasion, angiogenesis, and immunosuppression {1200}. When recruited to the glioma milieu, TAMs are reprogrammed to promote glioma homeostasis and progression using mechanisms that involve toll-like receptors and matrix metalloproteinases. Functionally, TAMs in glioblastoma are thought to exert predominantly immunosuppressive effects {2578}, including recruitment of CD4+, FOXP3+ T regulatory (Treg) cells and myeloid-derived suppressor cells {518,1100,2349}. Although cytotoxic CD8+ T cells are usually thought to be hypoactive through immune checkpoint signalling, mediated by receptors like PD1 {3478}, brisk cytotoxic T-cell infiltration has been associated with longer survival {3519}. Treg cells constitute about 10% of all intratumoural T cells in glioblastoma, and they are not associated with prognosis {3181,1284}.

Cytogenetics and numerical chromosome alterations
Whole chromosome 7 gain (trisomy 7) and whole chromosome 10 loss (monosomy 10) are the most frequent numerical chromosome alterations in glioblastoma and commonly occur in combination (+7/–10) {3036}; less common are gains restricted to 7q and/or losses restricted to 10q. The most common gene amplification involves the *EGFR* locus at 7p11.2 (see below) {3036}. The sensitivity and specificity for the diagnosis of IDH-wildtype glioblastoma were reported, respectively, as 59% and 98% for +7/–10, and as 36% and 100% for *EGFR* amplification {3036}. Other frequent numerical chromosome alterations in IDH-wildtype glioblastomas are losses on 9p (including homozygous deletion of the *CDKN2A* and/or *CDKN2B* locus at

9p21), 13q, 22q, and the sex chromosomes, as well as gains of chromosomes 19 and 20 {370,318}. Gene amplifications often manifest cytogenetically as extrachromosomal double-minute chromosomes and can be detected in as many as 50% of glioblastoma karyotypes {281}.

Epidermal growth factor receptor
The receptor tyrosine kinase (RTK) EGFR (HER1) is frequently altered in IDH-wildtype glioblastoma. Overall, about 60% of tumours show evidence of *EGFR* amplification, mutation, rearrangement, or altered splicing {370}. The most frequent of these alterations is *EGFR* amplification {1008}, which occurs in about 40% of all IDH-wildtype glioblastomas {370,3036} and in as many as 60% of glioblastomas in the DNA methylation group RTK2, but only in about 25% of RTK1 and mesenchymal glioblastomas {3060,3036}. In the majority of cases, *EGFR* amplifications are associated with a second *EGFR* alteration, such as extracellular domain mutations or in-frame intragenic deletions encoding either *EGFRvIII* or other alternative transcripts {370, 2868,3063}. *EGFR* gene fusions are discussed below.

PI3K–AKT–mTOR pathway
The PI3K pathway is important for regulating cell growth. Signalling is activated by RTKs and/or RAS and inhibited by PTEN. In IDH-wildtype glioblastoma, alterations of RTK genes, PI3K pathway genes, and *PTEN* are found in about 90% of cases{370,451}. Amplifications, truncations, and fusions of RTK genes are particularly frequent, typically involving *EGFR* (~60%, see above), *PDGFRA* (10–15%), *MET* (2–5%), or *FGFR3* (~3%) {2942,3315,370}. Mutations of *NF1* that activate the PI3K pathway via reduced RAS inhibition are present in approximately 10% of cases {370}. *PTEN*, which encodes the central inhibitor of the pathway, shows mutation/deletion in about 40% of glioblastomas, whereas mutations of *PIK3CA*, *PIK3R1*, or other PI3K pathway genes are observed in 25–30% {370}. RTK alterations may co-occur with PI3K or *PTEN* alterations in about 40% of cases, whereas PI3K mutations and *PTEN* mutations/deletions appear to be mutually exclusive {370}.

p14ARF–MDM2–MDM4–p53 pathway
The p53 pathway is central to the induction of DNA repair, cell-cycle arrest, and apoptosis. Genetic dysregulation of this pathway occurs in nearly 90% of glioblastomas {451,370}. MDM2 and MDM4 are both inhibitors of p53, and they are activated by amplification in about 15% of glioblastomas {370}. MDM2 is itself inhibited by p14ARF, which is an alternate reading frame protein encoded by the *CDKN2A* locus. This locus is deleted in about 60% of glioblastomas, resulting in inactivation of the p53 pathway and activation of the RB1 cell-cycle pathway (see below) {451,370}. *TP53* itself is mutated or deleted in 20–25% of IDH-wildtype glioblastomas {3564,370}. Genetic alterations affecting *CDKN2A* (*p14ARF*), *MDM2* or *MDM4*, and *TP53* are mostly exclusive of one another {370}.

CDK4/6–CDKN2A/B–RB1 cell-cycle pathway
CDK4 and CDK6 catalyse the phosphorylation of RB1 and thereby the release of E2F transcription factors, which then induce the expression of genes involved in the progression from G1 to S phase of the cell cycle. p16 (encoded by *CDKN2A*) is an inhibitor of CDK4. Approximately 80% of glioblastomas demonstrate one or more genetic alterations of the CDK4/6–RB1 cell-cycle pathway {451,370}. Most frequent are *CDKN2A* deletions that typically also involve nearby *CDKN2B* (~60%), amplifications of *CDK4* or *CDK6* (~15%), and mutations/deletions of *RB1* (~8%) {2259,2636,451,370}. *CDKN2A* deletion and *RB1* alterations are mutually exclusive {3249,451}, whereas *CDKN2A* deletion and *CDK4* amplification may occasionally coexist {2259, 451,370}. In rare cases, the cell-cycle pathway is alternatively activated by deletion of *CDKN2C* or amplifications of *CDK6* or *CCND2* {451,370}.

Gene fusions
Gene fusions in IDH-wildtype glioblastoma are mostly confined to members of the RTK family and recurrently involve *EGFR* (6–13%); *FGFR3* (~3%); *MET* (1–4%); or *NTRK1*, *NTRK2*, or *NTRK3* (1–2%) (see Table 2.02). *EGFR* fusions typically occur as part of complex rearrangements at chromosome band 7p11.2 {370}. Fusion partners are mostly neighbouring genes of

Table 2.02 Gene fusions with estimated frequencies of > 1% in IDH-wildtype glioblastoma

Gene	Frequent fusion partner(s)	Estimated frequency	Comment	References
EGFR	SEPTIN14, various others	~6–13%	Co-occurs with *EGFR* amplification and often results in EGFR C-terminal truncation	{981,370,1031,3192}
FGFR3	TACC3	~3%	Recurrently caused by chromosome 4p16.3 tandem duplication, associated with amplification of *CDK4* (22–44%) and *MDM2* (20–25%)	{2942,2400,370,193,751,907,752}
MET	PTPRZ1, various others	~1–4%	More typical for IDH-mutant high-grade astrocytoma and diffuse, paediatric-type high-grade glioma, H3-wildtype and IDH-wildtype	{193,907,1362}
NTRK1, NTRK2, NTRK3	Various	~1–2%	Fusions also observed in CNS WHO grade 1–3 gliomas; *NTRK3* fusion very rare	{981,3605,907,3192}

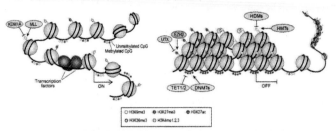

Active chromatin **Repressive chromatin**

Fig. 2.30 Glioblastoma, IDH-wildtype. DNA methylation, histone modifications, and numerous chromatin regulators determine the global structure of chromatin. Active chromatin (left) is globally accessible for transcriptional regulation. Repressive chromatin (right) sequesters portions of the genome, is enriched for characteristic histone modifications, and is refractory to regulatory activity. DNMTs, DNA methyltransferases; HDMs, histone demethylases; HMTs, histone methyltransferases.

EGFR (e.g. *SEPTIN14*, *PSPH*, *SEC61G*, *SDK1*), and the fusions frequently cause truncation of the *EGFR* C-terminal autophosphorylation domain {981,370,3192}, which has been shown to be transforming {579}. *EGFR* fusion co-occurs with *EGFR* amplification {981}. *FGFR3::TACC3* fusions and *EGFR* amplifications are mutually exclusive, and tumours with *FGFR3::TACC3* fusions have higher rates of *CDK4* and *MDM2* amplification {751,2942, 752,907}. The *FGFR3::TACC3* fusion is recurrently caused by a tandem duplication on 4p16.3 {2400}, which may allow screening by copy-number analysis {370}. The initially identified *FGFR1::TACC1* fusion {2942} was not observed in numerous follow-up studies and is therefore no longer considered typical of glioblastoma {2400,370,751,193}. *MET* fusions are more common in high-grade IDH-mutant astrocytomas {1362} and diffuse, paediatric-type high-grade glioma, H3-wildtype and IDH-wildtype {1415}, but they may also occur in adult-type IDH-wildtype glioblastomas {907,1362,193}. *NTRK1*, *NTRK2*, and *NTRK3* fusions occur infrequently {981,3605,907,3192}. *PDGFRA* fusions have been described but are exceedingly rare {65,370,907,2358}, whereas truncating deletion of exons 8 and 9 of *PDGFRA* recurrently occurs in *PDGFRA*-amplified tumours {2358}. Other potentially relevant fusions have been reported (e.g. *PTPRZ1::ETV1*, *KLHL7::BRAF*, *CEP85L::ROS1*, *CCDC127::TERT*) but require further validation {2038,3192}.

Tumour mutation burden

Tumour mutation burden has been proposed as a potential biomarker for estimating the abundance of neoantigens, which may have relevance for immunotherapy. In one study of IDH-wildtype glioblastoma, a high mutation burden (defined as > 20 mutations/1.4 Mb) was identified in 5 (2.7%) of 182 cases and was associated with mutation or loss of immunohistochemical expression of one or more mismatch repair markers (MLH1, MSH2, MSH6, PMS2) {1323}. Recurrent glioblastoma shows higher rates of mismatch repair deficiency (~10%), mostly due to acquired MSH6 loss, and this is associated with a dramatic increase of mutation burden {3372,1411}. A link between alkylating agent / temozolomide treatment and occurrence of *MSH6* mutation has been demonstrated {1380,435,451,3538}. Furthermore, *POLE*-mutated glioblastomas have a particularly high tumour mutation burden and may demonstrate a better response to immunotherapy than do other glioblastomas {1323, 1483,858}. A high tumour mutation burden has been linked

to shorter survival and a low rate of response to PD1 immune checkpoint inhibition in glioblastoma {3222}.

Epigenetics, chromatin, and promoter methylation

The interplay between epigenetic regulation and glioblastoma tumorigenesis has several modalities. Epigenetic modifiers can be bona fide oncogenes or tumour suppressors affected by gain- or loss-of-function genetic alterations, resulting in the disruption of epigenetic regulatory processes by affecting histone modifications, DNA methylation, and chromatin remodelling {3079}. Nearly half of 291 IDH-wildtype glioblastomas profiled by whole-exome sequencing harboured one or more nonsynonymous mutations affecting chromatin organization {370}. Even in the absence of direct genetic alterations, epigenetic modifiers can modulate gene expression and impact glioma-relevant processes {3058,3078}.

A key function of chromatin regulation is to maintain inactive portions of the genome in repressive structures. Canonical repressive states include heterochromatin marked by H3 p.K28me3 (K27me3), a mark deposited by PRC2 and its catalytic subunit, EZH2. EZH2 is overexpressed in IDH-wildtype glioblastoma and various other cancer types, presumably contributing to the silencing of key tumour suppressor genes {714}. Loss of function of EZH2 can also promote cancer in a context-dependent manner. Although loss-of-function mutations of *EZH2* in IDH-wildtype glioblastoma are rare (< 1%), inhibition of EZH2 enzymatic activity occurs through mutation of H3 genes in diffuse midline gliomas, resulting in p.K28M (K27M)-mutant protein {370,2867,3481}. Mutations in *ATRX*, which encodes a chromatin remodeller that deposits H3.3 in pericentromeric and subtelomeric regions, were observed in 13 (4.5%) of 291 IDH-wildtype glioblastomas {370}, in contrast to 60–70% of IDH-mutant gliomas and about 30% of paediatric high-grade gliomas {1474,2867,3482}.

Within chromatin, actively transcribed gene bodies are marked by H3 p.K37me3 (K36me3), a mark deposited by the methyltransferase SETD2. Mutations in *SETD2* occur in only about 2% of IDH-wildtype glioblastomas and are more common in paediatric and IDH-mutant gliomas {370,958}. Enhancers and promoters are marked by histone acetylation and H3 p.K5me (K4me). The methylation mark is catalysed by complexes that contain MLL homologues. Missense mutations in *KMT2B*, *KMT2C*, and *KMT2D* have been detected in rare cases (2–3%) of IDH-wildtype glioblastoma. Histone deacetylases and a range of histone demethylases are also infrequently mutated in IDH-wildtype glioblastoma, broadly affecting chromatin activity. Both histone and DNA demethylases are inhibited by IDH mutations {3058}.

Epigenetic gene silencing by DNA methylation is another common mechanism of inactivating genes {2543,1151,1796}. The *MGMT* gene encodes a DNA repair protein {598} and is transcriptionally silenced by promoter methylation in approximately 40–50% of IDH-wildtype glioblastomas {370,861,1279, 2588}. MGMT specifically removes promutagenic alkyl groups from the O6 position of guanine in DNA, thereby blunting the treatment effects of alkylating agents {860,1062}. *MGMT* promoter methylation is present in 40–50% of glioblastomas {370, 861,1279,2588} and is predictive of benefit from therapy with alkylating agents such as temozolomide (see below) {1279, 1998,3430}. A higher frequency of *MGMT* promoter methylation

(> 75%) is associated with tumours that have the glioma CpG island methylator phenotype (G-CIMP), which is characteristic of IDH-mutant gliomas {172,370,2313}. Distinct DNA methylation subclasses of glioblastoma have been suggested, partly correlated to tumour genotypes and potentially to developmental origins {370,3060,460}.

Macroscopic appearance

Glioblastomas are often large at presentation and can occupy much of a lobe. They are usually unilateral, but they can cross the corpus callosum and be bilateral (a butterfly lesion). Most hemispheric glioblastomas are clearly intraparenchymal and centred in the white matter. Infrequently, they are superficial and contact the leptomeninges and dura, sometimes mimicking a metastasis or meningioma. Cortical infiltration may produce a thickened tan cortex overlying a necrotic zone in the white matter.

Glioblastomas are poorly delineated; the cut surface is variable in colour, with peripheral greyish to pink masses and central areas of yellowish necrosis. In some areas, necrotic tissue may also border adjacent brain structures without an intermediate zone of macroscopically detectable tumour. Central necrosis can occupy as much as 80% of the total tumour. Glioblastomas are often stippled with red and brown foci of recent and remote haemorrhage. Extensive haemorrhages can occur and cause stroke-like symptoms, sometimes as the first sign of the tumour. Macroscopic cysts, when present, contain a turbid fluid of liquefied necrotic tumour tissue, in contrast to the well-delineated cysts present in lower-grade diffuse astrocytomas.

Epithelioid glioblastomas are typically single lesions, although at least one multifocal example has been reported, and metastatic disease may occur {1046}; leptomeningeal spread is also relatively common.

Histopathology

Glioblastoma, IDH-wildtype, is typically a diffusely infiltrating, highly cellular glioma composed of astrocytic, usually poorly differentiated tumour cells that show nuclear atypia and often marked pleomorphism. Mitotic activity is readily identifiable in most cases and is often brisk. Microvascular proliferation and necrosis, with or without perinecrotic palisading, are characteristic diagnostic features. In an IDH- and H3-wildtype diffuse glioma, at least one of these features (i.e. microvascular proliferation or necrosis) is sufficient for the diagnosis of glioblastoma. In specimens from treated patients, therapy-induced necrosis, in particular radionecrosis, must be distinguished from innate tumour necrosis.

As the outdated term "glioblastoma multiforme" suggests, the histopathology of this tumour is highly variable, which sometimes makes histopathological diagnosis difficult on specimens obtained by stereotactic needle biopsy {414}. Some lesions show a high degree of cellular and nuclear polymorphism, with numerous multinucleated giant cells; others are markedly cellular but relatively monomorphic. The astrocytic nature of the neoplasms is easily identifiable (at least focally) in some tumours, but it may be difficult to recognize in poorly differentiated lesions.

The distribution of histological features within a glioblastoma is variable, but large necrotic areas usually occupy the tumour centre, whereas viable tumour cells tend to be found in the

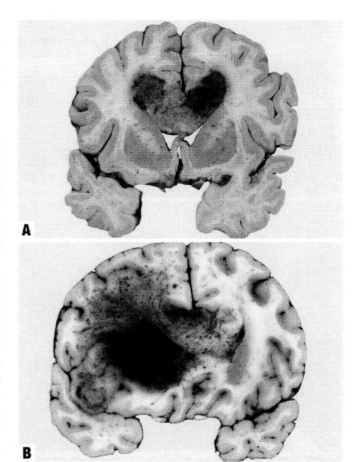

Fig. 2.31 Glioblastoma, IDH-wildtype. **A** Glioblastoma with bilateral, symmetrical invasion of the corpus callosum and adjacent white matter of the cerebral hemispheres (butterfly glioblastoma). **B** Large glioblastoma of the left frontal lobe with typical coloration: whitish-grey tumour tissue in the periphery, yellow areas of necrosis, and extensive haemorrhage. Note extension through the corpus callosum into the right hemisphere.

tumour periphery. The circumferential region of high cellularity and abnormal vessels corresponds to the contrast-enhancing ring seen radiologically and is therefore an appropriate target for biopsy. Microvascular proliferation is seen throughout the lesion but is usually most marked around necrotic foci and in the peripheral zone of infiltration.

Cellular heterogeneity and glioblastoma patterns

Few human neoplasms are as morphologically heterogeneous as glioblastoma. Poorly differentiated, fusiform, round, or pleomorphic cells may prevail, but better-differentiated neoplastic astrocytes are often discernible, at least focally {414}. The transition between areas that still have recognizable astrocytic differentiation and highly anaplastic (small, round, primitive-appearing) cells may be either continuous or abrupt. In gemistocytic lesions, anaplastic tumour cells may be diffusely mixed with differentiated gemistocytes. An abrupt change in morphology may reflect the emergence of a distinct tumour clone due to subclonal molecular diversification during tumour evolution (see *Primitive neuronal cells and glioblastoma with a primitive neuronal component*, below) {997}.

Cellular pleomorphism includes the formation of small, undifferentiated, spindled, lipidized, granular, epithelioid, and/or

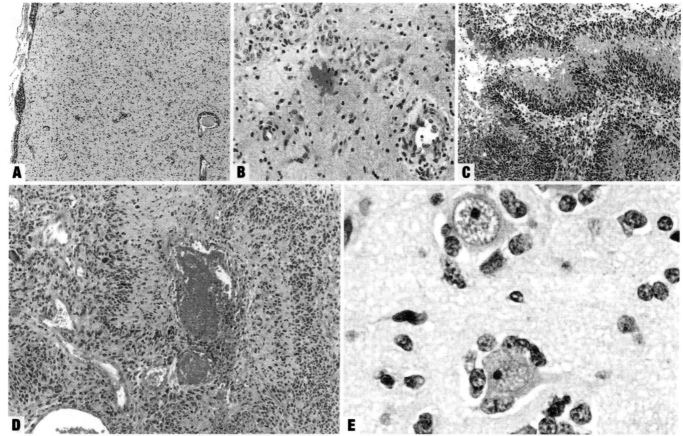

Fig. 2.32 Glioblastoma, IDH-wildtype. **A** Secondary structure formation with subpial, perivascular, and perineuronal accumulation of tumour cells. **B** Microvascular proliferation at the infiltrative edge of a glioblastoma, characterized by small blood vessels with prominent, multilayered cells sometimes forming glomeruloid structures. **C** Serpentine foci of palisading necrosis with tumour cells lining the ischaemic edges. **D** Thrombosis at the centre of palisading necrosis in a glioblastoma. **E** Secondary structures of migrating glioblastoma cells around neurons.

giant cells. In some tumours, these patterns can dominate, for example in areas of bipolar, fusiform cells that form intersecting bundles and fascicles resembling a spindle cell sarcoma. The accumulation of epithelioid tumour cells with well-delineated plasma membranes and a lack of cell processes, such as in epithelioid glioblastomas (see below), may mimic metastatic carcinoma or melanoma.

Some glioblastomas have well-recognized patterns that are characterized by a predominance of a particular cell type. These morphologies are discussed in the following subsections, along with the corresponding histological subtypes and patterns that can be established if a particular cellular morphology predominates.

Gemistocytes and gemistocytic astrocytic neoplasms
Gemistocytes are cells with copious, glassy, non-fibrillary cytoplasm that displaces the dark, angulated nucleus to the periphery of the cell. Processes radiate from the cytoplasm but are stubby, not elongated. GFAP staining is generally positive. Perivascular lymphocytes frequently populate gemistocytic regions, but they are inconspicuous in other regions in the same neoplasm. Gemistocytes may be present in IDH-wildtype glioblastoma as well as in IDH-mutant astrocytoma; the term "gemistocytic astrocytoma" describes a typically IDH-mutant astrocytoma that is characterized by a large proportion of

gemistocytic astrocytes (> 20% of tumour cells) (see *Astrocytoma, IDH-mutant*, p. 19).

Giant cells and giant cell glioblastoma
Large, multinucleated tumour cells may be present in glioblastoma and occur with a spectrum of increasing size and pleomorphism. Multinucleated giant cells are not found in all glioblastomas nor are they associated with a more aggressive clinical course {412}. The designation of a glioblastoma as a giant cell glioblastoma – a longstanding and established histopathological subtype of glioblastoma – should be reserved for those tumours in which bizarre, multinucleated giant cells are a dominant histopathological component. Glioblastomas arising from constitutional mismatch repair deficiency often exhibit severe nuclear atypia and multinucleation {1616}.

Giant cell glioblastomas are rare, accounting for < 1% of all glioblastomas {2333,284}, although they may be more common in paediatric populations {1561,1731,2098,2454}. The M:F ratio is 1.1–1.5:1 {1731,2333}. Giant cell glioblastomas typically develop de novo after a short preoperative history and without clinical or radiological evidence of a precursor lesion. They are often located subcortically in the temporal and parietal lobes, and they may be distinctive because of their circumscription, which on imaging and intraoperatively can mimic a metastasis.

Giant cell glioblastomas are frequently rich in reticulin, are firm and well circumscribed, and may be mistaken for a metastasis

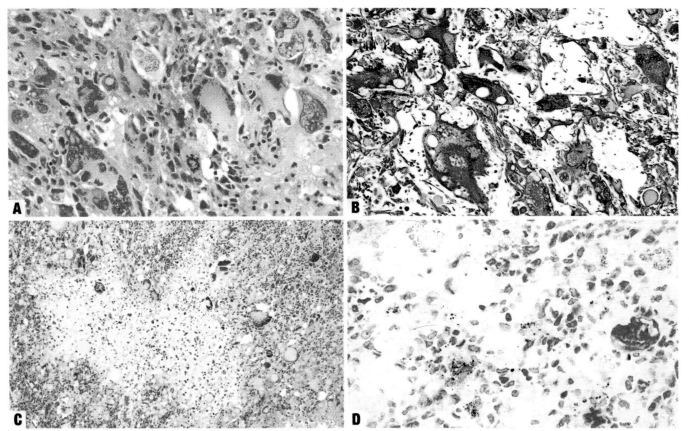

Fig. 2.33 Giant cell glioblastoma. **A** Numerous bizarre multinucleated giant cells. **B** GFAP immunoreactivity. **C,D** Giant cell glioblastoma in a patient with constitutional mismatch repair deficiency syndrome (CMMRD). **C** Next-generation sequencing of this tumour and matched blood showed a biallelic germline mutation of *PMS2*, consistent with a diagnosis of CMMRD. **D** This immunostain for PMS2 shows a lack of staining in both tumour cells and non-neoplastic cells, suggestive of CMMRD, which was subsequently confirmed by next-generation sequencing. Note that CMMRD-associated glioblastomas mostly occur in young children and epigenetically align with the paediatric-type diffuse high-grade gliomas (see *Constitutional mismatch repair deficiency syndrome*, p. 452).

or even a meningioma (when attached to the dura). They are characterized histologically by numerous multinucleated giant cells, in a background of small often fusiform cells {2012}. The giant cells are often extremely bizarre; they can be as large as 0.5 mm in diameter and contain anywhere from a few to > 20 nuclei. Mitoses are frequent and can be seen both in giant cells and in the smaller tumour cells. A typical although variable feature is the perivascular accumulation of tumour cells with the formation of a pseudorosette-like pattern {1937}. Occasionally, perivascular lymphocyte cuffing is observed. Palisading necrosis or large ischaemic necrotic zones may be present, whereas microvascular proliferation is not common. Giant cell glioblastoma shows consistent GFAP expression, although the level of expression is variable. OLIG2 expression is often found, either diffusely or focally, and more commonly in small tumour cells than in giant cells {1500}.

The giant cell phenotype typically reflects a state of genomic instability, often with superimposed *TP53* mutations and/or mismatch repair defects. Although most giant cell glioblastomas are IDH- and H3-wildtype, IDH-mutant gliomas and H3-mutant gliomas may show giant cell features {2235}. Genetically, giant cell glioblastoma does not seem to represent a distinct tumour entity, but it stratifies into different genotypes.

Especially in young patients, numerous multinucleated giant cells in glioblastomas may point to an underlying defect in DNA repair due to inherited or acquired mutations in *POLE* {858} or

DNA mismatch repair genes {205}. Immunohistochemistry may show loss of one or a pair of mismatch repair proteins in giant cell glioblastomas, which is associated with a mutation in the expected mismatch repair gene {205}.

The prognosis of giant cell glioblastoma is poor, but the clinical outcome may be slightly better than that of ordinary glioblastoma {418,1368,1731,2307,2333,2915}; for example, in two studies, median survival times of patients with giant cell glioblastoma were longer (11 and 13.5 months) than in standard glioblastoma (8 and 9.8 months) {1731,2333}.

Mesenchymal metaplasia and gliosarcoma

In general, "metaplasia" refers to the phenomenon whereby a differentiated cell acquires morphological features typical of another type of differentiated cell. The term is also used to designate aberrant differentiation in neoplasms. Metaplastic changes in glioblastoma may be mesenchymal or epithelial (see next subsection). Mesenchymal metaplasia may correspond to differentiation along various lineages, with spindled cells resembling fibroblast-like differentiation being most common. Patterns resembling osseous, chondroid, adipocytic, or myogenic differentiation are rare. Sarcomatous metaplasia is encountered most often within the setting of an IDH-wildtype glioblastoma, but metaplasia can also be seen rarely in IDH-mutant astrocytomas, H3-mutant gliomas, IDH-mutant and 1p/19q-codeleted oligodendrogliomas (oligosarcoma) {2699},

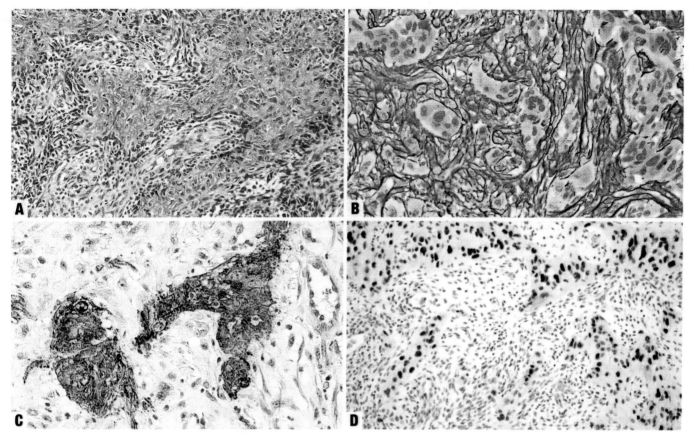

Fig. 2.34 Gliosarcoma. **A** Gliosarcoma with osteosarcoma-like foci. **B** Alternating areas of reticulin-poor glioma and reticulin-rich sarcoma. **C** GFAP highlights the glioma components. **D** The glioma regions are positive for OLIG2.

and ependymomas (ependymosarcoma) {2700}. It may be encountered either de novo at presentation or at the time of recurrence. The designation of gliosarcoma, also a long-standing and established histopathological subtype of glioblastoma, should be reserved for tumours showing prominent mesenchymal differentiation, characterized by a biphasic pattern with alternating areas displaying glial and mesenchymal differentiation.

Gliosarcomas are rare, accounting for approximately 2% of glioblastomas {1023,1730,1369}. Their age distribution is similar to that of glioblastoma overall, with preferential manifestation in patients aged 40–60 years (mean age: 52 years). Rare cases occur in children {1563}, and the M:F ratio is 1.4–1.8:1 {1227}. Gliosarcoma typically occurs de novo with symptoms of short duration that reflect the location of the tumour and increased intracranial pressure. Gliosarcoma can also arise secondarily after conventional adjuvant treatment of high-grade glioma {1226}. It usually occurs supratentorially, involving the temporal, frontal, parietal, and occipital lobes (in descending order of frequency). Posterior fossa {2240,2263}, lateral ventricles {2811}, and spinal cord {475} are rare locations, and some tumours are multifocal {2375}.

Because of its high connective-tissue content, gliosarcoma has the gross appearance of a firm, well-circumscribed mass, which can be mistaken for a metastasis or (when attached to the dura) a meningioma. Histologically, it is characterized by a mixture of gliomatous and sarcomatous tissues, which by definition show high-grade malignant features including mitotic

activity, microvascular proliferation, and/or necrosis. The sarcomatous component often demonstrates the pattern of a spindle cell sarcoma, with densely packed long bundles of spindle cells surrounded individually by reticulin fibres. The glial component, typically seen as reticulin-free nests or islands of fibrillary or gemistocytic astrocytoma cells, is positive for glial markers, including GFAP and OLIG2, which are negative or only focally positive in the sarcomatous component {2304,1500}. Occasionally, the sarcomatous component shows considerable pleomorphism {2240}. A subset of cases show additional lines of mesenchymal differentiation, such as the formation of cartilage {190}, bone {2036}, osteoid–chondroid tissue {669,1271, 3102}, smooth and striated muscle {1603,3084}, and even lipomatous features {1001}. Primitive neuronal components occur rarely {1554,3529}. The gliosarcoma subtype of IDH-wildtype glioblastoma is negative for IDH1 p.R132H and does not show *IDH1* or *IDH2* mutations.

The sarcomatous areas of gliosarcoma are thought to result from a phenotypic change in the glioblastoma cells (rather than from the coincidental development of two separate neoplasms, termed a "collision tumour", as originally hypothesized), and they may reflect the clonal evolution of a tumour. This hypothesis is supported by studies that have demonstrated common molecular abnormalities between the glial and sarcomatous components of the tumour, including gain of chromosome 7 and loss of chromosome 10 {312} and identical mutations in *TP53*, *PTEN*, and *TERT* {280,2646,3357}, as well as *CDKN2A* deletion and *MDM2* and *CDK4* co-amplification {2646}. Results from microarray-based comparative genomic hybridization analysis in the glial and mesenchymal tumour areas also suggest that the mesenchymal components may be derived from glial cells with additional genetic alterations in a subset of gliosarcomas {2190}.

Gliosarcomas have a genetic profile that is similar, but not identical, to that of IDH-wildtype glioblastoma: *PTEN* mutations, *CDKN2A* deletions, and *TP53* mutations, but infrequent *EGFR* amplification {17,2646}. Chromosomal imbalances are common, with frequent gains on chromosome 7 (up to 75%), and losses of chromosome 9 (mostly correlating to *CDKN2A* loss) and chromosome 10 (up to 72%) {17,1947}. At the protein level, expression of SNAI2, TWIST, MMP2, and MMP9 is characteristic of mesenchymal tumour areas, suggesting that the mechanisms involved in epithelial–mesenchymal transition in epithelial neoplasms may also pertain to mesenchymal differentiation in gliosarcomas {2191}.

The prognosis of patients with gliosarcoma is poor, with OS being similar to that of patients with histologically classic IDH-wildtype glioblastoma {1023}. There have been multiple reports of gliosarcomas with spinal and systemic metastases and even invasion of the skull {149,2841,227,2863,108}.

Epithelial metaplasia

Epithelial metaplasia in glioblastoma is rare and may comprise areas of squamous or adenomatous differentiation. Tumour cells can display features of squamous epithelial cells, including epithelial whorls with keratin pearls and immunohistochemical expression of squamous cell–associated markers like CK5/6 {416,2164,2698}. Other cases may contain foci with glandular and ribbon-like epithelioid structures that mimic metastatic adenocarcinoma {2728}. Some glioblastomas may contain so many of these structures that they are referred to as either adenoid glioblastoma (when they retain their glial immunophenotype) or glioblastoma with epithelial metaplasia (when they show a true epithelial immunophenotype) {2698}. Small cells with more marked epithelial features and more cohesiveness are less common {1591}. Adenoid features and true epithelial metaplasia are slightly more common in gliosarcoma than in ordinary glioblastoma {1591,2164,2698}.

Epithelioid glioblastoma

Epithelioid glioblastoma is a histological subtype of glioblastoma defined by a mostly sharply demarcated, loosely cohesive aggregate of large epithelioid to rhabdoid cells with abundant cytoplasm, large vesicular nuclei, and prominent macronucleoli, sometimes mimicking metastatic carcinoma or melanoma. Recent studies suggest that epithelioid features are most common in three distinct molecular subclasses: (1) a prognostically more favourable tumour of children and young adults that overlaps greatly with pleomorphic xanthoastrocytoma genetically (*BRAF* p.V600E mutation and homozygous *CDKN2A* deletions) and epigenetically (DNA methylation profile); (2) a poor-prognosis tumour of older adults that has features of conventional IDH-wildtype glioblastoma (albeit with more frequent *BRAF* p.V600E mutations); and (3) an intermediate-prognosis tumour with features of the RTK1-type paediatric high-grade glioma, frequently associated with *PDGFRA* amplification and chromothripsis {1716}. Rare examples of H3 K27–altered diffuse midline glioma also show epithelioid features {2988}, and other glioma types may occur with this pattern as well.

Epithelioid glioblastomas are dominated by a relatively uniform population of epithelioid cells showing focal loss of cohesion, scant intervening neuropil, a distinct cell membrane, abundant eosinophilic cytoplasm, and eccentric or centrally located nuclei. At least focal rhabdoid cytology is seen in most tumours. Exceptional cases have contained giant cells {1652}, lipidization {2698}, a desmoplastic response {2698}, or cytoplasmic vacuoles {2266}. Epithelioid glioblastoma may show areas with pleomorphic xanthoastrocytoma–like histology, although this appearance does not reliably associate with the pleomorphic xanthoastrocytoma–like molecular group {1716}.

Rosenthal fibres and eosinophilic granular bodies are uncommon. Necrosis is often present, but it is usually zonal rather than palisading. Some reports have noted a relative paucity of microvascular proliferation, but others found no substantial difference from classic glioblastoma in vascular patterns {384}.

Epithelioid glioblastomas show immunoreactivity for GFAP, although it is often patchy (and in a few cases, entirely absent); therefore, OLIG2 positivity may be helpful for establishing glial lineage {71}. Some tumours are focally immunoreactive

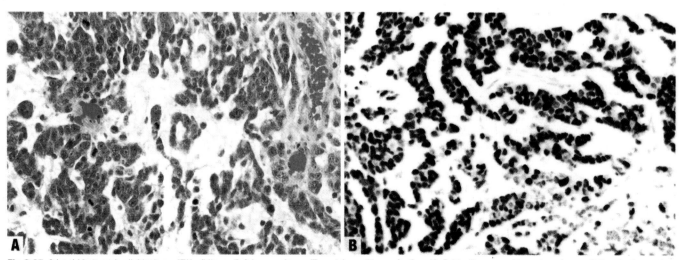

Fig. 2.35 Adenoid features in glioblastoma, IDH-wildtype. **A** Adenocarcinoma-like cytology with anaplastic epithelioid cells arranged in nests and rows. **B** Despite the carcinoma-like appearance, the glial histogenesis of this glioblastoma is supported by strong nuclear expression of OLIG2.

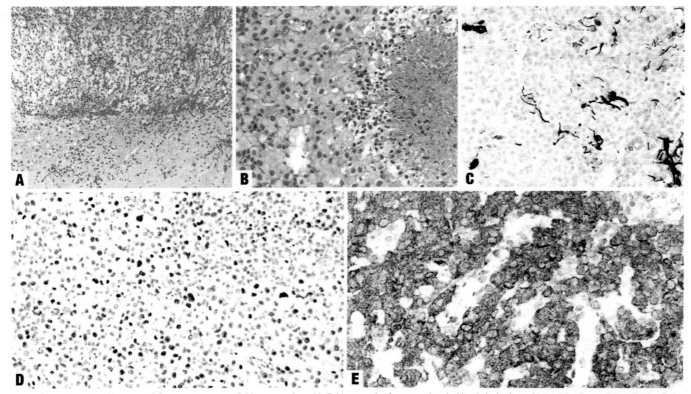

Fig. 2.36 Epithelioid glioblastoma. **A** In contrast to most glioblastomas, the epithelioid pattern is often associated with relatively sharp demarcation from adjacent brain. **B** Tumour cells are loosely cohesive and composed of large epithelioid to rhabdoid cells, often resembling metastatic melanoma or carcinoma. **C** Some examples show only limited GFAP expression. **D** A second glial marker (OLIG2) was positive in this case, helping to establish the diagnosis. **E** Immunoreactivity for BRAF p.V600E-mutant protein.

for EMA and cytokeratin cocktails (which is probably due to cross-reactivity with GFAP) {384,2698}, but CAM5.2 immunoreactivity is typically negative. Most authors have noted focal immunoreactivity for synaptophysin or neurofilaments. Expression of S100 and BRAF p.V600E may be mistaken for evidence of metastatic melanoma, but epithelioid glioblastomas do not express specific melanocytic markers such as HMB45 and melan-A. SMARCB1 expression and (in cases where it has been sought) SMARCA4 expression are retained {384}. Immunohistochemical staining for BRAF p.V600E is seen in roughly half of all cases of epithelioid glioblastoma, but it is most common in the pleomorphic xanthoastrocytoma–like molecular group and least common in the paediatric RTK1 molecular group {1652,1716}.

Oligodendrocyte-like cells

Occasional glioblastomas contain oligodendrocyte-like clear cells with round nuclei that mimic oligodendroglioma, sometimes including a chicken wire–like capillary network and microcalcifications. Oligodendroglioma-like foci may be focal or diffuse, although individual thresholds for identifying oligodendroglial features vary greatly. Notably, *FGFR3::TACC3* fusion–positive glioblastomas often show this pattern {276}. Two large studies of malignant gliomas in the pre-IDH era suggested that necrosis was associated with a significantly worse prognosis in the setting of anaplastic glioma with both oligodendroglial and astrocytic components {2113,3274}. Such tumours were also previously classified as glioblastomas with an oligodendroglial component and reported to have a better prognosis than classic glioblastoma {1273,1337,1734}.

However, more recent studies suggest that like lower-grade tumours with both oligodendroglial and astrocytic-appearing components (oligoastrocytomas), glioblastomas with oligodendroglial components are molecularly heterogeneous. Since 2016, the WHO classification has not considered glioblastoma with an oligodendroglioma component to be a distinct diagnostic entity; instead, such tumours genetically correspond to (1) IDH-wildtype glioblastoma (in particular the small cell pattern, given the morphological overlap with oligodendroglial cells), (2) IDH-mutant diffuse astrocytoma (CNS WHO grade 3 or 4), or (3) IDH-mutant and 1p/19q-codeleted CNS WHO grade 3 oligodendroglioma {1312}.

Small cells and small cell glioblastoma

Some IDH-wildtype glioblastomas feature a predominance of cells with highly monomorphic, small, round to slightly elongated, hyperchromatic nuclei and minimal discernible cytoplasm, little nuclear atypia, and (often) brisk mitotic activity. In the zone of infiltration, tumour cells can be difficult to identify, given their small size and bland cytology. GFAP immunoreactivity variably highlights delicate processes, and the Ki-67 proliferation index is typically high. Because of their nuclear regularity, clear haloes, microcalcifications, and chicken wire–like microvasculature, these tumours may resemble anaplastic oligodendrogliomas {2464}. But unlike oligodendrogliomas, small cell glioblastomas are uniformly IDH-wildtype, frequently showing *EGFR* amplification (in ~70% of cases) and chromosome 10 losses (in > 95%). IDH mutations are absent {1500,2464,3117}, as is 1p/19q codeletion {3117}. The clinical behaviour of the small cell pattern is similar to that of other

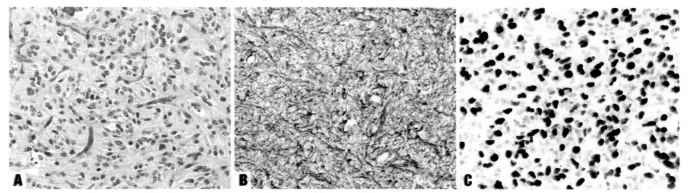

Fig. 2.37 Small cell glioblastoma. **A** A diffuse small cell glioma with monomorphic nuclei, delicate chromatin, and chicken wire–like capillaries (resembling oligodendroglioma), but with frequent mitoses despite only mild nuclear atypia. **B** Delicate processes are evident on a GFAP immunostain. **C** High Ki-67 labelling index despite the oligodendroglioma-like, cytologically bland nuclei.

glioblastomas, with an OS time of < 12 months in two series {2464,3117}. In one of these series, about a third of the tumours appeared as non-enhancing or minimally enhancing masses with no evidence of microvascular proliferation or necrosis on histology {2464}. However, follow-up imaging 2–3 months later often showed ring enhancement, and survival times were shorter for these patients (median: 6 months), consistent with such situations being early presentations of glioblastoma {2464}.

Primitive neuronal cells and glioblastoma with a primitive neuronal component

Rare glioblastomas may occur with one or more solid-looking primitive nodules showing immature cells with variable neuronal differentiation {2470}. The primitive foci are often sharply demarcated from the adjacent glioma, and they display markedly increased cellularity, with high N:C ratios and mitotic-karyorrhectic index values. More variable features include Homer Wright rosettes, cell wrapping, and anaplastic cytology similar

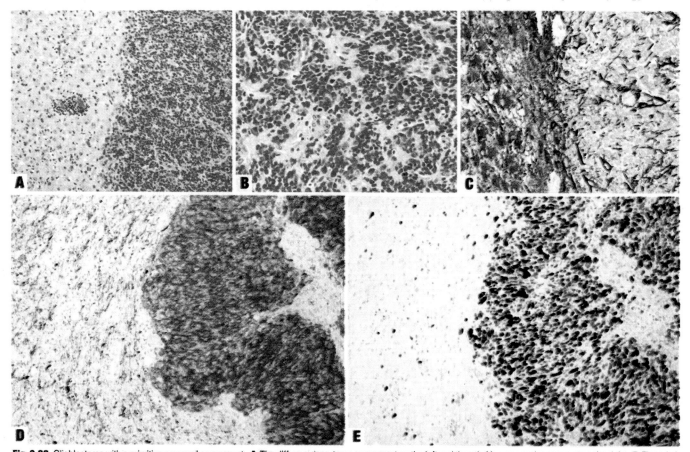

Fig. 2.38 Glioblastoma with a primitive neuronal component. **A** The diffuse astrocytoma component on the left and the primitive neuronal component on the right. **B** The primitive neuronal component has a small blue cell appearance, with high N:C ratios, nuclear moulding, cell wrapping, Homer Wright rosettes, and high mitotic count. **C** Extensive GFAP expression in the diffuse astrocytoma component, with loss of expression mostly in the primitive component. **D** Diffuse synaptophysin positivity in the primitive neuronal component, with staining of entrapped neuropil in the diffuse astrocytoma region. **E** Low Ki-67 labelling index in the diffuse astrocytoma component, with nearly 100% labelling in the primitive focus.

to that of medulloblastoma or other CNS embryonal neoplasms. Additional features include immunoreactivity for neuronal markers such as synaptophysin, reduction or loss of GFAP expression, and a markedly elevated Ki-67 proliferation index compared with that in adjacent areas of glioma. Survival time and genetic background are similar to those of glioblastoma in general {2470}. However, these tumours were reported to show a high rate (30–40%) of cerebrospinal fluid dissemination and increased frequency (~40%) of *MYCN* or *MYC* gene amplification. Spread to the lungs has also been reported {3119}. *MYC* amplifications are found only in the primitive-appearing nodules, and it is likely that such alterations drive the primitive-appearing clonal transformation at least in part, given that a similar phenotype has been observed in *Mycn*-driven murine forebrain tumours {3089}. A primitive neuronal component has also been reported in IDH-mutant high-grade astrocytic gliomas {1500,2991,3495} and to a lesser extent in H3 G34–mutant diffuse hemispheric gliomas, which were previously mistaken for supratentorial primitive neuroectodermal tumours in roughly half of all cases, even though they do not always show immunoreactivity for neuronal markers {1713}. Similarly, H3 K27–altered diffuse midline gliomas may also show primitive foci resembling an embryonal neoplasm {2988}.

Granular cells and granular cell astrocytoma/glioblastoma

Large cells with a granular, PAS-positive cytoplasm may be scattered within IDH-wildtype glioblastomas. In rare instances, they dominate and create an appearance similar to that of granular cell tumours in other parts of the body. Transitional forms between granular cells and neoplastic astrocytes can be identified in some cases, but in others it is difficult to identify any conventional astrocytoma component. Although larger and more coarsely granular, the tumour cells may resemble macrophages. Especially in the context of perivascular chronic inflammation, the tumour cells may be misinterpreted as a macrophage-rich lesion such as demyelinating disease. Given their lysosomal content, granular tumour cells are sometimes immunoreactive for macrophage markers such CD68, but not for lineage-specific markers such as CD163. Some cells may have peripheral immunopositivity for GFAP, or the cells may be completely GFAP-negative {364,1051}. When granular cell change is extensive, the tumours have been termed "granular cell astrocytoma" or "granular cell glioblastoma". These lesions have a distinct histological appearance and are typically characterized by aggressive glioblastoma-like clinical behaviour {364}, even when the histology otherwise suggests a lower-grade designation. A review of 59 reported patients found median survival times of 11 months for patients with CNS WHO grade 2 granular cell astrocytoma and 9 months for patients with CNS WHO grade 3–4 tumours {2843}. Another recent study of 39 patients (including patients with tumours histologically corresponding to CNS WHO grades 2, 3, and 4) showed a mean OS of only 11.3 months; notably, survival did not correlate significantly with CNS WHO grade, extent of granular cell change, sex, or Ki-67 (MIB1) index {3337}. That study did not find IDH mutations, but it identified *TERT* promoter mutations and +7/–10 copy-number changes in the majority of tumours, consistent with IDH-wildtype glioblastoma in general {3337}.

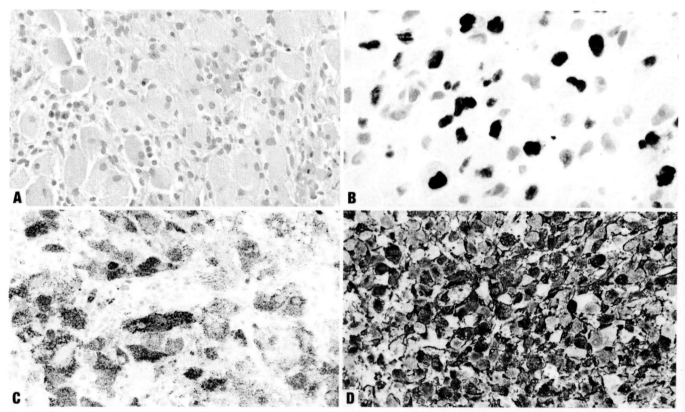

Fig. 2.39 Granular cell glioblastoma. **A** Eosinophilic cytoplasm, reminiscent of a granular cell tumour of the pituitary but invading the brain. When the cells are mostly vacuolated, they are often mistaken for macrophages. **B** OLIG2 immunoreactivity. **C** In contrast to most glioblastomas, the granular cell pattern often shows immunoreactivity for EMA. **D** GFAP immunoreactivity.

Lipidized cells and heavily lipidized glioblastoma

Cells with foamy cytoplasm are another feature occasionally observed in glioblastoma. The rare lesions in which they predominate have been designated malignant gliomas with heavily lipidized (foamy) tumour cells {1589,1594,2728,3129}. The lipidized cells may be grossly enlarged {1080}, and lobules of juxtaposed fully lipidized adipocyte-like cells can simulate adipose tissue. Pleomorphic xanthoastrocytoma should be considered in the differential diagnosis of such lesions.

Immunophenotype

By definition, IDH-wildtype glioblastomas lack immunostaining for IDH1 p.R132H and do not demonstrate positivity with mutation-specific antibodies against H3 p.K28M (K27M), H3.3 p.G35R (G34R), or H3.3 p.G35V (G34V). Nuclear immunostaining for ATRX is retained in the vast majority of tumours, and widespread nuclear positivity for p53 is seen in approximately 25–30% of tumours. Nuclear p53 positivity is particularly frequent in the giant cell glioblastoma subtype. Glioblastomas often express GFAP, but the degree of reactivity differs markedly between cases; for example, gemistocytic areas are frequently strongly positive, whereas primitive cellular components are often negative. S100 expression is also common. OLIG2 is a highly specific glioma marker and may be of diagnostic utility, being strongly positive more commonly in astrocytomas and oligodendrogliomas than in ependymomas and non-glial tumours {1421,2348,334,3225}; tumours with low nuclear expression of OLIG2 (< 30%) after adjuvant treatments may have a shorter time to recurrence and be associated with shorter survival {334}. Cytokeratin positivity may primarily indicate cross-reactivity with GFAP; immunostaining with the keratin antibody cocktail AE1/AE3 is most often positive, in contrast to the lack of positivity detected for most other keratins {3165}. However, glioblastomas with epithelial metaplasia may show expression of epithelial markers including cytokeratins in the epithelial component. Sarcomatous components in gliosarcoma typically lack expression of glial markers but react positively for vimentin. Rare cases may show expression of markers indicating differentiation along myogenic or other mesenchymal lineages (see *Gliosarcoma*, above). Cancer stem cell biomarkers such as CD133, CD44, SOX2, OCT4, and nestin may be found in glioblastomas {1260,132,54} but are of limited significance in diagnostic work. Notably, intratumoural heterogeneity for immunohistochemical positivity is common in glioblastomas, with differential expression of markers such as nestin, MAP2, and GFAP within different regions of the same tumour {249}. Expression of EGFR is frequent in IDH-wildtype glioblastoma and particularly strong in tumours with *EGFR* amplification, approximately half of which additionally show immunopositivity for EGFRvIII {906}.

Cytology

Intraoperative smear preparations of glioblastomas are valuable and complement the findings from histological sections. Cytological preparations usually demonstrate marked hypercellularity and nuclear pleomorphism, along with a discernible fibrillary background that is useful for establishing glial differentiation. Eosinophilic cytoplasm and processes vary, from naked nuclei lacking visible cytoplasm to gemistocytes showing elongated

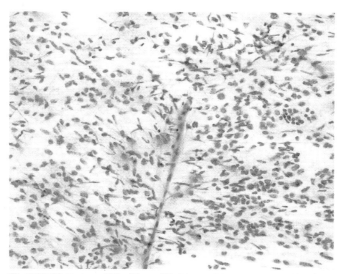

Fig. 2.40 Glioblastoma, IDH-wildtype. This intraoperative smear preparation shows elongated to irregular hyperchromatic nuclei, with thin eosinophilic cytoplasmic processes.

cellular extensions. Multinucleation can be seen and is prominent in some cases, as are mitotic figures.

Diagnostic molecular pathology

IDH-wildtype glioblastomas lack mutations in *IDH1* codon 132 and *IDH2* codon 172, and they do not carry H3 p.K28 (K27) or H3 p.G35 (G34) mutations. Absence of immunoreactivity for IDH1 p.R132H is sufficient (i.e. without further sequencing) to diagnose IDH-wildtype glioblastoma in a patient aged ≥ 55 years at diagnosis who has a histologically classic glioblastoma not located in midline structures and no history of a pre-existing lower-grade glioma {1940}. This practical approach is possible because the probability of a non-canonical IDH mutation is < 1% in glioblastomas from patients aged ≥ 55 years {539}. In patients aged < 55 years, or in patients with a history of lower-grade glioma and/or whose tumours show immunohistochemical loss of nuclear ATRX expression, negative IDH1 p.R132H immunostaining should be followed by DNA sequencing for less common *IDH1* or *IDH2* mutations. When no IDH mutations are detected by sequencing, such tumours are classified as glioblastoma, IDH-wildtype. However, tumours located in midline structures should additionally be evaluated for H3 p.K28M (K27M) mutation to exclude diffuse midline glioma, H3 K27–altered. In hemispheric tumours, particularly in younger patients, H3 G34–mutant diffuse hemispheric gliomas should be excluded by immunohistochemistry for H3.3 p.G35R (G34R) or H3.3 p.G35V (G34V) mutation or by *H3-3A* (*H3F3A*) sequencing.

Frequent and diagnostically relevant molecular alterations in IDH-wildtype glioblastomas include *TERT* promoter mutations, *EGFR* gene amplification, and a +7/−10 genotype {3036}. The presence of at least one of these aberrations in an IDH- and H3-wildtype diffuse glioma allows for the diagnosis of IDH-wildtype glioblastoma even in the absence of microvascular proliferation and/or necrosis {356,1944}.

In addition, demonstration of a DNA methylation profile of IDH-wildtype glioblastoma with a significant calibrated score is sufficient for the diagnosis {460}. DNA methylation profiles may further stratify molecular subgroups, with the RTK1, RTK2/classic, and mesenchymal subgroups being most common in adult patients {3060,460}. In this age group, the clinical relevance of methylation-based subgroups is still limited. In contrast, high-grade gliomas of children and adolescents may demonstrate less common DNA methylation profiles that have been linked to significantly longer survival {1721,1723}. DNA methylation profiling can also facilitate the diagnosis of challenging cases by helping to distinguish glioblastoma from histologically similar entities {1559,1458,463}.

BRAF p.V600E mutation is rare in IDH-wildtype glioblastoma {2842} but is detectable in as many as 50% of glioblastomas with epithelioid histology {1651}: *BRAF* p.V600E is found in 79% of pleomorphic xanthoastrocytoma–like tumours and 35% of adult-type IDH-wildtype glioblastomas, but 0% of paediatric RTK1 tumours {384,1651,1716}. *TP53* mutations are detectable in about a quarter of all IDH-wildtype glioblastomas but are found in > 80% of giant cell glioblastomas {2454}, which less commonly carry *EGFR* amplification and *TERT* promoter mutations {2304}. *EGFR* amplification appears to be frequent in small cell glioblastomas {415,2464}, whereas *MYC* or *MYCN* amplification has been linked to primitive neuronal components {2470}. However, none of these alterations is specific or sufficient for the respective morphological subtypes or patterns. Gliosarcomas rarely demonstrate *EGFR* amplification but otherwise lack distinguishing genetic alterations {17,2304}. Novel predictive biomarkers for molecularly targeted therapies in subsets of glioblastoma patients are under evaluation; these include high tumour mutation burden, *BRAF* p.V600E mutation, *NTRK* or *FGFR* gene family fusions, and *MET* amplification or fusions {1821}.

MGMT promoter methylation status is commonly determined in IDH-wildtype glioblastomas because it provides clinically relevant information on response to chemotherapy and survival of patients treated with temozolomide {1279,3431} or temozolomide plus lomustine (CCNU) {1299}. In elderly patients, *MGMT* promoter methylation status may guide decisions on chemotherapy or radiotherapy {2634,3430,1998}.

Gene expression patterns can be used to distinguish glioblastoma from pilocytic astrocytoma {2671}, other malignant astrocytomas {1009}, and oligodendroglioma {1009}, as well as IDH-mutant glioma from IDH-wildtype glioma, across grades and histology {370,1145,2287,3060}. Unsupervised analysis of expression profiles can be used to cluster gliomas into groups that correlate with histology and grade {1162,2293} and may be a better predictor of patient outcome {854}. A commonly used glioblastoma gene expression classifier defines proneural, classic, and mesenchymal subtypes, which correlate in part with mutations in *TP53*, mutation/amplification in *PDGFRA* or *EGFR*, and deletion/mutation in *NF1* {3315,3381}, but single-cell RNA sequencing showed that individual cells characteristic of different subtypes can be found within the same glioblastoma and that such expression subtypes may be related to malignant cell states reminiscent of neurodevelopmental cell types {2416,2226}. To date, gene expression profiles have not gained clear significance in clinical diagnostics.

Essential and desirable diagnostic criteria
See Box 2.03.

Staging
Not clinically relevant

Prognosis and prediction
Most glioblastoma patients die within 15–18 months after therapy with chemoradiation. The 5-year survival rate has been reported as 6.8% in the USA between 2012 and 2016 {2344} and as 10% in clinical trials with somewhat more favourable patient selection {3057}. Younger age (< 50 years), high performance status, and complete tumour resection are associated with longer survival, as is *MGMT* promoter methylation {3057, 2638}. Patients with IDH-wildtype glioblastomas have shorter survival times than patients with CNS WHO grade 4 IDH-mutant astrocytomas with similar histological features {1244}.

Some individuals with glioblastomas benefit from current treatments, including maximal safe surgery, radiation, alkylating chemotherapy, and bevacizumab (where approved), as well as experimental and immunological interventions. However, there is marked heterogeneity in treatment response, which probably reflects the biological heterogeneity of the disease. For example, more extensive surgery may be limited by the location of the tumour in an eloquent area and by the often diffusely infiltrative growth pattern {3409,3459}. And for most treatments, the basic molecular mechanisms for primary or acquired resistance are unknown or incompletely understood. Biological properties such as hypoxia, necrosis, DNA repair capacity, specific mutations (e.g. in *PTEN*), and volume of the disease may influence radiation response {3427,3439,3430,2476,1963}, but most such observations lack clinical validation.

Age
Clinical trials have shown that younger patients (< 50 years) with glioblastoma have longer survival times {3057,573,1104,1105}, with the age effect persisting through all age groups in a linear manner {2309}. In addition, coexisting medical and social conditions probably contribute to the poorer life expectancy of elderly patients (> 65 years) with glioblastoma. There are no validated age cut-off points for clinical decisions that are based on the distinction between fit and frail patients; however, fit older patients may benefit from chemoradiation {2476}, and for frail patients, *MGMT* promoter methylation status can influence the choice between chemotherapy and radiotherapy alone {2046, 3430,3427}.

Histopathology

Histological features do not confer significant prognostic information in IDH-wildtype glioblastoma, although necrosis has been associated with shorter survival {199,412,1337}. In some studies, giant cell glioblastoma has been noted to have a somewhat better prognosis than other types of glioblastoma {1731,2333,2908}; one study showed poorer prognosis for gliosarcoma than other glioblastomas {2960}, whereas another showed no survival difference for gliosarcomas {975}, and most studies of epithelioid glioblastoma have shown a poor prognosis {384,543,1653}. Tumours with a primitive neuronal component, particularly those with *MYC* or *MYCN* amplification, may have a greater tendency for cerebrospinal fluid spread {2470}.

Biomarkers

MGMT promoter methylation is an independent prognostic marker for longer OS in glioblastoma {3415} and a strong predictive marker for response to alkylating and methylating chemotherapy {1279,3416,3429,3430,3094}. More than 90% of longer-term surviving patients with glioblastoma have *MGMT* promoter methylation 19269895} versus only about 30% of the general patient population with glioblastoma {3056}. *MGMT* promoter methylation also correlates with longer progression-free survival and OS in elderly patients treated with temozolomide {3430, 1998}. Limitations for the general implementation of *MGMT* promoter methylation as a standardized test include variability of methods, determination of cut-off values, and reproducibility of test results {3431}. In addition, there are groups of patients who seemingly benefit from treatment despite having a non-methylated *MGMT* promoter {1279,2476}. Therefore, in some settings, *MGMT* promoter methylation testing has been restricted to trials that require stratification or inclusion of patients according to the test result.

TERT promoter mutation has been associated with more aggressive behaviour in IDH-wildtype glioblastoma {3022,

1780}, with IDH-wildtype and *TERT* promoter–wildtype glioblastomas tending to occur in younger patients and having more frequent PI3K pathway mutations {3448}. *EGFR* amplification and overexpression have been suggested as poor prognostic factors in glioblastomas {1870,2961,1779}, especially in highly amplified tumours {2175}, but a consistent relationship between *EGFR* amplification (or EGFRvIII status) and survival has not been found in other studies {2309,377,138,1325,906}. Allelic loss of 10q was associated with shorter survival in one report {2309}; however, *PTEN* mutation did not correlate with prognosis in other studies {2309,2850,2961,3415,408}.

Molecularly targeted therapies for patients with glioblastoma have been tested, but they have not yet yielded major successes {1821}. Patients with *BRAF* p.V600E mutations may respond to BRAF inhibitors {494,1544,3473}, and there are preliminary reports of patients with NTRK fusion–driven high-grade glioma responding to NTRK inhibitors {3615,1027}. Earlier attempts to target EGFR or EGFRvIII did not prove effective, but they have resulted in lessons learned. For example, EGFRvIII may be lost in a substantial proportion of glioblastomas at recurrence irrespective of treatment, thus mandating target assessment at the time of intended treatment {3414}. Targets should be prospectively validated, so efforts need to be directed to the parallel development of accurate, reproducible, and feasible tests {3428,67}. And, as mentioned, a general challenge in the development of molecularly targeted therapies is intratumoural and intertumoural heterogeneity {2416,2579}, including plasticity over time.

Tumour mutation burden serves as a biomarker in some solid cancers treated with checkpoint inhibitors, but it has not been shown to be useful in patients with glioblastoma {2797,3222}. However, the hypermutant phenotype may be predictive specifically for checkpoint inhibitor response in glioblastomas arising from genetically induced hypermutation {335} rather than the more common treatment-induced higher mutation load {3222}.

Diffuse astrocytoma, *MYB-* or *MYBL1*-altered

Hawkins CE
Blümcke I
Capper D
Ellison DW
Jones DTW
Najm I
Rosenblum MK

Definition

Diffuse astrocytoma, *MYB-* or *MYBL1*-altered, is a diffusely infiltrative astroglial neoplasm composed of monomorphic cells with genetic alterations in *MYB* or *MYBL1* (CNS WHO grade 1).

ICD-O coding

9421/1 Diffuse astrocytoma, *MYB-* or *MYBL1*-altered

ICD-11 coding

2A00.0Y & XH6PH6 Other specified gliomas of brain & Astrocytoma, NOS

Related terminology

Not recommended: isomorphic astrocytoma variant; isomorphic diffuse glioma.

Subtype(s)

Diffuse astrocytoma, *MYB*-altered; diffuse astrocytoma, *MYBL1*-altered

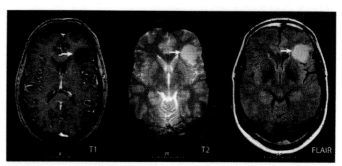

Fig. 2.41 Diffuse astrocytoma, *MYB-* or *MYBL1*-altered. MRI of a *MYBL1*-altered diffuse astrocytoma located in the inferior frontal gyrus in a 39-year-old patient with epilepsy since the age of 3 years. The tumour (white arrow) is T1-hypointense (left), T2-hyperintense (middle), and FLAIR-hyperintense (right).

Localization

Diffuse astrocytoma, *MYB-* or *MYBL1*-altered, is most commonly a cerebral tumour with cortical and subcortical components. In 40 reported cases, the tumour was centred in the temporal (42.5%), frontal (27.5%), occipital (20%), and parietal

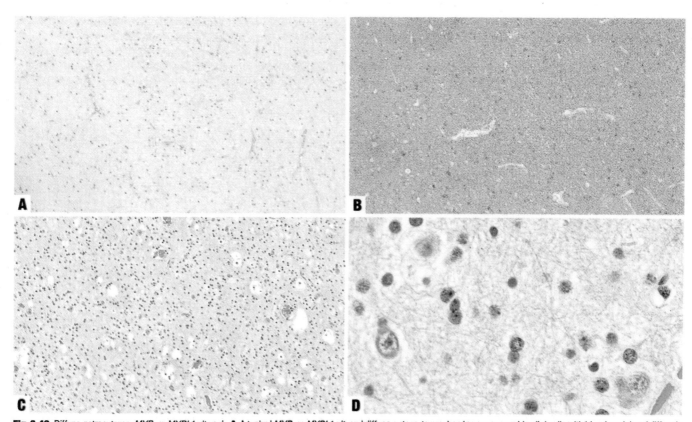

Fig. 2.42 Diffuse astrocytoma, *MYB-* or *MYBL1*-altered. **A** A typical *MYB-* or *MYBL1*-altered diffuse astrocytoma showing monomorphic glial cells with bland nuclei and diffusely permeating neuropil. **B** GFAP-immunostained section showing diffuse immunopositivity both of tumour cells and of the background neuropil. **C,D** Diffuse astrocytoma, *MYBL1*-altered. Infiltrative glioma with mild hypercellularity and atypia.

(10%) lobes {2953,304}. Rare brainstem cases have also been reported {2768}.

Clinical features

Patients typically present with drug-resistant epileptic seizures, which often have been present since childhood {2857,302, 3404}. Therefore, this neoplasm belongs within the broad category of long-term epilepsy-associated tumours {2953,3404, 302}. In one series, 81% of patients with MYB- or MYBL1-altered diffuse astrocytoma developed epilepsy during childhood, and the median age at onset of epilepsy was 10 years (range: 1–35 years) {3404}. However, only 23% of patients had a resection as children, with the median age at surgery being 29 years and the median time to operation after epilepsy onset being 15 years.

Imaging

Diffuse astrocytoma, MYB- or MYBL1-altered, is typically hypointense on T1, shows mixed signal or hyperintensity on T2-FLAIR, is non-enhancing, and does not show restricted diffusion {566,297,3404}. Tumours are mostly well defined, but they may show diffuse growth patterns, at least focally {566, 3404}. Large cysts are occasionally observed {3404}.

Epidemiology

Diffuse astrocytoma, MYB- or MYBL1-altered, is a rare tumour. In a population-based series of paediatric low-grade gliomas, tumours with MYB or MYBL1 alterations accounted for about 2% of cases {2768}, with the overall incidence among all brain tumours

likely to be < 0.5%. Paediatric series each described < 10 cases {3142,3597,2616,2584,188}, with no clear sex predilection. The largest series to date includes data on 20 patients with a MYB or MYBL1 alteration {3404}, with a median age of 29 years (range: 4–50 years) and a male preponderance (M:F ratio: 3:1).

Etiology

Unknown

Pathogenesis

MYB and its closely related family member MYBL1 are transcriptional transactivators that are important for cell proliferation and are downregulated with cellular differentiation {367}. In gliomas and other cancers, the genes encoding these proteins undergo structural rearrangements that result in truncation of the C-terminal negative-regulatory domains of the proteins, which, in many cases, leads to their overexpression {838}. These truncated proteins are oncogenic {2616}.

Macroscopic appearance

These tumours are typically unencapsulated, soft to friable, grey-white masses.

Histopathology

A proliferation of relatively monomorphic glial cells with bland, round to ovoid or spindled nuclei, diffusely disposed in a fibrillar matrix or permeating neuropil, is characteristic {2584,566, 3404}. Frequently, tumour cells barely raise the normal cell density of infiltrated parenchyma and may therefore be difficult

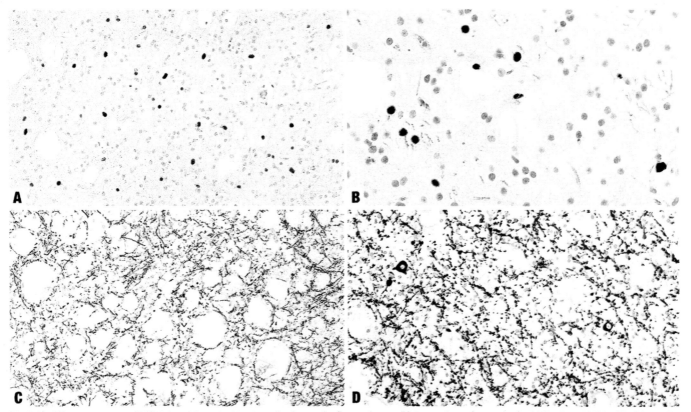

Fig. 2.43 Diffuse astrocytoma, MYBL1-altered. In contrast to most other low-grade glioma subtypes, this tumour is mostly negative for OLIG2 (**A**) and SOX10 (**B**). **C** Neurofilament immunostaining highlights numerous entrapped axons. **D** MAP2 immunostaining highlights entrapped ganglion cells and their processes, but most tumour cells are negative, unlike in most other low-grade astrocytic neoplasms.

to recognize as neoplastic {566,3404}. A vague angiocentric polarity may be regionally evident, particularly in the *MYB*-altered subtype. Entrapped neurons often attest to the infiltrative nature of these astrocytomas. Mitotic activity is typically absent or low, and microvascular proliferation and necrosis are not seen. Occasionally, cases with more pleomorphic nuclei and slightly elevated proliferation are observed, especially in paediatric patients.

Immunohistochemistry

Immunoreactivity for GFAP and low Ki-67 labelling index values are typical. One study reported that expression of MAP2 is limited to residual neurons and neuronal processes and that tumour cells are negative for OLIG2 and CD34 {3404}. IDH1 p.R132H is negative, and nuclear ATRX expression is retained {3404}.

Differential diagnosis

Some areas in angiocentric gliomas have the same architectural and cytological features that characterize *MYB*- or *MYBL1*-altered diffuse astrocytoma, and these two tumour types are considered to have overlapping morphology. A histogenetic relationship between these tumour types is reinforced at the genetic level; practically all angiocentric gliomas have a rearrangement of *MYB*, most commonly associated with a *MYB::QKI* fusion. It is more important to distinguish *MYB*- or *MYBL1*-altered diffuse astrocytoma from adult-type IDH-mutant or IDH-wildtype diffuse astrocytic gliomas, given their distinct biological behaviour.

Cytology

Not clinically relevant

Diagnostic molecular pathology

Sequencing demonstrates a structural variation that results in a fusion between *MYB* or *MYBL1* and a partner gene {838}. The most frequently reported partner genes are *PCDHGA1*, *MMP16*, and *MAML2* {3597,2584,3404,566}. *MYB* rarely partners with *QKI* in this tumour; a *MYB::QKI* fusion is typically found in angiocentric glioma {566}. Diffuse astrocytoma, *MYB*- or *MYBL1*-altered, is IDH- and H3-wildtype. Although sequencing determines the nature of the gene fusion, other methods (e.g. interphase FISH) can also demonstrate a rearrangement of *MYB* or *MYBL1*.

Essential and desirable diagnostic criteria

See Box 2.04.

Staging

Not applicable

Prognosis and prediction

Available outcome data are limited but suggest a benign clinical behaviour. In a series of 11 paediatric patients, 9 had stable disease or no evidence of disease after a median follow-up of 12 years {566}; 1 patient required surgery for recurrent disease after 17 months, and another patient died of the disease. In a second paediatric series of 16 patients with *MYB*- or *MYBL1*-altered gliomas, all were alive after a median follow-up of 6.2 years {2768}; 4 patients who did not receive an initial gross total resection required surgery for recurrence. In a series of 18 patients (predominantly adults) with a median follow-up of 2.5 years, only 1 patient required surgery for recurrence after 3 years, and none died {3404}. Of patients with epilepsy, about 90% became seizure-free after resection and the remainder had a reduction in seizure frequency {3404}.

Angiocentric glioma

Ellison DW
Jones DTW
Ligon KL
Preusser WM
Rosenblum MK

Definition
Angiocentric glioma is a diffuse glioma composed mainly of thin, cytologically bland, bipolar cells aggregating at least partly in perivascular spaces. Almost all angiocentric gliomas have a *MYB::QKI* gene fusion, and the remainder generally have another *MYB* alteration (CNS WHO grade 1).

ICD-O coding
9431/1 Angiocentric glioma

ICD-11 coding
2A00.0Y & XH41C5 Other specified gliomas of brain & Angiocentric glioma

Related terminology
Not recommended: angiocentric neuroepithelial tumour, monomorphous angiocentric glioma.

Subtype(s)
None

Localization
Angiocentric gliomas are typically located in the cerebral cortex, but the brainstem is an increasingly recognized site for this tumour {646,3399,510,678,566}.

Clinical features
Patients with angiocentric gliomas typically present with chronic and intractable partial epilepsy. Headache and visual impairment are other commonly reported symptoms {2953}.

Imaging
In the cerebral cortex, angiocentric gliomas are commonly located in the temporal or frontal lobes. Brainstem examples have also been reported {566}. On MRI, these tumours are often well-circumscribed, non–contrast-enhancing, and hyperintense on T2-weighted and FLAIR images. A rim-like hyperintensity

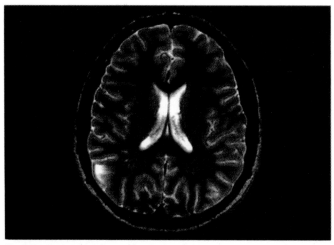

Fig. 2.44 Angiocentric glioma. T2-weighted MRI showing a mostly cortical parietal lesion on the right side, with minimal mass effect.

surrounding the tumour on T1-weighted MRI is present in some cases. A stalk-like extension to the adjacent lateral ventricle and dystrophic calcification are other variable features {1705,103}.

Epidemiology
Population-based epidemiological data are not yet available for this uncommon tumour. Most cases occur in children and young adults, with a median age of 13 years (range: 2–79 years) at presentation. No clear sex predilection is yet apparent, although slightly more male patients than female patients with angiocentric glioma are described in the literature {103}.

Etiology
The vast majority of angiocentric gliomas are sporadic and have not been associated with any specific risk factors. Only single cases have been reported in association with neurofibromatosis type 1 and Koolen–de Vries syndrome {2184,1792}, so it is unclear whether these are merely coincidental.

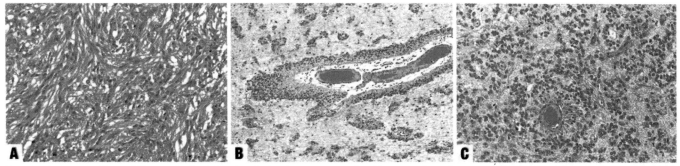

Fig. 2.45 Angiocentric glioma. **A** Elongated cells with bipolar cytoplasmic processes are found in most angiocentric gliomas, particularly in solid areas of the tumour. **B** Note both the pronounced angiocentric pattern and the entrapped neurons. **C** Entrapped neurons are present among tumour cells that show a syncytial pattern.

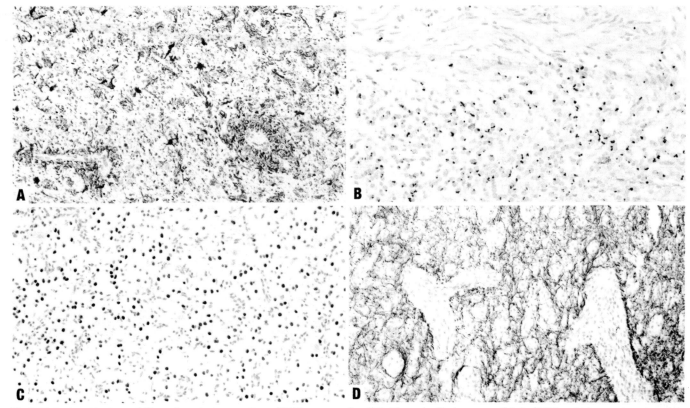

Fig. 2.46 Angiocentric glioma. **A** The perivascular tumour cells are GFAP-immunoreactive. **B** Dot-like or ring-like immunoreactivity for EMA is variably present across regions of most angiocentric gliomas. **C** Unlike in most low-grade astrocytomas, the tumour cells are predominantly OLIG2-negative, although there are many entrapped immunoreactive oligodendrocytes. **D** NFP staining highlights numerous entrapped axons, consistent with an infiltrative growth pattern.

Pathogenesis

Practically all angiocentric gliomas harbour rearrangements of the *MYB* transcription factor gene at the 6q23.3 locus. *MYB* is most commonly fused with *QKI*, in association with deletion of the intervening region. More rarely, *MYB* is fused with *ESR1*, *PCDHGA1*, or other genes {3597,2616,2584,2768}, or it is amplified {3142}. Angiocentric gliomas typically lack any other oncogenic mutations or copy-number alterations {396,3597, 2247}, although two cases have been reported to have both a *MYB::QKI* fusion and a *BRAF* p.V600E mutation {2584}. In DNA methylation profiling studies, angiocentric gliomas cluster with or close to other tumours that contain *MYB* alterations, such as paediatric diffuse astrocytomas and diffuse astrocytoma, *MYB*- or *MYBL1*-altered {2584,3404,566}.

MYB::QKI is oncogenic and has been proposed to drive tumorigenesis through simultaneous deletion of a negative-regulatory domain in *MYB*, functional deletion of the tumour suppressor *QKI*, and enhancer translocation forcing expression of the constitutively active *MYB::QKI* allele {188}. *MYB* activation appears to drive MAPK signalling, in common with almost all paediatric low-grade gliomas; one study showed higher activation of the MAPK pathway in *MYB*-altered tumours than in other low-grade gliomas, including those with a *BRAF* p.V600E mutation {2768}.

Macroscopic appearance

Angiocentric gliomas expand involved structures, with blurring of the cortical grey matter–white matter junction. They may produce induration {3377}, or they may be soft and gelatinous {2887}. Cystic changes may occur and solid components have been described as tan-grey in colour {2247}.

Histopathology

Typically, angiocentric gliomas have cytologically uniform, bipolar spindle cells with slender nuclei and granular chromatin oriented around blood vessels of every calibre; these cells are radially arrayed in a rosette-like pattern or form monolayered or multilayered sleeves lengthwise along vascular axes. Spindle cell elements can permeate the parenchyma extensively and at variable density, fashion compact nodules of schwannoma-like appearance, be disposed in tight and intersecting fascicles, and aggregate beneath the pial surface in horizontal streams or in a perpendicular and palisading alignment. Myxoid and micro-cystic alterations may be conspicuous. Entrapped neurons are not conspicuously dysmorphic {3377}. Some angiocentric gliomas harbour epithelioid elements that may contain rounded paranuclear structures with an internal granular stippling {2134}, which correspond to EMA-immunoreactive microlumina of the type seen in ependymomas and demonstrated in angiocentric gliomas at the ultrastructural level {3377}. Although histologically typical examples with apparent mitotic activity occur {2132, 1873}, mitoses are sparse in most cases, and neither microvascular proliferation nor necrosis is seen. Increased proliferative activity and other anaplastic features have been reported rarely, but the clinical significance of such findings is uncertain {1873, 2051,1883}.

Immunophenotype

On immunohistochemical study, GFAP expression is the rule, and a near-constant finding is at least regional EMA immunolabelling of the cytoplasm in a dot-like or ring-like (microlumen) pattern {3377,1852,2247}. Membranous EMA expression characterizes some epithelioid cells in perivascular and subpial locations. Tumour cells do not label for neuronal markers and are, in contrast to most other low-grade astrocytomas, predominantly OLIG2-negative. Ki-67 immunolabelling index values are generally < 5% (frequently < 1%), but a labelling index of 10% was found in an otherwise typical lesion that had not recurred 6 years after surgery {1873}.

Cytology
Not clinically relevant

Diagnostic molecular pathology
Practically all angiocentric gliomas show rearrangements and/ or copy-number alterations, including deletion or amplification {3142}, at the *MYB* locus on 6q23.3 {2616,2584}. Most rearrangements involve fusions between the *MYB* and *QKI* genes {566}. In data taken from several studies, a *MYB* alteration was found in 73 (99%) of 74 angiocentric gliomas {3142, 2584,188,510,678,566}. Where appropriate analyses could be undertaken, a *MYB::QKI* fusion was demonstrated in 41 (87%) of 47 tumours from these series. Rarely, *MYB* has been shown to fuse with several other genes, such as *PCDHGA1* {566}. Angiocentric gliomas lack mutations in *TP53*, *ATRX*, *IDH1*, *IDH2*, and histone H3 genes {2603,2584,566}. Another CNS tumour

with a relatively high frequency of *MYB* alterations is paediatric diffuse astrocytoma, *MYB*- or *MYBL1*-altered.

Essential and desirable diagnostic criteria
See Box 2.05.

Staging
Not applicable

Prognosis and prediction
Angiocentric gliomas usually have an indolent behaviour and are radiologically stable {2887,566}. In most cases, gross total resection can be achieved and is curative. Postoperative complications and tumour recurrence are uncommon {103}. There are no known prognostic or predictive factors.

Polymorphous low-grade neuroepithelial tumour of the young

Rosenblum MK
Blümcke I
Ellison DW
Huse JT

Definition

Polymorphous low-grade neuroepithelial tumour of the young (PLNTY) is an indolent cerebral neoplasm characterized by a strong association with seizures in young individuals, diffuse growth patterns, frequent presence of oligodendroglioma-like components, calcification, CD34 immunoreactivity, and MAPK pathway–activating genetic abnormalities (CNS WHO grade 1).

ICD-O coding

9413/0 Polymorphous low-grade neuroepithelial tumour of the young

ICD-11 coding

2A00.2Y Other specified tumours of neuroepithelial tissue of brain

Related terminology

Not recommended: diffuse glioneuronal tumour {74}; diffuse or nonspecific form of dysembryoplastic neuroepithelial tumour; massively calcified low-grade glioma {1189,1302}.

Polymorphous low-grade neuroepithelial tumours of the young have also been described under the generic designation of "long-term epilepsy–associated tumour" {3177,297}.

Subtype(s)

None

Localization

PLNTYs are cerebral tumours that usually have cortical and subcortical components. Approximately 80% have involved the temporal lobes, mostly on the right side and with frequent involvement of medial/posteroinferior structures {1384,1485, 549}. Other reported locations include the frontal, parietal, and occipital lobes as well as the third ventricular region {1485}.

Clinical features

PLNTYs typically cause seizures and are associated in many cases with refractory epilepsy (particularly partial complex epilepsy), but they can also cause headache or dizziness {1384, 288,2679,1193,549}. On neuroimaging, PLNTYs often have cystic, as well as solid, components, and they are often densely calcified on CT {1384,1485,549}. PLNTYs are FLAIR-hyperintense on MRI, often displaying signal heterogeneity, with calcified regions appearing T1/T2-hypointense, and non-calcified components appearing T2-hyperintense with variable T1 signal intensity {1384,1485,549}. Patchy or nodular contrast enhancement is observed in a minority of cases, but there is no substantial oedema or mass effect.

Epidemiology

Population-based incidence data are unavailable. PLNTYs have been reported in patients ranging in age from 4 to 57 years {1384,2679,549,1485}, with most occurring in the second and third decades of life (median age at diagnosis: 16 years). There is no clear sex predilection.

Etiology

Factors predisposing to the development of PLNTYs are unknown. An isolated example has been associated with germline *ATM* mutation {3075}.

Pathogenesis

Somatic MAPK pathway–activating genetic events (particularly *BRAF* mutations and FGFR fusions) clearly play a role in the development of PLNTYs, with the tumours' aberrant CD34 expression possibly reflecting an origin from developmentally dysregulated neural precursors {300,301,1384}. The specific mechanisms by which these genetic alterations contribute to the pathogenesis of PLNTYs are not clear.

Macroscopic appearance

PLNTYs have been described as unencapsulated, soft to friable, grey-white masses that are indistinctly demarcated from normal brain {2679,549}.

Histopathology

PLNTYs exhibit both infiltrative and compact growth patterns. Usually present and often dominant are oligodendroglioma-like components, which range from elements having uniformly small and round nuclei with perinuclear haloes to populations exhibiting obvious variation in nuclear size and shape with wrinkled or grooved nuclear membranes and intranuclear pseudoinclusions

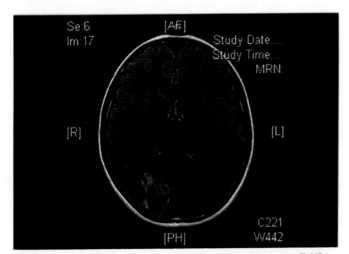

Fig. 2.47 Polymorphous low-grade neuroepithelial tumour of the young. FLAIR-hyperintense solid components, cystic changes, and the absence of mass effect are seen in this MRI.

{1384,2679,1485,549}. PLNTYs may also contain elements of astrocytic or morphologically ambiguous appearance, the former including fibrillary, spindled, and pleomorphic forms. Some examples display subtle perivascular pseudorosettes. Calcifications are present in the large majority and may be coarse and confluent. Generally absent are foci of necrosis, microvascular proliferation, gemistocytic elements, myxoid microcysts, neurocytic rosettes, and Rosenthal fibres. Eosinophilic granular bodies are only occasionally present {3075}. Patently neoplastic neuronal components are typically not in evidence, although modestly dysmorphic neurons in small numbers may be encountered. The nosological position of neoplasms otherwise qualifying as PLNTYs but having nodular ganglion cell aggregates is unclear. PLNTYs characteristically manifest little, if any, mitotic activity. However, one study described an example with increased mitotic activity and illustrated an unusually pleomorphic case with atypical mitoses {1485}.

Immunophenotype

On immunohistochemical assessment, PLNTYs exhibit expression of GFAP (this may be regional or generalized), OLIG2, and CD34 {1384,2679,1485,549}; the last may be patchy, or diffuse and intense. CD34 labelling is displayed both by tumour cells and by ramified neural elements in the associated cerebral cortex. There is retained tumour cell expression of ATRX but no labelling of IDH1 p.R132H. PLNTYs are typically negative for EMA, synaptophysin, chromogranin, NeuN, and HuC/HuD. Immunoreactivity for BRAF p.V600E may be encountered, reflecting the presence of these mutations in a subset of PLNTYs. Ki-67

labelling index values are generally low (≤ 1–2%), but higher values (up to 5%) have been reported {1384}.

Differential diagnosis

PLNTYs may be histologically indistinguishable from oligodendrogliomas or diffuse astrocytomas, but the latter are generally CD34-negative (whereas PLNTYs are CD34-positive) and PLNTYs do not manifest IDH mutations or 1p/19q codeletion like the other tumour types, and they display MAPK pathway–activating genetic abnormalities typically foreign to the adult-type infiltrating gliomas (see *Diagnostic molecular pathology*). An oligodendroglioma-like entity closely resembling PLNTY in morphology, immunophenotype, clinical presentation, and demonstration of *BRAF* p.V600E mutations, but manifesting chromosomal instability, has been described and could represent a PLNTY subtype {1003}. Also resembling PLNTYs at the morphological level, potentially expressing CD34 and (like select PLNTYs) exhibiting *FGFR3::TACC3* gene fusions (see *Diagnostic molecular pathology*), is a group of aggressive gliomas that principally arise in middle-aged and older adults, generally harbour high-grade components that would qualify as anaplastic astrocytoma or glioblastoma, and display copy-number abnormalities and other genetic alterations associated with IDH-wildtype glioblastomas {276}.

Cytology

PLNTYs cannot be identified on cytological grounds alone. In smear preparations, tumour cells may appear as rounded nuclei devoid of cytoplasm, or they may exhibit irregular nuclear

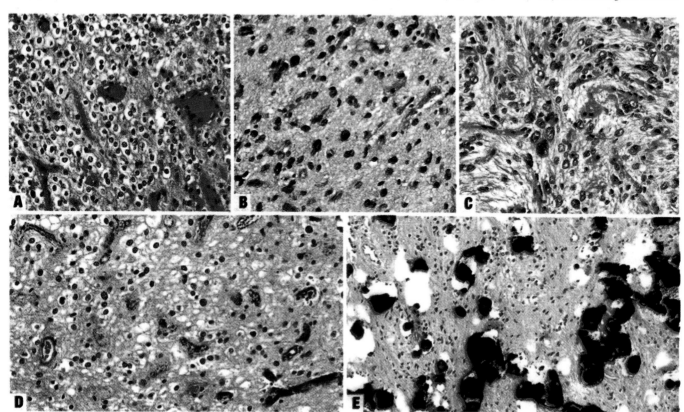

Fig. 2.48 Polymorphous low-grade neuroepithelial tumour of the young. **A** Oligodendroglioma-like features include small round nuclei, perinuclear haloes, and delicate branching capillaries. **B** Mild nuclear pleomorphism and membrane irregularities are common. **C** Astroglial elements here exhibit spindling and more conspicuous atypia without mitotic activity. **D** Vascular mineralization was evident in this example. **E** A diffuse growth pattern and conspicuous calcification are seen.

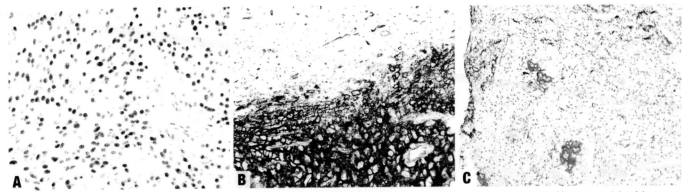

Fig. 2.49 Polymorphous low-grade neuroepithelial tumour of the young. **A** Extensive OLIG2 positivity in tumour cell nuclei. **B** Intense regional immunoreactivity of the tumour matrix for CD34 is seen in the lower half of this field. **C** Entrapped neurofilament-positive axons confirm that this tumour is at least partially infiltrative.

contours and cytoplasmic processes. The latter may anchor tumour cells to capillaries in a pseudorosette fashion {1384}.

Diagnostic molecular pathology

PLNTYs are consistently associated with MAPK pathway–activating abnormalities, which must be demonstrated for confident diagnosis. These specifically include *BRAF* p.V600E mutations {1384,288,1485,1193,3075}, as well as fusions involving *FGFR2* or *FGFR3* {1384,2679,1485,3075,549}. One such fusion, *FGFR2::CTNNA3*, has yet to be reported in any other CNS neoplasm {180}, whereas others, including *FGFR2::SHTN1* (*KIAA1598*), *FGFR2::INA*, and *FGFR3::TACC3*, are also encountered in various other entities. One *FGFR3::TACC3*–fused PLNTY also manifested low-level *FGFR3* amplification, but whether these changes involved the same allele was not clear {549}. A partial duplication of *NTRK2* was detected in a single case {1485}. PLNTYs do not harbour IDH or *ATRX* mutations, do not exhibit 1p/19q codeletion, and have a distinct DNA methylation profile most closely aligned to that of ganglioglioma {1384}.

Essential and desirable diagnostic criteria

See Box 2.06.

Staging

Not applicable

Prognosis and prediction

A series providing extended follow-up data suggests that PLNTYs generally behave in CNS WHO grade 1 fashion and are amenable to control by excision {1384}. At postoperative intervals of 12–89 months (mean: 47 months), only 1 of 9 patients had evidence of possible local recurrence after gross total resection. Tumour removal effected relief from seizures or reduced seizure frequency in most cases. One PLNTY reported

Box 2.06 Diagnostic criteria for polymorphous low-grade neuroepithelial tumour of the young

Essential:

Diffuse growth pattern (at least regionally)

AND

Oligodendroglioma-like components (although these may be minor)

AND

Few (if any) mitotic figures

AND

Regional CD34 expression by tumour cells and by ramified neural cells in associated cerebral cortex

AND

IDH-wildtype status

AND

Unequivocal expression of BRAF p.V600E on immunohistochemical assessment

OR

Molecular diagnostic evidence of *BRAF* p.V600E mutations, *FGFR2* or *FGFR3* fusions, or potentially other MAPK pathway–driving genetic abnormalities

Desirable:

Conspicuous calcification (characteristic, although not constant)

Absence of 1p/19q codeletion

as progressive at 60 months after complete resection occurred in the setting of germline *ATM* mutation and displayed unusually complex copy-number abnormalities {3075}, whereas an example displaying *FGFR3::TACC3* fusion coupled with uncharacteristic somatic mutations involving *TP53*, *ATRX*, *PTEN*, and *TEK* (as well as *RB1* mutation in a recurrence) underwent malignant transformation to glioblastoma-like histology {182}. Additional case identification and follow-up are required to determine the long-term risk of recurrence and biological progression associated with these neoplasms.

Diffuse low-grade glioma, MAPK pathway–altered

Jacques TS
Capper D
Giannini C
Orr BA
Tabori U

Definition

Diffuse low-grade glioma, MAPK pathway–altered, is a low-grade glioma with diffuse astrocytic or oligodendroglial morphology that generally occurs in childhood and is characterized by a pathogenic alteration in a gene that codes for a MAPK pathway protein. Typically, these tumours have an internal tandem duplication (ITD) or mutation in the tyrosine kinase domain (TKD) of *FGFR1*, or a *BRAF* p.V600E mutation. The tumour is IDH-wildtype and H3-wildtype and does not have a homozygous deletion of *CDKN2A*.

ICD-O coding

9421/1 Diffuse low-grade glioma, MAPK pathway–altered

ICD-11 coding

2A00.0Y Other specified gliomas of brain

Related terminology

Not recommended: diffuse astrocytoma; diffuse astrocytoma, IDH-wildtype; oligodendroglioma; paediatric-type oligodendroglioma.

Subtype(s)

Diffuse low-grade glioma, *FGFR1* tyrosine kinase domain–duplicated; diffuse low-grade glioma, *FGFR1*-mutant; diffuse low-grade glioma, *BRAF* p.V600E–mutant

Localization

MAPK pathway–altered diffuse low-grade gliomas are described throughout the craniospinal axis, particularly the cerebral hemispheres. Among paediatric low-grade gliomas, specific alterations are more common in specific locations {2768}, raising the possibility that there may be regional differences in subtypes.

Clinical features

Symptoms and signs depend on location. Epilepsy, sometimes longstanding, is common. Location-specific neurological deficits generally combine with more nonspecific manifestations of raised intracranial pressure. More detailed clinical data for these molecularly defined tumours are currently unavailable.

Imaging

On neuroimaging, diffuse low-grade gliomas may have a more diffuse picture with T2-FLAIR than do pilocytic astrocytomas, but both morphologies often appear as heterogeneously enhancing masses with cystic elements.

Epidemiology

There are no epidemiological studies of this specific tumour type. However, it is clearly rare. In a series of 843 patients aged < 19 years with low-grade gliomas and without neurofibromatosis type 1 (NF1), 5.9% of tumours had the morphology of a diffuse astrocytoma and 3.0% had that of an oligodendroglioma {2768}. Reports of this tumour have, by definition, focused on tumours affecting children.

Etiology

There are no definite causative factors. However, there are descriptions of diffuse low-grade astrocytomas in patients with NF1 {2704}, raising the possibility that NF1-associated gliomas may include tumours within the spectrum of MAPK pathway–altered diffuse low-grade glioma.

Pathogenesis

By definition, these tumours harbour an abnormality in the MAPK pathway, are IDH-wildtype and H3-wildtype, and do not show homozygous deletion of *CDKN2A* {838}. In the context

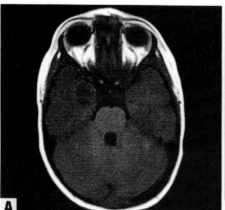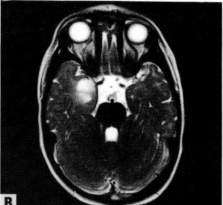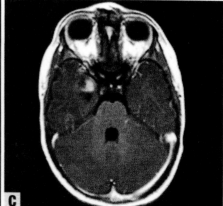

Fig. 2.50 Diffuse low-grade glioma, MAPK pathway–altered. Diffuse low-grade glioma in a 1-year-old girl. MRI shows a mass within the medial aspect of the right temporal lobe, with low T1 signal (**A**), high T2 signal (**B**), and heterogeneous enhancement with a cystic element on postcontrast T1-weighted imaging (**C**).

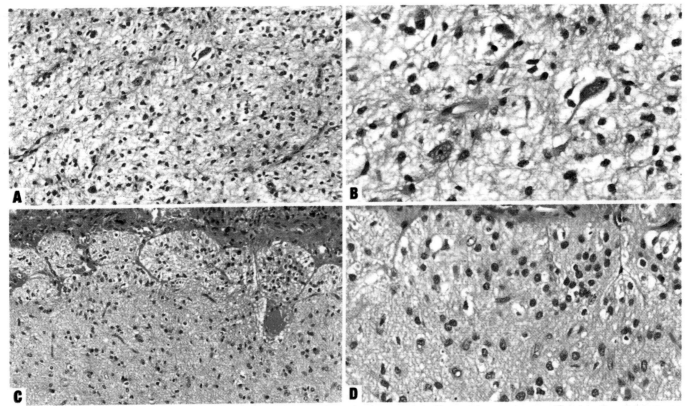

Fig. 2.51 Diffuse low-grade glioma, MAPK pathway–altered. A low-grade diffuse glioma of moderate cellularity (**A**) entrapping normal neurons (**B**) and showing subpial aggregation (**C**) typical of diffuse gliomas. The tumour cells have a bland appearance and are mildly atypical (**B,D**).

of paediatric diffuse low-grade gliomas, the MAPK alteration is most likely to be a *BRAF* p.V600E mutation or an alteration of *FGFR1* (duplication of the TKD, one or sometimes two single-nucleotide variants, or a fusion gene) {3597,2584,2768}.

Molecular alterations appear to associate with morphology; for example, alterations of *FGFR1* are frequent in oligoden-drogliomas but less so in diffuse astrocytomas {2584,2768}. However, aside from being diffuse low-grade gliomas, these MAPK pathway–altered tumours are not defined by a distinctive morphology or by a single DNA methylation or gene expression profile. In future, it is likely that a comprehensive analysis of this rare group of tumours will resolve their status and clinicopatho-logical associations.

Macroscopic appearance

Specific macroscopic appearances have not been described in the literature. However, these tumours are likely to have features similar to those of other (IDH-mutant) diffuse low-grade gliomas.

Histopathology

MAPK pathway–altered diffuse low-grade gliomas typically have a bland appearance, being composed of mildly atypi-cal glial cells at relatively low density and entrapped normal parenchyma. The pattern of infiltration is not as extensive as seen in some IDH-mutant low-grade gliomas; it is more in line with the degree of infiltration found in angiocentric gliomas and polymorphous low-grade neuroepithelial tumour of the young (PLNTY), yet exceeds the peripheral incorporation of normal cells sometimes found in other low-grade gliomas, such as pilo-cytic astrocytoma and pleomorphic xanthoastrocytoma.

Diffuse low-grade glioma, FGFR1 TKD–duplicated or FGFR1-mutant

Diffuse low-grade gliomas with *FGFR1* alterations typically have the morphological features of an oligodendroglioma {2584}, although astrocytomas can also have this genetic profile. A nodular architecture is occasionally present, and there is some overlap with the morphology of dysembryoplastic neuroepithe-lial tumour, which shares these genetic alterations {2584,2768}. Mitotic activity is rare or absent, and there is no microvascular proliferation or necrosis. These tumours are diffusely immu-nopositive for OLIG2 and show variable expression of GFAP. Immunoreactivity for CD34 is typically restricted to a few cells, unlike the widespread expression evident in PLNTY.

The differential diagnosis for diffuse low-grade glioma with *FGFR1* alterations includes dysembryoplastic neuroepithelial tumour, PLNTY, and adult-type IDH-mutant oligodendroglioma. Dysembryoplastic neuroepithelial tumours can only be distin-guished by the presence of their defining specific glioneuronal element and, in complex cases, glial nodules. PLNTYs have a distinctive cytology and show widespread strong expression of CD34. Adult-type oligodendroglioma is distinguished by the presence of an IDH mutation combined with 1p/19q codeletion.

Diffuse low-grade glioma, BRAF p.V600E–mutant

Diffuse low-grade gliomas with a *BRAF* p.V600E mutation are composed of well-differentiated glial cells with bland, ovoid to spindle-shaped nuclei and fine fibrillary processes. Neither Rosenthal fibres nor eosinophilic granular bodies are typically found. Subpial aggregation of tumour cells, a typical secondary structure of diffuse gliomas, may be present. Mitotic activity is

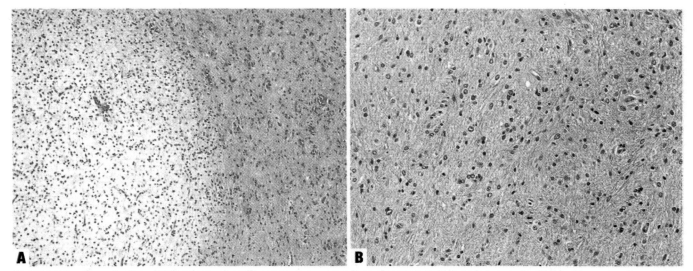

Fig. 2.52 Diffuse low-grade glioma, MAPK pathway–altered. Temporal lobe tumour in a 7-year-old patient. **A** Mildly atypical neoplastic glial cells with an astrocytic or oligodendrocytic morphology are diffusely distributed in cerebral cortex and underlying white matter. Nodule formation is rare. An *FGFR1* tyrosine kinase domain (TKD) duplication was detected. **B** A fibrillary matrix is found in some regions.

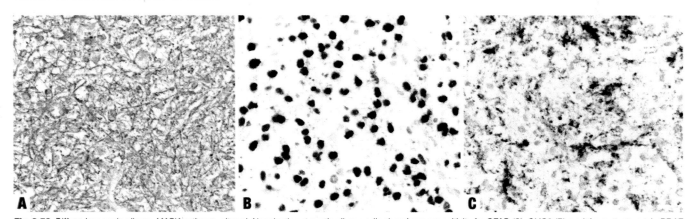

Fig. 2.53 Diffuse low-grade glioma, MAPK pathway–altered. Neoplastic astrocytic glioma cells show immunopositivity for GFAP (**A**), OLIG2 (**B**), and the mutant protein BRAF p.V600E (**C**).

rare or absent, and there is no microvascular proliferation or necrosis. Tumour cells are typically immunopositive for OLIG2 and GFAP, which highlights the fine cell processes. Immunoreactivity for BRAF p.V600E illustrates the *BRAF* mutation.

The differential diagnosis of diffuse low-grade glioma with a *BRAF* p.V600E mutation includes pilocytic astrocytoma, ganglioglioma, and pleomorphic xanthoastrocytoma. In addition, it is important to exclude IDH-mutant and H3 K27–altered diffuse midline gliomas, which can have histopathological features identical to those of a *BRAF* p.V600E–mutant diffuse low-grade glioma.

Despite its diffuse nature, this tumour type appears to have a better outcome than do CNS WHO grade 2 IDH-mutant diffuse gliomas (see *Prognosis and prediction*, below), and a CNS WHO grade has yet to be assigned.

Cytology

The intraoperative cytological features of MAPK pathway–altered diffuse low-grade gliomas have not been described, but these tumours are likely to show features of a low-grade astrocytoma or oligodendroglioma.

Diagnostic molecular pathology

The diagnosis requires evidence of a MAPK pathway alteration in the absence of an IDH or H3 p.K28M (K27M) mutation and without homozygous deletion of *CDKN2A*. The most commonly observed genetic alterations in these tumours occur in *BRAF* (generally a p.V600E mutation) and in *FGFR1* (TKD duplication, one or sometimes two single-nucleotide variants, or a fusion gene) {3597,2584,2768}. Further rare alterations are seen in a variety of other MAPK genes, including *FGFR2*, *NTRK1*, *NTRK2*, *NTRK3*, *MAP2K1*, and *MET* {2768}. Although there is emerging evidence that they may also result in MAPK pathway activation {2768}, diffuse astrocytomas with *MYB* or *MYBL1* alterations are listed separately under the family of paediatric-type diffuse low-grade gliomas.

DNA methylation profiling has not demonstrated a single cluster for MAPK pathway–altered diffuse low-grade gliomas. Instead, some data suggest that they cluster with other tumour types that have shared genetic alterations {2584,460}. Therefore, care is required to exclude other tumour types with distinct morphological features, and DNA methylation analysis can be helpful when histopathological examination is difficult or inconclusive {463}.

Box 2.07 Diagnostic criteria for diffuse low-grade glioma, MAPK pathway–altered

Essential:

Diffuse glioma with absent or minimal mitotic activity and neither microvascular proliferation nor necrosis

AND

Genetic alteration in the MAPK pathway

AND

IDH-wildtype and H3-wildtype

AND

Absence of homozygous deletion of *CDKN2A*

Desirable:

Onset in childhood, adolescence, or early adulthood

Absence of morphological features or DNA methylation profile suggestive of an alternative tumour type in which *FGFR* or *BRAF* abnormalities occur

Essential and desirable diagnostic criteria

See Box 2.07.

Staging

Not clinically relevant

Prognosis and prediction

It is currently uncertain to what extent MAPK-altered diffuse low-grade gliomas, as a group, will resolve into distinct tumour types, and the factors that best predict their outcome will probably evolve as the molecular nosology of this concept is resolved. Therefore, some caution is warranted when making clinical and prognostic correlations.

Although these are low-grade tumours, outcome will depend on location, morphology, and molecular alteration. IDH-wildtype diffuse low-grade gliomas in children rarely undergo anaplastic progression. However, some investigators have reported that a broad range of paediatric low-grade gliomas and glioneuronal tumours with a *BRAF* p.V600E mutation and *CDKN2A* deletion have a higher rate of progression and tendency for late transformation {2127,1806}.

The availability of novel targeted therapies for MAPK pathway–altered gliomas may change the prognostic and predictive value of the above alterations. Specifically, *BRAF* p.V600E–mutant diffuse gliomas respond favourably to BRAF inhibitors {1239}. Diffuse gliomas with *FGFR1* alterations and non-canonical *BRAF* mutations may also respond to MEK inhibitors.

Diffuse midline glioma, H3 K27–altered

Varlet P
Baker SJ
Ellison DW
Jabado N
Jones C
Jones DTW
Leske H
Orr BA
Solomon DA
Suvà ML
Warren KE

Definition

Diffuse midline glioma, H3 K27–altered, is an infiltrative midline glioma with loss of H3 p.K28me3 (K27me3) and usually either an H3 c.83A>T p.K28M (K27M) substitution in one of the histone H3 isoforms, aberrant overexpression of EZHIP, or an *EGFR* mutation (CNS WHO grade 4).

ICD-O coding

9385/3 Diffuse midline glioma, H3 K27–altered

ICD-11 coding

2A00.0Y & XH7692 Other specified gliomas of brain & Diffuse midline glioma, H3 K27M–mutant

Related terminology

Acceptable: diffuse intrinsic pontine glioma.

Subtype(s)

Diffuse midline glioma, H3.3 K27–mutant; diffuse midline glioma, H3.1 or H3.2 K27–mutant; diffuse midline glioma, H3-wildtype with EZHIP overexpression; diffuse midline glioma, *EGFR*-mutant

Localization

Paediatric diffuse midline gliomas (DMGs) are preferentially located in the brainstem or pons (the latter making it a diffuse intrinsic pontine glioma [DIPG]), or they are bithalamic, whereas DMGs in adolescents and adults predominantly arise unilaterally in the thalamus, or in the spinal cord {2738,2101}. Localization in other midline sites, such as the pineal region, hypothalamus, and cerebellum, is exceptional {1103,2101,2988}. Large autopsy-based studies of DIPG have described leptomeningeal involvement in 40% of cases, as well as diffuse spread to involve the thalamus, cervical cord, and even the frontal lobe {403}.

Clinical features

Most patients with DIPG present with a short medical history (< 2 months), with the classic triad: cranial nerve palsy (82%), long tract signs such as pyramidal tract impairment (51%), and ataxia (62%) {1329}. Common initial symptoms of thalamic DMGs include intracranial hypertension and motor or sensory deficit {3026}.

Imaging

On MRI, DIPGs classically have their epicentre in the pons and typically involve > 50% of its surface, often asymmetrically, with frequent encasement of the basilar artery {3024}. There may be an exophytic component and/or infiltration into the midbrain, the cerebellar peduncles, and the cerebellar hemispheres. Thalamic tumours may be unilateral or bilateral, the latter being more frequent in the *EGFR*-mutant subtype {383}. The lesions show T1 hypointensity or isointensity and T2 hyperintensity, but FLAIR sequences and contrast enhancement patterns can vary considerably, with many tumours not being contrast-enhancing {1083,2145}.

Epidemiology

Epidemiological data remain scarce for this recently described entity. The incidence of DIPG is estimated to be 0.54 cases per 1 million person-years overall, and 2.32 cases per 1 million person-years in people aged ≤ 20 years, with no sex predilection {1329}. DIPG represents 10–15% of all paediatric brain tumours and 75% of all paediatric brainstem tumours. Thalamic DMGs are rarer, representing 1–5% of paediatric brain tumours (25%

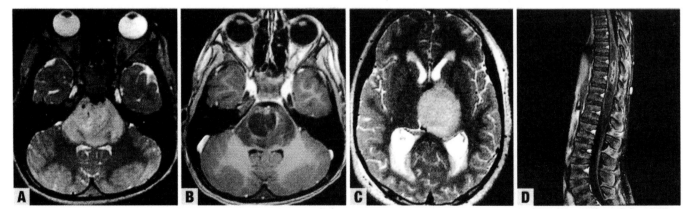

Fig. 2.54 Diffuse midline gliomas, H3 K27–altered, in classic midline locations. **A** Axial MRI demonstrates a T2-bright lesion expanding the pons and encasing the basilar artery. **B** MRI showing heterogeneous enhancement of a pontine lesion on a postgadolinium T1 sequence. **C** Axial MRI shows a left unithalamic T2-bright lesion with associated obstructive hydrocephalus. There is no peritumoural oedema. **D** Sagittal postgadolinium T1 sequence reveals an intramedullary tumour with heterogeneous annular enhancement.

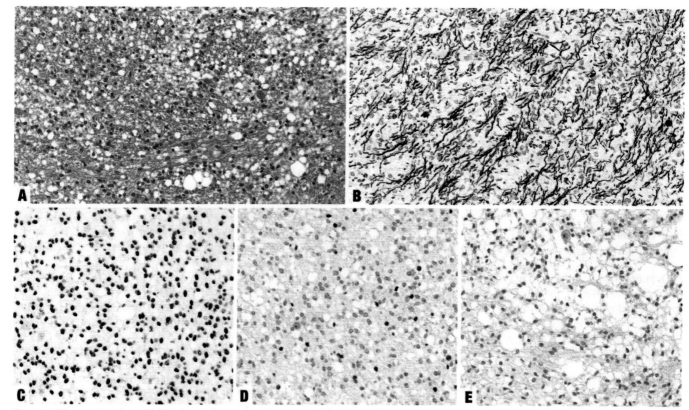

Fig. 2.55 Diffuse midline glioma, H3 K27–altered. **A** A pontine glioma showing infiltrative neoplastic cells in an oedematous background, with some residual neurons. **B** The neurofilament stain highlights the diffusely infiltrative growth. **C** Intense nuclear staining for H3 p.K28 (K27)-mutant protein, with internal negative controls in endothelial cells and neurons. **D** Immunohistochemical staining for H3 p.K28me3 (K27me3) shows loss of expression in tumour cells, with retention in endothelial cells and residual neurons. **E** Negativity for EZHIP immunostaining.

of thalamic tumours) {2766}. Spinal DMGs represent about 40% of spinal astrocytomas in paediatric and adult series {502,1070}.

EGFR-mutant DMGs most often occur during childhood, with a median patient age of 7–8 years {383,2145}. In the paediatric population, the occurrence of H3.3 p.K28M (K27M)-mutant DMGs and H3-wildtype DMGs with EZHIP overexpression peaks at about 7–8 years, whereas H3.1 or H3.2 p.K28M (K27M)-mutant DMGs occur in younger patients (median patient age: ~5 years) {1329,1976,483}.

Etiology

There is no known specific genetic susceptibility for DMG but, exceptionally, DMGs may occur in the setting of a cancer predisposition syndrome such as Li–Fraumeni syndrome or mismatch repair deficiency.

Pathogenesis

Loss of H3 p.K28me3 (K27me3)

Despite representing only a small proportion (3–17%) of the total cellular H3 pool, H3 p.K28 (K27) mutations occurring in either canonical (H3.1 or H3.2) or non-canonical (H3.3) sequence variants result in widespread loss of H3 p.K28me3 (K27me3) on the wildtype histone H3 {1862,237,514,3308}. The inhibitory interaction between H3 p.K28M (K27M) – and, rarely, H3 p.K28I (K27I) – and EZH2 (the methyltransferase catalytic subunit of PRC2) probably drives this dominant negative effect {1862,237, 1247,1519,1827,3014,3481}. In H3-wildtype cases, PRC2 inhibition is thought to be mediated by overexpression of EZHIP, which

acts as an endogenous H3 p.K28M (K27M) mimic {1448}. The marked decrease in H3 p.K28me3 (K27me3) is associated with gene expression changes resulting from the release of the poised state of bivalent promoters {1804,2937}. In some studies, changes in the transcriptome are relatively modest {636,1010,1247}.

Cell of origin and effects on differentiation

As PRC2 and its deposition of H3 p.K28me3 (K27me3) play critical roles in maintaining cell fate, H3 p.K28M (K27M) can enhance self-renewal and disrupt differentiation, with differing effects in different progenitor populations {1804,2193,1010}. Some studies indicate that the cell of origin, which could be neural stem cells, adopts an oligodendrocyte precursor cell–like transcriptome {932}.

Cooperating mutations

Somatic heterozygous H3 p.K28 (K27) mutations are invariably maintained during the disease, and they are generally found to be associated with collaborating mutations, which may also represent subclonal populations {2258,1327,3332}. These target canonical cancer-associated pathways have subtype-specific enrichment and include p53 (TP53, PPM1D, ATM), predominantly in H3.3 p.K28M (K27M)-mutant and EGFR-mutant cases, and PI3K or MAPK (PIK3CA, PIK3R1, PTEN), largely in the H3.1 or H3.2 p.K28M (K27M)-mutant subtype. Co-occurrence of H3.3 p.K28M (K27M) and BRAF p.V600E mutations may be observed {404,957,3482,3150}. Gain-of-function mutation and genetic amplification of growth factor receptors involved in

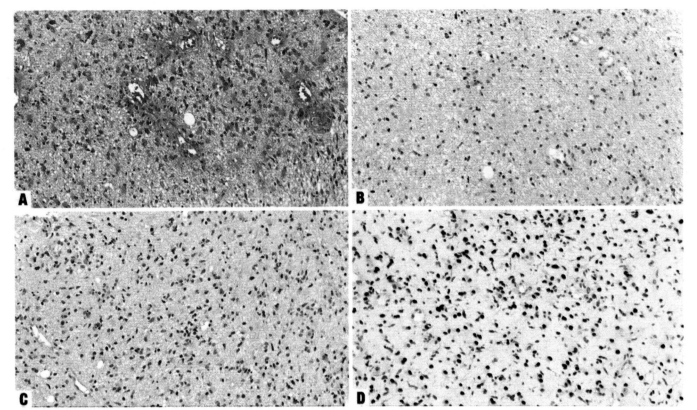

Fig. 2.56 Diffuse midline glioma, H3 K27–altered. A pontine glioma showing infiltrative tumour cells associated with vascular proliferation (**A**), loss of H3 p.K28me3 (K27me3) immunostaining in tumour cells with retention in endothelial cells (**B**), negative H3 p.K28M (K27M) immunoreactivity (**C**), and tumour cells with intense nuclear staining for EZHIP (internal negative controls represented by endothelial cells and residual neurons) (**D**).

brain development are common in p.K28M (K27M)-mutant subtypes, and they are found in *PDGFRA* (hindbrain, diencephalon, telencephalon), *FGFR1* (diencephalon), and *ACVR1* (hindbrain).

Macroscopic appearance

Diffuse infiltration of the parenchyma by neoplastic cells and related oedema causes enlargement and distortion of anatomical structures, as well as softening and discolouration of tissues with haemorrhagic or necrotic zones {403}.

Histopathology

DMGs diffusely infiltrate the CNS parenchyma, usually without particular perivascular or perineuronal tropism. Most cells are small and monomorphic, but they can be polymorphous, showing astrocytic, piloid, oligodendroglial, giant cell, undifferentiated, or epithelioid cytology {2988}. Even though mitotic figures are frequent and microvascular proliferation and/or necrosis may be observed, these features are not required for diagnosis and they are not independent predictors of survival {404,484, 1935,403}. Rosenthal fibres and eosinophilic granular bodies are not typically encountered.

In *EGFR*-mutant DMGs, mitotic activity is often present, but necrosis or microvascular proliferation is rare. DMGs are considered CNS WHO grade 4, irrespective of the presence of microvascular proliferation or necrosis.

Immunophenotype

DMGs typically express OLIG2, MAP2, and S100, whereas immunoreactivity for GFAP is variable apart from in the

EGFR-mutant subtype, which is typically GFAP-positive but may lack OLIG2 and SOX10. Neurofilament and synaptophysin stains highlight the infiltrated neuropil in the background, but they are negative in the tumour cells.

The combination of H3 p.K28M (K27M) and H3 p.K28me3 (K27me3) antibodies is highly effective as a diagnostic aid. Positive H3 p.K28M (K27M) nuclear staining (for the H3 K27–altered subtypes) in combination with the loss of nuclear H3 p.K28me3 (K27me3) immunoreactivity enables the detection of single tumour cells in infiltrating zones {1372,2988,3308}. Although no H3 p.K28M (K27M) staining is observed in DMGs with H3 p.K28I (K27I) mutation or EZHIP overexpression, these cases can be recognized by the loss of nuclear H3 p.K28me3 (K27me3) immunostaining and should be further evaluated by molecular analyses {2384}. In addition, EZHIP (CXorf67) antibodies are available that highlight EZHIP overexpression {483}, which is usually absent in H3 p.K28M (K27M)-altered DMGs. About 50% of cases show nuclear accumulation of p53, suggesting an underlying *TP53* mutation, and 15% of cases show a loss of nuclear ATRX expression {404,484}.

Differential diagnosis

Brainstem tumours constitute a heterogeneous group ranging from low-grade primary CNS tumours (e.g. pilocytic astrocytoma, ganglioglioma, and *MYB*- or *MYBL1*-altered diffuse astrocytoma) {2556} to high-grade tumours comprising H3 K27–altered DMG as well as H3-wildtype tumours (e.g. the diffuse paediatric-type high-grade glioma MYCN subtype, atypical teratoid/rhabdoid tumour, and embryonal tumour with

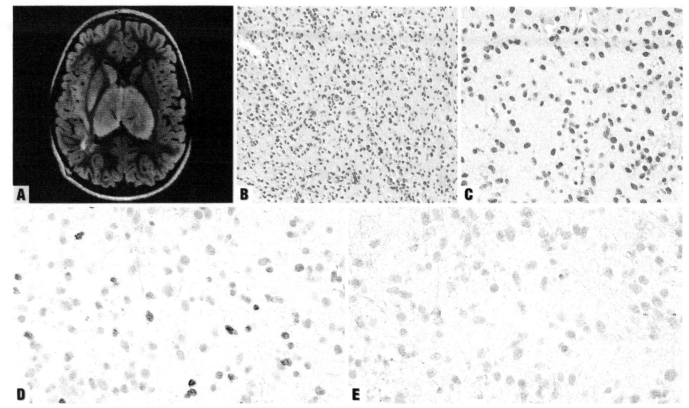

Fig. 2.57 Diffuse midline glioma, *EGFR*-mutant. **A** Axial FLAiR MRI of a bithalamic EGFR-mutant glioma in a child. **B,C** Histology of a bithalamic glioma harbouring a small in-frame insertion in exon 20 of the *EGFR* gene, demonstrating a diffuse astrocytic glioma. **D** Immunohistochemistry for H3 p.K28me3 (K27me3) showing loss in the majority of tumour cell nuclei in this bithalamic glioma with *EGFR* mutation that is H3-wildtype. **E** Immunohistochemistry for H3 p.K28M (K27M)-mutant protein is negative in the majority of bithalamic gliomas with *EGFR* mutation.

multilayered rosettes) {3145,404}. This reinforces the role of biopsy in the accurate diagnosis of brainstem tumours. Various midline circumscribed glial or glioneuronal tumours, including pilocytic astrocytomas {2556}, subependymomas {3528}, and gangliogliomas {2368}, have been described as having the same H3 p.K28 (K27) mutations; although the H3 p.K28M (K27M) mutation probably imparts a poorer prognosis in these entities, they should not be given a diagnosis of H3 K27–altered DMG. In posterior fossa group A (PFA) ependymomas, H3 p.K28 (K27) mutations are extremely rare {2556,2765}, but loss of H3 p.K28me3 (K27me3) or EZHIP overexpression occurs {2384,1448}; these tumours can be distinguished from DMGs on a morphological basis.

Exceedingly rare, non-midline, cortical or hemispheric diffuse gliomas with H3 p.K28M (K27M) mutation have been described {1976,1977,1927}. To date, the biology and prognosis for such tumours remain unknown, and the current recommendation is to report them as "diffuse hemispheric glioma with H3 p.K28M (K27M) mutation not elsewhere classified (NEC)".

EGFR-mutant DMG must be distinguished from pilocytic astrocytoma of the tectum (tectal glioma), which is an exophytic tumour emanating from the tectum of the midbrain into the posterior third ventricle. Tectal gliomas may occasionally show T2-FLAIR hyperintensity extending into the bilateral thalami, mimicking bithalamic glioma. Tectal gliomas can be distinguished from *EGFR*-mutant DMG on the basis of histological features and molecular signatures, with tectal gliomas typically displaying intact H3 p.K28me3 (K27me3) staining, wildtype

EGFR alleles, and frequent *KRAS* p.G12R mutations, often with accompanying *BRAF* mutation or fusion {567}.

Cytology
Not clinically relevant

Diagnostic molecular pathology
Distinct patterns of biological features (methylation profiling, gene expression, co-segregating mutations) and clinical correlations (age, location, outcome) suggest the presence of four subtypes of DMGs that are defined by the driving oncohistone alteration {483,485}: (1) H3.3 p.K28M (K27M)-mutant, (2) H3.1 or 3.2 p.K28M (K27M)-mutant, (3) H3-wildtype with EZHIP overexpression, and (4) *EGFR*-mutant (see *Pathogenesis*). No significant histological differences have been noted between these subtypes.

For the H3 K27–mutant subtypes, a somatic heterozygous mutation in one of the genes encoding histone H3 variants leads to the amino acid substitution of lysine (K) to methionine (M) or, rarely, isoleucine (I) at position 27 (as measured from the start of the processed H3, i.e. after the cleavage of the initiating methionine) {484}. However, genomic sequencing reports may list these mutations as H3 p.K28M (K27M) or H3 p.K28I (K27I). It is exceptional for H3 p.K28M (K27M) or H3 p.K28I (K27I) mutations to co-occur with mutations in *IDH1* or *IDH2* or with H3.3 p.G35R (G34R) or H3.3 p.G35V (G34V) mutations. Similarly, *CDKN2A* and/or *CDKN2B* deletions, *TERT* promoter mutations, and *MGMT* promoter methylation represent rare events in DMGs {1976,1977}.

EGFR-mutant DMG is genetically defined by abnormalities in the *EGFR* oncogene on chromosome band 7p11.2. Most tumours harbour small in-frame insertions/duplications within exon 20, which encodes the intracellular tyrosine kinase domain (TKD), whereas others harbour missense mutations in exons encoding parts of the extracellular domain, most commonly p.A289T or p.A289V. Rare instances of *EGFR* gene amplification occurring in the absence of an identifiable mutation have also been reported {2145,2933}.

H3-wildtype DMGs with EZHIP overexpression represent the rarest subtype {483}. In addition to immunohistochemical analyses, EZHIP overexpression can be measured by molecular analyses, such as RNA expression microarrays.

Essential and desirable diagnostic criteria
See Box 2.08.

Staging
Because of the diffusely infiltrative nature of this tumour, and the potential of leptomeningeal spread, imaging of the whole CNS is recommended.

Prognosis and prediction
Independently of the location, the prognosis of DMG is poor, with a 2-year survival rate of < 10% {1976}. Surgical options are limited due to tumour location. Patients with DMGs harbouring either an H3.1 or H3.2 p.K28M (K27M) mutation or showing EZHIP overexpression have slightly longer overall survival (16 months) than do patients with DMGs that bear an H3.3 p.K28M (K27M) mutation (11 months), respectively {483,485,1329}. Age (< 3 or > 10 years), longer symptom latency (> 24 weeks), and systemic therapy at diagnosis are predictors of longer survival {1329}.

Box 2.08 Diagnostic criteria for diffuse midline glioma, H3 K27–altered

Essential:

A diffuse glioma

AND

Loss of H3 p.K28me3 (K27me3) (immunohistochemistry)

AND

Midline location

AND

Presence of an H3 p.K28M (K27M) or p.K28I (K27I) mutation (for H3 K27–mutant subtypes)

OR

Presence of a pathogenic mutation or amplification of *EGFR* (for the *EGFR*-mutant subtype)

OR

Overexpression of EZHIP (for the H3-wildtype with EZHIP overexpression subtype)

OR

Methylation profile of one of the subtypes of diffuse midline glioma

Desirable:

Results from molecular analyses that enable discrimination of the H3.1 or H3.2 p.K28 (K27)-mutant subtype from the H3.3 p.K28 (K27)-mutant subtype

TP53 mutations have been shown to be associated with radioresistance {3419}. According to one study, the median survival for children with bithalamic gliomas with confirmed *EGFR* mutation was 10–14 months, with most children succumbing to their disease within 2 years {2145}. Historical outcomes have also been poor for children with either radiographically or histologically diagnosed bithalamic gliomas {3546,761,2086,1177,2596,1206, 2607,1447,2382,2479,3026,2894,383,2264}.

Diffuse hemispheric glioma, H3 G34–mutant

Korshunov A
Capper D
Jones DTW
Leske H
Orr BA

Rodriguez FJ
Solomon DA
Sturm D
Warren KE
Weller M

Definition

Diffuse hemispheric glioma, H3 G34–mutant, is an infiltrative glioma involving the cerebral hemispheres, with missense mutation of the *H3-3A* gene that results in one of the following substitutions of the histone H3 protein: c.103G>A p.G35R (G34R), c.103G>C p.G35R (G34R), or c.104G>T p.G35V (G34V) (CNS WHO grade 4).

ICD-O coding

9385/3 Diffuse hemispheric glioma, H3 G34–mutant

ICD-11 coding

2A00.0Y Other specified gliomas of brain

Related terminology

Not recommended: paediatric glioblastoma, H3.3 G34–mutant.

Subtype(s)

None

Localization

Diffuse hemispheric glioma, H3 G34–mutant, arises in the cerebral hemispheres. Occasional spread to midline structures and leptomeningeal dissemination have been observed {1713,1976}.

Clinical features

Patients develop clinical symptoms according to the anatomical structures involved, including seizures and motor or sensory deficits.

Imaging

MRI characteristics of H3 G34–mutant diffuse hemispheric glioma are similar to those of other high-grade non-midline gliomas. MRI typically reveals a contrast-enhancing tumour with mass effect in cortical areas, often involving the parietal or

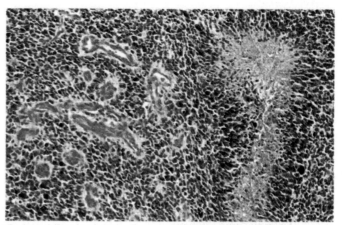

Fig. 2.58 Diffuse hemispheric glioma, H3 G34–mutant. Palisading necrosis.

temporal lobe, with occasional multifocal manifestation, including leptomeningeal dissemination. Necrosis, cystic changes, haemorrhage, and calcifications can be observed {3320}.

Epidemiology

H3 G34–mutant diffuse hemispheric gliomas typically affect adolescents and young adults (median age:15–19 years). Some studies have indicated that these tumours account for approximately 16% of hemispheric paediatric high-grade gliomas {1565,1976}, whereas others, including unpublished prospective studies, have indicated a lower incidence {2867}. There is a male predominance, with an M:F ratio of 1.4:1 {1713, 1976}.

Etiology

There is no known specific genetic susceptibility for H3 G34–mutant diffuse hemispheric glioma. No risk factors have been reported to date.

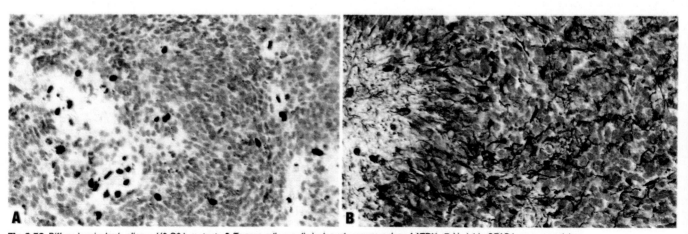

Fig. 2.59 Diffuse hemispheric glioma, H3 G34–mutant. **A** Tumour cells usually lack nuclear expression of ATRX. **B** Variable GFAP immunoreactivity.

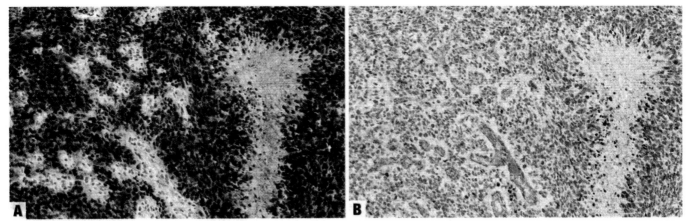

Fig. 2.60 Diffuse hemispheric glioma, H3 G34–mutant. **A** The tumour cells typically show nuclear accumulation of p53. **B** Tumour cells typically lack nuclear OLIG2 expression.

Pathogenesis

An acquired missense mutation in the *H3-3A* (*H3F3A*) gene, resulting in substitution at position p.G35 (G34) on the tail of the histone variant H3.3, plays a key oncogenic role in the pathogenesis of this entity. Several studies indicate that replacement of the amino acid glycine (G) with arginine (R) or valine (V) leads to steric hindrance and blocks the capacity of SETD2 {3523,3599,891} and KDM2A {554} to bind to the mutant histone H3.3 tail. Impaired binding of these H3 p.K37 (K36) methylation–modulating enzymes results in diminished levels of H3 p.K37me2 (K36me2) and H3 p.K37me3 (p.K36me3) on the mutant histone H3.3 tail.

Studies on H3.3 p.G35V (G34)-mutant cells demonstrate that differential binding of H3 p.K37me3 (K36me3) induces a transcriptional reprogramming, recapitulating that of the developing forebrain, and causes prominent upregulation of the protooncogene *MYCN* {289}.

Macroscopic appearance

Diffuse infiltration of the parenchyma generates enlargement and distortion of brain structures, as well as softening and discolouration with haemorrhagic and/or necrotic zones.

Histopathology

H3 G34–mutant diffuse hemispheric glioma typically has a glioblastoma-like pattern, characterized by a highly cellular, infiltrative astrocytic tumour with brisk mitotic activity. Additionally, microvascular proliferation and/or necrosis are usually seen, although the presence of these features is not required for the diagnosis. In some cases, multinucleated and pleomorphic cells can be observed. An alternative pattern resembles the morphology of CNS embryonal tumours, where tumour cells are rather small and monomorphic, with hyperchromatic nuclei and scant cytoplasm. Here, Homer Wright rosettes are occasionally present, whereas microvascular proliferation and necrosis are less prominent {1713}. Ganglion cell differentiation has also been reported in rare cases {111}.

Immunophenotype

The typical immunohistochemical pattern of H3 G34–mutant diffuse hemispheric glioma comprises MAP2 positivity, FOXG1

positivity, loss of ATRX expression, and nuclear accumulation of p53 in the majority of tumour cells. A further notable feature is OLIG2 negativity. GFAP expression is variable and can be negative, especially in cases with more primitive embryonal-like morphology {3060,1713}. The Ki-67 proliferation index is usually high. Mutation-specific antibodies against H3.3 p.G35R (G34R)- and p.G35V (G34V)-mutant proteins are available {1856A}. However, false negative immunoreactivity in H3 G34–mutant cases has been described {1097}.

Grading

H3 G34–mutant diffuse hemispheric glioma corresponds to CNS WHO grade 4, regardless of the presence or absence of necrosis or microvascular proliferation {1713}.

Cytology

Not clinically relevant

Diagnostic molecular pathology

The molecularly defining diagnostic criterion is a missense mutation replacing glycine (G) with arginine (R) (in > 94% of cases) or valine (V) (< 6%) at p.G35 (G34) of the histone variant H3.3, encoded by the *H3-3A* (*H3F3A*) gene: c.103G>A p.G35R (G34R), c.103G>C p.G35R (G34R), or c.104G>T p.G35V (G34V) {1857}. So far, the p.G35R (G34R) or p.G35V (G34V) substitution in diffuse hemispheric gliomas has been exclusively identified in *H3-3A* and not in other histone genes {1713,1976}. About 90% of tumours bear *TP53* mutations and approximately 95% have alterations in the *ATRX* gene {1713}. The H3.3 p.G35 (G34) mutations in diffuse hemispheric gliomas are mutually exclusive with *IDH1* or *IDH2* and H3 p.K28M (K27M) or p.K28I (K27I) mutations {3060}. DNA methylation patterns and gene expression signatures can be used to differentiate H3 G34–mutant diffuse hemispheric gliomas from other entities. Although H3 G34–mutant diffuse hemispheric gliomas show widespread DNA hypomethylation, *MGMT* is often methylated {3060,1976,3362}. So far, no differences between p.G35R (G34R) and p.G35V (G34V) mutations have been reported.

Box 2.09 Diagnostic criteria for diffuse hemispheric glioma, H3 G34–mutant

Essential:

Cellular, infiltrative glioma with mitotic activity

AND

H3.3 p.G35R (G34R) or p.G35V (G34V) mutation (*H3-3A* [*H3F3A*] c.103G>A, c.103G>C, or c.104G>T)

AND

Hemispheric location

AND (for unresolved lesions)

Methylation profile of diffuse hemispheric glioma, H3 G34–mutant

Desirable:

OLIG2 immunonegativity

Loss of ATRX expression

Diffuse p53 immunopositivity

Essential and desirable diagnostic criteria

See Box 2.09.

Staging

In addition to cerebral imaging, radiological investigation of the spine should be performed.

Prognosis and prediction

The prognosis for patients with H3 G34–mutant diffuse hemispheric glioma is poor, with a median progression-free survival of 9 months and a median overall survival of 18–22 months {1713, 1976}. Patients experience mainly local recurrences, although leptomeningeal dissemination can occur. *MGMT* methylation and the absence of oncogene amplifications (such as of *PDG-FRA*, *EGFR*, *CDK4*, *MDM2*, *CDK6*, *CCND2*, *MYC*, *MYCN*) may be associated with longer overall survival {1713}.

Diffuse paediatric-type high-grade glioma, H3-wildtype and IDH-wildtype

Capper D
Jones DTW
Tabori U
Varlet P

Definition

Diffuse paediatric-type high-grade glioma (pHGG), H3-wildtype and IDH-wildtype, is a diffuse glioma with histological features of malignancy, typically occurring in children, adolescents, or young adults, which is wildtype for histone H3, *IDH1*, and *IDH2* (CNS WHO grade 4).

ICD-O coding

9385/3 Diffuse paediatric-type high-grade glioma, H3-wildtype and IDH-wildtype

ICD-11 coding

2A00.0Y Other specified gliomas of brain

Related terminology

Not recommended: paediatric-type glioblastoma, H3-wildtype; paediatric glioblastoma, H3-wildtype; methylation class glioblastoma midline (MC GBM MID); diffuse high-grade glioma in childhood, H3-wildtype, group C (pHGG WT-C); methylation class glioblastoma RTK3 (MC GBM RTK III); diffuse high-grade glioma in childhood, H3-wildtype, group B (pHGG

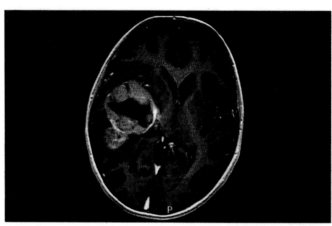

Fig. 2.61 Diffuse paediatric-type high-grade glioma, H3-wildtype and IDH-wildtype, MYCN subtype. Axial T1-weighted MRI demonstrating a well-circumscribed lesion in the left insular/temporal region with relatively homogeneous contrast enhancement and central cystic changes.

WT-B); methylation class glioblastoma MYCN (MC GBM MYCN).

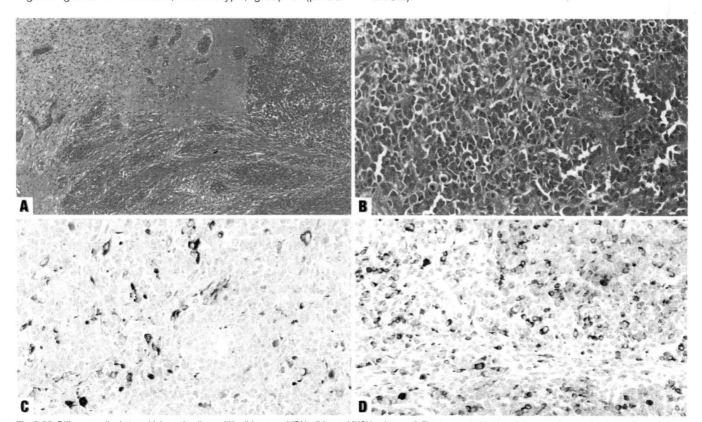

Fig. 2.62 Diffuse paediatric-type high-grade glioma, H3-wildtype and IDH-wildtype, MYCN subtype. **A** The tumour is highly cellular, reminiscent of embryonal morphology, and it shows areas of sharp demarcation from the brain tissue. **B** In addition to having glial areas, the tumour may show a prominent embryonal appearance. **C** GFAP may be expressed only in scattered cells. **D** Neuronal markers (here, neurofilament) may also be expressed.

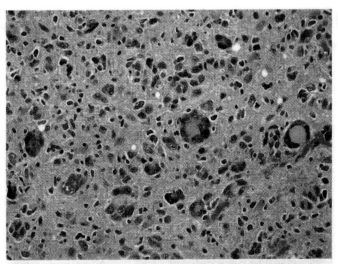

Fig. 2.63 Diffuse paediatric-type high-grade glioma, H3-wildtype and IDH-wildtype, RTK1 subtype, in Lynch syndrome. This glial tumour of a 10-year-old child shows numerous pleomorphic giant cells. Genetic analysis revealed a germline *MSH2* mutation and a high tumour mutation burden. Methylation profiling indicated the RTK1 subtype. Immunohistochemistry showed MSH2/MSH6 loss in tumour cells, and retention in normal cells, compatible with Lynch syndrome.

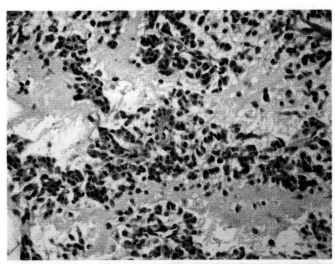

Fig. 2.64 Radiation-induced diffuse paediatric-type high-grade glioma, H3-wildtype and IDH-wildtype, RTK1 subtype. In areas, the tumour may show extensive myxoid change.

Subtype(s)

Diffuse paediatric-type high-grade glioma RTK2; diffuse paediatric-type high-grade glioma RTK1; diffuse paediatric-type high-grade glioma MYCN

Localization

pHGGs, H3-wildtype and IDH-wildtype, have been reported to arise throughout the supratentorial brain, brainstem, and cerebellum {1723}. The molecular subtypes have slightly different site predilections: pHGG RTK2 tumours mostly involve supratentorial structures (in 96% of cases), pHGG RTK1 tumours involve the supratentorial brain (in 82% of cases) and infratentorial/brainstem sites (in 18% of cases), and pHGG MYCN tumours involve the supratentorial brain (in 86% of cases) and infratentorial/brainstem structures (in 14% of cases) {1723}.

Clinical features

Like with other high-grade gliomas, patients develop clinical symptoms according to the anatomical structures involved. Symptoms can include seizures and motor or sensory deficits.

Imaging

The MRI characteristics of pHGGs, H3-wildtype and IDH-wildtype, are similar to those of other high-grade gliomas; MRI typically reveals a contrast-enhancing tumour with mass effect. pHGG MYCN tumours may be better circumscribed, with only slight perilesional oedema and homogeneous contrast enhancement {3146,3145}. Imaging characteristics for the other subtypes have not been reported.

Epidemiology

Epidemiological data for pHGG, H3-wildtype and IDH-wildtype, do not yet exist. In a clinical trial of non-brainstem paediatric high-grade gliomas in children aged 3–18 years, 32 (~40%) of 74 tumours with DNA methylation data corresponded to pHGG, H3-wildtype and IDH-wildtype {1977}. The median age of patients with pHGG, H3-wildtype and IDH-wildtype, is currently unclear because published series have focused on paediatric cases {1976,1723} and the occurrence in the adult population may therefore be underestimated.

Etiology

Gliomas arising after therapeutic radiation, or, as described above, in the context of germline mismatch repair deficiency, typically harbour molecular characteristics compatible with pHGG, H3-wildtype and IDH-wildtype {1928} and are predominantly of the pHGG RTK1 molecular subtype.

Gliomas arising in the context of constitutional mismatch repair deficiency syndrome (CMMRD), Lynch syndrome, or Li–Fraumeni syndrome should be recognized as distinct from spontaneously arising diffuse paediatric-type high-grade gliomas. For more details, see Chapter 14: *Genetic tumour syndromes involving the CNS*.

Pathogenesis

It is currently unclear why tumours arising subsequent to cranial irradiation and those occurring in the context of CMMRD and Lynch syndrome predominantly belong to the pHGG RTK1 subtype. It is likely that there are similarities in the cellular origins of these tumours and those of sporadically arising pHGG RTK1 tumours.

pHGGs, H3-wildtype and IDH-wildtype, harbour somatic alterations of known oncogenic drivers that are expected to play a central role in pathogenesis. Frequently observed are alterations in *TP53* (in 30–50% of cases), in genes encoding members of the RAS/MAPK and PI3K pathways, in *MYCN*, and/or in *ID2* {404,3059,1721,1976}.

Macroscopic appearance

Diffuse infiltration of the parenchyma causes enlargement and distortion of the brain structures, as well as softening and discolouration, with haemorrhagic/necrotic zones.

Histopathology

Histopathology typically shows features of either a glioblastoma-like malignant tumour (with mitotic activity, vascular proliferation,

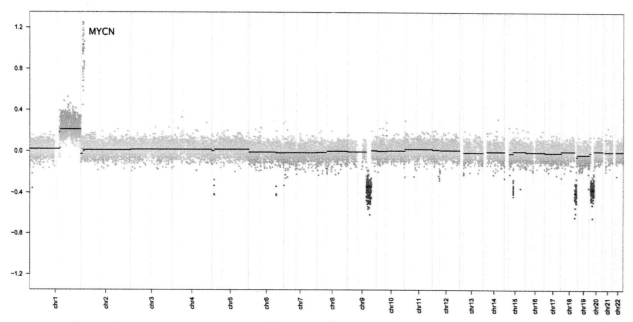

Fig. 2.65 Diffuse paediatric-type high-grade glioma, H3-wildtype and IDH-wildtype, MYCN subtype. Copy-number profile calculated from DNA methylation data, showing a *MYCN* amplification among other changes. Note that the adult-type +7/–10 chromosomal pattern is not present.

and necrosis) or a primitive, undifferentiated morphology. Areas of glial differentiation and primitive differentiation can often be found in the same specimen. In some cases, vascular proliferation and necrosis may be absent.

For the pHGG MYCN subtype, a biphasic pattern with areas of diffuse infiltration and highly cellular circumscribed nodules has been described {3146}. Tumours are often composed of large cells with distinct nucleoli and may show a mix of spindle-shaped and epithelioid cells {3146}.

Immunophenotype
Data on the immunophenotype of pHGG, H3-wildtype and IDH-wildtype, have not been specifically reported. Most reported cases were identified molecularly among series of paediatric glioblastomas or high-grade gliomas, and an immunophenotype compatible with such a diagnosis can therefore be expected, including at least focal positivity for GFAP and/or OLIG2 {1976,1721}. However, tumours of the pHGG MYCN molecular subtype may be largely negative for glial markers and instead express neuronal markers. All cases should have preserved expression of H3 p.K28me3 (K27me3) {3146}.

Differential diagnosis
Depending on the age of the patient and the location of the tumour, a large number of differential diagnoses should be considered. In particular, for infants, infant-type hemispheric glioma and desmoplastic infantile ganglioglioma / desmoplastic infantile astrocytoma should be excluded; these typically harbour alterations of *BRAF* or fusions involving NTRK genes, *ROS1*, *ALK*, or *MET*. H3 p.K28me3 (K27me3) is retained in pHGGs, H3-wildtype and IDH-wildtype, distinguishing them from diffuse midline gliomas. Tumours with glioblastoma morphology but the DNA methylation profile of pleomorphic xanthoastrocytoma or a combination of *BRAF* mutation and *CDKN2A* and/or *CDKN2B* deletion

are more likely to be adult-type epithelioid glioblastomas {1976, 1721}. The chromosomal pattern of +7/–10 and/or *EGFRvIII* mutations typical of adult-type glioblastoma are typically absent in pHGG, H3-wildtype and IDH-wildtype {3036}. Other differentials to consider include CNS embryonal tumours {3059} and, for posterior fossa tumours, medulloblastomas. Medulloblastomas are typically negative for OLIG2, whereas most pHGGs, H3-wildtype and IDH-wildtype, express this marker. CNS embryonal tumours should be considered less likely in older children and adults than in young children, and molecular alterations compatible with this diagnosis should be clearly demonstrated in these cases. In the postirradiation setting, the possibility of a pHGG versus relapse of an embryonal tumour should be considered {2493}.

Cytology
Not relevant

Diagnostic molecular pathology
Initial testing should exclude alterations in histone H3 and in *IDH1* or *IDH2*. Alterations frequently encountered in these tumours include *PDGFRA* amplification or mutation, *TP53* mutation, *NF1* alterations, *EGFR* amplification or mutation, or *MYCN* amplification. DNA methylation profiling is used for the identification of pHGG, H3-wildtype and IDH-wildtype, and it may be useful in guiding additional molecular testing {1723, 1976,1977}. Three molecular subgroups may be recognized by their distinct DNA methylation profiles or enrichment for molecular alterations: pHGG RTK1, pHGG RTK2, and pHGG MYCN. pHGG RTK1 is enriched for *PDGFRA* amplifications (~33% of cases), pHGG RTK2 is enriched for *EGFR* amplifications (~50% of cases) and *TERT* promoter mutations (~64% of cases) {1723}, and pHGG MYCN is enriched for *MYCN* amplifications (~50% of cases) {460,1723}. Tumours associated with CMMRD or Lynch syndrome are typically of the pHGG RTK1 subtype.

Essential and desirable diagnostic criteria

See Box 2.10.

Staging

Not relevant

Prognosis and prediction

pHGGs, H3-wildtype and IDH-wildtype, are aggressive tumours, and they are considered CNS WHO grade 4. Data from one multi-institutional series indicate a 2-year survival rate of 23.5% and a median overall survival (OS) of 17.2 months {1976}. Outcome was shown to be worst with pHGG MYCN (median OS: 14 months), intermediate with pHGG RTK1 (median OS: 21 months), and better with pHGG RTK2 (median OS: 44 months) {1723}. Unlike for adult high-grade gliomas, the finding of vascular endothelial proliferation and/or necrosis is not prognostic {3292}. Few data exist on potentially targetable alterations in pHGG, H3-wildtype and IDH-wildtype; recurrent alterations of *PDGFRA* and *EGFR* may be the most frequent of such alterations, but their predictive ability is yet to be demonstrated. Hypermutant tumours, most frequently arising in the context of CMMRD, may respond to immunotherapy {1977} (see *Constitutional mismatch repair deficiency syndrome*, p. 452).

Box 2.10 Diagnostic criteria for diffuse paediatric-type high-grade glioma (pHGG), H3-wildtype and IDH-wildtype

Essential:

A diffuse glioma with mitotic activity occurring in a child or young adult

AND

Absence of mutations in *IDH1* or *IDH2*

AND

Absence of mutations in H3 genes

AND

Methylation profile aligned with pHGG RTK1, pHGG RTK2, or pHGG MYCN

OR

Key molecular features: *PDGFRA* alteration, *EGFR* alteration, or *MYCN* amplification

Desirable:

Microvascular proliferation

Necrosis, typically palisading

H3 p.K28me3 (K27me3) retained

Infant-type hemispheric glioma

Jacques TS
Bandopadhayay P
Jones C
Tabori U
Varlet P

Definition
Infant-type hemispheric glioma is a cerebral hemispheric, high-grade cellular astrocytoma that arises in early childhood, typically with receptor tyrosine kinase (RTK) fusions including those in the NTRK family or in *ROS1*, *ALK*, or *MET*.

ICD-O coding
9385/3 Infant-type hemispheric glioma

ICD-11 coding
2A00.0Y Other specified gliomas of brain

Related terminology
None

Subtype(s)
Infant-type hemispheric glioma, NTRK-altered; infant-type hemispheric glioma, *ROS1*-altered; infant-type hemispheric glioma, *ALK*-altered; infant-type hemispheric glioma, *MET*-altered

Localization
These gliomas appear in the supratentorial compartment, usually as large masses {29,616,2322,3264,2238,603,1179}. There is frequently superficial involvement that includes the leptomeninges {603}.

Clinical features
The presentation is usually acute. During infancy, children with infant-type hemispheric glioma may present with nonspecific signs and symptoms ranging from agitation to lethargy. Head circumference may be large. Some tumours can be diagnosed antenatally.

Epidemiology
All reported cases have occurred early in childhood, mostly in the first year of life. In one cohort, the median age at presentation was 2.8 months (range: 0–12 months) {1179}.

Etiology
Unknown

Pathogenesis
Structural genomic variants, often driven by focal intragenic DNA copy-number changes, result in the acquisition of fusion genes involving numerous 5′ partners and the receptor tyrosine kinases *NTRK1*, *NTRK2*, *NTRK3*, *ALK*, *ROS1*, or *MET* at the 3′ end. These may be either interchromosomal or intrachromosomal and may result from small interstitial deletions or amplifications. They cause the aberrant expression of an active kinase domain, driving tumorigenesis via signalling through canonical PI3K and/or MAPK pathways. There are generally no other genetic alterations, rendering the tumours particularly sensitive to targeted inhibition of the relevant RTK {1179,603}.

Macroscopic appearance
There are few macroscopic pathology descriptions, but these tumours are large, and some have a cystic component and a solid portion. Necrosis or haemorrhage can occur {29,616, 2322,3264,2238,603,1179}.

Histopathology
The histological descriptions derive from two large studies {1179,603} and a few case reports {29,616,2322,3264,2238}. The original diagnoses were often glioblastomas or other high-grade gliomas (84%) {1179,603,29,616,3615} but also included anaplastic gangliogliomas, desmoplastic infantile

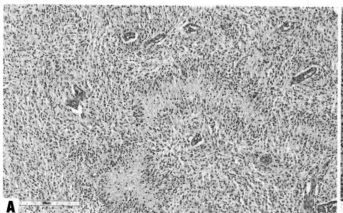
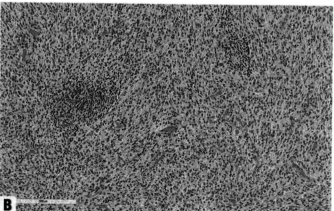

Fig. 2.66 Infant-type hemispheric glioma. **A** An infant-type hemispheric glioma showing classic features of a high-grade glioma including palisading necrosis and endothelial proliferation. **B** An infant-type hemispheric glioma with a *CLIP2::MET* fusion showing a cellular glioma with several clusters of more primitive-appearing cells.

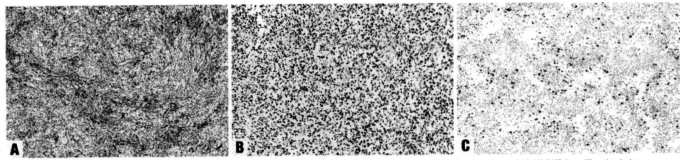

Fig. 2.67 Infant-type hemispheric glioma. **A** GFAP immunostaining. **B** OLIG2 immunostaining. **C** Immunostaining showing elevated Ki-67 (MIB1) proliferation index.

ganglioglioma/astrocytoma, ependymomas, and CNS primitive neuroectodermal tumours {603,2322}.

The tumours are frequently cellular, are well demarcated from the adjacent brain parenchyma, and involve the leptomeninges {603}. Astrocytic, often spindle-shaped, cells with mild to moderate pleomorphism are arranged in fascicles or uniform sheets. There is frequently palisading necrosis, mitotic activity, and microvascular proliferation. More rarely, a gemistocytic morphology is seen. Some tumours (including some with *ALK* fusions) may be more heterogeneous, with ependymal differentiation {603,2322} or a biphasic appearance with low-grade and high-grade components or occasional ganglion cells {603,1179, 3264,2238}. This tumour type is not currently graded.

Immunophenotype
The glial component shows immunoreactivity for GFAP but does not usually express neuronal markers {2322,3264,3615}. ALK immunostaining can be found in at least some tumours with *ALK* fusions {1179,2322}. NTRK immunostaining is not helpful because of the high level of NTRK expression in normal brain.

Differential diagnosis
The differential diagnosis includes other high-grade gliomas, desmoplastic infantile ganglioglioma/astrocytoma, ganglioglioma, and ependymomas in infants.

Cytology
Intraoperative cytology is not well described in genetically defined cases, but it is likely to mimic the features seen on paraffin histology.

Diagnostic molecular pathology
RTK fusions can be therapeutically targeted and are present in 60–80% of cases. Therefore, where possible, in infants, routine testing for such fusions should be considered {1179, 603}, both to establish the diagnosis and to provide options for therapy.

These tumours form a distinct subgroup by methylation array profiling regardless of formal tumour grading or RTK fusion type {603}. This can also be used to establish the diagnosis but it may not be sufficient to enable targeted therapy.

Essential and desirable diagnostic criteria
See Box 2.11.

Box 2.11 Diagnostic criteria for infant-type hemispheric glioma

Essential:

Cellular astrocytoma

AND

Presentation in early childhood

AND

Cerebral hemispheric location

AND

Presence of a typical receptor tyrosine kinase abnormality (e.g. fusion in an NTRK family gene or in *ROS1*, *MET1*, or *ALK*)

OR

Methylation profile aligned with infant-type hemispheric glioma

---

Staging
Occasional cases show leptomeningeal dissemination {2322}, so craniospinal imaging is prudent. However, a formal staging system is not available.

Prognosis and prediction
Prospective outcome data for this new entity are lacking. Historically, high-grade gliomas in infants have been recognized to have better outcomes than those in older children {801}. In this context, it is notable that most descriptions of infantile hemispheric gliomas report a higher survival rate than those of typical high-grade gliomas {29,616,2322,3264,2238,603,1179}. The total number of clinically annotated cases within each molecular subtype remains relatively small, but individual driver events may be associated with distinct clinical outcomes. In one study, patients with *ALK*-rearranged tumours appeared to have a better 5-year overall survival rate than patients with tumours that harboured *ROS1* alterations (53.8% vs 25%, respectively), and patients with NTRK fusion–positive tumours had an intermediate prognosis (5-year overall survival rate: 42.9%) {1179}. Patients with *ALK*-rearranged tumours with low-grade histology had survival rates superior to those of patients with *ALK*-altered high-grade gliomas. However, prospective studies across larger cohorts are needed to confirm these initial observations. Finally, the presence of RTK-activating fusions offers an opportunity for therapy with small-molecule inhibitors. Responses to specific inhibitors have been reported {603,786,3615} and may change the prognosis of infantile hemispheric gliomas. Further studies are needed to evaluate the efficacy of these inhibitors and the overall survival rates for each subtype.

Pilocytic astrocytoma

Tihan T
Figarella-Branger D
Giannini C
Gupta K
Hawkins CE
Jacques TS

Jones DTW
Pfister SM
Rodriguez FJ
Tabori U
Varlet P

Definition

Pilocytic astrocytoma is an astrocytic neoplasm with variable proportions of bipolar hair-like (pilocytic) cells, compact and loose or myxoid regions, Rosenthal fibres, and eosinophilic granular bodies. Pilocytic astrocytoma is associated with MAPK pathway gene alterations (most often *KIAA1549::BRAF* gene fusions) (CNS WHO grade 1).

ICD-O coding

9421/1 Pilocytic astrocytoma

ICD-11 coding

2A00.0Y & XH29Q5 Other specified gliomas of brain & Pilomyxoid astrocytoma

Related terminology

Not recommended (obsolete): juvenile pilocytic astrocytoma.

Subtype(s)

Pilomyxoid astrocytoma; pilocytic astrocytoma with histological features of anaplasia

Localization

Pilocytic astrocytomas can arise throughout the neuraxis, but they are most common in the cerebellum, especially in children {207,621}. Other preferred sites are the optic nerve, midline locations (brainstem, optic chiasm / hypothalamus, basal ganglia), and spinal cord. Tumours in the cerebral hemispheres are rare in children, but in adults they occur here with equal frequency as in the cerebellum {621}.

Clinical features

Presenting signs and symptoms, which are usually due to mass effect or ventricular obstruction, include macrocephaly, headache, endocrinopathy, and evidence of increased intracranial pressure. The slow growth sometimes leads to diagnostic delay because symptoms are subtle. Focal neurological signs relate to tumour location. Optic pathway tumours often produce visual loss {1360,1911}. Brainstem pilocytic astrocytomas most often cause hydrocephalus or signs of brainstem dysfunction. Patients with thalamic and other supratentorial tumours present with focal motor deficiencies or movement disorders, whereas spinal cord lesions are associated with back pain, paresis, and kyphoscoliosis. Hypothalamic/pituitary dysfunction, including obesity and diabetes insipidus, is often apparent in patients with large hypothalamic tumours {2706}. Especially in infants, midline tumours can be associated with emaciation and failure to thrive (diencephalic syndrome), with a poor clinical outcome {2125,2459}. Primary dissemination at diagnosis may also be more common in this age group {2125,2459}. However, neuraxis seeding does not necessarily indicate aggressive growth {2532}. Seeding may

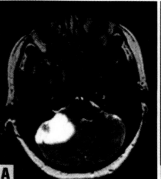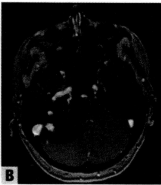

Fig. 2.68 Pilocytic astrocytoma. Typical MRI appearance of pilocytic astrocytoma in the posterior fossa of a 5-year-old boy, showing a large cystic lesion with an enhancing mural nodule. The tumour has *BRAF* kinase domain duplication with *KIAA1549::BRAF* gene fusion. **A** T2-weighted image. **B** Contrast-enhanced T1-weighted image.

be asymptomatic, and long-term survival is possible, even without adjuvant treatment {2532}.

Imaging

Pilocytic astrocytomas have a wide spectrum of imaging features, but about two thirds appear as a well-circumscribed cystic lesion with an enhancing mural nodule on MRI. The remainder often appear either as a cyst-like mass with a central non-enhancing zone or as a predominantly solid mass {612, 2451}. The cyst wall enhancement is variable, and enhancement does not necessarily indicate tumour involvement. Calcification may be present. Pilocytic astrocytomas are often contrast enhancing, with the solid tumour component typically isointense to hypointense on T1 imaging and hyperintense on T2. Imaging characteristics are often not specific enough to allow a diagnosis without biopsy. Imaging characteristics of optic nerve tumours vary, with neurofibromatosis type 1 (NF1)-associated tumours rarely extending beyond the optic pathway and often appearing solid, and non-NF1 counterparts involving the optic chiasm, extending beyond the optic pathway, and frequently being cystic {1711}.

Epidemiology

Pilocytic astrocytoma accounts for 5% of all primary brain tumours {2344}. It is most common during the first two decades of life, with an average annual age-adjusted incidence rate of 0.91 cases per 100 000 population {2344}. Pilocytic astrocytoma accounts for 17.6% of all childhood primary brain tumours and is the most common glioma in children. The incidence rate is highest in young children and decreases with advancing age {2344}. Pilocytic astrocytoma is rare in older adults {2344}.

Etiology

Although most cases are sporadic {3196}, pilocytic astrocytomas are also the principal CNS tumour type in a group of neurodevelopmental diseases with germline mutations in MAPK pathway genes, including NF1, Noonan syndrome, and encephalocraniocutaneous lipomatosis. NF1 (see *Neurofibromatosis type 1*, p. 426) is caused by *NF1* germline mutations, whereas Noonan syndrome is most frequently caused by mutations in *PTPN11* or *RAF1* {2859}, and encephalocraniocutaneous lipomatosis by *FGFR1* germline mutations {240,3263}.

Pathogenesis

Pilocytic astrocytomas are associated with genetic abnormalities in genes encoding members of the MAPK pathway. The most frequent abnormality (found in ~60% of all cases) is a duplication/rearrangement of approximately 2 Mb at 7q34, encompassing the *BRAF* gene {194,742,2491,2768} and resulting in gene fusions involving various combinations of *KIAA1549* and *BRAF* exons, which makes it difficult to comprehensively detect all possible fusions by RT-PCR.

Essentially all pilocytic astrocytomas studied genomically had a genetic alteration affecting the MAPK pathway {1493, 3597,1605}. These alterations include *NF1* mutations, which are mostly germline mutations in patients with NF1 {1201}; hotspot *BRAF* p.V600E mutations; *BRAF* fusions with partners other than *KIAA1549*; *BRAF* insertions; *KRAS* mutations; *FGFR1* mutations or fusions; very occasional NTRK family receptor tyrosine kinase fusions; and *RAF1* gene fusions, usually with *SRGAP3* but exceptionally with other partners {3532,2424}. NTRK genes fuse with several different 5′ partners that contain a dimerization domain. This is presumed to lead to constitutive dimerization of the NTRK fusion proteins and activation of the kinase {1493,3597}.

The *FGFR1* alterations seen in pilocytic astrocytomas overlap with those seen in other paediatric low-grade glial and glioneuronal tumours. They include hotspot point mutations (p.N546K and p.K656E) {3226}, *FGFR1::TACC1* fusions, and an internal tandem duplication of the kinase domain of *FGFR1* {1493}. The

incidence of MAPK pathway gene alterations identified to date is summarized in Table 2.03. Polysomies (in particular of chromosomes 5, 6, 7, 11, and 15) are reportedly more common in tumours of teenagers and adults {1494}.

The incidence of the various gene alterations varies with anatomical location {1493,3597}, and distinct anatomical subsets of tumours may be distinguished on the basis of gene expression and DNA methylation profiles {1795,2897,3157,460}. The *KIAA1549::BRAF* fusion is common in cerebellar tumours, but less common supratentorially. *FGFR1* alterations are widely distributed, whereas *BRAF* p.V600E mutations are more common in supratentorial tumours. Infratentorial and supratentorial tumours may also be distinguishable on the basis of their gene expression or DNA methylation signatures {1795,2897,3157}. The average mutation burden is low.

Macroscopic appearance

Most pilocytic astrocytomas are soft, grey, and relatively discrete. Intratumoural or paratumoural cyst formation, including mural tumour nodules, is common. Chronic lesions may be calcified. Spinal tumours may be associated with syrinx formation {2121}. Optic nerve tumours often circumferentially infiltrate the optic sheath {326}.

Histopathology

Pilocytic astrocytomas have low to moderate cellularity. Neoplastic cells range widely in their morphology and include varying proportions of piloid and oligodendrocyte-like cells. Nuclei are round to elongate. Multinucleated cells with horseshoe-shaped nuclear clusters (pennies-on-a-plate pattern) are often seen. In some cases, hyperchromasia and pleomorphism are obvious but mitotic figures are rare {1091}. Rare cases have brisk mitotic activity, which may imply aggressive behaviour {2697}. Rosenthal fibres and eosinophilic granular bodies are common, but they vary in prominence. Myxoid background

Table 2.03 Molecular alterations and their prevalence in pilocytic astrocytomas

Genetic alteration	% of tumours	Prevalence	References
KIAA1549::BRAF fusion	> 60%	Common, particularly cerebellar; rare in other tumour forms except diffuse leptomeningeal glioneuronal tumour	{1496,2936}
Other *BRAF* fusions	< 5%	Occasional; very rare in other entities	{1287}
BRAF mutations (especially p.V600E)	~5–10%	Occasional, mainly supratentorial; also in many other glial and glioneuronal tumours	{2842,1495}
NF1 mutation	~10–15%	Typically germline; common with optic pathway tumours	{1198,1201}
FGFR1 mutation	< 5%	Found mainly in midline tumours; also observed in other low-grade gliomas	{1493,3226,2932}
FGFR1 fusions (especially *FGFR1::TACC1*)	< 5%	*FGFR1::TACC1* fusion more common; also observed in other low-grade gliomas	{1493,2932}
NTRK family fusions	~2%	Rare; also observed in other glial/glioneuronal tumours	{1493,2424}
KRAS mutation	Single cases	Very rare in pilocytic astrocytoma; extremely rare in other entities	{2898,1454}
RAF1 fusion	Single cases	Very rare in pilocytic astrocytoma; extremely rare in other entities (with the possible exception of pleomorphic xanthoastrocytoma)	{1495,962,3532}
ROS1 fusions	Single cases	Very rare in pilocytic astrocytoma; more common in infantile hemispheric glioma; extremely rare in other entities	{2663,2768}
Other alterations (of *MET*, *RET*, etc.)	Single cases	Very rare in pilocytic astrocytoma; frequency in other entities not determined (probably extremely rare)	{2768}

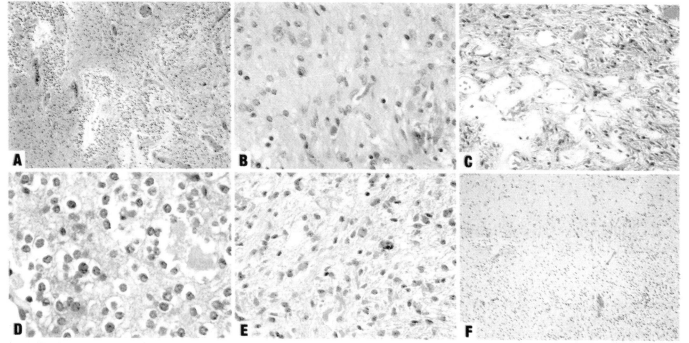

Fig. 2.69 Pilocytic astrocytoma. **A** Typical biphasic appearance of pilocytic astrocytoma. Compact areas that often harbour Rosenthal fibres alternate with loose and somewhat myxoid regions. **B** Rosenthal fibres and eosinophilic granular bodies. Typically, Rosenthal fibres are more abundant than eosinophilic granular bodies in pilocytic astrocytomas, but both can be observed, as in this case. **C** Hyaline vessels and Rosenthal fibres. In most pilocytic astrocytomas, vascular structures within the tumour demonstrate brisk hyalinization. Numerous Rosenthal fibres are also observed. **D** Tumour with oligodendrocyte-like cells. Even though this tumour resembles oligodendroglioma cytologically, the presence of eosinophilic granular bodies at higher magnification provides a useful diagnostic clue for pilocytic astrocytoma. **E** Pilocytic astrocytomas often harbour large cells with multiple nuclei (the pennies-on-a-plate appearance). **F** Infiltrative edge. In many pilocytic astrocytomas, infiltrative-appearing regions can be recognized. In small biopsies, these areas may evoke the impression of a diffuse astrocytoma.

with microcystic change is common, as are degenerative changes, including calcifications, hyalinized vessels, and haemorrhages {621}. Various histological patterns can be seen in pilocytic astrocytomas: (1) a biphasic pattern, in which compact areas rich in bipolar cells and Rosenthal fibres alternate with loose and microcystic regions rich in oligodendrocyte-like cells; (2) a predominantly compact, piloid pattern, with abundant Rosenthal fibres; and (3) a more dispersed pattern, rich in oligodendrocyte-like cells, mimicking oligodendroglioma. The biphasic pattern is common in cerebellar tumours. The compact pattern is often seen in adults, and the oligodendrocyte-like pattern may be associated with *FGFR1* alterations {2768}. Occasionally, typical pilocytic astrocytomas have foci that resemble pilomyxoid astrocytoma; these are called intermediate tumours. Rare examples also demonstrate the regimented palisaded (spongioblastoma) pattern. Pilocytic astrocytomas show highly vascular areas with thin glomerular capillaries often arranged in a linear fashion and associated with cystic structures, or they have thick-walled, hyalinized vessels and regressive changes. Glomeruloid microvascular proliferations line the cyst wall and should not prompt a higher grade designation. Infarct-like necrosis can occur, but palisading necrosis is exceptional. Leptomeningeal involvement can occur in any location, sometimes with extensive desmoplastic reaction. Some tumours may mimic diffuse astrocytomas on histopathology because of a surprising degree of infiltration, despite often appearing solid radiologically. Entrapped neurons can also be mistaken for a neuronal component (e.g. ganglioglioma).

Immunophenotype

Immunohistochemistry demonstrates strong diffuse positivity for GFAP, S100, and OLIG2. Many cases are positive for synaptophysin but negative for NFP, NeuN, and chromogranin. CD34 is usually negative, although expression has been reported in the hypothalamic/chiasmatic region {523}. IDH1 p.R132H expression is absent and the H3 p.K28M (K27M) stain is negative, with rare exceptions. Most tumours show strong and diffuse SOX10 and p16 staining, with SOX10 and OLIG2 positivity helping to distinguish pilocytic astrocytoma from ependymoma {1655}. The Ki-67 index is usually low, with only focal increases.

Subtypes
Pilomyxoid astrocytoma

Pilomyxoid astrocytoma {3197} shares many features with classic pilocytic astrocytoma but differs in some important clinicopathological respects {1694,910}. It is a tumour of infancy occurring in the hypothalamic/chiasmatic region, has a higher rate of recurrence and a poorer outcome than classic pilocytic astrocytoma, and shows a propensity for cerebrospinal dissemination {1694,1471}. Pilomyxoid astrocytoma is defined as a tumour with monomorphic piloid cytology, a diffusely myxoid background, and increased cellularity compared with that of classic pilocytic astrocytoma {3197}. It also has a prominent angiocentric arrangement of tumour cells and typically lacks Rosenthal fibres and eosinophilic granular bodies. On neuroimaging, pilomyxoid astrocytomas appear similar to classic pilocytic astrocytomas, but they are more often solid and uniformly

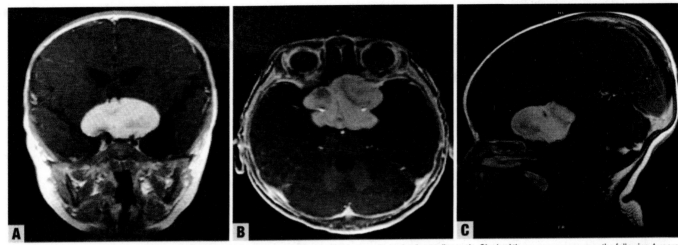

Fig. 2.70 Pilomyxoid astrocytoma. Tumour in a 7-month-old girl. There was spinal and brainstem dissemination at diagnosis. She had three recurrences over the following 4 years while being treated with trametinib with partial response. The tumour has *BRAF* kinase domain duplication with *KIAA1549::BRAF* gene fusion. Contrast-enhanced MRI. **A** Coronal. **B** Axial. **C** Sagittal.

enhancing {79,2188}. Some pilomyxoid astrocytomas develop into a classic pilocytic astrocytoma on recurrence. Rare hybrid pilomyxoid/pilocytic astrocytomas have been reported, but their biological behaviour is poorly defined {1487}. Molecular studies identify MAPK pathway gene alterations similar to those in classic pilocytic astrocytoma, but differences have been reported {1471,1656,1756}. Further studies are needed to elucidate the precise molecular profile of pilomyxoid astrocytomas {460}.

Pilocytic astrocytoma with histological features of anaplasia
Pilocytic astrocytomas are remarkable in that they maintain their CNS WHO grade 1 {421} status over decades. The terms "anaplastic pilocytic astrocytoma" and "pilocytic astrocytoma with histological anaplasia" have been proposed for tumours with morphological features of pilocytic astrocytoma but showing brisk mitotic activity with or without necrosis {2697}. Anaplastic changes may be present at initial diagnosis or at recurrence. In a study of 36 pilocytic astrocytomas with anaplasia defined histologically, they predominantly occurred in adults

(mean age: 32 years; range: 3–75 years), mostly involved the posterior fossa, and showed heterogeneous genetic features with alterations typical of pilocytic astrocytoma and other gliomas {2693}, including *BRAF* duplications (30%), germline or somatic *NF1* mutations (33%), loss of nuclear ATRX expression (57%), and an alternative-lengthening-of-telomeres phenotype (69%). Features associated with worse overall survival included necrosis, subtotal resection, alternative lengthening of telomeres, and ATRX loss (*P* < 0.05). The overlap between pilocytic astrocytoma with histological anaplasia and the rare midline pilocytic astrocytoma with double mutant *FGFR1*, *BRAF*, or *NF1* and H3 p.K28M (K27M) remains to be determined, although both have been associated with aggressive behaviour {2643,2693,1493}.

In a cohort of predominantly adult patients across > 20 institutions worldwide, who were considered to have histologically defined anaplastic pilocytic astrocytoma, 81% of the tumours harboured a distinct methylome signature, referred to as "DNA methylation class anaplastic astrocytoma with piloid features"

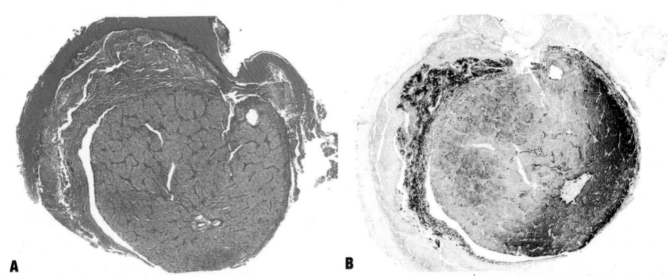

Fig. 2.71 Optic pathway glioma (pilocytic astrocytoma). **A** Cross-section reveals an expanded optic nerve with subarachnoid extension of the tumour. The latter is a common feature of pilocytic astrocytoma. **B** A GFAP stain highlights the regions of tumour involvement in this optic pathway glioma.

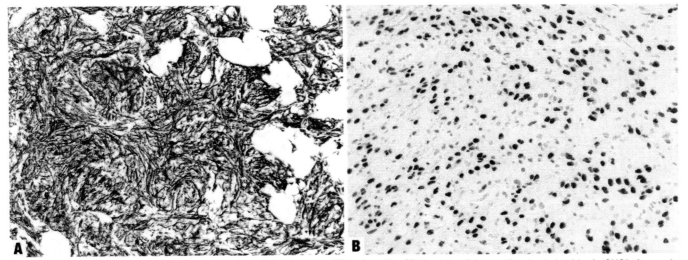

Fig. 2.72 Pilocytic astrocytoma. **A** Pilocytic astrocytomas typically show strong and diffusely positive GFAP staining. **B** Immunohistochemical staining for OLIG2 often results in diffuse nuclear positivity in pilocytic astrocytomas.

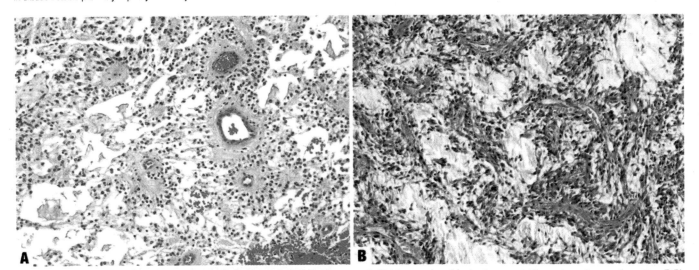

Fig. 2.73 Pilomyxoid astrocytoma. **A** Loose, mucin-rich arrangement of piloid cells, some of which form angiocentric structures resembling perivascular pseudorosettes. **B** Pilomyxoid astrocytoma in a 10-month-old boy, located in the hypothalamic region. The typical angiocentric and markedly myxoid pattern is seen throughout the tumour. The tumour has *BRAF* kinase domain duplication with *KIAA1549::BRAF* gene fusion.

{2643}. These tumours are now considered a distinct type, designated as "high-grade astrocytoma with piloid features". A similar DNA methylation profile was found in 36% of histologically defined cerebellar glioblastomas {2644}. Although this methylation class is enriched for neoplasms pathologically diagnosed as pilocytic astrocytoma with histological anaplasia, the two categories do not overlap completely and their relationship remains to be elucidated.

Histological and molecular diagnostic criteria established for pilocytic astrocytoma with anaplasia in adults may not be applicable to children. In one study of 31 paediatric patients (aged < 16 years), on multivariate analysis, only young age (< 6 years) and partial resection were associated with decreased progression-free survival {1040}. Necrosis and high mitotic activity were not significantly associated with survival. Nuclear ATRX expression was preserved in all tumours, and only one tumour matched the methylation class of high-grade astrocytoma with piloid features, with an additional case showing homozygous deletion of *CDKN2A* and/or *CDKN2B*.

Differential diagnosis

A relevant differential diagnosis in the presence of microvascular proliferation and/or necrosis is a high-grade astrocytic glioma including glioblastoma. Solid growth pattern, low mitotic activity, and bipolar cells, in addition to molecular features, help resolve this differential diagnosis. Rosenthal fibre–rich piloid gliosis may also mimic pilocytic astrocytoma, but it lacks the loose component. In the midline, an H3 K27–altered diffuse midline glioma must be excluded, although rare pilocytic astrocytomas acquire an H3 p.K28M (K27M) mutation in addition to their MAPK gene alteration. Other differential diagnoses include ganglioglioma, dysembryoplastic neuroepithelial tumour, pleomorphic xanthoastrocytoma, rosette-forming glioneuronal tumour, ependymoma (especially tanycytic), and diffuse leptomeningeal glioneuronal tumour. Some tumours of this last type may be virtually indistinguishable from pilocytic astrocytoma on routine histology.

A note of caution is warranted in regard to anaplastic transformation after radiation therapy, especially with a long interval

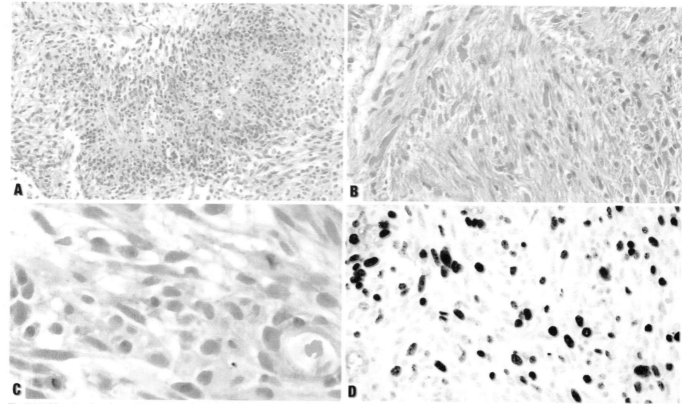

Fig. 2.74 Pilocytic astrocytoma with anaplastic features. **A** Region of tumour with anaplastic features, including increased cellularity and palisading necrosis. **B** Region of classic pilocytic astrocytoma with numerous Rosenthal fibres. **C** Region of tumour with anaplastic features including increased mitotic activity. **D** Region of tumour with anaplastic features including increased Ki-67 labelling index.

and without the presence of a pilocytic component: some of these tumours may instead be a second primary, i.e. radiation-induced high-grade glioma {1441}.

Cytology

Intraoperative smears of pilocytic astrocytoma are characterized by cells with long, fine, hair-like processes. The cells usually show uniform, round to spindled nuclei with minimal atypia. Rosenthal fibres, eosinophilic granular bodies, and glomeruloid vessels can be present. In some cases, there may be degenerative atypia, with multinucleated cells.

Diagnostic molecular pathology

The most frequent genetic alteration in pilocytic astrocytoma is a chromosome 7q34 rearrangement resulting in a *KIAA1549::BRAF* tandem duplication and fusion {1496,2491, 962}. In small numbers of cases, alternate *BRAF* fusions have also been identified, occurring by various genetic rearrangements (including deletions and translocations) but all resulting in loss of the N-terminal regulatory region of the BRAF protein, with retention of the kinase domain {1493,3597,1287,3211}. Other MAPK pathway gene alterations also occur (see Table 2.03, p. 84) {1493,3597}.

The presence of the *KIAA1549::BRAF* fusion (or other MAPK gene alterations) supports the diagnosis of pilocytic astrocytoma in an appropriate morphological context. However, the

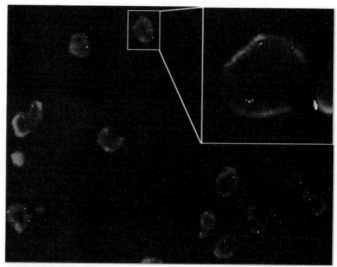

Fig. 2.75 Pilocytic astrocytoma. Interphase break-apart dual-colour FISH for the *BRAF* gene (red signal, 3′ end; green signal, 5′ end). The type of alteration to suggest fusion is duplication and splitting of the two probes. The duplication is considered positive if seen in > 30% of nuclei.

KIAA1549::BRAF fusion also occurs in diffuse leptomeningeal glioneuronal tumours {2702,736}. Other MAPK gene alterations similarly overlap with other tumour types.

Essential and desirable diagnostic criteria

See Box 2.12.

Staging

For infratentorial and spinal tumours, pilocytic astrocytoma staging involves cerebral and spinal MRI, whereas for supratentorial tumours, spinal MRI is only performed if there is evidence of intracranial dissemination. Cerebrospinal fluid cytology is only done if radiological findings indicate disseminated disease {1122}.

Prognosis and prediction

In most large series, pilocytic astrocytomas are associated with a favourable overall survival even after multiple progressions. When completely resected, pilocytic astrocytomas rarely recur {767,2230}. Because of the favourable overall outcome, radiation-sparing approaches are commonly recommended {1739}. And because the majority of tumours harbour alterations in MAPK pathway genes, they may favourably respond to targeted MEK inhibition. The overall long-term outcome of such approaches is yet to be determined. In cases of aggressive tumour behaviour and resistance to chemotherapy, a biopsy may be considered to allow for molecular characterization. A cautionary statement is warranted: pilomyxoid astrocytoma is

Box 2.12 Diagnostic criteria for classic pilocytic astrocytoma and pilomyxoid astrocytoma

Classic pilocytic astrocytoma

Essential:

Classic histological features of pilocytic astrocytoma, such as biphasic compact and loose growth patterns, piloid cytology, and low proliferative activity, with or without Rosenthal fibres and/or eosinophilic granular bodies

OR

A low-grade piloid astrocytic neoplasm with a solitary MAPK alteration, such as *KIAA1549::BRAF* fusion

Pilomyxoid astrocytoma

Essential:

A monomorphic, loose, myxoid neoplasm with piloid cytology and prominent angiocentric pattern, often without Rosenthal fibres and eosinophilic granular bodies

OR

An astrocytic neoplasm with pilomyxoid features and a solitary MAPK alteration, such as *KIAA1549::BRAF* fusion

likely to act aggressively {3197}. The prognostic significance of pilocytic astrocytoma with histological anaplasia needs to be determined.

High-grade astrocytoma with piloid features

Capper D
Jones DTW
Rodriguez FJ
Varlet P

Definition

High-grade astrocytoma with piloid features (HGAP) is an astrocytoma showing a distinct DNA methylation profile, often with high-grade piloid and/or glioblastoma-like histological features. Alterations of MAPK pathway genes are often combined with homozygous deletion involving the *CDKN2A* and/or *CDKN2B* locus, and/or *ATRX* mutation or loss of nuclear ATRX expression.

ICD-O coding

9421/3 High-grade astrocytoma with piloid features

ICD-11 coding

2A00.0Y & XH6PH6 Other specified gliomas of brain & Astrocytoma, NOS

Related terminology

Not recommended: anaplastic astrocytoma with piloid features; anaplastic pilocytic astrocytoma.

Subtype(s)

None

Localization

HGAP may occur throughout the entire CNS. Most frequently, tumours originate in the posterior fossa, where they typically affect the cerebellum (in 74% of cases). They can also be localized in the supratentorial (17%) and spinal (7%) regions {2643}.

Clinical features

Clinical signs and symptoms depend largely on tumour location. Clinical features distinct from those of other types of gliomas in the same locations have not been reported. On imaging, some tumours may appear as a ring-enhancing mass, mimicking the radiological appearance of glioblastoma.

Epidemiology

Comprehensive epidemiological data are not available, but several case series suggest that HGAPs are rare. In non–population-based case series, HGAPs (identified mostly in adults) have been estimated to account for about 1–3% of brain tumours {2573,1458,460}; however, the potential of selection bias in such series may mean this estimate is too high. In a population-based study of 306 paediatric brain tumours in the United Kingdom, not a single HGAP was identified {2505}. Furthermore, in a paediatric study of 31 anaplastic pilocytic astrocytomas, only 1 tumour (3%) was molecularly confirmed as HGAP {1040}. HGAP thus appears to be very rare in the paediatric population. In the combined data from three studies, the median age of reported patients was 40 years (range: 4–88 years), and the M:F ratio was balanced (1:1) {2643,1458,1040}.

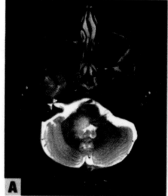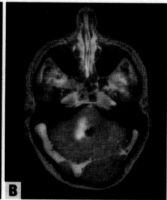

Fig. 2.76 High-grade astrocytoma with piloid features. **A** T2-weighted MRI shows a hyperintense lesion without sharp tumour margins in the dorsal pons and right cerebellar peduncle. **B** FET PET indicates highly increased amino acid metabolism in the tumour.

Etiology

Risk factors

In most patients, HGAP occurs de novo. In the remaining patients, the tumours may develop from a pre-existing lower-grade astrocytic tumour, including pilocytic astrocytoma. In one series, the precursor lesion dated back > 10 years in 4 (18%) of 22 cases {2643}. A prior history of cerebral irradiation is uncommon, reported in 4 (5%) of 83 patients {2643}, and no definite etiological role for irradiation has been established.

Genetic factors

Rare instances of HGAP have been reported in patients with neurofibromatosis type 1 (NF1) {2643}. Associations with other tumour predisposition syndromes have not been reported.

Pathogenesis

Molecular data imply that three pathways are centrally involved in the pathogenesis of HGAP: the MAPK pathway is frequently activated by mutations; the retinoblastoma tumour suppressor protein cell-cycle pathway is frequently deregulated by *CDKN2A* and/or *CDKN2B* inactivation or occasionally by *CDK4* amplification; and telomere maintenance is frequently activated by *ATRX* alterations and, rarely, *TERT* promoter mutations {2643}. In about half of all cases of HGAP, all three pathways are altered simultaneously; in the remaining cases, only one or two (or, very rarely, none) of these alterations are detectable {2643}.

The temporal order of these alterations is not known, but rare tumours developing in patients with NF1 may indicate that MAPK pathway gene alterations are an initiating genetic event. For a subset of HGAPs, lower-grade precursor lesions such as pilocytic astrocytomas have been reported, but a molecular workup of these potential precursors has not been performed {2643}.

HGAPs typically have numerous chromosomal alterations, with more than three structural aberrations found in 88% of cases {2643}. Besides frequent homozygous deletion of *CDKN2A* and/

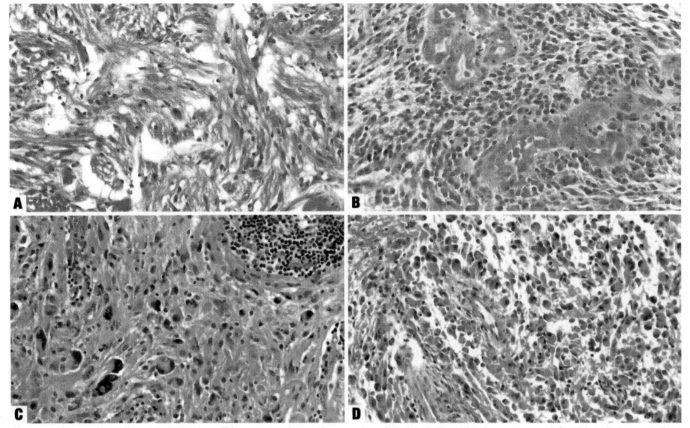

Fig. 2.77 High-grade astrocytoma with piloid features. This tumour type has a wide range of morphologies. **A** About 40% of cases have a mainly piloid morphology, sometimes with numerous Rosenthal fibres. **B** About 45% of cases show a mainly glioblastoma-like morphology. **C** About 10% of cases have features reminiscent of pleomorphic xanthoastrocytoma. **D** Tumours may rarely resemble epithelioid glioblastoma.

or *CDKN2B*, other chromosomal alterations that are recurrently seen and might play pathogenetic roles include partial gains of chromosome arms 12q and 17q (in ~30% of cases each), losses of 1p and 8p (in ~20% of cases each), and partial losses of chromosomes 14 and 19q (in ~20% of cases each) {2643}.

Macroscopic appearance

Macroscopic or imaging features specific for HGAP have not been reported. Some tumours may have areas of central necrosis mimicking glioblastoma.

Histopathology

The histological features of HGAP vary considerably and are not sufficiently distinct to diagnose this glioma type without additional molecular testing. In general, tumours appear as moderately cell-dense and moderately pleomorphic astrocytic gliomas. The growth pattern may resemble that of glioblastoma or pleomorphic xanthoastrocytoma, or the tissue may be enriched for thin, hair-like (piloid) cytoplasmic processes (hence the name "high-grade astrocytoma with piloid features"). In about a third of cases, eosinophilic granular bodies or Rosenthal fibres are observed. Almost 90% show alterations of vasculature, either in the form of hypertrophy and/or multilayering, or as glomeruloid proliferation. One third of the tumours show necrosis (with or without palisading), and about 80% have ≥ 0.42 mitoses/mm² (equating to ≥ 1 mitosis/10 HPF of 0.55 mm in diameter and 0.24 mm² in area).

Areas of solid tumour growth are frequent, but invasive growth into the adjacent parenchyma may also be observed {2643}.

Immunophenotype

A suggestive immunohistochemical marker observed in about 40% of HGAPs is loss of nuclear ATRX expression in the tumour cells, with non-neoplastic cell nuclei remaining ATRX-positive {2643}. IDH1 p.R132H immunohistochemistry is negative. Very rare tumours with expression of the H3 p.K28M (K27M)-mutant protein have been reported, but the definitive classification of these tumours has yet to be established {2643}.

Differential diagnosis

Because of the broad and diagnostically ambiguous spectrum of histological features, a wide range of gliomas represent relevant differential diagnoses, including IDH-wildtype glioblastoma, pleomorphic xanthoastrocytoma (CNS WHO grade 2 or 3), and pilocytic astrocytoma (especially tumours with histological features of anaplasia).

The first study of HGAP demonstrated that in a predominantly adult population, about 80% of tumours histologically considered to be anaplastic pilocytic astrocytomas represented HGAP upon DNA methylation analysis {2643}. In contrast, in a purely paediatric population of anaplastic pilocytic astrocytoma, only 1 (3%) of 31 tumours was molecularly confirmed as HGAP {1040}. It was further shown that about one third of

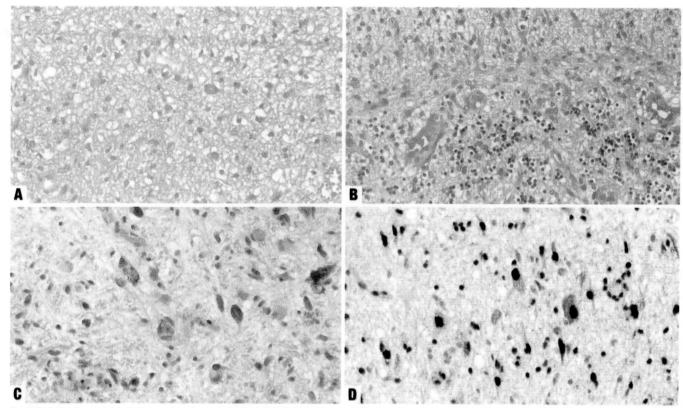

Fig. 2.78 Infiltration patterns of high-grade astrocytoma with piloid features. **A** Sparse infiltration of cerebellar white matter. Note the single pleomorphic cells. **B** Diffuse infiltration of the tumour into the granular layer of the cerebellar cortex. **C** Diffuse infiltration of the tumour into the pons, with residual pigmented neurons of the locus coeruleus. **D** ATRX immunohistochemistry of the same case as in C, with nuclear ATRX loss in tumour cells but retained staining in pre-existent cells.

histologically defined cerebellar glioblastomas molecularly represented HGAP {2644}.

Cytology
Not clinically relevant

Diagnostic molecular pathology
Currently, DNA methylation profiling is the only method for definitively establishing a diagnosis of HGAP {2643}. The

molecular class is included in widely used machine learning–based classifiers {460}. A combination of histology with certain genetic markers may be suggestive of the diagnosis but may not clearly distinguish these tumours from other gliomas such as pleomorphic xanthoastrocytoma or glioblastoma.

A variety of MAPK pathway gene alterations have been reported {1040,2643}, the most frequent being *NF1* alterations, *KIAA1549::BRAF* fusions, and *FGFR1* mutations (Table 2.04). In one tumour, an *NF1* alteration was combined with an *FGFR1*

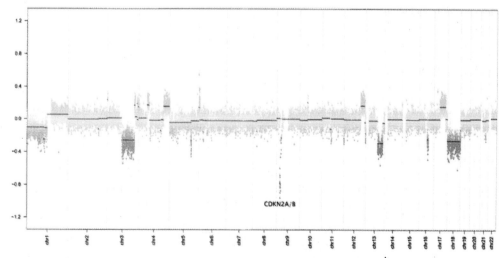

Fig. 2.79 High-grade astrocytoma with piloid features. The DNA copy-number profile of this case shows, among other changes, several chromosomal alterations that recurrently occur in this tumour type: homozygous deletion of *CDKN2A* and/or *CDKN2B* (observed in close to 80%), partial gain of 12q and 17q (each in ~30%), and 1p loss (in ~20%).

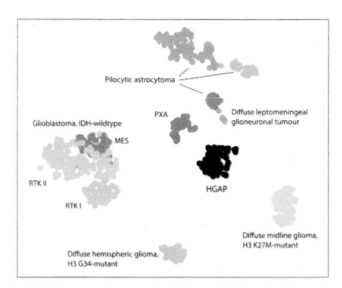

Fig. 2.80 High-grade astrocytoma with piloid features (HGAP) is defined by a specific DNA methylation profile. t-distributed stochastic neighbour embedding (t-SNE) of DNA methylation data of HGAP and several relevant differential diagnoses. HGAP forms a distinct molecular group. Data combined from {460} and {2643}. MES, mesenchymal; PXA, pleomorphic xanthoastrocytoma; RTK, receptor tyrosine kinase.

Table 2.04 Frequency of MAPK alterations detected to date in high-grade astrocytoma with piloid features

Type of MAPK alteration	Frequency
NF1 mutation[a]	19%
NF1 heterozygous deletion[a]	12%
KIAA1549::BRAF fusion	20%
BRAF p.V600E mutation	1%
FGFR1 p.K656E/N or p.N546D/K mutation	17%
FGFR1::TACC1 fusion	2%
KRAS mutation	3%

[a]Three cases had both an *NF1* mutation and an *NF1* heterozygous deletion.
Data from Reinhardt et al. {2643}.

mutation, but MAPK pathway gene mutations otherwise occur in a mutually exclusive fashion {2643}. The rate of occurrence of *BRAF* p.V600E is notably low, and the overall frequencies of reported MAPK pathway gene alterations are remarkably different from those of pleomorphic xanthoastrocytoma and pilocytic astrocytoma.

In one study of 74 cases, homozygous deletion (or, very rarely, mutation) of *CDKN2A* and/or *CDKN2B* occurred in about 80% of tumours {2643}. Alternatively, *CDK4* amplifications were

Box 2.13 Diagnostic criteria for high-grade astrocytoma with piloid features

Essential:

An astrocytic glioma

AND

A DNA methylation profile of high-grade astrocytoma with piloid features

Desirable:

MAPK pathway gene alteration

Homozygous deletion or mutation of *CDKN2A* and/or *CDKN2B*, or amplification of *CDK4*

Mutation of *ATRX* or loss of nuclear ATRX expression

Anaplastic histological features

observed in some cases {2643}. *ATRX* mutations and/or loss of ATRX expression was observed in 33 (45%) of cases. In rare instances without *ATRX* alteration, *TERT* promoter mutations were detected (2 [3%] of 74, both p.C228T mutations) {2643}. In 2 (3%) of the 74 tumours, H3 p.K28M (K27M) mutations were identified, but the definitive classification of these tumours has yet to be established {2643}.

Essential and desirable diagnostic criteria
See Box 2.13.

Staging
Not established

Prognosis and prediction
Prognostic data on patients diagnosed with HGAP are, to date, only available from a single retrospective study {2643}. In this study, the 5-year overall survival rate of patients diagnosed with HGAP was approximately 50%. Overall survival was shorter than that of patients with conventional pilocytic astrocytoma (CNS WHO grade 1) and IDH-mutant astrocytoma (CNS WHO grade 3), longer than that of patients with IDH-wildtype glioblastoma, and approximately comparable to that of patients with IDH-mutant astrocytoma (CNS WHO grade 4) {2643}. Associations of prognosis and histological features were not identified, and fatal outcomes were also seen in patients whose tumours lacked necrosis (8 of 28 patients died within 2 years of diagnosis) or lacked mitoses (3 of 10 patients died within 2 years). A methylated *MGMT* promoter was reported in 46% of HGAPs, without a statistical association with patient outcome; however, information on treatment of the patients by alkylating agent chemotherapy was not available {2643}. More data are required for assignment of a definitive CNS WHO grade, but current data suggest a clinical behaviour roughly corresponding to CNS WHO grade 3.

Pleomorphic xanthoastrocytoma

Giannini C
Capper D
Figarella-Branger D
Jacques TS

Jones DTW
Louis DN
Paulus W
Tabori U

Definition

Pleomorphic xanthoastrocytoma (PXA) is an astrocytoma with large pleomorphic (frequently multinucleated) cells, spindle cells, and lipidized cells, often with numerous eosinophilic granular bodies and reticulin deposition, and characteristically with *BRAF* p.V600E mutation (or other MAPK pathway gene alterations) and homozygous *CDKN2A* and/or *CDKN2B* deletion (CNS WHO grade 2 or 3).

ICD-O coding

9424/3 Pleomorphic xanthoastrocytoma

ICD-11 coding

2A00.0Y & XH99U2 Other specified gliomas of brain & Pleomorphic xanthoastrocytoma

Related terminology

Not recommended: pleomorphic xanthoastrocytoma with anaplastic features; anaplastic pleomorphic xanthoastrocytoma (for CNS WHO grade 3).

Subtype(s)

None

Localization

A superficial location involving the leptomeninges and cerebrum is typical. The majority of tumours (98%) occur supratentorially, most often in the temporal lobe {1400}. PXAs involving the cerebellum and spinal cord have been reported {1106,2202}, as well as 2 childhood cases in the retina {3582}.

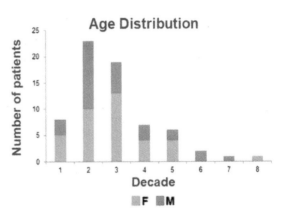

Fig. 2.81 Pleomorphic xanthoastrocytoma. Age and sex distribution in a recent series of 67 patients {3299}.

Clinical features

Many patients present with a long history of seizures. Cerebellar and spinal cord tumours have symptoms reflecting these sites of involvement. In cases with deep localization (e.g. brainstem) and/or wider infiltration, gross total resection cannot be achieved.

Imaging

On imaging, PXA is usually peripherally located and frequently cystic, involving the cerebral cortex and overlying leptomeninges. On CT, the tumour appearance is variable (hypodense, hyperdense, or mixed), with strong, sometimes heterogeneous, contrast enhancement {2337}. The tumour cysts are hypodense. On MRI, the solid portion of the tumour is either hypointense

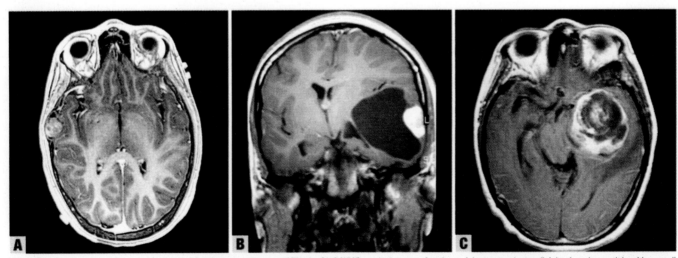

Fig. 2.82 Pleomorphic xanthoastrocytoma. **A** T1-weighted postcontrast MRI of a CNS WHO grade 2 tumour forming a right temporal superficial enhancing nodule with a small cystic component and scalloping of the bone. **B** T1-weighted postcontrast MRI of a CNS WHO grade 2 tumour showing a superficial enhancing mural nodule and a large cyst causing moderate midline shift. **C** T1-weighted postcontrast MRI of a CNS WHO grade 3 tumour forming a large, heterogeneously enhancing tumour with moderate surrounding oedema mass effect.

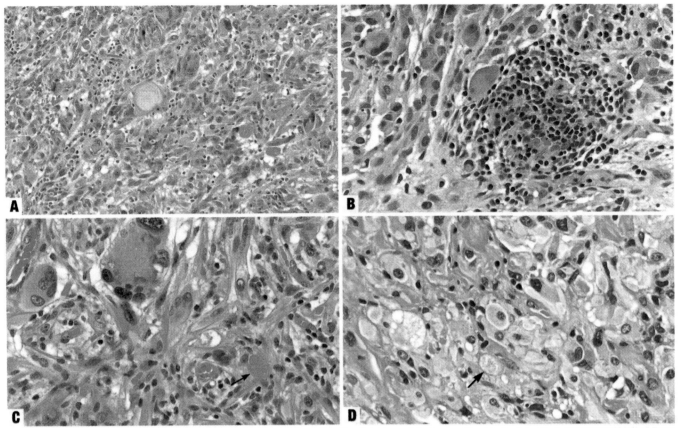

Fig. 2.83 Pleomorphic xanthoastrocytoma, classic histology. **A** Pleomorphic xanthoastrocytoma is a cellular tumour with marked cellular pleomorphism that is apparent even at low power. **B** Perivascular lymphocytic cuffing is common. **C** Tumour cells show marked cytoplasmic and nuclear pleomorphism with frequent intensely eosinophilic granular bodies (arrow). **D** There are frequent pale granular bodies (arrow) and cytoplasmic vacuolation with xanthomatous cells.

or isointense to grey matter on T1-weighted images and shows a hyperintense or mixed signal on T2-weighted and FLAIR images, whereas the cystic component is isointense to cerebrospinal fluid. Postcontrast enhancement is moderate or strong {2337}. Adjacent oedema is usually not pronounced.

Epidemiology

PXA accounts for < 0.3% of primary CNS tumours, with an annual incidence of < 0.7 cases per 100 000 population

{2344}. It occurs equally in male and female patients and typically develops in children and young adults {1092}. Mean age at diagnosis is 26.3 years (median: 20.5 years) {2460}. However, older patients (up to the eighth decade of life) may be affected {2460}. There are few data on the relative prevalence of CNS WHO grade 2 versus CNS WHO grade 3 tumours, but in one series, anaplasia was present in 31% of cases at first diagnosis (in 23% of paediatric patients and 37% of adult patients) {1400}.

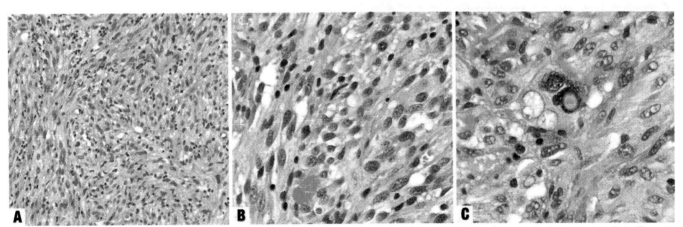

Fig. 2.84 Pleomorphic xanthoastrocytoma, spindle cell histology. Some tumours have a predominant cellular and spindle appearance with relative monomorphism (**A**), or with only rare eosinophilic granular bodies (**B**), or with large pleomorphic cells (**C**).

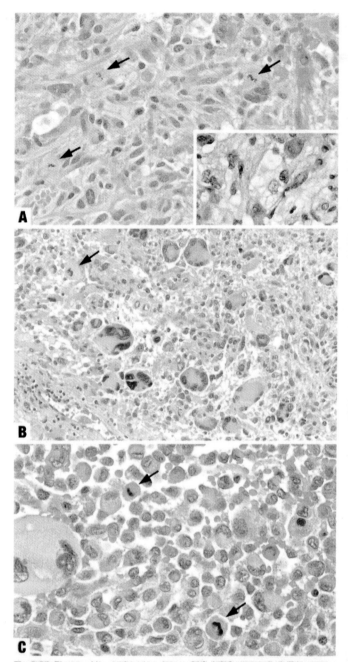

Fig. 2.85 Pleomorphic xanthoastrocytoma, CNS WHO grade 3. **A** This tumour shows classic features, with pleomorphic and xanthomatous cells (inset) and brisk mitotic activity (arrows). The tumour recurred 1 year later and showed remaining areas with pleomorphic morphology (**B**), transitioning to monomorphic areas with epithelioid and rhabdoid morphology (**C**).

Etiology

No specific etiology is known. PXA may be encountered in patients with neurofibromatosis type 1 {2560,20,1747,2224, 2359}, which is in keeping with the high frequency of MAPK pathway gene alterations in PXA. Rare cases have been reported in DiGeorge syndrome {2177}, familial melanoma-astrocytoma syndrome (with *CDKN2A* inactivation) {507}, Down syndrome {2484}, and Sturge–Weber syndrome {1612}.

Pathogenesis

It has been proposed that PXA originates from subpial astrocytes {1595}. This hypothesis would explain the superficial location of most tumours, and it is supported by the fact that subpial astrocytes and tumour cells in PXA have the same ultrastructural features.

PXA typically carries alterations in genes encoding members of the MAPK pathway (most frequently *BRAF* p.V600E mutation) combined with homozygous deletion of the tumour suppressor genes *CDKN2A* and/or *CDKN2B* at 9p21.3 {2499,3621,3098, 3299,2842,1680,3300,1361}. PXA may carry *TERT* promoter mutations or (less frequently) amplifications, and these *TERT* alterations may be more common in tumours with anaplasia {1678,1962,2499,3299}. *TP53* mutations are rare in PXAs {1090,1573,2430,2499}. Alterations in other genes (including *SMARCB1, BCOR, BCORL1, ARID1A, ATRX, PTEN, FANCA, FANCD2, FANCI, FANCM, PRKDC, NOTCH2, NOTCH3, NOTCH4,* and *BCL6* {2499,3299,3300}) have been described, but their pathogenetic significance is uncertain.

Macroscopic appearance

PXAs are sometimes yellow (from lipidization), partially cystic, superficial cortical masses, although their gross appearance may be nonspecific. They may extend into the adjacent leptomeninges.

Histopathology

PXA typically demonstrates a mostly solid, non-infiltrative growth pattern, although microscopic invasion at the periphery is common. Tumours are composed of a mixture of spindled, epithelioid, pleomorphic, and multinucleated astrocytes that are sometimes filled with lipid droplets (xanthomatous cells). Intranuclear pseudoinclusions, prominent nucleoli, and lymphocytic infiltration are frequent {1092}. Granular bodies, both pale and brightly eosinophilic, are characteristic {1092}. Reticulin fibres surrounding individual tumour cells are mainly encountered in leptomeningeal areas. Most PXAs have low mitotic activity. Anaplasia manifests as brisk mitotic activity, either focally or diffusely, and occurs at first diagnosis or at recurrence. Necrosis is frequent as well, whereas microvascular proliferation is uncommon {1092}. CNS WHO grade 3 PXAs may demonstrate less pleomorphism and a more diffusely infiltrative pattern than their grade 2 counterparts. Among the common cytological patterns of anaplasia, small cell, fibrillary, and epithelioid/rhabdoid subtypes have been reported {3300}.

Grading

CNS WHO grade 2 is assigned to tumours with < 2.5 mitoses/ mm² (equating to < 5 mitoses/10 HPF of 0.23 mm² in area and 0.54 mm in diameter). Tumours showing ≥ 2.5 mitoses/mm² (equating to ≥ 5 mitoses/10 HPF of 0.23 mm² in area and 0.54 mm in diameter) are CNS WHO grade 3 {1400,3300}. Necrosis is almost always seen in tumours with high mitotic activity, and its significance in isolation, if any, is indeterminate at present. In CNS WHO grade 3 tumours, a mean Ki-67 labelling index of 15% has been reported {2499}, whereas it is generally < 1% in CNS WHO grade 2 tumours {1092}. CNS WHO grade 3 tumours may occur de novo or at recurrence of a PXA that was initially CNS WHO grade 2 {3300}.

Immunophenotype

PXAs typically express GFAP and S100 {1092,1094,1314}. S100 is often diffusely positive, whereas at least focal positivity for GFAP is common. Most tumours are positive for CD34 {2635} and focally express neuronal markers (synaptophysin, neurofilament, class III β-tubulin, and MAP2) {1094,2548}, although the positive cells do not resemble neurons. BRAF p.V600E expression (VE1 antibody) is present in 60–80% of PXAs {1401, 2842,1680,3300,2499}. Focal SMARCB1 (INI1) loss has been reported in rare cases that transformed into malignant neoplasms resembling atypical teratoid/rhabdoid tumours {3300, 2268}.

Differential diagnosis

The most frequent differential diagnosis is ganglioglioma, which can have a glial component resembling PXA. Rare cases of composite tumours have also been reported {1706,2468}. Both PXA and ganglioglioma exhibit accumulation of eosinophilic granular bodies, lymphocytic infiltration, CD34 expression, and BRAF p.V600E; however, true ganglion cells are usually absent in PXA. Given this overlap, the diagnosis of ganglioglioma should be regarded with caution in cases with homozygous deletion of *CDKN2A* and/or *CDKN2B*.

PXA should be distinguished from giant cell glioblastoma, with which it shares the features of gross circumscription, reticulin deposition, marked pleomorphism, multinucleated giant cells, and lymphocytic infiltration. However, the immunophenotype – in particular p53 and neuronal antigen expression {2023} – and the molecular profile are markedly different (see *Glioblastoma, IDH-wildtype*, p. 39).

In cases showing a dominant population of epithelioid cells and frank anaplasia, especially in the absence of a history of a CNS WHO grade 2 PXA, the main differential diagnosis is epithelioid glioblastoma, because these tumours often carry a *BRAF* p.V600E mutation. Approximately 60% of epithelioid glioblastomas (the PXA-like epithelioid glioblastoma subset) were shown to cluster by methylation profiling with canonical PXAs {1716}. These tumours frequently carried a *BRAF* p.V600E mutation (79%), *CDKN2A* homozygous deletion (61%), and *TERT* promoter mutations (30%); they lacked oncogene amplifications and showed a low frequency of 10q loss. Although such tumours have a more favourable outcome than typical IDH-wildtype glioblastomas, it is unclear whether they are truly equivalent to PXA and will have similar outcomes.

Cytology

Intraoperative smears show a variable population of pleomorphic and spindled neoplastic cells with fibrillary processes {1475}. Large, bizarre cells with binucleation or trinucleation are common, whereas cells with cytoplasmic microvacuoles consistent with lipidized astrocytes are rare.

Diagnostic molecular pathology

MAPK pathway gene alterations

Essentially all PXAs harbour genetic alterations in a MAPK pathway gene causing aberrant activation of this pathway. By far the most frequent alteration is *BRAF* p.V600E (accounting for ~60% of cases in previous series {2842,756} and as many as 80% in combined data from two recent studies {2499,3299}). In most cases, this missense mutation is detectable using

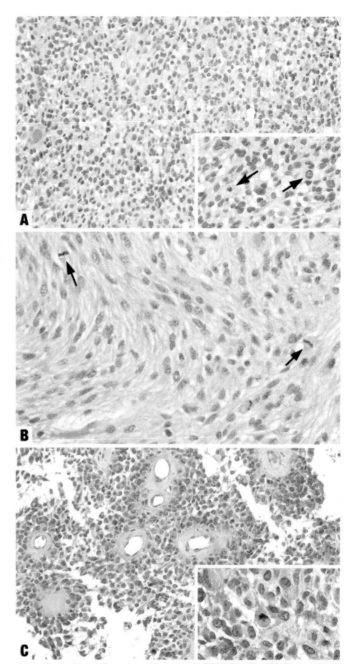

Fig. 2.86 Pleomorphic xanthoastrocytoma, CNS WHO grade 3. Additional patterns of anaplasia include monomorphic small cells (**A**) showing brisk mitoses (**inset**, arrows), fibrillary morphology showing brisk mitoses (**B**, arrows), and a pseudopapillary pattern (**C**) showing brisk mitoses (**inset**).

immunohistochemistry {1231}. Tumours without *BRAF* p.V600E mutation can harbour a wide variety of alternative MAPK pathway gene alterations, mostly affecting *BRAF* (non-p.V600E mutations, non–*KIAA1549::BRAF* fusions), *NTRK1*, *NTRK2*, *NTRK3*, *RAF1*, and *NF1*, and possibly additional genes. The frequency of *BRAF* mutation is unrelated to CNS WHO grade or elevated mitotic activity {2842,3300}.

CDKN2A and/or CDKN2B homozygous deletion

As many as 94% of PXAs harbour alterations of *CDKN2A* and/or *CDKN2B*, in most cases in the form of homozygous deletion

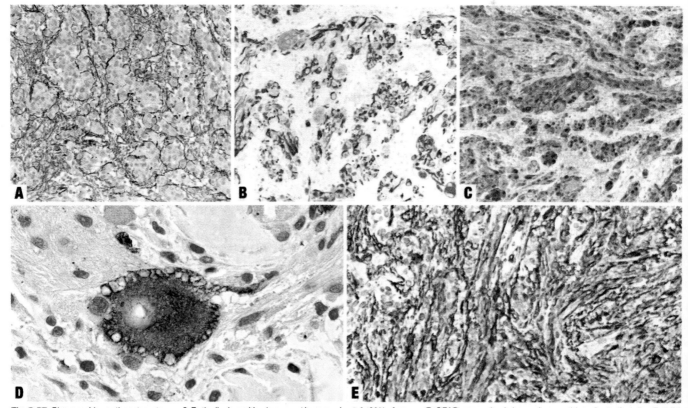

Fig. 2.87 Pleomorphic xanthoastrocytoma. **A** Reticulin deposition is present in approximately 60% of cases. **B** GFAP expression in large pleomorphic and spindle cells. **C** S100 is typically diffusely positive. **D** Neuronal markers are often expressed, in particular synaptophysin, shown here in a large pleomorphic and vacuolated tumour cell. **E** CD34 positivity is frequent but variable.

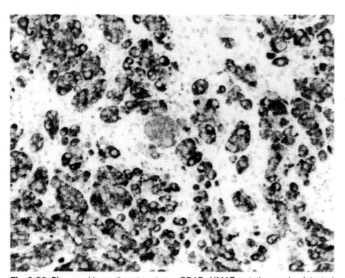

Fig. 2.88 Pleomorphic xanthoastrocytoma. *BRAF* p.V600E mutation can be detected by immunostaining.

{2499,3299}. In one study, 18 of 19 tumours showed homozygous *CDKN2A* and/or *CDKN2B* deletions, and the remaining tumour showed loss of protein expression, indicating that inactivation of *CDKN2A* and/or *CDKN2B* may be even more prevalent than previously thought, and possibly a defining molecular alteration of PXA {2499}. The combination of *BRAF* p.V600E mutation and *CDKN2A* and/or *CDKN2B* homozygous deletion

is highly suggestive of a diagnosis of PXA, although other rare examples of gangliogliomas, epithelioid glioblastomas, and high-grade astrocytomas with piloid features have also been reported to have this molecular constellation {2444,1716,2200, 2643}.

TERT alterations
TERT promoter mutation and (less frequently) *TERT* amplification have been identified in PXA in varying proportions; they are more common in anaplastic tumours than in other PXAs {1678, 1962,2499,3299}.

DNA methylation profiling
A DNA methylation profile for PXA has been reported {460}, which may be particularly useful in tumours with ambiguous morphology, but it is largely confirmatory in those with classic histology {463,3299}. Tumours with a methylation profile of PXA (and harbouring combined *BRAF* p.V600E mutation and *CDKN2A* and/or *CDKN2B* deletion) can be identified in substantial numbers among histological series of paediatric glioblastomas {1721,460}, epithelioid glioblastomas {1716,71}, and astroblastomas {317,1848,3474}, as well as in occasional embryonal tumours {3059}, gangliogliomas {460}, and atypical teratoid/rhabdoid tumours {460}. Although it has been suggested that the morphological spectrum of molecularly defined PXA could therefore be substantially wider than previously thought, further studies are required before a conclusion can be drawn regarding the definitive classification of such cases {463}.

Essential and desirable diagnostic criteria

See Box 2.14.

Staging

In contrast to most other types of circumscribed gliomas, PXAs tend to disseminate during tumour progression. MRI of the spine is recommended at the time of clinical progression.

Prognosis and prediction

PXA behaves in a less malignant fashion than might be suggested by its highly pleomorphic histology {1595}, but it frequently recurs and is associated with decreased survival compared with other CNS WHO grade 1 or grade 2 gliomas in children and young adults, in particular pilocytic astrocytoma. Furthermore, malignant progression is more common in PXA than in other RAS/MAPK-driven CNS WHO grade 1 or grade 2 gliomas {1400}. Upon progression, survival is markedly reduced, even with currently available therapy {2023,2127,2768}.

Extent of resection is the most significant prognostic factor associated with recurrence {1092,1400}. A consistent relationship has emerged between mitotic activity and outcome, and on this basis, tumours are divided into CNS WHO grades 2 and 3 {1092,1400}. In a retrospective series of 74 patients with PXA, the 5-year recurrence-free survival rates were 70.9% for patients with grade 2 tumours and 48.9% for those with grade 3 tumours ($P = 0.092$). The 5-year overall survival rate of patients with grade 2 tumours was also significantly higher than that of patients with grade 3 tumours (90.4% vs 57.1%, $P = 0.0003$). Tumour necrosis was significantly associated with lower 5-year overall survival rates (42.2% when present vs 90.2% when absent, $P = 0.0002$). But the dataset was too small to detect a difference in survival between patients whose tumours had high mitotic counts and necrosis versus those with only necrosis {1400}.

The prognostic significance of CNS WHO grading of PXA has recently been confirmed in two large independent studies {1004,3299}. When cases that clustered with "methylation cluster PXA" by DNA methylation profiling {460} were stratified by tumour grade, the prognostic value of grade was still significant {3299}. MAPK pathway gene aberrations, in particular BRAF p.V600E, as well as homozygous deletion of *CDKN2A* and/or *CDKN2B*, are central to the underlying genetics of PXA but are not associated with tumour grade or prognosis {3300, 3299}. Response to targeted BRAF p.V600E therapy, however, is not hampered by the presence of *CDKN2A* and/or *CDKN2B*

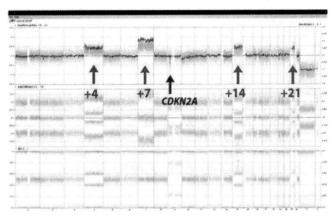

Fig. 2.89 Pleomorphic xanthoastrocytoma. Chromosomal microarray. Typical copy-number profile, demonstrating copy-neutral loss of heterozygosity of chromosome 9 with homozygous deletion of *CDKN2A* and/or *CDKN2B*. Additional whole-chromosome gains were present, including gains of chromosomes 4, 14, and 21 (three copies) and chromosome 7 (four copies).

homozygous deletion {1004}. *TERT* promoter alterations may be linked with a more aggressive phenotype and have been proposed as a marker of anaplastic transformation {2499,1353, 3299}.

Because CNS WHO grade 2 PXA tends to recur, disseminate, and progress to higher-grade PXA, early intervention with complete surgical resection is critical and may be followed by a watch-and-wait strategy after gross total resection {3417}. Patients with CNS WHO grade 3 PXA should be managed with additional therapy (adults probably with postoperative radiotherapy) {3417}. Targeted therapies are important to consider for patients, especially when gross total removal cannot be achieved, even while their tumours are still lower-grade.

Subependymal giant cell astrocytoma

Lopes MBS
Cotter JA
Rodriguez FJ
Santosh V
Sharma MC
Stemmer-Rachamimov AO

Definition

Subependymal giant cell astrocytoma (SEGA) is a periventricular tumour composed partly of large ganglion-like astrocytes, and strongly associated with tuberous sclerosis (TS) (CNS WHO grade 1).

ICD-O coding

9384/1 Subependymal giant cell astrocytoma

ICD-11 coding

2A00.0Y & XH1L48 Other specified gliomas of brain & Subependymal giant cell astrocytoma

Related terminology

Not recommended: subependymal giant cell tumour.

Subtype(s)

None

Localization

SEGAs typically arise from the subependymal tissue of the lateral ventricles adjacent to the foramen of Monro. Rare locations include the third ventricle {1925,2896} and the retina {2378}.

Clinical features

Most patients present with signs and symptoms of increased intracranial pressure. Tumour growth at the foramen of Monro can block cerebrospinal fluid circulation, leading to obstructive hydrocephalus {1127}. Massive spontaneous haemorrhage may be an acute manifestation {2731}. With the current practice of early screening of patients with TS, SEGAs may be diagnosed while still clinically asymptomatic {1745,2731}. Growth of subependymal nodule(s) (SENs) into a SEGA is usually a gradual process, which occurs at the highest rate in the first two decades of life {1127}. Marked growth in < 12 months has rarely been reported {2189}.

Imaging

On CT, SEGAs appear as solid, partially calcified masses located in the walls of the lateral ventricles, mostly near the foramen of Monro. Ipsilateral or bilateral ventricular enlargement may be apparent. On MRI, the tumours are usually heterogeneous, isointense, or slightly hypointense on T1-weighted images, and hyperintense on T2-weighted images, with marked contrast enhancement {1413}. Prominent signal voids, representing dilated vessels, are occasionally seen. SEGAs may show a high choline-to-creatinine ratio and a low ratio of N-acetylaspartate to creatinine on proton magnetic resonance spectroscopy, which seems to be a valuable tool for the early detection of neoplastic transformation of SEN to SEGA {2517}.

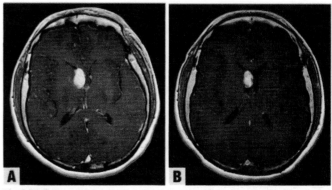

Fig. 2.90 Subependymal giant cell astrocytoma, postcontrast axial T1-weighted MRI. **A** A right subependymal giant cell astrocytoma near the foramen of Monro, with avid enhancement. **B** After 3 months of treatment with an mTOR inhibitor, the tumour shows decreased size and enhancement.

Spread

Leptomeningeal dissemination with drop metastases is rare, having been described only in two cases {3162,34}.

Epidemiology

Incidence

SEGA is the most common CNS neoplasm in patients with TS {37,2286,2731}. The incidence rate of SEGA among patients with TS is 5–15% {37,2286,2731}, and the tumour is one of the major diagnostic criteria of TS {2286}. The calculated overall incidence of SEGAs in the US Surveillance, Epidemiology, and End Results Program (SEER) 18 database is 0.027 cases per 100 000 person-years {2245}. It is uncertain whether the tumour also occurs outside the setting of TS or if it harbours currently undetectable TSC gene alterations {2286}.

Age and sex distribution

This tumour typically occurs during the first two decades of life and only infrequently arises de novo after the age of 20–25 years {2286}. SEGA can occur in infants, and several congenital cases diagnosed at birth or by antenatal MRI have been reported {1385,2061,2494,2608}.

Etiology

SEGA has a strong association with inherited TS (see *Tuberous sclerosis*, p. 441).

Pathogenesis

Evidence of biallelic inactivation of the *TSC1* or *TSC2* gene supports the hypothesis that SEGAs arise as a consequence of a second-hit mechanism {512}. Activation of the mTOR pathway has been shown in SEGAs, and clinical trials have shown reductions in tumour volumes using mTOR inhibitors {978}.

Cell of origin

SEGAs demonstrate glial, neuronal, and mixed neuroglial features (morphological, immunohistochemical, and ultrastructural), suggesting a cell of origin with the capacity to undergo differentiation along glial, neuronal, and neuroendocrine lines {2896,1925}. This hypothesis has been recently supported by data from mouse models in which loss of *Tsc1* or activation of the mTOR pathway in subventricular zone neural progenitor cells resulted in the formation of SEGA- and SEN-like lesions in the lateral ventricle {1984,2529}. SEGA and SEN also have similar histological and radiological features; the main distinction is based on size (SEGAs are ≥ 5 mm, SENs < 5 mm) and growth over time (which occurs only in SEGA). Radiological evidence supports the transition of some (5–15%) SENs into SEGAs over time, suggesting that these tumours represent a continuum {1127,604,327}. Several studies showed nuclear expression of thyroid transcription factor 1 (TTF1, also known as NKX2-1) in SEGAs. Given that TTF1 expression is transiently present in the medial ganglionic eminence in the fetal brain, this suggests a derivation of SEGAs from a regional progenitor cell {1229,1303}.

Genetic profile

SEGAs have a strong association with TS and typically show evidence of biallelic inactivation of *TSC1* (15%) or *TSC2* (56%), with the second hit frequently observed as deletion or loss of heterozygosity {1290,2137,319}. Lost or reduced tuberin and hamartin expression has been described in SEGAs from patients with either *TSC1* or *TSC2* germline mutations {1290,1507,1596,2137}.

Examples of SEGAs in the absence of TS have been reported, but these tumours may harbour currently undetectable TSC gene alterations (e.g. low-level somatic mosaicism or large deletions), or they may have other mechanisms of inactivation {226,319}.

BRAF p.V600E mutations were found in rare SEGAs in two case series {1828,2842}, including two patients with "definite" TS by clinical criteria. However, *BRAF* p.V600E mutations were not identified in a recent larger series of 58 SEGAs {319}. DNA methylation–based classification studies support SEGA as a distinct tumour entity {460}.

Macroscopic appearance

SEGAs are sharply demarcated, multinodular, solid tumours arising from the wall of the lateral ventricle, close to the foramen of Monro. Less frequently, they arise in the third ventricle {1925,2896}. Morphologically similar neoplasms may develop inside the eye in association with the retina in patients with TS, and outside the ventricles sporadically or in patients with TS or neurofibromatosis type 1 {2378}. The tumours show zones of calcification, often with cystic change and foci of haemorrhage.

Histopathology

Histologically, SEGAs are circumscribed, moderately cellular tumours composed of a wide spectrum of glial phenotypes. Typical appearances range from polygonal cells with abundant, glassy cytoplasm to smaller spindle cells and gemistocyte-like cells arranged in sweeping fascicles, sheets, or nests with

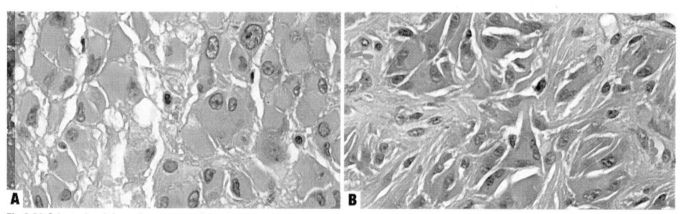

Fig. 2.91 Subependymal giant cell astrocytoma. **A** Large cells with voluminous cytoplasm and well-delineated borders may be present. **B** Elongated cytoplasmic profiles and a more ganglioid appearance may be a feature.

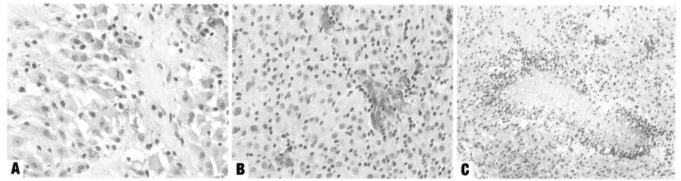

Fig. 2.92 Subependymal giant cell astrocytoma. The CNS WHO grade 1 designation is not changed by mitotic activity (**A**), by the rare presence of microvascular proliferation (**B**), or by necrosis (even if palisading) (**C**).

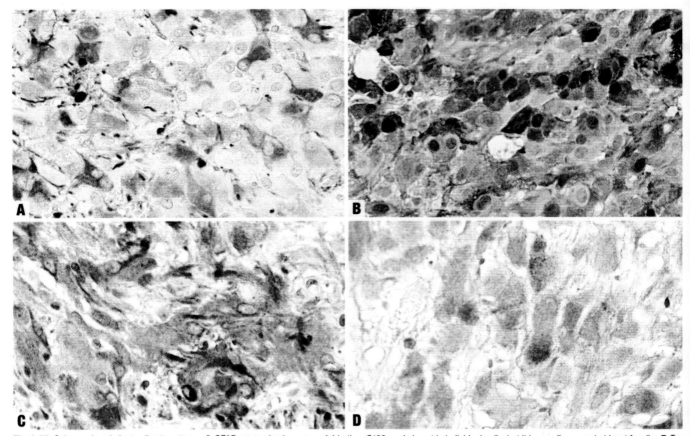

Fig. 2.93 Subependymal giant cell astrocytoma. **A** GFAP expression is more variable than S100, and absent in individual cells, but it is usually present at least focally. **B** Tumours uniformly express S100. **C** Class III β-tubulin (as recognized by TUJ1) is the most ubiquitous neuronal marker in these tumours. **D** Markers of neuronal differentiation, including synaptophysin, are frequently positive in these tumours.

intervening fibrillary septa. Giant pyramidal-like cells with a ganglionic-like appearance (without Nissl substance) are common; these large cells have often eccentric, vesicular nuclei with distinct nucleoli. Nuclear pseudoinclusions can be seen in some cases. Considerable nuclear pleomorphism and multinucleated cells are frequent. Clustering of tumour cells and a perivascular rosette-like pattern resembling that of ependymoma are common features. A rich vascular stroma with frequent hyalinized vessels and infiltration by mast cells and lymphocytes, predominantly T lymphocytes, is a constant feature {2896}. Parenchymal or vascular calcifications are frequently seen {2896,1161,2494}. The presence of mitoses, vascular proliferation, or necrosis does not indicate anaplastic progression {3509}.

Proliferation
The proliferation index as measured by Ki-67 (MIB1) immunostaining is generally low (mean: 3.0%), providing further support for the benign nature of these neoplasms {1205, 2895}. The topoisomerase II labelling index is also reportedly low (mean: 2.9%) {2895}. Although extremely uncommon, craniospinal dissemination has been reported in SEGAs with increased Ki-67 (MIB1) index values but without other malignant features {3162}.

Immunophenotype
SEGA has been designated as a distinctive, well-circumscribed astrocytoma, but because of its usually mixed glioneuronal

phenotype it has also been termed "subependymal giant cell tumour" {1925,398}. Tumour cells demonstrate variable immunoreactivity for GFAP and a uniform and intense immunoreactivity for S100 {1925,3550,2896}. Variable immunoreactivity for neuronal markers and neuropeptides has been detected. Neuron-associated class III β-tubulin appears more widespread in its distribution than any other neuronal epitope, whereas neurofilament is more restricted and mainly highlights cellular processes and a few ganglionic cells {1925}. SEGAs are variably immunoreactive for synaptophysin {2896}, NeuN {3550}, and neuropeptides {1925}. Neural stem cell markers including nestin and SOX2 are also expressed in SEGAs {2494}, but unlike in cortical dysplasias, CD34 immunoreactivity is not seen. Loss of either hamartin or tuberin immunoexpression alone is commonly seen in SEGAs, and rarely a combined loss may be present {2136}. In addition, SEGAs show strong immunoreactivity for phosphorylated S6, consistent with mTOR pathway activation {512}. SEGAs show nuclear immunoreactivity for TTF1, a feature shared by other tumours arising from ventral forebrain structures {1303,1658,277}. This helps differentiate SEGA from its close morphological mimics {1229}, thus widening the spectrum of TTF1-positive CNS tumours.

Ultrastructure
Ultrastructural features of neuronal differentiation, including microtubules, occasional dense-core granules, and (rarely) synapses, may be detectable; bundles of intermediate filaments

are seen in the cytoplasmic processes of the spindled astrocytic cells {1317,1506,398}.

Cytology

Cytological preparations of SEGAs show the diverse cellular elements that constitute the tumours, including elongated spindle-shaped and strap cells with long, thick cell processes to more pleomorphic binucleated or multinucleated cells. The combination of cytological features with clinical and radiological findings can be diagnostic of SEGAs in intraoperative consultations {1449,2213}.

Diagnostic molecular pathology

Molecular analyses are usually not needed to establish the diagnosis of SEGA. In histologically ambiguous cases, DNA methylome profiling and analyses for *TSC1* or *TSC2* alterations may help to establish the diagnosis.

Essential and desirable diagnostic criteria

See Box 2.15.

Staging

Not clinically relevant

Prognosis and prediction

Patients with SEGAs have a favourable prognosis when gross total resection of the tumour is achieved. Larger or symptomatic

Box 2.15 Diagnostic criteria for subependymal giant cell astrocytoma

Essential:

Characteristic histological features, with multiple glial phenotypes including polygonal cells, gemistocyte-like cells, spindle cells, and ganglionic-like cells

AND

Immunoreactivity for glial markers (GFAP, S100)

AND

Variable expression of neuronal markers (class III β-tubulin, neurofilament, synaptophysin, NeuN)

Desirable:

Nuclear immunoexpression of thyroid transcription factor 1 (TTF1)

Lost or reduced expression of tuberin and hamartin

Immunoexpression of phosphorylated S6

DNA methylome profile of subependymal giant cell astrocytoma

History of tuberous sclerosis

TSC1 or *TSC2* mutation

lesions tend to have greater morbidity {713}. Careful follow-up of residual tumour is recommended because of the potential for late recurrences. Optimal outcome is associated with early detection and treatment. In individuals with TS, surveillance by MRI every 1–3 years until the age of 25 years is recommended {713,1745}. Inhibition of mTOR with everolimus has been reported to result in significant reduction of tumour size and control of SEGA progression {976,977,978}.

Chordoid glioma

Fuller GN
Brat DJ
Kleinschmidt-DeMasters BK
Sanson M
Solomon DA

Definition

Chordoid glioma is a well-circumscribed glial neoplasm that arises in the anterior third ventricle, is histologically characterized by clusters and cords of GFAP-expressing epithelioid cells, and exhibits a recurrent p.D463H missense mutation in the *PRKCA* gene (CNS WHO grade 2).

ICD-O coding

9444/1 Chordoid glioma

ICD-11 coding

2A00.0Y & XH9HV1 Other specified gliomas of brain & Chordoid glioma

Related terminology

Not recommended: chordoid glioma of the third ventricle.

Subtype(s)

None

Localization

Chordoid gliomas have a stereotypical location in the anterior portion of the third ventricle, with larger tumours filling the middle and posterior aspects {2533}. They arise in the midline and displace normal structures as they enlarge. Neuroimaging findings suggest an origin in the region of the lamina terminalis in the ventral wall of the third ventricle {1844,2412}.

Clinical features

Presenting signs and symptoms typically reflect obstructive hydrocephalus, with headache, nausea, vomiting, and ataxia {366,743}. Other features may include endocrine abnormalities reflecting hypothalamic compression (hypothyroidism, amenorrhoea, diabetes insipidus); visual field disturbances due to compression of the optic chiasm; and personality changes, psychiatric symptoms, or memory abnormalities.

Imaging

Chordoid gliomas are well-circumscribed ovoid or multilobulated masses within the anterior third ventricle. MRI shows T1 isointensity to brain and strong homogeneous enhancement {2533}. Mass effect is distributed symmetrically, with vasogenic oedema in compressed adjacent CNS structures, including the optic tracts, basal ganglia, and internal capsules. Most tumours are continuous with the hypothalamus; some appear to have an intrinsic anterior hypothalamic component, suggesting a potential site of origin {1844}.

Epidemiology

Chordoid gliomas account for < 0.1% of primary brain tumours. They most frequently occur in adults, with a median age of

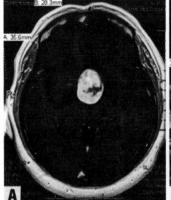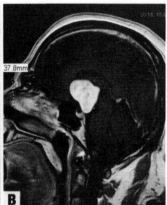

Fig. 2.94 Chordoid glioma. **A** Axial MRI from a tumour in a 67-year-old man shows the typical imaging features of chordoid glioma, including sharp circumscription, large size, contrast enhancement, and compression of nearby structures. **B** Sagittal MRI from the same patient shows the tumour located in the anterior third ventricle. Note the lack of involvement of the pituitary gland, lateral ventricle, and corpus callosum.

approximately 45 years, although age at presentation varies widely (5–71 years). A female predominance has been noted (M:F ratio: 1:2) {366,743,104}.

Etiology

No risk factors or inherited genetic susceptibility have been reported.

Pathogenesis

Two independent studies identified a novel missense mutation affecting codon 463 of the *PRKCA* gene as the molecular hallmark alteration {1139,2726}. *PRKCA* encodes the catalytic α-subunit of PKC, which functions in intracellular signalling downstream of multiple transmembrane receptors. Although *PRKCA* is occasionally mutated in other cancers, this specific p.D463H mutation has not been reported in other human tumour types to date. The mutation results in the substitution of histidine for aspartate at codon 463 within the active site of the kinase domain, where the side chain of aspartate normally functions as the proton acceptor during the ATP hydrolysis reaction. The precise oncogenic mechanisms of this mutation remain to be elucidated, but the mutation may modify substrate specificity or catalytic activity {1139,2726}. High levels of phosphorylated ERK have been found, suggesting that the *PRKCA* p.D463H mutation may function, at least in part, by activating the MAPK signalling pathway {1139}.

Cell of origin

On the basis of anatomical location, consistent immunoreactivity for thyroid transcription factor 1 (TTF1), and ependymoma-like ultrastructural features, chordoid gliomas are hypothesized to originate from specialized tanycytic ependymal cells of the organum vasculosum of the lamina terminalis {497,2412,277}.

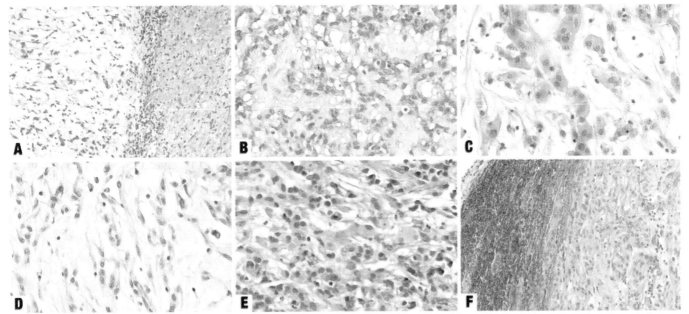

Fig. 2.95 Chordoid glioma. **A** The demarcation between the tumour and adjacent brain tissue is often sharp; individual cell infiltration is not seen. The adjacent brain tissue in this example shows chronic inflammation and numerous Rosenthal fibres. **B** Typical histological appearance of a chordoid glioma composed of cords and clusters of epithelioid tumour cells in a myxoid stroma, resembling the notochordal tumour chordoma. **C** This chordoid glioma is composed of plump epithelioid cells in a prominent myxoid stroma. **D** This chordoid glioma is composed of bipolar spindled cells in a prominent myxoid stroma. **E** The lymphoplasmacytic infiltrates in these tumours can have plasma cells containing eosinophilic small globular Russell bodies. **F** Chordoid glioma demonstrating a dense rim of lymphoplasmacytic inflammation at the periphery of the tumour.

Macroscopic appearance

Chordoid gliomas are well demarcated, often multilobulated, and typically soft, grey, and gelatinous.

Histopathology

Chordoid gliomas are solid neoplasms, most often composed of clusters and cords of epithelioid cells within a variably mucinous stroma. Three less common histological patterns have been reported: a solid pattern with sheets of polygonal epithelioid cells without appreciable mucinous stroma, a fusiform pattern with groups of spindle-shaped cells among loose collagen, and a fibrosing pattern with abundant collagenization. The fibrosing pattern tends to be more common in older patients {277}. Individual tumour cells have abundant eosinophilic cytoplasm. Nuclei are moderate in size, ovoid, and relatively uniform. Mitoses are usually rare or absent. A stromal lymphoplasmacytic infiltrate,

often containing numerous Russell bodies, is a common finding. Consistent with the imaging appearance, there is little tendency for brain infiltration. Reactive astrocytes, Rosenthal fibres, and chronic inflammatory cells may be seen in adjacent non-neoplastic tissue.

Immunophenotype

Chordoid gliomas show strong, diffuse expression of GFAP {366,2800} and consistently express the transcription factor TTF1 (NKX2-1). The percentage and intensity of nuclear TTF1 staining vary depending on the antibody clone used {277}, with rare examples showing minimal to no expression. Expression of vimentin and CD34 is strong. Expression of S100 and EMA is variable. Neuronal and neuroendocrine markers (synaptophysin, neurofilament, chromogranin A) are consistently negative {2639}. The Ki-67 proliferation index is usually < 2% {366}.

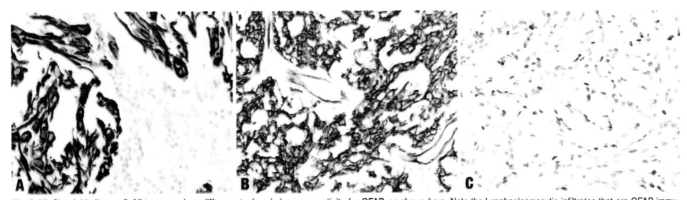

Fig. 2.96 Chordoid glioma. **A** All tumours show diffuse cytoplasmic immunoreactivity for GFAP, as shown here. Note the lymphoplasmacytic infiltrates that are GFAP-immunonegative, shown in the lower right of this image. **B** Strong diffuse cytoplasmic immunostaining for CD34 is typically seen in chordoid glioma. **C** Nuclear positivity for thyroid transcription factor 1 (TTF1, a homeobox transcription factor encoded by the gene *NKX2-1*) is typical of chordoid gliomas.

Differential diagnosis

The principal tumour types in the differential diagnosis are other chordoid neoplasms, including chordoma and chordoid meningioma.

Chordomas can be differentiated based on their consistent expression of brachyury and cytokeratins, with lack of GFAP and CD34 expression.

Chordoid meningiomas usually display small foci of whorl formation and psammoma bodies, and they are immunopositive for EMA and SSTR2A, but negative for GFAP and CD34 {2800}, as well as being negative for TTF1 {1740}.

The differential diagnosis also includes epithelioid haemangioendothelioma, which is composed of cords of cells, sometimes with a myxoid/mucinous background. Although both tumours share immunoreactivity for CD34, epithelioid haemangioendothelioma is additionally positive for CD31, VEGF, and factor VIII, but negative for GFAP {3077}.

Cytology

Not clinically relevant

Diagnostic molecular pathology

The p.D463H missense mutation in the *PRKCA* gene is nearly ubiquitous in chordoid glioma, having been found in 28 of 29 tumours studied to date {1139,2726}. This mutation has not been identified in any other human tumour, although the *PRKCA* gene is involved in fusions in papillary glioneuronal tumour {1354}. Therefore, the *PRKCA* p.D463H mutation is a diagnostic hallmark. Chordoid gliomas have lacked accompanying

pathogenic alterations in genes characteristic of other brain tumour entities (e.g. *IDH1*, *IDH2*, *H3-3A*, *H3C2* [*HIST1H3B*], *FGFR1*, *BRAF*, *NF1*, *CDKN2A*, *TP53*). A distinct epigenetic signature of chordoid glioma has also been identified, and DNA methylation profiling represents an ancillary method for diagnostic confirmation {463}.

Essential and desirable diagnostic criteria

See Box 2.16.

Staging

Not clinically relevant

Prognosis and prediction

Factors impacting morbidity, mortality, and recurrence have not been clearly elucidated. The treatment of chordoid glioma is based on maximal tumour resection while avoiding complications such as diabetes insipidus and other endocrine dysfunctions {104}. Radiotherapy may be considered in patients with subtotal resection, but the benefit is not well established.

Astroblastoma, *MN1*-altered

Brat DJ
Aldape KD
Idbaih A
Kool M

Orr BA
Rosenblum MK
Solomon DA
Sturm D

Definition
Astroblastoma, *MN1*-altered, is a circumscribed glial neoplasm with *MN1* alteration that is composed of round, cuboidal, or columnar cells with variable pseudopapillary or perivascular growth, perivascular anucleate zones, and vascular and pericellular hyalinization.

ICD-O coding
9430/3 Astroblastoma, *MN1*-altered

ICD-11 coding
2A00.4 & XH1DC5 Astroblastoma of the brain & Astroblastoma

Related terminology
Not recommended: CNS high-grade neuroepithelial tumour with *MN1* alteration.

Subtype(s)
None

Localization
Astroblastoma, *MN1*-altered, occurs predominantly in the cerebral hemispheres, most often in the frontal and parietal lobes, but also in occipital and temporal regions {546}. Intraventricular, brainstem, and spinal cord examples have been documented {3512,2914,546}.

Clinical features
Presenting symptoms include headache, seizures, paralysis, nausea, and vomiting {1315,2103}.

Imaging
On MRI, *MN1*-altered astroblastomas are well-demarcated, solid or cystic masses that are isointense or hypointense on T1 imaging and hyperintense on T2 imaging, with heterogeneous contrast enhancement and perilesional oedema {1315,2103}.

Epidemiology
Patient ages range from 3 months to 40 years at clinical presentation (median: 15 years) {546,3512}. These tumours have a striking female predominance, with women accounting for 39 of 41 reported cases included in a recent meta-analysis {546}.

Etiology
Acquired fusions involving the *MN1* gene play a key pathogenic role in this tumour type. There is no known specific genetic susceptibility for *MN1*-altered astroblastoma.

Pathogenesis
Elevated expression of *MN1* fusion partners *BEND2* and *CXXC5* suggests an activating, gain-of-function event {3059}, but the

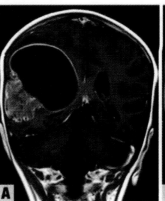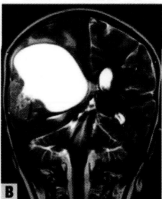

Fig. 2.97 Astroblastoma, *MN1*-altered. Postcontrast, T1-weighted MRI (**A**) and T2-weighted MRI (**B**) show a large, well-demarcated, contrast-enhancing, solid and cystic right temporoparietal mass.

specific mechanism by which *MN1* fusions drive tumour development remains unknown.

Macroscopic appearance
The gross appearance of *MN1*-altered astroblastoma has not been described. Histologically defined astroblastomas are greyish-pink or tan and have well-demarcated borders with adjacent brain. Foci of necrosis or haemorrhage may be present.

Histopathology
The histological hallmark of *MN1*-altered astroblastoma is the astroblastic pseudorosette, a perivascular structuring of neoplastic cells that appear radially arrayed, often forming papillary or pseudopapillary formations in cross-section, and regimented in ribbon-like/trabecular alignment in tangential views {360,3059,3474,1315,1848,2103}. In the classic form, tumour cells are anchored to centrally positioned blood vessels by eosinophilic cytoplasmic processes that are well defined, stout, or only slightly tapered. These lend inverted columnar or low cuboidal profiles to neoplastic elements. Round cell elements may also be found, which may mimic a primitive or embryonal neoplasm in hypercellular regions. Rhabdoid cytology can also be encountered {2914}. Astroblastic pseudorosettes may only focally emerge against a background of sheet-like tumour growth. Spindled cells forming fascicles may be encountered. A typical (though inconstant) and especially prominent feature of *MN1*-altered astroblastomas in some studies {1848} is vascular and stromal sclerosis, which may be limited or extensive, with broad regions of hyalinization containing only remnant tumour cell cords. Circumscription is the rule, with pushing borders or only limited CNS invasion being characteristic. Permeative growth in the manner of diffuse gliomas is not a feature. Mitotic activity is highly variable and some cases exhibit necrosis and microvascular proliferation. Histological features for grading

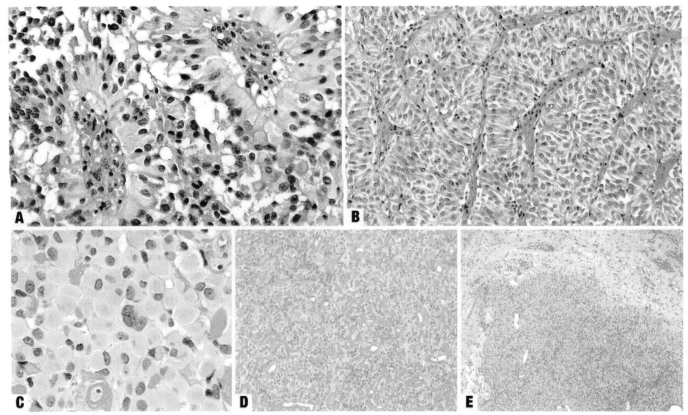

Fig. 2.98 Astroblastoma, *MN1*-altered. **A** The histological hallmark is the astroblastic rosette, characterized by radially oriented tumour cells with elongate, stout processes and distally located nuclei extending to a central vascular structure. **B** A ribbon-like or trabecular pattern is noted when elongated tumour cells oriented to central blood vessels are seen in cross-section. **C** This tumour included focal rhabdoid cytological features. **D** Perivascular and pericellular hyalinization is typical but varies considerably in its severity and extent. **E** Note the sharp demarcation from adjacent brain parenchyma.

have not been clearly defined and a definitive CNS WHO grade has not been established for *MN1*-altered astroblastoma.

Electron microscopy

An ultrastructural study of an *MN1*-altered astroblastoma revealed intercellular lumina containing microvilli and framed by elongated, zonula adherens–type cytoplasmic junctions {2914}. Such features have also been noted in histologically defined

astroblastomas, as have cell body polarization with investing basement membranes, lamellar cytoplasmic interdigitations (pleating), and apical cytoplasmic blebs with purse-string constrictions and capping microvilli {1754,1749}.

Immunophenotype

Cytoplasmic immunoreactivity for GFAP is characteristic, although the extent varies considerably. The large majority

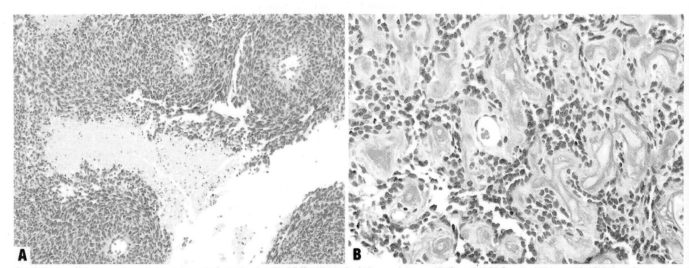

Fig. 2.99 Astroblastoma with primitive cytology. **A** The high cellularity, small round cell cytology, and geographical necrosis in this astroblastoma mimicked an embryonal neoplasm. Molecular testing revealed an *MN1::BEND2* fusion. **B** Other areas of this tumour featured perivascular and stromal sclerosis, more typical of astroblastoma.

of *MN1*-altered astroblastomas display at least focal nuclear OLIG2 expression {3474,1315,1848,2103,3147}. Cytoplasmic EMA labelling is regularly seen but varies in its distribution as diffuse, membranous, dot-like, or ring-like {3474,1315, 2103,3147}. Immunoreactivity for podoplanin (D2-40) is typical {1315}. The *MN1*-altered astroblastomas studied to date were not immunoreactive for L1CAM (a surrogate marker of *ZFTA* [*C11orf95*] fusion–positive ependymomas) {3474,1315}. A broad range of Ki-67 labelling index values has been communicated {360,1315,1848,2103}.

Differential diagnosis

The histological features noted in *MN1*-altered astroblastoma are not entity-specific and may be displayed focally or extensively by other tumours that are proved, on molecular diagnostic assessment, to represent *ZFTA* (*C11orf95*) fusion–positive ependymomas, *BRAF*-mutant epithelioid glioblastomas, *BRAF*-mutant pleomorphic xanthoastrocytomas, embryonal neoplasms, IDH-wildtype glioblastomas, or other gliomas {3474,1848,317,546,3147,3059}. *ZFTA* (*C11orf95*) fusion and *BRAF* mutation are mutually exclusive with *MN1* alterations and do not support a diagnosis of *MN1*-altered astroblastoma. Although a small subset of *MN1*-altered astroblastomas may harbour genetic alterations typical of IDH-wildtype glioblastoma (e.g. *EGFR* amplification, or homozygous deletion involving the *CDKN2A* and/or *CDKN2B* locus), IDH-wildtype glioblastomas are characterized by an infiltrative pattern of growth, distinctive cellular morphology, additional genetic alterations (e.g. *TERT* promoter mutations, gain of chromosome 7, loss of chromosome 10), and an absence of *MN1* alterations. A subset of histologically defined astroblastomas do not share a molecular signature with currently established molecular CNS tumour types {3474}.

Cytology

The intraoperative smear/squash preparation cytology of *MN1*-altered astroblastomas has not been described.

Diagnostic molecular pathology

Astroblastoma, *MN1*-altered, is characterized by structural rearrangements of the *MN1* gene at chromosome band 22q12.1. *MN1* fusions most often occur in-frame with *BEND2* at chromosome band Xp22.13, but other partners (including *CXXC5*) have also been described {3059,3474,2103,1315,1848}. *MN1* alterations can be detected by a variety of methodologies, including FISH, RT-PCR, RNA sequencing, and next-generation DNA sequencing {3059,3474,1315,1848,317}. Although *MN1* fusion is often the solitary pathogenic alteration identified, a subset of *MN1*-altered astroblastomas harbour accompanying *CDKN2A* homozygous deletion {3474,1848}. Recurrent chromosomal copy-number changes in *MN1*-altered astroblastoma include monosomy 16 and partial losses of 22q and X, probably reflecting the chromosomal rearrangement process leading to *MN1::BEND2* fusion {3059,3474,1315,1848}. Individual examples of astroblastoma-like tumours harbouring *EWSR1::BEND2* fusion instead of *MN1::BEND2* in the spinal cord have been reported {3512}. However, the biological nature and clinical outcomes of these rare cases have not been elucidated to date, and the designation "not elsewhere classified (NEC)" is recommended for such tumours at present. *MN1* fusions

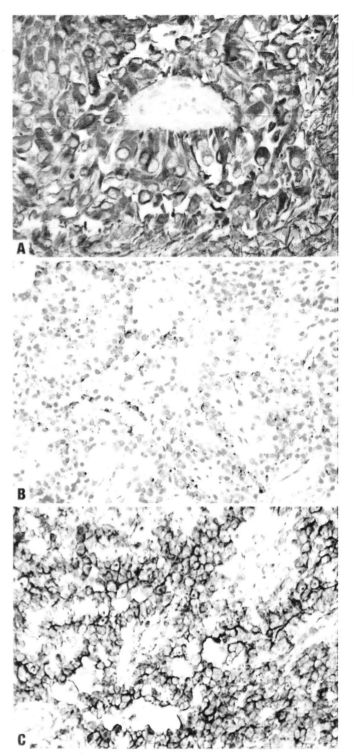

Fig. 2.100 Astroblastoma, *MN1*-altered. **A** Immunohistochemistry for GFAP often shows strong, diffuse immunoreactivity in astroblastoma, *MN1*-altered. **B** Patchy membranous and cytoplasmic dot-like immunostaining for EMA. **C** Membranous and cytoplasmic dot-like D2-40 (podoplanin) staining.

occur in as many as 70% of histologically defined astroblastomas, and > 60% of *MN1* fusion–positive CNS tumours show astroblastoma morphology {3059,3474,2103,1315,1848,546}. *MN1*-altered astroblastomas display a distinct DNA methylation pattern that reliably distinguishes them from other tumour types with astroblastomatous rosettes {3059,3474,1315,460,1848} (see *Differential diagnosis*, above).

Essential and desirable diagnostic criteria
See Box 2.17.

Staging
Not clinically relevant

Prognosis and prediction
Among histologically defined astroblastomas, high-grade histology has been found to be associated with recurrence, tumour progression, and worse prognosis {321,3174}. Outcome data for patients with *MN1*-altered astroblastoma are limited, and the relationship between specific clinical, histological, or molecular features and outcome has not been established. In the few cohorts with molecularly confirmed cases, *MN1*-altered astroblastomas are characterized by frequent local recurrence but good overall survival {3059,3474,1848}. Maximal safe surgery is associated with longer survival {3147}. Considering that the survival rates at 5 years and 10 years are close to 90% and 50%, respectively, conservative management may be warranted {1848,546}. Radiotherapy and chemotherapy seem beneficial when surgery is not feasible {411,2103,2078}. Aside from surgical resection, no additional prognostic factors have been identified {3147}.

Box 2.17 Diagnostic criteria for astroblastoma, *MN1*-altered

Essential:

A glial neoplasm with astroblastic perivascular pseudorosettes

AND

MN1 alteration

AND (for unresolved lesions)

DNA methylation profile of astroblastoma, *MN1*-altered

Desirable:

GFAP immunoreactivity

EMA immunoreactivity

Ganglioglioma

Solomon DA
Blümcke I
Capper D
Gupta K
Varlet P

Definition
Ganglioglioma is a well-differentiated, slow-growing glioneuronal neoplasm composed of a combination of neoplastic ganglion and glial cells, which is molecularly characterized by genetic alterations that cause MAPK pathway activation (CNS WHO grade 1).

ICD-O coding
9505/1 Ganglioglioma

ICD-11 coding
2A00.21 & XH5FJ3 Mixed neuronal-glial tumours & Ganglioglioma, NOS

Related terminology
None

Subtype(s)
None

Localization
These tumours can occur throughout the CNS, including in the cerebrum, brainstem, cerebellum, spinal cord, and optic nerves, as well as within the ventricular system, although the majority (> 70%) occur in the temporal lobes (Table 2.05) {2562, 3467,1801,1316,306}.

Clinical features
The symptoms vary according to tumour size and site. Tumours in the cerebrum are frequently associated with a history of focal seizures, which ranges in duration from 1 month to 50 years before diagnosis (typically 5–10 years) {2562,3467,1801}. For

Table 2.05 Localization of gangliogliomas

Localization	Total cases	Relative frequency
Temporal	604	77%
Frontal	58	7%
Parietal	24	3%
Occipital	22	3%
Multiple lobes	63	8%
Other sites	15	2%

Data from 786 surgical specimens submitted to the German Neuropathology Reference Center for Epilepsy Surgery.

tumours involving the brainstem and spinal cord, the mean duration of symptoms before diagnosis is 1.25 years and 1.4 years, respectively {1801}. Gangliogliomas have been reported in 10–25% of patients undergoing surgery for control of seizures {3177,304}. They are the tumours most commonly associated with chronic temporal lobe epilepsy {297,304}.

Imaging
The neuroimaging appearance of gangliogliomas is variable, but they often display a mix of solid and cystic components. The classic imaging features describe a well-delineated, T1-hypointense, T2-hyperintense cyst, with an enhancing nodule. However, the contrast enhancement pattern is variable. Scalloping of the calvaria may be seen in cortically based tumours. Calcifications may be detected. No imaging characteristics (cystic component, tumour size, contrast enhancement) have been shown to be significantly associated with morphological features or tumour genotype {2444}.

Epidemiology
A population-based study calculated a yearly incidence rate of ganglioglioma of 0.186 cases per 100 000 population worldwide, without significant ethnicity proclivity {677}. Gangliogliomas have been reported in patients ranging from 0 to 70 years of age, most occurring in the first and second decades of life (median age at diagnosis: 12 years) {1802,304}. In a single-centre study, ganglioglioma was more prevalent in male patients (59.8%) than in female patients (40.2%), and there was a similar ratio in the European Epilepsy Brain Bank cohort {799,304}.

Etiology
The vast majority of gangliogliomas are sporadic tumours. However, a small subset (< 2%) arise in the setting of neurofibromatosis type 1 due to germline mutations or deletions in the *NF1* tumour suppressor gene {2695,1114,2444}. No known risk factors or environmental exposures have been linked with ganglioglioma.

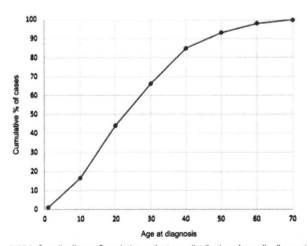

Fig. 2.101 Ganglioglioma. Cumulative patient age distribution of ganglioglioma at diagnosis, based on 887 cases from the German Neuropathology Reference Center for Epilepsy Surgery.

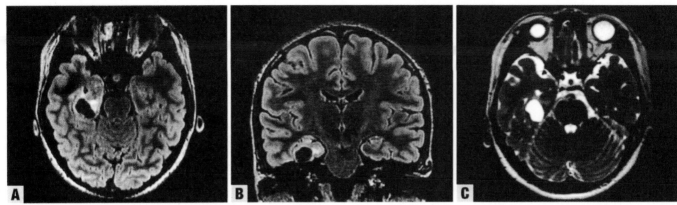

Fig. 2.102 Ganglioglioma. A solid and cystic neoplasm in the temporal lobe of the brain. **A** Axial FLAIR MRI. **B** Coronal FLAIR MRI. **C** Axial T2-weighted MRI.

Pathogenesis

Gangliogliomas result from genetic aberrations causing activation of the MAPK signalling pathway that drives cell proliferation. Most common are p.V600E hotspot mutations in the *BRAF* gene, which lead to the substitution of glutamic acid for valine at amino acid 600 within the P-loop of the serine/threonine kinase domain that causes constitutive activation. *BRAF* p.V600E mutation has been found in gangliogliomas at frequencies ranging from approximately 10% to 60% depending on the study and anatomical site, with the highest frequencies in cortical tumours and the lowest in spinal cord tumours {783,2842,1682, 523,3597,666,2616,780,1190,2584,1066,2368,548,3045,2444, 2768}. In gangliogliomas lacking p.V600E hotspot mutations,

other oncogenic mutations in the *BRAF* gene are often present, including recurrent small in-frame insertions at codon p.R506 in approximately 10% of cases {2444}. *BRAF* gene fusions are recurrently present in gangliogliomas lacking *BRAF* mutations, most commonly with *KIAA1549* as the fusion partner in spinal cord tumours, and with other fusion partners in tumours within the cerebral hemispheres {2444}. Gangliogliomas with wildtype *BRAF* alleles instead display a diverse array of other genetic alterations that similarly cause activation of the MAPK pathway, which include *RAF1* gene fusions, activating *KRAS* mutations, and inactivating *NF1* mutations or deletions {2444}.

The pathogenesis of ganglioglioma was addressed in a transgenic mouse model engineered to express *Braf* p.V600E mutations {1687}. When the mutation was successfully integrated into neuronal cell progenies, 90% of the mice showed spontaneous tonic–clonic seizures, which could be prevented with the small-molecule RAF inhibitor vemurafenib. The tumorigenic properties were mostly due to *Braf* p.V600E integration into the glial cell lineage. These studies experimentally confirmed the long-term observation that tumorigenesis in ganglioglioma is related to the glial component, whereas the epileptogenic phenotype associates with the neuronal component {306}.

Macroscopic appearance

Gangliogliomas are macroscopically well-delineated solid or cystic lesions, usually with little mass effect. Calcification may be observed. Haemorrhage and necrosis are rare.

Histopathology

Gangliogliomas are biphasic tumours composed of a variable admixture of neuronal and glial elements, which may exhibit marked heterogeneity. The two components may be intermixed or geographically separate. The neuronal element is composed of dysmorphic ganglion cells that may demonstrate abnormal clustering, a lack of cytoarchitectural organization, cytomegaly, perimembranous aggregation of Nissl substance, or binucleated forms (seen in < 50% of cases). The glial component, which constitutes the proliferative cell population of the tumour, may resemble fibrillary astrocytoma, oligodendroglioma, or pilocytic astrocytoma {1190,1066,2444}. Eosinophilic granular bodies are encountered more often than Rosenthal fibres {3467, 2444}. Although gangliogliomas are generally well demarcated on imaging, they often demonstrate an infiltrative growth pattern microscopically {1190,297,296,299,2953}. Extension into the

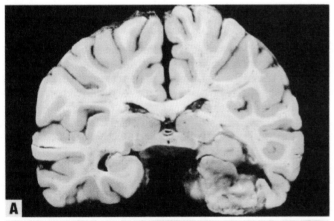

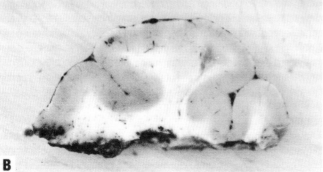

Fig. 2.103 Ganglioglioma. **A** Ganglioglioma of the right medial temporal lobe. Coronal postmortem section. **B** Surgical resection specimen of a ganglioglioma centred in the cerebral hemisphere, demonstrating a discrete mass lesion with a cystic component.

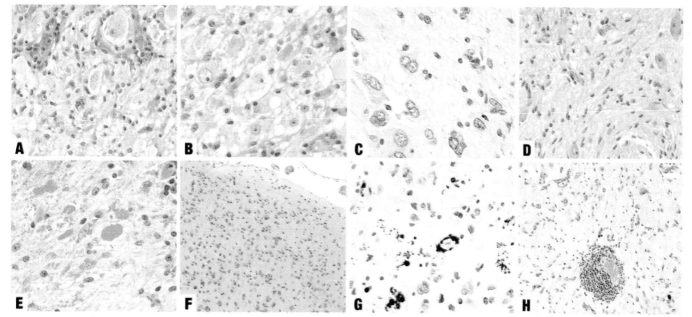

Fig. 2.104 Ganglioglioma. **A** Gangliogliomas are glioneuronal neoplasms composed of an admixture of neoplastic ganglion and glial cells. **B** The neoplastic ganglion cells in this ganglioglioma show abnormal clustering and cytomegaly. **C** The neoplastic ganglion cells in this example demonstrate frequent binucleated forms. **D** The neoplastic glial cells in this ganglioglioma feature astrocytic morphology. **E** Eosinophilic granular bodies are a common finding in gangliogliomas. **F** Despite a well-circumscribed appearance on radiological imaging, gangliogliomas often microscopically permeate into adjacent cerebral cortex. **G** This ganglioglioma shows dystrophic calcification that is encrusting capillaries and neuronal cell bodies. **H** Gangliogliomas frequently demonstrate perivascular lymphoplasmacytic infiltrates.

subarachnoid space is common. Gangliogliomas may uncommonly develop a reticulin fibre network apart from the vasculature (which is a feature more typical of pleomorphic xanthoastrocytoma). Mitotic activity is typically low or absent. Additional histopathological features frequently include dystrophic calcification, either within the matrix or as neuronal/capillary incrustation; extensive lymphoid infiltrates along perivascular spaces; and a prominent capillary network {306}.

Focal cortical dysplasia (FCD) arising in association with ganglioglioma is a frequently reported finding, but it remains controversial whether this actually represents infiltration of ganglioglioma or non-neoplastic dysplasia in most cases {305}. It should be diagnosed only in areas of cortical abnormalities without tumour cell infiltration and classified as FCD type 3b according to the classification proposed by the International League Against Epilepsy (ILAE) {305,200}.

Immunophenotype

Neuronal markers such as MAP2, neurofilament, chromogranin A, and synaptophysin highlight the neuronal component in gangliogliomas {303}. However, to date, there is no specific marker to unequivocally differentiate neoplastic neurons from their normal counterparts. Chromogranin A expression is usually very weak or absent in normal neurons, whereas diffuse and strong expression suggests a neoplastic neuron. Additionally, neoplastic neurons typically have low or absent NeuN expression, in contrast to normal cortical neurons. Immunohistochemistry for GFAP and OLIG2 highlights the neoplastic glial cell component {1316}. As many as 80% of gangliogliomas contain ramified cells either within the tumour or in the adjacent cortex that express the oncofetal epitope CD34, which is not normally expressed outside of vascular endothelial cells in the mature brain {300,306}. Ki-67 labelling is typically low (< 5%)

and usually limited to the glial component {2562,1316}. The VE1 antibody that recognizes BRAF p.V600E-mutant protein can be used with appropriate controls to identify the subset of gangliogliomas that are positive for this genetic alteration {1682}. However, the immunostaining intensity levels are typically lower than those observed in *BRAF*-mutant melanomas and other tumours, and in some gangliogliomas the positivity is most prominent in or exclusively limited to the ganglion cell component {1682}.

Grading

Ganglioglioma is a CNS WHO grade 1 neoplasm. However, gangliogliomas with anaplasia in the glial component (termed "anaplastic ganglioglioma"), with features including conspicuous mitotic activity, high Ki-67 proliferation index, necrosis, and microvascular proliferation, have been reported both at initial presentation and at time of recurrence {2562,1460,1801,1959, 1562,1955,1066,3578,3167}. However, most of these prior studies lacked molecular analysis to exclude other high-grade glioma subtypes. Further studies are needed to confirm the existence of anaplastic ganglioglioma and establish its diagnostic criteria.

Differential diagnosis

The diagnosis of ganglioglioma requires the histological identification of a neuronal component, but the near-normal morphology of the neuronal component in some cases remains a challenging issue because there is no specific marker protein for differentiating the neoplastic ganglion cells from native neurons. The diagnosis of ganglioglioma should be considered in all cases of low-grade neuroepithelial tumours associated with focal seizures that are difficult to classify, especially when located in the temporal lobe.

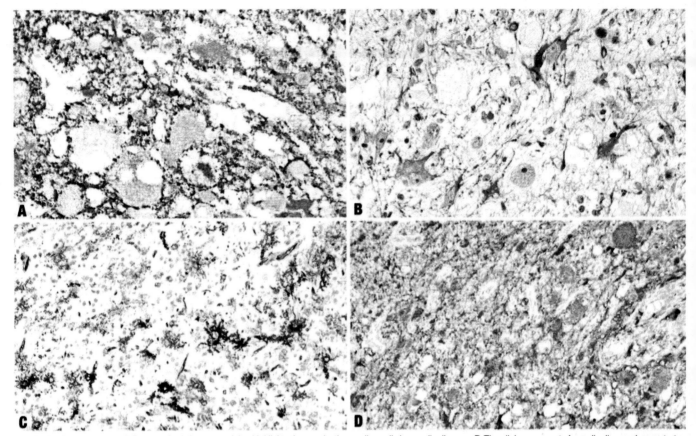

Fig. 2.105 Ganglioglioma. **A** Synaptophysin immunostaining highlights the neoplastic ganglion cells in gangliogliomas. **B** The glial component of gangliogliomas demonstrates labelling for GFAP. **C** Many gangliogliomas contain CD34-positive ramified or stellate cells either within the tumour or in the adjacent cerebral cortex. **D** This ganglioglioma demonstrates diffuse strong expression of BRAF p.V600E-mutant protein.

The differential diagnosis for ganglioglioma can include FCD, diffuse gliomas, and other glioneuronal tumours, specifically dysembryoplastic neuroepithelial tumour (DNT), polymorphous low-grade neuroepithelial tumour of the young (PLNTY), and multinodular and vacuolating neuronal tumour. The differentiation from FCD rests principally on the presence of a convincing neoplastic glial component in ganglioglioma; in challenging cases, the identification of *BRAF* p.V600E mutation or other MAPK pathway alterations provides support for a diagnosis of ganglioglioma, because FCD is genetically characterized by alterations in the PI3K/AKT/mTOR pathway and an absence of MAPK alterations {305,2016}. As discussed above, identifying the neoplastic neuronal component of ganglioglioma can be challenging, and diffuse gliomas with entrapped native neurons can enter the differential diagnosis in such cases. Reduced or absent NeuN expression in the neuronal cells, eosinophilic granular bodies, and CD34-positive ramified cells can all provide support for a diagnosis of ganglioglioma instead of diffuse glioma. Additionally, gangliogliomas harbour *BRAF* p.V600E mutation or other MAPK pathway alterations and lack the IDH mutation that characterizes IDH-mutant adult-type diffuse gliomas and the *MYB* or *MYBL1* fusion that characterizes angiocentric glioma and paediatric-type diffuse low-grade gliomas {1340,3404}. In low-grade glioneuronal tumours with an oligodendrocyte-like glial component, the differential diagnosis should include both DNT and PLNTY. Multinodular growth pattern, the presence of a specific glioneuronal element, absence

of CD34 immunoreactivity, and pathogenic *FGFR1* alteration all provide support for a diagnosis of DNT over ganglioglioma {299}. Abundant calcifications, diffuse strong CD34 staining of tumour cells, and *FGFR2* or *FGFR3* fusions all provide support for a diagnosis of PLNTY over ganglioglioma {1384}. Multinodular growth pattern, stromal and neuronal vacuolation, OLIG2 positivity of neoplastic neuronal cells, and *MAP2K1* mutation all provide support for a diagnosis of multinodular and vacuolating neuronal tumour over ganglioglioma {1383,2443}. Lastly, ganglion cell differentiation has been reported in a wide spectrum of CNS tumour entities (e.g. central and extraventricular neurocytoma, diffuse leptomeningeal glioneuronal tumour, papillary glioneuronal tumour, pleomorphic xanthoastrocytoma, paraganglioma of the cauda equina, H3 G34–mutant diffuse hemispheric glioma, CNS neuroblastoma), which require differentiation from ganglioglioma. The presence of xanthomatous tumour cells, intercellular basement membrane deposition (as highlighted by reticulin staining), and focal *CDKN2A* homozygous/biallelic deletion all provide support for a diagnosis of pleomorphic xanthoastrocytoma over ganglioglioma.

Cytology

Not clinically relevant

Diagnostic molecular pathology

For patients with ganglioglioma with a typical clinical and histological presentation, molecular testing may not be critical.

Diagnostic criteria for ganglioglioma

Essential:

Intra-axial low-grade glioneuronal tumour

AND

Combination of neoplastic ganglion and glial cells

AND (for unresolved lesions)

BRAF p.V600E mutation or other MAPK pathway alteration

OR

Methylation profile of ganglioglioma

Desirable:

Absence of IDH mutation

However, for cases with diagnostic uncertainty, the initial molecular workup should focus on *BRAF* p.V600E mutation testing either by sequencing or by immunohistochemistry using the mutant-specific antibody VE1 {1682}. Many gangliogliomas have low tumour cell content, so the selection of areas for molecular testing should be made cautiously, and sensitive sequencing methods capable of detecting variants at low allele frequencies should be employed. In gangliogliomas negative for *BRAF* p.V600E mutation, other *BRAF* alterations including mutations and fusions are commonly found, as well as various other genetic alterations causing activation of the MAPK signalling pathway, such as *RAF1* fusion, *KRAS* mutation, and *NF1* mutation or deletion {2444}. Most commonly, gangliogliomas harbour a solitary pathogenic alteration causing activation of the MAPK pathway. However, rare gangliogliomas have been reported with dual *BRAF* p.V600E mutation and *CDKN2A* homozygous deletion, which may potentially represent an adverse prognostic factor in ganglioglioma {2444}. However, this genetic pattern is far more common in pleomorphic xanthoastrocytoma and should prompt consideration of this alternative diagnosis {2499, 3299}. A small number of ganglioglioma-like tumours centred in midline structures of the CNS have been reported with dual *BRAF* p.V600E and H3 p.K28M (K27M) mutations {2368,1654, 2768}; however, the exact nature of these tumours is unknown at present. A small subset of histologically defined gangliogliomas have been reported with *FGFR1* or *FGFR2* mutations or fusions {2444}. However, *FGFR1* alterations are more characteristic of other glioneuronal tumour entities (e.g. DNT, rosette-forming glioneuronal tumour, and extraventricular neurocytoma), and the finding of *FGFR1* alteration in a low-grade neuroepithelial tumour should prompt consideration of these alternative entities. Additionally, *FGFR2* fusions are characteristic of PLNTY, and the finding of *FGFR2* fusion in a low-grade glioneuronal tumour should prompt consideration of this alternative diagnosis. *IDH* mutation (either *IDH1* p.R132 or *IDH2* p.R172), *MYB* or *MYBL1* fusion, and *PRKCA* fusion are not compatible with the diagnosis of ganglioglioma. Lastly, genome-wide DNA methylation profiling has established a distinct epigenetic signature of ganglioglioma that may aid in the classification of diagnostically challenging tumours {3045,460}. However, the low tumour cell content in ganglioglioma often limits the applicability of DNA methylation profiling {1004}.

Essential and desirable diagnostic criteria

See Box 2.18.

Staging

Not clinically relevant

Prognosis and prediction

Prognostic factors are difficult to define because of the complexity of the clinical picture, anatomical location, and molecular interrelationships in retrospective cohorts over the past few decades, as well as the small numbers of patients. However, ganglioglioma is generally a low-grade indolent tumour with excellent prognosis in combined paediatric and adult cohorts (15-year overall survival rate: 83–94%) {1959,624,3560}. The best prognostic indicator, including for better seizure outcome, is complete surgical resection {1959,624,3560}. The incidence of tumour progression is quite variable depending on the series (range: 16–35%) {3560,3577}, but no consistent correlations between histological features, imaging data, and clinical outcome have been found {1959,523,666,2444}. In a recent large series, *BRAF* p.V600E mutation conferred poor outcome relative to other genetic alterations (such as *BRAF* fusion in paediatric low-grade glioma) when considered as a group {2768}; however, the prognostic value of *BRAF* p.V600E mutation versus other alterations specifically in ganglioglioma was not clearly defined in that study. Prospective randomized studies testing small-molecule inhibitors of RAF and MEK will be important to validate the potential clinical benefit suggested by initial case reports {2753,725,35,2015,3221,1041}. The rare gangliogliomas with dual *BRAF* p.V600E mutation and *CDKN2A* homozygous deletion may potentially have an increased risk of recurrence compared with the vast majority of gangliogliomas without this accompanying *CDKN2A* homozygous deletion {1806,2444}. The ganglioglioma-like tumours centred in midline structures of the CNS with co-occurring *BRAF* p.V600E mutations and H3 p.K28M (K27M) mutation have been associated with poor outcomes {2368,1654,2768}.

Gangliocytoma

Giannini C
Blümcke I
Hawkins CE
Huse JT
Rosenblum MK

Definition
Gangliocytoma is a neuroepithelial neoplasm composed of irregular clusters of mostly mature neoplastic ganglion cells, often with dysplastic features (CNS WHO grade 1).

ICD-O coding
9492/0 Gangliocytoma

ICD-11 coding
2A00.21 & XH6KA6 Mixed neuronal-glial tumours & Gangliocytoma

Related terminology
None

Subtype(s)
None

Localization
Like gangliogliomas, these tumours can occur throughout the CNS. In a large series of seizure-associated tumours, > 80% of gangliocytomas were located in the temporal lobe {304}. Dysplastic cerebellar gangliocytoma is discussed in a separate section – see *Dysplastic cerebellar gangliocytoma (Lhermitte–Duclos disease)* (p. 146). Gangliocytoma of the pituitary is reviewed in the volume on tumours of endocrine organs {1919}.

Clinical features
Gangliocytomas have the same clinical features as gangliogliomas.

Epidemiology
Gangliocytomas are rare tumours that predominantly affect children. The relative incidence reported in epilepsy surgery series ranges from < 1% to 3.2% {3177,304}.

Etiology
No distinct genetic susceptibility factors have been reported for classic gangliocytoma. Dysplastic cerebellar gangliocytoma, which is associated with Cowden syndrome, is covered in a separate section – see *Dysplastic cerebellar gangliocytoma (Lhermitte–Duclos disease)* (p. 146).

Pathogenesis
Genetic data specifically addressing gangliocytomas have not been reported. A close genetic relationship with ganglioglioma seems possible.

Macroscopic appearance
Ganglion cell neoplasms are generally well-circumscribed, grey, solid or cystic lesions.

Histopathology
Gangliocytomas are composed of large, patently neuronal cells that lie singly or irregularly clustered in a matrix that may be indistinguishable from normal neuropil or may be more coarsely fibrillar and vacuolated. Binucleation and cytoplasmic ballooning or vacuolization are common. Microcalcifications can be present. The discrete micronodular substructure of the multinodular and vacuolating neuronal tumour is not seen. Glial elements are only sparsely represented and free of atypia. Because a variety of CNS tumours can exhibit gangliocytomatous maturation (including neuroblastomas, medulloblastomas, and embryonal tumours with multilayered rosettes), the presence of proliferative small cell components or neuroblasts must be excluded. Mitotic activity is absent and Ki-67 labelling is negligible.

Immunophenotype
Neoplastic ganglion cells exhibit variable immunoreactivity for synaptophysin, chromogranin, NFPs, and MAP2. NeuN

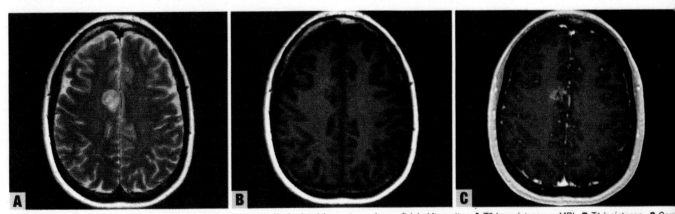

Fig. 2.106 Gangliocytoma. Right frontal lobe. Relatively circumscribed lesion involving cortex and superficial white matter. **A** T2-hyperintense on MRI. **B** T1-isointense. **C** Contrast enhancement is present after gadolinium administration.

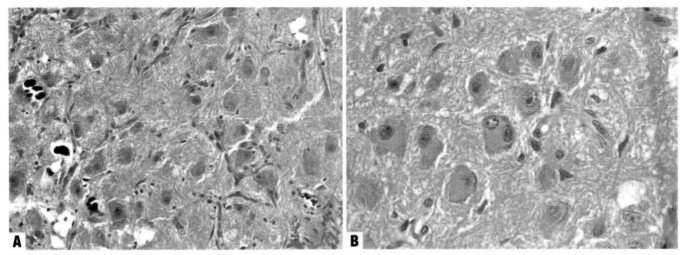

Fig. 2.107 Gangliocytoma. **A** Clusters of large ganglion cells in a matrix indistinguishable from normal neuropil. Microcalcifications are present. **B** Large ganglion cells with cytoplasmic ballooning; one is binucleated.

expression may be diminished or lost. GFAP labelling is restricted to reactive astroglia.

Grading

Gangliocytoma corresponds histologically to CNS WHO grade 1.

Differential diagnosis

Among non-neoplastic neuronal lesions, focal cortical dysplasia (FCD), primarily type 2, should be considered in the differential diagnosis of gangliocytoma. FCD type 2a is characterized by the disruption of cortical lamination with dysmorphic neurons that have enlarged cell bodies and prominent accumulation of Nissl substance and that lack anatomical orientation. The dysmorphic neurons in FCD show cytoplasmic accumulation of neurofilaments (SMI32) and, unlike in gangliocytoma, typically retain NeuN expression. In FCD type 2b, in addition to dysmorphic neurons, balloon cells with ample eosinophilic and glassy cytoplasm, at times multinucleated, are present, particularly in the deep layers of the cortex and

the underlying white matter. Balloon cells are highlighted by vimentin and αB-crystallin. Although FCD type 2b is associated with a thickening of the cortex and blurring of the grey matter–white matter junction macroscopically, it lacks the mass-like circumscribed appearance of gangliocytoma. In the suprasellar region, gangliocytoma should be distinguished from sporadic hypothalamic hamartoma (also referred to as "hamartoblastoma"), a congenital mass-like lesion that is characteristically located in the floor of the hypothalamus, involving the tuber cinereum and the mammillary bodies posteriorly and extending inferiorly into the interpeduncular cistern. Hypothalamic hamartoma consists of collections of small to medium-sized neurons typically arranged in nodules and separated by hypocellular neuropil resembling normal CNS neuropil. The glial/neuronal composition varies widely, with some lesions comprising predominantly neurons, and others predominantly glial cells (both astrocytes and oligodendrocytes) {634}. Hypothalamic hamartoma is the pathognomonic manifestation of Pallister–Hall syndrome, a rare autosomal dominant malformative disorder that includes (in addition to

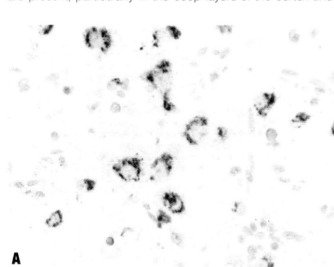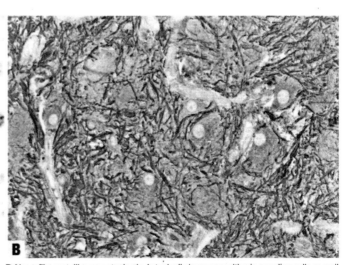

Fig. 2.108 Gangliocytoma. **A** Neoplastic ganglion cells are positive for chromogranin. **B** Neurofilament, like synaptophysin, is typically immunopositive in ganglion cells as well as (diffusely) in background neuropil.

hypothalamic hamartoma) polydactyly and imperforate anus as well as abnormalities of the pituitary, larynx, and genitourinary tract {805}. *GLI3* germline mutations have been associated with Pallister–Hall syndrome {733}. Mutations in *GLI3* and a variety of other genes often related to the SHH pathway have been reported in a subset of sporadic hypothalamic hamartomas {1308}. Mixed gangliocytoma–adenoma, also known as "pituitary adenoma with gangliocytic differentiation" or "pituitary adenoma–neuronal choristoma", typically involves the sella turcica and suprasellar region without connection with the hypothalamus. In addition to its gangliocytic component, mixed gangliocytoma–adenoma is characterized by the presence of an adenomatous component, most often a somatotroph adenoma manifesting as acromegaly or a mixed tumour producing prolactin and growth hormone {1926}.

Cytology
A characteristic profile in smear/squash preparations has not been described.

Diagnostic molecular pathology
To date, no signature molecular abnormalities have been ascribed to gangliocytoma specifically, although histopathologically related entities, including ganglioglioma and multinodular

Box 2.19 Diagnostic criteria for gangliocytoma

Essential:

A tumefactive lesion with presence of irregular groups of large, mature ganglion cells
AND

Matrix resembling normal neuropil, sometimes more coarsely fibrillar or vacuolated

Desirable:

Atypical and binucleated ganglion cells

Cytoplasmic ballooning or vacuolization

and vacuolating neuronal tumour, frequently harbour alterations in constituents of the RAS/MAPK signalling pathway.

Essential and desirable diagnostic criteria
See Box 2.19.

Staging
Not clinically relevant

Prognosis and prediction
Gangliocytomas are benign tumours with a favourable outcome. Specific prognostic or predictive factors have not been reported.

Desmoplastic infantile ganglioglioma / desmoplastic infantile astrocytoma

Figarella-Branger D
Gessi M
Reuss DE
Solomon DA
Varlet P

Definition

Desmoplastic infantile ganglioglioma (DIG) and desmoplastic infantile astrocytoma (DIA) are benign glioneuronal or glial tumours, occurring predominantly in the cerebral hemispheres of infants, that are driven by MAPK pathway activation and composed of a mixed astrocytic and neuronal component (DIG) or an astrocytic component only (DIA) embedded in an extensive desmoplastic stroma, often containing foci of undifferentiated embryonal-like tumour cells (CNS WHO grade 1).

ICD-O coding

9412/1 Desmoplastic infantile ganglioglioma
9412/1 Desmoplastic infantile astrocytoma

ICD-11 coding

2A00.21 & XH6TQ7 Mixed neuronal-glial tumours & Desmoplastic infantile ganglioglioma
2A00.21 & XH7M44 Mixed neuronal-glial tumours & Desmoplastic infantile astrocytoma

Related terminology

Not recommended: superficial cerebral astrocytoma attached to the dura.

Subtype(s)

None

Localization

DIG/DIAs typically arise in the cerebral hemispheres, involving the superficial cortex and leptomeninges, often with attachment to the dura. Rare cases have been reported in other locations (spinal, posterior fossa, intraventricular, suprasellar), but extensive genetic analysis of such cases has not been performed {2221,2210,3364}.

Clinical features

The most frequent clinical signs are increased head circumference, bulging of the fontanelles, lethargy, and the sunset sign {3136,3287}.

Imaging

The radiological aspects of DIG and DIA are similar: both appear as a large, superficially located, solid and cystic tumour that is enhancing after contrast administration. On CT, the solid part of the DIG/DIA is isodense or slightly hyperdense, with strong enhancement after iodine contrast administration; the cystic component is frequently hypodense or isodense {170,271}. On MRI, the cystic part is unilocular or multicystic, hypointense on T1-weighted sequences, and hyperintense on T2-weighted sequences, whereas the solid component is frequently dural based and appears hypointense on both T1- and T2-weighted sequences, with contrast enhancement after gadolinium injection {271}.

Epidemiology

DIG/DIAs are rare primary brain tumours, but their true incidence is not well defined, because they are usually included in the large group of glioneuronal tumours. DIG/DIAs account for 0.4% of brain tumours, with an M:F ratio of 1.8:1 {677,3288}. They represent 1.25% of intracranial tumours in children {3136} and 1.3–15.8% of infantile brain tumours {3622,1542}. The vast majority of cases occur before the age of 24 months. Rare non-infantile cases have been reported, but these were in the pre-genetic era and might represent misclassified tumour types {2453}.

Etiology

No risk factors have been reported for DIG/DIA, and no inherited genetic susceptibility or association with known tumour predisposition syndromes has been established. DIG/DIA is genetically driven by somatic alterations causing activation of the MAPK signalling pathway, most commonly via mutation or

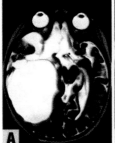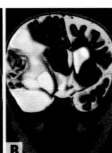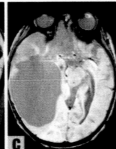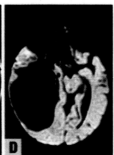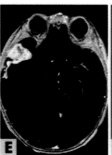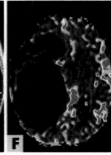

Fig. 2.109 Desmoplastic infantile ganglioglioma in the right hemisphere of an 18-month-old girl. Axial (**A**) and coronal (**B**) T2-weighted MRI shows multiple cystic components with cerebrospinal fluid–like signal, and a peripheral solid component that is isointense to grey matter. **C** Susceptibility-weighted MRI shows no blooming effect (pseudoenlargement of the lesion). **D** Diffusion-weighted MRI demonstrates a solid hyperintense portion, possibly due to desmoplastic reaction. **E** Contrast-enhanced T1-weighted MRI shows intense homogeneous enhancement of the solid component and no enhancement of the cyst walls. **F** Colour cerebral blood volume map (dynamic susceptibility contrast perfusion) shows relative hyperperfusion of the solid enhancing component compared with the contralateral white matter.

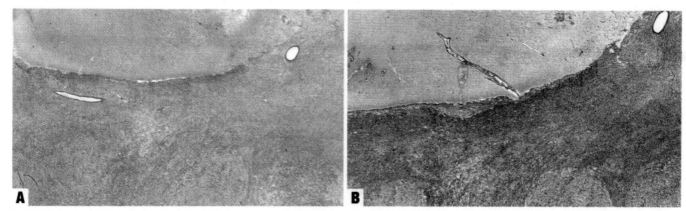

Fig. 2.110 Desmoplastic infantile ganglioglioma. **A** The tumour is superficial, with sharp demarcation from the cortex. **B** The tumour shows a marked desmoplastic component, evidenced by reticulin staining, whereas the adjacent cortex is negative.

fusion involving the *BRAF* or *RAF1* genes {1679,1163,525,3364, 295}. Most DIG/DIAs demonstrate a flat copy-number profile, and recurrent cytogenetic alterations have not been identified {1742,1077,3364}.

Pathogenesis

Although the exact cell of origin remains uncertain, DIG/DIA has been postulated to arise from a population of specialized sub-pial astrocytes in the developing brain {1942,164}. However, the presence of undifferentiated foci of embryonal-like tumour cells in most cases raises the possibility of an early progenitor cell that gives rise to a tumour with varying degrees of progressive maturation. DIG/DIA is genetically driven by the activation of the MAPK signalling pathway {1679,1163,525,3364,295}.

Macroscopic appearance

DIG/DIAs typically contain large uniloculated or multiloculated cysts filled with clear and colourless or xanthochromic fluid. The solid superficial portion is primarily extracerebral, involving the leptomeninges and superficial cortex. It is commonly attached to the dura, is firm or rubbery in consistency, and is grey or white in colour. There is typically no gross evidence of haemorrhage or necrosis {3136,3288}.

Histopathology

DIG/DIAs are biphasic tumours composed of a prominent des-moplastic leptomeningeal stroma and a variable proportion of neuroepithelial component. The desmoplastic leptomeningeal

component consists of a mixture of fibroblast-like, spindle-shaped cells intermixed with a collagen matrix. Reticulin-rich basal lamina classically surrounds almost every cell {3136, 3288}. In DIA, the neuroepithelial component comprises an astrocytic population only; in DIG, a neoplastic neuronal com-ponent with ganglionic differentiation is also observed {3288}. The neoplastic astrocytes are arranged in fascicles or dem-onstrate storiform or whorled patterns. In addition, DIG/DIAs often contain foci of primitive, embryonal-like tumour cells. This immature component, lacking desmoplasia, may predominate in some areas.

There is a sharp demarcation between the cortical surface and the desmoplastic tumour, although Virchow–Robin spaces are often filled with tumour cells. Calcifications are common, but perivascular mononuclear inflammatory infiltrates and xan-thomatous cells are usually absent. Necrosis is uncommon and is typically restricted to the foci of primitive, embryonal-like cells. Glomeruloid microvascular proliferation is usually absent {271}. In most cases, mitotic figures are limited to the foci of embryonal-like tumour cells and do not exceed 0.8 mitoses/ mm^2 (equating to < 2 mitoses/10 HPF of 0.55 mm in diameter and 0.24 mm^2 in area) in the desmoplastic component.

Immunohistochemistry

The glial component strongly expresses GFAP, whereas neuronal markers (synaptophysin, neurofilament, NeuN) are observed in neoplastic ganglion cells as well as in cells lack-ing obvious neuronal differentiation {2431,525}. The Ki-67

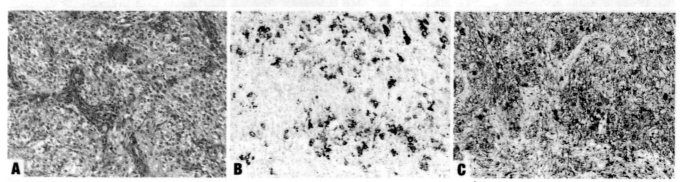

Fig. 2.111 Desmoplastic infantile ganglioglioma. **A** Advanced neuronal differentiation is associated with poorly differentiated cells. **B** Cells with advanced neuronal differentia-tion often express chromogranin. **C** Neuronal cells strongly express synaptophysin.

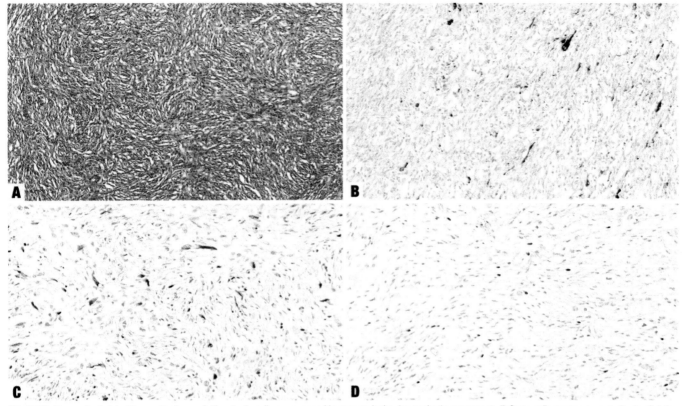

Fig. 2.112 Desmoplastic infantile ganglioglioma. **A** Neoplastic cells are arranged in streams in the desmoplastic component. **B** Some cells express synaptophysin. **C** A few cells are GFAP-positive. **D** The Ki-67 labelling index is very low in desmoplastic areas.

proliferation index within the desmoplastic component ranges from < 0.5% to 5%, with the majority of reported values being < 2% {1742,525}. However, the Ki-67 index can be significantly elevated (as high as 20%) in the foci of embryonal-like tumour cells {1077}. Immunohistochemistry using the VE1 clone is useful for detecting DIG/DIAs that harbour *BRAF* p.V600E mutation, but this mutation-specific antibody does not recognize the p.V600D mutation or any of the other *BRAF* mutations or rearrangements found in DIG/DIAs without p.V600E mutation {525,1679,1163}.

Differential diagnosis

The major differential diagnoses for DIG/DIA are ganglioglioma, pleomorphic xanthoastrocytoma, and the newly defined tumour type infant-type hemispheric glioma. Like DIG/DIA, ganglioglioma and pleomorphic xanthoastrocytoma are typically solid and cystic tumours with frequent *BRAF* mutations, but ganglioglioma and pleomorphic xanthoastrocytoma are typically much smaller and occur in older children, in contrast to the very large size and the infantile onset of DIG/DIA. Infant-type hemispheric glioma shares the characteristics of infantile onset and hemispheric location with DIG/DIA, but infant-type hemispheric gliomas usually lack desmoplasia and demonstrate an infiltrative growth pattern (unlike DIG/DIAs), and they are genetically characterized by fusions involving receptor tyrosine kinase genes (*ALK, ROS1, MET, NTRK1, NTRK2,* and/or *NTRK3*) {460, 463,3364}.

Cytology

Not clinically relevant

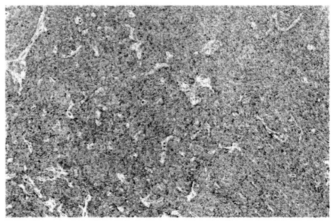

Fig. 2.113 Desmoplastic infantile astrocytoma. Diffuse BRAF p.V600E immunoexpression.

Diagnostic molecular pathology

DIG/DIAs are IDH- and histone H3-wildtype tumours characterized by genetic alterations causing activation of the MAPK signalling pathway, most commonly via mutation or fusion involving *BRAF* or *RAF1* {1679,1163,525,3364,295,2768}. *BRAF* mutations can include p.V600E and other variants at the same codon, such as p.V600D, in addition to variants at other locations or fusions involving partners other than *KIAA1549*. These *BRAF* or *RAF1* mutations or fusions are typically present as the sole pathogenic alteration identified, and DIG/DIAs lack the *CDKN2A* and/or *CDKN2B* homozygous deletion that commonly accompanies *BRAF* alterations in pleomorphic xanthoastrocytoma

{3364}. Although individual cases of histologically defined DIG/DIAs harbouring *ALK* or NTRK fusions have been reported {3364,295}, most hemispheric gliomas occurring in infants that harbour *ALK*, *ROS1*, *MET*, or NTRK fusions have been shown to epigenetically cluster with infant-type hemispheric glioma {1179,603}. Whether there are true DIG/DIAs that also harbour fusions in receptor tyrosine kinase genes (*ALK*, *ROS1*, *MET*, *NTRK1*, *NTRK2*, *NTRK3*, or *FGFR1*) remains to be established. DNA methylation profiling has revealed that DIG/DIAs have an epigenetic signature distinct from all other primary CNS tumour entities characterized to date, including pleomorphic xanthoastrocytoma and the aforementioned infant-type hemispheric glioma {460,463,3364}.

Essential and desirable diagnostic criteria
See Box 2.20.

Staging
Not clinically relevant

Prognosis and prediction
The prognosis of DIG/DIA is excellent when total surgical removal is achieved, with no relapse in most cases with follow-up ranging from 5 to 15 years {3136,3287,271}. Long-term outcome is better with hemispheric location than with suprasellar location {2221}, and leptomeningeal dissemination and/or multifocal disease, although rare, are most frequently associated with suprasellar location {2210}. In cases of subtotal resection or biopsy only, careful follow-up is mandatory to monitor for regrowth of the residual tumour, which typically remains stable or grows slowly over years {271,295}, but regression has also been documented {3116}. In cases of subtotal resection, adjuvant chemotherapy and/or radiotherapy is a therapeutic

Box 2.20 Essential and desirable diagnostic criteria for desmoplastic infantile astrocytoma (DIA) and desmoplastic infantile ganglioglioma (DIG)

Essential:

Biphasic morphology with a dominant desmoplastic leptomeningeal component admixed with a neuroepithelial component containing astrocytic cells only (DIA) or containing astrocytes and neuronal cells (DIG)

AND (for unresolved lesions)

Methylation profile of DIG/DIA

OR

BRAF or *RAF1* mutation or fusion, occurring in the absence of homozygous deletion of *CDKN2A* and/or *CDKN2B*

Desirable:

Tumour with a cystic component and a solid portion, with leptomeningeal involvement, usually attached to the dura

Infantile onset (typically at < 24 months)

consideration, especially for patients with progression of the residual tumour and/or leptomeningeal dissemination {3364, 3288}. Small-molecule tyrosine kinase inhibitors targeting the MAPK signalling pathway are also a therapeutic option in cases demonstrating *BRAF* mutations {294}. Although some DIG/DIAs demonstrate foci of frank anaplasia (e.g. high mitotic count, palisading necrosis), there is no clear relationship between anaplasia and clinical outcomes {711,3224,2492}. Rare cases of recurrence accompanied by malignant transformation of DIG/DIA occurring as late as 8–10 years after the first resection have been reported, accompanied by acquired *TP53*, *ATRX*, or *BCORL1* mutations in individual cases {1920, 2492,3364,2554}.

Despite the malignant transformation observed histologically, some patients remained alive for ≥ 3 years after the second surgery {1920,3364}.

Dysembryoplastic neuroepithelial tumour

Pietsch T
Ellison DW
Hirose T
Jacques TS
Schüller U
Varlet P

Definition

Dysembryoplastic neuroepithelial tumour (DNT) is a glioneuronal neoplasm in the cerebral cortex of children or young adults, characterized by the occurrence of a pathognomonic glioneuronal element that may be associated with glial nodules and activating mutations of *FGFR1* (CNS WHO grade 1).

ICD-O coding

9413/0 Dysembryoplastic neuroepithelial tumour

ICD-11 coding

2A00.21 & XH0H76 Mixed neuronal-glial tumours & Dysembryoplastic neuroepithelial tumour

Related terminology

None

Subtype(s)

None

Localization

DNTs can be located in any part of the cerebral cortex, but they show a predilection for the temporal lobe (67.3% of cases, preferentially involving mesial structures) {449,3180} and the frontal lobe (16.3% of cases); the remaining cases (16.4%) are located in other regions {3180}.

Clinical features

Patients with DNTs typically present with drug-resistant focal epilepsy with an onset in childhood, adolescence, or early adulthood.

Imaging

DNTs usually encompass the thickness of the normal cortex. The main distinctive characteristics for differentiating DNT from diffuse gliomas are a lobulated architecture, sharply defined margin, and absence of mass effect with no significant peritumoural oedema. DNTs appear as cystic or multicystic lesions, hypointense or nearly isointense to grey matter on T1-weighted MRI, and hyperintense on both T2-weighted and FLAIR MRI {449}. Marked high signal intensity within the mass (soap-bubble appearance) with intracystic septa, thin FLAIR hyperintensity surrounding the tumour (rim sign) {2403}, triangular cortical based, and remodelling of the adjacent inner table of bone (indicating a slow-growing lesion) are common findings {1423,74}. Calcifications and haemorrhage are rare {663}. About one third of complex DNTs exhibit enhancement after gadolinium administration, with a nodular pattern, peripheral rim-like enhancement, or both {663,74}.

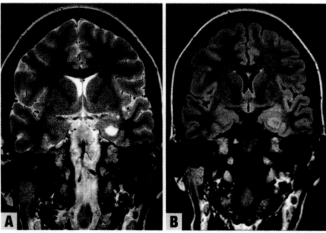

Fig. 2.114 Dysembryoplastic neuroepithelial tumour. **A** Coronal T2-weighted MRI of a temporal tumour. **B** Coronal FLAIR MRI of a temporal tumour.

Epidemiology

Incidence

The estimated incidence of DNT is 0.03 cases per 100 000 person-years. An analysis of SEER data from 2004–2013 found that the incidence of DNT was lower in the Black, American Indian / Alaskan Native, and Asian or Pacific Islander populations than in White people {2242}. In a large epilepsy surgery series, DNTs accounted for 5.9% of the cases {304}.

Age and sex distribution

In about 90% of patients with DNT, the first seizure occurs before the age of 20 years, with reported ages at seizure onset ranging from 1 week to 30 years {2628,2242}. There is a slight predominance of DNT in male patients (accounting for approximately 55% of cases in a large series) {304,2680}.

Etiology

Most DNTs are sporadic and caused by *FGFR1* alterations {2584,2680,934,3597,2040,2767,1828,3075}, although accumulating data suggest that they may also occur in the setting of RASopathies (a group of neurodevelopment diseases with germline mutations in the RAS signalling pathway), such as neurofibromatosis type 1 {1853,198} or Noonan syndrome {2926, 2059}, or in families with an *FGFR1* germline mutation {2680}.

Pathogenesis

Recent comprehensive genomic analyses revealed *FGFR1* alterations in approximately 40–80% of DNTs, with *BRAF* p.V600E mutation reported in as many as 50% of DNTs in some studies {2584, 2680,934,3597,523,2550,2040,2767,1828,3075}. *PDGFRA* and *NF1* mutations were also reported in a few cases {2584,3075}. These mutations are typically mutually exclusive {934,1528}. The FGFR genetic alterations induce autophosphorylation of FGFR1

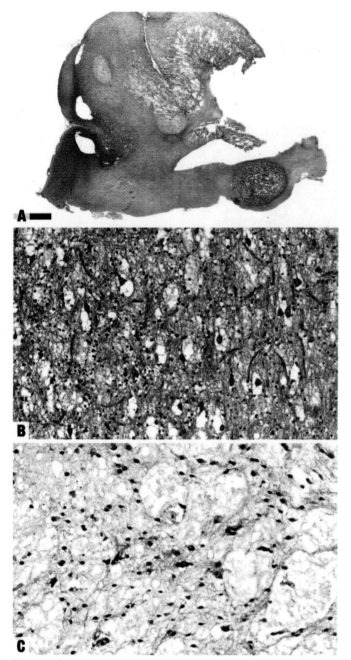

Fig. 2.115 Dysembryoplastic neuroepithelial tumour. **A** Low-power micrograph illustrating the multinodular intracortical growth pattern. **B** Specific glioneuronal element: bundles of axons lined by small oligodendroglia-like cells. Interspersed neurons appear to float in a mucoid matrix (floating neurons). **C** Large floating non-dysplastic neurons in an alcianophilic matrix (Alcian blue staining).

and then upregulate the MAPK and PI3K pathways {2680,2767, 1960}. FGFR1 activity is associated with inhibition of oligodendroglial precursor differentiation {3611}.

Macroscopic appearance
On the cut surface, DNTs are usually poorly defined and located mainly in the expanded grey matter and subcortical white matter. DNTs vary in size from a few millimetres to several centimetres {2411} and contain mucoid substances, solid areas, and small cysts in varying proportions {685,1338}.

Histopathology
The histopathological hallmarks are the multinodular intracortical growth pattern and the pathognomonic specific glioneuronal element, i.e. the presence of columns oriented perpendicularly to the cortical surface, formed by bundles of axons lined by small oligodendroglia-like cells. Between these columns, neurons with normal cytology appear to float in a mucoid matrix (floating neurons) {685}. Dysplastic ganglionic cells are absent. Intranodular glial components can be highly heterogeneous, with oligodendroglia-like, neuronal, or piloid or stellate astrocytic cells. The oligodendroglia-like component generally predominates {299,3045}. Mitoses are rare. High cellularity, necrosis, significant perivascular lymphoid infiltrates, and eosinophilic granular bodies are absent. The microvascular network is also heterogeneous, varying from meagre to extensive, and it may include glomerular formations as seen in pilocytic astrocytomas. Focal cortical dysplasia type 3b has been described in association with DNTs {683,3180} but remains controversial; it may be diagnosed only if areas of focal cortical dysplasia type 1 without tumour cell infiltration can be identified {305}.

Recognized histopathological patterns
Several histological forms of DNT, without clinical or therapeutic implications, have been described {687}.

The simple form consists of the unique glioneuronal element.

The complex form consists of the specific glioneuronal element in combination with glial nodules, and it resembles other gliomas such as pilocytic astrocytomas or oligodendrogliomas {569,3180,299,685}. Within the glial components, calcified vessels are common and can cause haemorrhage {3178}.

The diffuse/nonspecific form, which lacks the specific glioneuronal element {687,3180}, remains controversial; numerous terms have been used for it in the past, including "diffuse oligodendroglial tumour" {2584}, "DNT-like tumour" {2680}, "glioneuronal tumour NOS" {3045}, "paediatric oligodendroglioma" {2703}, and "diffuse glioneuronal tumour" {296,3180,74}. The variability of its histomorphological appearance is related to a low interobserver diagnostic concordance {299}. Recent data have shown that clear phenotype–genotype correlations are difficult to establish, even for experienced neuropathologists using advanced molecular techniques {3045}.

Immunohistochemistry
The small oligodendroglia-like cells express glial markers including S100, the glial transcription factor OLIG2, and PDGFRA, but not GFAP. MAP2 expression is typically faint in these cells; the strong perinuclear expression found in oligodendrogliomas is not detectable {303}. The floating normal neurons can be depicted by immunostaining for NeuN, but they are usually negative for chromogranin A. BRAF p.V600E-mutant protein and CD34 have been described with variable incidences in DNT {523,3180,299}, but they seem more characteristic of gangliogliomas {3045,299}. DNT cells do not label with antibodies against IDH1 p.R132H {461}.

Differential diagnosis
Sampling artefacts may make the diagnosis challenging. Clusters of abnormal neurons not otherwise explicable by anatomical localization may be focal and detectable only in some cases. In addition, the architectural heterogeneity of DNT (which

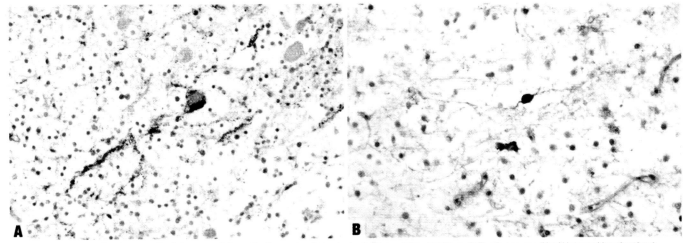

Fig. 2.116 Dysembryoplastic neuroepithelial tumour. **A** Large floating neuron (synaptophysin immunohistochemistry). **B** Floating neuron (NeuN immunohistochemistry).

generates inherent sampling bias) and the semiliquid consistency of the specific glioneuronal element, which can be lost during the neurosurgical procedure, pose further challenges.

DNTs do not contain dysplastic ganglion cells such as those described in gangliogliomas (i.e. binucleated neurons and large neuron clusters not otherwise explicable by anatomical region) {299}. Ganglioglioma should be suspected when the tumour shows perivascular lymphocytic infiltration, a desmoplastic component, eosinophilic granular bodies, a large cystic component, or a prominent component of CD34-positive satellite cells. The strong perinuclear expression of MAP2 found in diffuse oligodendrogliomas is not detectable in the oligodendroglia-like cells of DNT {303}.

Myxoid glioneuronal tumour, formerly known as DNT of the septum pellucidum {177,1072}, has been separated from conventional DNT because it harbours a specific molecular alteration (*PDGFRA* p.K385 mutation) not found in conventional DNT, and it has the potential for ventricular dissemination {1954,569}.

The spectrum of low-grade epilepsy-associated brain tumours is widening rapidly with new descriptions of various rare histomolecular tumour types; therefore, the differential diagnosis requires a combined histological, neuroradiological, and molecular diagnostic approach. Multinodular and vacuolating neuronal tumours have a multinodular architecture but a predominant neuronal (i.e. gangliocytoma-like) component with vacuolating cells, mainly in the subcortical white matter {2443}. *MAP2K1* mutation or (more rarely) *BRAF* mutations are found instead of the *FGFR1* alterations typical of DNT {2443,1383}. Polymorphous low-grade neuroepithelial tumour of the young is a morphologically variable entity and is mainly oligodendroglia-like, similar to DNT but with a more infiltrative growth pattern, calcifications, and intense CD34 immunopositivity of tumour cells. They harbour either *BRAF* p.V600E mutations or fusion events involving *FGFR2* or *FGFR3* {1384}. Diffuse astrocytoma, *MYB*- or *MYBL1*-altered, is a more monomorphic tumour, where the regular astrocytic cells are scattered in a fine bubbly neuropil. Unlike in angiocentric gliomas with *MYB::QKI* fusion transcripts, angiocentric patterns are absent or focal {3404}.

Cytology

Smear (squash) cytological findings typically reveal a spread of uniform rounded cells, without substantial pleomorphism or mitotic activity, set against a variably mucinous or fibrillary matrix. However, in more complex DNTs, there may be overlap with other glial tumours.

Diagnostic molecular pathology

Among *FGFR1* alterations, intragenic duplication (internal tandem duplication [ITD]) of the tyrosine kinase domain (TKD) of *FGFR1* is the most prevalent aberration (accounting for ~40–60% of cases) {2584,2680,934,2040}, followed by missense mutations at mutation hotspots in *FGFR1* {2680,934,2584, 3075}. *FGFR1* mutations were identified in both familial and sporadic cases, with double or multiple mutations often present on the same allele (in cis) {2680,2584}. *FGFR1::TACC1* fusion and complete duplication of *FGFR1* have also been reported {2680, 2584}. *FGFR1* alterations are characteristic of DNT (although not specific for it), and they are considered to be the main molecular driver of this tumour {2680,934,2040}. In particular, TKD duplication is known to be relatively specific to DNT {934, 2040,2584}.

BRAF p.V600E mutation has been reported in as many as 50% of DNTs in some studies. The wide range in incidence of the various alterations probably stems from differences in the morphological criteria used to make the diagnosis of DNT across the various studies; of note, several studies have shown marked variation in the reported frequencies of DNTs, as well as marked interobserver variability in making this diagnosis {299,296}. In contrast to *FGFR1* alterations, several studies failed to identify *BRAF* mutations in DNTs containing the specific glioneuronal element {2680,2040}. Therefore, alternative diagnoses, including ganglioglioma or MAPK pathway–altered diffuse low-grade glioma, should be carefully considered in the presence of a *BRAF* p.V600E mutation.

In support of this, DNA methylation or transcriptional profiling identifies different molecular groups of epilepsy-associated tumours {3046,299}, and although these groups correlate only partially with histological patterns, they separate epilepsy-associated tumours into those with *FGFR1* mutations and those with *BRAF* mutations, with the former being enriched for morphologically defined DNTs. These data suggest that, according to molecular criteria, DNTs have a distinct methylation and transcriptional profile, and most carry *FGFR1* mutations.

Box 2.21 Diagnostic criteria for dysembryoplastic neuroepithelial tumour

Essential:

Cortical glioneuronal tumour

AND

Presence of the specific glioneuronal element

AND (for unresolved lesions)

FGFR1 gene alteration (*FGFR1* internal tandem duplication [ITD], fusion, missense mutation)

OR

Methylation profile of dysembryoplastic neuroepithelial tumour

Desirable:

Early-onset focal epilepsy

Regarding copy-number aberrations, gains at chromosomes 5–7 and loss of chromosome 22 have been reported in a few cases {2551,2680}.

Essential and desirable diagnostic criteria

See Box 2.21.

Staging

Not clinically relevant

Prognosis and prediction

DNTs are considered benign lesions {3016}. Ischaemic or haemorrhagic changes may occur with or without an increase in size of the lesion or peritumoural oedema {686,911,1469, 2341,3016}. Risk factors for the development of recurrent seizures include a longer preoperative history of seizures {140, 1289}, the presence of residual tumour {2273}, and the presence of cortical dysplasia adjacent to DNT {2789}.

MRI may reveal tumour recurrence, but histopathology often remains benign. Malignant transformation has been documented in rare cases with {2756,2627} or without {2756,2627, 3180,522,1280,2039} radiation and/or chemotherapy.

Diffuse glioneuronal tumour with oligodendroglioma-like features and nuclear clusters

Sahm F
Haberler C
Pfister SM
Schüller U

Definition

Diffuse glioneuronal tumour with oligodendroglioma-like features and nuclear clusters (DGONC) is a provisional tumour type proposed as a neuroepithelial tumour characterized by variably differentiated cells frequently showing perinuclear haloes, scattered multinucleated cells, and nuclear clusters, with a distinct DNA methylation profile and frequent monosomy of chromosome 14.

ICD-O coding

None

ICD-11 coding

2A00.21 Mixed neuronal-glial tumours

Related terminology

None

Subtype(s)

None

Localization

All cases reported so far were supratentorial. Of 21 cases with data available, 11 were located in the temporal lobe, 4 in the parieto-occipital region, 5 in the frontal lobe, and 1 in a lateral ventricle {737,2506}.

Clinical features

There are currently no known tumour-specific symptoms. Patients present with symptoms characteristic for the tumour location within the brain.

Epidemiology

The majority of DGONC cases occur in paediatric patients, with a median age of 9 years in the 23 cases for which the age of initial diagnosis is known. However, the age range is wide (1 patient was aged 75 years). There is an equal sex distribution (13 male patients and 11 female patients reported) {737,2506}.

Etiology

Unknown

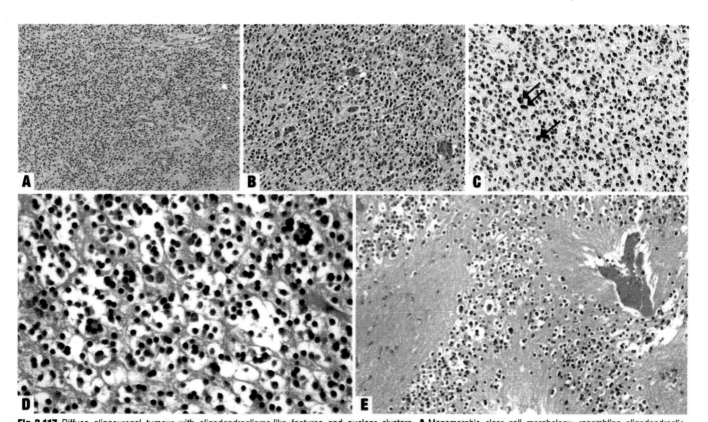

Fig. 2.117 Diffuse glioneuronal tumour with oligodendroglioma-like features and nuclear clusters. **A** Monomorphic clear cell morphology, resembling oligodendroglioma. **B** Clear cell histology can resemble oligodendroglioma. **C** Several nuclear clusters (some indicated by arrows). **D** Tumour with clear cell morphology and several ring- or C-shaped nuclear clusters. **E** Tumour with oligodendroglioma-like perinuclear haloes.

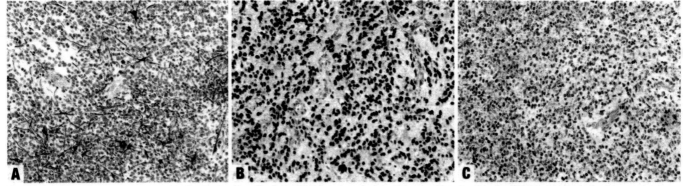

Fig. 2.118 Diffuse glioneuronal tumour with oligodendroglioma-like features and nuclear clusters. **A** Immunohistochemistry for GFAP is largely confined to reactive astrocytes. **B** Immunohistochemistry for OLIG2 is positive in the majority of tumour cells. **C** Immunohistochemistry for synaptophysin shows variable staining.

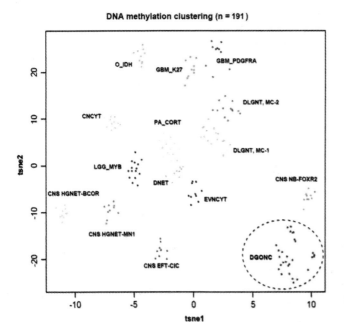

Fig. 2.119 Diffuse glioneuronal tumour with oligodendroglioma-like features and nuclear clusters (DGONC). DNA methylation profiling. DGONC samples (*n* = 31) were compared with 160 well-characterized reference samples representing CNS tumours of defined histological and/or molecular subgroups, confirming the distinct nature of the DGONC entity. Reference cohorts: central neurocytoma (CNCYT); CNS high-grade neuroepithelial tumour with *BCOR* alteration (CNS HGNET-BCOR); CNS Ewing sarcoma family tumour with *CIC* alteration (CNS EFT-CIC); CNS high-grade neuroepithelial tumour with *MN1* alteration (CNS HGNET-MN1); CNS neuroblastoma with *FOXR2* activation (CNS NB-FOXR2); diffuse leptomeningeal glioneuronal tumour, methylation class 1 and class 2 (DLGNT, MC-1 and MC-2); dysembryoplastic neuroepithelial tumour (DNET); extraventricular neurocytoma (EVNCYT); H3 K27M–mutant glioblastoma (GBM_K27); H3/IDH-wildtype glioblastoma RTK1 group (GBM_PDGFRA); low-grade glioma, *MYB-* or *MYBL1*-altered (LGG_MYB); IDH-mutant, 1p/19q-codeleted oligodendroglioma (O_IDH); hemispheric pilocytic astrocytoma (PA_CORT).

Pathogenesis

Monosomy 14 is probably a feature underlying the pathogenesis of this entity, having been found in 30 of 31 molecularly assessed cases. However, no other recurrent alterations on chromosome 14 that would result in a double hit of a specific gene have been found {737}. Because the morphological and immunohistochemical features of DGONC are similar to those of CNS neuroblastoma, it is possible that DGONC represents a type or subtype of a CNS embryonal tumour. Larger series are needed for a definite classification {2506}.

Macroscopic appearance

Not reported

Histopathology

DGONCs were described by Capper et al. in 2018, identified by the detection of a global DNA methylation profile that is distinct from that of all brain tumour entities previously analysed {460}. Subsequently, histological features were investigated in a supervised fashion on 13 samples of this cluster, for which histology slides were available. The histological characterization in the literature may therefore not cover the entire spectrum {737}. Another study reported 4 samples from 3 additional patients {2506}.

The tumours show a variation in differentiation and cellularity ranging from moderate to high in some cases. They are composed of small to medium-sized cells with scant cytoplasm, and they commonly show perinuclear haloes like in oligodendroglioma. In addition to small round nuclei, larger irregular nuclei are present, the latter showing marked nuclear pleomorphism in some cases. A characteristic feature is the presence of scattered multinucleated cells (pennies on a plate) and nuclear clusters composed of large pleomorphic nuclei. Mitotic frequency is variable, ranging from single mitotic figures in well-differentiated tumours to brisk mitotic activity in undifferentiated tumours. Microcalcifications and larger confluent calcifications are commonly encountered. The tumours infiltrate diffusely into the brain.

Immunohistochemistry

The tumour cells are diffusely OLIG2-positive in most cases, and GFAP-negative. Synaptophysin reveals a neuropil background. NeuN and MAP2 are expressed in a small proportion of cells {737}.

Cytology

Insufficient data available

Diagnostic molecular pathology

DGONCs show a distinct DNA methylation profile. In t-distributed stochastic neighbour embedding (t-SNE) analysis with the reference samples of Capper et al. {460}, DGONCs form a distinct cluster close to *FOXR2*-activated CNS neuroblastoma.

Monosomy of chromosome 14 has been reported in 30 of 31 investigated cases. No other specific recurrent alteration is known {737,2506}.

Essential and desirable diagnostic criteria
See Box 2.22.

Staging
Not clinically relevant

Prognosis and prediction
Outcome data are available for 26 patients. The 5-year progression-free survival rate was 81%, and the 5-year overall survival rate was 89% {737,2506}. Treatment data are available for 3 patients, all of whom received radiochemotherapy {2506}. The patients' initial diagnoses varied widely, from low-grade to high-grade, so some may have received aggressive therapy. It is therefore unclear to what extent treatment may have impacted the reported outcome data.

Box 2.22 Diagnostic criteria for diffuse glioneuronal tumour with oligodendroglioma-like features and nuclear clusters (DGONC)

Essential:

Methylation profile of DGONC

AND

Nuclear clusters of small to medium-sized cells exhibiting oligodendroglioma-like morphology

AND

Strong expression of both OLIG2 and synaptophysin

AND

Absence of widespread GFAP expression

Desirable:

Monosomy of chromosome 14

Caveat: DNA methylation profiling is so far the only method to clearly identify DGONC. If DNA methylation profiling is not available, morphological features may provide an approximation.

Papillary glioneuronal tumour

Varlet P
Komori T
Park SH
Rosenblum MK

Definition

Papillary glioneuronal tumour (PGNT) is a glioneuronal tumour exhibiting a biphasic pattern with variable representation of pseudopapillary glial structures and interpapillary neuronal components, and with *PRKCA* gene fusion (mainly *SLC44A1::PRKCA* fusion) (CNS WHO grade 1).

ICD-O coding

9509/1 Papillary glioneuronal tumour

ICD-11 coding

2A00.21 & XH3XU4 Mixed neuronal-glial tumours & Papillary glioneuronal tumour

Related terminology

Not recommended: pseudopapillary ganglioneurocytoma; pseudopapillary neurocytoma with glial differentiation.

Subtype(s)

None

Localization

PGNTs are supratentorial, most frequently affecting the temporal lobe (28%), and they are often in close proximity to the lateral ventricles (28%) {1354}.

Clinical features

Principal manifestations include headaches and seizures. Haemorrhagic presentation has been reported {399,243}.

Imaging

On MRI, the tumour is well demarcated, solid, and cystic, with a contrast-enhancing portion and little mass effect. The solid portion is isointense or hypointense on T1-weighted images and hyperintense on T2-weighted images or FLAIR. Most of the

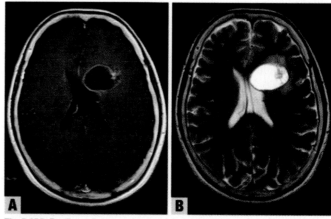

Fig. 2.120 Papillary glioneuronal tumour. **A** Contrast-enhanced T1-weighted image reveals peripheral enhancement in the cyst. **B** T2-weighted image shows a cystic mass pushing the anterior horn of the lateral ventricle.

tumours have no or only minimal peritumoural oedema, even when large {1867,3127}.

Epidemiology

PGNT is rare and the precise incidence remains to be determined. It is a tumour of young adults, with a median patient age at diagnosis of 16 years (range: 6–54 years) {1354}. No sex predilection was found in a cohort of patients with PGNT with *PRKCA* fusion {1354}.

Etiology

Unknown

Pathogenesis

The hallmark of PGNT is *PRKCA* gene fusion, mainly *SLC44A1::PRKCA* fusion; the only alternative *PRKCA* fusion partner that has been reported is *NOTCH1* {1354,2369,373}.

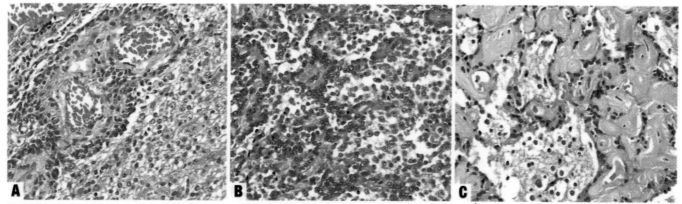

Fig. 2.121 Papillary glioneuronal tumour. **A** Biphasic appearance with pseudopapillary glial structures and interpapillary neuronal component. **B** Interpapillary component comprises neurocytes and ganglioid cells. **C** Hyalinized vessels can be prominent.

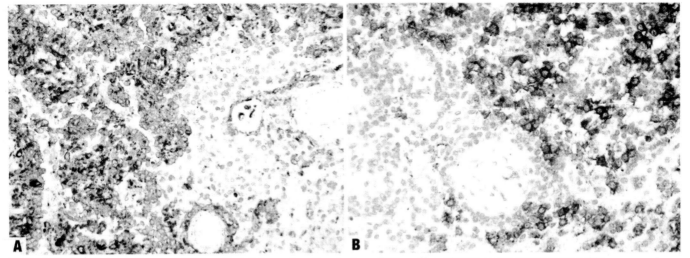

Fig. 2.122 Papillary glioneuronal tumour. **A** GFAP-positive cells in pseudopapillary structures. **B** Interpapillary cells show synaptophysin immunoreactivity.

The canonical *SLC44A1::PRKCA* fusion results from a reciprocal translocation t(9;17)(q31;q24), with consequent generation of a constitutively expressed oncoprotein {373}. *PRKCA* encodes protein kinase C alpha (PKCA), which is a member of the family of calcium- and phospholipid-dependent serine/threonine kinases that are involved in the MAPK signalling pathway.

Macroscopic appearance

PGNTs are well-delineated, solid, and cystic lesions. Calcification and haemorrhage may be observed.

Histopathology

PGNT is characterized by a distinctive biphasic pattern, consisting of (1) a glial pseudopapillary architecture and (2) an interpapillary component, heterogeneously distributed, with considerable variation in size between cases. In a series of 14 molecularly confirmed PGNTs, the pseudopapillary structures were constant except in 1 case {1354}. The cuboidal tumour cells cover hyalinized blood vessels in a single or pseudostratified layer. The glial cells have round nuclei and scant cytoplasm. Cellularity varies from case to case. Monomorphic neurocytes or medium-sized neurons are distributed in a neuropil background {1692}. Ganglion cells are not frequent (seen in 3 of the 14 cases), microcalcifications were present in 5 of 14 cases {1354}, and eosinophilic granular bodies are rare {1692}. Occasional mitoses may be seen, but microvascular proliferation and necrosis are absent {1354}. A few reports have described anaplastic features in PGNT, but those cases were not molecularly confirmed {1459,18}.

Immunophenotype

The immunophenotype is usually biphenotypic: glial in pseudopapillary structures and neuronal in interpapillary areas. The cuboidal glial cells draping vessels are positive for GFAP and S100. In some cases, oligodendrocyte-like cells that express OLIG2 but are GFAP-negative may be seen {3130}. The neuronal cells and fibrillary background (neuropil) express neuronal markers such as synaptophysin and NeuN. However, neurofilament is mostly confined to ganglioid cells, and chromogranin A is not widely expressed {1692}. Extravascular CD34 expression may be observed but only focally {2369}. The Ki-67 proliferation

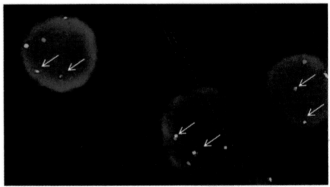

Fig. 2.123 Papillary glioneuronal tumour. Interphase FISH using a fusion probe for *SLC44A1* (green) and *PRKCA* (orange), showing *SLC44A1::PRKCA* fusion signals (arrows).

index generally does not exceed 2%, but elevated activity (ranging from 10% to > 50%) has been reported in non–molecularly confirmed cases {340,18}.

Differential diagnosis

PGNT diagnosis is challenging. In a series of 28 histologically diagnosed PGNTs {1354}, 17 (60%) clustered with an alternative methylation class (mainly dysembryoplastic neuroepithelial tumour, pilocytic astrocytoma, or pleomorphic xanthoastrocytoma). This may reflect the morphological heterogeneity of PGNT: the neuronal component may be limited, making it challenging to differentiate from astroblastoma, ependymoma, pilocytic astrocytoma, or pleomorphic xanthoastrocytoma; conversely, the neuronal component can be prominent with only focal papillary architecture (mimicking extraventricular neurocytoma or ganglioglioma). Moreover, perivascular tropism is not specific to PGNT and is shared by various glial or glioneuronal tumours such as pilomyxoid astrocytoma, astroblastoma, ependymoma, dysembryoplastic neuroepithelial tumour, ganglioglioma, and angiocentric glioma.

Cytology

Not clinically relevant

Diagnostic molecular pathology

PRKCA gene fusion (mainly *SLC44A1::PRKCA*) is the hallmark of PGNT {1354,2369,373}. To date, *SLC44A1::PRKCA* fusion has not been observed in other brain tumour types except one neurocytoma {1354}. Two alternative fusions, *PRKCA::FAT1* and *PRKCA::FAM91A1*, have been described in the diffuse glioma *MYB-* or *MYBL1*-altered methylation cluster {1354}. The fusion gene can be detected by simple interphase FISH on formalin-fixed, paraffin-embedded sections {2369}, but RNA sequencing can also be used {460}. No *PRKCA* recurrent mutation point has been reported in PGNT.

PGNTs exhibit a highly characteristic and diagnostic methylation profile {1354}. Copy-number variation analysis in the PGNT methylation group reveals flat profiles or only focal gains in a region of 17q that includes *PRKCA* (in 50% of cases) {1354}.

Essential and desirable diagnostic criteria

See Box 2.23.

Staging

Not clinically relevant

Prognosis and prediction

PGNTs correspond to CNS WHO grade 1, and gross total resection constitutes the main prognostic factor. One molecularly confirmed case has been described as recurrent {1354}. Morphologically diagnosed cases with a Ki-67 proliferation index > 20% or anaplastic features have been reported, with tumoural progression or dissemination {39,1459}. Such features have not been described in *PRKCA*-fused cases.

Rosette-forming glioneuronal tumour

Hainfellner JA
Jacques TS
Jones DTW
Rosenblum MK
Sievers P

Definition

Rosette-forming glioneuronal tumour (RGNT) is a glioneuronal tumour composed of two distinct histological components: one containing uniform neurocytes forming rosettes and/or perivascular pseudorosettes, and the other being glial in nature, with piloid and oligodendroglia-like cells, resembling pilocytic astrocytoma. These tumours are characterized by *FGFR1* mutation with frequent co-occurrence of a *PIK3CA* and/or *NF1* mutation (CNS WHO grade 1).

ICD-O coding

9509/1 Rosette-forming glioneuronal tumour

ICD-11 coding

2A00.21 & XH2JU8 Mixed neuronal-glial tumours & Rosette-forming glioneuronal tumour

Related terminology

None

Subtype(s)

None

Localization

RGNTs arise in the midline. They usually occupy the fourth ventricle and/or aqueduct and can involve adjacent brainstem, cerebellar vermis, quadrigeminal plate, pineal gland, or thalamus. Localization outside the fourth ventricle (e.g. in the pineal region, spinal cord, optic chiasm, septum pellucidum, and diencephalic region) has been described {105,3497,50}. In rare cases, dissemination throughout the ventricular system can occur {3386,81}.

Clinical features

Patients most commonly present with headache and diminished vision / papilloedema and/or ataxia, vertigo, diplopia, and dysarthria. Cervical pain is occasionally experienced. Rare cases are asymptomatic and discovered as incidental imaging findings.

Imaging

On CT, RGNTs appear hypodense. On MRI, RGNTs appear as relatively circumscribed, solid, cystic-solid, or multicystic tumours showing hypointensity on T1-weighted images and diffusion-weighted imaging, hyperintensity on T2-weighted images, and focal/multifocal and rim gadolinium enhancement. Contrast enhancement may fluctuate and spontaneously disappear. Haemorrhage and peripheral heterogeneous enhancement is common {2060,1030,3128}.

Epidemiology

RGNTs are slow-growing; they preferentially affect young adults, adolescents, and children; and they are rare. Specific population-based incidence rates are not available.

Etiology

Genetic susceptibility

RGNT has been described in patients with neurofibromatosis type 1 {91,1588,2925} or Noonan syndrome {1555,1896}.

Signalling pathways

The MAPK and PI3K signalling pathways appear to synergistically interact in the formation of RGNTs, and these tumours seem to be driven by constitutive activation of FGFR signalling together with frequent *PIK3CA* mutation {1896,2929}.

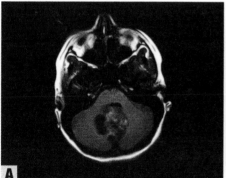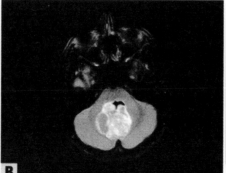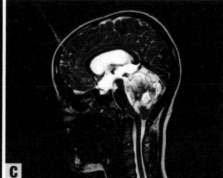

Fig. 2.124 Rosette-forming glioneuronal tumour. **A** Axial T1-weighted MRI without contrast showing a cerebellar midline mass with solid and cystic components. **B** Axial T2-weighted MRI with cerebrospinal fluid suppression demonstrating the heterogeneous signal of the partially solid, partially cystic midline mass. Note that the content of the cystic components is not isointense to cerebrospinal fluid. **C** Sagittal T2-weighted MRI showing compression of the fourth ventricle due to the cerebellar midline mass. As an effect of the obstructive hydrocephalus, the floor of the third ventricle is herniated into the suprasellar cistern.

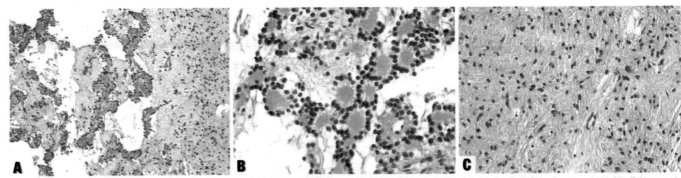

Fig. 2.125 Rosette-forming glioneuronal tumour. **A** Rosette-forming glioneuronal tumour consists of two components: neurocytic (left) and astrocytic (right). **B** Neurocytic rosettes: ring-like array of neurocytic tumour cell nuclei around eosinophilic neuropil cores. **C** Glial tumour component with piloid histomorphology.

Pathogenesis

Cell of origin

Neuroimaging, histological findings, and molecular evidence indicate that RGNT may arise from brain tissue surrounding the ventricular system. For cases affecting the fourth ventricle, an origin from the subependymal plate or the internal granule cell layer of cerebellum has been suggested {1693,3188}.

Genetic profile

Epigenetically, RGNTs display a distinct DNA methylation profile {2929}. At the genomic level, *FGFR1* hotspot mutations are typical, with co-occurrence of *PIK3CA* mutations in the majority of cases and additional loss-of-function mutation in *NF1* in a subset of cases {833,3188,1074,1643,2929}.

Macroscopic appearance

RGNTs are soft, gelatinous, generally well-demarcated tumours {1693}.

Histopathology

RGNTs are generally demarcated, but limited infiltration may be seen. They are characterized by a biphasic neurocytic and glial architecture {1693,2569,1438}. The neurocytic component consists of a uniform population of neurocytes forming neurocytic rosettes and/or perivascular pseudorosettes. Neurocytic rosettes feature ring-shaped arrays of neurocytic nuclei around delicate eosinophilic neuropil cores. Perivascular pseudorosettes feature delicate cell processes radiating towards vessels. Both patterns, when viewed longitudinally, may show a columnar arrangement. Neurocytic tumour cells

have spherical nuclei with finely granular chromatin and inconspicuous nucleoli, scant cytoplasm, and delicate cytoplasmic processes. These neurocytic structures may lie in a partly microcystic, mucinous matrix. The glial component of RGNT typically dominates and in most areas resembles pilocytic astrocytoma. Astrocytic tumour cells are spindle to stellate in shape, with elongated or oval nuclei and moderately dense chromatin. Cytoplasmic processes often form a compact to loosely textured fibrillary background. In some areas, the glial component may be microcystic, containing round to oval, oligodendrocyte-like cells with perinuclear haloes. Rosenthal fibres, eosinophilic granular bodies, microcalcifications, and haemosiderin deposits may be encountered. Overall, cellularity is low and necrosis is absent. Vessels may be thin-walled and dilated or hyalinized. Thrombosed vessels and glomeruloid vasculature may also be seen. Ganglion cells are occasionally present, but adjacent perilesional cerebellar cortex does not show dysplastic changes.

Proliferation

The Ki-67 proliferation index is low (< 3% in reported cases) and mitoses are usually absent.

Immunophenotype

Immunoreactivity for synaptophysin is present at the centres of neurocytic rosettes and in the neuropil of perivascular pseudorosettes {1693,2569,1438}. Both the cytoplasm and processes of neurocytic tumour cells may express MAP2. In some cases, NeuN positivity can be observed in neurocytic tumour cells. Tumour cells show nuclear expression of OLIG2. GFAP and

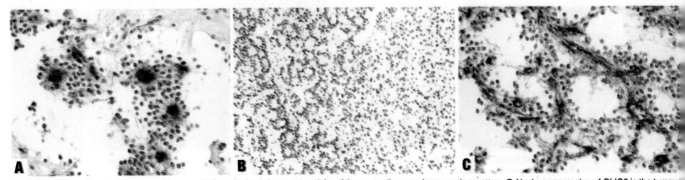

Fig. 2.126 Rosette-forming glioneuronal tumour. **A** Synaptophysin immunoreactivity of the neuropil cores of neurocytic rosettes. **B** Nuclear expression of OLIG2 in the tumour cell nuclei. **C** Synaptophysin immunoreactivity in the pericapillary area of perivascular pseudorosettes.

S100 immunoreactivity is present in the glial component but absent in rosettes and pseudorosettes.

Electron microscopy
Astrocytic cells of the glial component contain dense bundles of glial filaments. Rosette-forming neurocytic cells are intimately apposed and feature spherical nuclei with delicate chromatin, cytoplasm containing free ribosomes, scattered profiles of rough endoplasmic reticulum, prominent Golgi complexes, and occasional mitochondria. Loosely arranged cytoplasmic processes form the centres of rosettes and contain aligned microtubules as well as occasional dense-core granules. Presynaptic specializations may be seen, and mature synaptic terminals may form surface contacts with perikarya and other cytoplasmic processes {1693}.

Differential diagnosis
The main differential diagnosis is pilocytic astrocytoma. Diffuse leptomeningeal glioneuronal tumour may also be a differential diagnosis.

Cytology
In smear preparations, neurocytic cells feature round nuclei with granular chromatin, inconspicuous nucleoli, and scant cytoplasm. Cytological atypia is absent. Delicate, elongated processes are seen in the background. Piloid astrocytes with elongated nuclei and coarse bipolar processes may be evident. Clustering of tumour cells may be present {1693}.

Diagnostic molecular pathology
RGNTs are defined by a distinct DNA methylation profile. They are also characterized by *FGFR1* hotspot mutation (*FGFR1* p.N546 or p.K656) in combination with either *PIK3CA* or *PIK3R1*

Box 2.24 Diagnostic criteria for rosette-forming glioneuronal tumour

Essential:

Biphasic histomorphology with a neurocytic component and a glial component

AND

Uniform neurocytes forming rosettes and/or perivascular pseudorosettes associated with synaptophysin expression

AND (for unresolved lesions)

Small biopsies showing only one tumour component (neurocytic or glial) and a methylation profile of rosette-forming glioneuronal tumour

Desirable:

FGFR1 mutation with co-occurring *PIK3CA* and/or *NF1* mutation

---

mutation {2929,1953}. Accompanying *NF1* mutation can also occur, but this does not provide diagnostic specificity for RGNT because it can also be encountered in dysembryoplastic neuroepithelial tumour or pilocytic astrocytoma {2929,1953}. Because of the high number of misdiagnoses, molecular testing is highly recommended to confirm RGNT diagnosis {2929}.

Essential and desirable diagnostic criteria
See Box 2.24.

Staging
Not clinically relevant

Prognosis and prediction
The clinical outcome is favourable in terms of survival, but disabling postoperative deficits have been reported in approximately half of the cases. In rare cases, tumour dissemination, recurrence, or progression has been described {3191,2846,81}.

Myxoid glioneuronal tumour

Solomon DA
Blümcke I
Gessi M
Hawkins CE
Jones DTW

Definition

Myxoid glioneuronal tumour is a low-grade glioneuronal tumour typically arising in the septal nuclei, septum pellucidum, corpus callosum, or periventricular white matter. The tumour is characterized by a proliferation of oligodendrocyte-like tumour cells embedded in a prominent myxoid stroma, often including admixed floating neurons, neurocytic rosettes, and/or perivascular neuropil. There is a recurrent dinucleotide mutation at codon p.K385 in the *PDGFRA* gene (CNS WHO grade 1).

ICD-O coding

9509/1 Myxoid glioneuronal tumour

ICD-11 coding

2A00.21 Mixed neuronal-glial tumours

Related terminology

Not recommended: dysembryoplastic neuroepithelial tumour–like neoplasm of the septum pellucidum {177}; septal dysembryoplastic neuroepithelial tumour {569}.

Subtype(s)

None

Localization

Myxoid glioneuronal tumours are most commonly centred in the septal nuclei and septum pellucidum, but examples have also been reported in the genu of the corpus callosum and the periventricular white matter of the lateral ventricles {1954}.

This newly recognized tumour type probably encompasses a large subset of those neoplasms previously reported as dysembryoplastic neuroepithelial tumour and rosette-forming glioneuronal tumour centred within the deep periventricular white matter, lateral ventricles, and septum pellucidum {1184,1243, 2785,489,3493,3492,1072}.

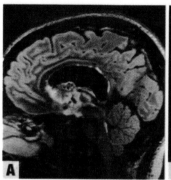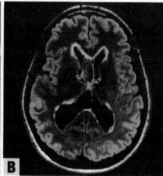

Fig. 2.127 Myxoid glioneuronal tumour. This tumour with characteristic *PDGFRA* p.K385 mutation is centred in the septal nuclei at the base of the septum pellucidum and is hyperintense on sagittal (**A**) and axial (**B**) T2-FLAIR MRI. There is also disseminated disease throughout the ventricular system, with hyperintense nodules along the ependymal surface of the lateral, third, and fourth ventricles (seen in **A**).

Clinical features

Presenting symptoms in patients with myxoid glioneuronal tumour are variable, but they most commonly include headaches, emesis, seizures, and behavioural disturbance {569}.

Imaging

On imaging, myxoid glioneuronal tumours are well-circumscribed lesions that are T1-hypointense and T2-hyperintense, without contrast enhancement or restricted diffusion. On susceptibility-weighted imaging, they occasionally demonstrate artefact suggestive of blood products from prior intratumoural haemorrhage. Tumours centred in the septal nuclei and septum pellucidum are often associated with obstructive hydrocephalus, whereas tumours centred in the corpus callosum and periventricular white matter have not been associated with hydrocephalus. A subset of patients have disseminated disease throughout the ventricular system at time of initial presentation {569,1954}.

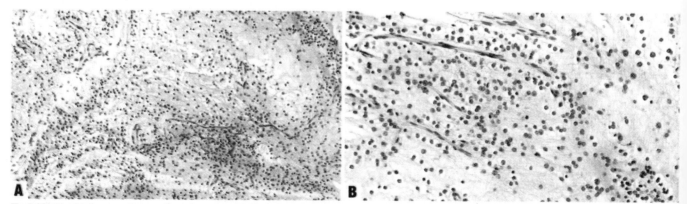

Fig. 2.128 Myxoid glioneuronal tumour. These tumours are histologically characterized by a proliferation of oligodendrocyte-like cells in a myxoid stroma with a delicate capillary network, occasionally containing floating neurons, neurocytic rosettes, and/or perivascular neuropil. **A** Low-power magnification. **B** High-power magnification.

Epidemiology

Myxoid glioneuronal tumours are rare primary brain tumours, with < 100 cases reported to date. They have an approximately equal sex distribution and predominantly occur in children and young adults, with a peak incidence in the second and third decades of life {569,1954}.

Etiology

No risk factors or inherited genetic susceptibility have been reported to date.

Pathogenesis

Myxoid glioneuronal tumours are genetically characterized by a recurrent dinucleotide mutation in the *PDGFRA* gene, which encodes platelet-derived growth factor receptor alpha (PDG-FRA), a transmembrane receptor tyrosine kinase. The characteristic mutation results in substitution of lysine with either leucine or isoleucine at codon 385 (p.K385L or p.K385I) in the vast majority of cases {2987,569,1954}. These p.K385L or p.K385I mutations have been somatic (tumour-specific) in all examined cases to date, and they typically occur in the absence of accompanying *PDGFRA* gene amplification. A single case has been described harbouring a *PDGFRA* p.E362delinsEW mutation instead of the canonical dinucleotide mutation at codon p.K385 {569}. The *PDGFRA* mutation is typically the solitary pathogenic alteration identified, with an absence of other accompanying genetic drivers in all cases studied to date. Most cases have had balanced diploid genomes without recurrent cytogenetic alterations. Although the functional impact of this specific p.K385L or p.K385I mutation in *PDGFRA* has not been studied to date, other mutations or intragenic deletions within the extracellular domain of the *PDGFRA* gene, which have been recurrently found in high-grade gliomas, have been shown to cause constitutive activation of the intracellular tyrosine kinase domain (TKD) and downstream activation of the PI3K and MAPK signalling pathways {2358,2425}.

Macroscopic appearance

Myxoid glioneuronal tumours are often soft, gelatinous, grey lesions.

Histopathology

Myxoid glioneuronal tumour is a mostly circumscribed, non-infiltrative glioneuronal neoplasm that is histologically characterized by a proliferation of oligodendrocyte-like tumour cells embedded in a prominent myxoid stroma. Some examples contain admixed floating neurons and perivascular neuropil resembling dysembryoplastic neuroepithelial tumour, whereas others contain neurocytic rosettes and perivascular neuropil resembling rosette-forming glioneuronal tumour. Myxoid glioneuronal tumours lack the multinodularity with patterned mucin-rich nodules that is characteristic of dysembryoplastic neuroepithelial tumours of the cerebral cortex. Rosenthal fibres, eosinophilic granular bodies, and microcalcifications typical of other low-grade neuroepithelial tumour entities are not commonly observed in myxoid glioneuronal tumours. Mitotic activity is typically very low or absent {569,1954}.

Immunophenotype

By immunohistochemistry, myxoid glioneuronal tumours are characterized by diffuse strong positivity for OLIG2, SOX10, GFAP, and MAP2 in the oligodendrocyte-like tumour cells. Synaptophysin staining is typically absent in the oligodendrocyte-like cells, but it is found in the floating neurons, neurocytic rosettes, and perivascular neuropil. CD34 staining is typically limited to the endothelial cells of the delicate capillary network. The Ki-67 labelling index is uniformly low (< 5%) {569,1954}.

Cytology

On intraoperative cytological preparation, these tumours are characterized by oligodendrocyte-like cells in a prominent myxoid background. Occasional neurons or neurocytic rosettes can be seen.

Diagnostic molecular pathology

Myxoid glioneuronal tumours are genetically characterized by a dinucleotide mutation in the *PDGFRA* gene that results in an amino acid substitution, either p.K385L or p.K385I, within the extracellular ligand-binding domain of the protein {2987, 569,1954}. Less commonly, other mutations in the extracellular domain of *PDGFRA* occur {569}. Most cases have had balanced

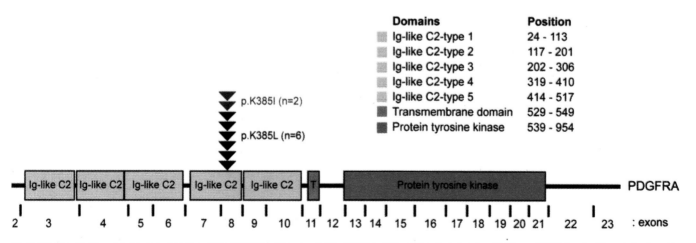

Domains	Position
Ig-like C2-type 1	24 - 113
Ig-like C2-type 2	117 - 201
Ig-like C2-type 3	202 - 306
Ig-like C2-type 4	319 - 410
Ig-like C2-type 5	414 - 517
Transmembrane domain	529 - 549
Protein tyrosine kinase	539 - 954

Fig. 2.129 Myxoid glioneuronal tumour. Diagram of the PDGFRA protein annotated with the location of the characteristic p.K385L or p.K385I dinucleotide mutation found in 8 cases of myxoid glioneuronal tumour {1954}.

diploid genomes without recurrent cytogenetic alterations. Myxoid glioneuronal tumours lack genetic alterations that are characteristic of other glioneuronal tumours and pilocytic astrocytoma (e.g. *BRAF*, *FGFR1*, *PIK3CA*, *PIK3R1*, *NF1*, *PTPN11*, or *MAP2K1* alterations). Genome-wide DNA methylation profiling has revealed that myxoid glioneuronal tumours harbour a distinct epigenetic signature that is closely related to that of dysembryoplastic neuroepithelial tumour of the cerebral cortex {2987, 569,565}.

Essential and desirable diagnostic criteria
See Box 2.25.

Staging
Not clinically relevant

Prognosis and prediction
Myxoid glioneuronal tumours are indolent, slow-growing tumours associated with favourable long-term outcomes in the absence of radiotherapy and chemotherapy {569,1954}. A subset of tumours can recur locally or disseminate throughout the ventricular system after subtotal resection, but they continue to be associated with indolent behaviour. High-grade transformation of myxoid glioneuronal tumours has not been described to date. Clinical experience for this rare tumour type remains limited, but the outcomes reported to date are favourable and equivalent to those of CNS WHO grade 1 tumour types such as pilocytic astrocytoma and rosette-forming glioneuronal tumour.

Box 2.25 Diagnostic criteria for myxoid glioneuronal tumour

Essential:

Oligodendrocyte-like tumour cells embedded in a prominent myxoid stroma

AND

Location in septal nuclei, septum pellucidum, corpus callosum, or periventricular white matter

Desirable:

PDGFRA p.K385L/I dinucleotide mutation or (less commonly) other mutations in the extracellular domain of *PDGFRA*

Methylation profile of myxoid glioneuronal tumour

Note: Desirable diagnostic criteria can be essential for unresolved cases.

Diffuse leptomeningeal glioneuronal tumour

Perry A
Capper D
Ellison DW
Jones DIW
Reifenberger G

Definition

Diffuse leptomeningeal glioneuronal tumour (DLGNT) is a glioneuronal neoplasm that commonly involves the leptomeninges diffusely, is composed of oligodendrocyte-like cells, and is molecularly characterized by chromosome arm 1p deletion and a mitogen-activated protein kinase (MAPK) pathway gene alteration, most commonly *KIAA1549::BRAF* fusion.

ICD-O coding

9509/3 Diffuse leptomeningeal glioneuronal tumour

ICD-11 coding

2A00.21 Mixed neuronal-glial tumours

Related terminology

Not recommended: disseminated oligodendroglioma-like leptomeningeal neoplasm; primary leptomeningeal oligodendrogliomatosis.

Subtype(s)

Diffuse leptomeningeal glioneuronal tumour with 1q gain; diffuse leptomeningeal glioneuronal tumour, methylation class 1 (DLGNT-MC-1); diffuse leptomeningeal glioneuronal tumour, methylation class 2 (DLGNT-MC-2)

Localization

These tumours preferentially involve the spinal and intracranial leptomeninges, although there are rare parenchymal examples without a leptomeningeal component, most often located in the spinal cord but occasionally also in the cerebral hemispheres {568,1545,125}. In the intracranial compartment, leptomeningeal growth is most commonly seen in the posterior fossa, around the brainstem, and along the base of the brain. One or more circumscribed, intraparenchymal, cystic or solid tumour nodules may be seen, with spinal intramedullary lesions being more common than intracerebral masses {2696}.

Clinical features

Patients often present with acute onset of signs and symptoms of increased intracranial pressure due to obstructive hydrocephalus, including headache, nausea, and vomiting. Opisthotonos and signs of spinal or cranial nerve damage may be present. Some patients show ataxia and signs of spinal cord compression. Rarely, patients present with epilepsy.

Imaging

In most cases, MRI shows widespread diffuse leptomeningeal enhancement and thickening along the spinal cord, often extending intracranially to the posterior fossa, brainstem, and basal cisterns. Small cystic or nodular T2-hyperintense lesions along the subpial surface of the spinal cord or brain are frequent.

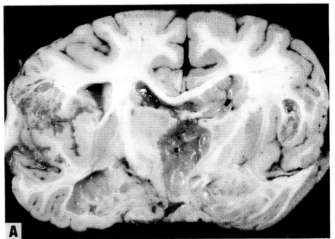

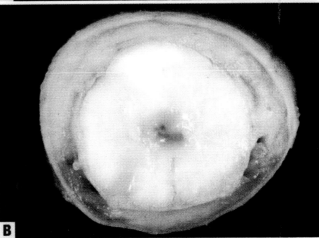

Fig. 2.130 Diffuse leptomeningeal glioneuronal tumour. **A** Note the extensive intraventricular involvement, as well as the parenchymal cysts. **B** Extensive spinal leptomeningeal involvement.

Discrete intraparenchymal lesions, most commonly in the spinal cord, were found in 25 (81%) of 31 patients in the largest reported cohort {2696}. Patients also commonly demonstrate obstructive hydrocephalus with associated periventricular T2 hyperintensity.

Epidemiology

DLGNTs are rare, and data on incidence are not available, but these tumours mostly affect paediatric patients. In the largest published series (36 patients) {2696}, the median age at diagnosis was 5 years (range: 5 months to 46 years). Another study found that the median age for DLGNT-MC-1 (5 years; range: 2–23 years) was lower than that for DLGNT-MC-2 (14 years; range: 5–47 years) {736}. The M:F ratio is roughly 1.6:1 {2659, 2696,2854,736}.

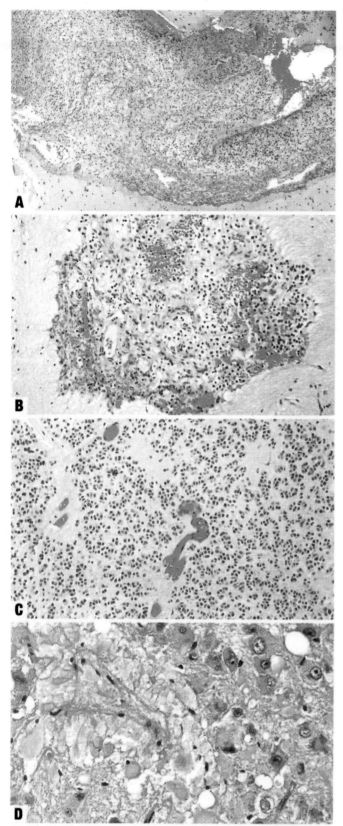

Fig. 2.131 Diffuse leptomeningeal glioneuronal tumour. **A** Marked expansion and hypercellularity of the leptomeninges. **B** Extension along the perivascular Virchow–Robin space is evident within the adjacent brain parenchyma of this tumour. **C** Neuronal differentiation is evident in the form of neurocytic rosettes and perivascular pseudorosettes. **D** Neuronal differentiation is evident in the form of ganglion cells.

Etiology

The etiology of DLGNT is unknown. The vast majority of tumours develop spontaneously, without evidence of genetic predisposition or exposure to specific carcinogens. In a series of 36 cases, no evidence of recognized genetic predisposing features or other tumour syndromes was observed, although 1 patient had a constitutional 5p deletion, 1 patient had a coexisting type 1 Chiari malformation, and 1 patient had a factor V Leiden mutation {2696}.

Pathogenesis

Cell of origin

The cellular origin of DLGNTs is unknown. The absence of obvious parenchymal lesions in some patients suggests an origin from displaced neuroepithelial cells within the meninges. However, an intraparenchymal origin is also possible, given that small intraparenchymal foci are frequently present in addition to the diffuse leptomeningeal tumour spread. Given the partial overlap in genetic features with oligodendroglioma and pilocytic astrocytoma, an origin from a precursor cell just upstream of this lineage segregation has also been speculated {736}.

Genetic profile

A frequent genetic alteration in DLGNTs reported to date is *KIAA1549::BRAF* fusion, found in 41 (72%) of 57 investigated cases from the combined data of four independent studies {2702}. Less common MAPK alterations include other *BRAF* alterations (including *BRAF* p.V600E mutations); *NTRK1*, *NTRK2*, or *NTRK3* gene fusions; *FGFR1* mutation; and *RAF1* rearrangements {768,814,736,125}. Deletions of chromosome arm 1p are also frequently observed in FISH analysis and were reported in 10 (59%) of 17 tumours in one series, and in 100% of tumours identified by DNA methylation profiling {24,342,1038, 2696,2702,736}. In cases with SNP array data or copy-number profiling from DNA methylation data, complete 1p arm loss was demonstrated {2696,2702,736}. Codeletion of 1p and 19q was observed at a frequency of 18% (3 of 17 tumours) in one series {2702} and in 10 (33%) of 30 tumours identified by DNA methylation profiling. In one case with 1p/19q codeletion, a t(1p;19q)(q10;p10) translocation was demonstrated by FISH {2730}. No mutations in *IDH1* or *IDH2* have been reported to date.

Within two distinct DNA methylation subclasses, 1q gain was found in all 13 cases of DLGNT-MC-2 and in 6 of 17 cases of DLGNT-MC-1 in one study (63% of all DLGNTs) {736}. Another group similarly found 1q gain in 14 (56%) of 25 DLGNTs {564}. Single cases with H3 p.K28M (K27M) mutation have been reported, but their relationship to H3 K27–altered diffuse midline glioma remains open {814,2208}.

Macroscopic appearance

DLGNT is generally characterized by a highly mucoid cut surface, whether present in the parenchyma, intraventricular spaces, or leptomeningeal spaces. Leptomeningeal tumour frequently extends along Virchow–Robin spaces, sometimes forming expansive cystic lesions. Obstructive hydrocephalus is common.

Histopathology

The diagnosis is most often made on meningeal biopsy or a biopsy taken from discrete intraparenchymal lesions. DLGNTs

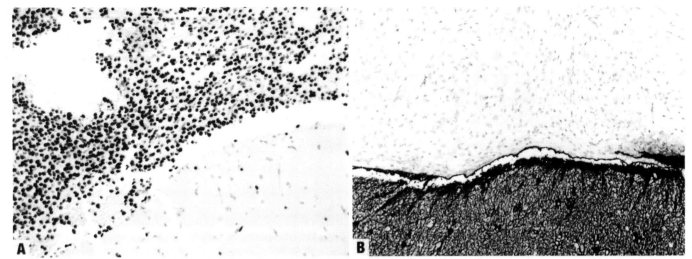

Fig. 2.132 Diffuse leptomeningeal glioneuronal tumour. **A** Tumour cells show extensive nuclear immunoreactivity for OLIG2. **B** The tumour cells are GFAP-negative.

are low- to moderate-cellularity neoplasms composed of relatively monomorphic oligodendrocyte-like tumour cells with uniform, medium-sized round nuclei and inconspicuous nucleoli. Like in oligodendrogliomas, clear perinuclear haloes are sometimes seen in DLGNTs as an artefact in formalin-fixed, paraffin-embedded tissue sections. The tumour cells grow diffusely or in small nests in the leptomeninges, with desmoplastic and myxoid changes commonly present. A storiform pattern may be observed in desmoplastic areas. Histological features of anaplasia are rare and include increased cytological atypia, brisk mitotic activity, microvascular proliferation, and/or palisading necrosis at primary presentation or after tumour progression {2696}; one example also featured a spongioblastic pattern with rhythmic nuclear palisades {3513}. A small subset of tumours contain overt neuronal differentiation, in the form of neurocytic rosettes, delicate perivascular pseudorosettes, neuropil-like islands, and/or ganglion cells. Rarely, eosinophilic granular bodies are observed. Rosenthal fibres are usually absent. The intraparenchymal component may resemble a dysembryoplastic neuroepithelial tumour or a diffusely infiltrative glioma, mostly oligodendroglioma, although astrocytic features occasionally predominate.

Grading

Histologically, the vast majority of DLGNTs are well-differentiated low-grade lesions. Nevertheless, a subset of tumours may show histological features of anaplasia or molecular alterations associated with shorter survival. The data for assigning distinct grades to this tumour type and its subtypes are still limited. Nevertheless, the clinical courses reported to date have been roughly similar to those of CNS WHO grade 2 entities for cases of conventional DLGNT and DLGNT-MC-1, and to those of CNS WHO grade 3 entities for tumours with anaplastic features, 1q gain, and/or the DLGNT-MC-2 profile.

Proliferation

Mitotic activity is sparse, and the Ki-67 proliferation index is usually low, with a median value of 1.5% reported in one series {2696}. However, some cases have an elevated Ki-67 proliferation index as evidence of anaplasia {2566}, with one study

reporting less favourable outcome associated with a proliferation index of > 4% {2696}. Brisk mitotic activity was defined as ≥ 1.7 mitoses/mm² (equating to ≥ 4 mitoses/10 HPF of 0.55 mm in diameter and 0.24 mm² in area) in one study {2696}.

Immunophenotype

The oligodendroglial-like tumour cells typically express OLIG2, MAP2, and S100 {2566}. GFAP immunoreactivity in tumour cells is seen in < 50% of cases and is often restricted to a minor proportion of neoplastic cells. Expression of synaptophysin is detectable in as many as two thirds of the tumours, and it is particularly common in those containing neuropil aggregates and ganglion cells. NeuN, neurofilament, and chromogranin stains are usually positive in only those tumours with more overt neuronal features on routine histopathology. EMA and IDH1 p.R132H stains are negative.

Differential diagnosis

The main differential diagnoses are intraparenchymal astrocytic or oligodendroglial gliomas with leptomeningeal dissemination; for instance, pilocytic astrocytoma may also show leptomeningeal dissemination. An absence of (or only focal) GFAP immunoreactivity, the presence of synaptophysin-positive cells, and the characteristic molecular profile of *KIAA1549::BRAF* fusion with isolated 1p deletion or 1p/19q codeletion in the absence of IDH mutation {2702,736} distinguish DLGNT from pilocytic astrocytoma, dysembryoplastic neuroepithelial tumour, oligodendroglioma, ganglioglioma, and diffuse astrocytoma. Pleomorphic xanthoastrocytomas can typically be distinguished by their pleomorphic histology, often with associated *BRAF* p.V600E mutation and *CDKN2A* and/or *CDKN2B* homozygous deletion {2702,3300}.

Cytology

Cerebrospinal fluid examination demonstrates elevated protein levels, although cytology is often negative {2696,2854}. Therefore, the diagnosis usually requires a biopsy. Intraoperative smear from a parenchymal lesion often resembles oligodendroglioma, whereas a meningeal biopsy is often less productive due to increased fibrous tissue.

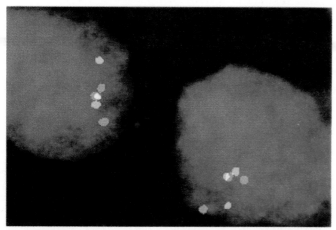

Fig. 2.133 Diffuse leptomeningeal glioneuronal tumour. FISH studies using *BRAF* (red) and *KIAA1549* (green) probes show increased copy numbers and yellow fusion signals.

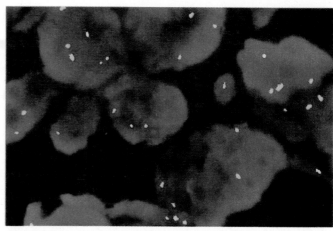

Fig. 2.134 Diffuse leptomeningeal glioneuronal tumour with 1q gain. FISH studies using chromosome 1p (orange) and 1q (green) probes show simultaneous 1p loss (only 1 signal) and 1q gain (> 2 signals) in most tumour nuclei.

Box 2.26 Diagnostic criteria for diffuse leptomeningeal glioneuronal tumour

Essential:

Oligodendroglioma-like morphology

AND

OLIG2 and synaptophysin immunoreactivity

AND

Chromosome arm 1p deletion

AND

MAPK pathway alteration (mostly *KIAA1549::BRAF* fusion)

AND (for unresolved lesions)

Methylation profile of diffuse leptomeningeal glioneuronal tumour

Desirable:

Childhood onset

Leptomeningeal dissemination

Caveat: This tumour type shows molecular overlap with pilocytic astrocytoma (*KIAA1549::BRAF* fusion) and oligodendroglioma (1p/19q codeletion). All diffuse leptomeningeal glioneuronal tumours are wildtype in *IDH1* and *IDH2*.

Diagnostic molecular pathology

For cases with typical clinical and histological features, molecular testing may be less critical. However, for any cases with diagnostic uncertainty, the initial molecular workup should include chromosome 1p status and *KIAA1549::BRAF* fusion testing. If 1p deletion is not detected, the diagnosis of DLGNT is unlikely. If *KIAA1549::BRAF* fusion is not detected, the possibility of less frequent MAPK alterations should be explored. For prognostic purposes, chromosome 1q status should also be tested. Alternatively, DNA methylation profiling can be performed for DLGNT class assignment, as well as for chromosome 1p and 1q copy-number alterations.

Essential and desirable diagnostic criteria

See Box 2.26.

Staging

Not clinically relevant

Prognosis and prediction

DLGNTs may go through periods of stability or slow progression over many years, although often with considerable morbidity {2696}. In a retrospective series of 24 cases with a median available follow-up of 5 years, 9 patients (38%) died between 3 months and 21 years after diagnosis (median: 3 years) {2696}, and 8 of the 24 patients lived for > 10 years after diagnosis {2696}. Mitotic activity, a Ki-67 proliferation index of ≥ 4%, and microvascular proliferation at the initial biopsy were each significantly associated with decreased overall survival {2696}. One study showed estimated 5-year overall survival rates of 100% and 43% in the DLGNT-MC-1 and DLGNT-MC-2 subclasses, respectively {736}. Another study showed substantially decreased progression-free and overall survival times for patients whose DLGNT harboured 1q gain versus those without this gain {564}.

Multinodular and vacuolating neuronal tumour

Rosenblum MK
Giangaspero F
Giannini C
Huse JT
Komori T
Pekmezci M

Definition

The multinodular and vacuolating neuronal tumour (MVNT) is composed of monomorphic neuronal elements distributed in discrete and coalescent nodules, with vacuolar changes in tumour cells and their matrix (CNS WHO grade 1).

ICD-O coding

9509/0 Multinodular and vacuolating neuronal tumour

ICD-11 coding

2A00.21 Mixed neuronal-glial tumours

Related terminology

Not recommended: diffuse gangliocytoma.

Subtype(s)

None

Localization

MVNTs typically involve the deep cortical ribbon and superficial white matter, predominantly of the temporal lobes (75–80%), followed by the frontal lobes (10–15%), and then the parietal and occipital lobes {1383,3179,2443,581}. A case involving the basal ganglia has been reported {3245}.

Clinical features

Seizures, particularly of complex partial type with or without secondary generalization, are the most common manifestation (~60% of cases), followed by headache (10–15%), episodic confusion, and dizziness. MVNTs may be incidentally discovered {307,2918}.

Imaging

Highly characteristic on MRI, although not always apparent, is the clustering of discrete or coalescent T2-FLAIR–hyperintense

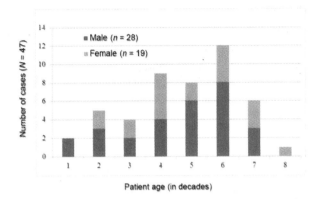

Fig. 2.135 Multinodular and vacuolating neuronal tumour. Distribution of cases by patient age at diagnosis.

nodules in deep cortex and superficial white matter, typically without associated mass effects, oedema, restricted diffusion, or contrast enhancement {1383,3179,2443,581}. Lesion stability on surveillance imaging is the rule.

Epidemiology

Population-based incidence data are not available. However, pathologically confirmed cases have been encountered mainly in adults (age range: 5–71 years; median: 42 years), with few paediatric examples recorded; the M:F ratio is 1.5:1 {1383,3179, 2443,581}.

Etiology

Factors predisposing individuals to the development of MVNTs have not been identified. An isolated lesion having the typical neuroradiological features of MVNT, but not biopsied, has been reported in a patient with Klinefelter syndrome {2147}.

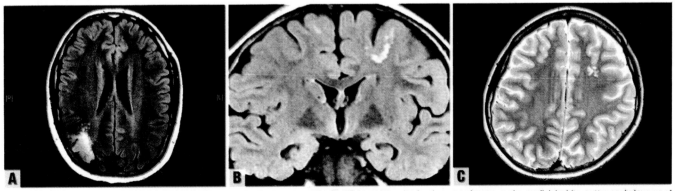

Fig. 2.136 Multinodular and vacuolating neuronal tumour. **A** Confluent and nodular FLAIR hyperintensity, involvement of cortex and superficial white matter, and absence of mass effect are characteristic on MRI. **B** MRI demonstrating FLAIR-hyperintense, clustered nodular lesions in the deep cortex and superficial subcortical white matter. **C** Axial MRI demonstrating clustered, T2-hyperintense nodular lesions in the superficial subcortical white matter.

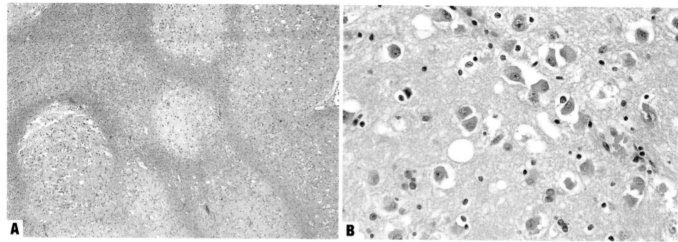

Fig. 2.137 Multinodular and vacuolating neuronal tumour. **A** Discrete tumour nodules with vacuolar changes are apparent. **B** Mature-appearing neurons of intermediate to large size populate this nodule with vacuolar matrix changes.

Pathogenesis

The clonal genetic abnormalities characterizing MVNTs indicate that these are neoplasms rather than malformations, but the precise role of MAPK pathway activation in this setting is not known. An origin from developmentally dysregulated, partially arrested neuronal or glioneuronal precursors destined for deep cortical layers could account for the characteristic localization {3179}. Somatic gene abnormalities that activate RAS/ RAF/MAPK signalling have been consistently identified, with *MAP2K1* and *BRAF* mutations (other than *BRAF* p.V600E) being recurrently identified {2443}.

Macroscopic appearance

MVNTs are characterized by multiple discrete or coalescent grey nodules involving the deep cortex, grey matter–white matter junction, and subcortical white matter {1383,307}.

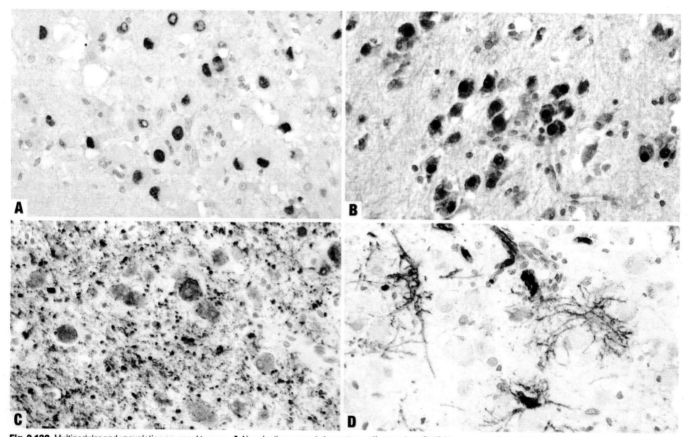

Fig. 2.138 Multinodular and vacuolating neuronal tumour. **A** Neoplastic neuronal elements manifest nuclear OLIG2 immunoreactivity. **B** Neoplastic neurons exhibit nuclear and cytoplasmic HuC/HuD immunoreactivity. **C** The neurons of this example are synaptophysin-immunoreactive (but most only weakly). **D** Ramified, CD34-immunoreactive neural elements are present in this example.

Box 2.27 Diagnostic criteria for multinodular and vacuolating neuronal tumour

Essential:

Multinodularity

AND

Neuronal cytological features or tumour cell immunoreactivity for synaptophysin, HuC/HuD, or non-phosphorylated 200-kDa NFP

AND

Absence of mitotic activity

AND

Tumour cell / matrix vacuolation (but may be minimal)

Desirable:

Immunoreactivity for OLIG2 and internexin A

Absence of NeuN or chromogranin expression

MAPK pathway–activating abnormalities

Histopathology

MVNTs are typically composed of pale, hypomyelinated nodules containing monomorphic neuronal elements that are most frequently of intermediate to large size (but generally not achieving ganglion cell proportions) with round and vesicular nuclei, distinct nucleoli, and amphophilic to eosinophilic cytoplasm {1383,307,2192,3179}. These lie in a delicate fibrillar matrix that usually exhibits conspicuous vacuolar change, with tumour cells often displaying cytoplasmic/pericellular vacuolization as well. A more diffuse distribution of neurons producing a band-like or gyriform expansion of the cortex or hippocampus may be evident, and some examples comprise small neuronal elements. Tumour cells are haphazardly distributed within nodules and some may align along capillary vessels. In select cases, small, oligodendrocyte-like cells are intermingled or clustered. Conspicuously dysmorphic and multinucleated neuronal forms are typically absent, as are Rosenthal fibres, eosinophilic granular bodies, myxoid microcysts and microcalcifications, although some tumours with MVNT-type and gangliogliomatous components have been described {3179,2443}. Mitotic figures, vascular proliferation, and necrosis have not been identified. MVNTs can be associated with regional cortical disorganization {1383} and hippocampal sclerosis {442}.

Immunophenotype

Tumour cells consistently express OLIG2, HuC/HuD, non-phosphorylated 200-kDa NFP, and doublecortin on immunohistochemistry, and they often express MAP2 and synaptophysin (although weakly, with much less labelling of the nodular matrix than the cortex) {1383,2192,3179,581}. Strong matrix labelling for α-internexin is present {2192,3179}, but tumour cells do not express phosphorylated NFPs or chromogranin, and they are negative or only weakly reactive for NeuN. Thus, they appear to have an incompletely matured neuronal immunophenotype. CD34 expression by ramified neural elements in associated cortex is common. GFAP labelling is restricted to reactive astrocytes.

Cytology

The identification of MVNTs requires examination of tissue sections. A characteristic profile in smear or squash preparations has not been described.

Diagnostic molecular pathology

MVNTs harbour MAPK pathway–activating abnormalities that most commonly involve small indels and hotspot mutations in *MAP2K1*, followed by pathogenic mutations in *BRAF* (excluding the common p.V600E mutations, which have not been documented in this tumour to date) and *FGFR2* fusions {2443,581}.

Essential and desirable diagnostic criteria

See Box 2.27.

Staging

Not clinically relevant

Prognosis and prediction

MVNTs are benign. Disease progression or recurrence have not been described after gross total excision, with subtotally resected tumours remaining stable {1383,3179,581}. The non-progressive nature of lesions exhibiting the characteristic neuroradiological features of MVNTs has prompted the suggestion that these can be safely followed without recourse to biopsy {2292,88}.

Hawkins CE
Blümcke I
Eberhart CG
Eng CE
Park SH

Dysplastic cerebellar gangliocytoma (Lhermitte–Duclos disease)

Definition

Dysplastic cerebellar gangliocytoma (Lhermitte–Duclos disease) is a cerebellar mass composed of dysplastic ganglion cells that conform to the existing cortical architecture and thicken the cerebellar folia (CNS WHO grade 1).

ICD-O coding

9493/0 Dysplastic cerebellar gangliocytoma (Lhermitte–Duclos disease)

ICD-11 coding

2A00.21 & XH6K00 Mixed neuronal-glial tumours & Dysplastic gangliocytoma of cerebellum (Lhermitte–Duclos)

Related terminology

Not recommended: cerebellar granule cell hypertrophy; diffuse hypertrophy of the cerebellar cortex; gangliomatosis of the cerebellum.

Subtype(s)

None

Localization

The tumour develops in the cerebellum, usually unilaterally (without preference for side) {1240,2758}. Rarely, bilateral tumours have been reported {1602,328}.

Clinical features

Dysplastic cerebellar gangliocytoma, or Lhermitte–Duclos disease, was first described in 1920 {1863,3012}. Patients with dysplastic cerebellar gangliocytoma most commonly present with dysmetria or other cerebellar signs, and/or signs and symptoms of obstructive hydrocephalus and increased intracranial pressure. Cranial nerve deficits, macrocephaly, and seizures are also often present. Variable periods of preoperative symptoms have been reported, with a mean duration of approximately 40 months {3331}.

Imaging

Neuroradiological studies demonstrate distorted architecture in the affected cerebellar hemisphere, with enlarged cerebellar folia and cystic changes in some cases. MRI is particularly sensitive in depicting the enlarged folia, with alternating T1-hypointense and T2-hyperintense tiger-stripe striations {1112,2111, 3408}. The lesions typically do not enhance. Infiltrating medulloblastomas may mimic dysplastic cerebellar gangliocytoma on imaging {784,2129}.

Epidemiology

Because of the rarity of dysplastic cerebellar gangliocytoma, there has not been a systematic study to determine the distribution of patient age at onset, but most cases have been identified

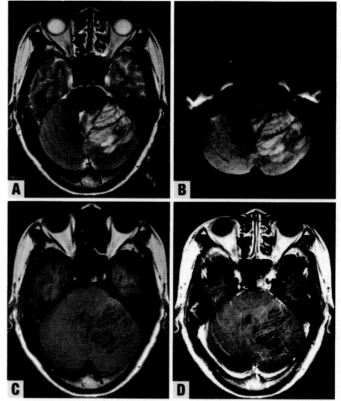

Fig. 2.139 Dysplastic cerebellar gangliocytoma. **A** T2-weighted MRI of a 37-year-old woman shows a mass of 56 mm in diameter with the typical tiger-stripe pattern of alternating inner hyperintense and outer hypointense layers in the left cerebellum. **B** Diffusion-weighted MRI reveals hyperintensity within the T2-hyperintense area of the tumour. **C,D** Precontrast (**C**) and postcontrast (**D**) T1-weighted MRI shows the vascular pattern of enhancement between the folia.

in adults. However, patients as young as 3 years and as old as in the eighth decade of life have been reported {849,1924, 3609}. *PTEN* mutations have been identified in virtually all cases of adult-onset dysplastic cerebellar gangliocytoma but not in childhood-onset cases {3609}, suggesting that the two differ in their biology.

Dysplastic cerebellar gangliocytoma is a component of Cowden syndrome. The single most comprehensive clinical epidemiological study estimated the prevalence of Cowden syndrome to be 1 case per 1 million person-years {3019}. However, after the identification of the gene for Cowden syndrome {1889}, a molecular-based estimate of prevalence in the same population was 1 case per 200 000 population {2227}. Because of difficulties in recognizing this syndrome, prevalence figures are likely to be underestimates. In one study of 211 patients with Cowden syndrome, 32% developed dysplastic cerebellar gangliocytoma {2672}.

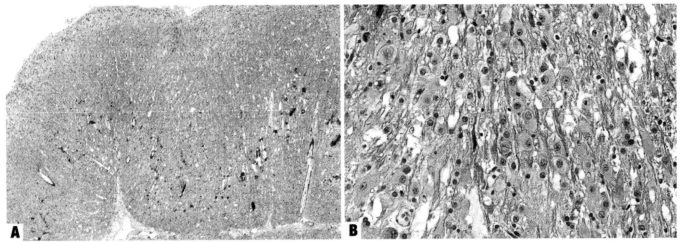

Fig. 2.140 Dysplastic cerebellar gangliocytoma (Lhermitte–Duclos disease). **A** Thickened cerebellar folium is replaced by large ganglion cells and disappearing inner granule cells. **B** Numerous large ganglion cells and abnormally myelinated axon bundles in the cerebellar cortex.

Etiology

Dysplastic cerebellar gangliocytoma is a component of Cowden syndrome, an autosomal dominant disorder characterized by multiple hamartomas involving tissues derived from all three germ cell layers {3125}. Approximately 85% of patients with Cowden syndrome have a germline mutation in *PTEN* (also called "*PTEN* hamartoma syndrome"), including intragenic mutations, promoter mutations, and large deletions/rearrangements {1889,2018,3610}. Patients without *PTEN* mutations may have germline variants of *SDHB* or *SDHD*, both of which have been shown to affect the same downstream signalling pathways as *PTEN* {2250}. Other alterations identified as predisposing to non-*PTEN* mutation–positive Cowden and Cowden-like syndromes include *SEC23B*, *USF3*, *KLLN*, and *WWP1* variants {3533}. WWP1 is an E3-ubiquitin ligase, and gain-of-function germline mutations increase ubiquitination and degradation of PTEN, mimicking germline *PTEN* mutations {1843}.

Pathogenesis

It remains unclear whether dysplastic cerebellar gangliocytoma is hamartomatous or neoplastic in nature. Malformative histopathological features, very low or absent proliferative activity, and the absence of progression support classification as hamartoma. However, recurrent growth has occasionally been noted, and dysplastic gangliocytomas can develop in adult patients with previously normal MRI findings {11,1218,2006}. It has been suggested that the primary cell of origin is the cerebellar granule neuron {1218}, and that a combination of aberrant migration and hypertrophy of granule cells is responsible for formation of the lesions {11}. Murine transgenic models with localized PTEN loss support this hypothesis {1776}.

Macroscopic appearance

The affected cerebellum displays a discrete region of hypertrophy and a coarse gyral pattern that extends into deeper layers.

Histopathology

Dysplastic cerebellar gangliocytoma causes diffuse enlargement of the molecular and internal granular layers of the cerebellum, which are filled by ganglionic cells of various sizes {11}. An important diagnostic feature is the relative preservation of the cerebellar architecture; the folia are enlarged and distorted but not obliterated. A layer of abnormally myelinated axon bundles in parallel arrays is often observed in the outer molecular

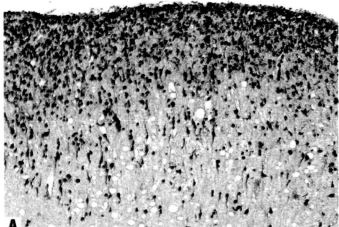
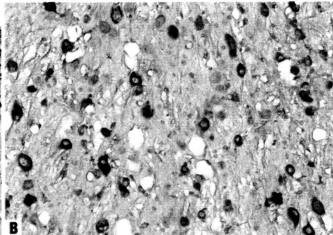

Fig. 2.141 Dysplastic cerebellar gangliocytoma (Lhermitte–Duclos disease). **A** NeuN immunohistochemistry reveals the abnormal arrangement of dysplastic ganglion cells, which are most densely present in the cerebellar molecular layer. **B** Some of the dysplastic ganglion cells are immunoreactive for phosphorylated mTOR.

layer. Scattered cells morphologically consistent with granule neurons are sometimes found under the pia or in the molecular layer. The resulting structure of these dysmorphic cerebellar folia has been referred to as inverted cerebellar cortex. Purkinje cells are reduced in number or absent. Calcification and ectatic vessels are commonly present within the lesion. Vacuoles are sometimes observed in the molecular layer and white matter {11}.

Immunophenotype

The dysplastic neuronal cells are immunopositive for synaptophysin. Antibodies specific to the Purkinje cell antigens CD3 (LEU4), PCP2, PCP4, and calbindin have been found to label a minor subpopulation of large atypical ganglion cells, but not to react with the majority of the neuronal elements, suggesting that only a small proportion of neurons are derived from a Purkinje cell source {1218,2919}. Immunohistochemistry also demonstrates loss of PTEN protein expression in most dysplastic cells and increased expression of phosphorylated AKT and S6, reflecting aberrant signalling that is predicted to result in increased cell size and lack of apoptosis {11,3609}. Undetectable or very low proliferative activity has been reported in the few cases analysed with proliferation markers {11,1218}.

Cytology

Not clinically relevant

Diagnostic molecular pathology

See *Pathogenesis*, above.

Essential and desirable diagnostic criteria

See Box 2.28.

Staging

Not clinically relevant

Prognosis and prediction

Although several recurrent dysplastic cerebellar gangliocytomas have been reported, most patients are cured by surgery, and no clear prognostic or predictive factors have emerged. Because cerebellar lesions may develop before the appearance of other features of Cowden syndrome, patients with dysplastic cerebellar gangliocytoma should be monitored for the development of additional malignant and benign tumours, including breast and thyroid cancers.

Central neurocytoma

Park SH
Giangaspero F
Honavar M
Sievers P

Definition
Central neurocytoma is an intraventricular neuroepithelial tumour composed of uniform round cells with a neuronal immunophenotype and low proliferation index (CNS WHO grade 2).

ICD-O coding
9506/1 Central neurocytoma

ICD-11 coding
2A00.3 & XH0C11 Central neurocytoma of brain & Central neurocytoma

Related terminology
None

Subtype(s)
None

Localization
Central neurocytomas are typically located supratentorially in the lateral ventricle(s) and/or the third ventricle. The most common site is the anterior portion of one of the lateral ventricles, followed by combined extension into the lateral and third ventricles, and then by a bilateral intraventricular location. Central neurocytoma is usually attached to the septum pellucidum near the foramen of Monro {1845,2585,3376}.

Clinical features
Most patients present with symptoms of increased intracranial pressure, rather than with a distinct neurological deficit. The clinical history is short (median: 1.7–3 months) {1845}.

Imaging
On CT, the masses are usually mixed solid and cystic (isodense/hyperdense). Calcifications may be seen {778}. On MRI, central neurocytomas are T1-isointense to the brain and have a soap-bubble (multicystic) appearance on T2-weighted images. They often exhibit FLAIR hyperintensity, with a well-defined margin. In all cases, heterogeneous enhancement after gadolinium injection is observed, and the tumour may show vascular flow voids. Haemorrhage may be seen {778,2257,3376}. An inverted alanine peak and a notable glycine peak on proton magnetic resonance spectroscopy are useful in the differential diagnosis of intraventricular neoplasms {778,1988}.

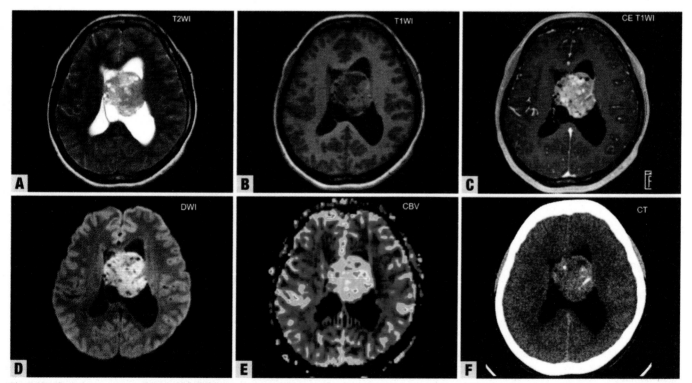

Fig. 2.142 Central neurocytoma. **A** T2-weighted MRI shows a mass of 52 mm in diameter in the left lateral ventricle; multifocal cystic portions can be seen. **B** T1-weighted MRI reveals a soap bubble–like multicystic appearance. The tumour is attached to the septum pellucidum. **C** The solid portions of the mass lesion reveal heterogeneous enhancement. **D** Diffusion-weighted MRI demonstrates diffusion restriction in the solid portions of the tumour, suggestive of high cellularity. **E** This mass has high cerebral blood volume, suggestive of hypervascularity. **F** CT reveals multifocal hyperattenuating calcifications within the tumour.

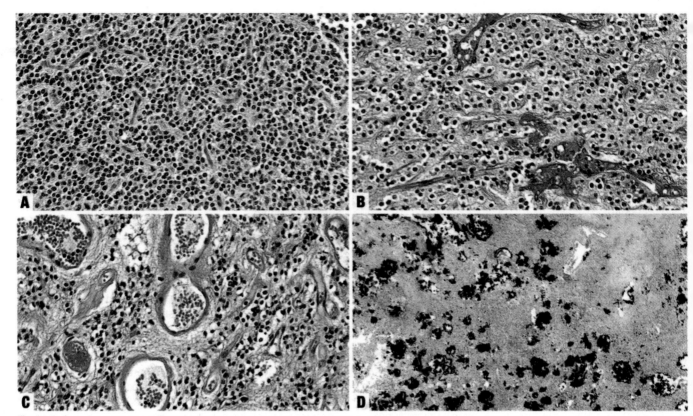

Fig. 2.143 Central neurocytoma. **A** Typical central neurocytoma shows a sheet of monotonous cells with round nuclei and salt-and-pepper chromatin patterns. **B** Sometimes cytoplasmic clearing is prominent. **C** Dilated and hyalinized blood vessels are sometimes prominent. **D** Numerous psammomatous calcifications may be present.

Spread

Craniospinal dissemination is exceptional and may occur in atypical central neurocytomas {851,3213,3017,2222}.

Epidemiology

In an analysis of > 100 cases, the mean patient age at clinical manifestation was 28.5 years; 46% of patients were diagnosed in the third decade of life and 70% were diagnosed between the ages of 20 and 40 years. Patient ages reported in the literature range from 8 days to 82 years, although paediatric cases are rare. Both sexes are equally affected, with an M:F ratio of 1.02:1. Population-based incidence rates for central neurocytoma are not available. In large surgical series, central neurocytomas account for 0.25–0.5% of all intracranial tumours {1262}.

Etiology

Unknown

Pathogenesis

Cell of origin

The cellular origin of central neurocytoma is unknown. Evidence of both glial and neuronal differentiation in some tumours suggests an origin from neuroglial precursor cells with the potentiality of dual differentiation {1419,2365,1695}. Central neurocytoma could originate from the subependymal plate of the lateral ventricles {3345}. However, an origin from circumventricular organs has also been proposed {1504}.

Genetic profile

The exact molecular features of this tumour are not known to date. Recurrent chromosomal alterations or mutations are not observed, and most cases show a flat disomy profile on copy-number analysis {463}. There was one report of central neurocytomas having numerous DNA copy-number alterations {1726}, including *MYCN* gain. Another transcriptomic study showed overexpression of genes involved in the WNT signalling pathway, calcium function, and maintenance of neural progenitors {3295}. Central neurocytomas have not been reported to exhibit 1p/19q codeletion.

Methylation profile

The methylation class of central neurocytomas exclusively comprises tumours with the histological diagnosis of central neurocytoma. A distinction between central neurocytoma and atypical central neurocytoma is currently not possible on the basis of methylation clustering {463}.

Macroscopic appearance

Grossly, central neurocytoma is greyish and friable. Calcifications and haemorrhage can be present.

Histopathology

Central neurocytoma is a neuroepithelial tumour composed of uniform round cells with a rounded nucleus with finely speckled chromatin and variably present nucleoli. Additional features include fibrillary areas mimicking neuropil, an oligodendroglioma-like honeycomb architecture, large fibrillary areas mimicking the irregular rosettes in pineocytomas, cells arranged in

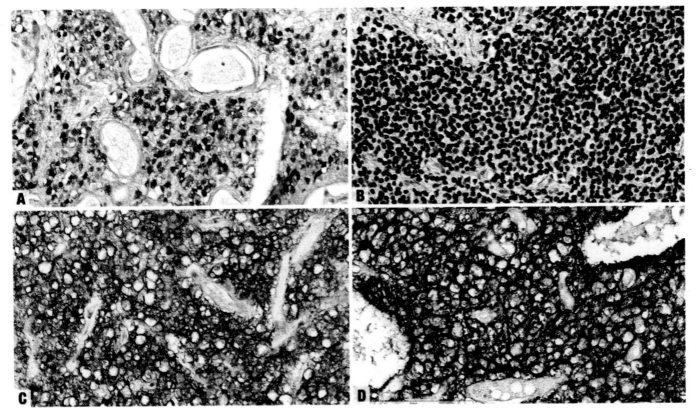

Fig. 2.144 Central neurocytoma. Immunohistochemically, the tumour cell nuclei in this particular case are robustly positive for NeuN (**A**) and for transcription factor 1 (TTF1) (**B**). The cytoplasm of the tumour cells is positive for synaptophysin (**C**) and for L1CAM (**D**).

straight lines, and perivascular pseudorosettes as observed in ependymomas. Capillary blood vessels, usually arranged in an arborizing pattern, give the tumours a neuroendocrine appearance. Calcifications are seen in half of all cases, usually distributed throughout the tumour. Occasionally, lipomatous changes can be observed {1054,3500,3498}. Rarer findings include Homer Wright rosettes and ganglioid cells {2684,3344}. Some cases show increased vascularity with substantial intratumoural haemorrhage (5–10% of cases), and early organizing haematoma can be present, which results in heterogeneity on T2-weighted images {3379}. In rare instances, anaplastic histological features (i.e. brisk mitotic activity, microvascular proliferation, and necrosis) can occur in combination, and tumours with these features are called atypical central neurocytomas {1262,3344,3531}.

Grading

Central neurocytoma corresponds histologically to CNS WHO grade 2. Tumours usually show a favourable behaviour, but some recur, even after total surgical removal. Moreover, several studies have shown increased aggressiveness in cases of atypical features and/or a Ki-67 (MIB1) proliferation index > 2–3% {1408,429,2592,2998}.

Proliferation

Mitoses are exceptional, and the Ki-67 (MIB1) proliferation index is usually low (< 2%). However, cases with a Ki-67 (MIB1) proliferation index as high as approximately 10% have been reported. The Ki-67 (MIB1) proliferation index is considered a powerful prognostic marker, but the optimal threshold of this index for predicting prognosis is still under debate {1408,429, 2592,2998}.

Electron microscopy

Electron microscopy shows regular round nuclei with finely dispersed chromatin and a small, distinct nucleolus in a few cells. The cytoplasm contains mitochondria, a prominent Golgi complex, and some cisternae of rough endoplasmic reticulum, often arranged in concentric lamellae. Numerous intermingled cell processes containing microtubules and dense-core or clear vesicles are always observed {496,1262}. Well-formed or abnormal synapses may be present, but they are not required for the diagnosis.

Immunophenotype

Synaptophysin expression is the most suitable and reliable diagnostic marker, with immunoreactivity diffusely present in the tumour matrix, especially in fibrillary zones and perivascular nucleus-free cuffs {930,1262}. Most cases are also immunoreactive for NeuN, although the intensity and extent of the labelling vary {2997,3296}. Thyroid transcription factor 1 (TTF1; clone SPT24) may also be positive in the tumour cell nuclei {1740}. Other neuronal epitopes (e.g. class III β-tubulin and MAP2) are usually expressed. In addition, L1CAM can be positive in the tumour cells. In contrast, expression of chromogranin A, NFP, and α-internexin is absent, except in sporadic cases showing gangliocytic differentiation. Although most studies have found GFAP to be expressed only in entrapped reactive astrocytes, this antigen has been reported in tumour cells by some authors {2998,3233,3344,3345}. OLIG2 is usually positive in occasional

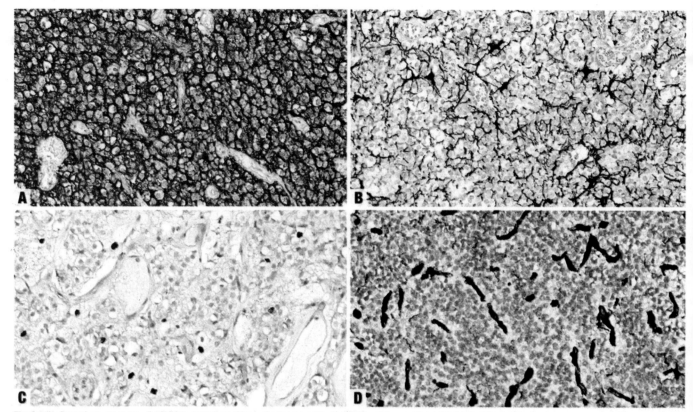

Fig. 2.145 Central neurocytoma. **A** MAP2 is strongly positive in the tumour cells. **B** GFAP-positive reactive astrocytes and cytoplasmic processes are variably present in the tumour. **C** OLIG2 stain reveals a few positive nuclei. **D** Vimentin is negative in tumour cells but stains blood vessels and fine cytoplasmic processes of reactive astrocytes.

Box 2.29 Diagnostic criteria for central neurocytoma

Essential:

Intraventricular localization

AND

Oligodendroglioma-like monomorphic cells

AND

Synaptophysin expression

AND (for unresolved lesions)

Methylation profile of central neurocytoma

Desirable:

Young adult patient

In most cases, no sign of malignancy

cells in central neurocytoma {1892}. However, a strong and diffuse OLIG2 immunoreactivity would favour a diagnosis of intraventricular oligodendroglioma {3489}.

Cytology

Intraoperative squash preparation shows a monotonous sheet of round cells with rounded nuclei and salt-and-pepper chromatin without cell aggregation or clustering, resembling the smear pattern of pituitary adenoma {2899}.

Diagnostic molecular pathology

See *Genetic profile* under *Pathogenesis*, above.

Essential and desirable diagnostic criteria

See Box 2.29.

Staging

Not clinically relevant

Prognosis and prediction

The clinical course of central neurocytoma is usually favourable, with the 5-year and 10-year overall survival rates estimated to be 96% and 82%, respectively {1408}. However, malignant behaviour with craniospinal dissemination has been reported {851, 3213,2222,3017}. The extent of resection is an important prognostic factor. Specifically, a pooled analysis of > 400 patients has demonstrated that gross total resection is superior to subtotal resection {2591}. Nevertheless, recent literature has not found statistically significant differences in overall survival between gross total and subtotal resection {1408,429}. Although gross total resection surgery should always be attempted, this procedure is not often feasible, because of the distinct location of the intraventricular area and vital neural structures in the periventricular region {429}. It is now well established that a higher Ki-67 (MIB1) labelling index is associated with more aggressive behaviour. A recent study reported a 2-year progression-free survival rate of 48% for cases with a Ki-67 (MIB1) labelling index > 4%, in contrast to 90% for those with a value ≤ 4% {1408}. However, the optimal threshold of this index is still a matter of debate {1408, 429,2592,2998}. Regardless of the threshold, there is evidence that adjuvant therapy should be considered for tumours with higher Ki-67 (MIB1) index values {1408}.

Extraventricular neurocytoma

Sievers P
Giangaspero F
Honavar M
Park SH
Soffietti R

Definition
Extraventricular neurocytoma is a usually well-circumscribed neuronal neoplasm that arises throughout the CNS outside the ventricular system, with histopathological characteristics resembling those of central neurocytoma but demonstrating a much wider morphological spectrum, and with frequent *FGFR1::TACC1* fusions (CNS WHO grade 2).

ICD-O coding
9506/1 Extraventricular neurocytoma

ICD-11 coding
2A00.3 & XH2HS1 Central neurocytoma of brain & Extraventricular neurocytoma

Related terminology
None

Subtype(s)
None

Localization
Extraventricular neurocytomas can arise in almost any location in the CNS without contact with the ventricular system. The most frequently documented locations are the cerebral hemispheres and cerebellum {3205,363,2935}. However, there are also reports of these tumours arising in the spinal cord, thalamus, hypothalamic region, and pons, with single cases reported in cranial nerves, the cauda equina, and even in the sellar region {1015,3091}, although these cases were reported in the pre-genetics era.

Clinical features
The clinical manifestation of extraventricular neurocytoma varies according to the multiple locations described for these tumours and whether the tumour exerts a mass effect. Patients may present with headache, seizures, visual disturbances, hemiparesis, and cognitive disturbances, but they can also display motor, sensory, and sphincter dysfunction, as well as epilepsy {363,1015,3091,3499,3590}.

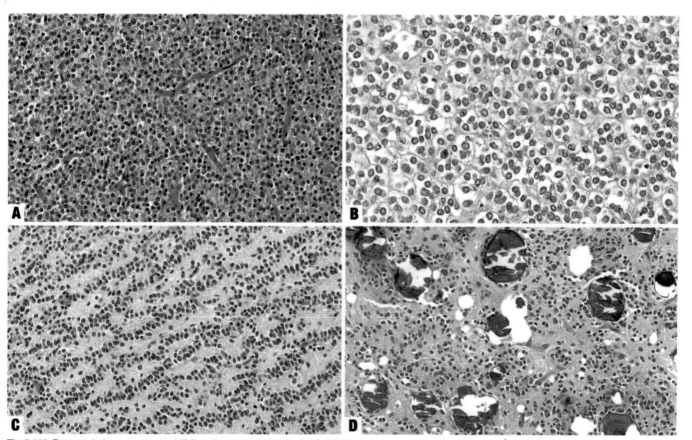

Fig. 2.146 Extraventricular neurocytoma. **A,B** Round, monomorphic, oligodendroglia-like tumour cells with small, uniform nuclei and sparse cytoplasm, frequently with clear perinuclear haloes, at low power (**A**) and high power (**B**). **C** Neoplastic cells arranged in rows or ribbons. **D** Microcalcifications may be present.

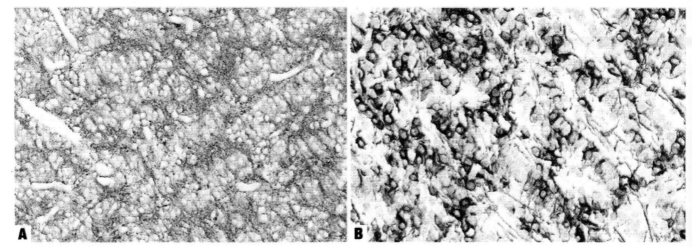

Fig. 2.147 Extraventricular neurocytoma. **A** Diffuse cytoplasmic immunoreactivity for synaptophysin is characteristic of extraventricular neurocytoma. **B** Variable proportions of GFAP-positive cells may be present in some tumours.

Imaging

Extraventricular neurocytomas exhibit a wide and variable imaging spectrum. They usually appear as large, well-demarcated, solitary, cystic-solid masses that are frequently associated with moderate peritumoural oedema and calcifications {363,1473, 2713}. Intratumoural haemorrhage may be present. On MRI, the solid portion is isointense to hypointense on T1-weighted images and predominantly hyperintense on T2-weighted images. In most cases, MRI shows heterogeneous contrast enhancement {1473,2713}.

Epidemiology

Extraventricular neurocytomas are rare, with an annual incidence rate in the USA of approximately 0.01 cases per 100 000 population {3205}. They generally affect patients of any age, with peak incidence in the third to fourth decades of life. There is no significant sex predilection {3205,2935,363}.

Etiology

The etiology of extraventricular neurocytoma is unknown. No risk factors or inherited genetic susceptibility have been reported to date.

Pathogenesis

Cell of origin

The cellular origin of extraventricular neurocytoma is unknown. The fact that extraventricular neurocytomas form a distinct molecular group suggests that these tumours may arise from a specific precursor cell population {2935}.

Genetic profile

The most frequent genetic alterations are *FGFR1::TACC1* fusions, which were found in 60% of cases in one large series of tumours identified by DNA methylation profiling. Less common alterations include other FGFR gene fusions {2935}. Neither IDH gene mutations nor *MGMT* promoter methylation has been reported to date {2187}.

Macroscopic appearance

Extraventricular neurocytomas are usually well circumscribed, sometimes with a cyst-mural nodule configuration, but they can occasionally be infiltrative.

Histopathology

Although some histopathological characteristics resemble central neurocytoma, a much wider morphological spectrum has been described in extraventricular neurocytomas. Histologically, extraventricular neurocytomas are usually moderate- to high-cellularity neoplasms often composed of relatively monomorphic oligodendroglia-like tumour cells with small, uniform nuclei and sparse cytoplasm, frequently with clear perinuclear haloes. Tumour cells are often arranged in sheets or cell clusters with neuropil islands; less frequent patterns include neurocytic rosettes or ribbons. A subset of tumours contain ganglion or ganglioid cells. Microcalcifications and hyalinized vessels may be present {1084,363,2935}. A rare case with lipomatous changes has been reported {436}. Mitotic activity is usually low. More recently, molecular investigations of extraventricular neurocytomas revealed a high rate of histologically misinterpreted cases and underlined the wide range of morphological heterogeneity in this entity {2935}.

Grading

The majority of extraventricular neurocytomas manifest histologically as low-grade tumours and correspond to CNS WHO grade 2. However, a subset of tumours (lacking genetic analyses) have been reported to show histopathological features of atypia or anaplasia, with increased mitotic and proliferative activity as well as microvascular proliferation and/or necrosis, suggestive of a more aggressive clinical behaviour {1540,3563, 1015}.

Immunophenotype

Diffuse cytoplasmic immunoreactivity for synaptophysin is characteristic of extraventricular neurocytoma and is present in the tumour cells and neuropil islands {363,2187,2935}. Chromogranin A and NeuN labelling in some cases confirms neuronal differentiation, but it might be very focal. In nearly half of the cases, immunopositivity for GFAP has been reported {363}. Expression of OLIG2 has been observed in a subset of extraventricular neurocytoma, but it is more typically negative in the neoplastic cells {2315,2187}. Immunohistochemistry for IDH1 p.R132H is negative {26,3535,461}. The Ki-67 proliferation index is usually low (1–3%), but it can be elevated in a subset of cases {1540, 363,2935}.

Differential diagnosis
Differential diagnostic considerations usually include oligodendroglioma and other glioneuronal and neuronal tumours. The diffuse cytoplasmic immunoreactivity for synaptophysin in the absence of IDH mutation and 1p/19q codeletion distinguishes extraventricular neurocytoma from oligodendroglioma. Central neurocytomas can typically be distinguished by their intraventricular localization. Because of a wide overlap with various glioneuronal entities, additional molecular analyses are highly recommended in cases with diagnostic uncertainty.

Cytology
Not clinically relevant

Diagnostic molecular pathology
Genome-wide DNA methylation profiling has provided evidence for a specific epigenetic signature of extraventricular neurocytoma that is clearly distinct from that of other CNS tumours; it has also indicated that many cases diagnosed histologically (without additional molecular analysis) may represent misdiagnoses. *FGFR1::TACC1* fusion is a highly frequent event in molecularly defined extraventricular neurocytoma, in addition to a small number of other FGFR alterations {2935}. Therefore,

Box 2.30 Diagnostic criteria for extraventricular neurocytoma

Essential:
Extraventricular neurocytic neoplasm without IDH alteration
AND
Synaptophysin expression
AND (for unresolved lesions)
Methylation profile of extraventricular neurocytoma

Desirable:
FGFR1 alteration (mostly *FGFR1::TACC1* fusion)

Caveat: Diagnosis should be heavily weighted towards molecular findings because morphological analyses frequently result in mistyping {2935}.

additional molecular analyses are strongly advised for a precise diagnosis of extraventricular neurocytoma.

Essential and desirable diagnostic criteria
See Box 2.30.

Staging
Not clinically relevant

Prognosis and prediction
Extraventricular neurocytoma is generally a low-grade tumour with a usually favourable prognosis {2935}. Gross total resection has been associated with a low rate of recurrence and good seizure control {1540,363,1015}. However, reports on the clinical courses and outcomes of these tumours vary considerably, not least because of a wide overlap with other entities and possible misdiagnosis in some cases.

Cerebellar liponeurocytoma

Giangaspero F
Chimelli L
Park SH
Sievers P

Definition

Cerebellar liponeurocytoma is a cerebellar neoplasm with advanced neuronal or neurocytic differentiation, variable glial differentiation, and focal lipoma-like changes (CNS WHO grade 2).

ICD-O coding

9506/1 Cerebellar liponeurocytoma

ICD-11 coding

2A00.3 & XH2GB0 Central neurocytoma of brain & Cerebellar liponeurocytoma

Related terminology

Not recommended: lipomatous medulloblastoma; lipidized medulloblastoma; neurolipocytoma; medullocytoma; lipomatous glioneurocytoma; lipidized mature neuroectodermal tumour of the cerebellum.

Subtype(s)

None

Localization

Cerebellar liponeurocytoma most commonly involves the cerebellar hemispheres, but it can also be located in the paramedian region or vermis and extend to the cerebellopontine angle or fourth ventricle {2260,1054,1606,570}. Recent reports {1054, 3500,3498,436} have described a series of cases of liponeurocytoma-like tumours occurring in the cerebellum and in supratentorial locations, causing confusion between bona fide cerebellar liponeurocytoma and central or extraventricular neurocytoma with lipomatous changes. There are also reports of multifocal tumours: a principal lesion with a satellite lesion in the opposite hemisphere {2447,1606}, multiple bilateral lesions {2875,2947}, and even a case associated with leptomeningeal spinal cord nodules at presentation {1699}.

Clinical features

Headache and other symptoms and signs of raised intracranial pressure (either from the lesion itself or due to obstructive hydrocephalus) are common presentations. Cerebellar signs, including ataxia and disturbed gait, are also common {2352}.

Imaging

On CT, the tumour is variably isodense or hypodense, with focal areas of marked hypoattenuation corresponding to high fat density {77,2260,1054}. On T1-weighted MRI, the tumour is isointense to hypointense, with patchy areas of hyperintensity corresponding to regions of high lipid content. Enhancement with gadolinium is usually heterogeneous, with areas of tumour showing variable degrees of enhancement. On T2-weighted and FLAIR imaging, the tumour is hyperintense to the adjacent brain {1054}. Associated oedema is minimal or absent {48}. Fat-suppressed images may be helpful in supporting a preoperative diagnosis {77}.

Epidemiology

More than 60 cases of cerebellar liponeurocytoma have been reported in the English-language literature {2260,1054,1606, 738}. The mean patient age is 50 years (range: 24–77 years), with peak incidence in the third to sixth decades of life. There is no significant sex predilection {1346,2417}. Familial predisposition has been reported {2513,3466}.

Etiology

Unknown

Pathogenesis

Cell of origin

One study demonstrated that the transcription factor NGN1, but not ATOH1, is expressed in cerebellar liponeurocytoma (unlike in normal adult cerebellum) and that adipocyte fatty acid–binding protein, typically found in adipocytes, is significantly

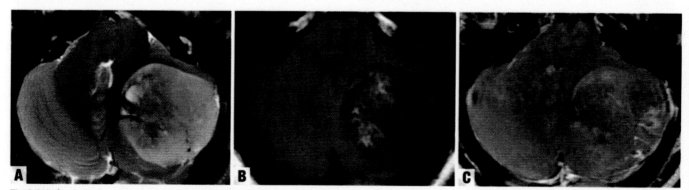

Fig. 2.148 Cerebellar liponeurocytoma. **A** T2-weighted MRI depicts the mass as well circumscribed and mildly heterogeneous, with small cystic areas medially. **B** Inherently bright signal on T1-weighted pre-contrast images corresponding to lipid within the tumour. **C** Postgadolinium T1-weighted imaging with fat saturation depicts mild diffuse enhancement of the mass, while the bright signal in fat-rich areas is lost with fat saturation.

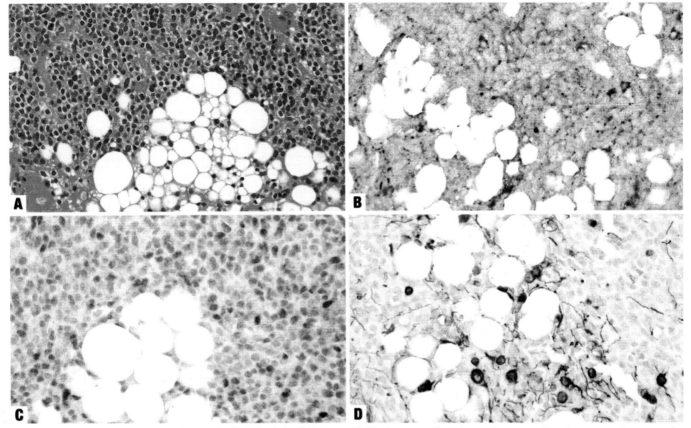

Fig. 2.149 Cerebellar liponeurocytoma. **A** Classic histology showing neurocytes and lipidized tumour cells. **B** Intense immunoreactivity of neurocytes for synaptophysin. **C** Liponeurocytomas also express NeuN. **D** GFAP-positive neoplastic cells can be present.

overexpressed in cerebellar liponeurocytoma compared with both normal adult cerebellum and human medulloblastoma. These findings suggest an origin of cerebellar liponeurocytoma from cerebellar progenitors, which are distinct from cerebellar granule progenitors and aberrantly differentiate into adipocyte-like tumour cells {115}.

Genetic profile

Genetic analyses indicate that this lesion is a rare but distinct clinicopathological entity {1346,2260,2999,1085,463}. Genome-wide DNA methylation analysis of cerebellar liponeurocytomas has shown that they are molecularly distinct and characterized by recurrent focal losses of chromosomes 14 and 2p {463}. These findings are supported by gene expression data indicating that cerebellar liponeurocytomas have profiles more similar to those of central neurocytoma than to those of medulloblastoma, and that they lack isochromosome 17q and mutations of *PTCH1*, *CTNNB1*, and *APC* {1346}, which are seen in a subset of medulloblastomas. *TP53* missense mutations were reported in 4 of 20 cases, which is a higher frequency than in medulloblastoma, and this is not an alteration typically seen in central neurocytoma {1346}. Although single reports suggest a possible inheritable predisposition {2513,3466}, no specific genetic susceptibility is known. Cerebellar liponeurocytoma displayed a unique epigenetic signature {460}.

Macroscopic appearance

Not reported

Histopathology

Cerebellar liponeurocytoma is composed of a uniform population of small neurocytic cells arranged in sheets and lobules and with regular round to oval nuclei, clear cytoplasm, and poorly defined cell membranes. The histological hallmark of this entity is focal accumulation of lipid-laden cells that resemble adipocytes but constitute lipid accumulation in neuroepithelial tumour cells. Features of anaplasia, such as nuclear atypia, necrosis, and microvascular proliferation, are typically absent in primary lesions, but they may be found in recurrent tumours {1085,2594}. The lipidized component may be markedly reduced or even absent {2594} in recurrent lesions. However, some tumour recurrences lack these atypical histopathological features {1467}.

Grading

Cerebellar liponeurocytoma corresponds histologically to CNS WHO grade 2.

Proliferation

The growth fraction as determined by the Ki-67 (MIB1) proliferation index is usually in the range of 1–4%, but it can be as high as 10% in cases of tumour recurrence {1054}.

Electron microscopy

Electron microscopy shows dense-core and clear vesicles, microtubule-containing neurites, and (occasionally)

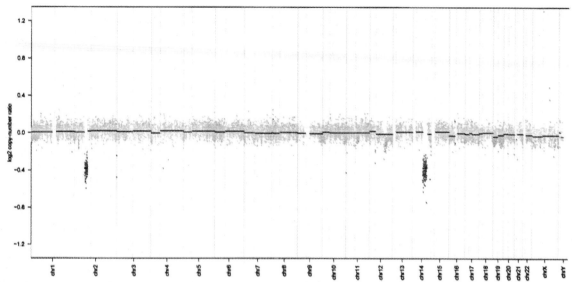

Fig. 2.150 Cerebellar liponeurocytoma. Copy-number analysis showing focal losses of chromosomes 14p and 2p.

synapse-like structures associated with non–membrane-bound lipid vacuoles of variable size {1529,1011,1085}.

Immunophenotype

Immunohistochemically, there is consistent expression of neuronal markers, including synaptophysin, NeuN, and MAP2. Focal GFAP expression by tumour cells, which indicates astrocytic differentiation, is observed in most cases {1054,2999}. One report mentioned immunoreactivity for desmin and morphological features of incipient myogenic differentiation {1137}.

Cytology

Not clinically relevant

Diagnostic molecular pathology

See *Genetic profile* under *Pathogenesis*, above.

Essential and desirable diagnostic criteria

See Box 2.31.

Staging

Not clinically relevant

Prognosis and prediction

This tumour has a favourable prognosis. Most patients with sufficient follow-up survived for > 5 years, and gross total resection and postoperative radiotherapy yield survival benefit {47,1467}. On meta-analysis, the postoperative 5-year survival rate was 71.3%, the 5-year progression-free survival rate was 60.8%, the mean overall survival was 16.3 years, and the median

Box 2.31 Diagnostic criteria for cerebellar liponeurocytoma

Essential:

Cerebellar localization

AND

Oligodendroglioma-like monomorphic cells associated with focal lipoma-like changes

AND

Synaptophysin expression

AND (for unresolved lesions)

Methylation profile of cerebellar liponeurocytoma

Desirable:

Adult patient

Focal GFAP immunoreactivity

Absence of histological features of malignancy

progression-free survival was 10 years (mean: 8.6 years) regardless of treatment {1504,77,433,47,1346,1895,2594,3500, 570}. Review of the literature showed that the tumour recurrence rate in patients treated by complete tumour resection (with or without adjuvant radiotherapy) was 15%, whereas the recurrence rate in patients treated by incomplete tumour resection (with or without radiotherapy) was 42% {1054}. Recurrent tumours may show increased mitotic activity (with an increased Ki-67 [MIB1] proliferation index as high as 30%), vascular proliferation, and necrosis {1085,2594}, although some tumour recurrences lack these atypical histopathological features {1467,1504}. All reported recurrences were confined to the posterior fossa {1433,2352,570}.

Ependymal tumours: Introduction

Ellison DW

Where possible, ependymal tumours should now be classified according to a combination of histopathological and molecular features and anatomical site {836}. DNA methylation profiling distinguishes types of ependymal tumours at different levels of the neuraxis, dividing them into molecular groups across the three main anatomical compartments of the CNS: the supratentorial region, posterior fossa, and spine {2374}. This pathobiological heterogeneity is now central to their classification.

One molecular group at each anatomical site consists almost entirely of tumours with the morphological features of subependymoma {2374}. Of the two remaining supratentorial molecular groups, one is dominated by ependymomas with fusion genes involving ZFTA (formerly known as C11orf95), and the other contains tumours with a high frequency of fusion genes involving YAP1 {113}. Methylation profiling divides the majority of posterior fossa ependymomas into two main groups, posterior fossa group A (PFA) and group B (PFB), which are also distinguished by global levels of H3 p.K28me3 (K27me3) {2374,2384}. Posterior fossa ependymomas generally lack recurrent mutations {2401},

but mutations in EZHIP and the histone H3 family resulting in H3 p.K28M (K27M), which are of uncertain clinicopathological significance, are found at frequencies of 9% and 4%, respectively {2373}. Two of the molecular groups of spinal ependymomas are dominated by tumours with either a classic or a myxopapillary morphology {2374}. There is also an aggressive type of spinal ependymoma characterized by high-grade histopathological features and MYCN amplification {1079}.

The new WHO classification of ependymal tumours lists two molecularly defined types of supratentorial ependymoma (with ZFTA or YAP1 fusion), two molecularly defined types of posterior fossa ependymoma (PFA and PFB), and a spinal tumour defined by the presence of MYCN amplification. Also listed are ependymomas defined by anatomical location but not by molecular alteration. These designations can be used either when molecular analysis reveals a different molecular alteration to one that defines ependymomas at a particular site (in such cases, the term "not elsewhere classified [NEC]" is used) or when molecular analysis fails or is unfeasible (in which case

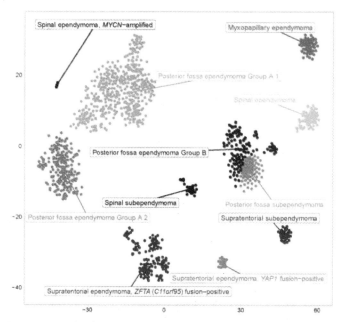

Fig. 2.151 Ependymal tumours: molecular groups. Unsupervised, non-linear t-distributed stochastic neighbour embedding (t-SNE) projection of methylation array profiles from ependymal tumours. Note that the posterior fossa group A (PFA) ependymal tumours split into two subgroups, which might reflect site of origin {2373}. Samples were selected from a large database of > 50 000 brain tumour datasets to serve as reference profiles for training a supervised classification model based on strict criteria: all these samples showed a high calibrated classification score (> 0.9) for ependymoma methylation classes when applying the brain tumour classifier available at https://www.molecularneuropathology.org. In a t-SNE projection like this, occasional samples of one subclass may fall closer to a different subclass because of the stochastic nature of the t-SNE algorithm and the gradual rather than strict boundaries between the subclasses.

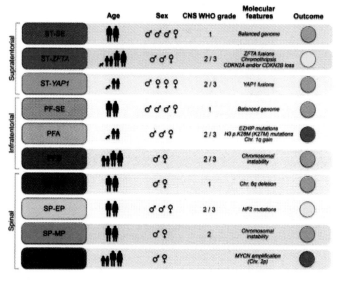

Fig. 2.152 Ependymal tumours: molecular groups. Group colours parallel those used in the t-distributed stochastic neighbour embedding (t-SNE) plot. Outcome colour code: green, good; yellow, intermediate; red, poor. Chr., chromosome; PFA, posterior fossa group A ependymoma; PFB, posterior fossa group B ependymoma; PF-SE, posterior fossa subependymoma; SP-EP, spinal ependymoma; SP-MP, myxopapillary ependymoma; SP-MYCN, spinal ependymoma, MYCN-amplified; SP-SE, spinal subependymoma; ST-SE, supratentorial subependymoma; ST-YAP1, supratentorial ependymoma, YAP1 fusion–positive; ST-ZFTA, supratentorial ependymoma, ZFTA (C11orf95) fusion–positive.

"not otherwise specified [NOS]" is used). Myxopapillary ependymoma and subependymoma remain listed as tumour types, like in the previous edition of the classification; currently, molecular classification does not provide added clinicopathological utility for these two tumours {836}.

Affording no clinicopathological utility, the papillary, clear cell, and tanycytic morphological patterns are no longer listed as subtypes of ependymoma; rather, they are included as patterns in the histopathological description of the classic tumour. Longstanding controversy surrounds the clinicopathological utility of grading ependymal tumours {840}, although use of CNS WHO grade in the therapeutic stratification of adult patients with supratentorial ependymoma remains established practice {3311}. The updated classification allows only a histologically defined diagnosis of "ependymoma" to be made at any of the three anatomical sites; "anaplastic ependymoma" is no longer listed {836}. However, as for other tumours in this edition of the classification, a pathologist can still choose to assign either CNS WHO grade 2 or CNS WHO grade 3 to an ependymoma, according to its histopathological features. In an integrated diagnosis, CNS WHO grade can be presented in a tier adjacent to one providing a histopathological diagnosis and another with molecular alterations and the methodologies used to determine them {1939}.

Supratentorial ependymoma

Pajtler KW
Aldape KD
Gilbertson RJ
Korshunov A

Pietsch T
Rudà R
Taylor MD
Venneti S

Definition

Supratentorial ependymoma is a circumscribed supratentorial glioma that focally demonstrates pseudorosettes or ependymal rosettes and comprises uniform small cells with round nuclei embedded in a fibrillary matrix. The diagnosis of supratentorial ependymoma should be used either when genetic analysis has not detected a pathogenic fusion gene involving *ZFTA* (*C11orf95*) or *YAP1* (not elsewhere classified; NEC) or when such analysis has been unsuccessful or is not feasible (not otherwise specified; NOS) (CNS WHO grade 2 or 3).

ICD-O coding

9391/3 Supratentorial ependymoma, NOS

ICD-11 coding

2A00.0Y & XH1511 Other specified gliomas of brain & Ependymoma, NOS

Related terminology

None

Subtype(s)

None

Localization

Supratentorial ependymomas are localized to the cerebral hemispheres and may or may not have an obvious connection to the ventricular system. They occur more frequently in the frontal or parietal lobe than in the temporal or occipital lobe {2818,3378}.

Clinical features

Common clinical manifestations include focal neurological deficits or seizures. Headache, nausea, and vomiting may occur due to raised intracranial pressure and hydrocephalus. Enlargement of the head or separation of the cranial sutures can be evident in infants. The interval between initial symptoms and diagnosis is generally ≤ 6 months {16}.

Imaging

On MRI, supratentorial ependymomas generally appear as masses with irregular contrast enhancement. They often demonstrate cysts or calcification and, more rarely, haemorrhage or necrosis. Diffusion-weighted MRI frequently shows reduced signal due to hypercellularity {728}.

Epidemiology

Supratentorial ependymomas of all types affect children and adults, and they account for approximately one third of intracranial ependymomas {3311,2073}. The proportion of ependymomas arising in the supratentorial compartment decreases with age: 41% in children, 27% in adolescents, 12% in young adults, and 11% in adults aged > 45 years {844}; the declining numbers

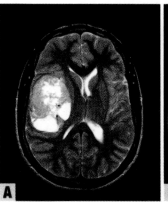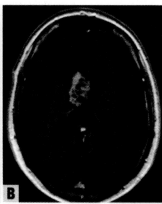

Fig. 2.153 Supratentorial ependymoma. **A** T2-weighted axial MRI showing a large circumscribed mass in the cerebral hemisphere. **B** T1-weighted gadolinium-enhanced axial MRI in an adult, showing an intraventricular nodular lesion with heterogeneous contrast enhancement and solid and cystic components.

reflect the increasing frequency of spinal ependymomas with age. The overall M:F ratio for supratentorial ependymomas is 1.32:1 {2347}.

Etiology

Radial glia are implicated in the histogenesis of supratentorial ependymoma {3155}. Genetic susceptibility for supratentorial ependymoma specifically has not been reported.

Pathogenesis

The precise pathogenic mechanisms leading to fusion-negative supratentorial ependymomas have yet to be elucidated {1002}.

Macroscopic appearance

Supratentorial ependymomas generally have a tan colour, are soft or spongy, and can exhibit a gritty texture if calcified.

Histopathology

The histopathological features of supratentorial ependymomas are quite heterogeneous. Most have a relatively abrupt interface with adjacent CNS parenchyma. Diffuse infiltration of adjacent normal tissue is rare and tends to be seen after multiple recurrences. Perivascular anucleate zones (pseudorosettes) are generally present, but they can be subtle in some examples. True ependymal rosettes are found in only a minority of cases. Hyalinization of blood vessels and calcification are frequent. A vascular pattern seen in supratentorial ependymomas, but not other ependymal tumours, manifests as a branching network of capillary blood vessels {926}. A clear cell phenotype is found more often in supratentorial ependymomas than in tumours in the posterior fossa or spinal cord. Tumour cells have round or oval nuclei, which generally show speckled chromatin. Ultrastructurally, ependymal features

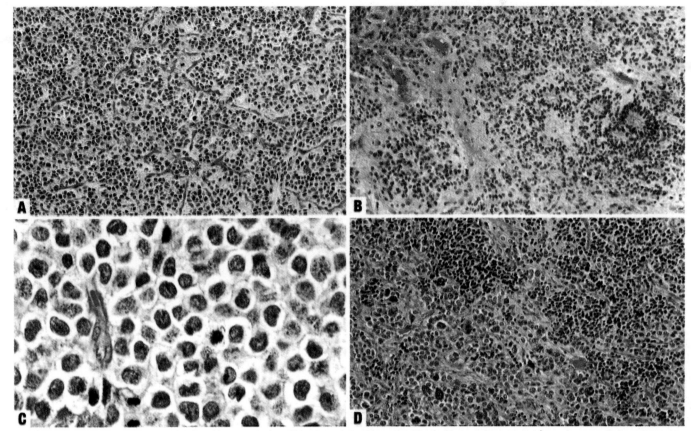

Fig. 2.154 Supratentorial ependymoma. **A** A branching network of small blood vessels is a frequent architectural feature of supratentorial ependymomas. Perivascular anucleate zones can be subtle. **B** Ependymal rosettes are present in a minority of cases. **C** Clear cell change is a frequent cytological feature of supratentorial ependymomas. Nuclear pleomorphism is mild in most cases, and the number of mitotic figures can be variable. **D** Nuclear pleomorphism is mild in most cases, but it can be marked in some cases.

(including intracytoplasmic villi, cilia, and complex intercellular zipper-like junctions) are present {3087,1079}.

Grading

The current classification allows only a histologically defined diagnosis of "ependymoma" to be made at any of the three anatomical sites; "anaplastic ependymoma" is no longer listed {836}. However, supratentorial ependymomas can be assigned CNS WHO grade 2 or 3, ideally in the context of an integrated diagnosis {1939}. High-grade features in ependymomas include brisk mitotic activity and microvascular proliferation. These are considered to have more prognostic impact than other histopathological features, such as nuclear pleomorphism or tumour necrosis {1123}. Supratentorial ependymomas with plentiful high-grade features are considered CNS WHO grade 3, with the caveat that the histopathological grading of ependymomas does not consistently relate to overall outcome {840,698}.

Immunophenotype

Most supratentorial ependymomas show immunoreactivity for S100 or GFAP, which is accentuated around blood vessels and perivascular pseudorosettes. Characteristic immunoreactivity for EMA, with a paranuclear dot-like pattern and along luminal surfaces of true ependymal rosettes, can be found in many, but not all, ependymomas. Expression of OLIG2 is usually present in only a small percentage of tumour cells {1579,2348,1633}.

Differential diagnosis

The differential diagnosis of fusion-negative supratentorial ependymomas includes histopathological mimics such as tumours with *BCOR* internal tandem duplication (ITD) and astroblastomas. These entities should be excluded by appropriate immunohistological and molecular analyses {2370,1002}.

Cytology

Cytological preparations generally show uniform cells with round nuclei and sparse delicate cytoplasmic processes. Nuclear pleomorphism is generally mild, but it is exaggerated in the rare giant cell phenotype {2376,1874}.

Diagnostic molecular pathology

Molecular analysis of supratentorial ependymomas should be directed towards determining *ZFTA* (*C11orf95*) and *YAP1* status and excluding tumours with similar histopathological features, such as *BCOR*-altered tumours and *MN1*-altered astroblastomas. A variety of diagnostic tests can be used to detect the presence or absence of *ZFTA* (*C11orf95*) or *YAP1* rearrangements, including interphase FISH, RT-PCR–based sequencing methods, and next-generation sequencing (including transcriptome sequencing) {2511,2374,2401,2370}. In 17–30% of supratentorial ependymomas, *ZFTA* (*C11orf95*) and *YAP1* fusion genes cannot be detected {1002,2288}; a diagnosis of supratentorial ependymoma can be used in this context. The detection of a genetic alteration not involving *ZFTA* (*C11orf95*) or *YAP1* should

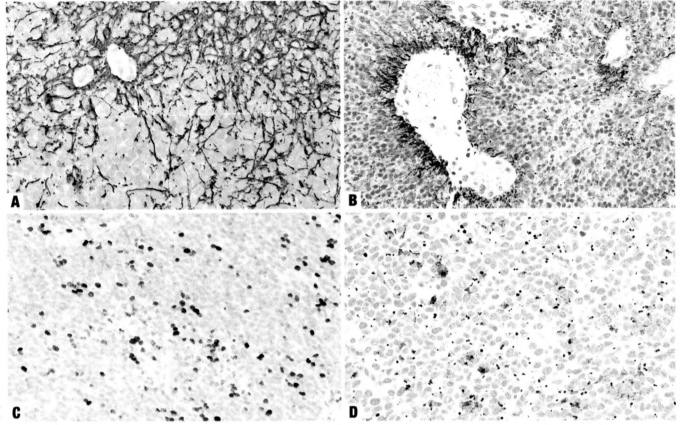

Fig. 2.155 Supratentorial ependymoma. **A,B** By immunohistochemistry, GFAP is variably expressed in supratentorial ependymomas. **C** OLIG2 is usually present in sparse tumour cells. **D** Immunoreactivity for EMA is present in a variable number of tumour cells and usually manifests as paranuclear dots or ring structures.

prompt the use of the suffix "NEC". An inability to perform the appropriate analysis prompts the addition of "NOS" {1946}.

Essential and desirable diagnostic criteria
See Box 2.32.

Staging
Not clinically relevant

Prognosis and prediction
Most outcome data for ependymomas are derived from retrospective studies in an era before molecular classification. Among adults, supratentorial location is associated with a poorer outcome than infratentorial location {3311}. The clinicopathological utility of grading for ependymal tumours remains controversial {840}, although the use of CNS WHO grade in the therapeutic stratification of adult patients with supratentorial ependymoma remains established practice {3311}. Infiltration of adjacent CNS parenchyma by ependymoma has been reported as an adverse prognostic indicator {1123}. Complete surgical resection is the best predictor of long-term survival both in

Box 2.32 Diagnostic criteria for supratentorial ependymoma NEC and supratentorial ependymoma NOS

Essential:

Supratentorial tumour with morphological and immunohistochemical features of ependymoma

AND

For NEC: the detected genetic alteration is not a fusion gene involving either *ZFTA* (*C11orf95*) or *YAP1*

OR

For NOS: genetic analysis was unsuccessful or unfeasible

children and in adults, and second-look surgery for resection of residual tumour is increasingly advocated. In addition to neurosurgical intervention, postoperative radiotherapy is considered the standard of care, in the absence of metastases, for lowering the risk of local recurrence {2074,2745}. The vast majority of tumour relapses are due to a lack of local control, and the number of late failures is substantial, especially in adults. Cerebrospinal fluid spread develops in as many as 15% of patients, more often in CNS WHO grade 3 tumours {2744}.

Supratentorial ependymoma, *ZFTA* fusion-positive

Pajtler KW
Aldape KD
Gilbertson RJ
Korshunov A
Pietsch T
Rudà R
Taylor MD
Venneti S

Definition

Supratentorial ependymoma, *ZFTA* fusion-positive, is a circumscribed supratentorial glioma with a *ZFTA* (formerly *C11orf95*) fusion gene, focally demonstrating pseudorosettes or ependymal rosettes and comprising uniform small cells with round nuclei embedded in a fibrillary matrix. In most of these supratentorial ependymomas, *ZFTA* is fused with *RELA*.

ICD-O coding

9396/3 Supratentorial ependymoma, *ZFTA* fusion-positive

ICD-11 coding

2A00.0Y & XH1511 Other specified gliomas of brain & Ependymoma, NOS

Related terminology

None

Subtype(s)

None

Localization

Most *ZFTA* fusion-positive cerebral ependymomas arise in the frontal or parietal lobe {2288,1893}. Less common sites are the thalamus or the region of the hypothalamus / third ventricle. Intracranial extra-axial *ZFTA* fusion-positive supratentorial ependymomas have been reported {1992,2288}.

Clinical features

Clinical symptoms and signs include focal neurological deficits or seizures, as well as features of raised intracranial pressure.

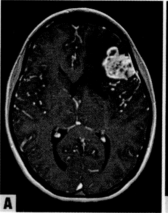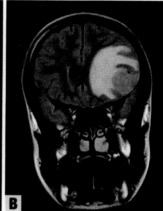

Fig. 2.156 Supratentorial ependymoma, *ZFTA* fusion-positive. **A** T1-weighted axial MRI with gadolinium, showing a well-demarcated left frontal lesion with heterogeneous contrast enhancement and areas of necrosis. **B** Coronal FLAIR MRI showing conspicuous surrounding oedema.

Imaging

On neuroimaging, intratumoural haemorrhage, cysts, and peritumoural oedema are common. High diffusion-weighted imaging signals with concomitant low signals in apparent diffusion coefficient or T2-weighted images suggest diffusion restriction. Most tumours show strong, but often inhomogeneous, enhancement in their solid components after intravenous gadolinium injection {2326,1625,2288,1028}.

Epidemiology

ZFTA fusion-positive tumours account for the majority of supratentorial ependymomas and may occur both in children

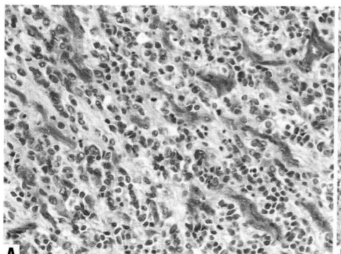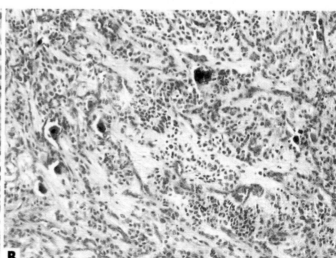

Fig. 2.157 Supratentorial ependymoma, *ZFTA* fusion-positive. Tumour cells with round nuclei set in a fibrillary matrix. Branching capillary blood vessels (**A**) or branching blood vessels and dystrophic calcification (**B**) can be seen.

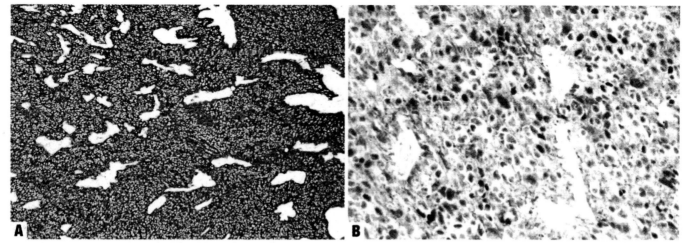

Fig. 2.158 Supratentorial ependymoma, *ZFTA* fusion–positive. **A** Universal cytoplasmic expression of L1CAM. **B** Nuclear immunoreactivity for p65 (encoded by *RELA*).

and in adults. The percentage of supratentorial ependymomas with a *ZFTA* fusion varies between retrospective studies: 20–58% in adults, 66–84% in children {2511,2374,3462,2370,3258}.

Etiology

Evidence from mouse modelling and cross-species genomics strongly suggests that *ZFTA* fusion–positive supratentorial ependymomas arise from radial glia {3155,2632,2357}. Genetic susceptibility in association with this molecular entity has not been reported.

Pathogenesis

Fusion of the *ZFTA* gene with partner genes, mainly *RELA*, is believed to be the principal oncogenic driver of the disease. Rearrangements containing *ZFTA* have been demonstrated to result from chromothriptic events on chromosome 11 {2401}. A pathological activation of NF-κB signalling has been demonstrated in supratentorial ependymomas with a *ZFTA::RELA* fusion {2511,2401}. Homozygous deletions of *CDKN2A* indicate a disruption of cell-cycle control in a subset of these tumours {1512}.

Macroscopic appearance

Generally, supratentorial ependymomas with a *ZFTA* fusion are sharply demarcated tumours of soft consistency. Dystrophic calcification and necrotic areas are common findings.

Histopathology

Supratentorial ependymomas with a *ZFTA* fusion are demarcated from adjacent brain and composed of cells characterized mainly by round uniform nuclei with speckled chromatin and poorly defined fibrillary cytoplasm. Pseudorosettes are not prominent in most cases, and true ependymal rosettes are rare. These tumours often have a network of branching capillary blood vessels and a clear cell phenotype.

Immunophenotype

The immunophenotype of *ZFTA* fusion–positive ependymomas is similar to that of other ependymomas. Ependymomas with a *ZFTA::RELA* fusion show nuclear accumulation of p65 protein (encoded by *RELA*) and universal cytoplasmic expression of L1CAM {2401,2511}. Immunoreactivity for p65 has been found

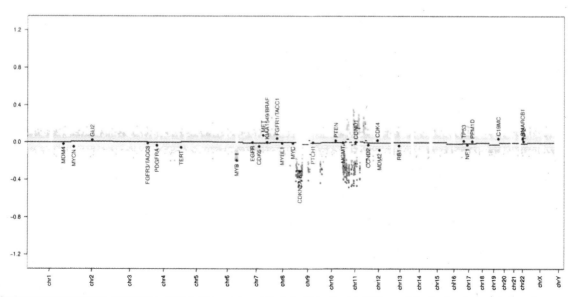

Fig. 2.159 Supratentorial ependymoma, *ZFTA* fusion–positive. Copy-number profile derived from Illumina 450K array data, showing chromothripsis on chromosome 11.

to have a slightly higher specificity for this molecularly defined ependymoma than does L1CAM expression {926}.

Grading
ZFTA-fused supratentorial ependymomas show varying degrees of anaplasia and have been regarded as CNS WHO grade 2 or 3 on this basis. Such information should be included in an integrated diagnosis {1939}.

Cytology
Cytological preparations generally show uniform cells with round nuclei and sparse delicate cytoplasmic processes. Nuclear pleomorphism is generally mild, but it is exaggerated in the rare giant cell phenotype {2376,1874}.

Diagnostic molecular pathology
Diagnostic tests for detecting *ZFTA* fusions include several sequencing methods, interphase FISH, and molecular inversion profiling {2401,2511,2374,2370,1002,2236,1512}. An RT-PCR method targeting the different types of *ZFTA::RELA* fusion has been proposed for detecting the most frequent fusions {2374, 1067,1992}. DNA methylation–based classification can be helpful, complementing assays directed towards identification of the fusion.

Essential and desirable diagnostic criteria
See Box 2.33.

Box 2.33 Diagnostic criteria for supratentorial ependymoma, *ZFTA* fusion–positive

Essential:

Supratentorial tumour with morphological and immunohistochemical features of ependymoma

AND

Gene fusion involving *ZFTA* (*C11orf95*)

Desirable:

DNA methylation profile aligned with supratentorial ependymoma, *ZFTA* fusion–positive

Immunoreactivity for p65 (RELA) or L1CAM

Staging
Not clinically relevant

Prognosis and prediction
Available clinical outcome data on molecularly defined supratentorial ependymomas suggest that *ZFTA* fusion–positive tumours have the poorest outcome. However, outcome data derived from retrospective studies show great variance, and validation of those findings needs to be undertaken in prospective therapeutic trials {2374,926,1893,3462,2370,1002,2073, 3258}. Homozygous deletion of *CDKN2A* and/or *CDKN2B* has been identified as an independent predictor of poor outcome (overall survival) in a series of ependymomas with *ZFTA::RELA* fusions {1512}.

Supratentorial ependymoma, *YAP1* fusion–positive

Pajtler KW
Aldape KD
Gilbertson RJ
Korshunov A

Pietsch T
Rudà R
Taylor MD
Vennetl S

Definition

Supratentorial ependymoma, *YAP1* fusion–positive, is a circum-scribed supratentorial glioma with a *YAP1* fusion gene, focally demonstrating pseudorosettes or ependymal rosettes and comprising uniform small cells with round nuclei embedded in a fibrillary matrix. In most of these supratentorial ependymomas, *YAP1* is fused with *MAMLD1*.

ICD-O coding

9396/3 Supratentorial ependymoma, *YAP1* fusion–positive

ICD-11 coding

2A00.0Y & XH1511 Other specified gliomas of brain & Ependy-moma, NOS

Related terminology

None

Subtype(s)

None

Localization

Most *YAP1* fusion–positive tumours are located within or adja-cent to the lateral ventricle.

Clinical features

YAP1 fusion–positive supratentorial ependymomas are often large by the time of presentation. Clinical features include symp-toms and signs of raised intracranial pressure, as well as focal neurological deficits or seizures.

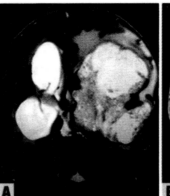
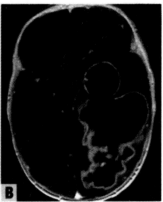

Fig. 2.160 Supratentorial ependymoma, *YAP1* fusion–positive. **A** T2-weighted coro-nal MRI showing a large cystic tumour. **B** Ependymoma with *YAP1::MAMLD1* fusion. T1-weighted axial MRI showing a large cystic tumour with contrast enhancement of solid tumour parts.

Imaging

Neuroimaging shows that tumours have sharp margins and prominent cystic components. They are mostly isointense on T1- and T2-weighted images. Contrast enhancement of solid tumour components is heterogeneous. Peritumoural oedema is variable {113}.

Epidemiology

YAP1 fusion–positive ependymomas are uncommon and appear to be restricted to young children. In paediatric cohorts, they account for 6–7.4% of supratentorial ependymomas. The M:F ratio is 0.3:1 {2374,3462,113,2370,3258}.

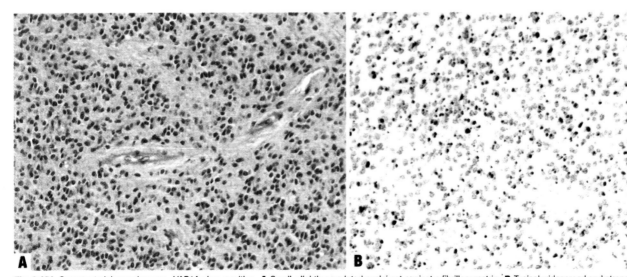

Fig. 2.161 Supratentorial ependymoma, *YAP1* fusion–positive. **A** Small, slightly angulated nuclei set against a fibrillary matrix. **B** Typical widespread and strong dot-like EMA immunoreactivity.

Etiology

Data suggest that *YAP1* fusion–positive ependymomas derive from PAX6-positive radial glial neural stem cells {2372,825}.

Pathogenesis

Genomic fusions of the *YAP1* gene with *MAMLD1* or other partner genes appear to be the principal oncogenic driver of the disease. Functional genomic analyses suggest that *YAP1::MAMLD1* fusions function as an oncogenic driver through the recruitment of nuclear factor I (NFI) and TEA domain (TEAD) family members {2372,825}.

Macroscopic appearance

Ependymomas with a *YAP1* fusion have macroscopic appearances similar to those of other supratentorial ependymomas. They are circumscribed and focally haemorrhagic, with a soft consistency.

Histopathology

Like other ependymal tumours, *YAP1*-fused supratentorial ependymomas are demarcated from adjacent brain. They are composed of relatively uniform cells with small to medium-sized round or angulated nuclei. Ependymal rosettes are present in some tumours. Clear cell, papillary, or tanycytic phenotypes have not been recorded. Mitotic activity is highly variable. In most cases, the fibrillary matrix contains PAS-positive eosinophilic granular bodies {113}. Frequent findings are vascular endothelial proliferation, dystrophic calcification, and necrosis.

Immunophenotype

Supratentorial ependymomas with a *YAP1* fusion show widespread and strong immunoreactivity for EMA {113}. There is no expression of L1CAM, and tumour cell nuclei are negative for p65 (RELA).

Grading

YAP1-fused supratentorial ependymomas show variable degrees of anaplasia, and such information should be included in an integrated diagnosis {1939}.

Box 2.34 Diagnostic criteria for supratentorial ependymoma, *YAP1* fusion–positive

Essential:

Supratentorial tumour with morphological and immunohistochemical features of ependymoma

AND

Gene fusion involving *YAP1*

Desirable:

DNA methylation profile aligned with supratentorial ependymoma, *YAP1* fusion–positive

No immunoreactivity for p65 (RELA) or L1CAM

PAS-positive eosinophilic granular bodies

Cytology

Cytological preparations generally show uniform cells with round nuclei and sparse delicate cytoplasmic processes. Nuclear pleomorphism is generally mild, but it is exaggerated in the rare giant cell phenotype {2376,1874}.

Diagnostic molecular pathology

Molecular testing for *YAP1* fusions includes several sequencing strategies and interphase FISH {1992,1002,2236}. DNA methylation–based classification can complement tests directed towards identification of the fusion.

Essential and desirable diagnostic criteria

See Box 2.34.

Staging

Not clinically relevant

Prognosis and prediction

Although often large at presentation and predominantly occurring in young children, ependymomas with a *YAP1* fusion carry a prognosis in retrospectively studied cohorts that appears to be favourable when compared with that of other supratentorial ependymal tumour types {113,2370,3258}. Molecular markers or clinical characteristics further defining prognosis in these tumours are currently unknown.

Posterior fossa ependymoma

Venneti S
Aldape KD
Pajtler KW
Pletsch T
Ramaswamy V
Taylor MD

Definition

Posterior fossa ependymoma is a circumscribed glioma in the posterior fossa, focally demonstrating pseudorosettes or ependymal rosettes and comprising uniform small cells with round nuclei embedded in a fibrillary matrix. The diagnosis of posterior fossa ependymoma should be used when molecular analysis either cannot assign a molecular group (not elsewhere classified; NEC) or is not feasible (not otherwise specified; NOS) (CNS WHO grade 2 or 3).

ICD-O coding

9391/3 Posterior fossa ependymoma, NOS

ICD-11 coding

2A00.0Y & XH1511 Other specified gliomas of brain & Ependymoma, NOS

Related terminology

None

Subtype(s)

None

Localization

Posterior fossa ependymomas mainly arise in the region of the fourth ventricle, including the floor, lateral aspect (cerebellar peduncles), and roof. They can also occur in the cerebellopontine angle {3463}.

Clinical features

Common clinical presentations relate to mass effect on surrounding posterior fossa structures and include secondary hydrocephalus. Clinical presentations vary by age and are often nonspecific (e.g. headache, vomiting, and lethargy). Babies can present with a rapidly growing head circumference.

Imaging

MRI usually demonstrates a homogeneous mass filling the fourth ventricle. Haemorrhages and punctate calcifications may be observed {2541}. The presence of intratumoural cysts and necrosis can result in variable enhancement on gadolinium injection. MRI can show lateral extension of the tumour via the foramina of Luschka and extension through the foramen of Magendie into the cisterna magna {2541}.

Epidemiology

Posterior fossa ependymomas of all types can develop at any age. However, they are most frequent in children, with a median age at presentation of 6 years. They are slightly more frequent in male patients (52–62%) {2054,2073,1043,2612,2032,3463}. According to the Central Brain Tumor Registry of the United States (CBTRUS), approximately 8% of all neuroepithelial

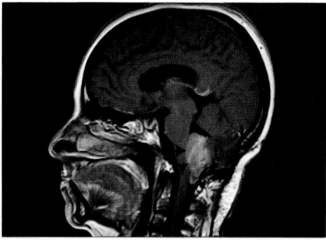

Fig. 2.162 Posterior fossa ependymoma. MRI shows a tumour in the fourth ventricle (arrows). Note that the aqueduct of Sylvius and the third ventricle are enlarged.

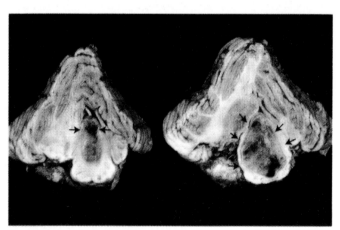

Fig. 2.163 Posterior fossa ependymoma. Ependymoma in the fourth ventricle (arrows) displacing adjacent posterior fossa structures.

neoplasms in children and adolescents (birth to 19 years) are ependymomas {2344}. In the USA, a higher incidence of ependymomas is reported in White people, including children with eastern European ancestry, than in the Black and Hispanic populations {2054,2344,3591}.

Etiology

The etiology is unknown. Associations with specific genetic susceptibilities have not been reported.

Pathogenesis

Across all types of posterior fossa ependymoma, copy-number alterations leading to altered gene expression are hypothesized to play an essential role in pathogenesis, as are epigenetic alterations, including aberrant DNA methylation patterns, *EZHIP* overexpression, and loss of H3 p.K28me3 (K27me3) {1975, 1974,2373,490}.

Macroscopic appearance

Posterior fossa ependymomas are usually circumscribed tumours arising in the fourth ventricle. They appear tan-coloured and are soft or spongy, with a gritty consistency if calcified. Tumour cells can grow through the foramina of Luschka to envelop the lower cranial nerves and the posterior inferior cerebellar artery.

Histopathology

Generally, posterior fossa ependymomas are circumscribed tumours composed of uniform small cells with indistinct cytoplasmic borders and round nuclei. Nodules of tumour cells, in which the cell density is higher than in surrounding syncytial areas, are common. Perivascular pseudorosettes are almost always present and are characterized by tumour cells arranged in a radial fashion around blood vessels to create an intervening anucleate zone. True ependymal rosettes are composed of columnar or cuboidal cells surrounding a central lumen. They are observed in a minority of cases. Regions of nuclear pleomorphism, increased mitotic activity in nodules, microcystic change, calcification, and hyalinization of blood vessels can be observed. Rarely, cartilaginous or osseous metaplasia is present.

Some posterior fossa ependymomas can have a focal papillary or pseudopapillary architecture, including finger-like projections lined by a single layer of cuboidal cells or papillae in which a central blood vessel is covered by layers of tumour cells. Clear cell change mimicking oligodendroglioma-like cytoplasmic clearing can be present, but this is more common in supratentorial ependymomas. Tumour cells with elongated nuclei focally arranged in fascicles represent the tanycytic pattern.

Grading

Posterior fossa ependymomas can be assigned CNS WHO grade 2 or 3, ideally in the context of an integrated diagnosis {1939}. High-grade features in ependymomas include brisk mitotic activity and microvascular proliferation. These are considered to have more prognostic impact than other histopathological features, such as nuclear pleomorphism or tumour necrosis {1123}. However, efforts to risk-stratify cases on the basis of histopathological grading criteria have yielded inconsistent results {840,1123,2032,2073}.

Immunophenotype

Most posterior fossa ependymomas show immunoreactivity for S100 or GFAP, which is accentuated around blood vessels in perivascular pseudorosettes. EMA expression can be seen in most ependymomas as a paranuclear dot-like pattern or ring-like structures. However, this is not an entirely specific finding {1256,1579}. OLIG2 expression is usually absent, and some tumours can show focal immunoreactivity for cytokeratins (including CK7 and CK20) {1421,2348,2567,3302}.

Ultrastructure

Ependymomas demonstrate characteristic ultrastructural features, including cilia (9 + 2 microtubular pattern), junctional complexes on lateral surfaces of cells, and microvilli on luminal surfaces {1124}.

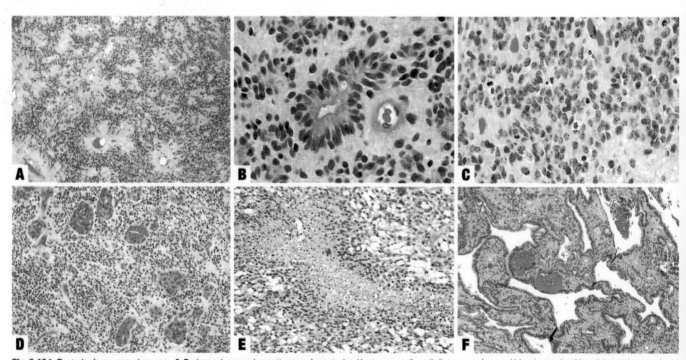

Fig. 2.164 Posterior fossa ependymoma. **A** Perivascular pseudorosettes are characterized by tumour cells radially arranged around blood vessels with an intervening anucleate zone. **B** True ependymal rosettes characterized by periluminal cuboidal or columnar cells without a basement membrane. **C** CNS WHO grade 3 posterior fossa ependymoma showing plentiful mitotic activity but little nuclear pleomorphism. **D** Microvascular proliferation typically characterized by multilayered endothelial cells. **E** Palisading necrosis. **F** A pseudopapillary pattern with finger-like projections lined by a single layer or multiple layers of cuboidal cells.

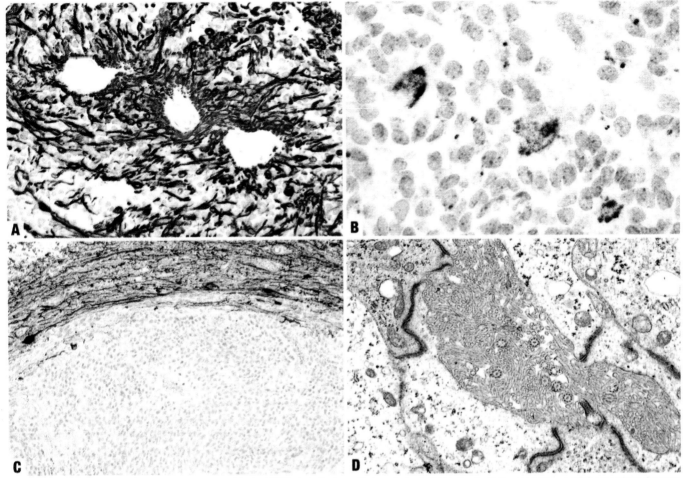

Fig. 2.165 Posterior fossa ependymoma. **A** Immunoreactivity for GFAP is typically present in many (but not all) tumour cells. Note accentuation of staining in perivascular pseudorosettes. **B** Immunoreactivity for EMA typically shows a paranuclear dot-like pattern and occurs along the luminal surface of true ependymal rosettes. **C** Immunoreactivity for NFP highlights axons in surrounding brain parenchyma and demonstrates the pushing border of the tumour. **D** At the ultrastructural level, the cells of an ependymoma typically show cilia with a 9 + 2 microtubular pattern and microvilli at luminal surfaces.

Box 2.35 Diagnostic criteria for posterior fossa ependymoma

Essential:

Posterior fossa tumour with morphological and immunohistochemical features of ependymoma

AND

Absence of morphological features of subependymoma

AND (for NOS lesions)

Molecular group evaluation was indeterminate, generated no result, or was not feasible

Cytology

Cytological preparations generally show uniform cells with round nuclei and sparse delicate cytoplasmic processes. Nuclear pleomorphism is generally mild, but it is exaggerated in the rare giant cell phenotype {2376}. Tumour cells can form clusters and palisades around vascular structures, reflecting the arrangement of perivascular pseudorosettes.

Diagnostic molecular pathology

If feasible, posterior fossa ependymomas should be assigned to a molecular group (PFA, PFB, or subependymoma) {2374}.

Absence of immunoreactivity for H3 p.K28me3 (K27me3) in the nuclei of tumour cells is a surrogate marker for PFA ependymoma {2384}, but classification using DNA methylation profiling is considered the standard method, because nuclear expression of H3 p.K28me3 (K27me3) is present in both PFB tumours and subependymomas. If appropriate molecular testing was successfully performed but did not assign a molecular group, a diagnosis of posterior fossa ependymoma can be used with the suffix "NEC" {1946}. An inability to perform the appropriate analysis prompts the addition of "NOS".

Essential and desirable diagnostic criteria

See Box 2.35.

Staging

Not clinically relevant

Prognosis and prediction

There is no robust relationship between histological grade and prognosis for posterior fossa ependymomas {840,1123}. However, the extent of surgical resection and the status of chromosome 1q are consistent outcome indicators {478,1611,1123,2612}.

Posterior fossa group A (PFA) ependymoma

Venneti S
Aldape KD
Korshunov A
Pajtler KW

Pietsch T
Ramaswamy V
Taylor MD

Definition

Posterior fossa group A (PFA) ependymoma is a circumscribed posterior fossa glioma aligned with the PFA molecular group of ependymomas, demonstrating pseudorosettes or ependymal rosettes and comprising uniform small cells with round nuclei embedded in a fibrillary matrix. An ependymoma can be classified as PFA by identifying a loss of nuclear H3 p.K28me3 (K27me3) expression in tumour cells or by DNA methylation profiling.

ICD-O coding

9396/3 Posterior fossa group A (PFA) ependymoma

ICD-11 coding

2A00.0Y & XH1511 Other specified gliomas of brain & Ependymoma, NOS

Related terminology

None

Subtype(s)

None

Localization

Studies correlating neuroimaging with molecular group have suggested that PFA ependymomas more frequently arise from the roof or lateral aspect of the fourth ventricle than from its floor {3463,2373}.

Clinical features

The clinical features of PFA ependymomas are similar to those described for posterior fossa ependymomas in general.

Epidemiology

PFA ependymomas predominantly occur in infants and children, with a median age of 3 years {3463,2373,2374,2612}. The proportion of posterior fossa ependymomas classified as PFA aligns with age: > 95% of posterior fossa ependymomas in children aged < 6 years are PFA tumours, and PFB ependymomas are rare in this age group; the proportion of posterior fossa ependymomas classified as PFA decreases to 45–50% in adolescents and 5–11% in adults {3463,2373,2374, 2612}. PFA ependymomas are slightly more prevalent in male patients (59–62%) than in female patients {3463,2373,2374, 2612}.

Etiology

Although the exact etiology of PFA ependymomas is unknown, it is hypothesized that aberrant epigenetic alterations may be central drivers. Associations with specific genetic susceptibilities have not been reported.

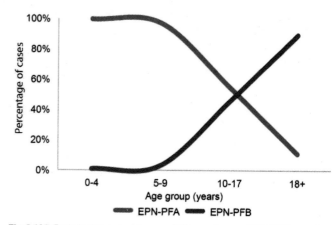

Fig. 2.166 Posterior fossa ependymoma. PFA ependymoma (EPN-PFA), sometimes referred to as "infantile posterior fossa ependymoma", predominantly occurs in infants and children. PFB ependymoma (EPN-PFB) occurs mainly in older children and young adults.

Pathogenesis

Cell of origin

PFA ependymomas are thought to arise from an undifferentiated glial stem or progenitor cell in the developing hindbrain {3338}.

Molecular profile

PFA ependymomas exhibit characteristic DNA methylation patterns, including hypermethylation of CpG islands and global DNA hypomethylation {1975,2374,223}. PFA ependymomas show a global reduction of the repressive histone mark H3 p.K28me3 (K27me3), which impacts several pathways, including neuroglial differentiation and cell-cycle regulation {223, 2373}, and is caused by overexpression of EZHIP {2373}. EZHIP phenotypically mimics the oncohistone H3 p.K28M (K27M) by binding to the H3 p.K28 (K27) methyltransferase EZH2 and inhibiting the function of PRC2 {1448,2597,2520,1374}. Although most PFA ependymomas do not carry recurrent genetic mutations, about 9% exhibit mutations in *EZHIP*. In addition, about 4% harbour H3 p.K28M (K27M) mutations, which are mutually exclusive with *EZHIP* mutations {260,1065,2373,2765}. A study that examined 675 PFA ependymomas by DNA methylation profiling identified 2 molecular subgroups and 9 molecular subtypes of PFA ependymomas {2373}. However, the clinicopathological implications of these findings have yet to be fully evaluated.

Macroscopic appearance

The macroscopic features of PFA ependymomas are similar to those described for posterior fossa ependymomas in general.

Histopathology

PFA ependymomas show the histopathological features described for posterior fossa ependymomas in general.

High-grade features, including prominent mitotic activity and microvascular proliferation, were observed in 64% of PFA ependymomas in one study {2373}. Clear cell, papillary, and tanycytic patterns can be focally present {2236}.

Immunophenotype

PFA ependymomas exhibit a reduction in H3 p.K28me3 (K27me3), which can be readily assessed by immunohistochemistry {2384,223,2373}. Retained H3 p.K28me3 (K27me3) immunoreactivity in endothelial cells can be used as an internal control for the method. In most PFA ependymomas, tumour cells show a global reduction in H3 p.K28me3 (K27me3) expression, but variability in the proportion of immunonegative cells can be encountered. A cut-off value of 80% immunopositive cells has been proposed, above which an ependymoma is more likely to fall into the PFB molecular group {2384,223,1002, 1228,3487,3580}.

Grading

PFA ependymomas show varying degrees of anaplasia and have been regarded as CNS WHO grade 2 or 3 on this basis. Such information should be included in an integrated diagnosis {1939}.

Cytology

Cytological preparations generally show uniform cells with round nuclei and sparse delicate cytoplasmic processes. Nuclear pleomorphism is generally mild, but it is exaggerated in the rare giant cell phenotype {2376}. Tumour cells can form clusters and palisades around vascular structures, reflecting the arrangement of perivascular pseudorosettes.

Diagnostic molecular pathology

Demonstration of loss of H3 p.K28me3 (K27me3) by immunohistochemistry, or assignment to the PFA molecular group by DNA methylation profiling, is required for a diagnosis of PFA

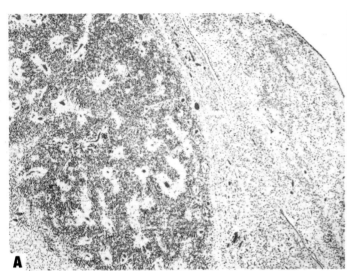
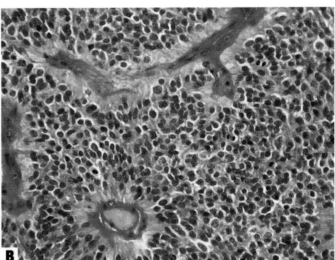

Fig. 2.167 Posterior fossa group A (PFA) ependymoma. **A** Nodules of high cell density are common in PFA ependymomas. **B** Subtle pseudorosette formation and a high cell density characterize some PFA ependymomas.

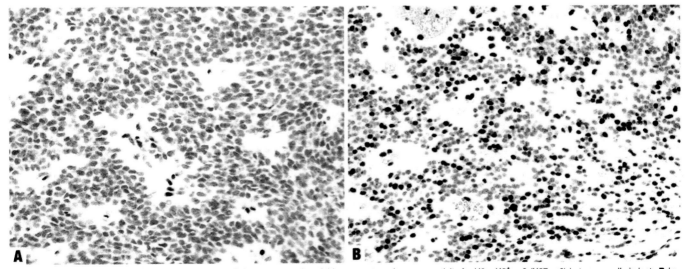

Fig. 2.168 Posterior fossa group A (PFA) ependymoma. **A** In most examples of this tumour type, immunoreactivity for H3 p.K28me3 (K27me3) in tumour cells is lost. **B** Immunoreactivity for H3 p.K28me3 (K27me3) can sometimes be retained in a variable proportion of tumour cells.

ependymoma. Because of its prognostic significance across all posterior fossa ependymomas {1123}, gain of chromosome 1q is often assessed in PFA ependymomas, even though molecular subtypes of PFA ependymoma with or without 1q gain can be associated with a poor outcome {2373}.

Essential and desirable diagnostic criteria
See Box 2.36.

Staging
Not clinically relevant

Prognosis and prediction
Extent of surgical resection is associated with outcome {1123}. PFA ependymomas have a poor prognosis compared with that of PFB ependymomas {2374}. Gain of chromosome 1q is a reproducible adverse prognostic indicator across all posterior fossa ependymomas {478,1611,1123}. However, among

Box 2.36 Diagnostic criteria for posterior fossa group A (PFA) ependymoma

Essential:

Posterior fossa tumour with morphological and immunohistochemical features of ependymoma

AND

Global reduction of H3 p.K28me3 (K27me3) in tumour cell nuclei

OR

DNA methylation profile aligned with PFA ependymoma

Desirable:

Stable genome on genome-wide copy-number analysis

molecular subtypes of PFA ependymoma, those with or without 1q gain can have an equally poor outcome {2373}. The prognostic significance of an H3 p.K28me3 (K27me3) mutation in a small proportion of PFA ependymomas is unknown.

Posterior fossa group B (PFB) ependymoma

Venneti S
Aldape KD
Pajtler KW
Pietsch T
Ramaswamy V
Taylor MD

Definition
Posterior fossa group B (PFB) ependymoma is a circumscribed posterior fossa glioma aligned with the PFB molecular group of ependymomas, demonstrating pseudorosettes or ependymal rosettes and comprising uniform small cells with round nuclei embedded in a fibrillary matrix. An ependymoma can be classified as PFB by DNA methylation profiling. Retention of nuclear H3 p.K28me3 (K27me3) expression is observed, but it is not specific for PFB ependymomas.

ICD-O coding
9396/3 Posterior fossa group B (PFB) ependymoma

ICD-11 coding
2A00.0Y & XH1511 Other specified gliomas of brain & Ependymoma, NOS

Related terminology
None

Subtype(s)
None

Localization
PFB ependymomas can occur anywhere in the region of the fourth ventricle and its exit foramina, but they are thought to arise more frequently from the floor of the fourth ventricle than from the roof or lateral recesses {3463}.

Clinical features
Clinical manifestations are similar to those observed in posterior fossa ependymomas in general.

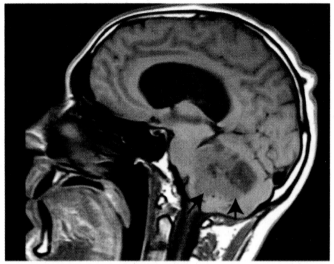

Fig. 2.169 Posterior fossa group B (PFB) ependymoma. T1-weighted MRI shows a large tumour in the fourth ventricle of a 37-year-old man.

Epidemiology
PFB ependymomas occur in adults and are more common in adolescents than in children and infants {3463,2374,2612,2373, 490,1513}. The median age at presentation is 30 years (range: 1–72 years). The relative frequency of the PFB molecular group among ependymomas is closely related to age: 90% in adults, 20–50% in adolescents, and < 5% in infants and children aged < 5 years {3463,2374,2612,490}. PFB ependymomas are slightly more prevalent in female patients (55–59%) {3463,2374,2612, 490}. Among the five molecular subgroups of PFB ependymoma {490}, PFB-1, PFB-2, and PFB-3 tumours tend to occur in patients aged 25–30 years. PFB-4 tumours arise in a younger age group

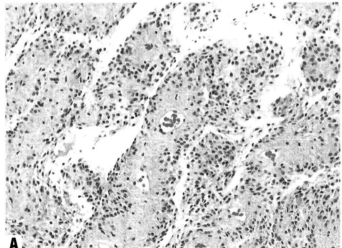
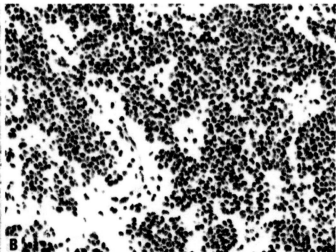

Fig. 2.170 Posterior fossa group B (PFB) ependymoma. **A** Pseudopapillary architectural pattern featuring finger-like projections and perivascular pseudorosettes. **B** Expression of H3 p.K28me3 (K27me3) is present in all tumour cells.

(median age: 15 years), whereas PFB-5 tumours occur in older individuals (median age: 40 years). PFB-2 and PFB-4 tumours are more common in male patients, whereas PFB-3 and PFB-5 tumours are more common in female patients {490}.

Etiology

The etiology of PFB ependymoma remains to be elucidated. No association with specific genetic susceptibilities has been reported.

Pathogenesis

The pathogenesis of PFB ependymomas is unclear, but it is thought to be driven by epigenetic changes and copy-number alterations that together produce aberrant gene expression.

Macroscopic appearance

The macroscopic features of PFB ependymomas are similar to those described for posterior fossa ependymomas in general.

Histopathology

PFB ependymomas show the histopathological features described for posterior fossa ependymomas in general. High-grade features, including prominent mitotic activity and microvascular proliferation, were observed in 41% of PFB ependymomas in a study of 51 patients {2374}.

Practically all PFB ependymomas exhibit retention of H3 p.K28me3 (K27me3), which can be readily assessed by immunohistochemistry {2384,223,2373}. Rare ependymomas with a DNA methylation profile that classifies them as PFB show reduced H3 p.K28me3 (K27me3), but the significance of these findings is unclear {2384,1002,2737}.

PFB ependymomas show varying degrees of anaplasia and have been regarded as CNS WHO grade 2 or 3 on this basis. Such information should be included in an integrated diagnosis {1939}.

Cytology

Cytological preparations generally show uniform cells with round nuclei and sparse delicate cytoplasmic processes. Nuclear pleomorphism is generally mild, but it is exaggerated in the rare giant cell phenotype {2376}. Tumour cells can form clusters and palisades around vascular structures, reflecting the arrangement of perivascular pseudorosettes.

Diagnostic molecular pathology

Demonstration of H3 p.K28me3 (K27me3) retention by immunohistochemistry or assignment to the PFB molecular group by DNA methylation profiling is required for a diagnosis of PFB ependymoma. Nuclear expression of H3 p.K28me3 (K27me3) is retained in PFB ependymomas, but this finding is not specific. PFB ependymomas exhibit widespread cytogenetic abnormalities, with many chromosomal aberrations {1975,2374,223,490}, the most common of which include loss of 22q, monosomy 6, and trisomy 18 (in 50–60% of cases).

Essential and desirable diagnostic criteria

See Box 2.37.

Staging

Not clinically relevant

Prognosis and prediction

Incomplete surgical resection and loss of 13q were associated with a poor prognosis in a cohort of 212 PFB ependymomas. Gain of 1q did not show a relationship with overall prognosis in these tumours {490}.

Spinal ependymoma

Pietsch T
Aldape KD
Korshunov A
Pajtlor KW
Taylor MD
Venneti S

Definition

Spinal ependymoma is a demarcated spinal glioma demonstrating pseudorosettes or ependymal rosettes and comprising uniform small cells with round nuclei embedded in a fibrillary matrix and, typically, a low level of mitotic activity. By definition, the tumour lacks features of myxopapillary ependymoma or subependymoma. When testing is feasible, *MYCN* amplification is absent.

ICD-O coding

9391/3 Spinal ependymoma, NOS

ICD-11 coding

2A00.0Z & XH1511 Other and unspecified neoplasms of brain or central nervous system & Ependymoma, NOS

Related terminology

None

Subtype(s)

None

Localization

Spinal ependymomas occur along the spinal canal and are intramedullary tumours {1674}. A cervical or cervicothoracic localization is common, in contrast to myxopapillary ependymomas, which nearly always arise in the lumbar region {1674}.

Clinical features

Spinal ependymomas do not have clinical features specific enough to differentiate them from other intramedullary spinal cord tumours. Patients often present with back pain and a myelopathy (motor and sensory deficits related to dysfunction of the spinal cord).

Imaging

On MRI examination, spinal ependymomas are intramedullary tumours. They are contrast-enhancing and mostly hypointense on T1-weighted images and hyperintense on T2-weighted images. They often display cystic changes, haemorrhage, necrosis, and/or calcification {1674}. Approximately 60% of ependymomas are associated with an intramedullary cyst (syringomyelia) rostral or caudal to the tumour {1674}.

Epidemiology

Ependymal tumours represent 20.6% of primary spinal tumours in children and adolescents and 17.6% of those in adults aged ≥ 20 years, according to a statistical report from the Central Brain Tumor Registry of the United States (CBTRUS) {2344}. Across various studies, the median age at diagnosis of patients with spinal ependymoma ranges from 25 to 45 years. The reported M:F ratio ranges from 1:1.3 to 2.16:1 {238}.

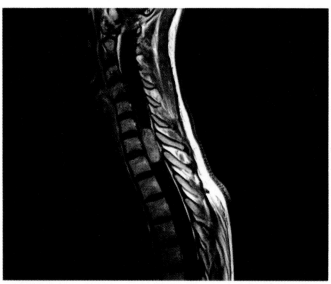

Fig. 2.171 Spinal ependymoma, CNS WHO grade 2. Sagittal T1-weighted MRI of a spinal ependymoma showing gadolinium contrast enhancement.

Etiology

Various studies have shown that 18–53% of patients with neurofibromatosis type 2 develop spinal ependymomas, but that clinical symptoms related to these are evident in < 20% of cases {153,2525,652}. Spinal ependymomas develop more frequently in patients with neurofibromatosis type 2 with germline nonsense and frameshift mutations in the *NF2* gene than in those with other types of *NF2* mutation {153}. A single Japanese family with 2 of 4 siblings affected by cervical spinal ependymomas has been described. Neurofibromatosis type 2 was excluded in this family, another tumour suppressor gene on chromosome 22q being considered causal {3540}.

Spinal ependymomas show frequent chromosomal alterations, the most common being chromosome 22 loss, which occurs in the majority of cases {2374}. Sporadic spinal ependymomas frequently have a somatic *NF2* mutation {820}.

Pathogenesis

Spinal ependymomas are hypothesized to originate from radial glia–like stem or progenitor cells {1490,3155}. Experimental *Nf2* inactivation in mice resulted in increased growth and reduced apoptosis of embryonal spinal cord neural progenitor cells, suggesting that *NF2* activation has an important role in the pathogenesis of spinal ependymomas {1035}.

Macroscopic appearance

Spinal ependymomas are generally circumscribed tumours. They appear soft and are mostly grey-white in colour. They can show cystic changes, calcification, and signs of haemorrhage.

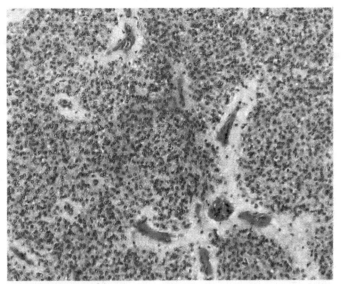

Fig. 2.172 Spinal ependymoma. Tumour showing characteristic perivascular anucleate areas (pseudorosettes).

Histopathology

The classic form of spinal ependymoma is composed of isomorphic glial cells with round to oval nuclei and indistinct cytoplasmic membranes. The cells are embedded in a fibrillary glial matrix and have a moderate to high cell density. A characteristic feature is the anucleate perivascular zone (pseudorosette); tumour cells are radially arranged around a blood vessel, with fibrillary processes creating the perivascular anucleate zone. True ependymal rosettes with a central lumen or ependymal tubules are present in only a minority of cases. Mitotic activity in the classic form is usually low. The rare tanycytic pattern with prominent spindle-shaped cells and bipolar processes, often in the absence of pseudorosettes, is overrepresented in spinal ependymomas and must be distinguished from pilocytic astrocytoma and schwannoma. Ependymomas can show calcification, haemorrhage, necrosis, cystic change, metaplastic cartilage, and bone and myxoid degeneration.

Grading

Although anaplastic ependymoma has been removed from the classification, a pathologist can still choose to assign either CNS WHO grade 2 or grade 3 to an ependymoma, according to its histopathological features {836}. Most spinal ependymomas are CNS WHO grade 2; CNS WHO grade 3 tumours are rare {852,495}. CNS WHO grade 3 spinal ependymomas show conspicuous mitotic activity, usually in the context of a high cell density, and they tend to invade adjacent spinal cord structures. Where possible, such tumours should be distinguished from *MYCN*-amplified spinal ependymoma and H3 K27–altered diffuse midline glioma.

Immunophenotype

Immunoreactivity for GFAP, S100, and vimentin is characteristic, as is focal dot-like or ring-like intracytoplasmic immunoreactivity for EMA. In contrast to astrocytic spinal neoplasms, spinal ependymomas are largely negative for OLIG2. They do not express SOX10, which is found in schwannoma, pilocytic astrocytoma, and most diffuse gliomas.

Electron microscopy

Ultrastructurally, ependymal features including intracytoplasmic villi, cilia, and complex intercellular zipper-like junctions are present {3087,1079}.

Cytology

Cytological preparations generally show uniform cells with round nuclei and sparse delicate cytoplasmic processes. Nuclear pleomorphism is generally mild but can be increased in some cases. Tumour cells can form clusters and palisades around vascular structures, reflecting the arrangement of perivascular pseudorosettes.

Diagnostic molecular pathology

Spinal ependymomas with a typical morphology are easily recognized. They are also readily distinguished from myxopapillary ependymomas, subependymomas, and *MYCN*-amplified spinal ependymoma by their DNA methylation profile {2374,3087}.

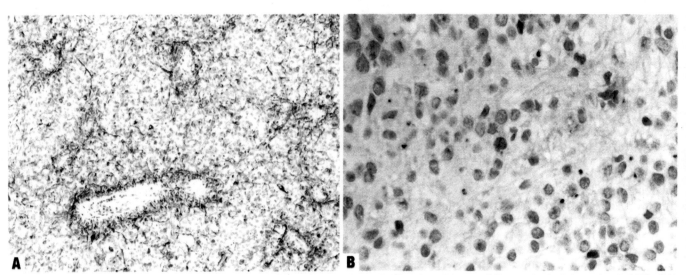

Fig. 2.173 Spinal ependymoma. **A** Tumour showing characteristic GFAP immunoreactivity, enriched in perivascular areas. **B** Tumour showing intracytoplasmic dot-like EMA immunoreactivity corresponding to microlumina.

Occasionally, a spinal ependymoma with a classic morphology exhibits the DNA methylation profile of myxopapillary ependymoma {3462}. The prognostic significance of a myxopapillary DNA methylation profile in the face of an ostensibly discordant morphological diagnosis remains to be clarified. Frequent loss of chromosome 22q and mutations of *NF2* are characteristic of spinal ependymomas {2374,1674}. By definition, *MYCN* amplification is absent.

Essential and desirable diagnostic criteria
See Box 2.38.

Staging
Not clinically relevant

Prognosis and prediction
Spinal ependymomas are associated with a favourable outcome in children and adults, with progression-free and overall survival rates of 70–90% and 90–100%, respectively, over 5–10 years {238}. However, progression-free survival declines over time,

Box 2.38 Diagnostic criteria for spinal ependymoma

Essential:

Spinal tumour with morphological and immunohistochemical features of ependymoma

AND

Absence of morphological features of myxopapillary ependymoma or subependymoma

Desirable:

DNA methylation profile aligned with spinal ependymoma

Loss of chromosome 22q

No *MYCN* amplification

reflecting a large number of late relapses {1131}. Extent of resection is a prognostic factor in most studies, patients with gross total resection having favourable progression-free survival {2306,330}. From the limited data available, it can be concluded that the prognosis of CNS WHO grade 3 spinal ependymoma is unfavourable {238}.

Spinal ependymoma, *MYCN*-amplified

Giannini C
Aldape KD
Korshunov A
Pajtler KW

Pietsch T
Ramaswamy V
Taylor MD
Venneti S

Definition

Spinal ependymoma, *MYCN*-amplified, is a well-demarcated spinal glioma demonstrating pseudorosettes or ependymal rosettes and comprising uniform, densely packed small cells with round nuclei embedded in a fibrillary matrix. Practically all tumours display microvascular proliferation, necrosis, and a high mitotic count. By definition, *MYCN* amplification is demonstrated in tumour cells.

ICD-O coding

9396/3 Spinal ependymoma, *MYCN*-amplified

ICD-11 coding

2A00.0Z & XH1511 Other and unspecified neoplasms of brain or central nervous system & Ependymoma, NOS

Related terminology

None

Subtype(s)

None

Localization

Tumours are localized to the spinal cord, primarily to the cervical or thoracic levels (in 78% of cases) and less frequently to lumbar levels (in 7% of cases) {2825,3087,1079,2595}.

Primary tumours may be intramedullary (sometimes with an exophytic component extending into the spinal canal {3087}) or mostly extramedullary {1079,2595}. They are generally large and involve multiple spinal segments. Leptomeningeal dissemination is frequent at diagnosis, or it occurs at some point during the course of the disease {2825,3087,1079,2595}.

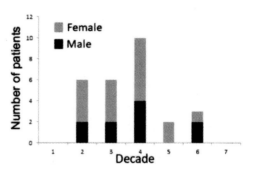

Fig. 2.174 Spinal ependymoma, *MYCN*-amplified. Age and sex distribution of patients with spinal ependymoma, *MYCN*-amplified (all published cases {2825,3087,1079,2595}).

Clinical features

Presenting symptoms depend on tumour location, but they typically include neck or back pain and progressive numbness and weakness in the extremities.

Epidemiology

MYCN-amplified spinal ependymoma is rare, with only 27 reported cases (17 in women and 10 in men; M:F ratio: 1:1.7). The median age at presentation was 31 years (range: 12–56 years) {2825,3087,1079,2595}.

Etiology

No specific etiology has been identified. However, multiple schwannomas were reported in 1 patient, raising the diagnostic possibility of neurofibromatosis type 2 {2825}. No other

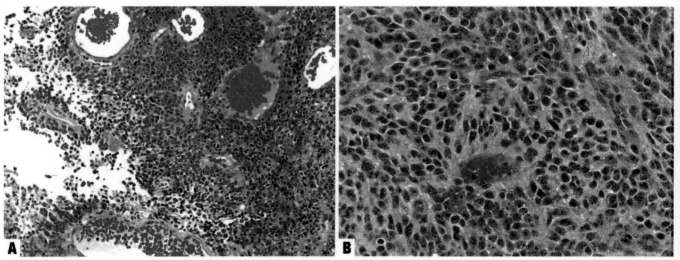

Fig. 2.175 Spinal ependymoma, *MYCN*-amplified. **A** Tumour with a focal pseudopapillary architecture and densely packed cells. **B** High cell density, mitotic activity, and vague pseudorosette formation are present.

patient has shown any signs of neurofibromatosis type 2, and no *NF2* mutation was found in the 4 analysed cases {3087, 1079}.

Pathogenesis

MYCN, a member of the MYC family of proto-oncogenes, encodes a transcription factor that regulates the expression of genes involved in cell growth {236}. How *MYCN* amplification contributes specifically to ependymoma development is unknown.

Macroscopic appearance

The macroscopic features of this specific tumour type have not been described, but they are unlikely to differ markedly from those reported for other circumscribed high-grade gliomas.

Histopathology

MYCN-amplified spinal ependymomas display perivascular anucleate zones (pseudorosettes) and can have a papillary or pseudopapillary architecture {3087,1079,2595}. Most have high-grade histopathological features, such as a high N:C ratio, plentiful mitotic activity, microvascular proliferation, and necrosis.

Two of four tumours with CNS WHO grade 2 histopathological features at presentation progressed to CNS WHO grade 3 at recurrence {2825,3087,1079}.

Immunophenotype

On immunohistochemistry, tumour cells express GFAP and show a focal cytoplasmic dot-like pattern of EMA expression {3087,1079}. MYCN protein expression can be detected by immunohistochemistry {1079,2595}. Cells are immunonegative for OLIG2 {3087}. Nuclear immunoreactivity for H3 p.K28me3 (K27me3) was variably present in the 4 tumours from one study {3087}, but was retained in all tumours from another {1079}.

Grading

Although nearly all *MYCN*-amplified spinal ependymomas show high-grade histopathological features and have a poor prognosis, this molecularly defined ependymal tumour has yet to be assigned a CNS WHO grade {836}.

Cytology

Tumour cells are generally small and have round hyperchromatic nuclei and scant cytoplasm.

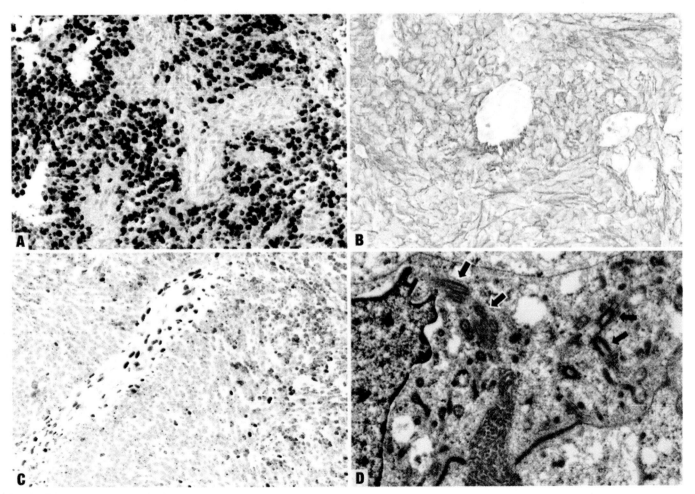

Fig. 2.176 Spinal ependymoma, *MYCN*-amplified. **A** Extensive nuclear expression of MYCN is detected by immunohistochemistry. **B** Immunohistochemistry shows many tumour cells expressing GFAP, which is typically present in perivascular radiating processes. **C** Nuclear immunoreactivity for H3 p.K28me3 (K27me3) can be completely lost, partially lost (as shown here), or retained. **D** Electron microscopy. Intercellular junctions end at a microlumen filled with microvilli, typical of ependymal differentiation. Cilia (black-and-white arrows) and basal bodies (black arrows) are also present.

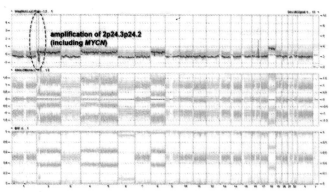

Fig. 2.177 Spinal ependymoma, *MYCN*-amplified. Chromosomal microarray showing amplification of 2p24.3-p24.2, including *MYCN*.

Box 2.39 Diagnostic criteria for spinal ependymoma, *MYCN*-amplified

Essential:

Spinal tumour with morphological and immunohistochemical features of ependymoma

AND

MYCN amplification

Desirable:

DNA methylation profile aligned with spinal ependymoma, *MYCN*-amplified

High-grade histopathological features

Diagnostic molecular pathology

High-level *MYCN* amplification is present and remains stable at relapse {2825,3087,1079,2595}. Additional chromosomal copy-number alterations occur with variable frequency and include loss of chromosome 10 (in 32% of cases) and focal losses on chromosome 11q (in 26% of cases). Demonstration of H3 p.K28me3 (K27me3) loss by immunohistochemistry requires assessment of histone H3 genes for genetic alterations, because *MYCN* amplification can be found in diffuse midline gliomas with H3 p.K28M (K27M) mutation {404}.

MYCN-amplified spinal ependymoma has a DNA methylation profile distinct from that of other ependymal tumour types, as well as from that of neuroblastoma and *MYCN*-amplified paediatric-type glioblastoma {1079,2595}.

Essential and desirable diagnostic criteria

See Box 2.39.

Staging

Not clinically relevant

Prognosis and prediction

MYCN-amplified spinal ependymoma is an aggressive tumour associated with poor progression-free and overall survival compared with that of other spinal ependymomas. Early metastasis and dissemination throughout the neuraxis are frequent. All patients with reported follow-up data have relapsed despite aggressive treatment {2825,3087,1079,2595}.

Myxopapillary ependymoma

Rosenblum MK
Korshunov A
Pajtler KW
Pietsch T
Taylor MD
Venneti S

Definition

Myxopapillary ependymoma is a glial neoplasm characterized by the radial arrangement of spindled or epithelioid tumour cells around blood vessels with perivascular myxoid change and microcyst formation (CNS WHO grade 2).

ICD-O coding

9394/1 Myxopapillary ependymoma

ICD-11 coding

2A00.0Y & XH15U1 Other specified gliomas of brain & Myxopapillary ependymoma

Related terminology

None

Subtype(s)

None

Localization

Myxopapillary ependymomas arise almost exclusively in, and are the most common tumours of, the conus medullaris and filum terminale, accounting for 83% of 320 filum terminale ependymomas in one study {500}. Multifocality has been described {2201}, as have examples originating in the cervicothoracic spinal cord {2993}, lateral ventricle {3390}, fourth ventricle {504}, and brain {2609}. Tumours outside the CNS are also recognized; these are most often sacrococcygeal (mimicking chordomas) or presacral in position, with rare examples described in the uterine adnexa, ischioanal fossa, mediastinum, and lung {3559}. A conus / filum terminale primary must be excluded when a myxopapillary ependymoma occurs at higher levels of the neuraxis {84}.

Clinical features

Lower back pain, often chronic, is an almost constant manifestation of myxopapillary ependymomas, and it can be accompanied by sciatica, sensorimotor deficits indicative of myelopathy, impotence, or urinary and faecal incontinence. Urgent neurosurgical intervention may be required to restore lower extremity function. Neuroimaging typically reveals an ovoid, sharply delimited, and contrast-enhancing mass. Cerebrospinal fluid–borne spread, particularly seeding of the distal thecal sac, may be evident at presentation.

Epidemiology

Incidence rates of 0.6–1.0 cases per 1 million person-years have been reported from the USA and Europe, with an M:F ratio of 1.4–2:1 {2345,3400,214}. Myxopapillary ependymomas occur at all ages but most commonly affect adults; peak case rates were found in patients aged 25–29 years and 45–59 years in one SEER Program analysis (USA, 2004–2012, n = 773) {214}. In another

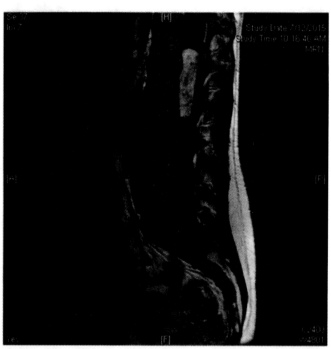

Fig. 2.178 Myxopapillary ependymoma. The well-circumscribed, contrast-enhancing primary tumour in the filum is associated with a drop metastasis in the low thecal sac.

SEER Program study (of cases in patients aged ≤ 21 years; USA, 1973–2012, n = 122), the median patient age was 16 years, and 63% of cases occurred in male patients {1956}.

Etiology

Unknown

Pathogenesis

The pathogenesis of myxopapillary ependymomas is unknown. A variety of recurring chromosomal copy-number abnormalities have been described in these tumours, but no consistent structural variants or other driving mutations {3462,2708}. Upregulation of key enzymes associated with the Warburg metabolic phenotype, including HK2, PKM2, and PDK, has been demonstrated {1973}.

Macroscopic appearance

Often encapsulated, myxopapillary ependymomas are soft and pink to tan-grey, may be grossly gelatinous, and can manifest cystic changes and haemorrhage.

Histopathology

Prototypical is the radial arrangement of cuboidal to elongated tumour cells around hyalinized fibrovascular cores in papillary fashion, with accumulation of basophilic, myxoid material around blood vessels and in microcysts. Myxoid material, highlighted

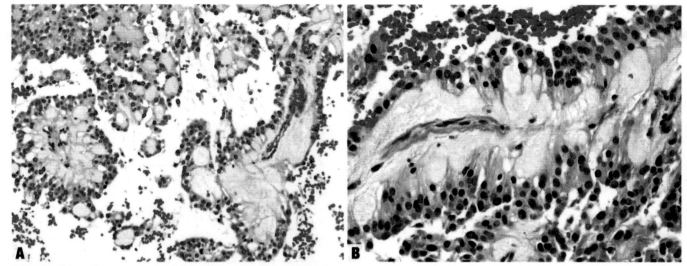

Fig. 2.179 Myxopapillary ependymoma. **A** Epithelioid tumour cells are arranged around fibrovascular cores and microcysts containing myxoid material. **B** Tapering tumour cell processes are oriented towards a fibrovascular core with collaring myxoid matrix.

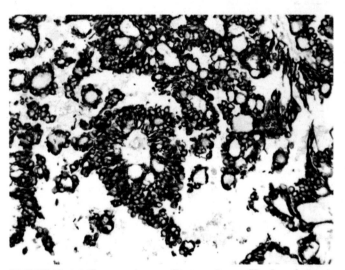

Fig. 2.180 Myxopapillary ependymoma. Tumour cells are diffusely and strongly GFAP-immunoreactive.

by PAS and Alcian blue positivity, is useful in the identification of examples manifesting little, if any, papillary structure and composed instead of epithelioid cells in confluent sheets. Tumour cell spindling and fascicular growth are common, and subpopulations of pleomorphic tumour giant cells can be seen in otherwise typical cases {3585}. Eosinophilic, PAS-positive spherules (balloons) that exhibit spiculated reticulin staining are an occasional feature. Common secondary alterations include fibrosis, haemorrhage, and haemosiderin deposition. Typical myxopapillary ependymomas show, at most, only low-level mitotic activity, and the Ki-67 labelling index usually does not exceed 2–3% {2559}. Exceptional examples termed "anaplastic myxopapillary ependymomas" manifest regional hypercellularity and reduced mucin in association with at least two of the following features: ≥ 2 mitoses/mm², Ki-67 labelling index ≥ 10%, microvascular proliferation, and spontaneous necrosis {1835}.

Immunophenotype
Diffuse immunoreactivity for GFAP distinguishes myxopapillary ependymomas from metastatic carcinomas, paragangliomas, schwannomas, chordomas, and myxoid chondrosarcomas {1799,3302}. Immunolabelling for S100 is also typical, and reactivity for CD99 and CD56 is frequent {1799}. Tumour cell nuclei are not immunoreactive for OLIG2, and dot-like cytoplasmic EMA labelling is typically absent. Myxopapillary ependymomas are often labelled by the AE1/AE3 pancytokeratin cocktail, but they are generally negative for CAM5.2, CK5/6, CK7, and CK20 {1799,3302}.

Cytology

Intraoperative squash and smear preparations of classic myxopapillary ependymomas show epithelioid to spindled cellular profiles, papillary structuring of tumour cells around blood vessels with perivascular myxoid change, and tumour cells arranged around myxoid microcysts. These features are diagnostic in the appropriate clinical setting. Such features may also be evident in fine-needle aspiration material, which may be assessed for confirmatory GFAP expression {41}.

Diagnostic molecular pathology

Myxopapillary ependymomas with a classic morphology are easily recognized, but these tumours also have a unique DNA methylation profile {2374,3462,2236}. However, tumours with the histopathological features of classic ependymoma, particularly lumbosacral lesions with tanycytic or papillary patterns, may also cluster with myxopapillary ependymomas {3462, 2236}. This reflects the fact that myxopapillary ependymomas can exhibit little myxoid change, form pseudorosettes of the usual ependymal type, and manifest spindle cell (tanycytic) features. The prognostic significance of a myxopapillary ependymoma methylation profile in the context of uncharacteristic histopathological features remains to be clarified. Recurrent gains of chromosome 16 and losses of chromosome 10 have been documented {3462}.

Box 2.40 Diagnostic criteria for myxopapillary ependymoma

Essential:

Glioma with papillary structures and perivascular myxoid change or at least focal myxoid microcyste

AND

Immunoreactivity for GFAP

AND (for unresolved lesions)

DNA methylation profile aligned with myxopapillary ependymoma

Desirable:

Papillary arrangements of tumour cells around vascularized fibromyxoid cores

Location in the filum terminale or conus medullaris

Essential and desirable diagnostic criteria
See Box 2.40.

Staging
Because myxopapillary ependymomas may exhibit leptomeningeal dissemination, some groups have recommended that craniospinal MRI and cerebrospinal fluid cytology should be performed after initial surgery and diagnosis {2745}.

Prognosis and prediction
Spinal myxopapillary ependymomas are associated with a relatively favourable prognosis in children and adults, with 10-year overall survival rates > 90% {3400,189,214,2481, 3}. Many patients, however, live with persistent disease and require repeated operations and adjuvant therapy, because myxopapillary ependymomas often resist complete removal owing to locally advanced growth and/or cerebrospinal fluid–borne seeding of the thecal sac or more rostral neuraxis. Paediatric patients are at heightened risk of such dissemination,

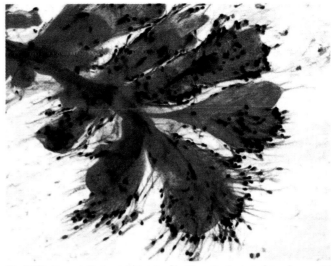

Fig. 2.181 Myxopapillary ependymoma. Papillary structure, perivascular myxoid change, and spindled tumour cells oriented towards fibromyxoid cores are evident in this smear preparation.

which may be evident at diagnosis in ≥ 50% of patients {189, 3}. Tumours arising in the conus have a poorer prognosis than cauda equina examples because the former adhere densely to the spinal cord and are less amenable to resection. Radiotherapy improves progression-free survival {3400}. Cytological atypia and modest mitotic activity do not appear to influence outcome {2993}. Tumours with anaplastic histology may carry an increased risk of aggressive behaviour {1835}. Spinal myxopapillary ependymomas rarely metastasize to extraneural sites, but metastasis frequently complicates the course of sacrococcygeal tumours {3559}.

Subependymoma

Rosenblum MK
Korshunov A
Pajtler KW
Pietsch T
Taylor MD
Venneti S

Definition

Subependymoma is a glioma characterized by the clustering of uniform to mildly pleomorphic tumour cell nuclei in an abundant fibrillary matrix prone to microcystic change (CNS WHO grade 1).

ICD-O coding

9383/1 Subependymoma

ICD-11 coding

2A00.0Y & XH8FZ9 Other specified gliomas of brain & Subependymoma

Related terminology

Not recommended: subependymal glomerate astrocytoma {346}.

Subtype(s)

None

Localization

The most frequent sites of origin are the fourth ventricle (in 50–60% of cases) and lateral ventricles (30–35%), followed distantly by the third ventricle and spinal cord, where subependymomas preferentially arise as eccentric masses in cervicothoracic segments {2755,269,3557,3293}. Cerebral, cerebellar, bulbar, and cerebellopontine angle examples have been reported {1626,269}.

Clinical features

Subependymomas are often asymptomatic and discovered only incidentally on neuroimaging for unrelated reasons or at autopsy. Symptomatic intracranial examples are typically associated with manifestations of ventricular obstruction and intracranial hypertension, occasionally showing evidence of intratumoural/intraventricular haemorrhage. Sensorimotor deficits indicative of myelopathy characterize intramedullary lesions.

Imaging

Most subependymomas are sharply demarcated, hypointense or isointense on T1-weighted MRI, and hyperintense on T2-weighted MRI; some exhibit calcification, cystic change, and foci of contrast enhancement {2755,269}.

Epidemiology

Because subependymomas are often clinically silent, reliable incidence figures are lacking. A SEER Program analysis of 466 intracranial cases (USA, 2004–2013) found an overall incidence of 0.055 cases per 100 000 person-years, an M:F ratio of approximately 2.5:1, and peak incidence in adults aged 40–84 years {2243}. Subependymomas account for approximately 8% of ependymal tumours and < 1% of intracranial neoplasms {2837,1765}.

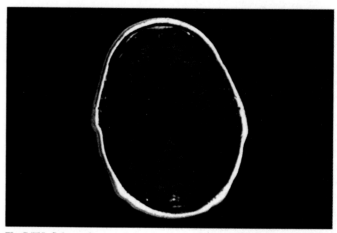

Fig. 2.182 Subependymoma. A sharply circumscribed, intraventricular mass with foci of wispy contrast enhancement is demonstrated in this T1-weighted MRI.

Etiology

Predisposing factors await further definition. Familial cases, including examples in monozygotic twins, are well documented but rare {2271}. These include examples associated with trichorhinophalangeal syndrome type 1 and germline *TRPS1* mutation; a subset of sporadic subependymomas also harbour *TRPS1* mutations {937}. Isolated cases have also been described in patients with hereditary aniridia and *PAX6* mutation {1982}, as well as Noonan syndrome with germline *PTPN11* mutation {323}. Patients with craniopharyngiomas have been reported to develop rare third-ventricular subependymomas {516}. Losses of chromosomes 19 and 6, the latter restricted to infratentorial tumours, appear to play a role in many sporadic cases {3462}.

Pathogenesis

How the chromosomal or genetic abnormalities displayed by subependymomas contribute to tumour development is currently unknown.

Macroscopic appearance

Subependymomas are firm, grey, and generally circumscribed; intracranial examples typically bulge into ventricles in an exophytic fashion. Cystic changes, calcification, and focal haemorrhage (unusual) may be apparent.

Histopathology

Typical is the clustering of small, euchromatic, and round to oval nuclei (resembling those of subependymal glia) in a voluminous matrix of fibrillary cytoplasmic processes. Microcystic changes are common, particularly in lateral ventricular subependymomas, as are calcifications. Nuclear pleomorphism and proliferative microvascular abnormalities may be encountered, with exceptional cases exhibiting low-level mitotic activity and even

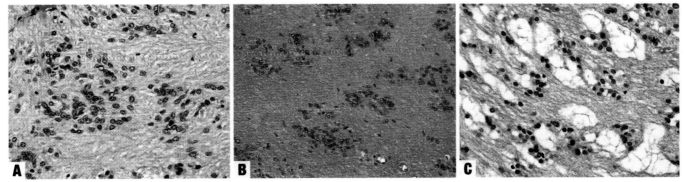

Fig. 2.183 Subependymoma. **A** Tumour cell nuclei are small, uniform, and without mitotic activity. **B** Tumour cell nuclei cluster in a dense fibrillary matrix. **C** Microcystic change in the fibrillary matrix is shown.

non-palisading necrosis {2755}. Just as classic ependymomas can focally exhibit subependymoma-type histology, so may subependymomas focally manifest perivascular pseudorosettes. Subependymoma-predominant neoplasms with nodules of classic ependymoma (termed "mixed ependymoma–subependymoma") are well recognized and mentioned below (see *Prognosis and prediction*). Otherwise typical examples may also harbour elements of fibrillary astroglial or (rarely) gemistocytic morphology. Sclerotic and ectatic blood vessels, haemorrhage, and haemosiderin deposits are common. Oddities include melanotic pigmentation {2727} and sarcomatous change {3212, 2700}.

Immunophenotype
Subependymomas manifest diffuse GFAP immunoreactivity and can display focal dot-like EMA expression, but they do so less frequently than ependymomas {2755,3528}. Some are reported to express OLIG2 or synaptophysin {269}, but this appears to be exceptional {3528}. SOX10 labelling, if present, is limited {1655}. Also reported is the expression of HIF1α, TOP2B, MDM2, nucleolin, and phosphorylated STAT3 {1697}, as well as aquaporin-1 and aquaporin-4 {2272}. Subependymomas retain ATRX expression, do not express the mutant IDH1 p.R132H or BRAF p.V600E gene products, and (except for rare bulbar lesions) are negative for H3 p.K28M (K27M), but they retain H3 p.K28me3 (K27me3) expression {3528}.

Cytology
The relatively uniform round or oval nuclear profiles, nuclear clustering, and fibrillary matrix of subependymomas are apparent in smear and squash preparations, which may also demonstrate myxoid and microcystic changes {3209}.

Diagnostic molecular pathology
Molecular analyses have shown subependymomas in the supratentorial, posterior fossa, and spinal anatomical compartments to have distinct DNA methylation profiles {2374,3462, 2236}. However, although tumours at each site with the histopathological features of subependymoma cluster together in these analyses and are not placed in other molecular groups, some tumours eliciting the morphological diagnosis of classic ependymoma may also cluster with typical subependymomas {3462,2236}. The prognostic significance of a subependymoma DNA methylation profile in the face of an ostensibly discordant morphological diagnosis remains to be clarified.

Box 2.41 Diagnostic criteria for subependymoma

Essential:

Circumscribed glioma with clustering of tumour cell nuclei within expansive, focally microcystic fibrillary matrix

AND

Lack of conspicuous nuclear atypia

AND

Absent or minimal mitotic activity

AND (for unresolved lesions)

DNA methylation profile aligned with subependymoma

Recurrent copy-number abnormalities are chromosome 19 loss and partial chromosome 6 loss (infratentorial cases) {3462}. *TRPS1* mutations have been documented {937}. Rare brainstem gliomas exhibiting subependymoma-type histology are H3 p.K28M (K27M)–mutant {3528}.

Essential and desirable diagnostic criteria
See Box 2.41.

Staging
Not clinically relevant

Prognosis and prediction
An excellent prognosis is associated with subependymomas {2755,269,2243,3557,3293}. Postsurgical recurrence is rare, even after subtotal resection, and only exceptional instances of subependymal seeding or anaplastic progression have been reported {2880,269}. Cytological pleomorphism, occasional mitoses, and necrosis have not proved prognostically significant {2558,2755}. A Ki-67 labelling index > 1% has characterized some subependymomas exhibiting recurrence {1729,3206} or dramatic interval growth on surveillance {2261}. The traditional grading of mixed ependymoma–subependymoma according to the histology of their ependymoma components is based on a historical series in which such lesions behaved more aggressively than pure subependymomas {2827}, but more recent analyses have not replicated this observation {2755,269}. Assessments of chromosome 19 status and DNA methylation profiling may prove useful in the risk stratification of patients with mixed or morphologically ambiguous lesions {3462}. The occurrence of H3 p.K28M (K27M) mutation in brainstem gliomas exhibiting subependymoma histology has not been associated with rapidly fatal progression {3528}.

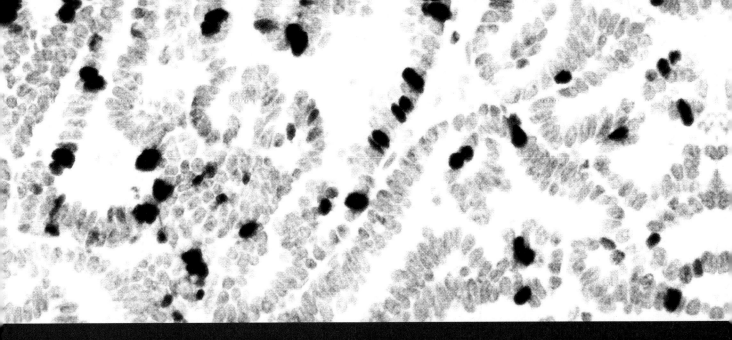

3

Choroid plexus tumours

Edited by: Hawkins CE

Choroid plexus papilloma
Atypical choroid plexus papilloma
Choroid plexus carcinoma

Choroid plexus papilloma

Pietsch T
Hasselblatt M
Malkin D
Paulus W

Definition

Choroid plexus papilloma is an intraventricular papillary neoplasm derived from choroid plexus epithelium, with very low or absent mitotic activity (CNS WHO grade 1).

ICD-O coding

9390/0 Choroid plexus papilloma

ICD-11 coding

2A00.22 & XH0RF9 Choroid plexus papilloma & Choroid plexus papilloma, NOS

Related terminology

None

Subtype(s)

None

Localization

Choroid plexus papillomas are located within the ventricular system where normal choroid plexus can be found. They occur most often in the lateral ventricles, followed by the fourth and third ventricles. Rare cases have been described within the spinal cord or in ectopic locations {2428}. Multifocal occurrence is exceptional {2486}.

Clinical features

By blocking cerebrospinal fluid (CSF) pathways, choroid plexus papillomas tend to cause hydrocephalus and increased intracranial pressure. It has been debated whether overproduction of CSF is a major contributing factor to hydrocephalus {259}.

Imaging

On CT and MRI, choroid plexus papillomas usually present as isodense or hyperdense, T1-isointense, T2-hyperintense, irregularly contrast-enhancing, well-delineated masses within the ventricles, but irregular tumour margins and disseminated disease may occur {1178}.

Spread

Even benign choroid plexus papilloma may seed cells into the CSF; in rare cases, this can result in drop metastases surrounding the cauda equina {3055}.

Epidemiology

Although choroid plexus tumours constitute 0.3–0.8% of all brain tumours overall, they account for 2–4% of those that occur in children aged < 15 years, and for 10–20% of those occurring in the first year of life {455}. The average annual incidence is 0.3 cases per 1 million population {1452,2667,3468}. Choroid plexus papillomas account for 58.2% of the choroid plexus tumours in the SEER database. The M:F ratio is 1.2:1. About 80% of lateral ventricular tumours are found in patients aged < 20 years, whereas fourth ventricle tumours are evenly distributed across all age groups {3468}.

Etiology

Environmental risk factors for the development of choroid plexus papilloma have not been confirmed. Earlier reports of a possible role of SV40 {1364} have not been confirmed in more recent studies. Genomic analysis of choroid plexus papilloma suggests a role for genes involved in the development and biology of plexus epithelium (e.g. *OTX2* and *TRPM3*). It is thought that their alteration may contribute to the initial steps of choroid plexus papilloma oncogenesis {1455}.

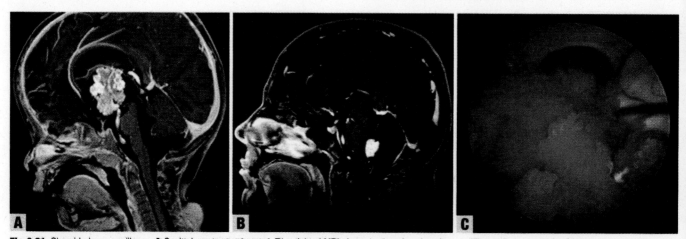

Fig. 3.01 Choroid plexus papilloma. **A** Sagittal, contrast-enhanced, T1-weighted MRI shows a strongly enhancing, cauliflower-like mass in the third ventricle of a 22-month-old girl. **B** Sagittal, contrast-enhanced, T1-weighted MRI shows a choroid plexus papilloma in the fourth ventricle of a 38-year-old man. **C** Intraoperative endoscopic view of a choroid plexus papilloma.

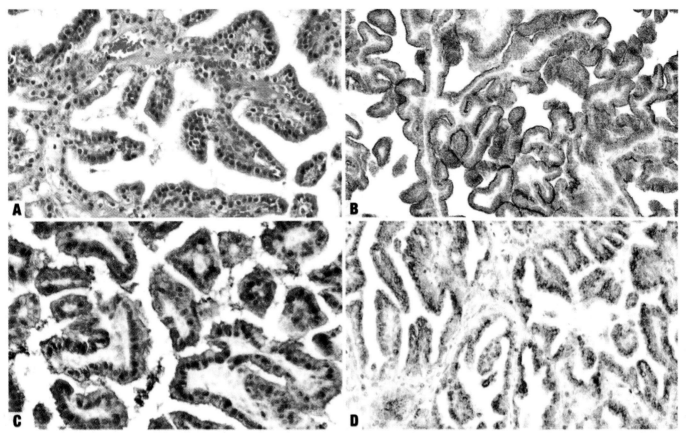

Fig. 3.02 Choroid plexus papilloma. **A** Papillary pattern with a single layer of monomorphic cuboidal cells. **B** Immunohistochemistry for the potassium channel Kir7.1 shows typical membranous labelling of the apical surface of tumour cells. **C** Immunohistochemistry for S100. **D** Immunohistochemistry for transthyretin (prealbumin).

Genetic susceptibility

Choroid plexus papilloma occurs in Aicardi syndrome, a disorder with lethality in males and presumably X-linked dominant inheritance, which is defined by the triad of agenesis of the corpus callosum, chorioretinal lacunae, and infantile spasms {43}. In the setting of an X;17(q12;p13) translocation, hypomelanosis of Ito has been associated with the development of choroid plexus papilloma in several cases {3574}. Gains of the short arm of chromosome 9, a rare constitutional abnormality, were shown to be associated with hyperplasia of the choroid plexus and with choroid plexus papilloma {2278,1012}.

Pathogenesis

Choroid plexus papillomas are believed to derive from monociliated progenitors of plexus epithelium located in the roof plate, and they show activation of the sonic hedgehog and Notch signalling pathways known to play a crucial role in the proliferation of plexus epithelial precursor cells {1876}. Notch signalling suppresses multiciliate differentiation of progenitor cells and may allow sonic hedgehog–mediated proliferative signals via the primary cilium in plexus papilloma cells {1876}.

Both classic cytogenetic and genome-wide array-based approaches demonstrated hyperdiploidy with whole-chromosome gains in choroid plexus papilloma {779,2669,2079,1455}. The pathogenetic impact of these chromosomal gains is not understood. Because constitutional trisomy or tetrasomy of chromosome 9p is linked to choroid plexus hyperplasia, it is speculated that this region, showing gains in 50% of sporadic plexus papillomas {2669}, contains genes that control the proliferation of choroid plexus progenitor cells {1012}. *TP53* mutations are rare in choroid plexus papillomas (present in < 10% of cases) {3097}. Epigenetic profiling identified three distinct methylation groups; cluster analysis showed separation of most choroid plexus papillomas from choroid plexus carcinomas {3184,2507}.

Macroscopic appearance

Choroid plexus papillomas are circumscribed, cauliflower-like intraventricular masses. Cysts and haemorrhage may occur.

Histopathology

The well-developed papillary pattern is composed of fibrovascular fronds that are covered by a single layer of uniform cuboidal to columnar epithelial cells with round or oval, monomorphic nuclei. Mitotic activity is absent or very low: < 1 mitosis/mm² (equating to < 2 mitoses/10 HPF of 0.23 mm²) {1463, 2927}. Brain invasion with cell clusters or single cells, high cellularity, necrosis, nuclear pleomorphism, and focal blurring of the papillary pattern may occasionally occur. Cells tend to be more crowded and nuclei more variable than in non-neoplastic choroid plexus. Choroid plexus papillomas can acquire unusual histological features, including oncocytic change, mucinous degeneration, melanization, tubular/glandular architecture (adenoma), neuropil-like islands, and degeneration of connective tissue (e.g. xanthomatous change; angioma-like increase of blood vessels; and bone, cartilage, or adipose tissue formation) {2563,395,1253,2002}.

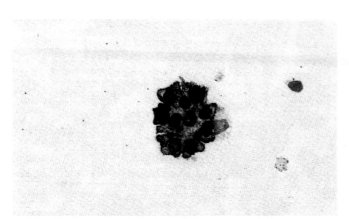

Fig. 3.03 Choroid plexus papilloma cells in cerebrospinal fluid. Immunohistochemistry for the potassium channel Kir7.1.

Box 3.01 Diagnostic criteria for choroid plexus papilloma

Essential:

Demonstration of choroid plexus differentiation by histopathological and immunophenotypic features

AND

Absent or low mitotic activity

AND

Intraventricular or cerebellopontine angle location

Immunophenotype

More than 90% of choroid plexus tumours are positive for cytokeratins (usually CK7-positive and CK20-negative), vimentin, and S100 {1204,2428}. GFAP and EMA may be expressed, but staining is often weak or focal {772,2207}. Membranous staining (mainly) of the apical border for the inward-rectifier potassium channel Kir7.1 is typical for non-neoplastic choroid plexus epithelium and is retained in > 80% of choroid plexus papillomas and about 50% of choroid plexus carcinomas, whereas it has not been described in other primary brain tumours or cerebral metastases {1250,582}. The glutamate transporter EAAT1 is expressed in most choroid plexus papillomas, whereas it is absent in endolymphatic sac tumours and in > 95% of non-neoplastic choroid plexus specimens {2844,258}. Transthyretin (prealbumin) is positive in normal choroid plexus, but staining may be negative or variable among choroid plexus papillomas, and it is also seen in some metastatic carcinomas {2428,59}. The Ki-67 proliferation index is usually < 5% and often < 1% {3244,3479}.

Cytology

In CSF samples and cytological imprints, clusters of choroid plexus papilloma cells show epithelioid morphology with isomorphic round nuclei and moderately developed cytoplasms {1641}.

Diagnostic molecular pathology

Choroid plexus papillomas are easily recognized by their histology. Genome-wide chromosomal copy-number analysis can demonstrate characteristic hyperploidy {1455}. Choroid plexus papillomas also show typical epigenetic signatures {460}.

Essential and desirable diagnostic criteria

See Box 3.01.

Staging

Not relevant

Prognosis and prediction

Prognosis is excellent, especially upon gross total resection. In a series of 41 patients with choroid plexus papilloma, the 5-year overall survival rate was 97% {1738}. Similar results were obtained in another series {1463}. Choroid plexus papillomas in children aged < 36 months also have an excellent prognosis after surgery alone {1786}. Malignant progression of choroid plexus papilloma is rare {589,1464}.

Atypical choroid plexus papilloma

Pietsch T
Hasselblatt M
Malkin D
Paulus W

Definition

Atypical choroid plexus papilloma is a choroid plexus papilloma that has increased mitotic activity but does not fulfil the criteria for choroid plexus carcinoma (CNS WHO grade 2).

ICD-O coding

9390/1 Atypical choroid plexus papilloma

ICD-11 coding

2A00.22 & XH3Y57 Choroid plexus papilloma & Atypical choroid plexus papilloma

Related terminology

None

Subtype(s)

None

Localization

Atypical choroid plexus papillomas arise in locations where normal choroid plexus can be found. In contrast to choroid plexus papillomas (CNS WHO grade 1), which occur in the supratentorial and infratentorial regions with nearly equal frequency, atypical choroid plexus papillomas are more common in the lateral ventricles {1463,3479}.

Clinical features

Like choroid plexus papillomas, atypical choroid plexus papillomas tend to block cerebrospinal fluid pathways, and patients present with hydrocephalus and raised intracranial pressure.

Imaging

No differences in MRI characteristics have been reported between choroid plexus papilloma and atypical choroid plexus papilloma {3479}.

Spread

Atypical choroid plexus papilloma has been reported with metastasis at diagnosis in 17% of cases {3479}.

Epidemiology

In two paediatric studies of choroid plexus tumours, patients with atypical choroid plexus papilloma were on average younger (median age: 8 months in one study, 0.84 years in the other) than those with choroid plexus papilloma (median age: 35 months in one, 2.18 years in the other) {3183,2927}. Although both studies included patients of up to 18 years of age, the oldest patients with atypical choroid plexus papilloma were 10- and 11-year-olds.

Etiology

No differences have been established between the etiology of atypical choroid plexus papilloma and that of choroid plexus papilloma.

Pathogenesis

Genetic profile

Atypical choroid plexus papillomas are genetically highly similar to choroid plexus papilloma but different from choroid plexus carcinoma {2079}. Consistent with the entity's defining histological feature (i.e. increased mitotic activity), a higher RNA expression

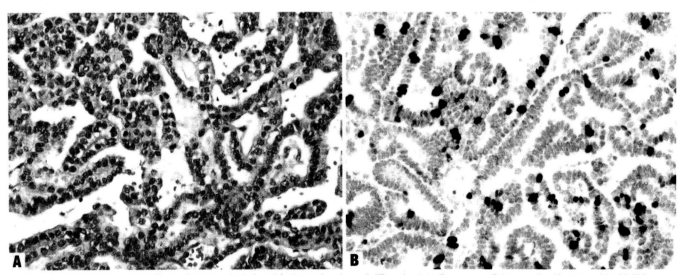

Fig.3.04 Atypical choroid plexus papilloma. **A** Increased mitotic activity in an otherwise well-differentiated papillary tumour. **B** Increased proliferative activity (Ki-67 immunohistochemistry).

of cell cycle–related genes was found in atypical choroid plexus papilloma than in choroid plexus papilloma {1455}.

Macroscopic appearance

Intraoperative observations in atypical choroid plexus papillomas demonstrate a highly vascular tumour with a propensity to bleed {3107}, similar to choroid plexus papillomas.

Histopathology

Atypical choroid plexus papilloma is a choroid plexus papilloma with increased mitotic activity. A mitotic count of ≥ 1 mitosis/mm^2 (equating to ≥ 2 mitoses/10 HPF of 0.23 mm^2) has been used to establish this diagnosis {1463,2927}. One or two of the following four features may also be present: increased cellularity, nuclear pleomorphism, blurring of the papillary pattern (solid growth), and areas of necrosis; however, these features are not required for a diagnosis of atypical choroid plexus papilloma.

Immunophenotype

The expression pattern corresponds to that of choroid plexus papilloma. Prognostic correlates have been described for various antigens, such as S100, transthyretin, and CD44, but these markers are not helpful in grading choroid plexus tumours in individual cases. The median Ki-67 index is 9.1% {3479}.

Cytology

Cytological features are similar to those of choroid plexus papillomas {1641}.

Diagnostic molecular pathology

Atypical choroid plexus papillomas are recognized by their histology. Genome-wide chromosomal copy-number analysis can demonstrate characteristic hyperploidy {1455}, which may be helpful in the diagnostic differentiation from choroid plexus carcinomas.

Essential and desirable diagnostic criteria

See Box 3.02.

Box 3.02 Diagnostic criteria for atypical choroid plexus papilloma

Essential:

Intraventricular or cerebellopontine angle location

AND

Demonstration of choroid plexus differentiation by histopathological and immunophenotypic features

AND

Demonstration of ≥ 1 mitosis/mm^2 in a minimum of 2.3 mm^2 (equating to ≥ 2 mitoses/10 HPF of 0.23 mm^2)

AND

Absence of criteria qualifying for the diagnosis of choroid plexus carcinoma

Desirable:

In select cases: demonstration of hyperploidy by genome-wide chromosomal copy-number analysis

---

Staging

Not relevant

Prognosis and prediction

The 5-year overall survival and event-free survival rates for atypical choroid plexus papillomas (89% and 83%, respectively) are intermediate between those for choroid plexus papilloma and choroid plexus carcinoma {3479}. In a series of 124 atypical choroid plexus papillomas, increased mitotic activity was the only histological feature independently associated with recurrence. Tumours with ≥ 1 mitosis/mm^2 in a minimum of 2.3 mm^2 (equating to ≥ 2 mitoses/10 HPF), which constituted the definition of atypical choroid plexus papilloma, were 4.9 times as likely to recur after 5 years of follow-up as were those with lower mitotic counts {1463}. Children aged < 3 years harbouring atypical choroid plexus papilloma seem to have a good prognosis {3183}. In older patients, choroid plexus papilloma is more likely to recur; there is evidence that the diagnosis of atypical choroid plexus papilloma is prognostically relevant in children aged > 3 years and adults.

Choroid plexus carcinoma

Pietsch T
Hasselblatt M
Malkin D
Paulus W

Definition

Choroid plexus carcinoma (CPC) is a malignant epithelial neoplasm of the choroid plexus that shows at least four of the following five histological features: frequent mitoses, increased cellular density, nuclear pleomorphism, blurring of the papillary pattern with poorly structured sheets of tumour cells, and necrotic areas (CNS WHO grade 3).

ICD-O coding

9390/3 Choroid plexus carcinoma

ICD-11 coding

2A00 & XH3M77 Primary neoplasms of brain & Choroid plexus carcinoma

Related terminology

None

Subtype(s)

None

Localization

Most CPCs are located in the lateral ventricles {1786}.

Clinical features

CPCs tend to block cerebrospinal fluid pathways and cause symptoms related to hydrocephalus, such as increased intracranial pressure, increased head size, nausea, and vomiting {259}.

Imaging

On MRI, CPCs typically appear as large intraventricular lesions with irregular enhancing margins, a heterogeneous signal on T2- and T1-weighted images, oedema in adjacent brain, hydrocephalus, and disseminated tumour {2100}.

Epidemiology

In the SEER database, CPCs accounted for 34.4% of choroid plexus tumours {455}. About 80% of all CPCs occur in children.

Etiology

Most CPCs occur sporadically, but about 40% occur in the context of Li–Fraumeni syndrome with germline *TP53* pathogenic sequence variants {1746,3097}. It is recommended that any patient with a CPC, and their family, be offered genetic counselling and testing for *TP53* germline mutations {1134,336}. CPC has also been described in Aicardi syndrome {3103}.

Pathogenesis

CPCs are believed to derive from monociliated progenitors of plexus epithelium located in the roof plate, and they show activation of the sonic hedgehog and Notch signalling pathways

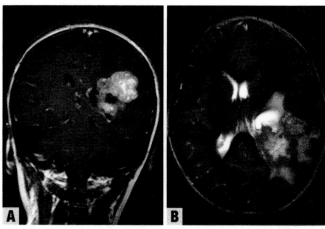

Fig. 3.05 Choroid plexus carcinoma. **A** This T1-weighted coronal MRI of a 5-year-old girl shows a contrast-enhancing tumour related to the lateral ventricle. **B** Axial T2-weighted MRI of a 5-year-old girl.

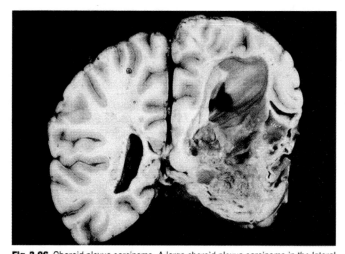

Fig. 3.06 Choroid plexus carcinoma. A large choroid plexus carcinoma in the lateral ventricle with extensive invasion of brain tissue.

known to play a crucial role in the proliferation of these cells {1876}. About 50% of CPCs carry *TP53* mutations. In > 90% of *TP53*-wildtype CPCs, the combination of the *TP53* p.R72 variant and the *MDM2* SNP309 polymorphism, which is associated with reduced *TP53* activity, was observed {3097}, implicating p53 dysfunction in virtually all CPCs. *TP53* mutations in CPC are associated with increased genomic instability {3097}, with aneuploidy demonstrable by both classic cytogenetic and genome-wide array-based approaches {2079,2669,3575,2748, 1455}. These complex chromosomal alterations are related to patient age {2748}, with childhood CPCs showing marked hypodiploidy {1455}. *TAF12*, *NFYC*, and *RAD54L* oncogenes, within chromosomal gains at 1p35.3-p32, cooperate in disease

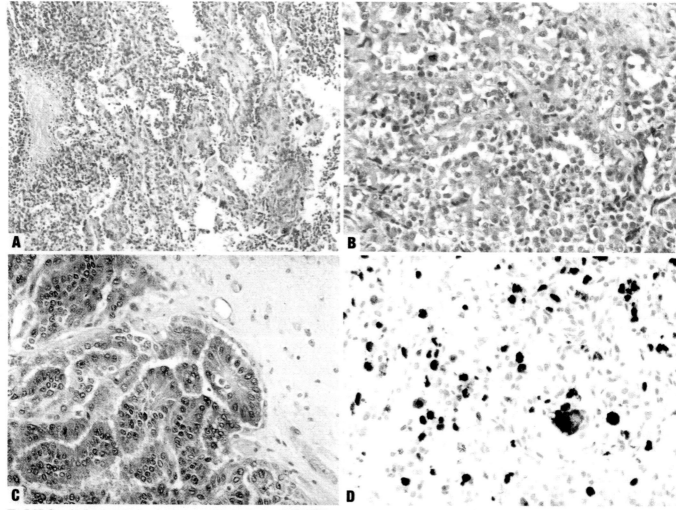

Fig. 3.07 Choroid plexus carcinoma. **A** Increased cellularity, blurring of the papillary pattern, and necrosis. **B** Increased cellularity, nuclear pleomorphism, and mitotic activity. **C** Immunohistochemistry for transthyretin highlights infiltration of surrounding brain tissue. **D** Ki-67 immunohistochemical staining shows high proliferative activity.

initiation and progression and suggest potential therapeutic targets {3214}.

Macroscopic appearance

CPCs are highly vascular tumours that may appear solid, haemorrhagic, or necrotic, and that show invasive growth.

Histopathology

CPCs demonstrate frank signs of malignancy, defined as showing at least four of the following five histological features: increased cellular density; nuclear pleomorphism; blurring of the papillary pattern with poorly structured sheets of tumour cells; necrotic areas; and frequent mitoses, usually > 2.5 mitoses/mm²

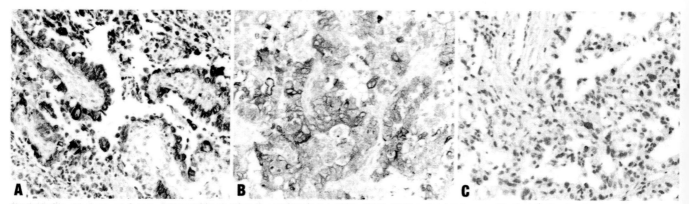

Fig. 3.08 Choroid plexus carcinoma. **A** Immunohistochemistry for cytokeratin is positive. **B** Immunohistochemisty for transthyretin (prealbumin). **C** Immunohistochemistry demonstrates a lack of expression of epithelial membrane antigen (EMA).

(equating to > 5 mitoses/10 HPF of 0.23 mm²) {1463,2927}. Diffuse brain invasion is common.

Immunophenotype

Like choroid plexus papillomas, CPCs express cytokeratins, but they are less frequently positive for S100 and transthyretin. There is usually no membranous positivity for EMA. Distinct membranous staining for the potassium channel Kir7.1 is seen in about 50% of CPCs. Nuclear accumulation of p53 has been reported in CPCs that harboured *TP53* mutation {3097}. CPCs retain nuclear positivity for SMARCB1 and SMARCA4. The median Ki-67 index is reported as 20.3% (range: 7.8–42.5%) {3479}.

Cytology

On touch preparation, CPC cells show high nuclear variance and a high N:C ratio.

Diagnostic molecular pathology

CPCs can usually be identified by histological and immunophenotypic analysis. Genome-wide chromosomal copy-number analysis shows complex chromosomal alterations and characteristic hypoploidy {1455}, which may be helpful in the diagnostic differentiation from atypical choroid plexus papillomas. *TP53* mutations can be found in about 50% of cases by sequencing. Methylome analysis has revealed three clinically distinct subgroups of choroid plexus tumours, with all CPCs clustering within the same subgroup, together with prognostically unfavourable grade 1 and 2 choroid plexus tumours {3184}.

Essential and desirable diagnostic criteria

See Box 3.03.

Staging

Patients with CPC present with metastasis at diagnosis in 21% of cases {3479}, so investigation for the presence of metastases is recommended.

Prognosis and prediction

The 5-year progression-free and overall survival rates in patients with CPC have been reported as 38% and 62%, respectively {3576}. The extent of surgery has a significant impact on survival {455}. Several studies have suggested that the presence of *TP53* mutations, as identified by immunohistochemical staining, is associated with a less favourable outcome {1157,3097,3576}.

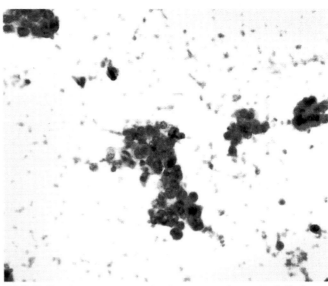

Fig. 3.09 Choroid plexus carcinoma. Touch preparation shows epithelioid cells with pleomorphism.

Box 3.03 Diagnostic criteria for choroid plexus carcinoma

Essential:

Demonstration of choroid plexus differentiation by histopathological and immunophenotypic features

AND

Presence of at least four of the following five histological features:

- Increased cellular density
- Nuclear pleomorphism
- Blurring of the papillary pattern with poorly structured sheets of tumour cells
- Necrotic areas
- Frequent mitoses, usually > 2.5 mitoses/mm² in a minimum of 2.3 mm² (equating to > 5 mitoses/10 HPF of 0.23 mm²)

AND

Intraventricular location

Desirable:

TP53 mutation analysis

Methylation profile of choroid plexus carcinoma

In select cases: demonstration of hypoploidy by genome-wide chromosomal copy-number analysis

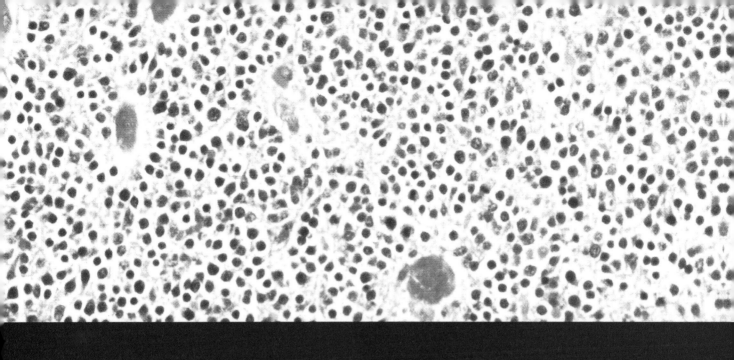

4

Embryonal tumours

Edited by: Ellison DW, Figarella-Branger D, Pfister SM, von Deimling A, Wesseling P

Medulloblastoma: Introduction

Ellison DW
Taylor MD

Medulloblastomas display considerable biological heterogeneity, which is evident across the diverse types of molecularly defined medulloblastomas listed in this classification and among the morphological patterns shown by these tumours.

Medulloblastoma as a unitary disease

Medulloblastoma can arise at all ages but most commonly occurs in childhood. It is the second most common CNS malignant tumour in childhood, after high-grade glioma, and it accounts for approximately 20% of all intracranial neoplasms in this age group {1604,2344}. The annual overall incidence of medulloblastoma is 1.8 cases per 1 million population, whereas the annual childhood incidence is 6 cases per 1 million. These rates have not changed over time {2406}.

The median patient age at diagnosis of medulloblastoma is 9 years, with peaks in incidence at 3 and 7 years of age {2686}. As many as one quarter of all medulloblastomas occur in adults, but < 1% of adult intracranial tumours are medulloblastomas {2075}. The tumour has an overall M:F ratio of 1.7:1.

As with other high-grade brain tumours, the incidence of medulloblastoma differs across ethnic groups. In the USA, overall annual incidence is highest among White non-Hispanic people (2.2 cases per 1 million population), followed by among Hispanic people (2.1 per 1 million) and African-American people (1.5 per 1 million) {2344}.

Medulloblastomas occur in the setting of several inherited cancer syndromes {3392}. Germline mutations can occur in ELP1 {3393}, SUFU and PTCH1 (naevoid basal cell carcinoma syndrome / Gorlin syndrome) {1381}, TP53 (Li–Fraumeni syndrome) {2331}, APC (familial adenomatous polyposis) {1616}, CREBBP (Rubinstein–Taybi syndrome) {339}, NBN (NBS1) (Nijmegen breakage syndrome) {1366}, PALB2, and BRCA2, among others {3392,3234}.

Medulloblastomas grow into the fourth ventricle or are located in the cerebellar parenchyma {293}. Some cerebellar tumours can be laterally located in a hemisphere, and almost all of these belong to the sonic hedgehog (SHH)-activated molecular group {3164}. Wingless/INT1 (WNT)-activated medulloblastomas are thought to arise from cells in the dorsal brainstem {1099,1472}, although not all brainstem embryonal tumours are WNT-activated medulloblastomas.

All types of medulloblastomas are considered to be embryonal tumours and CNS WHO grade 4, even though some molecular groups and subgroups of medulloblastoma, such as WNT-activated tumours, show a very good response to current therapeutic regimens and almost all of these patients can be cured. Small, poorly differentiated cells with a high N:C ratio and high levels of mitotic activity and apoptosis dominate the histopathology. However, architectural and cytological diversity can manifest as nodule formation, neurocytic or ganglion

Table 4.01 Characteristics of medulloblastoma molecular groups

	Medulloblastoma molecular group				
	WNT-activated	**SHH-activated TP53-wildtype**	**SHH-activated TP53-mutant**	**Non-WNT/non-SHH group 3**	**Non-WNT/non-SHH group 4**
Subgroups		SHH-1 to SHH-4	SHH-3	Group 3/4 subgroups 1–8	
Relative frequency	10%	20%	10%	25%	35%
Predominant age group	Childhood	Infancy/adulthood	Childhood	Infancy/childhood	All age groups
M:F ratio	1:2	1:1	3:1	2:1	3:1
Predominant morphology	Classic	Desmoplastic/nodular	Large cell / anaplastic	Classic	Classic
Frequent copy-number alterations	Monosomy 6	PTCH1 deletion; 10q loss	MYCN amplification; GLI2 amplification; 17p loss	MYC, MYCN amplification; 1q, 7q gain; 10q, 16q loss; isodicentric 17q	MYCN, OTX2 amplification; CDK6 amplification; 7 gain; 8, 11 loss; isodicentric 17q
Frequent genetic alterations	CTNNB1, DDX3X mutation	PTCH1, SMO, SUFU, ELP1, DDX3X, KMT2D, U1 snRNA mutation	TP53, DDX3X, U1 snRNA, TERT mutation	GFI1, GFI1B activation; SMARCA4, KBTBD4, CTDNEP1, KMT2D mutation	GFI1, GFI1B activation; PRDM6 activation; KDM6A, ZMYM3, KMT2C, KMT2D, KBTBD4 mutation
Genes with germline mutation	APC	PTCH1, SUFU, ELP1	TP53	Rare BRCA2, PALB2	Rare BRCA2, PALB2

SHH, sonic hedgehog; snRNA, small nuclear RNA.

cell differentiation, or even myogenic and/or melanotic differentiation {971,2057,2770,2497,2973}. Such varied morphological features can be seen across medulloblastoma molecular groups.

Molecular heterogeneity

Medulloblastomas should now be classified according to a combination of molecular and histopathological features. Their molecular classification reflects biological heterogeneity that can be demonstrated by the clustering of medulloblastomas into groups using transcriptome or DNA methylation profiling {2280}. Initially, consensus that was built upon several datasets established four principal molecular groups: WNT-activated, SHH-activated, group 3, and group 4 {3153}. Tumours in the WNT and SHH groups show activation of their respective cell signalling pathways. WNT and SHH medulloblastomas were included in the 2016 WHO classification of CNS tumours, and SHH tumours were divided on the basis of TP53 status (TP53-mutant and TP53-wildtype tumours having very different clinicopathological and biological characteristics). Non-WNT/non-SHH medulloblastomas comprise group 3 and group 4 tumours (see Table 4.01).

These groups are represented in the current classification; however, new subgroups have emerged at a more granular level, within the four principal molecular groups, having been discovered through the analysis of large numbers of tumours {2865, 491,2279,2900,1757,1355}. These new subgroups are introduced in the sections on molecularly defined medulloblastomas that follow. There are four subgroups of SHH medulloblastoma and eight subgroups of non-WNT/non-SHH medulloblastoma {2865,491,2900,1757,1355}. Like the four principal molecular groups of medulloblastoma, some of these subgroups are associated with clinicopathological and genetic features that provide

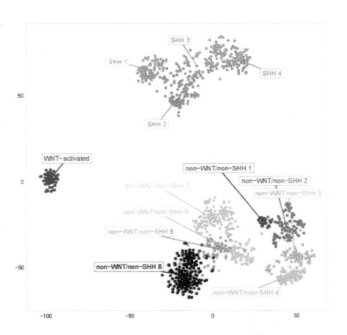

Fig. 4.01 Medulloblastoma molecular groups and subgroups. Unsupervised, non-linear t-distributed stochastic neighbour embedding (t-SNE) projection of methylation array profiles of 1089 medulloblastoma samples. Samples were selected from a large database of > 50 000 brain tumour datasets to serve as reference profiles for training a supervised classification model based on strict criteria: all these samples showed a high calibrated classification score (> 0.9) for medulloblastoma methylation class when applying the brain tumour classifier available at https://www.molecularneuropathology.org. In a t-SNE projection like this, occasional samples of one subclass may fall closer to a different subclass because of the stochastic nature of the t-SNE algorithm and the gradual, rather than strict, boundaries between the subclasses.

Group	SHH			
Subgroup	1	2	3	4
Related terminology	SHH-I, SHH-beta, SHH-infant	SHH-II, SHH-gamma, SHH-infant	SHH-alpha, SHH-child TP53-wildtype / TP53-mutated	SHH-delta, SHH-adult
Frequency	15–20%	15–20%	20–25% / 10–15%	30–35%
Age				
Sex	♂ ♀	♂♂ ♀♀♀	♂ ♀ / ♂♂♂♂ ♀	♂♂♂♂ ♀♀♀
Histology	Desmoplastic > Classic	Desmoplastic/MBEN > Classic	Classic > LCA / LCA > Classic	Desmoplastic > Classic
Outcome	heterogeneous prognosis	good prognosis	good prognosis / poor prognosis	intermediate prognosis
Cytogenetics	2+	9q– 10q–	9p+ 9q– / 17p– 3p– 3q+ 10q– 14q–	3q+ 9q– 10q– 14q–
Driver events	PTCH1, SUFU mutation/deletion SMO, KMT2D mutation	PTCH1, SUFU mutation/deletion SMO mutation	PTCH1, ELP1, DDX3X, KMT2D mutation PPM1D amplification / TP53, DDX3X, U1 snRNA, TERT mutation MYCN, GLI2 amplification	U1 snRNA, TERT, PTCH1, DDX3X, SMO, CREBBP, GSE1, FBXW7 mutation

Fig. 4.02 SHH-activated medulloblastoma subgroups. Demographic, clinical, and molecular features of the four molecular subgroups of SHH-activated medulloblastoma. LCA, large cell / anaplastic; MBEN, medulloblastoma with extensive nodularity; SHH, sonic hedgehog.

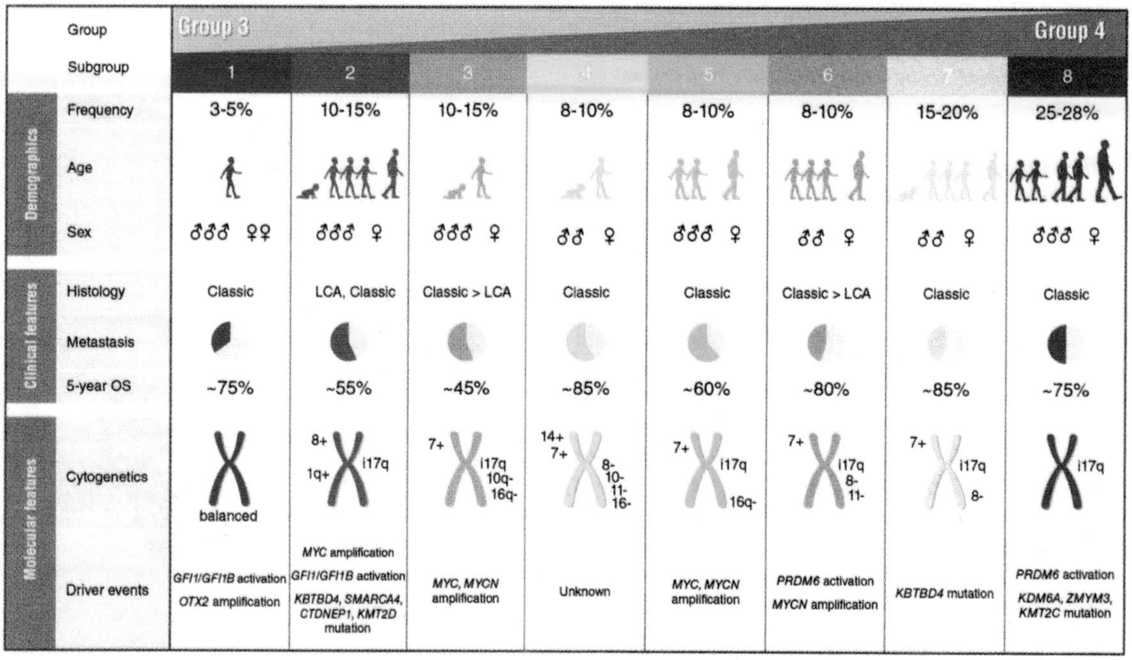

Group	Group 3							Group 4
Subgroup	1	2	3	4	5	6	7	8
Demographics								
Frequency	3-5%	10-15%	10-15%	8-10%	8-10%	8-10%	15-20%	25-28%
Sex	♂♂♂ ♀♀	♂♂♂ ♀	♂♂♂ ♀	♂♂ ♀	♂♂♂ ♀	♂♂ ♀	♂♂ ♀	♂♂♂ ♀
Clinical features								
Histology	Classic	LCA, Classic	Classic > LCA	Classic	Classic	Classic > LCA	Classic	Classic
5-year OS	~75%	~55%	~45%	~85%	~60%	~80%	~85%	~75%
Molecular features								
Cytogenetics	balanced	8+ 1q+ i17q	7+ i17q 10q- 16q-	14+ 7+ 8- 10- 11- 16-	7+ i17q 16q-	7+ i17q 8- 11-	7+ i17q 8-	i17q
Driver events	GFI1/GFI1B activation; OTX2 amplification	MYC amplification; GFI1/GFI1B activation; KBTBD4, SMARCA4, CTDNEP1, KMT2D mutation	MYC, MYCN amplification	Unknown	MYC, MYCN amplification	PRDM6 activation; MYCN amplification	KBTBD4 mutation	PRDM6 activation; KDM6A, ZMYM3, KMT2C mutation

Fig. 4.03 Non-WNT/non-SHH medulloblastoma subgroups. Demographic, clinical, and molecular features of the eight molecular subgroups of group 3/4 medulloblastomas. LCA, large cell / anaplastic; OS, overall survival; SHH, sonic hedgehog.

clinical utility, either being of diagnostic or prognostic value or having implications for therapy. One example is the delineation of two SHH subgroups, SHH-1 and SHH-2, both dominated by medulloblastomas from young children {2691,1355,1303A}. Cases in these subgroups have statistically significantly different outcomes, and recent clinical trial data suggest that specific chemotherapeutic regimens can help those patients with tumours in the poorer prognosis subgroup (SHH-1) {2186,2690, 1303A}.

The histopathological classification of medulloblastomas listed in the 2016 WHO classification of CNS tumours, comprising four morphological types (classic, desmoplastic/nodular, medulloblastoma with extensive nodularity, and large cell / anaplastic), has now been combined into one section that describes the morphological variation as patterns of a single tumour type: medulloblastoma, histologically defined. The morphological patterns have their own specific clinical associations {818,2056,2057,2031}, and molecularly defined medulloblastomas demonstrate specific associations with the morphological patterns. All true desmoplastic/nodular medulloblastomas and medulloblastomas with extensive nodularity align with the SHH molecular group {837}, and most are in the SHH-1 and SHH-2 subgroups {1355}. Nearly all WNT tumours have classic morphology, and most large cell / anaplastic tumours belong either to the SHH-3 subgroup or to the non-WNT/non-SHH (i.e. group 3/4) subgroup 2 {1757}.

Recent studies have described the detailed genomic landscape of medulloblastoma {2279,2283}. Some driver genes aligned to a particular molecular group – such as PTCH1 (SHH-activated group), CTNNB1 (WNT-activated group), and MYC (non-WNT/non-SHH subgroup 3) – are found to be altered at a relatively high frequency when sought in large tumour cohorts. Although other genetic alterations might be recorded at low frequency, they often converge on key biological pathways, such as histone modification {2282}.

Integrated diagnosis

A classification listing molecularly defined medulloblastomas while also recognizing morphological patterns with clinicopathological utility is intended to encourage an integrated approach to diagnosis {1939}. A combination of molecular analysis (e.g. DNA methylation profiling) and morphological interpretation provides optimal prognostic and predictive information. Integrating information on genetic alterations further enhances the level of diagnostic precision, for example by allowing SHH-activated medulloblastomas to be divided into tumours with wildtype or mutant TP53. Other genetic alterations currently used in the risk stratification of medulloblastomas but not included in the classification, such as MYC amplification, could also be placed into an integrated diagnosis to enhance precision. An integrated approach to diagnosis, with commentary, also offers an opportunity to list the methodologies used to provide molecular results and to highlight the clinical significance of germline mutations when a medulloblastoma arises in the setting of a hereditary tumour syndrome, such as naevoid basal cell carcinoma syndrome (Gorlin syndrome) or Li–Fraumeni syndrome.

Medulloblastoma, WNT-activated

Ellison DW
Clifford SC
Kaur K
Korshunov A
Northcott PA
Taylor MD

Definition

Medulloblastoma, WNT-activated, is an embryonal tumour arising from the dorsal brainstem demonstrating activation of the WNT signalling pathway.

ICD-O coding

9475/3 Medulloblastoma, WNT-activated

ICD-11 coding

2A00.10 & XH0ZP6 Medulloblastoma of brain & Medulloblastoma, WNT-activated, NOS

Related terminology

None

Subtype(s)

None

Localization

WNT-activated medulloblastomas are located either around the foramen of Luschka, appearing to arise from the brainstem or cerebellum, or in the cerebellar midline, generally contiguous with the brainstem {1099,3164}. Extension towards the cerebellopontine angle or cerebellar peduncle is noted in a clinically significant number of cases {2463,2415,620}.

Clinical features

Most patients present with symptoms and signs of raised intracranial pressure from non-communicating hydrocephalus due to occlusion of the fourth ventricle by the primary tumour.

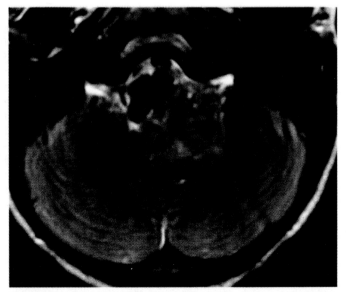

Fig. 4.04 Medulloblastoma, WNT-activated. MRI of WNT-activated medulloblastoma arising in the cerebellopontine angle.

Imaging

Neuroimaging of WNT-activated medulloblastomas shows tumours located in the cerebellar midline or cerebellopontine angle, with many in close contact with the brainstem {1099}. WNT-activated medulloblastomas have a relatively porous blood–brain barrier when compared with other types of medulloblastoma, and therefore enhance very brightly {2500}.

Spread

It is rare for a patient with a WNT-activated medulloblastoma to present with leptomeningeal metastases.

Epidemiology

WNT-activated tumours account for about 10% of all medulloblastomas {841,1022,2509}. They typically occur in children aged between 7 and 14 years, and they also account for 15–20% of adult medulloblastomas {3472}. Slightly more female than male patients have this type of medulloblastoma. WNT-activated medulloblastomas hardly ever occur in infants {1757}.

Etiology

The vast majority of WNT-activated medulloblastomas are sporadic, and little is known about their etiology. A rare subset of WNT-activated medulloblastomas are diagnosed within the setting of constitutional mismatch repair deficiency syndrome, in individuals with germline *APC* mutations and a predisposition to colon cancer {3392,3076}.

Pathogenesis

WNT-activated medulloblastomas transcriptionally resemble normal progenitor cells from the lower rhombic lip–derived mossy fibre neuron lineage, consistent with an extracerebellar (dorsal brainstem) origin {1099,1472}. The DNA methylation profile and transcriptional signatures of these tumours, which might be the best evidence for the cell of origin in human tissues, indicate that WNT-activated medulloblastoma has a profile distinct from those of tumours in other medulloblastoma molecular groups {1356,2509,491,2279}.

Genetic profile

Large next-generation sequencing studies have confirmed that 86–89% of WNT-activated medulloblastomas harbour somatic mutations in exon 3 of *CTNNB1* {2284,2279,3392}. Among WNT-activated medulloblastomas lacking somatic *CTNNB1* mutations, most arise in children carrying pathogenic germline *APC* mutations {3392}. Other genes with somatic mutations in WNT-activated medulloblastomas include those encoding subunits of the SWI/SNF nucleosome-remodelling complex (*SMARCA4, ARID1A, ARID2*; in 33% of cases), *DDX3X* (in 36%), *CSNK2B* (in 14%), *TP53* (in 14%), *KMT2D* (in 14%), and *PIK3CA* (in 11%) {2279}. Cytogenetically, monosomy 6 occurring on the background of an otherwise diploid genome is a characteristic

Chapter 4

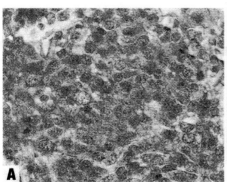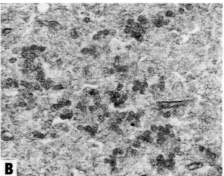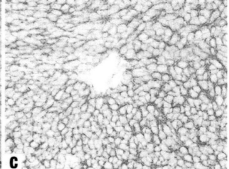

Fig. 4.05 Medulloblastoma. WNT-activated medulloblastomas show diffuse (**A**) or patchy (**B**) nuclear immunoreactivity for β-catenin. **C** Non-WNT/non-SHH medulloblastoma showing cytoplasmic, but not nuclear, immunoreactivity for β-catenin.

genetic feature of WNT-activated medulloblastomas and is observed in approximately 83% of cases {609,1703,2279}.

Macroscopic appearance
Medulloblastomas appear as friable pink masses. At surgery, intratumoural haemorrhage is particularly associated with WNT-activated medulloblastomas {2500}.

Histopathology
Nearly all WNT-activated medulloblastomas have a classic morphology. Anaplastic WNT-activated tumours have been reported but are rare {837,1575}. Desmoplastic/nodular medulloblastomas do not occur in this group.

Immunophenotype
Activation of the WNT pathway can be demonstrated by universal or patchy β-catenin immunoreactivity in tumour cell nuclei {837,1576}. Medulloblastomas in other molecular groups show cytoplasmic expression of β-catenin.

Grading
WNT-activated medulloblastomas are assigned CNS WHO grade 4.

Cytology
Evaluation of the presence of tumour cells in cerebrospinal fluid is required for staging.

Diagnostic molecular pathology
CTNNB1 exon 3 mutations and monosomy 6 on the background of a diploid genome are present in > 80% of WNT-activated medulloblastomas {609}. These alterations have been used to identify WNT-activated medulloblastomas, but DNA methylation profiling is considered the standard method for determining medulloblastoma group or subgroup status {1356,2866}. Array-based DNA methylation analysis, array- and sequencing-based RNA expression analysis, NanoString analysis, and minimal methylation classifier assays have all been used for assignment of molecular group {2864,1715}. In addition, immunohistochemistry can be used to discriminate between WNT, sonic hedgehog (SHH), and non-WNT/non-SHH medulloblastomas {837}.

Two molecular subgroups of WNT-activated medulloblastoma have been suggested: WNT-α and WNT-β {491}. WNT-α tumours show monosomy 6 and arise in children. WNT-β tumours are

Box 4.01 Diagnostic criteria for medulloblastoma, WNT-activated

> **Essential:**
> A medulloblastoma
> **AND**
>> WNT pathway activation
>> **OR**
>> A DNA methylation profile aligned with medulloblastoma, WNT-activated

commonly diploid for chromosome 6 and arise in older children and young adults.

Essential and desirable diagnostic criteria
See Box 4.01.

Staging
Clinical staging procedures include MRI examinations of the CNS with contrast agent. This is complemented by lumbar puncture postoperative cerebrospinal fluid cytology. The postoperative staging system developed by Chang and others in 1969 {519}, which defines the following degrees of metastatic spread, is still being used:

M0   No evidence of subarachnoid or haematogenous metastasis
M1   Microscopic tumour cells found in the cerebrospinal fluid
M2   Gross nodular seeding demonstrated in the cerebellar/cerebral subarachnoid space or in the third or lateral ventricles
M3   Gross nodular seeding in the spinal subarachnoid space
M4   Metastasis outside the cerebrospinal axis

Prognosis and prediction
The prognosis of children with WNT-activated medulloblastoma is excellent despite the CNS WHO grade; with current surgical approaches and adjuvant therapeutic regimens, the overall survival rate is close to 100% {841,2283}. The excellent outcome is expected for tumours with germline *APC* mutations, as well as those with *CTNNB1* mutations {3076}. Adult patients with WNT-activated medulloblastoma do not have such a favourable outcome {2649,2913,1148}. Unlike *TP53* mutations in SHH-activated medulloblastomas, *TP53* mutations in WNT-activated medulloblastomas, which are all somatic and most commonly heterozygous, do not confer a poor prognosis {3614}.

Medulloblastoma, SHH-activated and *TP53*-wildtype

Ellison DW
Clifford SC
Kaur K
Korshunov A
Northcott PA
Taylor MD

Definition

Medulloblastoma, SHH-activated and *TP53*-wildtype, is an embryonal tumour of the cerebellum demonstrating activation of the sonic hedgehog (SHH) signalling pathway in combination with a wildtype *TP53* gene (CNS WHO grade 4).

ICD-O coding

9471/3 Medulloblastoma, SHH-activated and *TP53*-wildtype

ICD-11 coding

2A00.10 & XH9M38 Medulloblastoma of brain & Medulloblastoma, SHH-activated and *TP53*-wildtype

Related terminology

None

Subtype(s)

SHH-activated medulloblastomas comprise four provisional molecular subgroups (SHH-1, SHH-2, SHH-3, SHH-4), which can be demonstrated by DNA methylation or transcriptome profiling (see Fig. 4.02, p. 201).

Localization

SHH-activated medulloblastomas arise in the cerebellar hemisphere or vermis and can sometimes involve both structures. However, localization of this tumour type is related to age. Tumours in infants frequently involve the vermis, whereas hemispheric tumours are relatively infrequent in this age group. In older children and young adults, SHH-activated medulloblastomas arise mainly in the cerebellar hemispheres {1099,2463, 3164,3405,3601}.

Clinical features

Most patients present with symptoms and signs of raised intracranial pressure from non-communicating hydrocephalus due to occlusion of the fourth ventricle by the primary tumour.

Imaging

Neuroimaging shows SHH-activated medulloblastomas as solid, intensely contrast-enhancing masses. Oedema was relatively common in one imaging series that included 12 desmoplastic/nodular medulloblastomas and 9 medulloblastomas with extensive nodularity (MBENs) {991}. A grape-like pattern on MRI generally characterizes MBEN {1088,2197}. Rarely, medulloblastomas involving the lateral cerebellum occur as extra-axial masses resembling meningiomas or acoustic nerve schwannomas {230}.

Spread

Medulloblastomas have the potential to invade locally, metastasize to the leptomeninges, or (rarely) spread outside the CNS. Most metastases are found on the surface of the CNS, attached to the pia mater. Mechanisms of metastasis for SHH-activated medulloblastoma are unclear, with spread to the leptomeninges through the cerebrospinal fluid (CSF) or via a haematogenous route with return to the leptomeninges {1044}. The molecular groups of medulloblastoma, including SHH-activated tumours, have been shown to remain stable in comparisons of primary and metastatic lesions {3382}. Whereas non-WNT/non-SHH medulloblastomas occur almost exclusively with distant CNS metastases at the time of recurrence, a large proportion of SHH medulloblastomas demonstrate isolated recurrences in the tumour bed {2614,1309A}.

Epidemiology

SEER data from 1973–2007 show annual medulloblastoma incidence rates of 6 cases per 1 million children aged 1–9 years and 0.6 cases per 1 million adults aged > 19 years {2972}. SHH-activated medulloblastomas in general show a bimodal age distribution, being most common in infants and adults, with an M:F ratio of approximately 1.5:1 {2280,1757}.

Etiology

There are several hereditary tumour syndromes that predispose to the development of SHH-activated medulloblastoma {3392}. The canonical inherited syndrome associated with SHH-activated and *TP53*-wildtype medulloblastoma is naevoid basal cell carcinoma syndrome (Gorlin syndrome). Medulloblastomas in the setting of naevoid basal cell carcinoma syndrome are always classified in the SHH molecular group, and most are due to inactivating germline mutations in *PTCH1*, the gene that encodes the receptor for the SHH protein. Naevoid basal cell carcinoma syndrome due to a *SUFU* or *PTCH2* mutation is rare. Germline *SUFU* mutations are largely restricted to infants, who exhibit developmental anomalies and predisposition to additional malignancies. Germline mutations in *ELP1*, which is close to *PTCH1* on chromosome 9q, have also been reported in SHH-activated medulloblastoma {3393}. Heterozygous germline mutations in *GPR161* are exclusively associated with SHH-activated medulloblastoma and account for approximately 5% of subtype 1 tumours {232}. The frequency of germline mutations in patients with SHH-activated medulloblastoma is estimated to be ≥ 40% {3393}.

Pathogenesis

Cell of origin

SHH-activated medulloblastomas are thought to derive from an ATOH1-positive cell in the external granule cell lineage of the cerebellum {2860,3526}. These cells are unusual among neurons in that they continue to divide after birth {3402}. The mitogen that primarily drives the expansion of the external granule cell layer is the SHH protein, and many of the mutational events in this type of medulloblastoma lead to constitutive SHH activation {1702}.

Genetic profile

Germline or somatic mutations in SHH signalling pathway genes are characteristic of most SHH-activated medulloblastomas and cause SHH pathway activation. They include mutations in *PTCH1* (~40% of tumours) and *SMO* (~10%), the protein products of which form the receptor for the SHH protein, and in *SUFU* (~10%), a cytoplasmic mediator of GLI transcription factors. Amplifications of *GLI1* or *GLI2* (~10%) and other downstream SHH target genes (*MYCN*, *MYCL*, and *YAP1*; < 10%) have also been found {2279}. Alterations involving known SHH pathway genes were reported in 116 (87%) of 133 SHH-activated tumours in one study {1702}.

Other genes commonly mutated in SHH-activated medulloblastoma, but not directly involved in the SHH signalling pathway, include *DDX3X* (~20%), *KMT2D* (10–15%), and *CREBBP* (~10%) {2279}. Non-coding somatic *TERT* promoter alterations, which affect telomere maintenance, are frequent among non-infant SHH medulloblastomas. Most adult tumours (> 80%) harbour *TERT* promoter mutations, compared with about 15% and 20% of tumours in infants and children, respectively. Hypermethylation of the *TERT* promoter is seen in most childhood SHH-activated medulloblastomas without *TERT* promoter mutation, and both *TERT*-mutant and *TERT*-wildtype SHH-activated medulloblastomas are associated with elevated *TERT* expression {2650,1903}. Mutations in the U1 spliceosomal small nuclear RNA (snRNA) are found in about 15% of SHH-activated medulloblastomas {3083}. Like *TERT* alterations, U1 mutations are found in almost all SHH medulloblastomas in adults and a subset of SHH medulloblastomas in adolescents, but rarely in children or infants {3393}. Common copy-number variations in SHH-activated medulloblastoma include losses of chromosome 9q and 10q, which harbour the *PTCH1* (9q22) and *SUFU* (10q24) tumour suppressor gene loci, respectively {2284}.

Molecular subgroups

Four provisional molecular subgroups of SHH-activated medulloblastoma can be demonstrated by DNA methylation or transcriptome profiling (see Fig. 4.02, p. 201) {2865,491,2691, 3083,3393,1303A}. Two occur mainly in infants: one (SHH-1) is enriched with somatic and germline *SUFU* mutations and chromosome 2 gain, and the other (SHH-2) is characterized by 9q loss and extensive nodular morphology. The other two subgroups arise in older patients: one (SHH-3) is associated with *TP53* and *ELP1* mutations {3393}, and the other (SHH-4) occurs mainly in adults and is associated with near-universal U1 and *TERT* mutations and frequent somatic *PTCH1* or *SMO* alterations {2650,1903,1702,973,3393}. Consensus on molecular subgroup nomenclature and defining features has not yet been achieved through an international cooperative meta-analysis of SHH subgroups as it has for non-WNT/non-SHH medulloblastomas {2900}.

Macroscopic appearance

SHH-activated and *TP53*-wildtype medulloblastomas tend to be firm (reflecting intratumoural desmoplasia) and circumscribed.

Histopathology

Most SHH-activated and *TP53*-wildtype medulloblastomas have a desmoplastic/nodular morphology or are MBENs {837, 1722}. Others are classic or large cell / anaplastic, although the latter is rare {837,3153}. However, recurrence of desmoplastic/nodular SHH-activated and *TP53*-wildtype tumours can be associated with transformation to a focal anaplastic morphology {1718}.

Immunophenotype

A panel of immunohistochemical markers can be used to identify SHH-activated tumours among medulloblastomas (but not other embryonal tumours) {837,1576}. SHH-activated tumours express GAB1. Both SHH-activated and WNT-activated medulloblastomas express YAP1, but SHH-activated medulloblastomas do not show nuclear immunoreactivity for β-catenin. Typically, weak to moderate nuclear immunoreactivity for p53 is present in a few scattered tumour cells when *TP53* is wildtype.

Cytology

Evaluation of the presence of tumour cells in CSF is required for staging.

Diagnostic molecular pathology

DNA methylation profiling is considered the gold-standard method for determining medulloblastoma group or subgroup status {1356,2866}. Array-based DNA methylation analysis, array- and sequencing-based RNA expression analysis, NanoString analysis, and minimal methylation classifier assays have all been used for assignment of molecular group {2864, 1715}. In addition, immunohistochemistry can be used to discriminate between WNT-activated, SHH-activated, and non-WNT/non-SHH medulloblastomas {837}.

TP53 sequencing allows SHH-activated medulloblastomas to be classified as wildtype or mutant, and analysis of SHH pathway genes (*PTCH1*, *SMO*, *SUFU*) provides further diagnostic information. *TP53* mutation and *MYCN* amplification (and large cell / anaplastic morphology) are important for therapeutic stratification, as these markers are associated with a poor prognosis among SHH-activated medulloblastomas {2865,2279}. Given the high incidence of germline predisposition among patients with SHH-activated medulloblastoma, germline analysis of *PTCH1*, *SUFU*, *TP53*, *ELP1*, and *GPR161* is recommended {3392}.

Essential and desirable diagnostic criteria

See Box 4.02.

Staging

Clinical staging procedures include MRI examinations of the CNS with contrast agent. This is complemented by lumbar puncture postoperative CSF cytology. The postoperative staging system developed by Chang and others in 1969 {519}, which defines the following degrees of metastatic spread, is still being used:

M0 No evidence of subarachnoid or haematogenous metastasis
M1 Microscopic tumour cells found in the CSF
M2 Gross nodular seeding demonstrated in the cerebellar/ cerebral subarachnoid space or in the third or lateral ventricles
M3 Gross nodular seeding in the spinal subarachnoid space
M4 Metastasis outside the cerebrospinal axis

Prognosis and prediction

The prognosis for all SHH-activated medulloblastomas is intermediate, between those for WNT-activated and group 3 medulloblastomas. However, prognosis is highly variable among patients with SHH tumours and is associated with the specific clinicopathological and molecular features.

In infants, desmoplastic/nodular tumours and MBENs are typically SHH-activated and *TP53*-wildtype {2865,1702}. Such tumours are associated with favourable outcomes, even when radiation-sparing treatment protocols are used at presentation {2763,2764}. Among infants with SHH-activated medulloblastomas in one clinical trial {2691}, SHH-1 tumours were associated with a worse progression-free survival than SHH-2 tumours, which are enriched for MBEN pathology; however, results from other trials differ or are equivocal {1783,2186}, probably reflecting differences in cohort composition and treatment strategies (e.g. different schedules of intrathecal methotrexate).

Metastatic disease and *MYCN* amplification are independently associated with a poor prognosis in non-infant children

Box 4.02 Diagnostic criteria for medulloblastoma, SHH-activated and *TP53*-wildtype

> *Essential:*
>
> A medulloblastoma
>
> **AND**
>
> Wildtype *TP53* gene
>
> **AND**
>
> SHH pathway activation
>
> **OR**
>
> A DNA methylation profile aligned with SHH-activated medulloblastoma

and adolescents {2865,3614}. In the absence of these high-risk features, patients in this age group have better outcomes (> 80% survival rate) {2865,1148}. Adult SHH-activated medulloblastomas have a relatively favourable prognosis, although molecularly defined and clinically controlled trial cohorts in this patient group are rare {973}.

Medulloblastoma, SHH-activated and *TP53*-mutant

Ellison DW
Clifford SC
Kaur K
Korshunov A
Northcott PA
Taylor MD

Definition

Medulloblastoma, SHH-activated and *TP53*-mutant, is an embryonal tumour of the cerebellum demonstrating activation of the sonic hedgehog (SHH) signalling pathway in combination with a mutant *TP53* gene (CNS WHO grade 4).

ICD-O coding

9476/3 Medulloblastoma, SHH-activated and *TP53*-mutant

ICD-11 coding

2A00.10 & XH1SH4 Medulloblastoma of brain & Medulloblastoma, SHH-activated and *TP53*-mutant

Related terminology

None

Subtype(s)

SHH-activated medulloblastomas comprise four provisional molecular subgroups (SHH-1, SHH-2, SHH-3, SHH-4), which can be demonstrated by DNA methylation or transcriptome profiling (see Fig. 4.02, p. 201).

Localization

Insufficient data exist to derive confident conclusions about the localization of *TP53*-mutant, SHH-activated medulloblastomas. However, *TP53*-mutant tumours tend to occur in children aged 5–14 years, and most medulloblastomas arising within this age range are found in the cerebellar hemispheres {2463,3164, 3405}.

Clinical features

Most patients present with symptoms and signs of raised intracranial pressure from non-communicating hydrocephalus due to occlusion of the fourth ventricle by the primary tumour.

Imaging

On CT and MRI, medulloblastomas appear as solid, intensely contrast-enhancing masses. SHH-activated medulloblastomas are most often identified in the lateral hemispheres but can also involve midline structures. *TP53*-mutant tumours are more likely to be midline {1099,3164}.

Spread

Medulloblastomas have the potential to invade locally, metastasize to the leptomeninges, or (rarely) spread outside the CNS. Most metastases are found on the surface of the CNS, attached to the pia mater. Mechanisms of metastasis for SHH-activated medulloblastoma are unclear, with spread to the leptomeninges through the cerebrospinal fluid (CSF) or via a haematogenous route with return to the leptomeninges {1044}. SHH-activated medulloblastomas are less frequently metastatic at presentation than molecular group 3 tumours, but leptomeningeal spread is often a presenting feature of SHH-activated and *TP53*-mutant medulloblastomas {2615,2865}.

Epidemiology

SEER data from 1973–2007 show annual medulloblastoma incidence rates of 6 cases per 1 million children aged 1–9 years and 0.6 cases per 1 million adults aged > 19 years {2972}. SHH-activated medulloblastomas in general show a bimodal age distribution, being most common in infants and young adults, with an M:F ratio of approximately 1.5:1 {2280}. In contrast, SHH-activated and *TP53*-mutant tumours are generally found in children aged 4–17 years {1702}. In one study that included 133 SHH-activated medulloblastomas, 28 patients (21%) had a *TP53* mutation, and the median age of these patients at presentation was approximately 15 years {3614}.

Etiology

There are several hereditary tumour syndromes that predispose to the development of SHH-activated medulloblastoma {3392}. Germline *TP53* point mutations (Li–Fraumeni syndrome) predispose to medulloblastoma, and these tumours belong to the SHH-activated group {2622}. More than half of all SHH-activated and *TP53*-mutant medulloblastomas have germline rather than somatic *TP53* alterations. Mutations in *TP53* are most commonly found in the DNA-binding regions encoded by exons 4 through 8 {3614}. Although some WNT-activated medulloblastomas have mutations in *TP53*, these have so far been somatic, and *TP53* mutations do not portend a negative prognosis in WNT-activated medulloblastoma {3614}.

Pathogenesis

TP53 mutations are reported in 10–15% of SHH-activated medulloblastomas, and more than half of these are germline. *MYCN* amplification is observed in 5–10% of SHH-activated medulloblastomas {1702,2865,2279,3614}. *TP53* mutations and *MYCN* amplifications occur as part of a constellation of associated features alongside *GLI2* amplification and chromothriptic rearrangements {1702,2865,2279,2622}. Isolated chromosome 17p deletion and loss of heterozygosity at the mutant *TP53* locus are characteristic of SHH-activated *TP53*-mutant tumours.

SHH-3 subgroup medulloblastomas characterized by *TP53* mutation, *MYCN* amplification, and/or large cell / anaplastic morphology are reported not to have *ELP1* mutations {3393}. *TP53*-mutant tumours do not form a discrete molecular subgroup upon class discovery analysis using genome-wide expression and DNA methylation–based techniques {1702,491, 2865}.

See also *Medulloblastoma, SHH-activated and TP53-wildtype* (p. 205).

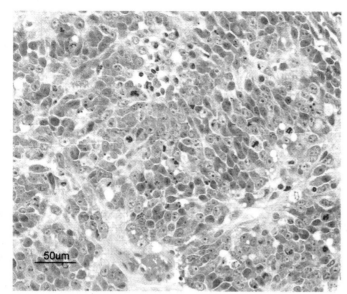

Fig. 4.06 SHH-activated and *TP53*-mutant medulloblastoma. Marked anaplasia and mitotic activity, consistent with large cell / anaplastic medulloblastoma.

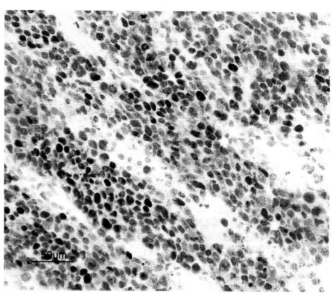

Fig. 4.07 SHH-activated and *TP53*-mutant medulloblastoma. Widespread strong nuclear immunoreactivity for p53, reflecting the presence of a *TP53* mutation.

Macroscopic appearance

In general, medulloblastomas appear as friable pink masses. No data exist to suggest that tumours of this specific type have any characteristic macroscopic feature.

Histopathology

Diffuse anaplasia accompanied by a substantial large-cell phenotype occurs in approximately 70% of SHH-activated and *TP53*-mutant medulloblastomas. Other tumours are generally desmoplastic/nodular with focal anaplasia {2613}.

Immunophenotype

A panel of immunohistochemical markers can be used to identify SHH-activated tumours among medulloblastomas (but not other embryonal tumours) {837,1576}. SHH-activated tumours express GAB1. Both SHH-activated and WNT-activated medulloblastomas express YAP1, but SHH-activated medulloblastomas do not show nuclear immunoreactivity for β-catenin. The presence of a *TP53* mutation is suggested by widespread strong immunoreactivity for p53 protein in tumour cell nuclei.

Cytology

Evaluation of the presence of tumour cells in CSF is required for staging.

Diagnostic molecular pathology

SHH-activated medulloblastomas comprise four provisional molecular subgroups (SHH-1, SHH-2, SHH-3, SHH-4), which can be demonstrated by DNA methylation or transcriptome profiling (see Fig. 4.02, p. 201). SHH-activated and *TP53*-mutant medulloblastomas almost always belong to subgroup SHH-3 {2865,491,2691,3083,3393}.

Groups and subgroups of medulloblastoma may be identified using DNA methylation profiling or gene expression profiling and associated minimal classifier assays {2866,1356, 1715,2864}, as well as by immunohistochemistry {837,2117}.

Box 4.03 Diagnostic criteria for medulloblastoma, SHH-activated and *TP53*-mutant

> *Essential:*
>
> A medulloblastoma
>
> **AND**
>
> Mutant *TP53* gene
>
> **AND**
>
> SHH pathway activation
>
> **OR**
>
> A DNA methylation profile aligned with SHH-activated medulloblastoma

Mutation analysis of mutated SHH pathway genes (*PTCH1, SUFU, SMO*) provides further diagnostic markers for SHH-activated tumours.

For identification of a *TP53*-mutant and/or *MYCN*-amplified SHH-activated medulloblastoma, assessment of *TP53* mutation and *MYCN* amplification status are essential. Large cell / anaplastic morphology and chromothriptic rearrangements are also associated with this tumour type and provide useful supplementary assessments {2865,2279}. Given the association of SHH-activated *TP53*-mutant medulloblastoma with Li–Fraumeni syndrome, and the high overall incidence of germline predisposition within SHH-activated medulloblastoma, mutation analysis of tumour and blood samples for *PTCH1, SUFU, TP53, ELP1,* and *GPR161* and genetic counselling are recommended for all patients with SHH-activated medulloblastoma {3392}.

MYCN amplification is also associated with group 4 non-WNT/non-SHH medulloblastoma, and *TP53* mutation with WNT-activated medulloblastoma. However, neither alteration is associated with a poor outcome when they arise in these specific contexts {3614,2279,2865,2913,1148}.

Essential and desirable diagnostic criteria

See Box 4.03.

Staging

Clinical staging procedures include MRI examinations of the CNS with contrast agent. This is complemented by lumbar puncture postoperative CSF cytology. The postoperative staging system developed by Chang and others in 1969 {519}, which defines the following degrees of metastatic spread, is still being used:

M0 No evidence of subarachnoid or haematogenous metastasis
M1 Microscopic tumour cells found in the CSF
M2 Gross nodular seeding demonstrated in the cerebellar/ cerebral subarachnoid space or in the third or lateral ventricles
M3 Gross nodular seeding in the spinal subarachnoid space
M4 Metastasis outside the cerebrospinal axis

Prognosis and prediction

In non-infant children and adolescents with SHH-activated medulloblastoma, *TP53* mutation and *MYCN* amplification are associated with each other and with a very poor outcome {1702, 3614,2865,1148}. Among SHH group tumours, both alterations are consistently associated with poor outcomes in univariate survival analyses and are independent predictors of poor outcomes when considered together in multivariate analyses {3614,2913,2865,1148}.

Medulloblastoma, non-WNT/non-SHH

Ellison DW
Clifford SC
Kaur K
Korshunov A
Northcott PA
Taylor MD

Definition

Medulloblastoma, non-WNT/non-SHH, is an embryonal tumour of the cerebellum without a molecular signature associated with activation of the WNT or sonic hedgehog (SHH) signalling pathway. Non-WNT/non-SHH medulloblastomas are classified as group 3 or group 4 tumours and comprise eight molecular subgroups, demonstrated by DNA methylation profiling.

ICD-O coding

9477/3 Medulloblastoma, non-WNT/non-SHH

ICD-11 coding

2A00.10 & XH87Q5 Medulloblastoma of brain & Medulloblastoma, non-WNT/non-SHH

Related terminology

None

Subtype(s)

Non-WNT/non-SHH medulloblastomas comprise eight molecular subgroups (group 3/4 subgroups 1–8), which can be demonstrated by DNA methylation profiling analysis of non-WNT/non-SHH group 3 and group 4 medulloblastomas {2865,491, 2279,2900}.

Localization

Non-WNT/non-SHH medulloblastomas arise exclusively in the cerebellum (usually in the midline), and almost always in its inferior portion.

Clinical features

Most patients present with symptoms and signs of raised intracranial pressure from non-communicating hydrocephalus due to occlusion of the fourth ventricle by the primary tumour.

Spread

Mechanisms of metastasis for medulloblastoma are unclear, with spread to the leptomeninges through the cerebrospinal fluid (CSF) or via a haematogenous route with return to the leptomeninges {1044}. Patients with non-WNT/non-SHH medulloblastomas present almost universally with distant CNS metastases at the time of recurrence {2614,1309A}. Metastatic disease is present at diagnosis in about 40% of group 3 tumours in infants and affects > 50% of patients with non-WNT/non-SHH (group 3/4) subgroups 2–5 {1703,2280}. An isolated local recurrence of a group 3 or group 4 medulloblastoma should be considered a radiation-induced neoplasm until proved otherwise by biopsy.

Epidemiology

Group 3 tumours account for approximately 25% of all medulloblastomas, and for a higher proportion of cases (~40%) in infants. Group 3 medulloblastomas are exceedingly rare in adults {1703,491}. Group 4 medulloblastomas are the largest molecular group, accounting for about 40% of all medulloblastomas. Peak incidence occurs in patients aged 5–15 years, with lower incidence in infants and adults {1703,491}.

Etiology

Very little is known about the molecular etiology of group 3 and group 4 medulloblastomas; generally, they are not associated with known hereditary tumour syndromes. Rare cases of group 3 or group 4 medulloblastoma have been reported in individuals with a germline CREBBP mutation (Rubinstein–Taybi syndrome) {689}. Germline mutations of the DNA repair genes PALB2 and BRCA2 have also been identified in non-WNT/non-SHH medulloblastoma {2206}.

Pathogenesis

Cross-species single-cell transcriptomic studies have discerned putative cellular origins of group 4 medulloblastoma, including upper rhombic lip–derived glutamatergic neurons from cerebellar nuclei and unipolar brush cells {3338,1357}. The pathogenesis of group 3 tumours remains less clear. Primitive nestin-positive cerebellar stem or progenitor cells are implicated by single-cell transcriptomics {3338}, and various neural stem or progenitor cell populations demonstrate vulnerability to transformation in mouse tumour modelling studies {1580,3134,2437}.

Genetics

Overexpression of MYC is a common feature of group 3 medulloblastomas, and MYC amplification, often accompanied by PVT1::MYC fusion {2284}, occurs in 17% of group 3 tumours {839,2279}. Other recurrently mutated or focally amplified genes include SMARCA4 (mutated in 9% of cases), CTDNEP1 (mutated in 5%), KMT2D (mutated in 5%), MYCN (amplified in 5%), and OTX2 (amplified in 3%) {2279}. Two oncogenes in medulloblastomas from groups 3 and 4 are the homologues GFI1 and GFI1B, which are aberrantly overexpressed through a mechanism called enhancer hijacking in 15% and 12% of group 3 and group 4 tumours, respectively {2281,2279}. The most common cytogenetic aberrations in medulloblastoma (occurring in 55–58% of group 3 and 80–85% of group 4 tumours) involve chromosome 17 copy-number alterations: 17p deletion, 17q gain, or a combination of these in the form of an isodicentric 17q {837,1703,2280,2279}.

The most frequently mutated or focally amplified genes in group 3 and 4 tumours are KDM6A (mutated in 7% of cases), OTX2 (amplified in 6%), ZMYM3 (mutated in 6%), KMT2C (mutated in 6%), KBTBD4 (mutated in 6%), MYCN (amplified in 6%), ZIC1 (mutated in 4%), CDK6 (amplified in 4%), KMT2D (mutated in 3%), and TBR1 (mutated in 3%) {2279}. Enhancer hijacking of the SNCAIP gene locus leading to aberrant overexpression of PRDM6 is specific to group 4 medulloblastoma and is seen in about 17% of tumours {2284,2279}. Deleterious heterozygous germline mutations in *BRCA2* and *PALB2* are present in 1–2% of patients, substantiated by tumour-associated mutation signatures typical of homologous recombination repair deficiency {3392}. Medulloblastomas from both group 3 and group 4 show recurrent somatic genetic events that converge on the posttranslational modifications of histones, particularly H3 p.K28 (K27) and H3 p.K5 (K4) {2689,795,1497}.

Macroscopic appearance
Medulloblastomas appear as friable pink masses, occasionally with macroscopic foci of necrosis. At surgery, non-WNT/non-SHH medulloblastomas show brainstem invasion more often than do other types of medulloblastomas {2463}. Group 3 tumours are more likely to contain macrocysts and are usually smaller at presentation than group 4 tumours. {3601,3581,681}.

Histopathology
Most non-WNT/non-SHH medulloblastomas have a classic morphology. Such tumours occasionally exhibit areas of Homer Wright (neuroblastic) rosette formation, or a palisading pattern of tumour cell nuclei or even nodule formation, in the absence of desmoplasia (which has been termed "biphasic classic" morphology) {2057}. Large cell / anaplastic tumours can belong to either group 3 or group 4. However, they are present at a higher frequency in group 3 {837,676} and are relatively enriched in group 3/4 subgroup 2 tumours {1355}. Very rarely, desmoplastic/nodular medulloblastomas have been assigned to the non-WNT/non-SHH group {2865}.

Immunophenotype
A panel of immunohistochemical markers can be used to identify non-WNT/non-SHH tumours among medulloblastomas {837, 1576}. Unlike WNT and SHH medulloblastomas, non-WNT/non-SHH tumours do not express YAP1. They do not express GAB1 and show no nuclear immunoreactivity for β-catenin.

Cytology
Evaluation of the presence of tumour cells in CSF is required for staging.

Diagnostic molecular pathology
Analysis of DNA methylation profiles, either alone or in combination with transcriptomic data, has identified molecularly heterogeneous subgroups among group 3 and group 4 medulloblastomas with distinct clinical and genetic associations {2279,2865,491}. A large meta-analysis of 1501 medulloblastomas studied by DNA methylation profiling supports the existence of eight robust group 3 or group 4 subgroups, designated group 3/4 subgroups 1–8 {2900} (see Fig. 4.03, p. 202). Subgroups 2, 3, and 4 consist exclusively of group 3 medulloblastomas, whereas subgroups 6, 7, and 8 predominantly comprise group 4 medulloblastomas. Subgroups 1 and 5 are intermediate subgroups, exhibiting molecular and cellular attributes characteristic of both group 3 and group 4 medulloblastomas {2279, 2900,1357}. Most non-WNT/non-SHH medulloblastomas have a classic morphology, but large cell / anaplastic tumours are more

Box 4.04 Diagnostic criteria for medulloblastoma, non-WNT/non-SHH

Essential:

A medulloblastoma

AND

> No WNT or SHH pathway activation
>
> **OR**
>
> A DNA methylation profile aligned with group 3 or group 4 medulloblastoma

frequent in subgroup 2. Metastatic disease at presentation is relatively frequent in subgroups 2–5. A relatively poor outcome is associated with tumours in subgroups 2 and 3.

Essential and desirable diagnostic criteria
See Box 4.04.

Staging
Clinical staging procedures include MRI examinations of the CNS with contrast agent. This is complemented by lumbar puncture postoperative CSF cytology. The postoperative staging system developed by Chang and others in 1969 {519}, which defines the following degrees of metastatic spread, is still being used:

M0 No evidence of subarachnoid or haematogenous metastasis
M1 Microscopic tumour cells found in the CSF
M2 Gross nodular seeding demonstrated in the cerebellar/cerebral subarachnoid space or in the third or lateral ventricles
M3 Gross nodular seeding in the spinal subarachnoid space
M4 Metastasis outside the cerebrospinal axis

Prognosis and prediction
MYC amplification has long been established as a genetic alteration associated with poor outcome in patients with medulloblastoma {2832,819,839}. This observation is reflected in the relatively poor outcomes ascribed to group 3 medulloblastomas overall, but *MYC* amplification, isodicentric 17q, and metastatic disease at diagnosis all have prognostic significance among group 3 tumours {2913,2865}. Metastatic disease at the time of presentation, which is associated with poor outcome, is currently the most robust prognostic marker among group 4 tumours {2913}. High-risk DNA methylation patterns are also associated with a poor prognosis {2865}. In contrast, chromosome 7 gain, chromosome 8 loss, chromosome 11 loss, and chromosome 17 gain have been implicated as markers of favourable outcome among group 4 medulloblastomas in retrospective clinical studies {2913,2865,1148}. The DNA methylation subgroups of non-WNT/non-SHH tumours exhibit disparate outcomes, with subgroups 2 and 3 exhibiting particularly poor outcomes {2900}. Favourable-risk cytogenetic aberrations (i.e. chromosome 7 gain, chromosome 8 loss, and chromosome 11 loss) are associated with subgroups 6 and 7, whereas poor-prognosis tumours, with isochromosome 17q and otherwise quiet genomes, are commonly associated with subgroup 8 {1148,2900}.

Medulloblastoma, histologically defined

Korshunov A
Ellison DW
Giangaspero F
Orr RA
Pietsch T
Taylor MD

Definition

Medulloblastoma is an embryonal neuroepithelial tumour arising in the posterior fossa, histologically characterized by small, poorly differentiated cells with a high N:C ratio and high levels of mitotic activity and apoptosis.

ICD-O coding

9470/3 Medulloblastoma, histologically defined
9471/3 Desmoplastic nodular medulloblastoma
9471/3 Medulloblastoma with extensive nodularity
9474/3 Large cell medulloblastoma
9474/3 Anaplastic medulloblastoma

ICD-11 coding

2A00.10 & XH0RY1 Medulloblastoma of brain & Classic medulloblastoma
2A00.10 & XH7PN5 Medulloblastoma of brain & Desmoplastic nodular medulloblastoma
2A00.10 & XH6JN6 Medulloblastoma of brain & Medulloblastoma with extensive nodularity
2A00.10 & XH0H95 Medulloblastoma of brain & Anaplastic medulloblastoma

Related terminology

Not recommended: cerebellar neuroblastoma.

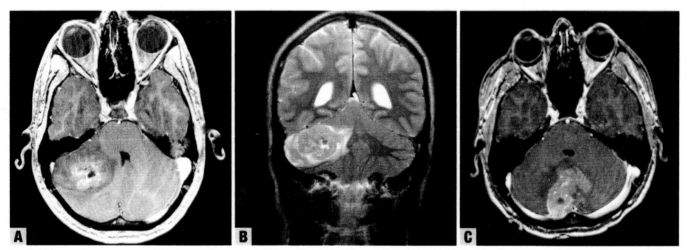

Fig. 4.08 Desmoplastic/nodular medulloblastoma. T1-weighted (**A**), and T2-weighted (**B**), contrast-enhanced MRI of tumours in the cerebellar hemisphere. **C** T1-weighted, contrast-enhanced MRI of a tumour in the vermis.

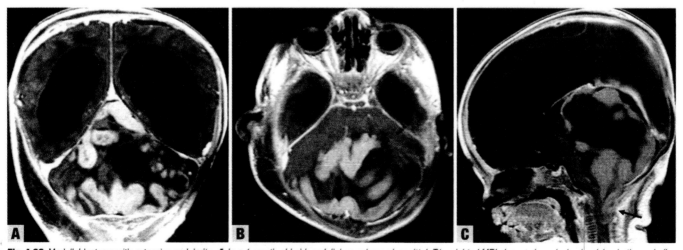

Fig. 4.09 Medulloblastoma with extensive nodularity. **A** In a 1-month-old girl, gadolinium-enhanced, sagittal, T1-weighted MRI shows a huge lesion involving both cerebellar hemispheres and the vermis. The lesion has a multinodular and gyriform pattern of enhancement. There is also supratentorial hydrocephalus and macrocrania. **B** Multinodular and gyriform pattern. **C** Note the downward herniation of the tumour through the foramen magnum (arrow) and the marked effacement of the cisternal spaces of the posterior fossa. There is also supratentorial hydrocephalus and macrocrania.

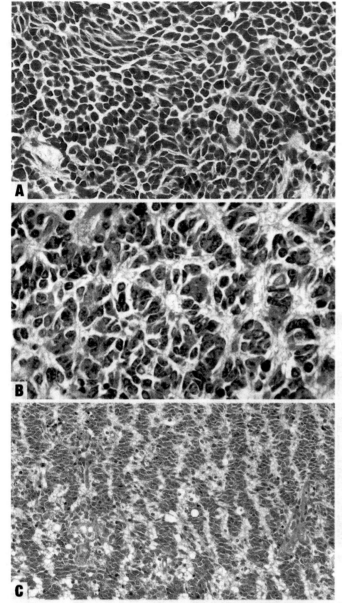

Fig. 4.10 Histopathological features of classic medulloblastoma. **A** Typical syncytial arrangement of undifferentiated tumour cells. **B** Area with Homer Wright (neuroblastic) rosettes. **C** Arrangement of tumour cells in parallel rows (spongioblastic pattern).

Subtype(s)

Classic medulloblastoma; desmoplastic/nodular medulloblastoma; medulloblastoma with extensive nodularity; large cell / anaplastic medulloblastoma

Localization

Classic medulloblastomas are typically located in the cerebellar midline, involving the fourth ventricle cavity, with or without close contact with the brainstem. Some classic (WNT- or sonic hedgehog [SHH]-activated) medulloblastomas are localized laterally, involving the cerebellar peduncle and hemisphere {3153,3164,2463,3405,3601}.

Desmoplastic/nodular (D/N) medulloblastomas may arise both in the cerebellar hemisphere and in the vermis. Most

medulloblastomas occurring in the cerebellar hemispheres are of the D/N type, especially in adults {3153,3164,2463,3405,3601}.

Medulloblastomas with extensive nodularity (MBENs) are located in the vermis, with involvement of both hemispheres. This localization contrasts with that of D/N medulloblastoma, which more frequently involves the cerebellar hemispheres {1099,3164,3405,2463,3601}.

Large cell / anaplastic (LC/A) medulloblastomas are typically located in the cerebellar midline and involve the fourth ventricle cavity and adjacent brainstem and cerebellar structures. LC/A medulloblastomas with SHH activation can show lateral localization with extracerebellar extension {1089,3405,3601}.

Clinical features

Most patients present with symptoms and signs of raised intracranial pressure from non-communicating hydrocephalus due to occlusion of the fourth ventricle by the primary tumour.

Imaging

On MRI, classic medulloblastomas generally appear as hyperintense, homogeneous, contrast-enhancing masses with midline localization. Some medulloblastomas (frequently non-WNT/non-SHH group 4 medulloblastomas) enhance inhomogeneously. WNT-activated medulloblastomas are typically located in the cerebellar midline / cerebellopontine angle, with many in close contact with the brainstem {3164,2463,3405}.

D/N medulloblastomas appear as solid, frequently contrast-enhancing masses. Tumours originating peripherally in a cerebellar hemisphere in adults occasionally occur as extra-axial lesions {2463,3405,3601}. Infants frequently present with a very superficial lesion of the lateral cerebellar hemisphere, which is densely enhancing and nearly pathognomonic for SHH-activated medulloblastoma.

MBENs appear as very large multinodular lesions with an enhancing bunch-of-grapes structure involving the vermis and sometimes the adjacent cerebellar hemispheres {1088,2197}. Rare cases have a peculiar gyriform appearance, in which the cerebellar folia are well delineated and enlarged, with contrast enhancement {32}. Downward herniation of the cerebellar tonsils and effacement of the cisternal spaces of the posterior fossa can be observed.

LC/A medulloblastomas appear as heterogeneously contrast-enhancing masses with foci suggestive of necrosis and peritumoural oedema {1089,3405,3601}.

Spread

At diagnosis, classic medulloblastoma has disseminated to the leptomeningeal compartment of the CNS in as many as 40% of classic medulloblastomas {3153,1703}.

Leptomeningeal metastases are found in 20% of D/N medulloblastomas at diagnosis. Most recurrences of D/N medulloblastoma are found locally in the tumour bed, in the posterior fossa, whereas metastatic spread to the leptomeninges or systemically is less common among patients with these tumours {3153,1703}.

MBEN can relapse locally or (rarely) metastasize via cerebrospinal fluid (CSF) pathways. However, such cases seem to respond well to subsequent treatment and have a favourable prognosis {2614}.

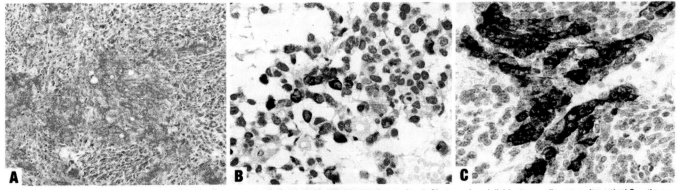

Fig. 4.11 Medulloblastoma. **A** Focal expression of synaptophysin. **B** Focal GFAP staining of tumour cells. **C** Clusters of medulloblastoma cells expressing retinal S-antigen.

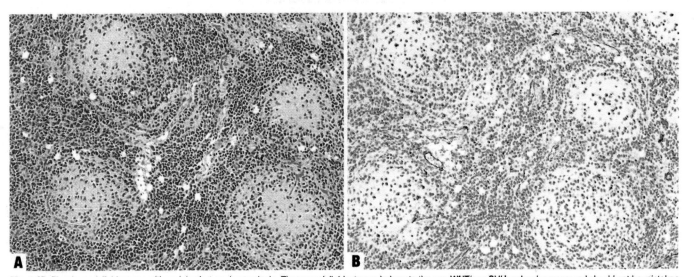

Fig. 4.12 Classic medulloblastoma with nodules but no desmoplasia. These medulloblastomas belong to the non-WNT/non-SHH molecular group and should not be mistaken for desmoplastic/nodular medulloblastomas. **A** H&E stain. **B** Reticulin stain.

At diagnosis, metastatic disease is found in as many as 60–70% of patients with LC/A medulloblastomas. Tumours recur frequently and metastasize via CSF pathways {1089, 3405,3601}.

Epidemiology

Classic medulloblastomas account for 70–80% of all medulloblastomas {818,819,834}. They can occur at any age, from infancy to adulthood, but predominantly arise in childhood (60–70% of cases), and they are found in all four genetically defined medulloblastoma types but predominantly in WNT-activated and non-WNT/non-SHH medulloblastomas {1720, 3153,1703}.

D/N medulloblastomas are estimated to account for 20% of all medulloblastomas. In children aged < 3 years, D/N medulloblastomas account for 40–60% of all cases. In adult patients, D/N medulloblastomas constitute 20–40% of all histological subtypes {1720,3153,1703}

In large series, MBENs account for 3.2–4.2% of all medulloblastoma subtypes overall, but in children aged < 3 years (in whom D/N medulloblastomas account for as many as 50% of cases), MBENs have been reported to account for 20% of all cases {1088,1703,1722,1719}. Both D/N medulloblastoma and MBEN belong to the SHH-activated molecular medulloblastoma type.

LC/A medulloblastomas can occur in patients of any age and account for about 10% of all tumours. Considered separately, anaplastic medulloblastomas are about 10 times as prevalent as large cell medulloblastomas. They are most frequent among medulloblastomas in the non-WNT/non-SHH (group 3) and SHH-activated, *TP53*-mutant groups, but very rare in the WNT-activated group {839,3153,1703,1355}.

Etiology

Medulloblastomas occurring in the context of naevoid basal cell carcinoma syndrome are mainly desmoplastic subtypes (D/N medulloblastoma or MBEN). This syndrome is diagnosed in 5.8% of all patients with medulloblastoma, in contrast to 22.7% of patients with a D/N medulloblastoma and 41% of patients with an MBEN {1702,5,3392,1722,1718,1719,2510}. Conversely, the risk of medulloblastoma is approximately 2% in *PTCH1*-related naevoid basal cell carcinoma syndrome and 20 times higher in *SUFU*-related naevoid basal cell carcinoma syndrome {3152, 100,1042,391,2963,1182}. Recurrent germline alterations in *ELP1* or *GPR161* also predispose to medulloblastomas in this (SHH-activated) group {3392,232,3393}. Because of the frequency of predisposing germline mutations in this patient population, genetic counselling is indicated for children and their families diagnosed with D/N medulloblastoma or MBEN {1042}.

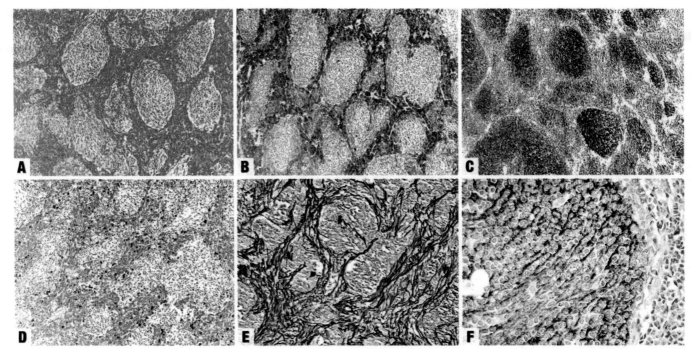

Fig. 4.13 Desmoplastic/nodular medulloblastoma. **A** Pale nodular areas surrounded by densely packed hyperchromatic cells. **B** Sonic hedgehog (SHH) activation can be visualized by immunohistochemistry with antibodies against SHH targets, in this case, with antibodies against p75-NGFR (TNFRSF16) {407,1776}, which is strongly expressed in the synaptophysin-negative internodular areas. **C** Neuronal differentiation, shown by immunoreactivity for NSE, occurs mainly in the pale islands. **D** MIB1 monoclonal antibody staining shows that proliferative activity predominates in the highly cellular, internodular areas. **E** Reticulin silver impregnation showing the reticulin-free pale islands. **F** The nodules represent zones of neuronal maturation and show intense immunoreactivity for synaptophysin.

In rare cases, classic medulloblastomas are diagnosed within the setting of constitutional mismatch repair deficiency syndrome or Rubinstein–Taybi syndrome, or in individuals with germline *APC*, *BRCA2*, or *PALB2* mutations.

The vast majority of LC/A medulloblastomas are sporadic, and little is known about their etiology. SHH-activated, *TP53*-mutant medulloblastomas are often diagnosed within the setting of Li–Fraumeni syndrome.

Pathogenesis

See also the sections on *Medulloblastomas, molecularly defined* (p. 203).

D/N medulloblastomas are derived from granule cell progenitor cells forming the external granule cell layer during cerebellar development {3402,2860}. These progenitors are dependent on SHH (produced by Purkinje cells) as a mitogen. Recently, single-cell RNA sequencing revealed that these tumours contain cells resembling different stages of granule cell precursor development (granule cell progenitor–like cells) {1355}. D/N medulloblastomas in adults contain a higher proportion of undifferentiated granule cell progenitor–like cells than do tumours in infants.

Like D/N medulloblastomas, MBENs are believed to derive from cerebellar precursor cells of the granule cell lineage {3402, 2860}.

Non-WNT/non-SHH group 3 LC/A medulloblastomas probably arise from a stem cell–like population in the early developing cerebellum {3338}.

Macroscopic appearance

Classic medulloblastomas appear as friable pink masses, occasionally with macroscopic foci of necrosis {2463}.

D/N medulloblastomas tend to be firm and circumscribed, reflecting intratumoural desmoplasia.

MBENs tend to be firm, grape-like, and well circumscribed.

LC/A medulloblastomas appear as friable greyish-pink masses, occasionally with macroscopic foci of necrosis. At surgery, LC/A medulloblastomas often show cerebellar and brainstem invasion {2463}.

Histopathology

There are four established morphological subtypes of medulloblastoma. Each of these histologically defined subtypes has particular clinical and molecular associations {818,2056,2057, 2031}. Architectural and cytological diversity can manifest not only as nodule formation but also as neurocytic or ganglion cell differentiation. Rarely, any histological subtype of medulloblastoma may show myogenic and/or melanotic differentiation; the terms "medullomyoblastoma" and "melanocytic medulloblastoma", respectively, have been used to describe these patterns {971,2057,2770,2497,2973}.

Classic medulloblastoma

Classic medulloblastomas are the archetypal CNS small blue round cell tumour. They consist of densely packed, poorly differentiated embryonal cells with hyperchromatic nuclei of various shapes. Mitotic activity is increased and apoptotic bodies can be found. Intratumoural desmoplasia is absent, but a desmoplastic reaction can be induced where tumour cells invade the leptomeninges. Homer Wright rosettes are found in some classic medulloblastomas. Occasionally, nodules of neurocytic differentiation and reduced cell proliferation are locally present in classic tumours, but these are never associated with

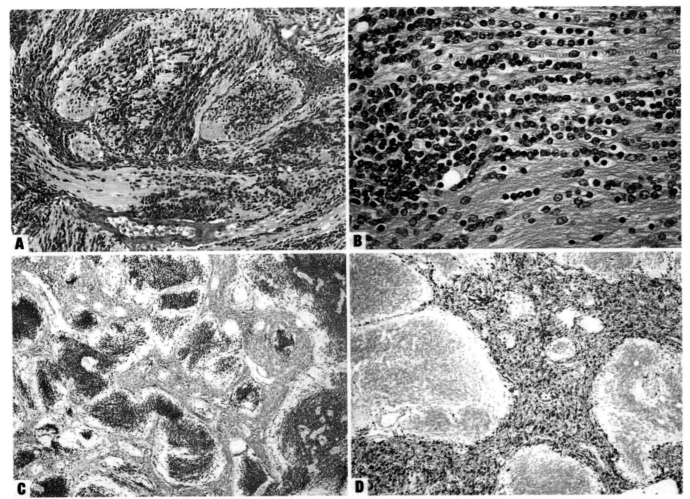

Fig. 4.14 Medulloblastoma with extensive nodularity. **A** Lobular architecture with large, elongated, reticulin-free zones. **B** Elongated, reticulin-free zones containing streams of small round neurocytic cells on a fibrillary background. **C** Strong immunoreactivity for NeuN in the neurocytic cells of the pale islands. **D** Strong MIB1 immunolabelling in the internodular regions, contrasting with minimal proliferation in the pale islands.

internodular desmoplasia or perinodular collagen when examined in a reticulin preparation. Such non-desmoplastic nodular medulloblastomas correspond to non-WNT/non-SHH tumours, unlike the typical D/N medulloblastomas, which belong to the SHH-activated type. WNT-activated classic medulloblastomas often show intense vascularization and blood–brain barrier disruption {3153,1703}.

Desmoplastic/nodular (D/N) medulloblastoma

D/N medulloblastoma is characterized by a bicompartmental arrangement of nodular, reticulin-free zones (pale islands) surrounded by densely packed, poorly differentiated, highly proliferative cells with hyperchromatic and moderately pleomorphic nuclei, which produce an extensive network of intercellular reticulin fibres {818,2057,1086,837,2031}. In rare cases, this defining pattern is not present throughout the entire sample, with some areas instead having a more syncytial arrangement of non-desmoplastic embryonal cells. The nodules contain tumour cells with features of variable neurocytic maturation embedded in a neuropil-like fibrillary matrix. Homer Wright rosettes are generally not found in D/N medulloblastoma. Tumours with small nodules can easily be overlooked if no reticulin staining is performed. The level of mitotic activity and the Ki-67 proliferation

index are much higher in the internodular areas than in the nodules.

Focal frank anaplasia can be seen occasionally within the internodular areas, especially in SHH-activated and *TP53*-mutant tumours. Medulloblastomas that show only an increased amount of reticulin (without a nodular pattern) or that show a focal nodular pattern but without complete perinodular encircling by reticulin are not classified as D/N medulloblastoma (see *Classic medulloblastoma*, above); the two characteristic features must occur together for a diagnosis of D/N medulloblastoma. However, posttreatment progression-associated anaplasia with loss of the key diagnostic features has been described in D/N medulloblastomas, especially in patients with germline *PTCH1* aberrations {1718}.

Medulloblastoma with extensive nodularity (MBEN)

MBEN differs from the related D/N subtype in that it has an expanded lobular architecture due to the reticulin-free zones being substantially larger and richer in neuropil-like matrix {1088,1722,1719}. These zones contain a population of small cells with round nuclei, which show various degrees of neurocytic differentiation and can exhibit a streaming pattern. The internodular component can vary from one area to another and

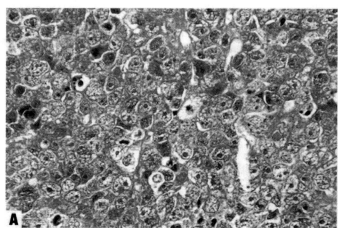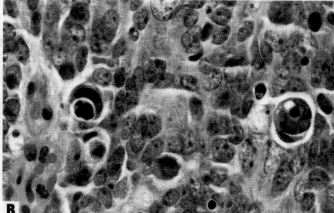

Fig. 4.15 Large cell / anaplastic medulloblastoma. **A** Increased nuclear size, pleomorphism, and prominent nucleoli. **B** Tumour cell wrapping is also evident.

appear markedly reduced in some places. Like in D/N medulloblastomas, mitotic activity and Ki-67 proliferation index is low or absent in the neurocytic areas and much higher in the internodular areas. After radiotherapy and/or chemotherapy, MBENs occasionally undergo further maturation into tumours dominated by ganglion cells {533,700}.

Large cell / anaplastic (LC/A) medulloblastoma

Most LC/A medulloblastomas show a combination of large cell and anaplastic features. Anaplasia as a feature of embryonal tumours was first proposed for medulloblastomas with marked nuclear pleomorphism accompanied by particularly high mitotic and apoptotic counts {818,1089}. Nuclear moulding, cytoplasmic pseudoinclusions, and cell wrapping are typical features. The large cell phenotype manifests more uniform round nuclei with prominent nucleoli, lacking the variability in cell size and shape that characterizes the anaplastic phenotype; its cells are relatively large and monomorphic but show the high rate of turnover seen in anaplastic tumours.

Immunophenotype

Classic medulloblastomas express various nonspecific neural markers, such as CD56 (NCAM1), MAP2, and NSE. Most cases are immunopositive for synaptophysin and NeuN, but these neuronal markers may also be absent. Immunoreactivity for NFPs is very rare. Embryonal tumour cells showing GFAP expression can be observed in rare cases. Some classic medulloblastomas express the transcription factor OTX2, with the exception of classic medulloblastomas with SHH activation {2508}.

In D/N medulloblastomas, activation of the SHH pathway can be inferred by immunohistochemistry for specific targets, such as GAB1 and p75-NGFR {834,3153,837,1703}. These markers are predominantly expressed in internodular areas. The transcription factor OTX2 is negative, unlike in non-SHH medulloblastomas {2508}. Widespread and strong nuclear accumulation of p53, suggesting a *TP53* mutation, can be detected in rare D/N medulloblastomas, frequently in association with signs of cytological anaplasia. This finding can accompany either somatic or germline *TP53* alteration (Li–Fraumeni syndrome) {3096,3614,1718}. The nodules in D/N medulloblastoma show variable expression of neuronal markers, including synaptophysin and NeuN. Nodules with very strong NeuN expression, which is an indicator of advanced neurocytic differentiation, are

typical of MBEN, but they can also occur in D/N medulloblastoma. GFAP expression can be frequently found in both components, most often in the internodular cells. D/N medulloblastomas express GAB1, YAP1, and the low-affinity nerve growth factor receptor p75-NGFR (particularly in internodular areas), whereas OTX2 immunohistochemistry is consistently negative {2508}.

In MBENs, the neuropil-like tissue matrix and the differentiated neurocytic cells within nodules are strongly immunoreactive for synaptophysin. These latter cells are also strongly (and less variably than in D/N medulloblastomas) immunoreactive for NeuN {1722,1719}. Like D/N medulloblastomas, MBENs are negative for OTX2 and positive for GAB1 and p75-NGFR in internodular areas {1722,1719}.

Differential diagnosis

Embryonal tumours with multilayered rosettes and atypical teratoid/rhabdoid tumours may show histomorphological overlap with medulloblastomas. Unlike medulloblastomas, embryonal tumours with multilayered rosettes are typically LIN28A-immunoreactive. Nuclear SMARCB1 and SMARCA4 expression is retained in all medulloblastoma types; the loss of expression of one of these SWI/SNF complex proteins is diagnostic of atypical teratoid/rhabdoid tumours.

Cytology

Evaluation of CSF cytology is required for staging. In CSF samples and touch preparations, small clusters of poorly differentiated cells with mostly round hyperchromatic nuclei and scant cytoplasm can be seen {3113}. In samples of D/N medulloblastoma, neurocytic differentiation – characterized by smaller cell size and round nuclei – may be observed, whereas samples of LC/A medulloblastoma may reveal small clusters of poorly differentiated cells with large, atypical nuclei and scant cytoplasm; nuclear moulding and wrapping; and visible nucleoli {3113}.

Diagnostic molecular pathology

See the sections on *Medulloblastomas, molecularly defined* (p. 203).

In most cases, the molecular type of medulloblastoma can be identified by immunohistochemistry, particularly for β-catenin, GAB1, YAP1, OTX2, p75-NGFR, and p53 (see *Immunophenotype*, above).

Essential and desirable diagnostic criteria

See Box 4.05.

Staging

Clinical staging procedures include MRI examinations of the CNS with contrast agent. This is complemented by lumbar puncture postoperative CSF cytology. The postoperative staging system developed by Chang and others in 1969 {519}, which defines the following degrees of metastatic spread, is still being used:

M0 No evidence of subarachnoid or haematogenous metastasis
M1 Microscopic tumour cells found in the CSF
M2 Gross nodular seeding demonstrated in the cerebellar/cerebral subarachnoid space or in the third or lateral ventricles
M3 Gross nodular seeding in the spinal subarachnoid space
M4 Metastasis outside the cerebrospinal axis

Prognosis and prediction

See also the sections on *Medulloblastomas, molecularly defined* (p. 203).

In most cases, D/N medulloblastoma in early childhood has an excellent outcome with surgery and chemotherapy alone. In a meta-analysis of prognostic factors in infant medulloblastoma, progression-free survival and overall survival were significantly better for desmoplastic subtypes than for other medulloblastomas {2057,839,2764,2031,2691}. However, no difference in survival between D/N medulloblastoma and classic medulloblastoma was found in a European multicentre trial involving older children with standard-risk medulloblastoma {2763}.

MBENs are typically associated with good to excellent outcomes, reaching an overall survival rate of almost 100% in representative series, although some cases have been reported

Box 4.05 Diagnostic criteria for classic medulloblastoma, histologically defined

> **Essential:**
>
> A medulloblastoma
>
> **AND**
>
> Absence of histological features qualifying for the diagnosis of desmoplastic/nodular medulloblastoma or medulloblastoma with extensive nodularity
>
> **AND**
>
> Absence of predominant areas with severe cytological anaplasia and/or large cell cytology
>
> **AND**
>
> Retained expression of SMARCB1 (INI1)

to show an unfavourable clinical course {2057,839,2764,2031,2691}. Metastatic disease at presentation did not affect the favourable prognosis, suggesting that a diagnosis of MBEN confers a better outcome regardless of adverse clinical features. However, germline *PTCH1* or *SUFU* alterations accompanied by cancer-associated transcriptome signatures have recently been identified as molecular hallmarks of MBEN progression {1722, 1719}.

At the time the tumours were first described, LC/A medulloblastomas were strongly suspected to behave more aggressively than other histological subtypes, with metastatic disease often evident at presentation. In retrospective studies of patients in trial cohorts, LC/A morphology has been shown to be an independent prognostic indicator of outcome. In contemporary trials, LC/A histology is regarded as a high-risk pattern warranting intensified adjuvant therapy {819,2913,839,2832}. The 5-year progression-free survival rate for LC/A medulloblastomas is 30–40%, although more aggressive behaviour can be shown by SHH-activated LC/A tumours with a *TP53* mutation and by non-WNT/non-SHH group 3 tumours with *MYC* amplification {1702,3614,2865,1148}.

Other CNS embryonal tumours: Introduction

Wesseling P
Pfister SM

CNS embryonal tumours encompass a heterogeneous group of malignant tumours that are composed of immature cells resembling neural progenitors. They are mainly, but not exclusively, a disease of childhood. Among CNS embryonal tumours, medulloblastomas are relatively common; other CNS embryonal tumours are rare. In contrast to medulloblastomas, which by definition originate from the cerebellum or dorsal brainstem, other CNS embryonal tumours may arise across the neuraxis.

The overarching term "CNS primitive neuroectodermal tumour" previously encompassed many of the embryonal tumours described in the following sections. However, this term is now obsolete, thanks to an increased understanding of the heterogeneity and biology of these tumours and the emergence of a classification based on molecular characteristics {3059,1944}.

The tumours discussed in the following sections include atypical teratoid/rhabdoid tumour (AT/RT), embryonal tumour with multilayered rosettes (ETMR), *FOXR2*-activated CNS neuroblastoma, and CNS tumour with *BCOR* internal tandem duplication (ITD). Whereas AT/RT and ETMR were included in previous editions of this classification, *FOXR2*-activated CNS neuroblastoma and CNS tumour with *BCOR* ITD are new. In addition, cribriform neuroepithelial tumour has been introduced as a provisional entity within this category, and CNS embryonal tumour is included for embryonal tumours that defy a more specific diagnosis. The designation "not elsewhere classified (NEC)" can be added to a CNS embryonal tumour diagnosis in cases where adequate testing does not reveal signature molecular aberrations, and "not otherwise specified (NOS)" is used for cases where molecular analysis could not be (successfully) performed {1946,1934}.

Assessment of molecular characteristics is now considered the standard of care for CNS embryonal tumours and is exemplified by the evaluation of medulloblastoma molecular group and genetic profile {3153,835}. For other CNS embryonal tumours, a diagnostic approach should seek the following: (1) biallelic inactivation of the *SMARCB1* (or rarely *SMARCA4*) gene in AT/RT {1840,1252,1481,2853}, (2) C19MC alteration or *DICER1* mutation in ETMR {1650,1797}, (3) *FOXR2* activation in CNS neuroblastoma, and (4) a heterozygous ITD in *BCOR* exon 15 in CNS tumour with *BCOR* ITD {3059,460}. Immunohistochemistry serves as a helpful surrogate for analysis of the actual molecular alterations in some of these tumours, most notably AT/RT. DNA methylation profiling is another useful alternative diagnostic approach to this family of tumours. An integrated diagnosis using tiers of histological and molecular information in the pathology report is helpful for transparent and effective communication of relevant tumour characteristics {1939,1945}.

Patients presenting with CNS embryonal tumours may have an inherited cancer syndrome and require genetic counselling.

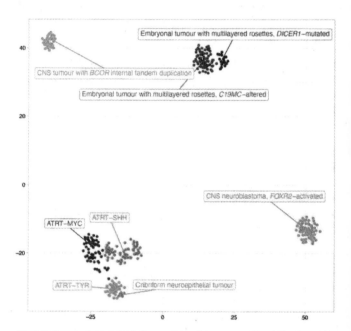

Fig. 4.16 Other CNS embryonal tumour molecular groups. Unsupervised, non-linear t-distributed stochastic neighbour embedding (t-SNE) projection of methylation array profiles from non-medulloblastoma CNS embryonal tumours. Samples were selected from a large database of > 50 000 brain tumour datasets to serve as reference profiles for training a supervised classification model based on strict criteria: all these samples showed a high calibrated classification score (> 0.9) for tumours listed in the category of "other CNS embryonal tumours" when applying the brain tumour classifier available at https://www.molecularneuropathology.org. ATRT, atypical teratoid/rhabdoid tumour.

Among the syndromes associated with non-medulloblastoma CNS embryonal tumours, the risk of rhabdoid tumour predisposition syndrome 1 in a patient diagnosed with a SMARCB1-deficient tumour is reported to be between 26% and 41%, and the risk of rhabdoid tumour predisposition syndrome 2 in a patient with a SMARCA4-deficient tumour appears to be much higher {2885,1453,273,816,992,1254}. Almost all patients with a *DICER1*-mutant ETMR carry a pathogenic *DICER1* germline alteration.

Like previous editions of the WHO classification of CNS tumours, this fifth edition should be regarded as a work in progress. For example, we have included CNS tumours with *BCOR* ITD under the heading *Other CNS embryonal tumours*; however, these tumours are not definitively neural, and exon 15 *BCOR* ITDs have been reported in several sarcomas. There is currently no consensus as to whether these tumours should be considered neuroepithelial or mesenchymal neoplasms, and our perception of the nosology of such tumour types may need to change as new findings emerge.

Atypical teratoid/rhabdoid tumour

Haberler C
Hasselblatt M
Huang A
Judkins AR
Kool M
Wesseling P

Definition

Atypical teratoid/rhabdoid tumour (AT/RT) is a high-grade malignancy composed of poorly differentiated cells and a variable number of rhabdoid cells, with the potential to differentiate along neuroepithelial, epithelial, and mesenchymal lines. Genetically, these tumours are characterized by biallelic inactivation of *SMARCB1* (also known as *hSNF5*, *INI1*, or *BAF47*) or rarely (in < 5% of cases) of *SMARCA4* (*BRG1*) (CNS WHO grade 4).

ICD-O coding

9508/3 Atypical teratoid/rhabdoid tumour

ICD-11 coding

2A00.1Y & XH7ZQ4 Other specified embryonal tumours of brain & Atypical teratoid/rhabdoid tumour

Related terminology

None

Subtype(s)

DNA methylation profiling and gene expression profiling demonstrate three molecular groups of AT/RT, each demonstrating upregulation of gene profiles that have contributed to their nomenclature.

These three sets of tumours can be regarded as subtypes of AT/RT: AT/RT-SHH, AT/RT-TYR, and AT/RT-MYC.

Localization

AT/RTs occur throughout the neuraxis. Supratentorial tumours, which are more common with increasing age {2343}, are often located in the cerebral hemispheres and less frequently in the ventricular system, suprasellar region, or pineal gland. Infratentorial tumours can arise in the cerebellar hemispheres, cerebellopontine angle, and brainstem. Spinal cord localization is rare {1785,992}. Rare AT/RTs affecting adults tend to occur in the cerebral hemispheres and sellar region {515}.

Clinical features

The clinical presentation is variable, depending on the age of the patient and on the location and size of the tumour. Infants, in particular, present with nonspecific signs of lethargy, vomiting, and/or failure to thrive. More specific signs include head tilt and cranial nerve palsy, most commonly sixth and seventh nerve paresis. Headache and hemiplegia are more commonly reported in children aged > 3 years.

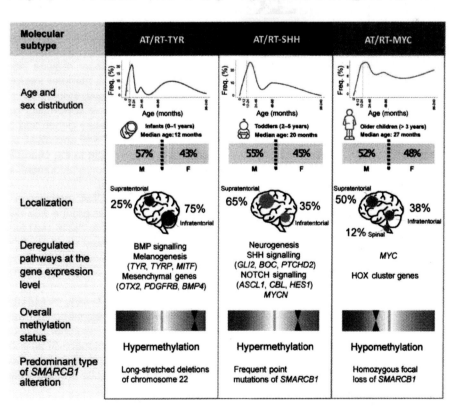

Fig. 4.17 Atypical teratoid/rhabdoid tumour (AT/RT) consensus subtypes. Summary of demographic and molecular features of AT/RT subtypes.

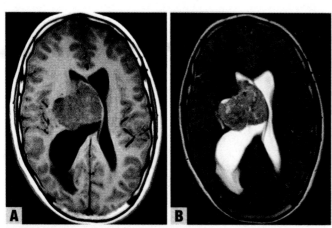

Fig.4.18 Atypical teratoid/rhabdoid tumour. **A** Axial T1-weighted MRI. **B** Axial T2-weighted MRI demonstrating tumour heterogeneity.

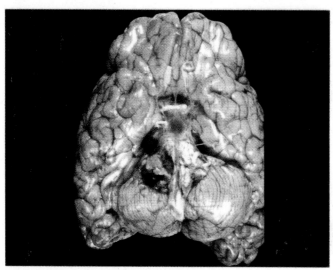

Fig.4.19 Atypical teratoid/rhabdoid tumour. Tumour with multiple haemorrhagic areas, arising in the right cerebellopontine angle.

Imaging

MRI findings for AT/RTs are similar to those for other embryonal tumours. Almost all tumours are variably contrast-enhancing and show isointense or hyperintense signal intensity on FLAIR images and restricted diffusion {2099}. Differences in contrast enhancement, peripheral tumour cysts, and peritumoural oedema have been described across the molecular groups {2289}.

Spread

Seeding of AT/RT via the cerebrospinal fluid (CSF) pathways is common and found in approximately one third of all patients at presentation {1785,992}.

Epidemiology

In a US study using data from the Central Brain Tumor Registry of the United States (CBTRUS), AT/RTs accounted for 1.6% of all paediatric CNS tumours and for 10.1% of CNS tumours in children aged < 1 year, with an M:F ratio of 1.2:1 {2343}. The majority of patients are aged < 2 years, with 33% aged ≤ 1 year at diagnosis {964,2343}. Occurrence in adults is rare {515}.

Etiology

Familial cases arise in the setting of rhabdoid tumour predisposition syndrome 1 (*SMARCB1* gene) or 2 (*SMARCA4* gene) {2885,1453,1254}. The risk of germline mutations is reported to be between 26% and 41% in *SMARCB1*-deficient tumours {273,816,992} and may be substantially higher in *SMARCA4*-deficient tumours {1254}. De novo germline mutations have been described {816,338}, and they accounted for two thirds of germline mutations in one study {816}. Unaffected adult carriers {1453,101} and gonadal mosaicism {2885} have been reported.

Pathogenesis

Mutation or loss of the *SMARCB1* locus at 22q11.2 is a genetic hallmark of this tumour {3318,275}. Whole-genome and whole-exome sequencing demonstrate remarkably simple genomes and a mean mutation rate of 0.19 mutations/Mb, with loss of *SMARCB1* being the primary recurrent alteration (> 95% of cases) {1840,1252,1481}. SMARCB1 is a component of the mammalian SWI/SNF complex, which remodels chromatin, affecting transcriptional regulation and mediating cell differentiation and lineage specification {3383,92,2130}. Inactivation of *SMARCB1* is caused by structural variants (partial or complete deletion, copy-neutral loss of heterozygosity, exon duplication, gene fusion, or chromosomal inversion) and mutations (insertion/deletion, point mutation, or frameshift mutation) {273,1053,1481,3215}.

Rare tumours (< 5% of AT/RTs) with histopathological features of AT/RT but retained SMARCB1 protein expression harbour biallelic inactivation and no expression of the SMARCA4 protein, another SWI/SNF complex component {2853}. These tumours are associated with very young age and poor prognosis {1254}.

The specific functions of SMARCB1 and SMARCA4, and their roles in malignant transformation, are still not entirely clear. Loss of SMARCB1 disturbs the balance between activating SWI/SNF complex members and the repressive polycomb complex PRC2 at promoter and enhancer regions {1522,3383}. Analyses of chromatin states show a complex interplay and divergent roles for SWI/SNF and polycomb that results in repression of neuronal differentiation and tumour suppressor genes as well as activation of cell-cycle regulatory genes and oncogenes {1522,856}. Alterations in SWI/SNF BAF and pBAF subunit complexes have been shown to contribute to the characteristic multilineage differentiation, immune microenvironment, and potential prognosis of these tumours {2385}.

Transcriptome and DNA methylation profiling separate AT/RTs into three molecular groups with different methylation and transcriptional signatures {3216,1481,3215}, which by consensus have been designated as AT/RT-TYR, AT/RT-SHH, and AT/RT-MYC {595,1320}. These groups show differences in patient age, localization, and *SMARCB1* / chromosome 22 alteration patterns.

AT/RT-SHH tumours (~44% of AT/RTs) overexpress proteins in the SHH and Notch signalling pathways and genes involved in axonal guidance or neuronal development. Localization is most commonly infratentorial (~67%) and otherwise supratentorial. Median patient age is 20 months. Compound heterozygous *SMARCB1* point mutations are frequently present in this group {1320}.

AT/RT-TYR tumours (~34%) demonstrate upregulation of proteins in the melanosomal pathway, including tyrosinase; proteins

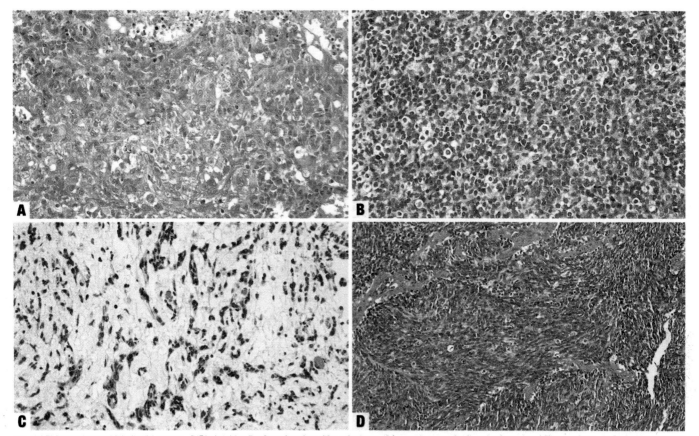

Fig. 4.20 Atypical teratoid/rhabdoid tumour. **A** Rhabdoid cells of varying size with vesicular nuclei, prominent nucleoli, and pale eosinophilic cytoplasm. **B** Lesions composed of small embryonal cells without typical rhabdoid cells raise the diagnostic possibility of other CNS embryonal tumours. **C** Mesenchymal area composed of loosely arranged elongated cells. **D** Compact area with fascicular growth pattern.

in the BMP pathway; and development-related transcription factors, including OTX2. Localization is predominantly infratentorial, and patients with AT/RT-TYR tumours have the youngest age at presentation (median age: ~12 months). *SMARCB1* is inactivated mostly by mutation in one allele and whole or partial chromosome 22 loss removing the second allele {1320}.

AT/RT-MYC tumours (~22%) are characterized by expression of the *MYC* oncogene and HOXC cluster genes. Localization is more commonly supratentorial than infratentorial. Rare spinal AT/RTs are generally AT/RT-MYC, and sellar AT/RTs in adults also belong to this group {1480}. Patients with AT/RT-MYC tumours are significantly older (median age: ~27 months) than patients with AT/RT-SHH or AT/RT-TYR {1320}.

The histogenesis of rhabdoid tumours is unknown. They also occur outside the CNS (in kidneys and soft tissues). Recent studies propose a cell of origin for AT/RT-SHH among neural progenitors and for AT/RT-TYR and AT/RT-MYC from cells outside the neuroectoderm {1472}. Single AT/RTs arising in the setting of low-grade glial/glioneuronal tumours, high-grade glioma, and ependymoma suggest the possibility of progression from other tumour types {80,2267,347,257}.

Macroscopic appearance

The macroscopic appearance of AT/RTs is similar to that of other CNS embryonal tumours. AT/RTs tend to be soft and pink-red, and they often appear to be demarcated from adjacent parenchyma. Those with substantial amounts of mesenchymal tissue

may be firm and tan-white in some regions. Tumours arising in the cerebellopontine angle wrap themselves around cranial nerves and vessels and invade brainstem and cerebellum to various extents. Areas of haemorrhage and necrosis may be observed.

Histopathology

AT/RTs are heterogeneous tumours that can be difficult to recognize solely on the basis of histopathological findings {419, 2721}. Characteristically, a population of rhabdoid cells and variable components with primitive neuroectodermal, mesenchymal, and epithelial features are present. Rhabdoid cells fall along a spectrum from small cells with scant cytoplasm to large, typical rhabdoid cells with eccentrically located nuclei and extensive homogeneously eosinophilic cytoplasm. Occasionally, intracytoplasmic globular eosinophilic inclusions are present. Nuclei are round and contain vesicular chromatin and prominent eosinophilic nucleoli. Binucleated elements may be found. Cell borders are generally well defined. A frequently encountered artefact is cytoplasmic vacuolation.

Rhabdoid cells are the exclusive or predominant histopathological finding in only a minority of cases and may be very rare or even completely lacking in some cases {1208}. Small embryonal (medulloblastoma-like) cells can be present, rarely alongside Homer Wright or Flexner–Wintersteiner rosettes. Mesenchymal differentiation typically demonstrates a spindle cell morphology, with cells either being dispersed in a pale or basophilic

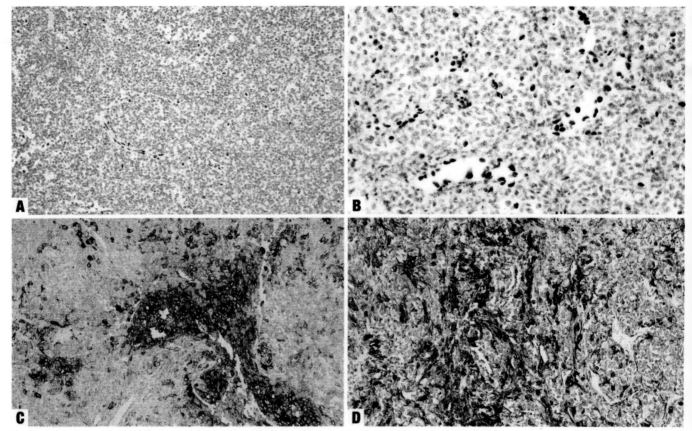

Fig. 4.21 Atypical teratoid/rhabdoid tumour. **A** Loss of nuclear immunoreactivity for SMARCB1 in tumour cells, with retained expression in endothelial cells. **B** Rare cases manifest loss of SMARCA4 (BRG1) immunoreactivity, as illustrated here, but retain expression of SMARCB1 (INI1). **C** Patchy expression of EMA. **D** SMA positivity.

mucopolysaccharide-rich matrix or having a compact arrangement reminiscent of fibrosarcoma. Epithelial differentiation is the least common histopathological feature. It can take the form of papillary structures, adenomatous areas, or poorly differentiated ribbons and cords. Mitotic figures are usually abundant. Extensive geographical necrosis and haemorrhage are commonly encountered.

Immunophenotype

AT/RTs demonstrate a broad spectrum of immunoreactivities. Rhabdoid cells characteristically demonstrate expression of EMA, SMA, and vimentin. Immunoreactivity for GFAP, NFP, synaptophysin, and cytokeratins is also commonly observed. Germ cell markers and markers of skeletal muscle differentiation are not typically expressed. Nuclear loss of SMARCB1 (INI1) protein expression is a highly sensitive marker for the diagnosis of AT/RT. Expression in non-neoplastic nuclei (e.g. within vascular endothelial cells) serves as an internal positive control {1511}. CNS embryonal tumours without rhabdoid features but with loss of nuclear SMARCB1 expression qualify as AT/RTs {1208}.

SMARCB1 protein loss may also occur in poorly differentiated chordomas and, with a mosaic expression pattern, in schwannomatosis-associated schwannomas {1258,1378}. Tumours suspected on morphological grounds of being AT/RT but showing retained SMARCB1 expression should be examined for loss of nuclear SMARCA4 protein {1251}. However, single AT/RTs with biallelic *SMARCA4* inactivation but retained protein expression

have been reported {1254,2029}. Rare *SMARCB1*-deficient non-rhabdoid tumours forming cribriform strands, trabeculae, and well-defined surfaces are recognized as cribriform neuroepithelial tumours {1255}.

Cytology

Most AT/RTs are dominated by embryonal cells with hyperchromatic round or oval nuclei and minimal cytoplasm. Rhabdoid cells are slightly larger than embryonal cells and have an eccentrically located nucleus and brightly eosinophilic cytoplasm. Evaluation of CSF cytology is required for staging.

Diagnostic molecular pathology

Due to the high risk of germline mutations in the setting of AT/RT, particularly with very young children, molecular analyses of *SMARCB1* or *SMARCA4* should be performed and genetic counselling and germline analysis recommended. *SMARCB1* alterations comprise biallelic structural variations, a structural variation combined with a mutation, or compound heterozygous mutations {1053,1320}.

The three AT/RT subtypes can be identified as distinct molecular groups using gene expression or DNA methylation profiling {1481,1856}. ASCL1 and tyrosinase immunoreactivities are potential surrogate markers for AT/RT-SHH and AT/RT-TYR, respectively {3216,1259}, pending validation studies.

Essential and desirable diagnostic criteria

See Box 4.06.

Staging

Clinical staging procedures include MRI examinations of the CNS with contrast agent. This is complemented by lumbar puncture postoperative CSF cytology. The postoperative staging system developed by Chang and others in 1969 {519}, which defines the following degrees of metastatic spread, is still being used:

M0 No evidence of subarachnoid or haematogenous metastasis
M1 Microscopic tumour cells found in the CSF
M2 Gross nodular seeding demonstrated in the cerebellar/ cerebral subarachnoid space or in the third or lateral ventricles
M3 Gross nodular seeding in the spinal subarachnoid space
M4 Metastasis outside the cerebrospinal axis

Prognosis and prediction

Overall, the prognosis of patients with AT/RT is poor. However, data from retrospective studies and clinical trials have shown that AT/RTs do not always have a dismal outcome. In the Children's Oncology Group (COG) ACNS0333 trial, a regimen of high-dose chemotherapy with stem cell rescue and radiotherapy was associated with a 4-year event-free survival rate of 37% and an overall survival rate of 43% {2630}. A retrospective study of children enrolled in the German HIT trial demonstrated a 3-year overall survival rate of 22% and an event-free survival rate of 13%, but also identified a subset of patients (14%) who were long-term event-free survivors {3347}. In a small prospective trial incorporating intensive multimodal treatment, including chemotherapy and irradiation, a 2-year progression-free survival rate of 53% ± 13% (standard error) and a projected overall survival rate of 70% ± 10% (standard error) were found {563}. Similarly, a retrospective Canadian Brain Tumour Consortium study reported that high-dose chemotherapy, in some cases without radiation, resulted in a 2-year overall survival rate of 60% ± 12.6% (standard error) {1785}. The European Rhabdoid Registry (EU-RHAB) protocol, using an anthracycline-based induction and either radiotherapy or high-dose chemotherapy, demonstrated 5-year overall and event-free survival rates of 34.7% and 30.5%, respectively {992}.

The different epigenomic landscapes of AT/RT subtypes could be associated with distinct therapeutic vulnerabilities {3215,1328, 2130}. Both the COG ACNS0333 trial and the EU-RHAB study analysed the prognostic impact of molecular group. In the EU-RHAB cohort, a non-AT/RT-TYR profile was identified as an independent negative prognostic marker. In the COG trial, the 4-year survival rate was higher in patients with AT/RT-SHH tumours. Thus, although the impact of molecular group on patient outcome awaits further validation, it may ultimately be possible to stratify patients with AT/RT on the basis of molecular group, age, tumour site, and extent of resection. Significant immune cell infiltration has been reported in AT/RT-MYC and AT/RT-TYR tumours {595, 1856}, suggesting that immune checkpoint inhibition is a potential therapeutic strategy for these tumours.

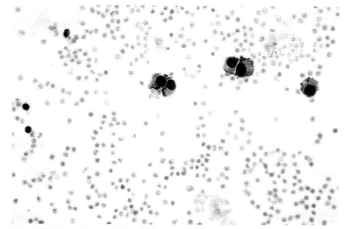

Fig. 4.22 Atypical teratoid/rhabdoid tumour. Leptomeningeal tumour spread. Cerebrospinal fluid cytology shows large tumour cells with rhabdoid features (extensive cytoplasm with eccentric nuclei). May–Grünwald–Giemsa staining.

Box 4.06 Diagnostic criteria for atypical teratoid/rhabdoid tumour

Essential:

A CNS embryonal tumour with a polyimmunophenotype

AND

Loss of nuclear SMARCB1 or SMARCA4 expression in tumour cells

OR (for unresolved lesions)

A DNA methylation profile aligned with atypical teratoid/rhabdoid tumour

Desirable:

Rhabdoid cells

SMARCB1 or *SMARCA4* alteration

Cribriform neuroepithelial tumour

Hasselblatt M
Capper D
Jones DTW
Pietsch T

Definition
Cribriform neuroepithelial tumour (CRINET) is provisionally defined as a non-rhabdoid neuroectodermal tumour characterized by cribriform strands and ribbons, and showing loss of nuclear SMARCB1 expression.

ICD-O coding
None

ICD-11 coding
2A00.2Y Other specified tumours of neuroepithelial tissue of brain

Related terminology
None

Subtype(s)
None

Localization
CRINET is located in the vicinity of the fourth, third, or lateral ventricles {1255,2399,139,1073}.

Clinical features
The clinical features of CRINET are nonspecific and related to tumour location.

Epidemiology
The median age of 10 children harbouring CRINET was 20 months (range: 10–129 months). The M:F ratio was 1.5:1 {1482}.

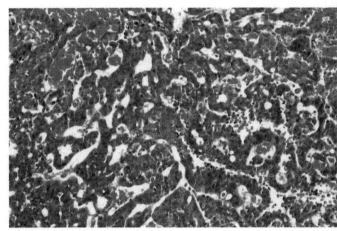

Fig. 4.23 Cribriform neuroepithelial tumour. A highly cellular tumour composed of relatively small cells arranged in cribriform strands, and trabeculae of varying thickness, forming well-defined surfaces.

Etiology
SMARCB1 germline alterations (including familial cases with unaffected adult carriers) have been reported {1395,1482}.

Pathogenesis
Losses on chromosome 22q affecting the SMARCB1 region are the only recurrent chromosomal alteration {1073,1482} so far described. SMARCB1 point mutations, as well as deletions of exons 7 and 8 {1073} or duplication of exon 6 {1395}, may represent the second hit.

On unsupervised clustering analysis of DNA methylation profiles, CRINET grouped within the atypical teratoid/rhabdoid

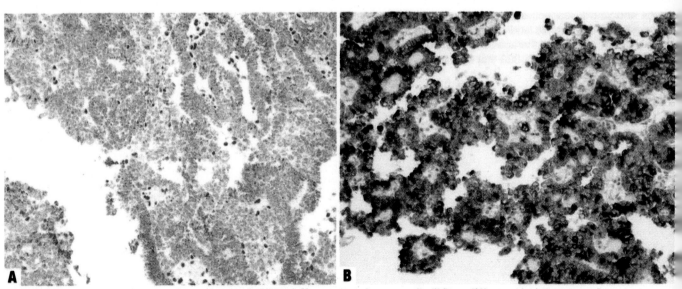

Fig. 4.24 Cribriform neuroepithelial tumour. **A** Loss of nuclear SMARCB1 (INI1) expression in the tumour cells. **B** Strong EMA expression in the tumour cells.

tumour (AT/RT) molecular subtype AT/RT-TYR {1482}. The observation that expression of tyrosinase is present not only in AT/RT-TYR but also in CRINET suggests similarities also at the protein expression level {1259,1482}.

Macroscopic appearance
Insufficient data have been reported on the macroscopic appearance of CRINET specifically.

Histopathology
CRINET is a highly cellular tumour characterized by the presence of cribriform strands and ribbons. In more compact areas, small lumina and true rosettes are also present, but rhabdoid tumour cells showing eosinophilic cytoplasms and eccentric nuclei with prominent nucleoli are not encountered.

Immunophenotype
Loss of nuclear SMARCB1 protein expression in tumour cells is a feature shared with AT/RT {1073,1255}. There is distinct expression of EMA {1073,1255}, and there is frequent expression of tyrosinase {1482}, MAP2, and synaptophysin as well as vimentin. Expression of S100, GFAP, and cytokeratins is variable {1073,1255}. Many CRINETs had initially been diagnosed as choroid plexus carcinoma {1482}, but staining for choroid plexus marker Kir7.1 is generally absent {1255}.

Proliferation
Ki-67/MIB1 proliferation index values between 5% and 35% have been reported {1073,1482}. In the largest series reported to date, the median Ki-67/MIB1 proliferation index was 29% (range: 15–35%) {1482}.

Box 4.07 Diagnostic criteria for cribriform neuroepithelial tumour (CRINET)

Essential:
Highly cellular tumour characterized by the presence of cribriform strands and ribbons
AND
Loss of nuclear SMARCB1 protein expression of tumour cells

Desirable:
Distinct expression of EMA highlighting cell surfaces

Caveat: The distinction of CRINET from the AT/RT-TYR subgroup is not fully established.

Cytology
Not clinically relevant

Diagnostic molecular pathology
CRINETs should be assessed for SMARCB1 deficiency.

Essential and desirable diagnostic criteria
See Box 4.07.

Staging
None validated

Prognosis and prediction
Many patients with CRINET respond well to therapy and experience long-term survival. In a retrospective series, the overall survival of 10 patients with CRINET was found to be significantly longer than that of 27 patients with AT/RT-TYR {1482}.

Embryonal tumour with multilayered rosettes

Korshunov A
Fuller GN
Haberler C
Huang A

Kool M
Sturm D
von Hoff K
Wesseling P

Definition

A CNS embryonal tumour with multilayered rosettes (ETMR) is an embryonal neoplasm conforming to one of three morphological patterns – embryonal tumour with abundant neuropil and true rosettes, ependymoblastoma, or medulloepithelioma – and typically having a C19MC alteration or (rarely) a *DICER1* mutation (CNS WHO grade 4).

ICD-O coding

9478/3 Embryonal tumour with multilayered rosettes

ICD-11 coding

2A00.1Y & XH0KZ2 Other specified embryonal tumours of brain & Embryonal tumour with multilayered rosettes, NOS

2A00.1Y & XH51C5 Other specified embryonal tumours of brain & Embryonal tumours with multilayered rosettes with C19MC alteration

Related terminology

Not recommended: embryonal tumour with abundant neuropil and true rosettes (ETANTR); embryonal tumour with abundant neuropil and ependymoblastic rosettes (ETANER); ependymoblastoma; medulloepithelioma.

Subtype(s)

Embryonal tumour with multilayered rosettes, C19MC-altered; embryonal tumour with multilayered rosettes, *DICER1*-mutated

Localization

Most ETMRs are intracranial; examples in the spinal cord are rare. The most common site is the cerebral hemisphere, although 45% arise in non-hemispheric locations. Occasionally, ETMRs are very large, involving multiple cerebral lobes and even both hemispheres. Posterior fossa ETMRs occur in both cerebellum and brainstem, occasionally involving the cerebellopontine cistern {3005,2290,1798}.

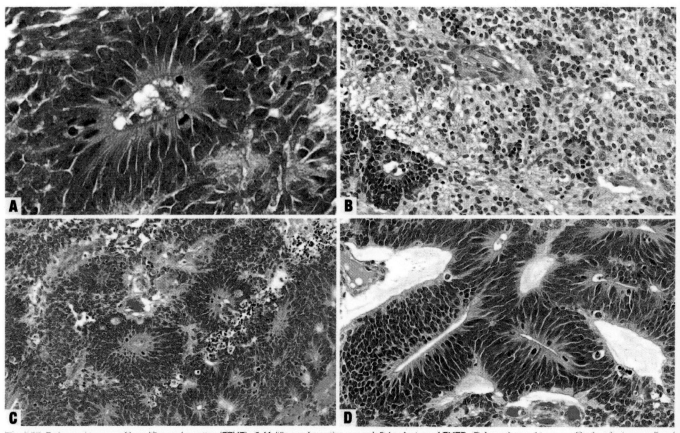

Fig. 4.25 Embryonal tumour with multilayered rosettes (ETMR). **A** Multilayered rosettes are a defining feature of EMTR. **B** An embryonal tumour with abundant neuropil and true rosettes pattern. Groups of densely packed embryonal cells, some including multilayered rosettes, contrast with neuropil-like areas that typically contain neoplastic neurocytic cells. **C** ETMR with ependymoblastoma morphology. Multilayered rosettes are abundant. **D** ETMR with medulloepithelioma morphology. Tubular structures resemble embryonic neural tube or elongated multilayered rosettes.

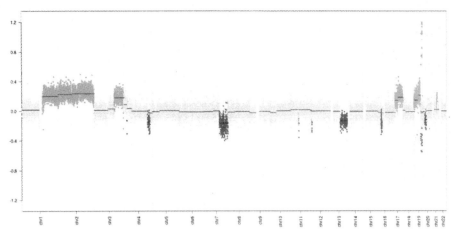

Fig. 4.26 Embryonal tumour with multilayered rosettes. Panchromosomal copy-number alterations shown by DNA methylation array. Amplification and rearrangement of the C19MC locus on chromosome 19q and gain of chromosome 2 are prominent.

Clinical features

ETMRs commonly produce symptoms and signs of raised intracranial pressure (e.g. headache, nausea, vomiting, and visual disturbances). A few patients present with epilepsy due to a small cortical tumour. Focal neurological signs are more common in older children and in patients with infratentorial tumours.

Imaging

The neuroimaging characteristics of ETMR vary; for example, large cerebral tumours frequently enhance, whereas smaller, cortical tumours may be non-enhancing. Tumours may contain cysts or calcification {2290}. Radiologically, brainstem ETMRs may mimic diffuse midline glioma, although they tend to be more circumscribed.

Spread

Most tumours (75%) are localized at presentation, with the remainder showing a range of tumour dissemination (stage M2–M4). Rarely, ETMRs with extracranial invasive growth and extradural metastases have been reported {2886}.

Epidemiology

The true incidence of ETMR is difficult to determine because of its rarity. In addition, before its defining genetic alteration was discovered, multiple diagnostic terms were used for its varied morphological features. With few exceptions, ETMRs affect children aged < 4 years, the vast majority of cases occurring during the first 2 years of life. In larger cohorts, the incidence seems to be equally balanced between male and female patients {1798}.

Etiology

No genetic susceptibility for patients with C19MC-altered ETMRs has been reported. In contrast, almost all patients with DICER1-mutant ETMRs carry a pathogenic DICER1 germline alteration, which should prompt genetic testing and counselling {1797}. No other risk factors have been reported to date.

Pathogenesis

Cell of origin

Distinct histological patterns of ETMR share a molecular signature, which suggests that they have a common histogenesis.

Single-cell RNA sequencing data have identified clusters of stem cell–like, oligodendrocyte precursor–like, and astrocyte-like tumour cell populations {1797}.

Genetic profile

Approximately 90% of ETMRs harbour specific structural alterations of a microRNA cluster on chromosome 19q13.42 (C19MC), including focal high-level amplification, fusion to TTYH1, and other rare rearrangements (e.g. fusion to MYO9B or MIRLET7BHG), all of which produce strong upregulation of this microRNA cluster as a driving event {1650,1797}.

Rare ETMRs (5%) have a DICER1 mutation, and almost all of these are in the setting of a DICER1 genetic tumour syndrome {705}. Typically, the germline mutation is associated with a second mutation in the (hotspot) RNase IIIb domain that is important for microRNA processing {1798}. Other ETMRs without a C19MC alteration or DICER1 mutation may be driven by amplification of the miR-17–92 microRNA cluster on chromosome 13 {1798}.

Despite ETMR subtypes having different mechanisms for deregulating microRNA processing, microRNA expression profiles are nevertheless very similar across ETMRs. In

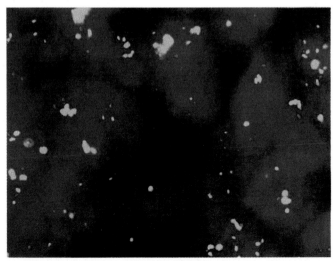

Fig. 4.27 Embryonal tumour with multilayered rosettes. Interphase FISH. Amplification (green signals) of the C19MC locus at 19q13.42.

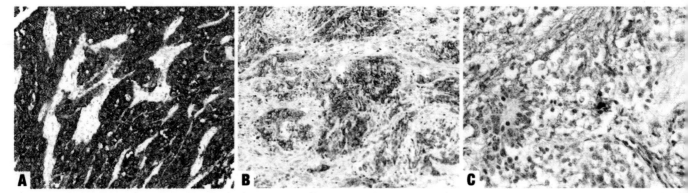

Fig. 4.28 Embryonal tumour with multilayered rosettes (ETMR). **A** Tumour cells are strongly immunopositive for LIN28A. **B** Many cells are immunopositive for vimentin. **C** The neuropil-like matrix of ETMRs with an abundant neuropil and true rosettes pattern is synaptophysin-immunopositive.

a recent study, R loop–associated chromosomal instability was suggested as a key factor in ETMR pathogenesis {1797}. Other recurrently mutated genes, such as *CTNNB1* (10%) and *TP53* (7%), are likely to play a role during ETMR development. Relapsed ETMRs can acquire additional copy-number aberrations (loss of 6q, gains of 1q or 17q) and increased polyploidy accompanied by chromosomal instability, and they show a large increase in somatic single-nucleotide variants {1797}.

Macroscopic appearance
ETMR is a grey to pink, well-circumscribed tumour, with areas of necrosis and haemorrhage and, sometimes, minute calcifications. Some tumours are cystic. Widespread leptomeningeal dissemination and extradural metastases are frequent in the terminal stage of disease.

Histopathology
By definition, rosettes are a characteristic histological feature of ETMRs. They are multilayered structures consisting of embryonal cells in a pseudostratified neuroepithelium with a central round or slit-like lumen. The cells facing the lumen have a defined apical surface, with a prominent internal limiting membrane. The nuclei of the rosette-forming cells tend to be located away from the lumen towards the outer cell border. In most tumours, a defined outer membrane around the rosettes is absent. Mitotic figures are commonly observed in the embryonal cells of rosettes. ETMRs have three histological patterns: embryonal tumour with abundant neuropil and true rosettes, ependymoblastoma, and medulloepithelioma. On the basis of their molecular commonality, all three are now considered to constitute various points along a morphological spectrum of diverse differentiation within a single tumour entity, rather than distinct nosological tumour types {1510,1725}.

Embryonal tumour with abundant neuropil and true rosettes
This pattern of ETMR shows a biphasic architecture featuring densely packed, small embryonal cells with round or polygonal nuclei and scant cytoplasm, as well as large, neuropil-like areas with sparse neoplastic neurocytic and ganglion cells {817,1068}. In some cases, the neuropil has a fascicular quality. Multilayered rosettes are often present among the embryonal cells, although in some cases they are observed in the otherwise paucicellular neuropil-like areas.

Ependymoblastoma
This pattern of ETMR features sheets of embryonal cells incorporating numerous multilayered rosettes, but it typically lacks a neuropil-like matrix and ganglion cell element.

Medulloepithelioma
This pattern of ETMR is characterized by papillary, tubular, or trabecular arrangements of neoplastic pseudostratified neuroepithelium with an external (PAS-positive) limiting membrane, resembling the primitive neural tube. On the luminal surface of these tubules, cilia and blepharoplasts are absent. In zones away from tubular and papillary structures, there are large sheets of embryonal cells. Rare tumours display epithelial, myeloid, osteoid, myoid, or other mesenchymal differentiation, or they contain melanin pigment {75,397}.

All morphological patterns of ETMR show abundant mitotic figures and apoptotic bodies, indicating a high rate of cell turnover. The Ki-67 proliferation index ranges from 20% to 80%. After therapy, some ETMRs show neuronal and glial differentiation resembling a low-grade glioneuronal tumour {806,1784,119}. During progression, other tumours show complete loss of recognizable ETMR patterns and instead resemble other embryonal neoplasms {3465}.

Immunophenotype
Most of the embryonal component of ETMR (the rosettes and tubular structures) is intensely immunoreactive for nestin and vimentin {817,1068}. Embryonal cells and rosettes may also show focal expression of cytokeratins (particularly in the medulloepithelioma pattern), EMA, and CD99, but they are usually negative for neuronal and glial markers. In contrast, the neuropil-like matrix is strongly immunopositive for synaptophysin, NFP, and NeuN. Immunoreactivity for GFAP highlights scattered cells resembling reactive astrocytes, but it may also be present in a few embryonal cells. ETMRs show strong and diffuse nuclear immunoreactivity for SMARCB1 (INI1) throughout all components. Strong and diffuse cytoplasmic immunoreactivity for LIN28A is found in ETMRs irrespective of their morphological pattern {1725,3005}. However, LIN28A expression also occurs in some gliomas, atypical teratoid/rhabdoid tumours, germ cell tumours, teratomas, and some non-CNS neoplasms {3005,3411}.

Differential diagnosis

Intraocular medulloepithelioma and sacrococcygeal ependymoblastoma share some histopathological features with CNS ETMR but harbour striking molecular differences and consequently deserve a separate nosological designation.

Cytology

Evaluation of tumour cell presence in cerebrospinal fluid cytology is required for staging.

Diagnostic molecular pathology

A limited range of recurrent molecular alterations is displayed by ETMRs. To date, structural variants of the C19MC microRNA cluster at 19q13.42 have been found only in ETMRs, occurring in approximately 90% of cases. These are usually focal amplifications, but fusions can also occur, generally with *TTYH1*. C19MC alterations can be detected by array-based copy-number profiling or interphase FISH. It should be borne in mind that the characteristic morphological features of ETMR, including rosettes, might not always be present in tissue submitted for histopathological examination. The combination of LIN28A immunoreactivity and C19MC alterations by interphase FISH can be helpful in this situation. However, although C19MC alterations are specific for ETMR, immunoreactivity for LIN28A is not.

About half of the ETMRs without a C19MC alteration harbour *DICER1* mutations. These are generally compound heterozygous mutations, combining one somatic mutation (usually in exon 24 or 25) and a second mutation in the patient's germline. Germline testing for a *DICER1* mutation should be undertaken in patients with an ETMR that lacks a C19MC alteration. Not all high-grade neuroepithelial tumours with a *DICER1* mutation are ETMRs; a *DICER1* mutation can be found in other embryonal tumours and gliomas. Rare ETMRs without a C19MC alteration or *DICER1* mutation should be classified as ETMR not elsewhere classified (NEC).

Essential and desirable diagnostic criteria

See Box 4.08.

Staging

Clinical staging procedures include MRI examinations of the CNS with contrast agent. This is complemented by lumbar puncture postoperative cerebrospinal fluid cytology. The

Box 4.08 Diagnostic criteria for embryonal tumour with multilayered rosettes (ETMR)

Essential:

A CNS embryonal tumour with the morphological and immunohistochemical features of one of the three ETMR morphological patterns:

- Embryonal tumour with abundant neuropil and true rosettes
- Ependymoblastoma
- Medulloepithelioma

AND

Genetic alteration defining one of the two ETMR molecular subtypes:

- C19MC alteration
- *DICER1* mutation

AND (for unresolved lesions)

A DNA methylation profile aligned with ETMR

postoperative staging system developed by Chang and others in 1969 {519}, which defines the following degrees of metastatic spread, is still being used:

M0 No evidence of subarachnoid or haematogenous metastasis
M1 Microscopic tumour cells found in the cerebrospinal fluid
M2 Gross nodular seeding demonstrated in the cerebellar/cerebral subarachnoid space or in the third or lateral ventricles
M3 Gross nodular seeding in the spinal subarachnoid space
M4 Metastasis outside the cerebrospinal axis

Prognosis and prediction

ETMRs demonstrate rapid growth and are associated with an aggressive clinical course, with reported survival times averaging 12 months after intensive combination therapies {1068, 1060,3004,1725,1352}. Few prognostic indicators have been reliably identified. Gross total resection, radiotherapy, and high-dose chemotherapy probably prolong overall survival {1456}. Metastatic disease at presentation and brainstem tumours have been significantly associated with an adverse outcome. Patient survival does not differ significantly between the three morphological patterns of ETMR. From extremely rare cases with long-term survival, posttreatment neuronal differentiation has been proposed as a favourable indicator of outcome {806,1784,119}.

CNS neuroblastoma, *FOXR2*-activated

Wesseling P
Haberler C
Huang A
Kool M

Korshunov A
Sturm D
von Hoff K

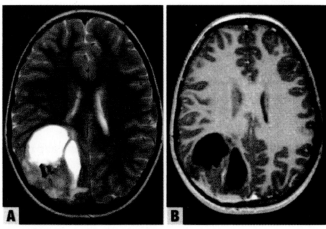

Fig. 4.29 CNS neuroblastoma, *FOXR2*-activated. **A** Axial T2-weighted image showing a large, partially cystic mass involving the right parietal lobe (left). **B** Postcontrast T1-weighted image showing thickening and enhancement of overlying meninges as well as inhomogeneous enhancement of solid tumour components.

Definition

CNS neuroblastoma, *FOXR2*-activated, is an embryonal neoplasm exhibiting varying degrees of neuroblastic and/or neuronal differentiation, including foci of ganglion cells and neuropil-rich stroma. It is characterized by activation of the transcription factor *FOXR2* by structural rearrangements (CNS WHO grade 4).

ICD-O coding

9500/3 CNS neuroblastoma, *FOXR2*-activated

ICD-11 coding

2A00.1Y & XH85Z0 Other specified embryonal tumours of brain & Neuroblastoma, NOS

Related terminology

None

Subtype(s)

None

Localization

FOXR2-activated CNS neuroblastoma is typically located in the cerebral hemisphere, with intraventricular location observed in occasional cases {3059,2502}.

Clinical features

Clinical data on *FOXR2*-activated CNS neuroblastoma, as diagnosed by current molecular criteria, are limited. Leptomeningeal metastasis develops in some cases {3059,2502}.

Imaging

FOXR2-activated CNS neuroblastoma usually appears as a demarcated mass in a cerebral hemisphere. There may be a prominent cystic component. The solid component may show moderate and heterogeneous enhancement {3059,2502,1016, 1450,1336}.

Epidemiology

FOXR2-activated CNS neuroblastoma is a rare, recently described tumour, and epidemiological data are incomplete.

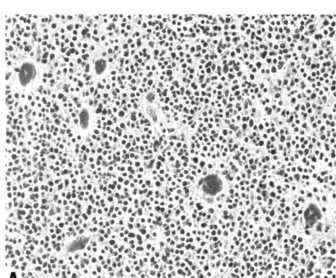
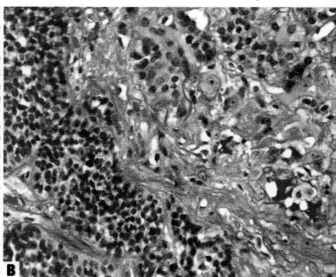

Fig. 4.30 CNS neuroblastoma, *FOXR2*-activated. **A** Neurocytic and neuroblastic cells are set in a neuropil-like matrix. **B** Some tumours show focal ganglion cell formation (ganglioneuroblastoma phenotype).

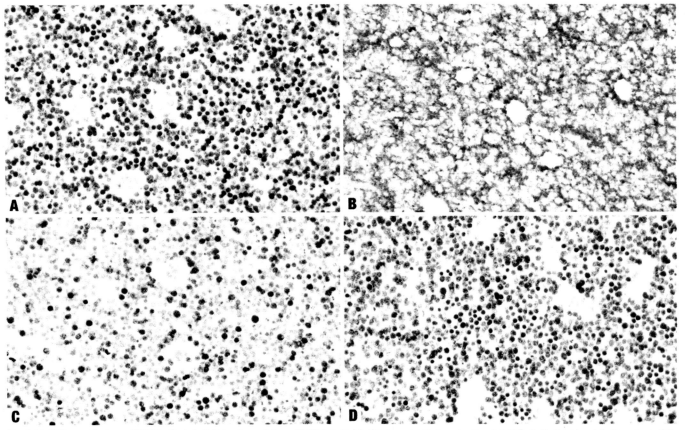

Fig. 4.31 CNS neuroblastoma, *FOXR2*-activated. **A** Extensive and strong OLIG2 immunolabelling is present in tumour cell nuclei. **B** Typically, there is patchy immunoreactivity for synaptophysin, although expression is widespread in this example. **C** The Ki-67 proliferation index is high. **D** Widespread and strong immunoreactivity for thyroid transcription factor 1 (TTF1, also called NKX2-1) may be found.

However, these tumours usually occur in childhood, with a slight female preponderance {3059}. *FOXR2*-activated CNS neuroblastoma may represent approximately 10% of tumours previously classified as primitive neuroectodermal tumour of the CNS {3059,1389}.

Etiology
No risk factors have been reported to date.

Pathogenesis
The exact cellular origin of CNS neuroblastomas remains unknown. The most frequent genetic alterations in tumours classified morphologically as CNS neuroblastoma are complex interchromosomal and intrachromosomal rearrangements converging on the transcription factor gene *FOXR2*, producing a fusion between the entire *FOXR2* gene and different gene partners {3059}. The elevated *FOXR2* expression levels in CNS neuroblastomas, compared with its expression in other CNS tumour types and non-neoplastic brain tissue, are suggestive of *FOXR2* activation facilitated by promoters of active genes (possibly through enhancer hijacking) {3059}. Although *FOXR2* has been demonstrated to play a causative role in the formation of CNS embryonal tumours, the exact underlying mechanisms have yet to be elucidated {2528}.

Macroscopic appearance
Insufficient data have been reported on the macroscopic appearance of *FOXR2*-activated CNS neuroblastoma specifically. However, CNS embryonal tumours are typically well-circumscribed pink masses. They are soft, unless they contain a prominent desmoplastic component, in which case they are firm and often have a tan colour.

Histopathology
In many microscopic regions, *FOXR2*-activated CNS neuroblastoma consists of sheets of poorly differentiated cells with a high N:C ratio; round, oval, or angulated hyperchromatic nuclei; and abundant mitotic activity. Infiltration of adjacent CNS parenchyma is variable. Areas of necrosis are common. Palisades of embryonal cells and Homer Wright (neuroblastic) rosettes may be evident. Cells showing neurocytic differentiation and mature ganglion cells may be present, often in clusters (known as ganglioneuroblastomas).

Immunophenotype
Most cells in *FOXR2*-activated CNS neuroblastomas strongly express OLIG2. Immunoreactivity for synaptophysin can be found in some embryonal cells, but its expression is accentuated in regions of neurocytic or ganglion cell differentiation {1336}. Immunoreactivities for GFAP and vimentin are generally absent, although staining for the former can pick out reactive astrocytes. The Ki-67 proliferation index is high.

Cytology

Evaluation of cerebrospinal fluid for the presence of tumour cells is required for staging.

Diagnostic molecular pathology

Structural rearrangements of *FOXR2* are frequent and usually complex, requiring next-generation sequencing methods for detection. Furthermore, alterations affecting the *FOXR2* locus on chromosome Xp11.21 may be visible by copy-number analysis. Gain of chromosome 1q is present in most tumours {3059}.

Most CNS embryonal tumours that are not classified as medulloblastoma, embryonal tumour with multilayered rosettes, atypical teratoid/rhabdoid tumour, or pineoblastoma are *FOXR2*-activated CNS neuroblastomas. However, high *FOXR2* expression also occurs in a subset of high-grade gliomas and (rarely) in medulloblastoma. The DNA methylation cluster that includes *FOXR2*-activated CNS neuroblastomas is distinct; therefore, DNA methylation profiling can facilitate the diagnosis of these tumours {3059,460}.

Essential and desirable diagnostic criteria

See Box 4.09.

Staging

Clinical staging procedures include MRI examinations of the CNS with contrast agent. This is complemented by lumbar puncture postoperative cerebrospinal fluid cytology. The postoperative staging system developed by Chang and others in 1969 {519}, which defines the following degrees of metastatic spread, is still being used:

M0 No evidence of subarachnoid or haematogenous metastasis
M1 Microscopic tumour cells found in the cerebrospinal fluid
M2 Gross nodular seeding demonstrated in the cerebellar/cerebral subarachnoid space or in the third or lateral ventricles
M3 Gross nodular seeding in the spinal subarachnoid space
M4 Metastasis outside the cerebrospinal axis

Prognosis and prediction

Limited information is available on the prognosis of *FOXR2*-activated CNS neuroblastoma.

CNS tumour with
BCOR internal tandem duplication

Wesseling P
Haberler C
Huang A
Kool M

Korshunov A
Solomon DA
Sturm D
von Hoff K

Definition
CNS tumour with *BCOR* internal tandem duplication (ITD) is a malignant CNS tumour characterized by a predominantly solid growth pattern, uniform oval or spindle-shaped cells with round to oval nuclei, a dense capillary network, focal pseudorosette formation, and an ITD in exon 15 of the *BCOR* gene.

ICD-O coding
9500/3 CNS tumour with *BCOR* internal tandem duplication

ICD-11 coding
2A00.1Y Other specified embryonal tumours of brain

Related terminology
Not recommended: CNS high-grade neuroepithelial tumour with *BCOR* internal tandem duplication.

Subtype(s)
None

Localization
CNS tumour with *BCOR* ITD most commonly occurs in a cerebral or cerebellar hemisphere. Occurrence in the basal ganglia, cerebellopontine angle, brainstem, or spinal cord has rarely been described {3059,124,3547,918,710}.

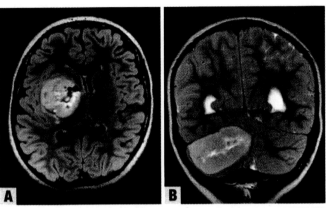

Fig. 4.32 CNS tumour with *BCOR* internal tandem duplication. **A** Axial MRI/FLAIR image of a tumour in the basal ganglia. **B** Coronal T2-weighted MRI of a tumour located in the cerebellar hemisphere.

Clinical features
The clinical presentation is based on the location of the tumour and encompasses symptoms of raised intracranial pressure (e.g. headache, vomiting, nausea, visual disturbances), focal neurological deficits, and seizures.

Imaging
On MRI, these tumours are typically well demarcated. They often have a central cystic component and variable, inhomogeneous

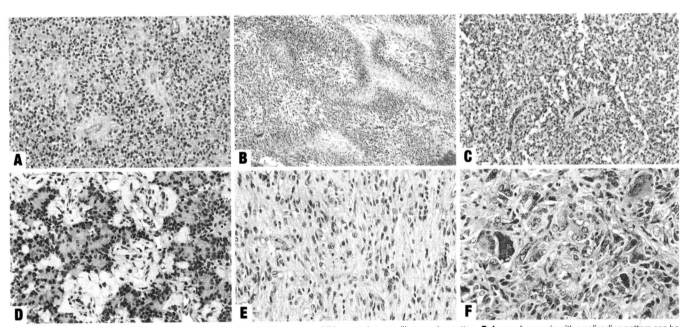

Fig. 4.33 CNS tumour with *BCOR* internal tandem duplication. **A** This tumour exhibits ependymoma-like pseudorosettes. **B** Areas of necrosis with a palisading pattern can be present. **C** This field shows a high cell density and brisk mitotic activity. **D** A collagenous stroma and rosette formation are occasionally seen. **E** Some tumours demonstrate a glioma-like fibrillarity. **F** Marked cytological pleomorphism may occasionally be found.

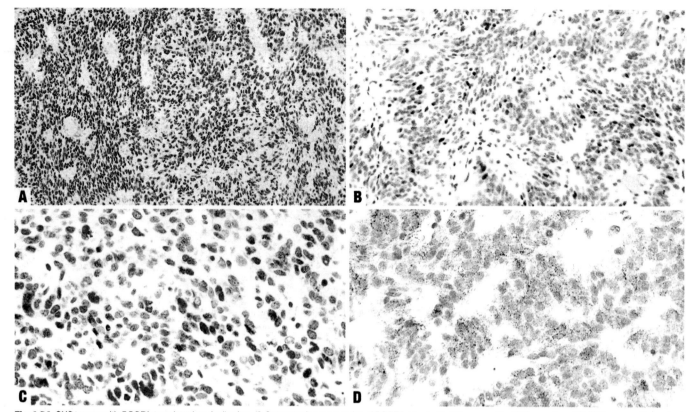

Fig. 4.34 CNS tumour with *BCOR* internal tandem duplication. **A** Strong nuclear expression of BCOR is present in all tumour cells. **B** Expression of OLIG2 is present in a subset of tumour cell nuclei. **C** Expression of NeuN is variable. **D** Weak, granular, cytoplasmic immunoreactivity for EMA is occasionally found.

contrast enhancement. Tumours can be very large at presentation, involving multiple lobes and both cerebral hemispheres {918,368}. Location adjacent to the dura has been described for most of the neuroradiologically annotated cases, although definite dural infiltration has not been observed {918}.

Spread
So far, no patient with metastatic disease at presentation has been described. At relapse, leptomeningeal metastases, as well as metastases to the bone and inoculation metastases along the neurosurgical access route, have been observed {124,2392,1638,918}.

Epidemiology
Limited data are available, but the median age at presentation of reported patients is 3.5 years (range: 0–22 years), with a balanced M:F ratio {918}.

Etiology
There is no known specific risk factor or genetic susceptibility for CNS tumours with *BCOR* ITD {918}.

Pathogenesis
A somatic heterozygous ITD in the *BCOR* gene plays a key oncogenic role in the pathogenesis of this tumour type {3059}. The majority of tumours harbour a *BCOR* ITD as the solitary pathogenic alteration. Although it is very likely that the ITD in *BCOR* produces an activating, gain-of-function event, the specific mechanism by which this recurrent alteration drives tumour development remains unknown. Additional genetic alterations

that probably contribute to pathogenesis in some cases include inactivating mutations in other genes, such as *EP300*, *SMARCA2*, *STAG2*, and *BCORL1* {918}. *BCOR* expression is higher in this tumour type than in most other CNS tumours, and activation of the WNT signalling pathway is frequently observed {3059}.

The exact nature of CNS tumours with *BCOR* ITD is not clear. The duplicated region in exon 15 of *BCOR* is identical to that of *BCOR* ITDs in clear cell sarcomas of the kidney, undifferentiated round cell sarcomas in infants, and primitive myxoid mesenchymal tumour of infancy {3250,1553,2807}. There is currently no consensus as to whether CNS tumours should be considered mesenchymal or neuroepithelial neoplasms.

Macroscopic appearance
Insufficient data have been published on this tumour's macroscopic appearance.

Histopathology
CNS tumours with *BCOR* ITD are generally demarcated at the interface with adjacent CNS parenchyma, although infiltration of the brain may sometimes occur {3547,918}. Histological features can be variable {124,3547,918,1808}. Tumours are generally composed of uniform oval or spindle-shaped cells, with round or oval nuclei showing a delicate chromatin pattern. The cytoplasm is weakly stained with eosin. Most cases demonstrate dispersed glioma-like fibrillary processes, but a compact fascicular pattern can occur. A characteristic feature is the formation of ependymoma-like perivascular pseudorosettes. A myxoid or microcystic matrix is often encountered. A branching

capillary network is often present. Glomeruloid microvascular proliferation is not a typical feature. Necrosis, which is often palisading, is commonly observed. Mitoses are frequently encountered, including foci with brisk mitotic activity. The differential diagnosis includes glioma, ependymoma, and other embryonal tumours.

Immunophenotype

In the immunohistochemical assessment of CNS tumours with BCOR ITD, expression of vimentin and CD56 is universal. A few tumour cells can be immunopositive for OLIG2, GFAP, or S100 {918}, but their widespread expression, as found in gliomas, is absent. Perivascular pseudorosettes are GFAP-negative, unlike in ependymomas. Variable expression of NeuN is detected in a few tumours {1662,124,3547}. Neuronal markers are generally not expressed. Widespread strong nuclear expression of BCOR is a sensitive marker, but it is not specific because it may also occur in other tumours, such as solitary fibrous tumour {124,3547,1209,918}. The Ki-67 labelling index is elevated and ranges between 15% and 60% {918,124}.

Grading

Insufficient data currently exist to assign a CNS WHO grade to this tumour.

Cytology

Evaluation of cerebrospinal fluid for the presence of tumour cells is required for staging.

Diagnostic molecular pathology

The defining diagnostic finding is a heterozygous ITD in exon 15 of the BCOR gene. This BCOR ITD appears to be mutually exclusive with BCOR or BCORL1 fusions and hotspot mutations in H3 or IDH genes (as found in infiltrating gliomas), ZFTA (C11orf95) or YAP1 fusions (as found in supratentorial ependymomas), or alterations in FOXR2 or MN1 (as found in other neuroepithelial tumours) {3059,3218}. DNA methylation and gene expression profiles can be reliably used to differentiate CNS tumours with BCOR ITD from other CNS tumours {3059,460}.

Box 4.10 Diagnostic criteria for CNS tumour with BCOR internal tandem duplication

Essential:

A malignant primary CNS tumour with a predominantly solid growth pattern, uniform oval or spindle-shaped cells with round to oval nuclei, and a dense capillary network

AND

An internal tandem duplication in exon 15 of BCOR

AND (for unresolved lesions)

A DNA methylation profile aligned with CNS tumour with BCOR internal tandem duplication

Essential and desirable diagnostic criteria

See Box 4.10.

Staging

Clinical staging procedures include MRI examinations of the CNS with contrast agent. This is complemented by lumbar puncture postoperative cerebrospinal fluid cytology. The postoperative staging system developed by Chang and others in 1969 {519}, which defines the following degrees of metastatic spread, is still being used:

M0   No evidence of subarachnoid or haematogenous metastasis

M1   Microscopic tumour cells found in the cerebrospinal fluid

M2   Gross nodular seeding demonstrated in the cerebellar/cerebral subarachnoid space or in the third or lateral ventricles

M3   Gross nodular seeding in the spinal subarachnoid space

M4   Metastasis outside the cerebrospinal axis

Prognosis and prediction

Clinical data are limited, but most reported patients relapsed. In a cohort of 24 patients, overall survival was poor {918}. However, time to relapse can be prolonged, and recurrence up to 5 years after initial diagnosis has been reported {918,368}.

CNS embryonal tumour NEC/NOS

Wesseling P
Haberler C
Huang A
Kool M
Korshunov A
Sturm D
von Hoff K

Definition

CNS embryonal tumour NEC/NOS is a tumour arising in the CNS with embryonal morphology and immunophenotype and either lacking an alteration that would classify it as one of the molecularly defined CNS embryonal tumours (not elsewhere classified; NEC) or not susceptible to further analysis (not otherwise specified; NOS).

ICD-O coding

9473/3 CNS embryonal tumour, NEC/NOS

ICD-11 coding

2A00.1Y & XH8SH6 Other specified embryonal tumours of brain & CNS embryonal tumour, NOS

Related terminology

Not recommended: primitive neuroectodermal tumour.

Subtype(s)

None

Localization

CNS embryonal tumours occur throughout the neuraxis, but most are supratentorial.

Clinical features

Patients with CNS embryonal tumours generally present acutely with symptoms and signs of raised intracranial pressure, epilepsy, or focal neurological deficit. Metastatic dissemination is evident in 25–35% of CNS embryonal tumours at presentation {1347}.

Imaging

Appearances on MRI can vary, depending on the site of origin. CNS embryonal tumours often appear solid but may contain

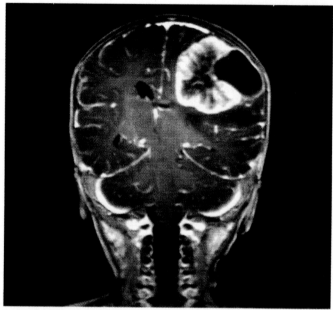

Fig. 4.35 CNS embryonal tumour. Postcontrast, T1-weighted MRI showing a large, partly solid, partly cystic tumour in the left frontal lobe of an infant. This is the same patient of whom the histology and copy-number variation profile are shown in Fig. 4.36.

cystic or necrotic areas. Most tumours show contrast enhancement and restricted diffusion {1450}.

Epidemiology

Shifting diagnostic criteria and nomenclature complicate analysis of the epidemiology of the spectrum of CNS embryonal tumours. Although most of these tumours occur in infancy and childhood, some are diagnosed in adults {1618,233,1076}.

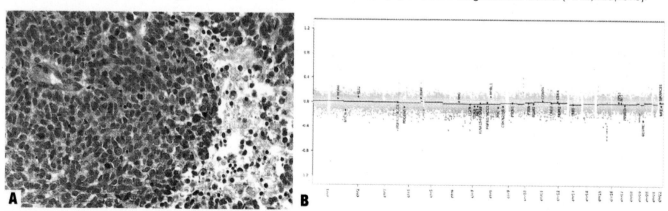

Fig. 4.36 CNS embryonal tumour. **A** CNS embryonal tumour (from the same patient shown in Fig. 4.35) consisting of densely packed, small, poorly differentiated cells with a high mitotic count. RNA sequencing revealed a *BRD4::CREBBP* fusion gene. Methylation profiling did not result in a match using the brain tumour classifier available at https://www.molecularneuropathology.org. **B** The copy-number variation profile of the tumour in panel A (derived from genome-wide methylome analysis) did not reveal large chromosomal gains or losses. The tumour was classified as CNS embryonal tumour not elsewhere classified (NEC).

Etiology

No risk factors have been reported to date.

Pathogenesis

By definition, CNS embryonal tumours NEC/NOS are distinct from those with specific genetic alterations; molecular drivers for this heterogeneous group of tumours remain to be elucidated.

Macroscopic appearance

CNS embryonal tumours are often circumscribed and solid, but they can contain cystic areas, haemorrhage, and necrosis.

Histopathology

CNS embryonal tumours are characterized by sheets of densely packed, immature cells that have a high N:C ratio and round, oval, or angulated hyperchromatic nuclei. Foci of neurocytic or ganglion cell differentiation can be present. Mitotic activity is typically high. Infiltration of adjacent CNS parenchyma is variable. Areas of necrosis and haemorrhage may be present. The heterogeneous nature of these high-grade tumours and their variable behaviours do not readily allow distinction between CNS WHO grades 3 and 4.

Immunophenotype

The neoplastic cells in CNS embryonal tumours are variably immunopositive for synaptophysin and OLIG2. They demonstrate a high Ki-67 proliferation index. GFAP and vimentin are generally absent, although staining for the former can pick out reactive astrocytes.

Differential diagnosis

The differential diagnosis of CNS embryonal tumours encompasses many poorly differentiated embryonal tumours and high-grade gliomas with specific molecular alterations. Just a few examples are *FOXR2*-activated CNS neuroblastoma, atypical teratoid/rhabdoid tumour, and H3 G34–mutant diffuse hemispheric glioma, all of which can have similar morphological features, especially in limited biopsies. Ideally, the diagnosis of CNS embryonal tumour should be made by excluding other morphologically similar but molecularly distinct tumour types.

Cytology

Evaluation of cerebrospinal fluid for the presence of tumour cells is required for staging.

Diagnostic molecular pathology

CNS embryonal tumour NEC/NOS shares a morphology and immunophenotype with many other poorly differentiated embryonal tumours and high-grade gliomas and is a diagnosis

Box 4.11 Diagnostic criteria for CNS embryonal tumour NEC/NOS

Essential:

An embryonal tumour originating in the CNS

AND

Absence of criteria qualifying for the diagnosis of a more specific type of embryonal CNS tumour

Desirable:

Focal expression of neuronal markers and absence of glial markers

of exclusion, pending a greater understanding of the molecular alterations that characterize this heterogeneous group of tumours. Examples with rare gene fusions are emerging, such as tumours with a *BRD4::CREBBP* fusion or ganglioneuroblastomas with a *MYO5A::NTRK3* fusion {1425}. However, when molecular analysis of CNS embryonal tumours fails to detect an alteration that allows specific classification or is unsuccessful, the designations "not elsewhere classified (NEC)" or "not otherwise specified (NOS)", respectively, should be applied {1946, 1934}.

Essential and desirable diagnostic criteria

See Box 4.11.

Staging

Clinical staging procedures include MRI examinations of the CNS with contrast agent. This is complemented by lumbar puncture postoperative cerebrospinal fluid cytology. The postoperative staging system developed by Chang and others in 1969 {519}, which defines the following degrees of metastatic spread, is still being used:

M0 No evidence of subarachnoid or haematogenous metastasis
M1 Microscopic tumour cells found in the cerebrospinal fluid
M2 Gross nodular seeding demonstrated in the cerebellar/cerebral subarachnoid space or in the third or lateral ventricles
M3 Gross nodular seeding in the spinal subarachnoid space
M4 Metastasis outside the cerebrospinal axis

Prognosis and prediction

As we understand more about the heterogeneity of tumours with an embryonal morphology, historical data on the outcome of patients with these tumours (which have included types of poorly differentiated high-grade glioma) become less representative of specific tumour types {3059,1389}.

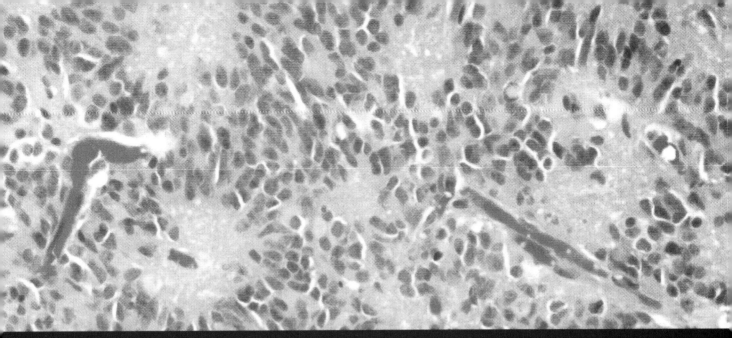

5

Pineal tumours

Edited by: Figarella-Branger D

Pineocytoma
Pineal parenchymal tumour of intermediate differentiation
Pineoblastoma
Papillary tumour of the pineal region
Desmoplastic myxoid tumour of the pineal region, *SMARCB1*-mutant

Pineal region tumours encompass a heterogeneous group of relatively rare neoplasms affecting different age groups. Pineal parenchymal tumours include pineocytoma (CNS WHO grade 1), pineal parenchymal tumour of intermediate differentiation (PPTID; CNS WHO grade 2–3), and pineoblastoma (CNS WHO grade 4). Papillary tumour of the pineal region (CNS WHO grade 2–3), a neuroepithelial tumour thought to originate from specialized ependymal cells of the subcommissural organ, had already been included in previous editions of the WHO classification of CNS tumours {1502}, but desmoplastic myxoid tumour, *SMARCB1*-mutant, a rare *SMARCB1*-mutant tumour lacking histopathological signs of malignancy {3185}, is new to this edition and has not yet had a CNS WHO grade assigned.

While histological grading criteria for PPTID; papillary tumour of the pineal region; and desmoplastic myxoid tumour, *SMARCB1*-mutant, remain to be defined, molecular studies play a more important role in the diagnosis of pineal region tumours. This is exemplified by the demonstration of *KBTBD4* in-frame insertions, which is now a desirable criterion for the diagnosis of PPTID {1834}.

Molecular profiling may also provide important prognostic information. An example is the segregation of pineoblastoma into four subtypes showing distinct molecular and clinical features: (1) pineoblastoma, miRNA processing-altered_1, arises in children and is characterized by mutations of *DICER1*, *DROSHA*, or *DGCR8*, as well as by intermediate outcome; (2) pineoblastoma, miRNA processing-altered_2, mainly occurs in older children and is also characterized by *DICER1*, *DROSHA*, or *DGCR8* mutations, but in this subgroup, outcome is excellent; (3) pineoblastoma, MYC/FOXR2-activated, arises in infants and is characterized by MYC activation and FOXR2 overexpression, as well as by a generally poor prognosis; and (4) pineoblastoma, *RB1*-altered, arises in infants and shows similarities with retinoblastoma, with frequent metastatic spread and a very poor prognosis {2490,1865,1913}.

The main clinical features of the pineoblastoma subtypes and PPTID, as well as their genetic alterations and associated hereditary cancer predisposition syndromes, are summarized in Fig. 5.01. The distinct subtypes are illustrated in the t-distributed stochastic neighbour embedding (t-SNE) representation of pineal tumour DNA methylation profiles in Fig. 5.02.

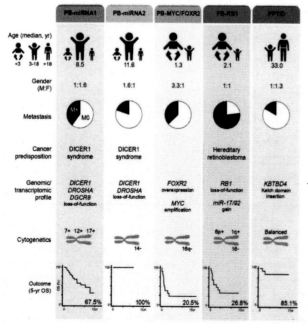

Fig. 5.01 Pineoblastoma subtypes and pineal parenchymal tumour of intermediate differentiation (PPTID). Main clinical features, genetic alterations, and association with hereditary cancer predisposition syndromes. OS, overall survival; PB-miRNA1, pineoblastoma, miRNA processing-altered_1; PB-miRNA2, pineoblastoma, miRNA processing-altered_2; PB-MYC/FOXR2, pineoblastoma, MYC/FOXR2-activated; PB-RB1, pineoblastoma, *RB1*-altered.

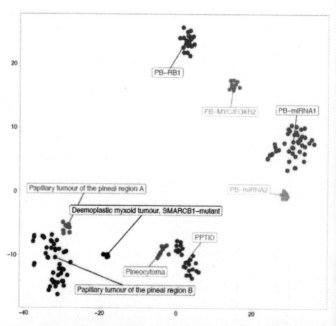

Fig. 5.02 Pineal tumours. t-distributed stochastic neighbour embedding (t-SNE) representation of DNA methylation profiles. PB-miRNA1, pineoblastoma, miRNA processing-altered_1; PB-miRNA2, pineoblastoma, miRNA processing-altered_2; PB-MYC/FOXR2, pineoblastoma, MYC/FOXR2-activated; PB-RB1, pineoblastoma, *RB1*-altered; PPTID, pineal parenchymal tumour of intermediate differentiation.

Pineocytoma

Hasselblatt M
Huang A
Jones DTW
Orr BA
Snuderl M
Vasiljevic A

Definition

Pineocytoma is a well-differentiated pineal parenchymal neoplasm composed of (1) uniform cells forming large pineocytomatous rosettes and/or (2) pleomorphic cells showing gangliocytic differentiation (CNS WHO grade 1).

ICD-O coding

9361/1 Pineocytoma

ICD-11 coding

2A00.20 & XH1K94 Tumours of the pineal gland or pineal region & Pineocytoma

Related terminology

None

Subtype(s)

None

Localization

Pineocytomas typically remain localized in the pineal area. Compression of adjacent structures and protrusion into the posterior third ventricle are common.

Clinical features

Patients with pineocytomas present with signs and symptoms related to increased intracranial pressure due to aqueductal obstruction, neuro-ophthalmological dysfunction (Parinaud syndrome), and brainstem or cerebellar dysfunction {325,578, 600,1219,2839}.

Imaging

On CT, pineocytomas are usually globular, well-delineated masses that appear hypodense and homogeneous, some harbouring calcification {571}. On MRI, the tumours tend to be hypointense or isointense on T1-weighted images and

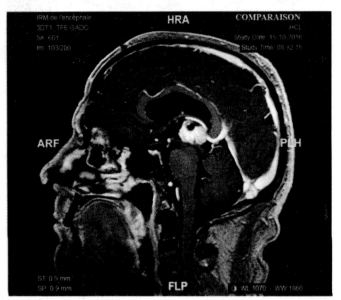

Fig. 5.03 Pineocytoma. Sagittal, gadolinium-enhanced, T1-weighted MRI showing a well-delineated tumour with strong contrast enhancement.

hyperintense on T2-weighted images, with strong, homogeneous contrast enhancement {2203}. They can usually be easily distinguished from pineal cysts {885}.

Spread

Pineocytomas grow locally and are not associated with cerebrospinal fluid seeding {896}.

Epidemiology

Pineal region tumours are rare and account for < 1% of all intracranial neoplasms; approximately 27% of pineal region tumours are of pineal parenchymal origin {1700,3074}, and approximately 25% of these are pineocytomas {137,1505,2839,3510}. Pineocytomas can occur at any age, but they most frequently

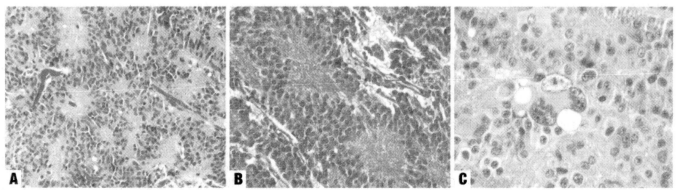

Fig. 5.04 Pineocytoma. **A** Large fibrillary pineocytomatous rosettes are a characteristic feature. **B** Pineocytomatous rosettes are large irregular eosinophilic fibrillary areas surrounded by pinealocyte-like neoplastic cells. **C** Pleomorphic pineocytoma. Multinucleated pleomorphic cell.

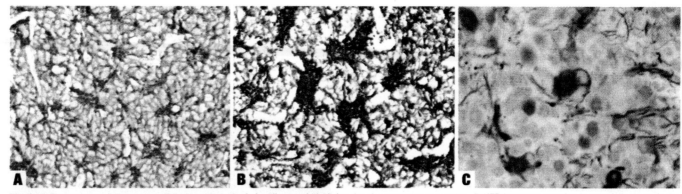

Fig. 5.05 Pineocytoma. **A** Immunoreactivity for synaptophysin is diffuse and highlights the pineocytomatous rosettes. **B** NFP immunoexpression is especially strong in the pineocytomatous rosettes. **C** Pleomorphic pineocytoma. Pleomorphic cells often show immunoreactivity for NFP.

affect adults, with a median patient age of 44 years (range: 1.1–85 years) {137,1505,2119,2839,3510}. There is a female predominance, with an M:F ratio of 0.6:1.

Etiology

There are no syndromic associations or genetic susceptibilities reported. Occurrence of pineocytoma in siblings has been reported in one family {1056}.

Pathogenesis

Cell of origin

The histogenesis of pineal parenchymal tumours has been linked to the pinealocyte, a cell with photosensory and neuroendocrine functions. Microarray analysis of pineocytoma showed high-level expression of genes coding for enzymes related to melatonin synthesis and genes involved in retinal phototransduction {922}.

Genetic profile

No chromosomal gains or losses were found by comparative genomic hybridization {2668}. On DNA methylation profiling, cases diagnosed as pineocytoma grouped within a distinct subgroup, which was in close proximity to normal pineal gland tissue {2490}.

Macroscopic appearance

Pineocytomas are well-circumscribed lesions with a greyish-tan, homogeneous or granular cut surface {325,1297,2826}. Degenerative changes, including cyst formation and foci of haemorrhage, may occur {2067}.

Histopathology

Pineocytoma is a well-differentiated, moderately cellular neoplasm composed of relatively small, uniform, mature cells resembling pinealocytes. It grows primarily in sheets, and it often features large pineocytomatous rosettes composed of abundant delicate tumour cell processes. Pineocytomatous rosettes are not seen in the normal pineal gland. In pineocytoma, poorly defined lobules may be seen, but a conspicuous lobular architecture is instead a feature of normal pineal gland. Most nuclei are round to oval, with inconspicuous nucleoli and finely dispersed chromatin. Cytoplasm is moderate in quantity and homogeneously eosinophilic. Processes are conspicuous, often ending in club-shaped expansions that are

optimally demonstrated by neurofilament immunostaining or silver impregnation. Pineocytomatous rosettes vary in number and size. Their anucleate centres are composed of delicate, enmeshed cytoplasmic processes resembling neuropil {325, 1505,2291,2839}. The nuclei surrounding the periphery of the rosette are not regimented.

A pleomorphic cytological pattern is encountered in some pineocytomas {924}. This pattern is characterized by large ganglion cells and/or multinucleated giant cells with bizarre nuclei {1751,2067,2839}. The stroma of pineocytoma consists of a delicate network of vascular channels lined with a single layer of endothelial cells and supported by scant reticulin fibres. Microcalcifications are occasionally seen but usually correspond to calcifications of the remaining pineal gland.

Proliferation

Mitotic figures are rare or absent {1505,1548}, even in pleomorphic cases {924}. The mean Ki-67 proliferation index is < 1% {137,925,1548}.

Electron microscopy

Ultrastructurally, pineocytomas are composed of clear cells and various numbers of dark cells joined with zonulae adherentes {1261,1297,1503,2119}. The cells extend tapering processes that occasionally terminate in bulbous ends. Their cytoplasm is relatively abundant and contains well-developed organelles. Pineocytoma cells share numerous ultrastructural features with normal mammalian pinealocytes, such as paired twisted filaments, annulate lamellae, cilia with a 9 + 0 microtubular pattern, microtubular sheaves, fibrous bodies, vesicle-crowned rodlets, heterogeneous cytoplasmic inclusions, and membrane whorls, as well as mitochondrial and centriolar clusters. Membrane-bound dense-core granules and clear vesicles are present in the cytoplasm and cellular processes. The cellular processes show occasional synapse-like junctions.

Immunophenotype

Pineocytomas usually show strong immunoreactivity for synaptophysin, NSE, and NFP. Variable staining has also been reported for other neuronal markers, including class III β-tubulin, the microtubule-associated protein tau, chromogranin A, and the neurotransmitter serotonin (5-HT) {615,1503,1505,1751, 2291,3510}. In pleomorphic cases, the gangliocytic cells usually express multiple neuronal markers, especially NFP. Expression of CRX, a transcription factor involved in the development and differentiation of pineal cell lineage, is an additional indication that these tumours are biologically linked to pinealocytes {2806, 650}.

Differential diagnosis

The wall of a pineal cyst may masquerade as a pineocytoma, especially when the pineal parenchyma has lost its normal lobular architecture and is distorted. The distinction may be difficult in small specimens. However, normal pineal parenchyma does not show pineocytomatous rosettes. Immunohistochemistry may be helpful in highlighting the typical layered architecture of the pineal cyst wall: an inner GFAP-positive piloid gliotic layer and an outer synaptophysin/NFP-positive pineal parenchymal layer. Unlike pineal parenchymal tumour of intermediate differentiation, pineocytoma does not show *KBTBD4* alterations {2490,1834}. The pleomorphic pattern of pineocytoma may be misinterpreted as ganglioglioma. However, pleomorphic pineocytoma does not show a neoplastic glial component, tumoural CD34 expression, or *BRAF* p.V600E mutation.

Cytology
Limited clinical relevance

Diagnostic molecular pathology
Pineocytomas do not show any recurrent genetic alterations but do have a distinct DNA methylation profile.

Box 5.01 Diagnostic criteria for pineocytoma

> *Essential:*
>
> Demonstration of pineal parenchymal differentiation by histopathological and immunophenotypic features (e.g. positivity for synaptophysin)
>
> **AND**
>
> Absence of criteria qualifying for the diagnosis of pineal parenchymal tumour of intermediate differentiation or pineoblastoma
>
> **AND**
>
> Low proliferative/mitotic activity
>
> **AND**
>
> Pineal region location

Essential and desirable diagnostic criteria
See Box 5.01.

Staging
Not relevant

Prognosis and prediction
The clinical course of pineocytomas is characterized by a long interval between onset of symptoms and surgery {325}. The reported 5-year survival rate of patients with pineocytoma ranges from 86% to 91% {896,2838}. In one series, the 5-year event-free survival rate was 100% {896}. Extent of surgical resection is considered to be the major prognostic factor {600}.

Pineal parenchymal tumour of intermediate differentiation

Hasselblatt M
Huang A
Jones DTW
Orr BA
Snuderl M
Vasiljevic A

Definition

Pineal parenchymal tumour of intermediate differentiation (PPTID) is a tumour of the pineal parenchyma that is intermediate in malignancy between pineocytoma and pineoblastoma, composed of diffuse sheets or large lobules of monomorphic round cells that appear more differentiated than those observed in pineoblastoma (CNS WHO grade 2 or 3).

ICD-O coding

9362/3 Pineal parenchymal tumour of intermediate differentiation

ICD-11 coding

2A00.20 & XH1S48 Tumours of the pineal gland or pineal region & Pineal parenchymal tumour of intermediate differentiation

Related terminology

Not recommended: malignant pineocytoma; pineocytoma with anaplasia; pineoblastoma with lobules.

Subtype(s)

None

Localization

PPTIDs occur in the pineal region.

Clinical features

The clinical presentation is similar to that of other tumours of the pineal parenchyma (see under *Pineocytoma*, p. 243).

Imaging

PPTIDs usually appear larger and more heterogeneous than pineocytomas, and they often demonstrate local invasion {1690}.

Spread

PPTIDs have the potential for local recurrence and craniospinal dissemination {896,1427,3396,3554}.

Epidemiology

PPTIDs account for approximately 45% of all pineal parenchymal tumours {137,1427,3510,3612}. Median patient age is 33 years (range: 3.5–64 years). There is a slight female preponderance (M:F ratio: 0.8:1) {999,1427,1505,3510}.

Etiology

No syndromic associations or genetic susceptibilities have been reported.

Pathogenesis

Cell of origin

The histogenesis of PPTID has been linked to the pinealocyte.

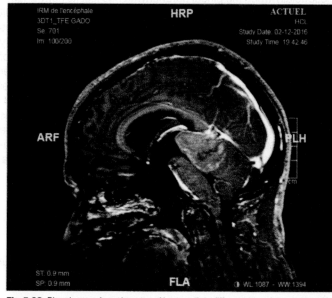

Fig. 5.06 Pineal parenchymal tumour of intermediate differentiation. A tumour located in the pineal region shows mild and heterogeneous contrast enhancement with invasion of the tectal plate and compression of the aqueduct of Sylvius, mesencephalon, pons, and cerebellar vermis (T1 gadolinium).

Genetic profile

Small in-frame insertions of *KBTBD4* are recurrent and characteristic {1834}. PPTIDs have relatively flat copy-number profiles, with some cases showing broad gains or losses {2490,2668}.

On DNA methylation profiling, PPTID as a distinct molecular subgroup can be separated into two further subtypes: PPTID-A and PPTID-B {2490}. The prognostic significance of these molecular subgroups requires further evaluation.

Macroscopic appearance

The macroscopic appearance is similar to that of pineocytomas.

Histopathology

PPTID may exhibit two architectural patterns: diffuse (neurocytoma- or oligodendroglioma-like) and/or lobulated (with vessels delineating vague lobules) {1505}. PPTID is a potentially aggressive neoplasm and is characterized by moderate to high cellularity. The neoplastic cells usually harbour round nuclei showing mild to moderate atypia and salt-and-pepper chromatin. The cytoplasm of cells in PPTID is more easily distinguishable than in pineoblastoma.

Grading

The biological behaviour of PPTIDs is variable. Although the majority correspond to CNS WHO grade 2, more aggressive cases may correspond to grade 3, but definite histological grading criteria remain to be defined.

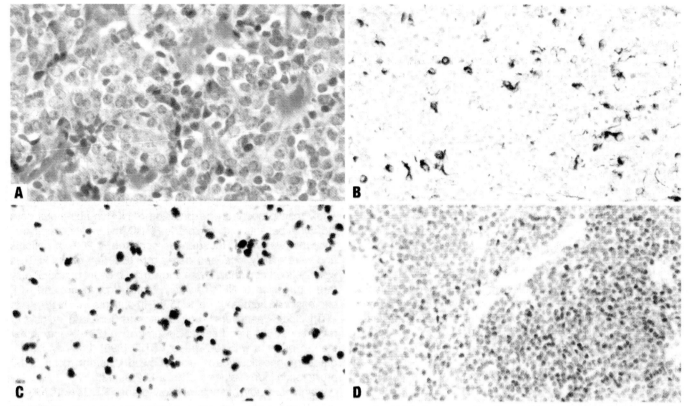

Fig. 5.07 Pineal parenchymal tumour of intermediate differentiation. **A** Tumour cells are round and relatively monomorphic, with a conspicuous cytoplasm. Nuclei are round to oval with a finely dispersed chromatin and a small nucleolus. **B** A few neoplastic cells show cytoplasmic immunoexpression of NFP. **C** In this example, the Ki-67 proliferation index is about 15%. **D** Diffuse nuclear immunoexpression of CRX, consistent with pineal differentiation.

Proliferation

Mitotic activity is low to moderate {1505}. The Ki-67 proliferation index ranges from 3.5% to 16.1% {137,1427,2668,3554,3612}.

Immunophenotype

PPTIDs usually stain positively for synaptophysin {137,999,1427, 1505}. Labelling for NFP and chromogranin A is variable {1503, 1505,3235,3510}. PPTIDs typically show diffuse (> 50% of cells) nuclear expression of CRX, a transcription factor involved in the differentiation of retinal and pineal lineages {650}.

Differential diagnosis

Histologically, PPTID may resemble central neurocytoma. Both have a sheet-like architecture, monomorphic round cells, and diffuse synaptophysin immunopositivity. However, PPTID does not express NeuN. Checking the imaging is critical, because a tumour in the pineal region resembling neurocytoma is most likely a primary pineal parenchymal tumour.

The histology of PPTID may also be confused with that of oligodendroglioma. PPTID does not express OLIG2 or show the typical molecular alterations of oligodendroglioma, such as IDH mutations and 1p/19q codeletion.

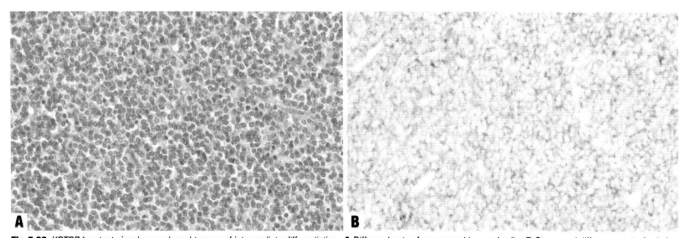

Fig. 5.08 *KBTBD4*-mutant pineal parenchymal tumour of intermediate differentiation. **A** Diffuse sheets of monomorphic round cells. **B** Strong and diffuse synaptophysin immunopositivity.

Box 5.02 Diagnostic criteria for pineal parenchymal tumour of intermediate differentiation

---

Essential:

Demonstration of pineal parenchymal differentiation by histopathological and immunophenotypic features (e.g. positivity for synaptophysin)

AND

Increased proliferative/mitotic activity

AND

Absence of criteria qualifying for the diagnosis of pineoblastoma

AND

Pineal region location

AND (for unresolved cases)

DNA methylation profiling

Desirable:

Molecular demonstration of *KBTBD4* in-frame insertions

Mixed pineocytoma–pineoblastoma, composed of clearly delineated areas of pineoblastoma admixed with well-demarcated areas of pineocytoma {2067,2839}, should not be diagnosed as PPTID (see *Pineoblastoma*, p. 249).

Cytology

Insufficient data available

Diagnostic molecular pathology

Although a morphological diagnosis is still acceptable in the absence of molecular data, evidence of a *KBTBD4* alteration is considered highly desirable for the diagnosis of PPTID. The finding of this alteration in what appears to be another pineal parenchymal tumour type histologically, or conversely the absence of this alteration in a tumour otherwise resembling PPTID, should prompt careful consideration as to whether an alternative diagnosis may be more suitable.

Essential and desirable diagnostic criteria

See Box 5.02.

Staging

No staging system has been defined.

Prognosis and prediction

In 29 studies including 127 patients with PPTID, median overall survival was 14 years, and the 5-year overall survival rate was 84% {1996}. Median progression-free survival was 5.2 years, and the 5-year progression-free survival rate was 52% {1996}; recurrences often involved spinal/leptomeningeal dissemination {1996}.

In one study, low-grade PPTIDs were defined as tumours with a low mitotic count and expression of NFP in numerous cells {1505}. In patients with low-grade PPTID, the 5-year overall survival rate was 74%. Recurrences occurred in 26% of patients and were mainly local and delayed {896}. High-grade PPTIDs were defined as tumours with a low mitotic count but no or only rare expression of NFP, or with a high mitotic count and NFP expression in numerous cells {1505}. In patients with high-grade PPTID, the 5-year overall survival rate was 39%, and the risks of recurrence (56%) and spinal dissemination (28%) were higher than in patients with low-grade PPTID {896}. Low- and high-grade prognostic groups also showed different mean Ki-67 proliferation index values (5.2% vs 11.2%) {925}.

In another study, patients with low-grade PPTIDs (with a Ki-67 proliferation index of < 5%) had better overall survival and progression-free survival than did those with high-grade PPTIDs (with a Ki-67 proliferation index of ≥ 5%) {3554}.

The prognostic role of mitotic count, NFP immunopositivity, and Ki-67 proliferation index requires confirmation by further studies, and the prognostic role of molecular subgrouping remains to be determined; consequently, there are currently no recommended grading criteria for PPTID.

Pineoblastoma

Hasselblatt M
Huang A
Jones DTW
Orr BA
Snuderl M
Vasiljevic A

Definition
Pineoblastoma is a poorly differentiated cellular embryonal neoplasm arising in the pineal parenchyma (CNS WHO grade 4).

ICD-O coding
9362/3 Pineoblastoma

ICD-11 coding
2A00.20 & XH1ZH1 Tumours of the pineal gland or pineal region & Pineoblastoma

Related terminology
None

Subtype(s)
Pineoblastoma, miRNA processing-altered_1; pineoblastoma, miRNA processing-altered_2; pineoblastoma, *RB1*-altered (pineal retinoblastoma); pineoblastoma, MYC/FOXR2-activated

Localization
Pineoblastomas are found in the pineal region.

Clinical features
The clinical presentation is similar to that of other tumours of the pineal parenchyma (see under *Pineocytoma*, p. 243).

Imaging
Pineoblastomas are often detected as large tumours, frequently showing invasion of surrounding structures and resulting in obstructive hydrocephalus {571,2203,2958,2645,3195}. On CT, pineoblastomas are usually slightly hyperdense with postcontrast enhancement {571,2203}. On T1-weighted MRI, tumours are often hypointense to isointense, with heterogeneous contrast

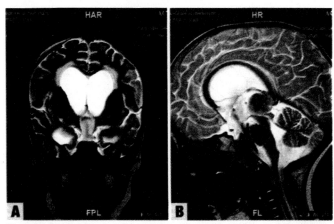

Fig. 5.09 Pineoblastoma. **A** This patient has obstructive triventricular hydrocephalus (T2-weighted MRI). **B** A tumour located in the pineal region appears mildly hypointense on T2-weighted MRI.

enhancement. On T2-weighted images they are typically isointense to mildly hyperintense {571,2203,2645,3195}.

Spread
Craniospinal dissemination is observed in 25–33% of patients {896,1838,3139,3325}.

Epidemiology
Pineoblastomas account for approximately 35% of all pineal parenchymal tumours {137,1505,2839,3325,3510}. They can arise at any age but mostly occur in children. The median patient age reported in a recent consensus paper {1913A} was 6 years (range: 0–41.5 years), in contrast to 33 years for pineal parenchymal tumour of intermediate differentiation. The median patient ages for the molecularly defined subtypes of

Table 5.01 Clinical and molecular features of pineoblastoma subtypes

	Pineoblastoma subtype			
	miRNA processing-altered_1	**miRNA processing-altered_2**	**RB1-altered (pineal retinoblastoma)**	**MYC/FOXR2-activated**
Median patient age	8.5 years	11.6 years	2.1 years	1.3 years
Cancer predisposition	*DICER1* syndrome	*DICER1* syndrome	Hereditary retinoblastoma	None
Molecular features	Copy-number alterations; mutually exclusive mutations targeting *DICER1, DROSHA,* or *DGCR8*	Copy-number alterations; mutually exclusive mutations targeting *DICER1, DROSHA,* or *DGCR8*	*RB1* alterations	*MYC* amplification and activation; chromosome 16q losses; FOXR2 overexpression
Median OS	10.4 years	Not reached	2.8 years	1.2 years
5-year OS rate	68%	100%	29%	23%
5-year PFS rate	54%	93%	27%	13%

PFS, progression-free survival; OS, overall survival.

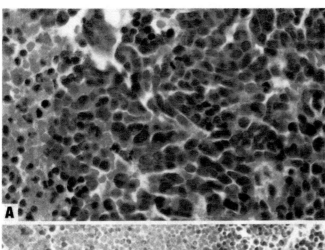

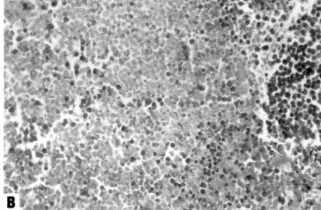

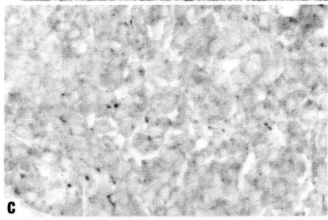

Fig. 5.10 Pineoblastoma. **A** This is a highly cellular tumour composed of small cells with a high N:C ratio; atypical, angular, hyperchromatic nuclei; and frequent mitoses and apoptotic bodies. **B** These tumours frequently show areas of necrosis. **C** There is diffuse expression of synaptophysin with paranuclear dot–like reactivity.

pineoblastoma are shown in Table 5.01 (p. 249). There is a slight female predominance, with an M:F ratio of 0.7:1.

Etiology

Genetic susceptibility

Pineoblastomas can occur in patients with familial (bilateral) retinoblastoma – a condition called trilateral retinoblastoma {703} – and there is a strong association with *DICER1* germline mutations {706,2769}. Cases in patients with familial adenomatous polyposis have also been reported {1020,1404}.

Pathogenesis

Cell of origin

Pineoblastomas share morphological and immunohistochemical features with cells of the developing human pineal gland and retina.

Genetic profile

Cytogenetic studies have shown structural alterations of chromosome 1 and losses involving chromosomes 9, 13, and 16 {385,2115,2668,2761} (see the *Diagnostic molecular pathology* subsection below).

Macroscopic appearance

Pineoblastomas are soft, friable, and pinkish grey {325,2826}. Haemorrhage and/or necrosis may be present.

Histopathology

Pineoblastomas resemble other embryonal tumours of the CNS and are composed of highly cellular, patternless sheets of densely packed small cells. The cells feature somewhat irregular nuclear shapes, a high N:C ratio, hyperchromatic nuclei with an occasional small nucleolus, scant cytoplasm, and indistinct cell borders. The diffuse growth pattern is interrupted only by occasional rosettes. Pineocytomatous rosettes are absent, but Homer Wright and Flexner–Wintersteiner rosettes may be seen. Flexner–Wintersteiner rosettes indicate retinoblastic differentiation, as do highly distinctive but infrequently occurring fleurettes. Necrosis is common and mitotic activity is generally high {1297,1505,2119,2839}. The mean Ki-67 proliferation index in pineoblastoma ranges from 23.5% to 50.1% {137,925,999, 2668}.

Mixed pineocytoma–pineoblastoma

Mixed pineocytoma–pineoblastoma is a somewhat controversial neoplasm showing a biphasic pattern with distinct alternating areas resembling pineoblastoma and pineocytoma. Areas resembling pineocytoma must be distinguished from overrun normal parenchyma {1297,2067,2291,2839}.

Pineal anlage tumours

Pineal anlage tumours are extremely rare neoplasms of the pineal region. They are often considered a subtype of pineoblastoma because of their pineal region localization, a pineoblastoma-like tumour component, and an aggressive clinical course. Historically, pineal anlage tumours were named after the histological features they share with melanotic neuroectodermal tumour of infancy (or retinal anlage tumour, a benign tumour typically located in the maxilla). Pineal anlage tumours are characterized by a combination of neuroectodermal and heterologous ectomesenchymal components. The neuroepithelial component is characterized by pineoblastoma-like sheets or nests of small round blue cells, neuronal ganglionic/glial differentiation, and/or melanin-containing epithelioid cells. The ectomesenchymal component contains rhabdomyoblasts, striated muscle, and/or cartilaginous islands {42,253,2849}. Two cases diagnosed as pineal anlage tumour were classified by DNA methylation profiling in the "pineoblastoma, MYC/FOXR2-activated" group {1865,1913A} and another showed molecular features of an infantile cerebellar tumour resembling embryonal tumour with multilayered rosettes, with *DICER1* mutation {3259}.

Immunophenotype

Pineoblastomas stain positively for synaptophysin and NSE. Staining for NFP and chromogranin A is less frequent than in pineocytomas {1505,2067,3510}. SMARCB1 staining is consistently retained {2116}

Differential diagnosis

The histopathology of pineoblastomas is not distinctive, as they are composed of sheets of poorly differentiated embryonal neoplastic cells. Confirming the location of the tumour in the pineal region is thus a first critical step in ruling out other non-pineal embryonal tumours, especially medulloblastomas. Nuclear expression of SMARCB1 (INI1) and SMARCA4 (BRG1) is retained in pineoblastomas, allowing their distinction from atypical teratoid/rhabdoid tumour. Pineoblastomas are typically negative for LIN28A, a marker of embryonal tumour with multilayered rosettes. Pineoblastomas typically show diffuse (> 50% of cells) nuclear expression of CRX, a transcription factor involved in the differentiation of retinal and pineal lineages {650}. Unlike pineal parenchymal tumours of intermediate differentiation, pineoblastomas do not show *KBTBD4* alterations {2490,1834}.

Cytology

Cerebrospinal fluid cytology is used in staging. Cerebrospinal fluid dissemination is characterized by clusters of poorly differentiated cells with round, hyperchromatic nuclei and scant cytoplasm {3325}.

Diagnostic molecular pathology

Copy-number alterations and/or mutually exclusive mutations targeting *DICER1*, *DROSHA*, or *DGCR8* have been described {706,2976,1865,2490,1913}. DNA methylation profiling segregates pineoblastoma into four molecular subgroups showing distinct genetic and clinical features {1865,2490,1913}:

Pineoblastoma, miRNA processing-altered_1 arises in children and is characterized by copy-number alterations and/or mutually exclusive mutations targeting *DICER1*, *DROSHA*, or *DGCR8*, which cause aberrant microRNA processing {1865, 2490,1913}.

Pineoblastoma, miRNA processing-altered_2 arises mainly in somewhat older children and is also characterized by copy-number alterations and/or mutually exclusive mutations targeting *DICER1*, *DROSHA*, or *DGCR8*, which cause aberrant microRNA processing {1865,2490,1913}.

Pineoblastoma, *RB1*-altered arises in infants, shows similarities with retinoblastoma, and includes cases of trilateral retinoblastoma as well as sporadic pineal tumours with *RB1* alterations {1865,2490}.

Pineoblastoma, MYC/FOXR2-activated arises in infants and exhibits recurrent focal gains or amplifications affecting the *MYC* region as well as chromosome 16q losses {1865,2490}. *MYC* activation and overexpression of FOXR2 are characteristic features {2490}.

Recently, WNT-activated embryonal tumours of the pineal region have been reported. Whether these tumours represent a novel pineoblastoma subgroup or ectopic WNT medulloblastomas remains uncertain {1914}.

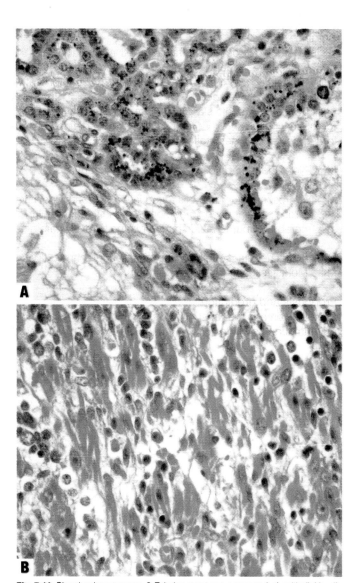

Fig. 5.11 Pineal anlage tumour. **A** Tubular structures composed of epithelioid cells containing melanin pigment. **B** Striated muscle cells.

Box 5.03 Diagnostic criteria for pineoblastoma

Essential:

Histopathological features of an embryonal tumour

AND

High proliferative/mitotic activity

AND

Pineal region location

Desirable:

Retained nuclear SMARCB1 (INI1) staining

DNA methylation profile of pineoblastoma subtype

Essential and desirable diagnostic criteria

See Box 5.03.

Staging

Clinical staging procedures include MRI examinations of the CNS with contrast agent. This is complemented by cerebrospinal fluid cytology at the time of diagnosis. The postoperative staging system developed by Chang and others in 1969 {519} (included in the Toronto staging system, endorsed by the Union for International Cancer Control [UICC]), which defines the following degrees of metastatic spread, is still being used:

M0 No evidence of gross subarachnoid or haematogenous metastasis
M1 Microscopic tumour cells found in the cerebrospinal fluid
M2 Gross nodular seeding demonstrated in the cerebellar/cerebral subarachnoid space or in the third or lateral ventricles
M3 Gross nodular seeding in the spinal subarachnoid space
M4 Metastasis outside the cerebrospinal axis

Prognosis and prediction

Pineoblastoma is the most aggressive of the pineal parenchymal tumours, as evidenced by the occurrence of craniospinal seeding and (rarely) extracranial metastasis {896,1297,1435, 2839}. Overall survival is short; older studies reported median values ranging from 1.3 to 2.5 years {521,896,2067}, but recent studies have reported improved median overall survival times reaching 4.1–8.7 years {893,1451}. Similarly, reported 5-year overall survival rates vary from 10% to 81%. Disseminated disease at the time of diagnosis (as determined by cerebrospinal fluid examination and MRI of the spine) {521,893,3139}, young patient age {801,1311,3139}, and partial surgical resection {1451,1838,3139} are negative prognostic predictors. Radiotherapy seems to positively affect prognosis {893,1838,2839}. The 5-year survival of patients with trilateral retinoblastoma syndrome has increased over the past few decades, probably due to better chemotherapy regimens and earlier detection of pineal disease {703}.

The prognostic value of molecular subgrouping is high, as shown in Table 5.01 (p. 249) {1865,2490,1913}.

The recently described WNT-activated embryonal tumours of the pineal region have a good prognosis. At median follow-up of 3 years (range: 0.8–12.8 years), all patients were alive without disease ($n = 5$) or with stable residual disease ($n = 2$) {1914}.

Papillary tumour of the pineal region

Hasselblatt M
Huang A
Jones DTW
Orr BA
Snuderl M
Vasiljevic A

Definition
Papillary tumour of the pineal region (PTPR) is a neuroepithelial tumour characterized by a combination of papillary and solid areas, with epithelial-like cells and immunoreactivity for cytokeratins (CNS WHO grade 2 or 3).

ICD-O coding
9395/3 Papillary tumour of the pineal region

ICD-11 coding
2A00.20 & XH3904 Tumours of the pineal gland or pineal region & Papillary tumour of the pineal region

Related terminology
None

Subtype(s)
None

Localization
PTPRs are located in the pineal region.

Clinical features
The clinical features of PTPRs are similar to those of other pineal parenchymal tumours (see under *Pineocytoma*, p. 243).

Imaging
PTPRs appear as well-circumscribed heterogeneous masses composed of cystic and solid portions. Aqueductal obstruction with hydrocephalus is a frequent associated finding {97,2547, 2664,2816}. Intrinsic T1 hyperintensity {499,517,2816} may be related to secretory material {517}, but this association remains controversial {97,1627}. Postcontrast enhancement is heterogeneous.

Spread
PTPRs are characterized by frequent local recurrence. Spinal dissemination may occur {895,1627}.

Epidemiology
There are no incidence data for these rare tumours. PTPRs occur in children and adults. Reported patient ages range from 1 to 71 years, with a median of 35 years. There is no sex predilection {921,923,1146,1249,1281}.

Etiology
Unknown

Pathogenesis
Cell of origin
Immunohistochemical findings and ultrastructural demonstration of ependymal, secretory, and neuroendocrine organelles suggest that PTPR may originate from remnants of the specialized ependymal cells of the subcommissural organ {1502}. Further evidence for a putative origin from specialized ependymocytes of the subcommissural organ comes from high levels of expression of genes expressed in the subcommissural organ, including *SPDEF*, *ZFHX4*, *RFX3*, *TTR*, and *CALCA* {922,1283}.

Genetic profile
Recurrent chromosomal imbalances include losses from chromosome 10 as well as gains on chromosomes 4 and 9 {1196, 1249,1283}. Genetic alterations of *PTEN* have been reported {1146}.

On DNA methylation profiling, PTPR as a distinct molecular subgroup can be separated into two further subtypes: PTPR-A and PTPR-B {1283,2490}. The prognostic significance of these molecular subgroups needs further evaluation.

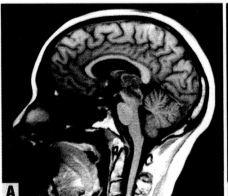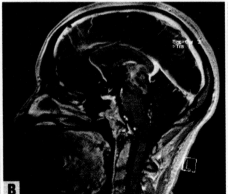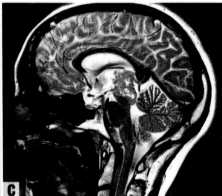

Fig. 5.12 Papillary tumour of the pineal region. **A** Sagittal, T1-weighted MRI showing a heterogeneous tumour in the pineal region. **B** Sagittal, contrast-enhanced, T1-weighted MRI showing a heterogeneously enhancing tumour of the pineal region. **C** Sagittal, T2-weighted MRI showing some cystic areas in a tumour of the pineal region.

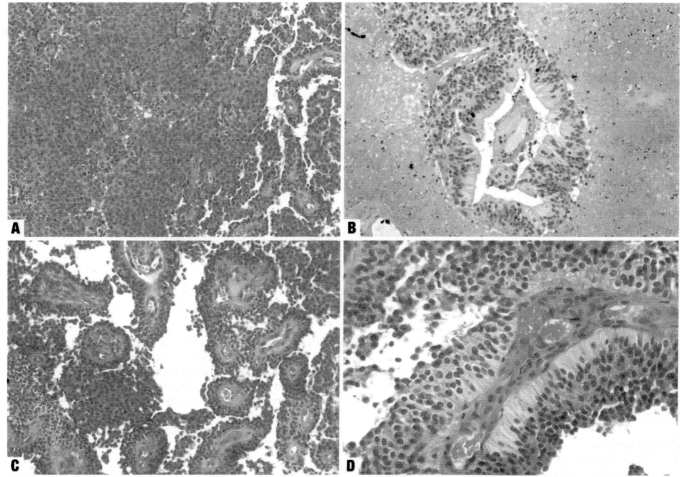

Fig. 5.13 Papillary tumour of the pineal region. **A** Papillary structures, which may alternate with diffuse solid areas. **B** Neoplastic cells, detached from the papillary vascularized core, create an apparent clear perivascular space. Note the extensive necrosis in this case. **C** Tumour architecture is characterized by a variable number of papillary structures. **D** Papillae are covered by large, columnar, epithelial-like cells.

Macroscopic appearance

PTPRs appear as well-circumscribed tumours, grossly indistinguishable from pineocytomas.

Histopathology

PTPR is an epithelial-looking tumour with papillary features and more densely cellular areas, often exhibiting ependymal-like differentiation (true rosettes and tubes). PTPR may exhibit a prominent papillary architecture or, conversely, a more solid morphology in which papillae are barely recognizable {920,1281}. In papillary areas, the vessels are covered by layers of large, pale to eosinophilic, columnar cells. In cellular areas, cells with a somewhat clear or vacuolated cytoplasm (and occasionally with an eosinophilic PAS-positive cytoplasmic mass) may also be seen. The nuclei are round to oval, with stippled chromatin; pleomorphic nuclei may be present. Necrotic foci may be seen. Vessels are hyalinized and often have a pseudoangiomatous morphology, with multiple lumina {920}. There is clear demarcation between the tumour and the adjacent pineal gland.

Grading

The biological behaviour of PTPRs is variable. Although the majority correspond to CNS WHO grade 2, more aggressive cases may correspond to grade 3, but definite histological grading criteria remain to be defined.

Proliferation

Mitotic activity is moderate in most cases {1146,1502,920,1282}. In one series, the Ki-67 proliferation index ranged from 1.0% to 29.7% (median: 7.5%), and increased proliferative activity (defined as a Ki-67 proliferation index of ≥ 10%) was observed in 39% of cases {920}; in another series, Ki-67 ≥ 10% was observed in 40% of cases {1281}. High proliferative activity has been linked to younger patient age {923}.

Immunophenotype

The most distinctive immunohistochemical feature of PTPRs is their reactivity for cytokeratins (especially CK18), particularly in papillary structures. SPDEF is frequently expressed and has been proposed as a diagnostic marker {1283}. PTPRs also stain for vimentin, S100, NSE, MAP2, CD56, and transthyretin {1249, 2909}. GFAP expression is less common than in ependymomas, and focal membrane or dot-like EMA staining as encountered in ependymomas is rare {1249,1502,1750}. Neurofilament immunolabelling is never seen, whereas the neuroendocrine markers synaptophysin and chromogranin A are sometimes weakly and focally expressed {1502}. Most PTPRs are negative for Kir7.1,

E-cadherin (cadherin 1), and claudin-2, i.e. markers frequently present in choroid plexus tumours {920,923,1249}.

Differential diagnosis

Because of its epithelioid cytology and papillary architecture, PTPR may mimic pineal metastasis of adenocarcinoma. In this situation, clinical history and imaging workup of the patient should be carefully assessed and immunohistochemical studies performed accordingly (e.g. thyroid transcription factor 1 [TTF1], GATA3). Choroid plexus papilloma differs from PTPR by its straightforward epithelial morphology and conspicuous basement membrane. Unlike PTPR, choroid plexus tumours show frequent immunoexpression of E-cadherin and are typically CD56-immunonegative or only weakly positive {927}. Membranous staining for Kir7.1 is frequent in choroid plexus tumours, but rare in PTPR {1249}. In contrast to PTPRs, ependymomas usually stain positively for GFAP and lack CK18 expression. The diagnosis of a pineal parenchymal tumour may be considered in small specimens or solid forms of PTPR. The strong expression of synaptophysin and CRX in pineal parenchymal tumours allows their distinction from PTPR {650}.

Cytology
Limited clinical relevance

Diagnostic molecular pathology
DNA methylation profiling clearly distinguishes PTPR from ependymomas and pineal parenchymal tumours {1283}.

Essential and desirable diagnostic criteria
See Box 5.04.

Staging
Not relevant

Prognosis and prediction
The clinical course of PTPR is often complicated by local recurrences. In a retrospective multicentre study of 31 patients, tumour progression occurred in 72% of cases, and the estimated 5-year overall and progression-free survival rates were 73% and 27%, respectively {923}. Leptomeningeal seeding through the cerebrospinal fluid has been rarely reported {895}. Incomplete resection tended to be associated with decreased survival and with recurrence {923}. In an updated retrospective series of 44 patients, only gross total resection and younger patient age were associated with overall survival; radiotherapy and chemotherapy had no significant impact {895}. Another study, of 19 patients, also found no significant effect of clinical

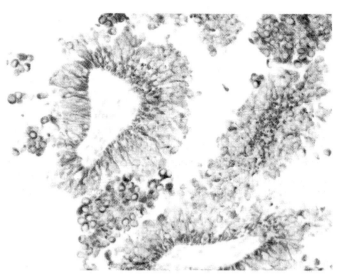

Fig. 5.14 Papillary tumour of the pineal region. Immunoexpression for CK18 typically predominates in perivascular areas.

Box 5.04 Diagnostic criteria for papillary tumour of the pineal region

Essential:

Papillary growth pattern with epithelial-like cells

AND

Characteristic immunohistochemical staining pattern (e.g. positivity for cytokeratins, SPDEF, CD56)

AND

Pineal region location

AND (for unresolved cases)

Confirmatory DNA methylation profiling

factors on overall or progression-free survival {1281}. In that series, increased mitotic activity was significantly associated with shorter progression-free survival. Increased proliferative activity was also associated with shorter progression-free survival: patients whose tumours had a Ki-67 proliferation index of ≥ 10% had a median progression-free survival time of 29 months (range: 0–64 months), versus 67 months (range: 44–90 months) for those whose tumours had a Ki-67 proliferation index of < 10%. The tumours of the 3 patients who succumbed to disease all showed increased mitotic and proliferative activity {1281}. The usefulness of mitotic count or proliferation index in defining a more aggressive subset of PTPRs requires confirmation in further studies. Recurrences may show higher proliferative activity {1196,1825}.

Desmoplastic myxoid tumour of the pineal region, *SMARCB1*-mutant

Hasselblatt M
Huang A
Jones DTW
Orr BA
Snuderl M
Vasiljevic A

Definition

Desmoplastic myxoid tumour (DMT) of the pineal region, *SMARCB1*-mutant, is a tumour showing desmoplasia and myxoid changes but lacking histopathological signs of malignancy, with alterations of the *SMARCB1* region on chromosome 22q11.

ICD-O coding

None

ICD-11 coding

2A00.20 Tumours of the pineal gland or pineal region

Related terminology

None

Subtype(s)

None

Localization

All 7 cases reported to date were localized in the pineal region.

Clinical features

The clinical features are similar to those of pineal parenchymal tumours (see under *Pineocytoma*, p. 243).

Epidemiology

The median age of 4 female and 3 male patients was 40 years (range: 15–61 years) {3185}.

Etiology

Unknown

Pathogenesis

Cell of origin

Unknown

Genetic profile

Apart from alterations affecting the *SMARCB1* region on 22q11, chromosomal alterations are rare and non-recurrent {3185}.

On DNA methylation profiling, DMT, *SMARCB1*-mutant, forms a distinct group located in close proximity to one of the molecular subgroups of atypical teratoid/rhabdoid tumour (AT/RT-MYC) and to poorly differentiated chordoma {3185}.

Macroscopic appearance

Insufficient data available

Histopathology

DMT, *SMARCB1*-mutant, is characterized by an admixture of variably dense cords of small to medium-sized oval to spindled and epithelioid cells embedded in a heavily collagenized matrix. Tumour cells are dispersed to a variable extent within a loose pale basophilic myxoid matrix. Fascicular and whorling growth patterns may be encountered, and irregularly shaped and elongated blood vessels with marked fibrosis are frequent. Scattered rhabdoid tumour cells are rare. Mitotic activity is exceptional (< 1 mitosis/mm²) {3185}

Grading

The biological behaviour of DMT, *SMARCB1*-mutant, seems to be less aggressive than that of atypical teratoid/rhabdoid tumour {3185}, but grading remains to be defined.

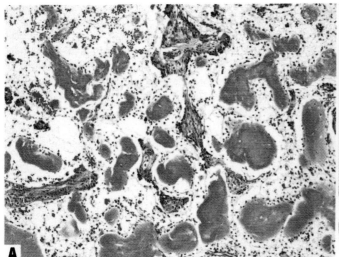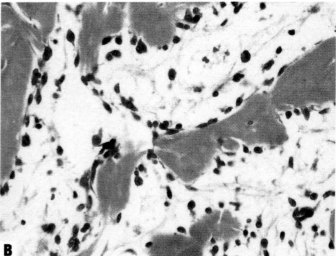

Fig. 5.15 Desmoplastic myxoid tumour of the pineal region, *SMARCB1*-mutant. **A** Tumour cells embedded in loose, pale basophilic myxoid matrix with dispersed heavily collagenized material. **B** Small to medium-sized oval to spindled and epithelioid cells.

Proliferation

The Ki-67 (MIB1) proliferation index is low (median: 3%), and only one tumour in a young patient showed higher proliferative activity (15%) {3185}.

Immunophenotype

Tumour cells show loss of nuclear SMARCB1 (INI1) expression. Expression of CD34 and EMA is often present {3185}.

Cytology

Insufficient data available

Diagnostic molecular pathology

Tumours should be assessed for SMARCB1 deficiency {3185}.

Essential and desirable diagnostic criteria

See Box 5.05.

Staging

Not relevant

Prognosis and prediction

Gross total resection was achieved in 4 of 7 patients, and 3 of 7 patients did not show evidence of residual disease on postoperative MRI {3185}. There was no evidence of metastatic disease in any patient. After a median observation time of 48 months, 3 patients were alive with stable disease, 1 patient had experienced tumour progression, and 3 patients had died from the disease {3185}. Prognostic markers have not yet been reported.

Box 5.05 Diagnostic criteria for desmoplastic myxoid tumour of the pineal region, *SMARCB1*-mutant

> **Essential:**
>
> Desmoplasia and myxoid changes
>
> **AND**
>
> Lack of histopathological signs of malignancy
>
> **AND**
>
> Loss of tumoural SMARCB1 expression
>
> **AND (for unresolved cases)**
>
> > Confirmatory DNA methylation profiling

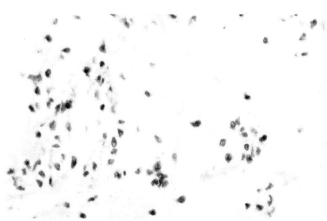

Fig. 5.16 Desmoplastic myxoid tumour of the pineal region, *SMARCB1*-mutant. Note loss of nuclear SMARCB1 staining in the tumour cells but not the non-neoplastic cells.

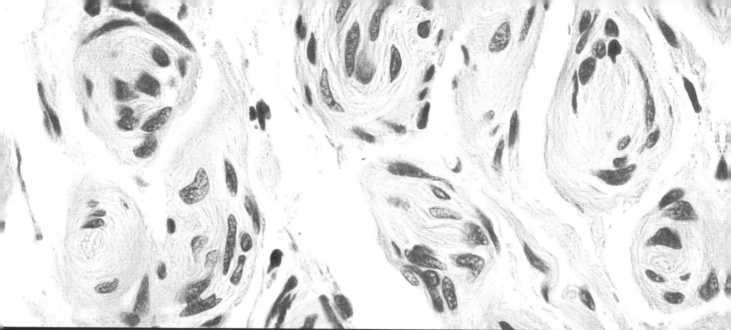

6

Cranial and paraspinal nerve tumours

Edited by: Figarella-Branger D, Lazar AJ, Perry A, von Deimling A

Schwannoma
Neurofibroma
Perineurioma
Hybrid nerve sheath tumours
Malignant melanotic nerve sheath tumour
Malignant peripheral nerve sheath tumour
Cauda equina neuroendocrine tumour (previously paraganglioma)

Cranial and paraspinal nerve tumours: Introduction

Perry A

Nerve sheath tumours are common throughout the craniospinal axis and may be encountered either sporadically or as part of a wide variety of tumour predisposition syndromes, including neurofibromatosis type 1 and type 2, schwannomatosis, and Carney complex. Whereas most are thought to arise from classic peripheral nervous system elements (such as Schwann cells and, less commonly, perineurial cells), the paragangliomas involve specialized neuroendocrine cells of the sympathetic and parasympathetic nervous system. Therefore, cauda equina neuroendocrine tumours (previously termed "CNS paragangliomas") are now discussed within this chapter, rather than with neuronal and mixed neuronal-glial tumours as done previously. We now know that a wide variety of pathogenic germline alterations predispose to familial paragangliomas, although those arising in the filum terminale / cauda equina region appear to be the exception to that rule, with recent data suggesting that they are biologically distinct from paragangliomas elsewhere in the body. Since the last edition of the WHO Classification of Tumours, it has similarly been appreciated that melanotic schwannoma is a highly distinct and frequently aggressive tumour type with unique genetic underpinnings that distinguish it from all other nerve sheath tumours, including schwannomas. Therefore, and in keeping with the changes in the soft tissue classification scheme, its name has been changed to "malignant melanotic nerve sheath tumour". The majority of both sporadic and Carney complex–associated malignant melanotic nerve sheath tumours have an inactivated *PRKAR1A* gene, so immunohistochemical loss of its protein product serves as a useful diagnostic surrogate. The current chapter also updates the genetic advances in malignant peripheral nerve sheath tumour, including useful biomarkers recently translated into molecular diagnostic tools. A growing body of evidence now suggests that epithelioid malignant peripheral nerve sheath tumour is also genetically unique. Therefore, it could potentially be separated out in future iterations, but for now it continues to be treated as a subtype of malignant peripheral nerve sheath tumour.

Schwannoma

Stemmer-Rachamimov AO
Jo VY
Reuss DE
Rodriguez FJ

Definition
Schwannoma is a benign nerve sheath tumour composed entirely or nearly entirely of differentiated neoplastic Schwann cells (CNS WHO grade 1).

ICD-O coding
9560/0 Schwannoma

ICD-11 coding
2A02.3 & XH98Z3 Benign neoplasm of cranial nerves & Schwannoma

Related terminology
Not recommended: neurilemmoma.

Subtype(s)
Ancient schwannoma; cellular schwannoma; plexiform schwannoma; epithelioid schwannoma; microcystic/reticular schwannoma

Localization
Common sites of origin are peripheral nerves in the skin and subcutaneous tissues of the head and neck, or along the flexor surfaces of the extremities. Spinal intradural extramedullary examples are also common and form dumbbell tumours when growing through neural foramina. Multiple paraspinal schwannomas are common in neurofibromatosis type 2 (NF2). Another frequent location is the vestibular division of the eighth cranial nerve, and bilateral involvement is a definitional criterion for NF2 {862}. Spinal intramedullary and CNS sites are rare {480}, as are cases involving viscera (such as the gastrointestinal tract) or bone {3343}.

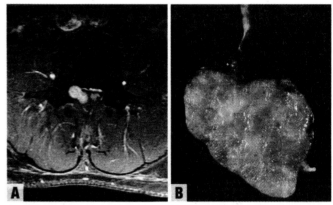

Fig. 6.01 Schwannoma. **A** T1-weighted MRI showing the characteristic dumbbell shape of a spinal root schwannoma. **B** Cut surface showing a globoid encapsulated tan-grey tumour with areas of xanthic change (yellow) and attached nerve.

Clinical features
Schwannomas are slow-growing tumours, often appearing as asymptomatic masses or incidental findings on imaging studies. Spinal schwannomas may elicit sensory or, less frequently, motor symptoms. Vestibular schwannomas often come to clinical attention with hearing loss and vertigo. Painful schwannomas may be associated with schwannomatosis.

Epidemiology
More than 90% of schwannomas are solitary and sporadic. Schwannomas affect people of all ages, but the peak incidence is in the fourth to sixth decades of life. There is no known sex or race predisposition.

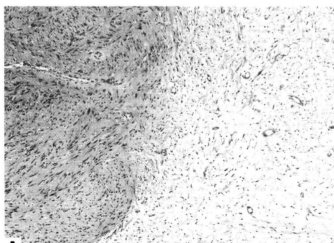
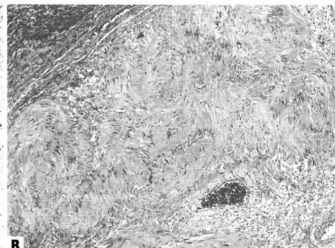

Fig. 6.02 Conventional schwannoma. **A** Compact Antoni A tissue (left) adjacent to loose Antoni B tissue (right). **B** Nuclear palisades, known as Verocay bodies, are a typical feature of schwannoma in Antoni A areas.

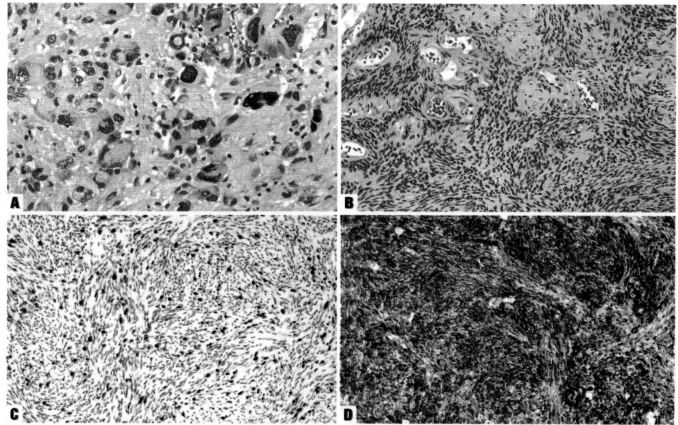

Fig. 6.03 Schwannoma. **A** Ancient schwannoma. Scattered bizarre, atypical nuclei are often considered to represent a degenerative change that does not impact prognosis. **B–D** Cellular schwannoma. **B** Marked hypercellularity and compact arrangement, which may prompt the consideration of sarcoma in the differential diagnosis. **C** The Ki-67 proliferation index is < 20% in most cases. **D** Diffuse S100 positivity helps distinguish the cellular schwannoma subtype from malignant peripheral nerve sheath tumour.

Etiology

The etiology of most sporadic schwannomas is unknown, although there is an established increased incidence associated with prior irradiation {2716,2565}. There is an association with NF2 or schwannomatosis in some cases (see *Pathogenesis*, below, as well as *Neurofibromatosis type 1*, p. 426; *Neurofibromatosis type 2*, p. 429; and *Schwannomatosis*, p. 434).

Pathogenesis

A causal relationship exists between schwannoma tumorigenesis and loss of expression of merlin (also called NF2 or schwannomin), the growth inhibitory protein product of the *NF2* tumour suppressor gene located at 22q12.2 {3031}. *NF2*-inactivating mutations have been detected in approximately 50–75% of sporadic cases {1437,1807,2305,1268}. Underlying genetic events are predominantly frameshift and nonsense mutations, with loss of the remaining wildtype allele on chromosome 22. Other common mutations involve the *LATS1*, *LATS2*, *ARID1A*, *ARID1B*, and *DDR1* genes, whereas a recurrent in-frame *SH3PXD2A::HTRA1* fusion is found in roughly 10% of cases {2305,31}.

Multiple schwannomas are a feature of NF2 and schwannomatosis, both of which can also occur in mosaic or segmental forms {292,1583}.

NF2-associated schwannomas commonly occur before the age of 30 years, whereas tumours in schwannomatosis usually manifest later. Bilateral vestibular schwannoma is a hallmark of NF2, often showing multifocal nerve involvement and a distinct nodular growth pattern. Patients may also develop multiple meningiomas (which are associated with increased morbidity and mortality) and spinal ependymomas {862}. NF2 is inherited in an autosomal dominant manner, with 50% of cases representing new or sporadic mutations.

Schwannomatosis is characterized by the presence of multiple schwannomas, mostly (but not invariably) in the absence of vestibular nerve involvement. Cranial and cutaneous nerves are infrequently affected. Tumours are often associated with pain. Germline mutations of either the *SMARCB1* or the *LZTR1* tumour suppressor gene are found in 69–86% of patients with familial schwannomatosis {2518,2966,2366} and 40% of patients with sporadic schwannomatosis {1583}. The tumorigenesis appears to be complex, given that these tumours arise from a four-hit mechanism that involves two genes: a germline *SMARCB1* or *LZTR1* mutation is followed by a somatic *NF2* mutation on the same chromosome 22, along with a deletion of the entire other chromosome 22, leading to biallelic inactivation of both tumour suppressor genes simultaneously. Not surprisingly, therefore, the somatic *NF2* mutation often differs among schwannomas from any one patient, as well as between the schwannomas of different family members.

Macroscopic appearance

Schwannomas are mainly solitary and globoid, with a smooth surface. Most measure < 100 mm in greatest dimension, but giant schwannomas (which are mostly encountered in the lumbosacral region) are larger. Fewer than half of all schwanno-mas have an evident attached nerve, which is most often small and draped over the tumour capsule. Except for those arising in CNS parenchyma, skin, viscera, and bone, the tumours are usually encapsulated. Sectioned tumours reveal firm, light-tan, glistening tissue, interrupted by white/yellow areas and/or patches of haemorrhage.

Histopathology

Conventional schwannoma is usually an encapsulated spin-dle cell tumour composed nearly entirely of well-differentiated Schwann cells. Schwannomas have a broad morphological range. The large majority are biphasic tumours with compact areas (Antoni A tissue) showing occasional nuclear palisad-ing (Verocay bodies), alternating with loosely arranged foci (Antoni B tissue). Cells of Antoni A tissue have modest eosino-philic cytoplasm; no discernible cell borders; and normochro-mic, elongated, tapered nuclei. Cytoplasmic nuclear inclu-sions, nuclear pleomorphism, and mitotic figures may be seen. Palisading (Verocay bodies) takes the form of parallel rows of Schwann cell nuclei separated by their aligned cell processes. Antoni B tissue commonly contains a cobweb-like network of tumour processes with collections of lipid-laden histiocytes and thick-walled, hyalinized blood vessels. Lymphoid aggregates are often present in a subcapsular distribution or at the periph-ery in unencapsulated tumours. A minority of schwannomas deviate from the description above. Eighth cranial nerve and intestinal schwannomas predominantly show Antoni A tissue. The most extreme deviation is seen in the morphological sub-types (see below).

Diffuse staining for S100 in cell nuclei and cytoplasm, which is more prominent in Antoni A areas than in Antoni B areas, is found in all tumours and subtypes. Similarly, SOX10 immunore-activity is usually extensive {2276,1556}. Expression of GFAP is less frequent and more variable. Retroperitoneal and mediastinal lesions are commonly positive for keratin AE1/AE3 due to cross-reactivity with GFAP {890}. In contrast to the lattice-like stain-ing pattern in neurofibromas, CD34 is commonly positive only in subcapsular areas, although a small subset of cases show more extensive positivity. Staining for NFP is helpful in identi-fying entrapped intratumoural axons, found in many sporadic

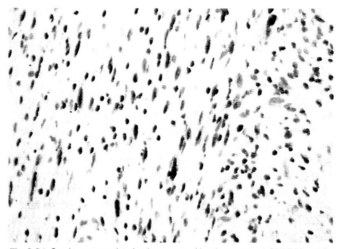

Fig. 6.04 Syndrome-associated schwannoma. Mosaic pattern of SMARCB1 (INI1) immunostaining, suggestive of a schwannoma arising in neurofibromatosis type 2 or schwannomatosis.

schwannomas, albeit most often at their periphery {2212}. EMA highlights perineurial cells in the capsule, if present.

Ancient schwannoma: This subtype differs from conven-tional schwannoma only by the presence of scattered atypical to bizarre-appearing nuclei, a feature that is often considered degenerative. Such cases may show extensive hyalinization or central ischaemic changes.

Cellular schwannoma: This subtype is composed exclusively or predominantly of Antoni A tissue and is devoid of Verocay bodies. The tumours most commonly involve large nerves and nerve plexuses at paravertebral sites and in the mediastinum, retroperitoneum, and pelvis {3475,3425,2441}. Cranial nerves are rarely affected {857}. In addition to the cells being closely packed, they are often hyperchromatic and mitotically active. Small areas of necrosis may be seen. These features may raise suspicion for malignant peripheral nerve sheath tumour (MPNST); however, the presence of conventional features of schwannoma (encapsulation, subcapsular lymphocytes, hya-linized blood vessels, and Schwannian whorls) aid in this dis-tinction. Cellular schwannoma shows Ki-67 labelling hotspots (rather than diffuse increases), often with an index of < 20% (but

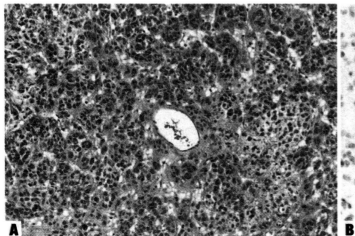
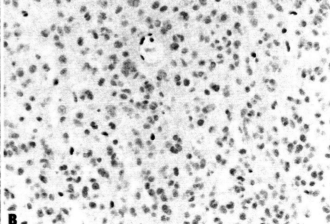

Fig. 6.05 Epithelioid schwannoma. **A** Multilobular growth pattern at low magnification. **B** Loss of SMARCB1 expression, which occurs in 40% of cases.

index values > 20% do not exclude the diagnosis), and p16 and H3 p.K28me3 (K27me3) positivity are retained {2441}.

Plexiform schwannoma: Tumours of this subtype, which can be conventional or cellular, often arise in skin or subcutaneous tissue, growing as thinly encapsulated plexiform or multinodular tumours {244,947}. Less frequently, these tumours can occur in the deep soft tissues {25}. The tumours come to clinical attention early in life, often in childhood and even at birth {3476}, with some predilection for the trunk and the head and neck region. Most are sporadic, but some occur in patients with NF2 or schwannomatosis. Biphasic plexiform schwannomas are more readily identifiable pathologically than are cellular examples. The tumours generally differ from conventional schwannoma in that they lack a well-formed capsule and thick-walled vessels.

Epithelioid schwannoma: Most epithelioid schwannomas arise as sporadic tumours, although some may be multiple and/ or arise in the setting of schwannomatosis {1242,1479}. Tumours show multilobulated growth of epithelioid cells arranged singly or in nests, set within a variably myxoid or hyalinized stroma. Tumour cells have amphophilic to eosinophilic cytoplasm and uniform, round nuclei with small or inconspicuous nucleoli, occasionally with pseudoinclusions. Some tumours may show conventional areas of spindled morphology, Antoni A or Antoni B tissue, and hyalinized vessels. Loss of SMARCB1 (INI1) expression is observed in approximately 40% of cases, associated with *SMARCB1* inactivation {1479,2820}. Some examples show increased cytological atypia, and rare cases undergo malignant transformation to epithelioid MPNST {1478}.

Microcystic/reticular schwannoma: This is the rarest subtype of schwannoma, and these tumours seem to preferentially arise in visceral sites, most commonly in the gastrointestinal tract {1891}. In visceral sites, lesions are often unencapsulated. Microscopically, tumours are characterized by a microcyst-rich network of interconnected bland spindle cells with eosinophilic cytoplasm, associated with a myxoid, fibrillary, and/or hyalinized collagenous stroma. Antoni A tissue is frequent, and tumours show strong and diffuse expression of S100. However, conventional features of hyalinized blood vessels, foamy histiocytes, and Verocay bodies are generally absent.

Other patterns: Although most syndrome-associated schwannomas are not histologically distinguishable from their sporadic counterparts, several clinicopathological clues may indicate a setting of NF2 or schwannomatosis: young patient age, multiple tumours, extensive longitudinal involvement of a nerve, a discontinuous or multinodular growth pattern, and a mosaic SMARCB1 immunostaining pattern (an admixture of positive and negative nuclei) {2421,443}. Some schwannomas feature predominantly small blue round cells, and may or may not have structures resembling Homer Wright rosettes or giant rosettes, which surround collagen fibres resembling those of low-grade fibromyxoid sarcoma; these cases are often referred to as neuroblastoma-like, although they lack increased proliferative activity and show a typical schwannoma immunoprofile {1728}. Another rare pitfall is a schwannoma with neuromelanin-like pigment accumulation that is positive on Fontana–Masson staining. Nevertheless, the histology is otherwise typical of

Box 6.01 Diagnostic criteria for schwannoma

Essential:

Histopathology of schwannoma, such as Antoni A or Antoni B areas

AND

Extensive S100 or SOX10 expression

Desirable:

Verocay bodies

Subcapsular lymphocytes

Hyalinized blood vessels

Lack of a lattice-like pattern of CD34 staining

Loss of SMARCB1 (INI1) expression (epithelioid schwannoma), or a mosaic pattern of SMARCB1 (INI1) expression (syndrome-associated schwannoma)

schwannoma, and the tumour cells are negative for more specific melanocytic markers, such as HMB45 {1000}; therefore, these should not be equated with the more aggressive, Carney complex / PRKAR1A–associated malignant melanotic nerve sheath tumour (previously termed "melanotic schwannoma").

Cytology

Aspirate smears of schwannoma typically yield cohesive syncytial fragments of spindle cells {532}. Within the fragments, variably wavy and bent tumour cell nuclei with tapered edges and fibrillary cytoplasm are seen. Nuclear pleomorphism or degenerative atypia and intranuclear inclusions may be seen. Schwannomas may be difficult to distinguish from other spindle cell neoplasms on cytological preparation alone, and their diagnosis requires correlation with core biopsy and/or immunohistochemical staining {40}.

Diagnostic molecular pathology

Loss of chromosome 22q and/or mutation of *NF2* in schwannomas are frequent but nonspecific molecular alterations. Schwannomas exhibit a distinct DNA methylation pattern {460, 2709,1676,31}.

Essential and desirable diagnostic criteria

See Box 6.01.

Staging

Not clinically relevant

Prognosis and prediction

Schwannomas are benign and do not usually recur if treated by gross total resection. Cellular and plexiform examples are least amenable to total removal and sometimes can only be debulked. Malignant transformation of conventional schwannoma is exceptionally rare; in the small number of cases reported to date, it has most often taken the form of epithelioid MPNST {3477,2058,476}. Less common examples feature foci of conventional MPNST, primitive neuroectodermal cells, rhabdomyosarcoma, and/or angiosarcoma {3477,3223,2058,1766, 476,27}.

Neurofibroma

Rodriguez FJ
Reuss DE
Stemmer-Rachamimov AO

Definition

Neurofibroma is a benign peripheral nerve sheath tumour consisting of mature neoplastic Schwann cells intermixed with non-neoplastic cell types. All subtypes are considered CNS WHO grade 1, except atypical neurofibromatous neoplasm of uncertain biological potential (ANNUBP), which is not assigned a grade.

ICD-O coding

9540/0 Neurofibroma
9550/0 Plexiform neurofibroma

ICD-11 coding

2A02.3 & XH87J5 Benign neoplasm of cranial nerves & Neurofibroma, NOS

Related terminology

None

Subtype(s)

Cellular neurofibroma; atypical neurofibroma / atypical neurofibromatous neoplasm of uncertain biological potential; plexiform neurofibroma; diffuse neurofibroma; nodular neurofibroma; massive soft tissue neurofibroma

Localization

The most common site is the skin, with predominant dermal involvement. Less often involved are more-deeply situated medium-sized nerves, a nerve plexus, or a major nerve trunk. Tumours may also arise from spinal nerve roots. Bilateral involvement of multiple spinal roots is typical of neurofibromatosis type 1 (NF1). Involvement of dorsal root ganglia may be present. Cranial nerve examples are exceptional.

Clinical features

Cutaneous neurofibromas are usually asymptomatic and most commonly occur as a mass. They are soft, mobile lesions without a particular anatomical predilection. Patients with deep tumours often present with motor or sensory symptoms in the distribution of the affected nerve. Least commonly, the tumour appears as a plaque-like, cutaneous and subcutaneous mass, mainly in the head and neck region, or as massive soft tissue enlargement of a body region such as the shoulder or pelvic girdle in patients with NF1. The presence of multiple neurofibromas, a plexiform neurofibroma, or a massive soft tissue neurofibroma should raise suspicion of underlying NF1.

Epidemiology

Neurofibromas are the most common peripheral nerve sheath tumours, and the majority are sporadic solitary lesions. Less often, they are multiple in individuals with NF1. Plexiform tumours are often congenital {2450}, whereas the localized cutaneous and localized intraneural neurofibromas in NF1 begin to appear at about 5–10 years of age. All demographic groups are affected and there is no sex predilection.

Etiology

Unknown

Pathogenesis

Conventional neurofibromas (including subtypes)
A biallelic genetic inactivation of the tumour suppressor gene *NF1* in a Schwann cell subpopulation is generally the only recurrent somatic event detectable {846,2450}. Complete loss of function of the *NF1* gene product, neurofibromin (NF1), is considered a prerequisite for tumour development. Neurofibromin (NF1) is a negative regulator of RAS signalling and

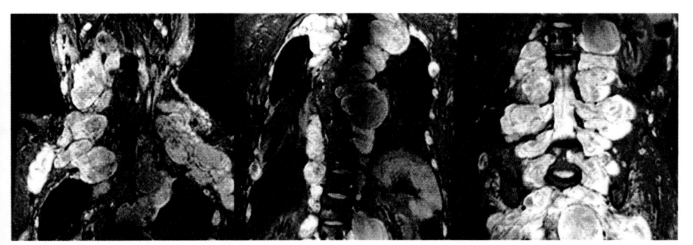

Fig. 6.06 Neurofibroma. Total spine MRI in a patient with neurofibromatosis type 1 with extensive bilateral paraspinal disease burden. Neurofibromas involve nearly every nerve root; also note the thoracic spine curvature defect (scoliosis).

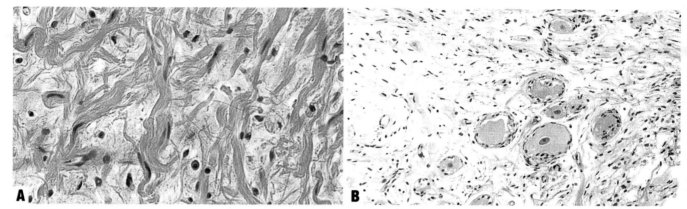

Fig. 6.07 Neurofibroma. **A** Note the wavy nuclei and cytoplasmic processes within a mucin-rich matrix and variable collagen. **B** Neurofibromas associated with the nerve root frequently extend to sensory ganglia, a finding that should not be mistaken for ganglioneuroma.

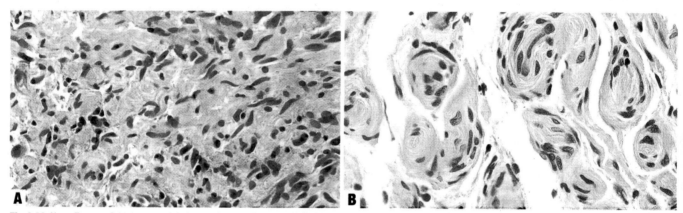

Fig. 6.08 Neurofibroma. **A** Increased cellularity (cellular neurofibroma) may be present usually as a focal finding in large, longstanding neurofibromas, but it lacks prognostic significance in the absence of other atypical features. **B** Concentric arrangements (whorls) of Schwann cells around axons, resembling onion bulbs.

acts as a RAS-GAP {2938}. The best-characterized signalling pathways active in the context of NF1 tumorigenesis are the RAS/RAF/MEK/ERK and PI3K/AKT/mTOR pathways, which play important roles in cell growth, survival, (de)differentiation, and migration {1923}. However, inactivation of *Nf1* alone was insufficient for neurofibroma development in several mouse models, because a contribution of the microenvironment is also required. There is increasing evidence that inflammatory signals mediated by various components of the microenvironment (e.g. mast cells, macrophages, lymphocytes, and dendritic cells), as well as Schwann cell interactions with axons, are important for tumour development {2552,948,1888,1887}. *NF1* haploinsufficiency of the microenvironment and nerve injury may promote tumorigenesis {1887,2660}. Dermal and plexiform neurofibromas exhibit distinct DNA methylation profiles, suggesting that they have different cells of origin {2709}. Consistent with this assumption, dermal skin–derived and Schwann cell precursors in embryonic nerve roots were identified as cells of origin for dermal and plexiform neurofibromas, respectively, in transgenic mouse models {552,1819}. More recently, it has been shown that *Nf1* loss in a neural crest–derived HOXB7 lineage cell population leads to both dermal and plexiform neurofibroma development in mice, and Hippo pathway activation acts as a modifier {553}.

Atypical neurofibroma / atypical neurofibromatous neoplasm of uncertain biological potential

Histological features of atypical neurofibroma (AN)/ANNUBP described in the setting of NF1 are strongly associated with deletions of the *CDKN2A* and/or *CDKN2B* locus encoding cell-cycle regulators p16 (p16INK4a), p14ARF (both encoded by *CDKN2A*), and/or p15 (p15INK4b; encoded by *CDKN2B*) {231, 2709,2109,474,2449}. One study showed an association of heterozygous *CDKN2A* and/or *CDKN2B* deletion with cytological atypia alone, and of homozygous *CDKN2A* and/or *CDKN2B* deletion with AN/ANNUBP histology, in different parts of the same tumour {474}. Another study showed additional heterozygous loss of *SMARCA2* in a portion of AN/ANNUBP, either as part of a larger deletion together with *CDKN2A* and/or *CDKN2B* or in the form of a separate, smaller deletion event {2449}.

Macroscopic appearance

Five macroscopic forms are distinguished: localized/nodular cutaneous, diffuse cutaneous, localized/nodular intraneural, plexiform intraneural, and massive diffuse soft tissue neurofibroma. Localized cutaneous neurofibromas can have a variety of gross appearances, including flat, sessile, globular, and pedunculated, whereas diffuse neurofibromas typically form large plaques {2335}. Intraneural neurofibromas occur as solitary fusiform masses or as ropy to worm-like growths when plexiform. Massive soft tissue neurofibromas range in shape from a relatively uniform regional soft tissue enlargement to

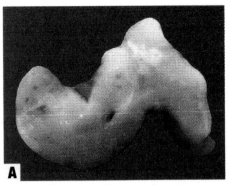
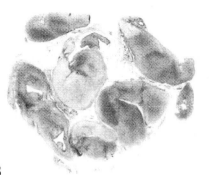
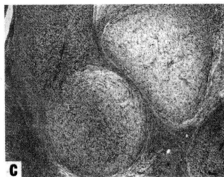

Fig. 6.09 Plexiform neurofibroma. **A** Gross appearance, demonstrating a tortuous architecture and a yellow, slightly heterogeneous cut surface. **B** By definition, involvement of multiple fascicles must be present, which imparts a multinodular appearance on low magnification. **C** Higher-power view of the adjacent enlarged nerve fibres.

pendulous bag-like or cape-like masses. The skin overlying massive tumours commonly shows hyperpigmentation. Cut surfaces of neurofibromas are most often uniformly tan or greyish-tan, glistening, mucoid, semitranslucent, and firm. On neuroimaging, ANNUBP or malignant peripheral nerve sheath tumour (MPNST) arising from a plexiform neurofibroma is suspected when there is a distinct growing nodule and/or increased PET activity {1307}.

Histopathology

Neurofibromas are characterized by cytologically bland spindle cells with thin, wavy nuclei representing the neoplastic Schwann cell, immersed in a variably loose myxoid stroma. The tumour cells are typically smaller than those of schwannoma. Stromal collagen is characteristic, colourfully likened in classic pathology descriptions to shredded carrots. A variety of other cells are also identifiable in neurofibroma, including perineurial and perineurial-like cells, fibroblasts, and mast cells. Even when localized at the gross level, neurofibromas typically lack a capsule and tend to infiltrate adjacent soft tissues and parent nerves, in contrast to the more circumscribed schwannoma. Nerve fibres are easily identifiable in intraneural subtypes, which are characterized by expansion of single (localized) or multiple (plexiform) nerve fascicles, but they may be rare in cutaneous and soft tissue locations. Entrapped ganglion cells may be conspicuous in neurofibromas that infiltrate dorsal root ganglia, and these should not be mistaken for ganglioneuroma. The individual fascicles are recognized by the outlining perineurium that is composed of EMA-positive cells.

Neurofibroma with atypia (ancient neurofibroma) is characterized by scattered bizarre nuclei with smudgy chromatin in the absence of other worrisome histological features. This is not considered a premalignant change, and should therefore not be confused with AN/ANNUBP as described below.

Cellular neurofibroma is defined by hypercellularity in the absence of other worrisome features. Increased cell crowding leads to a generally blue appearance at low magnification. These cellular neurofibromas may even show a fascicular growth pattern, but they lack the uniform cytological atypia, chromatin morphology, and mitotic activity seen in MPNST.

Plexiform neurofibroma is defined by its involvement of multiple nerve fascicles, each surrounded by perineurium. It most often involves a large nerve or plexus, imparting a bag-of-worms or ropy gross appearance. It is highly associated with NF1 and an increased risk of transformation to MPNST {2641}.

Pseudomeissnerian bodies or corpuscles are most often seen in diffuse and plexiform neurofibromas. They are delicate, round, layered structures and are strongly labelled by S100 immunohistochemistry. In the rare massive soft tissue subtype limited to individuals with neurofibromatosis, extensive infiltration of soft tissue and even skeletal muscle may be present. Pseudomeissnerian corpuscles are frequent in this subtype, as are cellular areas containing cells with high N:C ratios. Although they may be alarming at first glance, proliferative activity is very low. Other histological features that may be identifiable in individual neurofibromas include Schwann cell nodules, S100-positive onion bulb–like Schwann cell proliferations, melanin pigment,

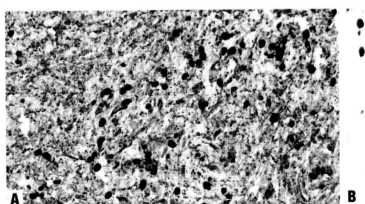

Fig. 6.10 Neurofibroma. Immunohistochemistry for Schwann cell markers usually labels most, but not all, cells in neurofibromas. **A** S100 cytoplasmic and nuclear staining. **B** SOX10 nuclear staining.

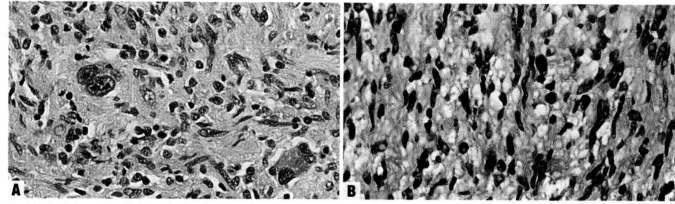

Fig. 6.11 Atypical neurofibromatous neoplasm of uncertain biological potential (ANNUBP). **A** Tumours designated as ANNUBP in patients with neurofibromatosis type 1 may have several worrisome features, including cytological atypia. **B** ANNUBP with increased cellularity and mitotic activity, but otherwise falling short of a malignant diagnosis.

metaplastic bone, epithelioid change, and even glandular differentiation.

Markers of mature Schwann cells highlight the neoplastic component, including S100, SOX10, and collagen IV, albeit to a lesser extent than in schwannomas. Non-neoplastic components are also intermixed, including scattered EMA-positive and GLUT1-positive perineurial cells, as well as CD34-positive stromal cells. Immunostaining for p16 typically highlights a subset of tumour cells of neurofibroma, whereas complete loss of expression is often seen in foci of ANNUBP and MPNST. NFP highlights entrapped axons. Staining for p53 is usually negative, and the Ki-67 proliferation index is low. H3 p.K28me3 (K27me3) is retained in neurofibroma and ANNUBP, but it is frequently lost in MPNST.

AN/ANNUBP is characterized by at least two of the following worrisome features: cytological atypia, hypercellularity, loss of neurofibroma architecture (on H&E and/or CD34 staining), and a mitotic count of > 0.2 mitoses/mm^2 and < 1.5 mitoses/mm^2 (equating to > 1 mitosis/50 HPF and < 3 mitoses/10 HPF of 0.51 mm in diameter and 0.2 mm^2 in area) {2109}. This is considered a premalignant or early malignant change that falls short of the diagnostic criteria for MPNST but is associated with increased risk of progression to MPNST {1307}. The term "ANNUBP" is applied to NF1-associated tumours and is not currently applicable to sporadic lesions.

Cytology
Intraoperative smears and FNA specimens are often paucicellular due to the increased collagen stroma in neurofibromas. Nevertheless, the presence of a mucin-rich background and small spindled cells with thin, wavy nuclei can provide diagnostic clues. Identification of mitoses is a worrisome finding.

Diagnostic molecular pathology
Molecular analyses do not have an established role in the diagnosis of neurofibroma. However, chromosomal copy-number profiling may be helpful for the evaluation of AN/ANNUBP (*CDKN2A* and/or *CDKN2B* deletion) and its differentiation from MPNST (complex, highly rearranged genome). Of

Box 6.02 Diagnostic criteria for neurofibroma

Essential:

Infiltrative, low-cellularity spindle cell neoplasm associated with a variably myxoid to collagenous stroma and a mixed cell population

Desirable:

S100 positivity in the Schwann cell population, with a lattice-like CD34 pattern, highlighting the stromal component

Intraneural localization

Patient has neurofibromatosis type 1

Atypical histological features (nuclear enlargement, hypercellularity, architectural loss, mitoses) for atypical neurofibroma / atypical neurofibromatous neoplasm of uncertain biological potential in the setting of neurofibromatosis type 1, often with loss of p16 expression

note, conventional dermal and plexiform neurofibromas, AN/ANNUBP, and MPNST all exhibit distinct DNA methylation profiles {2709}. The presence of *SUZ12* or *EED* mutations, leading to H3 p.K28me3 (K27me3) loss, is restricted to MPNST.

Essential and desirable diagnostic criteria
See Box 6.02.

Staging
Staging is not applicable, although one study showed that AN/ANNUBP is associated with low recurrence rates even when surgical margins are positive, suggesting that an overly aggressive surgical approach may not be necessary {255}.

Prognosis and prediction
Localized cutaneous neurofibromas are consistently benign. Plexiform neurofibroma, ANNUBP, and solitary intraneural neurofibroma arising in sizeable nerves can be precursor lesions of MPNST. The lifetime risk for MPNST in patients with NF1 is estimated at 9–13% {870}. Diffuse cutaneous neurofibromas rarely undergo malignant transformation {2821}. Massive soft tissue neurofibromas, invariably benign, may nevertheless overlie an intraneural or plexiform neurofibroma–derived MPNST.

Perineurioma

Paulus W
Reuss DE
Stemmer-Rachamimov AO

Definition
Perineurioma is a benign tumour composed of neoplastic perineurial cells (CNS WHO grade 1).

ICD-O coding
9571/0 Perineurioma

ICD-11 coding
2A02.3 & XH0XF7 Benign neoplasm of cranial nerves & Perineurioma, NOS

Related terminology
Not recommended: localized hypertrophic neuropathy (for intraneural perineurioma).

Subtype(s)
Soft tissue perineurioma; intraneural perineurioma; reticular perineurioma; sclerosing perineurioma

Localization
Intraneural perineuriomas primarily affect peripheral nerves of the extremities; cranial nerve lesions are rare {82,593}. Soft tissue perineuriomas are located in the deep soft tissue and are grossly not associated with nerves. One example involving the CNS arose within a lateral ventricle {1095}.

Clinical features
In intraneural perineurioma, progressive muscle weakness (with or without atrophy) is more frequent than sensory disturbances. Patients with soft tissue perineurioma present with nonspecific mass effects. Both intraneural and soft tissue perineuriomas have been described in patients with neurofibromatosis type 1 (NF1) and type 2 (NF2); however, these are rare cases and it is unclear whether there is a true association {2823,51,3423,2452}.

Epidemiology
Intraneural perineurioma typically affects young adults and adolescents {78}, although rarely it occurs in children {913}. There is no sex predilection. The incidence of soft tissue perineurioma peaks in middle-aged adults, and the M:F ratio is 1:2 {1345}. Both the intraneural and soft tissue subtypes of perineurioma are rare, accounting for approximately 1% of nerve sheath and soft tissue neoplasms, respectively. More than 50 cases of intraneural perineurioma and more than 300 cases of soft tissue perineurioma have been described {919,1093,1158,1345,2618}.

Etiology
Unknown

Pathogenesis
Like meningiomas, the majority of intraneural perineuriomas harbour missense mutations in *TRAF7*, affecting the WD40 domains of the protein. Some *TRAF7*-wildtype intraneural perineuriomas were shown to carry large genomic deletions/duplications, including deletions of 22q {1649}.

Soft tissue perineuriomas do not carry *TRAF7* mutations but commonly show chromosomal alterations. The most frequently observed alterations are deletions of 22q (including the *NF2* tumour suppressor gene) and deletions of 17q11 (encompassing the *NF1* tumour suppressor gene) as well as 2p deletions {477}. The sclerosing subtype of soft tissue perineurioma shows recurrent rearrangements or deletions of chromosome 10q {379}.

Macroscopic appearance
Intraneural perineurioma produces a segmental, several-fold enlargement of the affected nerve. Individual nerve fascicles appear coarse and pale. Most lesions are < 100 mm long, but one 400-mm-long sciatic nerve example has been reported {847}. Although multiple fascicles are often involved, a bag-of-worms plexiform growth is not seen. Involvement of two neighbouring spinal nerves has been reported {847}.

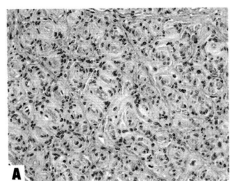 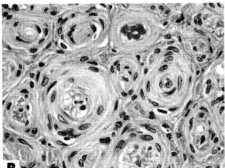 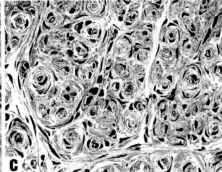

Fig. 6.12 Intraneural perineurioma. **A** Pseudo–onion bulbs and variable collagenization on cross-section. **B** High magnification view of pseudo–onion bulb formation. **C** On a toluidine blue–stained plastic section, myelinated axons are surrounded by concentric rings of perineurial cell processes (pseudo–onion bulbs).

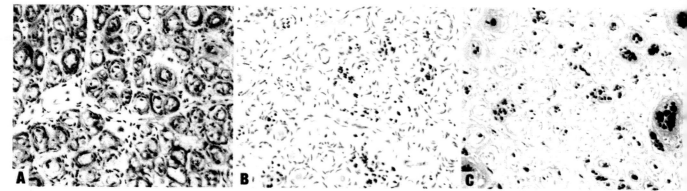

Fig. 6.13 Intraneural perineurioma. EMA staining highlights concentric layers of perineurial cells (**A**), NFP staining highlights entrapped centrally located axons (**B**), and S100 staining shows entrapped centrally located Schwann cells (**C**) in pseudo–onion bulbs.

Soft tissue perineurioma is solitary, generally small (< 70 mm), and well circumscribed but unencapsulated. The cut surface is firm and greyish white and occasionally myxoid.

Histopathology

Intraneural perineurioma consists of concentric layers of perineurial cells around axons, forming characteristic pseudo–onion bulbs. This distinctive architectural feature is best seen on cross-section, wherein fascicles vary in cellularity. Perineurial cells accumulate in the endoneurium, but the perineurium is often affected as well. Particularly large whorls can envelop numerous nerve fibres. In early lesions, axonal density and myelination may be almost normal, whereas in fully developed lesions, when most fibres are surrounded by perineurial cells and therefore widely separated, myelin is often scant or absent. At late stages, only Schwann cells without accompanying axons may remain at the centre of the perineurial whorls. Hyalinization may be prominent.

Soft tissue perineuriomas are composed of spindle cells with wavy or tapering nuclei, indistinct nucleoli, and bipolar cytoplasmic processes. They typically exhibit a storiform or whorled growth pattern. The stroma is usually collagenous. Mitoses are very rare to absent. Necrosis is typically absent. Degenerative features may include nuclear pleomorphism, multinucleated cells, and a myxoid matrix {1345}.

Immunohistochemically, tumour cells of intraneural and soft tissue perineurioma are consistently positive for EMA, which ranges from weak and focal to strong and diffuse {1345}; claudin-1 and GLUT1 are also often positive {951,3508}. CD34 is expressed in about 60% of soft tissue perineuriomas {1345}. Staining for S100, SOX10, and GFAP is negative.

Some rare subtypes such as reticular and sclerosing perineuriomas are described in the *Soft tissue and bone tumours* volume of this series. The very rare malignant perineurioma is usually considered a malignant peripheral nerve sheath tumour with perineurial differentiation {1318,2128} and is discussed in *Malignant peripheral nerve sheath tumour* (p. 273). Hybrid nerve sheath tumours may include a perineurioma component.

Cytology

There is little experience with cytological diagnosis of these lesions, but FNA specimens are said to be paucicellular, with smears containing fragments of myxoid stroma {1839}.

Diagnostic molecular pathology

Molecular analyses do not have an established role in the diagnosis of perineurioma. Because of the rareness of perineurioma, a reference group for its DNA methylation–based classification is not currently available.

Essential and desirable diagnostic criteria

See Box 6.03.

Staging

Not relevant

Prognosis and prediction

Long-term follow-up of intraneural perineuriomas indicates that they do not have a tendency to recur or metastasize. Radiological follow-up studies have shown that intraneural perineuriomas only rarely grow in length and do not grow to involve new nerves or nerve divisions, and that growth does not correlate with clinical progression {3456}.

Soft tissue perineuriomas are usually amenable to gross total removal. Recurrences are very infrequent, even in cases with histological atypia/degeneration, and there have been no reported metastases {919,1158}. Malignant progression of soft tissue perineurioma has not been documented. Malignant perineurial tumours with high mitotic activity and poor prognosis including metastases correspond to malignant peripheral nerve sheath tumours {1318}.

Hybrid nerve sheath tumours

Stemmer-Rachamimov AO
Reuss DE

Definition
Hybrid nerve sheath tumours are benign peripheral nerve sheath tumours with combined features of more than one conventional type (neurofibroma, schwannoma, perineurioma).

ICD-O coding
9563/0 Hybrid nerve sheath tumour

ICD-11 coding
2A02.3 & XH01G0 Benign neoplasm of cranial nerves & Hybrid nerve sheath tumour

Related terminology
Acceptable: benign peripheral nerve sheath tumour NOS.

Subtype(s)
Schwannoma/perineurioma; neurofibroma/schwannoma; neurofibroma/perineurioma

Localization
Tumours show a wide anatomical distribution in somatic soft tissue, most commonly occurring in the dermis or subcutaneous tissue {1344,898}. Rare cases arise in cranial nerves. The most commonly reported site for hybrid schwannoma / reticular perineurioma is the fingers {2105}.

Clinical features
Hybrid nerve sheath tumours occur as painless masses in subcutaneous tissue or dermis. When large peripheral nerves or spinal nerves are involved, the tumours may be associated with pain or neurological deficit.

Epidemiology
Hybrid nerve sheath tumours are rare. The most common subtypes show hybrid features of schwannoma and perineurioma, followed by hybrid neurofibroma/schwannoma. These tumours occur over a wide age range, with a peak in young adults and an equal sex distribution {1344}. Hybrid neurofibroma/perineurioma is the rarest.

Etiology
Hybrid schwannoma/perineurioma occurs sporadically {1344}, whereas hybrid neurofibroma/schwannoma is strongly associated with neurofibromatosis type 1 (NF1), neurofibromatosis type 2 (NF2), and schwannomatosis {1237}. A high prevalence of hybrid neurofibroma/schwannoma morphology (71%) is found in tumours from patients with schwannomatosis, often leading to misdiagnosis as neurofibroma {1237,1967}. Hybrid neurofibroma/perineurioma has been described in association with NF1 {1410,1521}.

Pathogenesis
The pathogenesis of the dual-differentiation characteristic of the hybrid tumour is unknown. Activating *ERBB2* mutations have been identified in a subset of neurofibroma/schwannoma hybrid tumours, which fall in a DNA methylation subcluster containing the majority of neurofibroma/schwannoma hybrid tumours associated with sporadic schwannomatosis {2719}.

Macroscopic appearance
Grossly, the tumours are well circumscribed, with a firm cut surface. Their appearance is similar to that of other benign peripheral nerve sheath tumours.

Histopathology
Hybrid schwannoma/perineurioma shows a storiform or fascicular growth and is composed of Schwann cells with plump nuclei and eosinophilic cytoplasm admixed with perineurial cells with slender nuclei and delicate, elongated cytoplasmic processes. The Schwann cell component is often prominent. The tumours

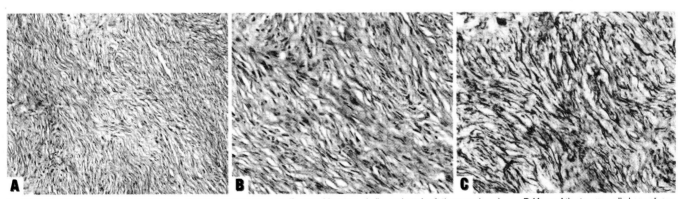

Fig. 6.14 Hybrid schwannoma/perineurioma. **A** The tumour shows a storiform architecture, similar to that of soft tissue perineurioma. **B** Many of the tumour cells have plump, tapering nuclei and eosinophilic cytoplasm, typical of Schwann cells. The perineurial cell component is often inconspicuous. **C** Double immunolabelling for S100 (red) and EMA (brown) highlights alternating Schwann cells and perineurial cells, respectively.

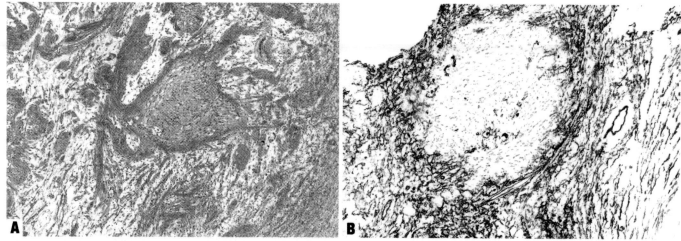

Fig. 6.15 Hybrid neurofibroma/schwannoma. **A** Solid schwannomatous nodule surrounded by loose, hypocellular neurofibromatous tumour. **B** CD34 stain reveals a lattice-like fibroblastic network in the neurofibromatous component, which is absent in the solid Schwann cell nodule.

Box 6.04 Diagnostic criteria for hybrid nerve sheath tumours

> *Essential:*
>
> Intermingled features of two types of benign nerve sheath tumours
>
> **AND**
>
> Appropriate immunohistochemical staining for each component

may show degenerative nuclear atypia (ancient change). Mitoses are rare. Rare cases show a biphasic appearance and a lobulated growth pattern, either with separate schwannomatous and perineurial nodules or with schwannomatous nodules surrounded by a perineurial component with a reticular growth pattern and myxoid stroma. The two components can be highlighted by immunohistochemistry: S100-positive Schwann cells and EMA-positive perineurial cells. Perineurial cells may also be immunoreactive for claudin-1 and GLUT1 {1344}.

Hybrid neurofibroma/schwannoma is composed of schwannomatous nodules within an otherwise typical neurofibroma, or of Schwann cell bundles dispersed in a myxoid background. The tumours may have a plexiform architecture. The Schwann cell nodular proliferations may exhibit Verocay body formation or fascicular growth, and the neurofibroma component may demonstrate myxoid change, collagen bundles, and mixed cellular composition. Tumours may contain entrapped NFP-positive axons. Immunostaining highlights the mixed population of cells in the neurofibromatous component, including fibroblasts (CD34), Schwann cells (S100 and SOX10), and perineurial cells (EMA, claudin-1, and GLUT1), whereas there

is a monomorphic Schwann cell population in the schwannomatous component (diffuse expression of S100 and SOX10) {898,1237}.

Hybrid neurofibroma/perineurioma contains a plexiform neurofibroma with areas of perineurial differentiation. These areas are often only recognizable with the aid of immunohistochemistry. The perineuriomatous areas are immunopositive for EMA, GLUT1, and claudin-1, and the neurofibromatous areas show a mixed population of cells that includes fibroblasts (CD34), Schwann cells (S100 and SOX10), and perineurial cells (EMA, claudin-1, and GLUT1) {1521,23}.

Cytology
Not clinically relevant

Diagnostic molecular pathology
Not clinically relevant

Essential and desirable diagnostic criteria
See Box 6.04.

Staging
Not clinically relevant

Prognosis and prediction
The tumours are benign and rarely recur locally {1344}. *ERBB2* mutations in a subset of neurofibroma/schwannoma hybrid tumours have been proposed as a potential therapeutic target in unresectable tumours {2719}.

Malignant melanotic nerve sheath tumour

Reuss DE
Folpe AL
Jo VY
Stemmer-Rachamimov AO

Definition

Malignant melanotic nerve sheath tumour (MMNST) is a peripheral nerve sheath tumour composed uniformly of tumour cells with features of both Schwann cell and melanocytic differentiation, usually arising in association with spinal or autonomic nerves. It is variably associated with Carney complex and frequently shows aggressive clinical behaviour. *PRKAR1A* mutations and loss of PRKAR1A protein expression are seen in the overwhelming majority of cases.

ICD-O coding

9540/3 Malignant melanotic nerve sheath tumour

ICD-11 coding

2A02.0Y Other specified gliomas of spinal cord, cranial nerves, or other parts of the central nervous system

Related terminology

Acceptable: malignant melanotic Schwannian tumour.
Not recommended: melanotic schwannoma; psammomatous melanotic schwannoma.

Subtype(s)

None

Localization

MMNST most often arises from spinal or autonomic nerves near the midline. However, cases have been reported in the gastrointestinal tract {551,557}, as well as in bone, soft tissues, heart, bronchus, liver, and skin.

Clinical features

Presenting symptoms include pain, sensory abnormalities, and mass effect. Bone erosion may be seen in spinal nerve root tumours. Systemic symptoms, such as respiratory and liver failure, may be seen in patients with metastatic disease. Although it was once thought that psammoma bodies were more likely in familial tumours, there are no clinical differences between psammomatous and non-psammomatous MMNSTs, with both showing a variable association with Carney complex, loss of PRKAR1A expression, and similar clinical behaviour {3219, 3375}.

Epidemiology

MMNST is rare and occurs chiefly in adults. The tumour typically develops at an earlier age (average: 22.5 years) in patients with Carney complex than in sporadic cases (average: 33.2 years) {470,3219}. Multiple tumours are seen in about 20% of patients; in such patients, there is a higher probability that other manifestations of Carney complex will also be present than in patients with a single tumour {470,3219}.

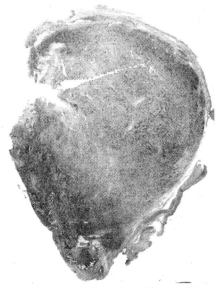

Fig. 6.16 Malignant melanotic nerve sheath tumour. Tumour arising in a spinal nerve root. The tumour is heavily pigmented and partially encapsulated.

Etiology

In some series, > 50% of patients with MMNSTs have evidence of Carney complex, an autosomal dominant, sometimes familial, multiple neoplasia syndrome {470}. However, other series have noted an association with Carney complex in ≤ 5% of affected patients {3266,3219,3594,3375}. Other cases are considered sporadic and of unknown etiology.

Pathogenesis

Two genetic loci have been identified in Carney complex: *PRKAR1A* (*CNC1*) and *CNC2*, mapping to 17q24.2 and 2p16, respectively. *PRKAR1A* inactivation is seen in roughly 50% of Carney complex kindreds {2043,1639}. *PRKAR1A* encodes the type 1A regulatory (R1α) subunit of PKA, which inhibits PKA activity by binding to active catalytic subunits. *PRKAR1A* acts as a tumour suppressor gene. Loss of R1α leads to increased PKA activity, which has been associated with secondary dysregulation of the ERK, TGF-β, and WNT signalling pathways {2830}.

PRKAR1A mutations and loss of PRKAR1A protein expression are seen in the overwhelming majority of studied MMNSTs, most of which have occurred in patients lacking other stigmata of Carney complex {3219,3375}. Chromosomal copy-number profiling of MMNST revealed recurrent whole-chromosome losses and gains. The most frequent alterations are monosomies of chromosomes 1, 2, 17, 21, and 22q and whole-chromosome gains variably involving chromosomes 5, 6, 7, 8, and 9 {3375,1676, 463}. Inactivation of both alleles of *PRKAR1A* through mutations and/or loss of heterozygosity of 17q has been reported {3375}.

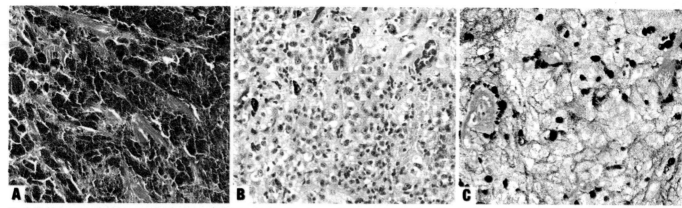

Fig. 6.17 Malignant melanotic nerve sheath tumour. **A** Cellular detail is often obscured by heavy pigment deposition. **B** Sheets of vaguely syncytial epithelioid cells. **C** Tumour cell–specific loss of PRKAR1A expression (immunohistochemistry for PRKAR1A with red chromogen).

Box 6.05 Diagnostic criteria for malignant melanotic nerve sheath tumour

Essential:

Fascicular to sheet-like proliferation of variably pigmented, relatively uniform, plump, spindled to epithelioid cells

AND

Coexpression of S100/SOX10 and melanocytic markers (e.g. HMB45, melan-A)

OR

Loss of PRKAR1A expression, or *PRKAR1A* mutation

AND (for unresolved lesions)

Methylation profile of malignant melanotic nerve sheath tumour

Desirable:

Origin from a paraspinal or visceral autonomic nerve

Gene expression analyses show MMNST to clearly segregate from conventional schwannomas and melanomas {3219}. The molecular distinctiveness of MMNST is further corroborated by DNA methylation profiling {1676}.

Macroscopic appearance
Most MMNSTs are solitary, although multiple and multicentric tumours may be seen in patients with Carney complex. Grossly, the tumours appear circumscribed or partially encapsulated, and they are frequently heavily pigmented, with the appearance of dried tar.

Histopathology
The neoplastic cells grow in short fascicles or sheets, vary in shape from polygonal to spindled, and often have a syncytial appearance. Vague palisading or formation of whorled structures may be present. Cellular detail is often difficult to discern, owing to the heavy pigment deposits. The melanin pigment may be coarsely clumped or finely granular and varies from area to area. It stains positively with the Fontana stain and negatively for iron and PAS. In less pigmented areas, the tumour cells have eosinophilic to amphophilic cytoplasm, round to ovoid nuclei (often with nuclear grooves and pseudoinclusions), and usually small nucleoli. Occasional tumours show marked nuclear atypia with prominent macronucleoli. Mitoses and necrosis can be present, but they are not clearly associated with outcome. Psammoma bodies are present in roughly 50% of cases, although extensive sampling may be required to identify them.

Immunohistochemically, MMNSTs strongly express S100 and SOX10, as well as various melanocytic markers, including HMB45, melan-A, and tyrosinase. Basement membrane markers (collagen IV, laminin) often show increased intercellular deposition compared with melanoma, although there are many exceptions. PRKAR1A expression is typically lost {3219,3375}. Ultrastructurally, the cells resemble Schwann cells with elaborate cytoplasmic processes that interdigitate or spiral in the manner of mesaxons; however, pre-melanosomes and melanosomes are also present {3594,1365}.

Cytology
Not clinically relevant

Diagnostic molecular pathology
PRKAR1A immunoexpression is typically lost, corresponding to gene inactivation {3219,3375}. MMNSTs show a distinct DNA methylation pattern {1676} and do not harbour mutations in *GNAQ* or *GNA11*, which is useful for their differentiation from primary CNS melanocytomas and melanomas. MMNSTs also do not harbour *BRAF*, *NRAS*, or *TERT* promoter mutations, which is useful for their differentiation from metastatic cutaneous melanomas {1676,1770,3268}.

Essential and desirable diagnostic criteria
See Box 6.05.

Staging
Not available

Prognosis and prediction
The behaviour of MMNST is difficult to predict and metastases can occur in the absence of morphologically malignant features. In the past, it was thought that most of these lesions had a benign, indolent course, with < 15% metastatic risk {470}. However, more recent reports have shown frequently aggressive behaviour, with local recurrence and metastatic rates of 26–44% {3266,3219,3375,1607}. Additionally, only 53% of patients followed for > 5 years have been reported to have remained disease-free, suggesting that long-term follow-up is required. In general, histopathological features are not predictive of outcome, although there are limited data suggesting more aggressive behaviour in mitotically active tumours {3219}.

Malignant peripheral nerve sheath tumour

Reuss DE
Hirose T
Jo VY
Rodriguez FJ
Stemmer-Rachamimov AO

Definition
Malignant peripheral nerve sheath tumour (MPNST) is a malignant spindle cell tumour often arising from a peripheral nerve, from a pre-existing benign nerve sheath tumour, or in a patient with neurofibromatosis type 1 (NF1), and often showing limited Schwannian differentiation. Molecular hallmarks are the combined genetic inactivation of *NF1*, *CDKN2A* and/or *CDKN2B*, and *SUZ12* or *EED* genes, as well as complex genomic rearrangements.

ICD-O coding
9540/3 Malignant peripheral nerve sheath tumour

ICD-11 coding
2A02.0Y & XH2XP8 Other specified gliomas of spinal cord, cranial nerves, or other parts of the central nervous system & Malignant peripheral nerve sheath tumour

Related terminology
Not recommended: malignant schwannoma, neurofibrosarcoma, neurogenic sarcoma.

Subtype(s)
Epithelioid malignant peripheral nerve sheath tumour; perineurial malignant peripheral nerve sheath tumour

Localization
The most common locations are extremities, the trunk, and the head and neck area {1817,796}.

Clinical features
MPNST occurs most commonly in patients aged 20–50 years. MPNSTs in children are usually associated with NF1. The mean age of patients with NF1-associated MPNST is about a decade younger than that of patients with sporadic tumours. Patients with MPNSTs often present with enlarging masses that may cause pain or other neuropathic symptoms {912,3034}. PET-CT

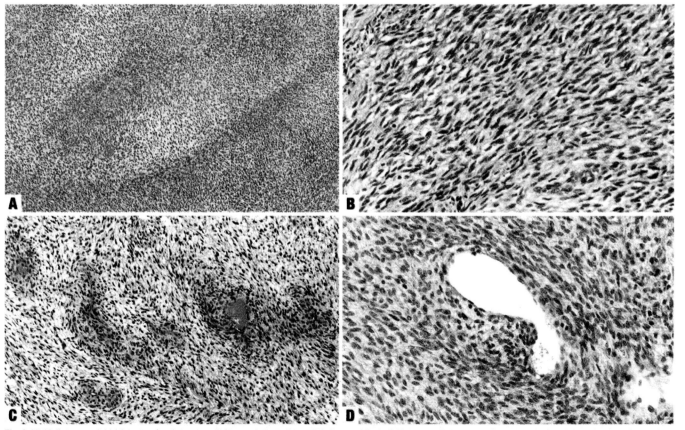

Fig. 6.18 Malignant peripheral nerve sheath tumour. **A** Areas of alternating cellularity (marbling). **B** Tumour cells have spindle-shaped nuclei, often with tapered ends, that frequently appear wavy or buckled. The cytoplasm is palely eosinophilic and fibrillary. **C** Accentuated perivascular cellularity. **D** Nodular herniation of tumour cells into the vessel lumen.

Chapter 6

imaging is sensitive but not specific for the detection of MPNST in patients with NF1 {375}.

Epidemiology

MPNSTs account for approximately 2–10% of soft tissue sarcomas {371,3434}, with epithelioid MPNST being particularly rare (~5% of all cases). The estimated overall incidence is 1.46 cases per 1 million person-years; there is slightly greater risk in Black people and lower risk in Asian and Latino/a people than in White people; the M:F ratio is roughly 1.2:1 {215,2435}.

Etiology

About 50% of all MPNSTs are associated with NF1. In this setting, they most commonly arise from deep-seated plexiform neurofibromas or large intraneural neurofibromas {912}. The lifetime risk for MPNST in patients with NF1 is 10% {863,2052}. About 10% of all MPNSTs are associated with previous irradiation {950}. Epithelioid MPNST is not associated with NF1, but it has been associated with malignant transformation of schwannoma and has histological and molecular features in common with epithelioid schwannoma {2058,2820}.

Pathogenesis

The pathogenesis of MPNST is complex and incompletely understood. Most available data are for NF1-associated tumours. In that setting, MPNSTs commonly develop from plexiform neurofibromas or localized intraneural neurofibromas,

in which a subpopulation of Schwann cells already carries a biallelic inactivation of *NF1* {1923}. An intermediate lesion is the atypical neurofibromatous neoplasm of uncertain biological potential (ANNUBP), which frequently harbours homozygous *CDKN2A* and/or *CDKN2B* deletions {2109,474}. MPNSTs are molecularly characterized by two additional hallmarks: inactivation of *SUZ12* or *EED* (core components of PRC2) {217,3598, 1842} as well as complex genomic rearrangements including numerous chromosomal deletions and oncogene amplifications {1670,2709}. In addition, some MPNSTs harbour mutations in *TP53* {3313,381,2984}.

PRC2 mediates the deposition of H3 p.K28me3 (K27me3), an important repressive mark that plays a critical role in cellular differentiation and cellular identity {630,2013}. Inactivation of PRC2 leads to a complete global loss of H3 p.K28me3 (K27me3) in tumour cells, which can be demonstrated by immunohistochemistry. About 80% of conventional high-grade MPNSTs show loss of H3 p.K28me3 (K27me3) {2822}. Conventional MPNSTs with loss of H3 p.K28me3 (K27me3) and those with retained H3 p.K28me3 (K27me3) form two distinct DNA methylation classes {2709}. Those with loss of H3 p.K28me3 (K27me3) frequently display losses of 1p, 9p, 10q, 11, 17p, and segments of 17q including *NF1* and *SUZ12*. The most frequent gains involve 7p, 8q, and larger parts of 17q. Amplified oncogenes include *EGFR*, *PDGFRA*, and *MET*. Tumours with retained H3 p.K28me3 (K27me3) are predominately paraspinal and show more frequent losses of 3q and gains of 5p {2709}.

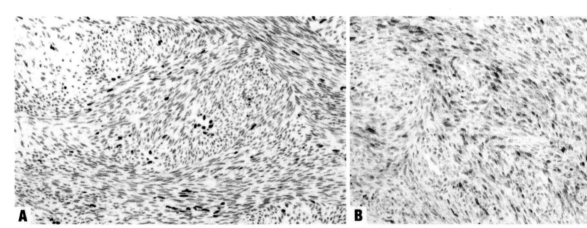

Fig. 6.19 Malignant peripheral nerve sheath tumour. **A** H3 p.K28me3 (K27me3) stain showing complete loss of expression in tumour cells but retained expression in non-neoplastic elements. **B** Patchy S100 expression.

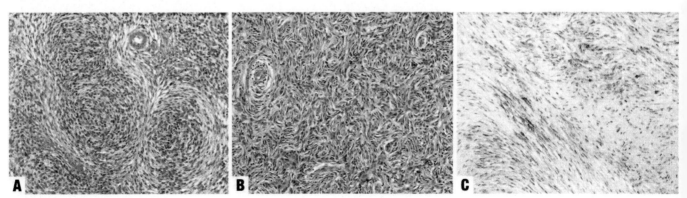

Fig. 6.20 Perineurial malignant peripheral nerve sheath tumour. **A** Cellular whorls showing concentric arrangement of tumour cells. **B** Storiform and whorling pattern. **C** Immunoreactivity for EMA.

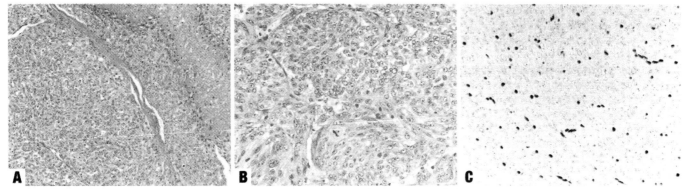

Fig. 6.21 Epithelioid malignant peripheral nerve sheath tumour. **A** Lobulated growth of epithelioid cells. **B** Epithelioid cells have atypical nuclei with prominent nucleoli and eosinophilic cytoplasm. **C** Loss of SMARCB1 staining is a feature of epithelioid malignant peripheral nerve sheath tumour.

The pathogenesis of epithelioid MPNST is distinct from that of conventional MPNST. Epithelioid MPNSTs are not associated with NF1 and do not harbour most of the genetic alterations present in conventional MPNST; they retain H3 p.K28me3 (K27me3) and are driven by genetic inactivation of *SMARCB1* in the vast majority of cases {1842,1478,2820}. Recurrent chromosomal alterations in epithelioid MPNST include loss of 22q, deletion of 9p including *CDKN2A* and/or *CDKN2B*, and gain of 2q {2820}.

The pathogenesis of perineurial MPNST is currently unknown.

Macroscopic appearance

Most MPNSTs are > 50 mm in diameter at diagnosis. They have a tan-white, fleshy cut surface, often with areas of haemorrhage and necrosis. They may occur with fusiform enlargement of a peripheral nerve and may include a precursor neurofibroma.

Histopathology

Conventional high-grade MPNST appears as a hypercellular spindle cell tumour, with tumour cells arranged in interlacing fascicles. The nuclei are wavy or buckled and considerably larger and more atypical than in neurofibroma. There is pale eosinophilic and often indistinct cytoplasm. The cell density often alternates between highly cellular and less cellular areas, creating a marbled appearance. The cellularity around vessels

may be increased, and tumour cell herniation into blood vessels is a common feature. Mitotic activity is usually brisk {2109}. Well-demarcated areas of necrosis are frequently present. About 15% of MPNSTs show evidence of divergent differentiation. There may be mesenchymal osseous, cartilaginous, or rhabdomyosarcomatous (skeletal muscle) heterologous elements, or epithelial elements such as mucinous glands or islands of squamous differentiation. Conventional MPNST with prominent rhabdomyosarcomatous differentiation has been termed "malignant triton tumour". Additionally, MPNST may show a broader morphological range and occasionally resemble various mesenchymal tumours, including synovial sarcoma, solitary fibrous tumour, and undifferentiated pleomorphic sarcoma. MPNST may diffusely infiltrate peripheral nerve tissue as well as precursor neurofibromas. Therefore, it is not uncommon to find areas with different degrees of malignant progression in the same tumour mass (e.g. neurofibroma, ANNUBP, low-grade MPNST, high-grade MPNST), especially in NF1-associated tumours.

To improve reproducibility and association with clinical and molecular parameters, a consensus nomenclature for the spectrum of NF1-associated nerve sheath tumours has been proposed (Table 6.01). The extent of mitotic activity and the presence of necrosis is critical both for the distinction of ANNUBP from MPNST and for the grading of MPNST (low-grade or high-grade) {2109}.

Table 6.01 Proposed nomenclature for the spectrum of nerve sheath tumours associated with neurofibromatosis type 1

Diagnosis	Proposed definition
Neurofibroma	Benign Schwann cell neoplasm with thin (often wavy) nuclei, wispy cell processes, and a myxoid to collagenous (shredded carrots) matrix; immunohistochemistry includes extensive but not diffuse S100 and SOX10 positivity and a lattice-like CD34+ fibroblastic network
Plexiform neurofibroma	Neurofibroma diffusely enlarging and replacing a nerve, often involving multiple nerve fascicles, delineated by EMA+ perineurial cells
Neurofibroma with atypia (ancient neurofibroma)	Neurofibroma with atypia alone, most commonly manifesting as scattered bizarre nuclei
Cellular neurofibroma	Neurofibroma with hypercellularity but retained neurofibroma architecture and no mitoses
ANNUBP	Schwann cell neoplasm with at least two of the following four features: cytological atypia, loss of neurofibroma architecture, hypercellularity, and a mitotic count of > 0.2 mitoses/mm² and < 1.5 mitoses/mm² (> 1 mitosis/50 HPF and < 3 mitoses/10 HPF[a])
MPNST, low-grade	Features of ANNUBP, but with a mitotic count of 1.5–4.5 mitoses/mm² (3–9 mitoses/10 HPF[a]) and no necrosis
MPNST, high-grade	MPNST with a mitotic count of ≥ 5 mitoses/mm² (≥ 10 mitoses/10 HPF[a]), or with a mitotic count of 1.5–4.5 mitoses/mm² combined with necrosis

ANNUBP, atypical neurofibromatous neoplasm of uncertain biological potential; MPNST, malignant peripheral nerve sheath tumour.
[a]1 mm² ≈ 5 HPF of 0.51 mm in diameter and 0.20 mm² in area.

Immunohistochemically, the majority of MPNSTs are negative for Schwann cell markers like S100, SOX10, and GFAP. Importantly, if positivity is present, the staining is typically not diffuse but patchy or restricted to a subpopulation of cells, sometimes attributable to entrapped neural remnants. Only a minority of MPNSTs retain a Schwann cell phenotype. Surrogate molecular immunostains are often more helpful than lineage markers. As many as 90% of conventional MPNSTs show loss of neurofibromin {2654,2441,2709}, although a commercial antibody is not currently available. Complete loss of H3 p.K28me3 (K27me3) is detectable in 50–80% of all MPNSTs, with the highest frequencies reported in high-grade and radiation-induced MPNSTs {2822,2576}. A small subset of MPNSTs demonstrate ATRX loss and an alternative-lengthening-of-telomeres phenotype {2694, 1949}.

The tumour cells of epithelioid MPNST are predominantly epithelioid with abundant eosinophilic cytoplasm and nuclei with visible nucleoli. They often show a lobulated growth pattern and a fibrotic or myxoid matrix. Immunohistochemically, they are consistently strongly and diffusely positive for S100 and SOX10 but negative for melanocytic markers. Epithelioid MPNSTs retain H3 p.K28me3 (K27me3), but most show a loss of SMARCB1 expression {2820}.

Very rare malignant tumours with perineurial features have been described and termed "perineurial MPNST". They are composed of spindle cells arranged in intersecting fascicles or whorls and exhibit frank histological signs of malignancy, such as frequent mitoses and necrosis. Immunohistochemically, tumour cells are S100-negative but express EMA and (variably) CD34 {1318}. Perineurial MPNST is not associated with NF1.

Cytology
Not clinically relevant

Diagnostic molecular pathology
DNA methylation–based classification may unequivocally define a tumour as MPNST, especially one with retained H3 p.K28me3 (K27me3). Other molecular data may provide supportive information for the diagnosis of MPNST, such as mutations in *NF1*, *SUZ12*, or *EED*, or the chromosomal copy-number profile. Chromosomal alterations are particularly helpful in borderline cases to distinguish between ANNUBP (*CDKN2A* and/or *CDKN2B* deletion and no or very few other alterations) and MPNST (complex genomic profile).

Essential and desirable diagnostic criteria
See Box 6.06.

Staging
Not clinically relevant

Prognosis and prediction
In a recent study, the 5-year overall survival rate of MPNST associated with NF1 was 35%, whereas it was 65% for sporadic

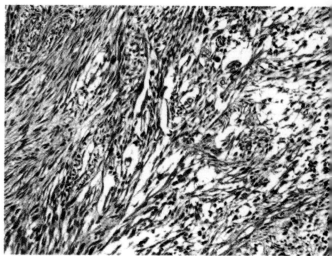

Fig. 6.22 Malignant peripheral nerve sheath tumour. Rhabdomyoblastic differentiation.

Box 6.06 Diagnostic criteria for conventional malignant peripheral nerve sheath tumour (MPNST)

Essential:

Histopathologically consistent malignant spindle cell tumour in a patient with NF1[a] **OR** in a pre-existing neurofibroma

OR

Malignant spindle cell tumour associated with a peripheral nerve **AND** no more than focal/patchy S100/SOX10 expression **AND** no *SS18::SSX* (*SSX1, SSX2,* or *SSX4*) fusion gene present

OR

Malignant spindle cell tumour associated with a peripheral nerve **AND** evidence of PRC2 inactivation (molecularly or via loss of H3 p.K28me3 [K27me3] immunostaining)

OR

Tumour with features of ANNUBP in a patient with NF1, but with a mitotic count of at least 1.5–4.5 mitoses/mm² (3–9 mitoses/10 HPF of 0.51 mm in diameter and 0.20 mm² in area)

OR

Unresolved lesion with the methylation profile of MPNST

Desirable:

Loss of H3 p.K28me3 (K27me3)

Loss of neurofibromin expression

ANNUBP, atypical neurofibromatous neoplasm of uncertain biological potential; NF1, neurofibromatosis type 1.
[a]In the setting of NF1, a diagnosis other than conventional MPNST demands strong molecular evidence (e.g. detection of a fusion gene pathognomonic for another tumour type).

MPNST. Deep location, positive surgical margins, and high-grade histology were additional factors associated with a poorer outcome {1817}. The prognosis of radiation-induced MPNST is even worse, with a reported 5-year overall survival rate of 23.5% {2104}. Epithelioid and perineurial MPNSTs seem to be less aggressive than conventional MPNST {1478,1318}.

Cauda equina neuroendocrine tumour (previously paraganglioma)

Brandner S
Kleinschmidt-DeMasters BK
Sarkar C

Definition

Cauda equina neuroendocrine tumour is a neuroendocrine neoplasm arising from specialized neural crest cells in the cauda equina / filum terminale region.

ICD-O coding

8693/3 Cauda equina neuroendocrine tumour (previously paraganglioma)

ICD-11 coding

2A02.0Y & XH1X68 Other specified gliomas of spinal cord, cranial nerves, or other parts of the central nervous system & Paraganglioma, benign

2A02.0Y & XH0EW6 Other specified gliomas of spinal cord, cranial nerves, or other parts of the central nervous system & Paraganglioma, NOS

Related terminology

Acceptable: paraganglioma of the cauda equina; cauda equina paraganglioma.

Subtype(s)

None

Localization

The majority of spinal paragangliomas / neuroendocrine tumours are located in the cauda equina region {1052}. Most neuroendocrine tumours of the cauda equina are entirely intradural and are attached either to the filum terminale or (less often) to a caudal nerve root {2992}.

Clinical features

Cauda equina neuroendocrine tumours exhibit no clinical features that allow their distinction from other spinal cord tumours. The most common presenting symptoms include a history of low back pain and sciatica. Less common manifestations are numbness, paraparesis, and sphincter symptoms {1052}. Fully developed cauda equina syndrome is uncommon, as are signs of increased intracranial pressure and papilloedema {21, 1052}. Endocrinologically functional neuroendocrine tumours of the cauda equina region, which are extremely rare {1052}, can lead to signs and symptoms of catecholamine hypersecretion such as episodic or sustained hypertension, palpitations, diaphoresis, and headache. Subarachnoid haemorrhage is another unusual presentation of cauda equina neuroendocrine tumours {1878}. Cerebrospinal fluid protein is usually markedly increased {2981,2992}.

Imaging

MRI findings are nonspecific {21}, and the appearance of paraganglioma is indistinguishable from that of schwannoma or ependymoma {2126}. Tumours are sharply circumscribed and

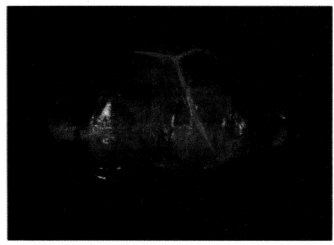

Fig. 6.23 Cauda equina neuroendocrine tumour. A well-circumscribed, encapsulated tumour with prominent vasculature on the surface.

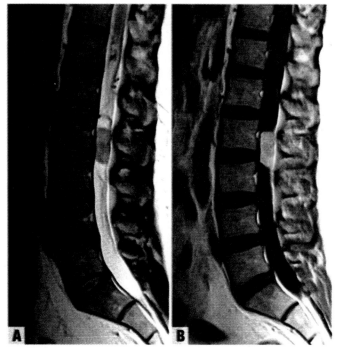

Fig. 6.24 Cauda equina neuroendocrine tumour. **A** Hypointense tumour on T2-weighted image with prominent flow voids from enlarged draining veins superiorly. **B** T1-weighted image with marked contrast enhancement.

occasionally partly cystic, and they can be hypointense, isointense, or hyperintense on T1- and T2-weighted images. Gadolinium enhancement may be present or absent. A low signal intensity rim (cap sign) on T2-weighted images can be caused by subcapsular haemosiderin {1861,3524,3517}. The hypervascular architecture can give a salt-and-pepper appearance on T2-weighted images. Serpentine flow voids along the tumour surface or spinal cord margin may also be seen at MRI {732, 2068}.

Epidemiology

Neuroendocrine tumours of the cauda equina region are uncommon, but nearly 300 cases have been reported since their initial description in 1970 {1339,2112}. In a series of 430 spinal tumours, < 3% were paragangliomas / neuroendocrine tumours {852,133}, and of cauda equina region tumours, 3.4–3.8% are neuroendocrine tumours {3460,3524}. Cauda equina neuroendocrine tumours generally affect adults, with a peak incidence in the fourth through sixth decades of life. Patient age ranges from 9 to 75 years (mean: 46–47 years) {3517,1339}, with a slight predominance in male patients (M:F ratio: 1.5:1) {1052,1339}.

Etiology

Almost all neuroendocrine tumours of the cauda equina are sporadic. In contrast, as many as half of all phaeochromocytomas/paragangliomas outside the CNS in adults, and > 80% of these tumours in children, are inherited {1109}. The role of germline mutations in the pathogenesis of paragangliomas outside the cauda equina region is discussed in Chapter 14: *Genetic tumour syndromes involving the CNS*.

Pathogenesis

Cauda equina neuroendocrine tumours are histogenetically and molecularly distinct from paragangliomas and phaeochromocytomas outside the CNS. They overexpress the transcription factor HOXB13 {306A}, which is developmentally expressed in the caudal extent of the spinal cord and in the urogenital sinus. It coincides with dynamic changes associated with the formation of the secondary neural tube {3585A,824A}, providing circumstantial evidence of a cell of origin. Cauda equina neuroendocrine tumours have not been seen in people with hereditary paraganglioma/phaeochromocytoma syndrome due to mutations in SDH subunit genes {2165A}.

Genetic profile

The molecular alterations that drive tumorigenesis in cauda equina neuroendocrine tumours are unknown. The mutations found in paragangliomas outside the cauda equina region are described in Chapter 14: *Genetic tumour syndromes involving the CNS*. The genetic and epigenetic profiles (i.e. methylation, expression {1222,1858}, microRNA {701}, and metabolomics {488,1409}) of phaeochromocytomas/paragangliomas with succinate dehydrogenase defects differ substantially from those with other genetic causes.

Macroscopic appearance

Tumours are oval to sausage-shaped, delicately encapsulated, soft, red-brown masses that bleed freely; in 5 series

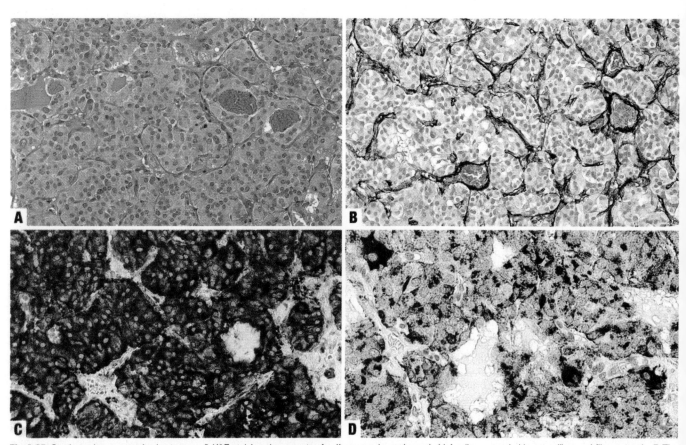

Fig. 6.25 Cauda equina neuroendocrine tumour. **A** H&E staining shows nests of uniform round or polygonal chief cells surrounded by a capillary and fibre network. **B** The nests of tumour cells are surrounded by a delicate supporting reticulin fibre network (reticulin silver stain). **C** Synaptophysin immunostaining labels the neuroendocrine (chief) cells. **D** Chromogranin A immunostaining labels the neuroendocrine (chief) cells.

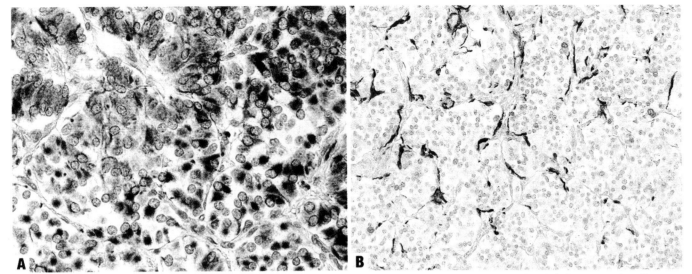

Fig. 6.26 Neuroendocrine tumour / paraganglioma. **A** Spinal neuroendocrine tumours can express cytokeratin. **B** S100 immunostaining labels the sustentacular cells, encompassing the lobules.

of 59 spinal tumours, size ranged from 10 mm to 112 mm in greatest dimension {2126,3517,2037}. Capsular calcification and cystic components may be found. An occasional tumour penetrates the dura to invade bone. For tumours in the cauda equina, a macroscopically identifiable attachment may be found, either to the filum terminale or (less often) to a caudal nerve root {2992}.

Histopathology

Cauda equina neuroendocrine tumours / paragangliomas are well-differentiated. They are composed of chief (type I) cells disposed in nests or lobules (Zellballen), surrounded by an inconspicuous, single layer of sustentacular (type II) cells. The Zellballen are surrounded by a delicate capillary network and a delicate supporting reticulin fibre network that may undergo sclerosis. The uniform round or polygonal chief cells have central, round to oval nuclei with finely stippled chromatin and inconspicuous nucleoli. Degenerative nuclear pleomorphism (endocrine anaplasia) is generally mild. Cytoplasm is usually eosinophilic and finely granular; in some instances, it is amphophilic or clear. Sustentacular cells are spindle-shaped; encompassing the lobules, their long processes are often so attenuated as to be undetectable by routine light microscopy and visible only on immunostains for S100. Approximately 25% of cauda equina neuroendocrine tumours contain mature ganglion cells and a Schwann cell component (gangliocytic neuroendocrine tumours). Ependymoma-like perivascular formations are also common. Some tumours show architectural features reminiscent of carcinoid tumours, including angiomatous, adenomatous, and pseudorosette patterns {2992}. Tumours composed predominantly of spindle cells {2162} and melanin-containing cells (melanotic neuroendocrine tumours) {2162} have also been described at this site, as have oncocytic neuroendocrine tumours {1021,2395}. Foci of haemorrhagic necrosis may occur, and scattered mitotic figures can be seen, but neither these features nor nuclear pleomorphism is of prognostic significance {2992}.

The neuroendocrine chief cells are immunoreactive for chromogranin A and synaptophysin {1661,2992,2095}, and they show variable S100 immunoreactivity. Immunoreactivity for cytokeratins (especially CAM5.2, AE1/AE3, and MNF116) has been described in the majority of cauda equina neuroendocrine tumours {2332,556,3053,2095,1176,739,2610}, but it has also been described in other locations {739}.

Furthermore, gangliocytic neuroendocrine tumours / paragangliomas containing a variable mixture of epithelioid neuroendocrine cells, Schwann-like cells, and scattered ganglion-like cells can show cytokeratin positivity in the epithelioid cells {2889,2583}. Expression of serotonin (5-HT) and of various neuropeptides (somatostatin, leu-enkephalin, and met-enkephalin) has been demonstrated in neuroendocrine tumour of the cauda equina region {2162,2992}.

Sustentacular cells show inconsistent S100 protein reactivity {2978,3241} and occasionally express GFAP {2996}. They often express the neural crest transcription factor SOX10 {2276}. The value of proliferation markers in cauda equina neuroendocrine tumours has not been established.

Unlike paragangliomas of the autonomic nervous system {2978}, cauda equina neuroendocrine tumours do not express the zinc finger transcription factor GATA3 {2610}. They express HOXB13 (a transcription factor that is developmentally expressed in progenitor cells of the caudal spinal cord), a feature they share with myxopapillary ependymoma {306A}.

Grading

Neuroendocrine tumours of the cauda equina correspond to CNS WHO grade 1.

Cytology

Not clinically relevant

Diagnostic molecular pathology

The DNA methylation profiles and chromosomal copy-number profiles of cauda equina neuroendocrine tumours are distinct from those of paragangliomas arising from other locations {2610,2871}.

Essential and desirable diagnostic criteria

See Box 6.07.

Staging

Not relevant

Prognosis and prediction

The vast majority of cauda equina neuroendocrine tumours are slow-growing and curable by total excision; only 4% recur after gross total removal {3053}. Cerebrospinal fluid seeding of spinal paragangliomas has occasionally been documented {627,2692, 3053,3176,3190}, and metastasis outside the CNS (to the bone) from cauda equina neuroendocrine tumours has been reported only once {2162}. In contrast, 10–20% of paragangliomas outside the CNS have metastatic potential {1811,639}.

Box 6.07 Diagnostic criteria for cauda equina neuroendocrine tumour

Essential:

Well-demarcated tumour with Zellballen architecture

AND

Synaptophysin or chromogranin immunoreactivity in chief cells

AND

Cauda equina location

AND (for unresolved lesions)

Methylation profile of cauda equina neuroendocrine tumour

Desirable:

S100-positive sustentacular cells

Cytokeratin-positive chief cells

Reticulin silver stain showing typical architecture

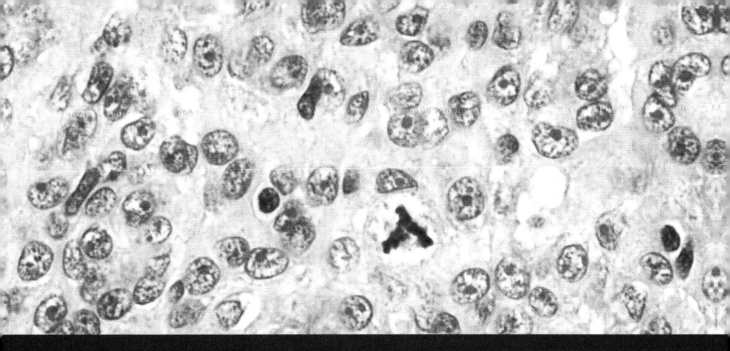

7

Meningioma

Edited by: Louis DN

Meningioma

Sahm F
Brastianos PK
Claus EB
Mawrin C

Perry A
Santagata S
von Deimling A

Definition
Meningiomas comprise a family of neoplasms that are most likely derived from the meningothelial cells of the arachnoid mater (CNS WHO grade 1, 2, or 3).

ICD-O coding
9530/0 Meningioma

ICD-11 coding
2A01.0Z Meningiomas, unspecified

Related terminology
None

Subtype(s)
See Box 7.01.

Localization
Meningiomas typically arise in intracranial, intraspinal, or orbital locations. The most common sites include the cerebral convexities (with tumours often located parasagittally, in association with the falx cerebri and/or venous sinuses), olfactory grooves, sphenoid ridges, parasellar/suprasellar regions, optic nerve sheath, petrous ridges, tentorium, and posterior fossa. Intraventricular and epidural localization is uncommon. Most spinal meningiomas occur in the thoracic region. Tumour location is strongly associated with the mutation spectrum: convexity meningiomas and the majority of spinal meningiomas often carry a 22q deletion and/or *NF2* mutations, whereas skull base meningiomas harbour mutations in *AKT1*, *TRAF7*, *SMO*, and/or *PIK3CA* {601,3451,3052,9,2777,353}. Higher-grade meningiomas most commonly arise from the convexity and other

Box 7.01 Subtypes of meningioma

Meningothelial meningioma

Fibrous meningioma

Transitional meningioma

Psammomatous meningioma

Angiomatous meningioma

Microcystic meningioma

Secretory meningioma

Lymphoplasmacyte-rich meningioma

Metaplastic meningioma

Chordoid meningioma

Clear cell meningioma

Rhabdoid meningioma

Papillary meningioma

Atypical meningioma

Anaplastic (malignant) meningioma

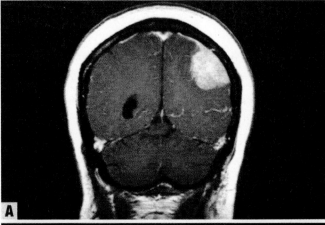
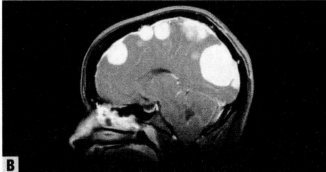

Fig. 7.01 Meningioma. **A** Postcontrast T1-weighted MRI showing an extra-axial, left convexity mass with homogeneous contrast enhancement and a dural tail sign. **B** Multiple meningiomas. Postcontrast MRI shows several dural-based masses in the same patient, consistent with multiple meningiomas. Most such cases arise from a single clone and are thought to represent dural spread.

non–skull base sites. Rare primary meningiomas arise outside the neuraxis (e.g. in the lung).

Clinical features
Meningiomas are usually slow-growing, occurring with neurological deficits that vary depending on tumour location. Clinical signs and symptoms can arise from compression of adjacent structures. Headaches, weakness, and seizures are common, although not specific for meningiomas. Higher-grade tumours and those with molecular biomarkers of aggressive behaviour progress more rapidly.

Imaging
Meningiomas characteristically appear as isodense, uniformly contrast-enhancing dural masses on MRI. Calcification is common and is best visualized on CT. A frequent imaging feature is a contrast-enhancing dural tail sign at the tumour perimeter, which often corresponds to reactive fibrovascular tissue and does not necessarily predict dural involvement. Peritumoural

cerebral oedema can be prominent with certain histological subtypes, such as secretory {3552}, angiomatous/microcystic, lymphoplasmacyte-rich, and high-grade meningiomas {2336}. Cyst formation may occur within or at the periphery of a meningioma. Neuroimaging features are not always specific for the diagnosis of meningioma or for estimating prognosis; however, quantitative and qualitative imaging features from gadolinium-enhanced MRI can suggest the histological grade of meningiomas and predict more-likely patient outcomes {638,2163}.

Spread

Meningiomas commonly invade adjacent anatomical structures (especially the dura), although the rate and extent of local spread are often greater in the more aggressive subtypes. Thus, depending on their location and grade, some meningiomas produce considerable patient morbidity and mortality. Extracranial metastases (e.g. to lung, pleura, bone, and/or liver) are rare and most often associated with CNS WHO grade 3 meningiomas. In one series, the incidence of metastases from all meningiomas was 0.67%, with a greater incidence in CNS WHO grade 2 (2%) and grade 3 (9%) meningiomas {670}.

Epidemiology
Incidence

Meningioma occurs in the USA at an average annual age-adjusted rate of 8.58 cases per 100 000 population, accounting for 37.6% of CNS tumours {2344}. It is the most common primary brain tumour in adults (estimated to occur in up to 1% of the population) {3316} but the least common in children aged 0–19 years.

Age, sex, and race distribution

The risk of meningioma increases with age; the median age at diagnosis is 66 years {2344}. Across all ages, the incidence of grade 1 meningioma is 2.32 times greater in women than in men, with the greatest risk differential (3.28) seen before menopause and decreasing thereafter. The incidence is significantly higher in Black people than in White people (9.25 vs 7.88 cases per 100 000 person-years) {2344}.

Etiology

Exposure to ionizing radiation is the primary established environmental risk factor for meningioma. The risk is higher in people who were exposed to ionizing radiation in childhood than in those exposed in adulthood, and in people exposed to high levels of ionizing radiation, such as atomic bomb survivors and patients treated with therapeutic radiation to the head. There is evidence that lower doses of ionizing radiation also increase the risk of meningioma, including exposure to CT in childhood or adolescence {2035,2434}. The *Tinea capitis* cohort study provided strong evidence of genetic susceptibility to the development of meningioma after exposure to ionizing radiation {949}.

Evidence of an association between hormones and meningioma risk is suggested by a number of findings, including the greater incidence of the disease in women than in men and the presence of hormone receptors in some meningiomas, as well as reports of a modestly increased risk associated with endogenous/exogenous hormone use, body mass index, and current smoking, and a decreased risk associated with breastfeeding

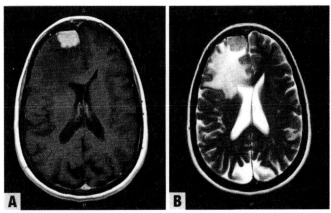

Fig. 7.02 Secretory meningioma. A small secretory meningioma on postcontrast T1-weighted (**A**) and T2-weighted (**B**) MRI, showing extensive peritumoural brain oedema.

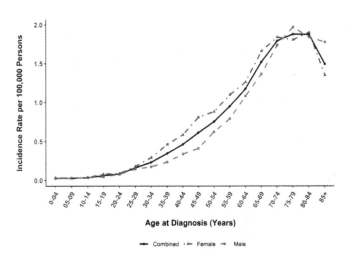

Fig. 7.03 Meningioma. Incidence (number of cases per 100 000 person-years) of non-malignant meningioma by age at diagnosis and sex. Data are from the Central Brain Tumor Registry of the United States (CBTRUS), 2012–2016, and include all 50 states and Puerto Rico. Meningioma is defined by ICD-O-3 codes 9530–9534 and 9537–9539.

for ≥ 6 months {605,3435}. One study found enrichment of *PIK3CA* mutations in meningiomas of patients treated with progestin {792}. A large case–control study showed that women with meningioma were more likely than those without to report hormone-related conditions: uterine fibroids (odds ratio: 1.2; 95% CI: 1.0–1.5), endometriosis (odds ratio: 1.5; 95% CI: 1.5–2.1), and breast cancer (odds ratio: 1.4; 95% CI: 0.8–2.3) {605}.

Attempts to link specific chemicals, diet, occupation, head trauma, and mobile phone use with meningioma have been inconclusive. However, allergic diseases such as asthma and eczema have been fairly consistently associated with a reduced risk of meningioma {3380}.

Several syndromes increase the risk of meningioma development, most notably neurofibromatosis type 2, and rare associations with naevoid basal cell carcinoma syndrome (Gorlin syndrome) have been reported. Meningiomas have also been reported in families with germline defects in *NF1*, *VHL*, *PTEN*, *PTCH1*, *BAP1*, *SUFU*, *SMARCE1*, and *CREBBP* {152,876,2,1610, 1597,2888,2968,3503,3297,1154,1549,3319}. Many of these

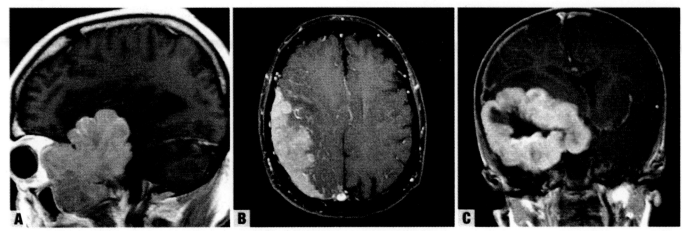

Fig. 7.04 Meningioma. Postcontrast T1-weighted MRI. **A** Papillary meningioma. Occasional papillary meningiomas feature a cauliflower-like imaging appearance. **B** Atypical meningioma. An irregular interface between the atypical meningioma and adjacent brain. **C** Anaplastic meningioma. A centrally necrotic, contrast-enhancing tumour with marked mass effects.

syndromes are associated with increased radiosensitivity. Family history studies suggest that inherited susceptibility not attributable to established syndromes plays a role, with a positive family history associated with up to a four-fold personal risk of developing meningioma {606,644}. Genome-wide association studies have recently detected SNPs on chromosomes 10 and 11 that are significantly associated with meningioma risk {764,607,828}. The 10p12 SNP is located in the *MLLT10* gene, a component in several gene fusions resulting in forms of leukaemia {764}.

Pathogenesis

Monosomy of chromosome 22 is the most frequently reported genetic abnormality in meningioma, with > 50% of tumours showing allelic losses in 22q12.2, the region encoding the *NF2* gene. Higher-grade meningiomas exhibit more complex genetic changes, with losses on 1p, 6p/q, 10q, 14q, and 18p/q, and (less frequently) losses on 2p/q, 3p, 4p/q, 7p, and 8p/q, as well as heterozygous or homozygous deletions of *CDKN2A* and/or *CDKN2B*. Gains of chromosomal arms are less common and mostly found in angiomatous, metaplastic, and microcystic meningiomas.

Genomic sequencing of two series of sporadic meningiomas {353,601} identified similar meningioma subsets, notable for their distinct and mutually exclusive mutation distributions as well as for their correlation with clinical behaviours and anatomical locations. The first subset of meningiomas was defined by *NF2* mutations and loss of chromosome 22. The second subset lacked *NF2* mutations and was characterized by recurrent oncogenic (p.E17K) mutations in *AKT1*, as well as alterations in *TRAF7* {601}, *KLF4* {601}, or *SMO* {353}. These findings have been confirmed and expanded, with oncogenic *PIK3CA* mutations also identified {9,602,3052}. The accumulation of additional copy-number losses, general genomic instability, and emergence of *TERT* promoter mutations was largely restricted to the group with *NF2* mutation and/or loss of chromosome 22q, whereas cases with *AKT1*, *KLF4*, *SMO*, *PIK3CA*, and/or *TRAF7* mutations had balanced copy-number profiles {1153,601,353,1152,2488,1516,2390}. *YAP1* alterations occur in a subset of predominantly paediatric meningiomas that do not have *NF2* mutations, possibly resulting in activation of the Hippo pathway {2930}.

Initiation and malignant progression of *NF2*-driven meningiomas has been confirmed in genetically engineered mouse models. Inactivation of *Nf2* by injection of an adenovirus-encoding recombinant Cre into the subdural space of mice harbouring floxed *Nf2* alleles (Nf2flox/flox) with arachnoid-specific deletion of *Nf2* results in the induction of meningiomas, proving that inactivation of *NF2* is an essential initial step for meningioma development {1530}. *NF2* alterations are found in meningiomas of all CNS WHO grades and thus represent an early event in meningioma development {1153}. Progression of meningiomas to CNS WHO grades 2 and 3 has been achieved in mice by combined arachnoid-specific deletion of *Nf2* along with *Cdkn2a* and *Cdkn2b* {2489}.

In contrast, tumour initiation of non-*NF2* meningiomas has not been adequately modelled to date, but experimental evidence supports their role in oncogenesis. The meningioma hotspot mutation *AKT1* p.E17K, which is also found in breast and urinary bladder cancer, leads to constitutive activation of AKT1 and induces leukaemia in mice (which cannot be induced by wildtype *AKT1* alone), suggesting that the *AKT1* p.E17K mutation is an oncogenic driver {472,690,1991}. The *SMO* hotspot mutations p.L412F and p.W535L are associated with increased SMO transactivating activity and development of basal cell carcinoma {1530,3490}. *KLF4* has been associated with context-dependent tumour suppression or oncogenesis {2740}, and it may act as a tumour suppressor in meningioma {3132}. Functionally, the *KLF4* p.K409Q mutation triggers the induction of HIF1α {3348}. TRAF7 interacts with MAP3K3 (MEKK3) and is involved in the regulation of the TNF-α/NF-κB signal transduction pathway {344}. Non-*NF2* meningiomas with *TRAF7* mutation show upregulation of the inhibitory immune checkpoint molecules PDL1, IDO, and TDO (TDO2) {1233}, linking this mutation with suppressed immune response in meningiomas. The oncogenic potential of *PIK3CA* mutations has been demonstrated in several tumour types {1403}, and *PIK3CA* mutations activate several proliferation-associated signalling pathways in meningiomas {831}. Moreover, *PIK3CA* mutations are convincingly linked to antihormone treatment. Women with meningioma who are under long-term progestin therapy carry *PIK3CA* mutations more frequently than those not under hormone therapy, and high-dose antiandrogen treatment with cyproterone leads to an enrichment of *PIK3CA*-mutated skull base meningiomas {2487,2544}. *POLR2A* mutations may drive meningioma development by altering the transcriptional machinery and essential meningeal genes {602}.

Macroscopic appearance

Meningiomas are generally solid, globular, circumscribed masses that have broad dural attachment. Some are lobulated or bilobed and others grow in a flat, carpet-like, en plaque pattern, such as those growing along the dura of the sphenoid bone. Meningiomas are firm, rubbery, or (sometimes) gelatinous or cystic. Some meningiomas, particularly the spinal psammomatous subtype, can have a gritty texture due to an abundance of psammoma bodies; others, such as the fibrous subtype, can have a smooth surface. Most grade 1 meningiomas displace and compress the adjacent brain but are not adherent or invasive and can be separated readily from the brain. Higher-grade meningiomas, however, can be broadly adherent and invasive and may also feature areas of necrosis. Meningiomas can also invade the dural sinuses, for example, parasagittal meningiomas that can partly or completely obstruct the superior sagittal sinus. Occasionally, meningiomas invade the skull and induce reactive hyperostosis of areas such as the skull vault, the sphenoid bone, or the bones of the orbit. Meningiomas may also attach or encase cerebral arteries and/or cranial nerves, but they rarely infiltrate these structures. They may infiltrate through the cranium into the soft tissues of the scalp and skin, and into extracranial compartments, such as the orbit.

Histopathology

The wide morphological spectrum of meningiomas is reflected by the 15 subtypes described in Box 7.01 (p. 284). The most commonly encountered subtypes are meningothelial, fibrous, and transitional meningiomas. Most subtypes have a benign clinical course and correspond to CNS WHO grade 1. However, features of more aggressive growth can arise in any of these morphological patterns; in other words, the criteria defining atypical or anaplastic meningioma (see Box 7.02) should be applied regardless of the underlying subtype. Notably, two subtypes – chordoid and clear cell meningiomas – have been reported to have a higher likelihood of recurrence than the average CNS WHO grade 1 meningioma and have therefore been assigned to CNS WHO grade 2, independent of the criteria otherwise applied for CNS WHO grade 2 atypical meningioma; nonetheless, larger and prospective studies would be helpful to validate these proposed CNS WHO grade 2 assignments and to suggest additional prognostic biomarkers. In addition, historically, rhabdoid and papillary morphology qualified for CNS WHO grade 3 irrespective of any other indications for malignancy. Although papillary and rhabdoid features are often seen in combination with other aggressive features, more recent studies suggest that the CNS WHO grade should be assigned by applying the criteria for CNS WHO grade 2 atypical or CNS WHO grade 3 anaplastic meningioma, not on the basis of rhabdoid or papillary histology alone {3301}. Issues relating to grading meningiomas, as well as recommendations for the use of particular biomarkers, are discussed in the description of each subtype below.

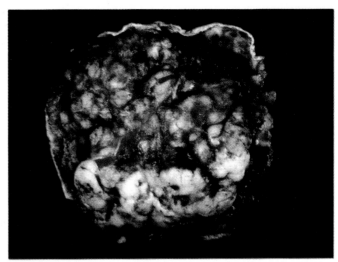

Fig. 7.05 Meningioma. This surgically resected meningioma shows the typical bosselated surface and dural attachment.

Box 7.02 Criteria for assigning meningiomas to CNS WHO grades 2 and 3; these criteria can be applied across all meningioma subtypes, but the CNS WHO grade 2 criteria must be met for a diagnosis of atypical meningioma, and the CNS WHO grade 3 criteria must be met for a diagnosis of anaplastic (malignant) meningioma

CNS WHO grade 2

4 to 19 mitotic figures in 10 consecutive HPF of each 0.16 mm² (at least 2.5/mm²)

OR

Unequivocal brain invasion (not only perivascular spread or indentation of brain without pial breach)

OR

Specific morphological subtype (chordoid or clear cell; see text)

OR

At least three of the following:

- Increased cellularity
- Small cells with high N:C ratio
- Prominent nucleoli
- Sheeting (uninterrupted patternless or sheet-like growth)
- Foci of spontaneous (non-iatrogenic) necrosis

CNS WHO grade 3

20 or more mitotic figures in 10 consecutive HPF of each 0.16 mm² (at least 12.5/mm²)

OR

Frank anaplasia (sarcoma-, carcinoma-, or melanoma-like appearance)

OR

TERT promoter mutation

OR

Homozygous deletion of *CDKN2A* and/or *CDKN2B*

Immunohistochemistry and proliferation

Immunohistochemistry can assist in establishing a meningioma diagnosis and can exclude other differential considerations. Meningiomas typically express EMA and vimentin. However, the EMA staining can be faint, focal, or even absent, particularly in fibrous and higher-grade subtypes, and vimentin positivity has low specificity. SSTR2A is expressed strongly and diffusely in almost all cases, but it can also be expressed in neuroendocrine neoplasms.

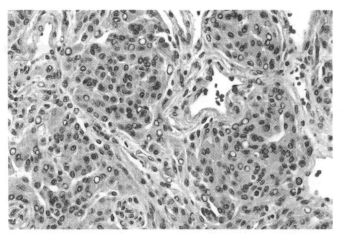

Fig. 7.06 Meningothelial meningioma. Lobular growth pattern, syncytium-like appearance due to poorly defined cell borders, and frequent clear nuclear holes, with occasional intranuclear pseudoinclusions.

Immunohistochemistry for Ki-67 can highlight an uneven distribution of proliferation and guide assessment of mitotic counts. Studies suggest that cases with a proliferation index > 4% have recurrence rates similar to those of CNS WHO grade 2 (atypical) meningiomas, and that cases with an index > 20% are associated with mortality rates similar to those of CNS WHO grade 3 (anaplastic) meningiomas. One study found that staining for the mitosis marker phosphohistone H3 can stratify meningiomas into three risk groups, defined by 0–2, 3–4, and ≥ 5 labelled mitoses per 1000 tumour cells {2319}; however, interlaboratory differences that affect staining and interpretation limit the translation of these findings.

Meningothelial meningioma

In the meningothelial subtype of meningioma, epithelioid cells form syncytia-like lobules, with some nuclei appearing to have nuclear holes and pseudoinclusions.

Meningothelial meningioma cells resemble the morphology of arachnoid cap cells. They are largely monomorphic, with abundant eosinophilic cytoplasm, and are arranged in lobules that can be demarcated by fine collagen septa. Borders between the cells are hardly appreciable with light microscopy, giving the impression of a syncytium, although ultrastructural investigations have revealed that the tumour cells have separate delicate processes, demonstrating that the pattern is a pseudosyncytium. The round to oval nuclei can have internal empty spaces (nuclear holes) and pseudoinclusions (cytoplasmic invaginations). Whorls and psammoma bodies are rare compared with their occurrence in transitional, fibrous, and psammomatous meningiomas.

The similarity to arachnoid cap cells warrants caution when encountering small fragments that may also be compatible with meningothelial hyperplasia, which can occur in the vicinity of other neoplasms such as optic gliomas.

Meningothelial meningiomas often harbour *AKT1* p.E17K mutations, frequently combined with *TRAF7* mutations (also common in secretory meningioma), or *SMO* and *PIK3CA* mutations {601,353,9,2777}. *AKT1*, *SMO*, and *PIK3CA* mutations are virtually absent in other subtypes. Conversely, *NF2* mutations are rare in meningothelial meningioma, as are deletions of chromosomal arm 22q or other chromosomal alterations. The DNA methylation profile of meningothelial meningiomas is similar to that of secretory meningioma {2783}. Meningiomas of this subtype are more common at the skull base than other subtypes, and the frequencies of *AKT1*, *TRAF7*, *SMO*, and/or *PIK3CA* mutations in meningothelial meningioma at this location are particularly high.

Fibrous meningioma

The fibrous subtype of meningioma has spindle cells in parallel, storiform, or interlacing bundles in a collagen-rich matrix.

Tumour cells form fascicles with varying amounts of intercellular collagen. The collagen deposition can be extensive and suggest the differential diagnosis of solitary fibrous tumour, but only solitary fibrous tumour shows nuclear staining for STAT6. EMA expression can be weak or absent, whereas S100 staining can be surprisingly strong. In contrast to that seen in schwannoma, though, SSTR2A expression is often strong and diffuse in fibrous meningioma.

Fibrous meningiomas typically show 22q deletion and mutation of the retained *NF2* allele, similar to transitional and

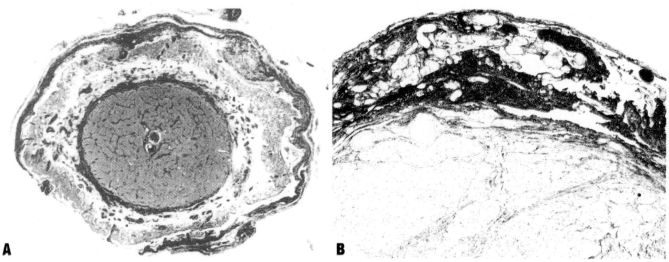

A **B**

Fig. 7.07 Meningothelial hyperplasia. **A** An optic nerve glioma surrounded by meningothelial hyperplasia. On biopsy, this may be mistaken for meningioma, but it differs in its smaller size, multicentricity, and lack of dural invasion. **B** EMA immunostaining highlights the meningothelial hyperplasia surrounding this paraspinal neurofibroma.

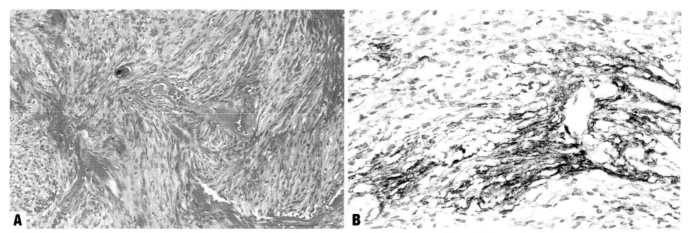

Fig. 7.08 Fibrous meningioma. **A** Fascicular spindle cell tumour with variable collagen deposition. **B** There is only focal EMA expression in this tumour.

psammomatous meningiomas. Their DNA methylation features overlap those of transitional and psammomatous meningiomas. They are frequently found at the convexity.

Transitional meningioma

The transitional subtype of meningioma contains meningothelial and fibrous patterns as well as transitional features.

Lobular and fascicular areas appear side by side, with some areas not clearly attributable to one or the other of the two patterns (hence "transitional"). Whorl formation and psammoma bodies are frequent in this subtype. Transitional meningiomas share with fibrous and psammomatous meningiomas the features of frequent 22q deletions and *NF2* mutations, and they have similar DNA methylation characteristics. They often arise from the convexity.

Psammomatous meningioma

In the psammomatous subtype of meningioma, psammoma bodies predominate over the viable tumour cells.

The overlap of individual psammoma bodies can result in large, confluent, calcified masses. Actual meningioma cells can be rare to virtually absent, but they can be highlighted by

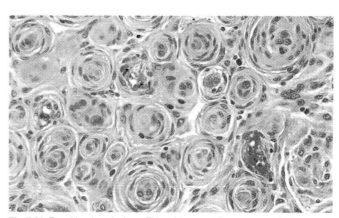

Fig. 7.09 Transitional meningioma. This subtype contains numerous whorls.

immunohistochemistry for EMA or SSTR2A. Non-calcified foci typically conform to the fibrous or transitional subtypes. Psammomatous meningiomas share molecular features with fibrous and transitional meningiomas, particularly 22q deletions, *NF2* mutations, and epigenetic profiles. This subtype often occurs in the thoracic spine region of middle-aged to elderly women.

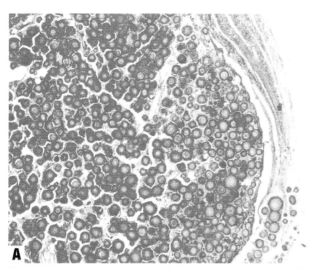

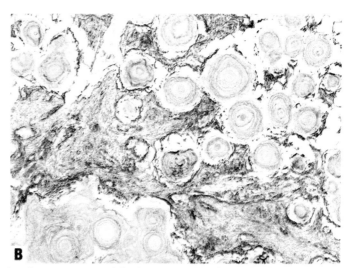

Fig. 7.10 Psammomatous meningioma. **A** Almost complete replacement of the meningioma by psammomatous calcifications (postdecalcification specimen). **B** EMA immunostaining reveals meningioma cells between psammoma bodies.

Chapter 7

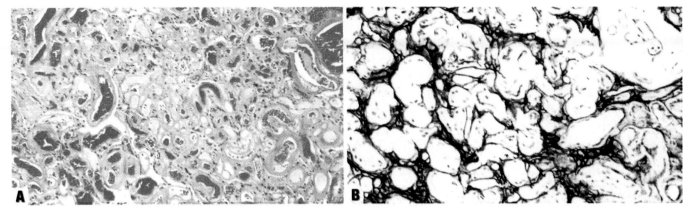

Fig. 7.11 Angiomatous meningioma. **A** Blood vessels constitute most of the cross-sectional area of this tumour. **B** The tumour cells between blood vessels are highlighted on SSTR2A immunohistochemistry.

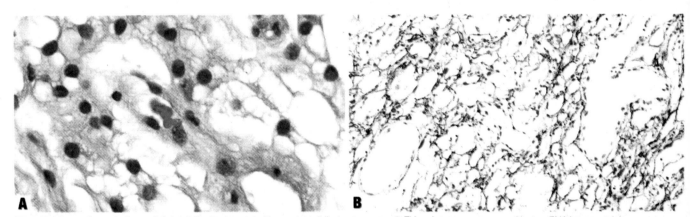

Fig. 7.12 Microcystic meningioma. **A** Cobweb-like background with numerous delicate processes. **B** Thin, wispy processes are evident on EMA immunostaining.

Angiomatous meningioma

In the angiomatous subtype of meningioma, often-hyalinized small blood vessels predominate over the intermixed meningioma cells.

Between the numerous vessels, the actual tumour cells may be hard to find and to identify as meningioma cells. Blood vessels can be thin- or thick-walled, and variably hyalinized. Angiomatous areas can also be intermixed with microcystic or even metaplastic areas, and, like in these subtypes, the cells can show degenerative nuclear atypia. Hypervascular examples may mimic haemangioblastoma but are typically inhibin-negative and SSTR2A-positive.

Angiomatous, microcystic, and metaplastic meningiomas all have a high frequency of chromosome 5 gain {10}.

Like secretory and microcystic meningiomas, angiomatous meningiomas are often associated with cerebral oedema beyond that expected for the tumour size.

Microcystic meningioma

The microcystic subtype of meningioma has microcysts formed by cells with thin, elongated processes, creating a cobweb-like background on histology.

The cysts can expand to macroscopically or radiologically detectable macrocysts. Like in angiomatous meningioma, the presence of degenerative nuclear atypia in microcystic meningioma can raise the suspicion of a higher grade. However, microcystic meningiomas are typically benign. Gain of chromosome 5 is common, as it is in angiomatous and metaplastic meningiomas, with which microcystic areas can be combined {1599}. Cerebral oedema is frequent, as it is in angiomatous and secretory meningiomas.

Secretory meningioma

The secretory subtype of meningioma is characterized by foci of gland-like epithelial differentiation with PAS-positive eosinophilic secretions and/or combined *KLF4* and *TRAF7* mutations.

The eosinophilic secretions (pseudopsammoma bodies) are positive for a variety of epithelial and secretory markers, including CEA. The surrounding cells can also be positive for CEA and cytokeratins. Elevated CEA levels in the blood can occasionally be observed {1936}, which drop with resection and rise in the rare cases of recurrence. Peritumoural oedema is common.

Combined *KLF4* p.K409Q and *TRAF7* (distributed across the WD40 domain) mutations genetically characterize this subtype {601,2656}. In a few instances, the *KLF4* mutations may be isolated.

Lymphoplasmacyte-rich meningioma

Lymphoplasmacyte-rich meningioma is a rare subtype in which extensive chronic inflammatory infiltrates predominate over the meningothelial component.

Despite the name, plasma cells may be scant, and macrophages often predominate {1793}. In some cases, it may be challenging to distinguish this subtype from inflammatory disorders with patchy meningothelial hyperplasia.

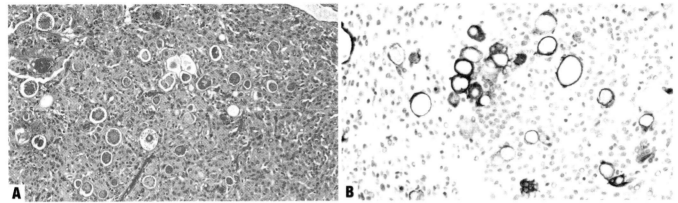

Fig. 7.13 Secretory meningioma. **A** The presence of gland-like spaces filled with pseudopsammoma bodies characterizes this as a secretory meningioma. **B** The cells surrounding gland-like spaces are positive for cytokeratin.

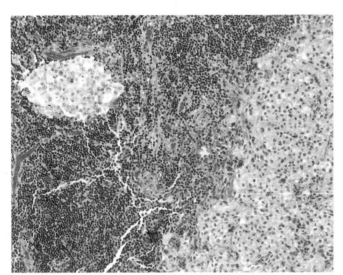

Fig. 7.14 Lymphoplasmacyte-rich meningioma. Marked tumour-associated chronic inflammation.

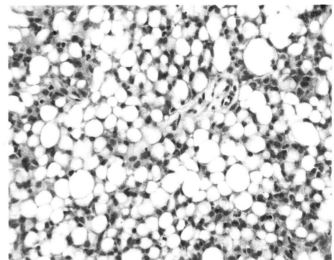

Fig. 7.15 Lipoma-like metaplastic meningioma. Lipidized meningioma cells resemble lipoma.

Metaplastic meningioma

The metaplastic subtype of meningioma has focal or extensive mesenchymal components, including osseous, cartilaginous, lipomatous, myxoid, and xanthomatous tissue, either singly or in combinations.

These alterations have no known clinical relevance, and most do not constitute true metaplasia (e.g. a lipomatous appearance as a result of lipid accumulation rather than true lipomatous metaplasia). The morphological features of metaplastic meningioma can overlap with those of angiomatous and microcystic meningiomas, and gain of chromosome 5 is frequent in all three subtypes {2783}.

Ossification in metaplastic meningioma can be hard to distinguish from dystrophic ossification of psammoma bodies in psammomatous meningioma, or from bone invasion. Remnants of the concentric inner structure of psammoma bodies or radiographic imaging of adjacent bone, respectively, may assist in differentiation.

Chordoid meningioma

The chordoid subtype of meningioma predominantly resembles chordoma, featuring cords or trabeculae of small, epithelioid (or less often spindled), variably vacuolated cells embedded in a mucin-rich matrix.

Chordoid areas are often interspersed with more typical meningioma; however, pure examples are also encountered. Chronic inflammatory infiltrates are often patchy when present, but they may be prominent. Chordoid meningiomas are characteristically large, supratentorial tumours, and the patients may be younger, with an average age at presentation of about 45 years {590}. Chordoid meningiomas often lack any other high-grade histopathological features, but they have recurrence rates analogous to those of atypical meningiomas and have therefore been designated CNS WHO grade 2 {642, 2934}. One study reported frequent epithelial differentiation with NHERF1-immunoreactive cytoplasmic microlumina, similar to that in secretory meningiomas {1059}. Rarely, patients have associated haematological conditions, such as anaemia or Castleman disease {1590}. Chromosome 2p deletions are overrepresented, but DNA methylation profiles overlap with those of other meningioma subtypes {2934}.

Clear cell meningioma

The clear cell subtype of meningioma has a predominantly patternless or sheeting architecture containing round to polygonal

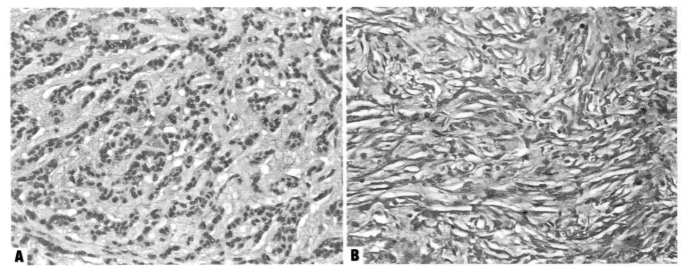

Fig. 7.16 Chordoid meningioma. **A** Cords of small epithelioid to vacuolated tumour cells embedded in a mucin-rich matrix. **B** Alcian blue highlights the mucin-rich matrix.

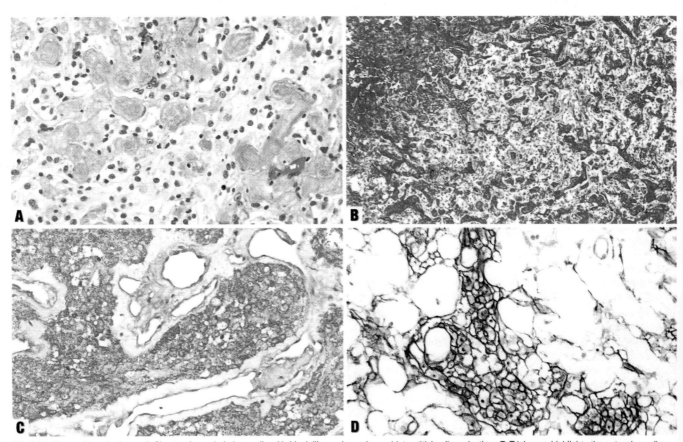

Fig. 7.17 Clear cell meningioma. **A** Sheets of rounded clear cells with block-like perivascular and interstitial collagenization. **B** Trichrome highlights the extensive collagen deposits, including larger coalescent forms. **C** Abundant intracytoplasmic glycogen is noted on PAS histochemistry. **D** SSTR2A-immunoreactive tumour cells.

cells with clear, glycogen-rich cytoplasm and prominent perivascular and interstitial collagen.

The perivascular and interstitial collagen occasionally coalesces into large acellular zones of collagen or forms brightly eosinophilic, amianthoid-like collagen. It shows prominent PAS-positive and diastase-sensitive cytoplasmic glycogen. Whorl formation is vague and psammoma bodies are inconspicuous. Clear cell meningioma has a proclivity for the cerebellopontine

angle and spine, especially the cauda equina region. It also tends to affect younger patients, including children and young adults (mean age in one series: 24 years) {3593}. Clear cell meningiomas are associated with more aggressive behaviour, including recurrence and occasional cerebrospinal fluid seeding, and have therefore been designated CNS WHO grade 2, pending larger studies to confirm the higher rates of recurrence {3620}. Both germline (familial examples) and somatic

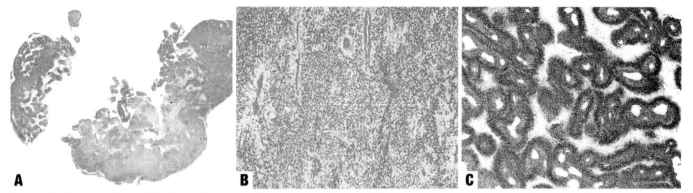

Fig. 7.18 Papillary meningioma. **A** Papillary architecture is evident at low magnification. **B** Nucleus-free perivascular zones resemble the pseudorosettes of ependymoma. **C** SSTR2A immunoreactivity highlights the perivascular aggregation of tumour cells.

SMARCE1 mutations are common, with virtually all cases showing loss of nuclear SMARCE1 expression by immunohistochemistry {1061,3148,575}.

Papillary meningioma

The papillary subtype of meningioma is defined by the presence of a predominant perivascular pseudopapillary pattern.

In the papillary subtype, meningioma tumour cells surround thin-walled blood vessels in a perivascular, pseudorosette-like pattern (i.e. a perivascular nucleus-free region). Some meningiomas have cells with rhabdoid cytomorphology arranged in a papillary architecture, consistent with a molecular and genetic link between the papillary and rhabdoid subtypes {3485,3301, 2888,3449}. Papillary meningiomas have been reported in children {1957} and adults {1864,3592}. These tumours are commonly associated with peritumoural oedema and bone hyperostosis or destruction; cyst formation can be seen {1910,1864, 3555}. A papillary growth pattern has been associated with brain invasion and aggressive clinical behaviour including dissemination and metastasis, predominantly to the lung {2410,1957,2593, 3485,1864}. Focal papillary architecture, in the absence of any other features of higher grades, does not suffice for designating tumours as CNS WHO grade 2 or 3.

Some meningiomas have cells with rhabdoid cytomorphology arranged in a papillary architecture {3485,3301}. Consistent with this occasionally observed morphological overlap, papillary and rhabdoid meningiomas have the same genetic alterations:

PBRM1 is predominantly mutant or deleted in papillary meningioma, but it is also altered in single rhabdoid meningioma cases {3449}. Similarly, *BAP1* mutations or deletions, typically found in rhabdoid meningiomas, have also been reported in papillary meningiomas or rhabdoid meningiomas with partly papillary features, which are then usually combined with alterations of *PBRM1* {3449,2888}.

Rhabdoid meningioma

The rhabdoid subtype of meningioma is defined by the presence of rhabdoid cells, which are plump cells with eccentric nuclei, open chromatin, macronucleoli, and prominent eosinophilic paranuclear inclusions appearing either as discernible whorled fibrils or compact and waxy spheres.

Rhabdoid features are usually present at primary resection but can become increasingly evident upon recurrence. Most rhabdoid meningiomas are highly proliferative and have other histological features of malignancy. Original cohorts of rhabdoid meningiomas comprised tumours with high rates of recurrence and death {1592,2474}, supporting the designation as a CNS WHO grade 3 malignancy. Most of the tumours in those cohorts otherwise fulfilled the criteria for classification as CNS WHO grade 3 anaplastic/malignant meningioma, irrespective of rhabdoid cytology. A large portion of rhabdoid meningiomas, however, have since been diagnosed on the basis of rhabdoid cells alone, not fulfilling other criteria for CNS WHO grade 3 classification; of those, 50% have CNS WHO grade 1 features and

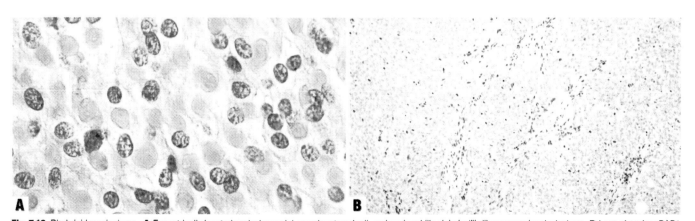

Fig. 7.19 Rhabdoid meningioma. **A** Eccentrically located vesicular nuclei, prominent nucleoli, and eosinophilic globular/fibrillar paranuclear inclusions. **B** Loss of nuclear BAP1 immunoreactivity, which has been associated with a more aggressive biology.

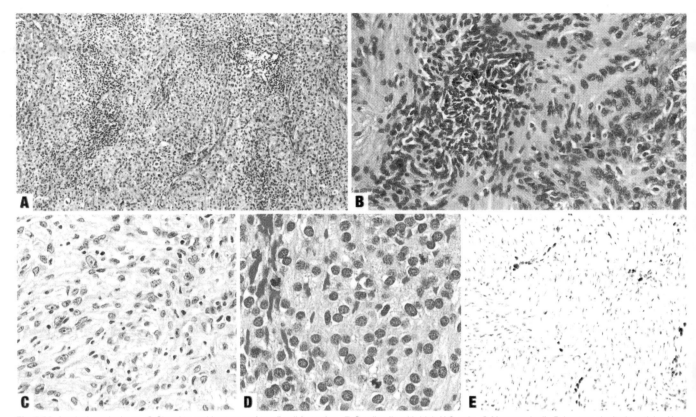

Fig. 7.20 Atypical meningioma. **A** Sheeting architecture and small cell formation. **B** Small cells with high N:C ratio. **C** Macronucleoli. **D** Increased mitotic activity. Note the lack of nuclear atypia, despite the name "atypical meningioma". **E** Loss of nuclear H3 p.K28me3 (K27me3) immunostaining, which has been associated with a worse prognosis.

50% have CNS WHO grade 2 features {3301}. A meta-analysis showed that patient outcome is strongly correlated with CNS WHO grade, independent of the rhabdoid features; this work suggests that rhabdoid meningiomas should be graded similarly to non-rhabdoid meningiomas, but the authors cautioned that some of these tumours may still behave aggressively and that close patient follow-up is required {3301}. Some meningiomas have cells with rhabdoid cytomorphology arranged in a papillary architecture, suggesting a relationship between these two subtypes {3485,3301,2888,3449}. A subset of rhabdoid and/or papillary meningiomas arise in patients with germline mutations in the *BAP1* gene as part of the *BAP1* tumour predisposition syndrome, in which family members may develop uveal and cutaneous melanoma, mesothelioma, and renal cell carcinoma, among other tumours. Importantly, in this context, immunohistochemical loss of BAP1 expression was associated with aggressive (consistent with CNS WHO grade 3) clinical behaviour in these tumours {2888}. In addition, as discussed above under *Papillary meningioma*, there may be overlap between the histological and genetic features of rhabdoid and papillary meningiomas.

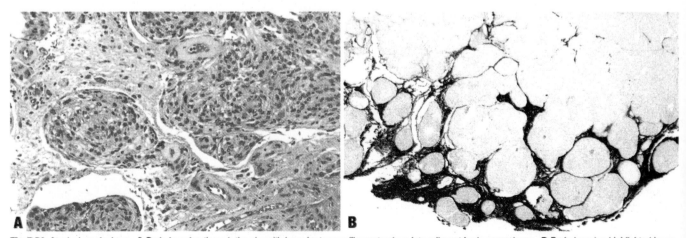

Fig. 7.21 Atypical meningioma. **A** Brain invasion through the pia, with irregular tongue-like protrusions into adjacent brain parenchyma. **B** Brain invasion highlighted by entrapped GFAP-positive islands of gliotic brain parenchyma at the tumour periphery.

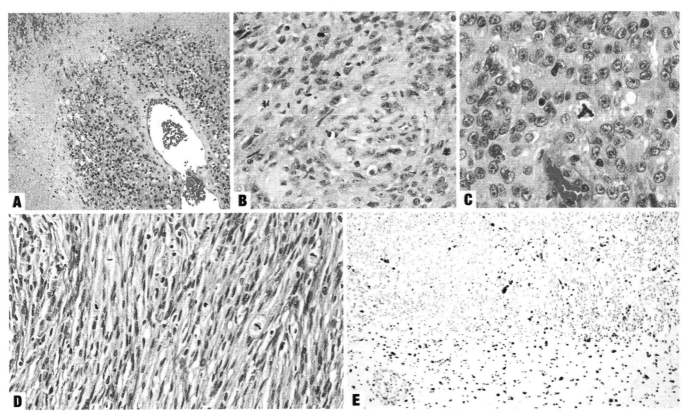

Fig. 7.22 Anaplastic meningioma. **A** Extensive geographical necrosis. **B** Poorly differentiated neoplasm with markedly elevated mitotic count. **C** Carcinoma- or melanoma-like cytology with an atypical mitotic figure. **D** Fibrosarcoma-like (sarcomatoid) meningioma with markedly elevated mitotic count. **E** Loss of nuclear H3 p.K28me3 (K27me3) staining in tumour cells.

Atypical meningioma

Atypical meningioma is an intermediate-grade meningioma with increased mitotic activity, brain invasion, and/or at least three of the following: high cellularity, small cells with a high N:C ratio, prominent nucleoli, sheeting (uninterrupted patternless or sheet-like growth), and foci of spontaneous (non-iatrogenic) necrosis.

Increased mitotic activity was defined in one large clinicopathological series as ≥ 2.5 mitoses/mm² (equating to ≥ 4 mitoses per/10 HPF of 0.16 mm², as originally described) {2475}. Despite the name "atypical meningioma", nuclear atypia is not a useful criterion, as it is often considered degenerative in nature and not associated with patient outcome. Clinical risk factors for atypical meningioma include male sex, non–skull base location, and prior surgery {1539}. Atypical meningiomas have been associated with high recurrence rates despite gross total resection {30}, and bone involvement may be associated with a further increase in recurrence risk {1018}. Brain invasion by meningioma is characterized by irregular, tongue-like protrusions of tumour cells into underlying GFAP-positive parenchyma, without intervening leptomeninges. Extension along perivascular Virchow–Robin spaces does not constitute brain invasion because the pia is not breached. Such perivascular spread and hyalinization is most commonly encountered in children and can mimic meningioangiomatosis {1087, 2469}. Brain invasion occurs most often in meningiomas with additional high-grade features. Nonetheless, the presence of brain invasion in clinically totally resected, otherwise benign-appearing meningiomas remains controversial, as it has been associated with recurrence rates similar to those of other CNS

WHO grade 2 meningiomas in some, but not all, studies {2473, 220,272}. Larger series with longer follow-up times may be needed to resolve this issue. Atypical meningiomas can be further risk stratified based on the inclusion of various additional clinicopathological and genetic factors {773,2782,2783, 547,1569,405,206,936,1018}. However, some genetic changes (e.g. *TERT* promoter mutation or homozygous *CDKN2A* and/ or *CDKN2B* deletion) are evidence for diagnosing CNS WHO grade 3 meningioma (see below), so consideration should be given to *TERT*, *CDKN2A*, and *CDKN2B* analysis in clinically aggressive atypical meningiomas or those with borderline CNS WHO grade 2/3 features.

Anaplastic (malignant) meningioma

Anaplastic (malignant) meningioma is a high-grade meningioma with overtly malignant cytomorphology (anaplasia) that can (1) resemble carcinoma, high-grade sarcoma, or melanoma; (2) display markedly elevated mitotic activity; (3) harbour a *TERT* promoter mutation; and/or (4) have a homozygous *CDKN2A* and/or *CDKN2B* deletion.

A mitotic count of ≥ 12.5 mitoses/mm² (equating to ≥ 20 mitoses/10 HPF of 0.16 mm², as originally described) was used to define markedly elevated mitotic activity in a study of 116 patients {2473}. Anaplastic meningiomas account for 1–3% of meningiomas. Most of these tumours display extensive necrosis and can invade brain. In some anaplastic cases, meningothelial origin can be confirmed using immunohistochemistry {2070,791} or genetic testing {2783,266,2390,2214}. Because malignant progression in meningiomas is a continuum

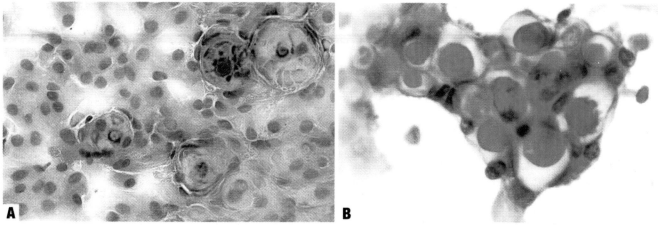

Fig. 7.23 Meningioma. **A** Intraoperative touch preparation of meningioma. Whorls and small psammoma bodies can be appreciated. **B** Secretory meningioma. Pseudopsammoma bodies are evident on intraoperative smear.

of increasing anaplasia, determining the cut-off point between atypical and anaplastic meningioma can be challenging. Inter-observer reproducibility is good for mitotic count but only fair for overt anaplasia {1048}. The presence of a *TERT* promoter mutation confers a high risk of recurrence and short interval to progression, irrespective of other histological features {1152, 2782,1517}. Similarly, homozygous deletion of *CDKN2A* and/or *CDKN2B* is associated with high-grade histopathology, elevated risk of recurrence, and shorter time to progression {331,2939, 2465,1724,2931}. Loss of H3 p.K28me3 (K27me3) is observed in about 10–20% of anaplastic meningiomas and is associated with shorter overall survival {1569,1048}.

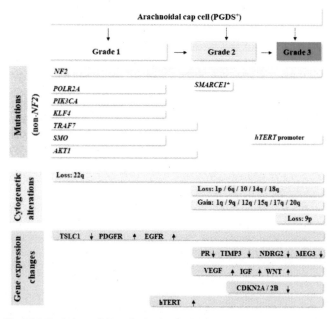

Fig. 7.24 Meningioma. Schematic showing the distribution and evolution of genomic and expression characteristics in meningioma grades. Mutations are listed in the grey bars, with light grey indicating mutations occurring in meningiomas without *NF2* alterations. Cytogenetic alterations are listed in the blue bars, and gene expression changes in green. Bar length indicates the relative frequency of an alteration within the given tumour grade. **SMARCE1* mutations have been found nearly exclusively in clear cell meningiomas. PGDS⁺, prostaglandin D2 synthase–positive precursor cells in murine meningioma models.

Other histopathological patterns

The large number of subtypes covered above already illustrates the wide morphological spectrum of meningiomas. However, meningiomas can have a variety of morphological characteristics that even exceed those of the established subtypes. These include meningiomas with oncocytic, mucinous, sclerosing, whorling–sclerosing, GFAP-expressing, and granulofilamentous inclusion–bearing features, or the occurrence of meningothelial rosettes {2717,1025,1207,1342,250,69}. These patterns are rare, and the data on biological and clinical correlations are too scarce to identify any relevant implications.

Cytology

On intraoperative smear and touch preparations, characteristic cytological features of meningioma are often apparent, with oval, euchromatic nuclei (sometimes with intranuclear pseudoinclusions) and delicate cytoplasm visible. Whorls may be prominent on touch preparations. Adequate smears may be difficult in meningiomas with more copious collagen.

Diagnostic molecular pathology

Genetic changes (e.g. in *AKT1*, *SMO*, *PIK3CA*) are strongly related to the subtypes of meningioma, but do not define them. The status of most genetic alterations immediately relevant to subtyping and grading (including *TERT* promoter, *SMARCE1*, *KLF4* and *TRAF7*, and other alterations) can be assessed by DNA sequencing. Because *TERT* mutations can arise during progression, selection of tissue for DNA extraction should focus on the most malignant-appearing and proliferative regions. Homozygous deletion of *CDKN2A* and/or *CDKN2B* can be assessed by in situ hybridization or calculated from various high-throughput sequencing or hybridization assays; however, FISH probes are large, so small deletions can sometimes be missed by this technique. Rare events such as *TERT* activation by gene fusion or such as gene fusions involving *YAP1* may in some cases be inferred from high-resolution copy-number plots, but they can typically only be proved by RNA sequencing or in situ hybridization. *BAP1* and *PBRM1* can be affected by both mutation and deletion, thus requiring DNA sequencing and, if not already provided within the sequencing approach, independent copy-number assessment. Alternatively to DNA-based methods, surrogate immunohistochemical stains can be used to detect some genetic alterations, including SMARCE1 loss (clear cell meningioma), BAP1 loss (rhabdoid meningioma), or posttranslational modifications including H3 p.K28me3 (K27me3) status (trimethylation is lost in a subset of aggressive meningiomas).

Methylome profiling can provide information about tumour type in histologically challenging cases and define the epigenetic subgroup; in addition, copy-number alterations are reported in parallel with the DNA methylation results.

Essential and desirable diagnostic criteria
See Box 7.03.

Staging
Brain invasion is a criterion for the diagnosis of CNS WHO grade 2 meningioma, and bone invasion has been associated with worse prognosis in atypical meningioma {1018}.

Prognosis and prediction
The major prognostic questions regarding meningiomas involve estimates of recurrence, progression-free survival, and overall survival.

Clinical factors
A major clinical predictor of recurrence and overall survival is the extent of resection {45}, which is influenced by the tumour site, extent of invasion, attachment to critical intracranial structures, and availability of expert neurosurgical services. In most cases, meningiomas can be removed entirely, as assessed by operative or neuroradiological criteria; however, recurrence can occur even after complete resection. In one series, 20% of gross totally resected benign meningiomas recurred within 20 years {1429}. Rates of recurrence are significantly higher in CNS WHO grade 2 and 3 meningiomas than in CNS WHO grade 1 meningiomas {1430}; mortality rates are also higher, and especially so in patients with CNS WHO grade 3 tumours.

Histopathology and grading
Overall, CNS WHO grade is the most useful histopathological predictor of recurrence, and (as mentioned above) some histological subtypes of meningioma are more likely to recur. CNS WHO grade 1 meningiomas have recurrence rates of about 7–25%, whereas CNS WHO grade 2 meningiomas recur in 29–52% of cases and CNS WHO grade 3 meningiomas in 50–94%. Even among CNS WHO grade 1 meningiomas, however, the presence of some atypical features increases the risk of subsequent progression/recurrence {2009}. Malignant histological features are associated with shorter survival times {45, 622,2473}. Anaplastic meningioma is often fatal, with median survival times ranging from < 2 years to > 5 years, depending on the extent of resection and the use of radiation therapy {2473,3064,1045,2334}. In one study, which found a median overall survival of 2.6 years and a 5-year survival rate of 10%, de novo anaplastic meningiomas had a better outcome than did secondary anaplastic meningiomas {2488}. Patients with meningiomas that show high mitotic counts have significantly shorter overall survival than patients with meningiomas showing overt anaplasia without a high mitotic count, and those tumours are associated with significantly lower patient survival rates than atypical meningiomas {2488,1048}.

Molecular features
A number of molecular features have prognostic significance in meningiomas. Higher-grade meningiomas are associated with more complex copy-number changes and chromosomal abnormalities {266,353,1851}. DNA methylation patterns separate subgroups of meningiomas, including those with higher risk of recurrence {1569,2390,2783}. Meningiomas that have *TERT* promoter mutations have a higher rate of malignant transformation, a shorter time to recurrence, and a lower overall survival rate than those without {1152,2782,1517}. In a meta-analysis comprising 677 patients, the median overall survival was 58 months in patients with meningiomas harbouring *TERT* mutations versus 160 months in the *TERT*-wildtype group {2124}. Intragenic deletions in the dystrophin-encoding and muscular dystrophy–associated *DMD* gene are common in progressive/high-grade meningiomas and are associated with shorter overall survival {1516}. A subset of meningiomas with rhabdoid features have inactivation of *BAP1* and a shorter time to recurrence than other meningiomas {2888}. In papillary meningiomas, mutations in the chromatin modifier *PBRM1* are enriched, suggesting that such mutations may be linked with aggressive tumour behaviour {3449}. Alterations in *CDKN2A* and/or *CDKN2B* (which are cell-cycle regulator genes) are frequently found in recurrent and progressive meningiomas and are associated with a poor prognosis {1202,1153,2465}.

Several potentially clinically actionable mutations have been described in meningiomas, including mutations in *SMO, AKT1,* and *PIK3CA* {353,9,601,2777}, for which targeted therapies have shown efficacy in other tumour types. Furthermore, PDL1 (which is associated with response to immune checkpoint blockade in other cancers) may be overexpressed in high-grade meningiomas {790}. Efficacy of immune checkpoint blockade has been described in rare meningiomas with high tumour mutation burdens due to the inactivation of components of the mismatch repair apparatus {806A}. Ongoing precision medicine trials for meningiomas will help us understand the importance of these alterations for predicting response to therapy.

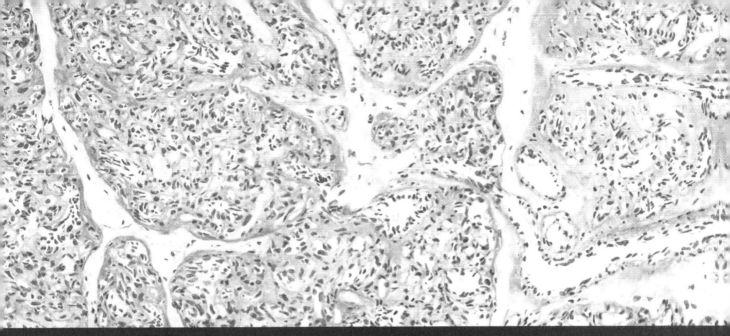

8

Mesenchymal, non-meningothelial tumours involving the CNS

Edited by: Lazar AJ, Ng HK

Mesenchymal, non-meningothelial tumours involving the CNS: Introduction

Ng HK

The terminology and histological features of benign and malignant mesenchymal, non-meningothelial tumours originating in the CNS correspond to those of their soft tissue and bone counterparts, and we have attempted to harmonize the terminology and diagnostic criteria presented in this classification with those in the *Soft tissue and bone tumours* volume of this series. Mesenchymal tumours arise more commonly in the meninges than in the CNS parenchyma or choroid plexus. In general, any mesenchymal tumour may arise within or have an effect on the nervous system, but primary mesenchymal CNS tumours are very rare. They can occur in patients of any age, and they arise more commonly in supratentorial locations than in infratentorial or spinal locations. The clinical symptoms and neuroradiological appearance of most tumours are nonspecific. Please refer to the relevant sections in this chapter for details on individual lesions.

This chapter covers only those entities that have special histological or molecular features, occur uniquely in the CNS, or (although similar to their soft tissue counterparts) are relatively common in the CNS compared with other tissues. Some common soft tissue tumours that can exceptionally be found in the CNS (e.g. leiomyoma, fibrosarcoma) and that were covered in previous editions are no longer included in this edition because their histological and diagnostic features are identical to those of their soft tissue counterparts. Please refer to the fifth-edition *Soft tissue and bone tumours* volume of this series for these entities {3426}. New lesions that have been added are intracranial mesenchymal tumour, FET::CREB fusion–positive; *CIC*-rearranged sarcoma; and primary intracranial sarcoma, *DICER1*-mutant. Tumours of the peripheral nerves are covered in Chapter 6: *Cranial and paraspinal nerve tumours*. Antiquated nosological terms, such as "spindle cell sarcoma", "pleomorphic sarcoma", "myxosarcoma", and "haemangiopericytoma", are discouraged. Two relatively common vascular lesions in the CNS, arteriovenous malformation and cavernous haemangioma, are covered in the section on haemangiomas because there was debate as to whether arteriovenous malformation is truly neoplastic.

Solitary fibrous tumour

Giannini C
Bouvier C
Demicco EG
Figarella-Branger D

Fritchie KJ
Macagno N
Perry A

Definition

Solitary fibrous tumour (SFT) is a fibroblastic neoplasm with a genomic inversion at the 12q13 locus, leading to *NAB2* and *STAT6* gene fusion as well as STAT6 nuclear expression.

ICD-O coding

8815/1 Solitary fibrous tumour

ICD-11 coding

2F7C & XH7E62 Neoplasms of uncertain behaviour of connective or other soft tissue & Solitary fibrous tumour, NOS
2B5Y & XH1HP3 Other specified malignant mesenchymal neoplasms & Solitary fibrous tumour, malignant

Related terminology

Not recommended: solitary fibrous tumour / haemangiopericytoma; haemangiopericytoma.

Subtype(s)

None

Localization

Most SFTs are dural based (often supratentorial), and about 10% are spinal. Skull base, parasagittal, and falcine locations are especially common {2066,2833}. Uncommon locations include the cerebellopontine angle {3138}, pineal gland {3595}, and sellar region {1508}.

Clinical features

In most cases, the symptoms and signs are consistent with the localization, mass effect, and increased intracranial pressure due to tumour size {1125,2066}. Massive intracranial haemorrhage {2027} and hypoglycaemia from tumours that release insulin-like growth factor {2983} are rare complications.

Imaging

Plain CT images show solitary, irregularly contoured masses without calcifications or hyperostosis of the adjacent skull. On MRI, the tumours are isointense on T1-weighted images, show high or mixed intensity on T2-weighted images, and have variable contrast enhancement. Dural contrast enhancement at the periphery of the lesion (dural tail) and flow voids may be observed {3384}. At present, no specific features on CT or MRI can be used to distinguish SFT from meningiomas {544}.

Epidemiology

The true incidence and prevalence of this entity are difficult to ascertain because of its inconsistent nomenclature. In the 2019 statistical report published by the Central Brain Tumor Registry of the United States (CBTRUS), SFT is grouped with other mesenchymal tumours of the meninges because of its rarity; as a group, mesenchymal tumours of the meninges have an average annual age-adjusted incidence rate of 0.12 cases per 100 000 population {2344}. Data from large series suggest that SFTs constitute < 1% of all CNS tumours {672,2066,2833}.

Age and sex distribution

In two recently published series comprising 265 patients, peak incidence occurred between the fifth and the seventh decades of life, with 18% of cases occurring in patients aged < 40 years. The sex distribution was nearly equal (M:F ratio: 1.08:1) {1966,988}. Primary CNS SFT has been reported in the paediatric population, but it is exceedingly rare {2055,3193, 3530}.

Etiology

Genetic susceptibility

There is no evidence of familial clustering of meningeal SFT.

Pathogenesis

The histogenesis of CNS SFT remains a matter of debate. Its fibroblastic nature and the presence of a common *NAB2::STAT6* gene fusion {577,2688,2870} are strong arguments for grouping CNS SFT with its pleural and soft tissue counterparts; nevertheless, the precise cell of origin has not been determined.

The genetic hallmark of SFT at all anatomical sites is a paracentric inversion involving chromosome 12q13, resulting in the fusion of the *NAB2* and *STAT6* genes {577,2688}. Demonstration

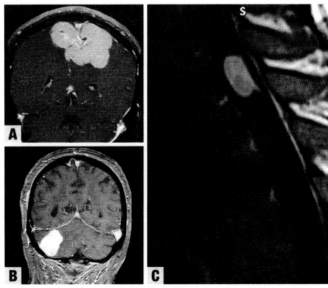

Fig. 8.01 Solitary fibrous tumour (SFT). **A** This large and multiloculated falcine tumour in a 74-year-old man shows diffuse postgadolinium enhancement. **B** This dural-based posterior fossa tumour in a 73-year-old man is strongly and diffusely enhancing, and it has a small dural tail. **C** A dural tail (16 mm in length) is visible in this tumour of the upper thoracic spine in a 45-year-old man. On imaging, SFTs may mimic meningioma.

Chapter 8

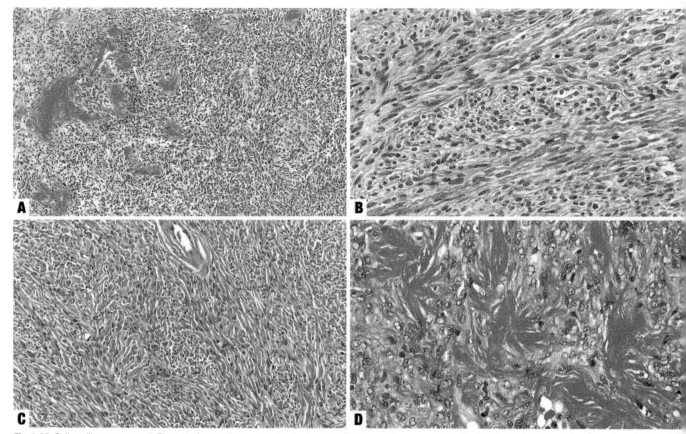

Fig. 8.02 Solitary fibrous tumour. **A** The typical patternless architecture is shown. **B** This tumour is composed of cells with bland spindle-shaped nuclei and scant eosinophili cytoplasm immersed in a collagenous background. **C** There is often stromal and perivascular hyaline collagen deposition. **D** This tumour shows keloidal or amianthoid collagen

of *NAB2::STAT6* gene fusion is virtually pathognomonic of SFT. Like their counterparts at other sites, CNS SFTs with fusions between *NAB2* exon 5, 6, or 7 and *STAT6* exon 16 or 17 tend to have a more cellular and more mitotically active phenotype (corresponding to a higher grade) than do CNS SFTs with fusions between *NAB2* exon 4 and *STAT6* exon 2 or 3 (which have a hypocellular grade 1 phenotype) {989,3340,988,3561, 209,3104}. *TERT* promoter mutations have been identified in 10–30% of meningeal SFTs {3340,731}. *TP53* mutation and overexpression of p16 have been reported in more aggressive tumours {2396,1886}.

Macroscopic appearance

SFTs are usually dural-based, well-circumscribed, firm, white to reddish-brown masses, depending on the degree of collagenous stroma and cellularity. Occasionally, they show infiltrative growth or they lack dural attachment {469,482,2096}. Variable myxoid or haemorrhagic changes may be present.

Histopathology

SFT is composed of haphazardly arranged spindled to ovoid monomorphic cells admixed with hyalinized, dilated, thin-walled, branching (staghorn-shaped) blood vessels. SFT has a wide histological spectrum, ranging from a hypocellular phenotype to a highly cellular phenotype in a patternless architecture, and multiple phenotypes may coexist. The paucicellular end of the spectrum shows abundant stromal keloidal-type collagen, whereas cellular tumours display densely packed round to

ovoid cells with little or no intervening stroma and less conspic uous vasculature, albeit often interspersed with pale zones o foci of necrosis. Nuclei are monotonous and round to oval, anc they lack the pseudoinclusions typical of meningioma. Invasior of brain parenchyma or engulfment of vessels or nerves ma be present {2096}. Calcifications, including psammoma bodies are not seen. Myxoid stroma, giant cells, and/or a variably prom inent adipocytic component (lipomatous SFT), as described in soft tissue and other extracranial sites {741,952,1186,2254,550} can be seen in meningeal SFT, but only rarely. Papillary anc pseudopapillary patterns have also been reported {1422,3530} Dedifferentiated (anaplastic) SFT, in which conventional SF areas are admixed with focal high-grade pleomorphic sarcoma forming eosinophilic amorphous osteoid (osteosarcoma), has recently been reported in a case of recurrent meningeal tumou {1981,1533}.

In two separate studies, histological grading based on a combination of mitotic activity and tumoural necrosis has beer found to correlate with prognosis {988,1966}. In both studies mitotic activity was evaluated in 10 adjacent high-power fields (400×; 1 HPF = 0.22 mm²) in the most proliferative zones. The following grades were identified:

- **CNS WHO grade 1:** < 2.5 mitoses/mm² (< 5 mitoses/10 HPF
- **CNS WHO grade 2:** ≥ 2.5 mitoses/mm² (≥ 5 mitoses/10 HPF without necrosis
- **CNS WHO grade 3:** ≥ 2.5 mitoses/mm² (≥ 5 mitoses/10 HPF with necrosis

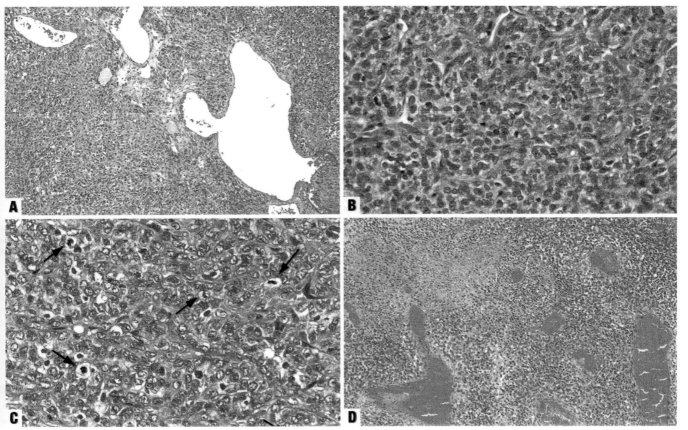

Fig. 8.03 Solitary fibrous tumour. **A** A highly cellular tumour with thin-walled, branching (staghorn) vessels. **B** There may be closely apposed cells with round to ovoid nuclei arranged in a haphazard pattern, with limited intervening stroma. **C** Numerous mitoses (arrows) are present in this tumour. **D** Focal necrosis is present in this tumour.

As a consequence of *NAB2::STAT6* fusion, diffuse and intense nuclear expression of STAT6 (C-terminal epitopes) constitutes the immunohistochemical hallmark of SFT, with very high sensitivity and specificity {1681,2351,2870}. STAT6 immunohistochemistry reliably differentiates meningeal SFT from a variety of neoplasms, including meningioma, meningeal Ewing sarcoma, mesenchymal chondrosarcoma, malignant peripheral nerve sheath tumour, synovial sarcoma, and other sarcomas that may occur in the meninges {1965,531}. Rare cases, including dedifferentiated SFTs, may require further molecular or immunohistochemical workup because they may partially or completely lack STAT6 nuclear expression by immunohistochemistry {664,2852,988}. CD34 is typically diffusely positive in grade 1 SFT, although little to no expression is common in higher-grade tumours {2472}. ALDH1 is a robust and specific marker, staining > 84% of meningeal SFTs compared with only 1% of meningiomas {343,1965}. Other markers, such as desmin, SMA, cytokeratin, EMA, and PR, may be rarely encountered as a focal finding {2096,2472,2606,3458}.

Differential diagnosis

The differential diagnosis includes both meningothelial and soft tissue neoplasms. Fibrous meningioma is a close mimic of SFT {469}, but it typically expresses EMA and is negative for CD34 and nuclear STAT6 expression. Dural-based Ewing sarcoma / peripheral primitive neuroectodermal tumour shares the hypercellularity and CD99 positivity of SFT, but it lacks nuclear STAT6 staining, and it is characterized by *EWSR1* gene rearrangement

in the great majority of cases {721}. Both primary and metastatic monophasic synovial sarcomas can simulate SFT. Immunoreactivity for EMA and TLE1, and/or *SS18* gene rearrangement detected by FISH analysis, supports this diagnosis {1900}. Mesenchymal chondrosarcoma, a rare malignant tumour with a biphasic pattern, is composed of sheets and nests of poorly differentiated small round cells interrupted by islands of well-differentiated hyaline cartilage and a branching vasculature. Because the cartilage islands can be extremely focal, this entity may be mistaken for malignant SFT if insufficiently sampled {3426}. Malignant peripheral nerve sheath tumour rarely occurs in the meninges and may resemble SFT, but it is usually negative for CD34 and STAT6 and may show focal expression of S100 and SOX10.

Cytology

Not clinically relevant

Diagnostic molecular pathology

The *NAB2::STAT6* fusion can be detected by sequencing techniques, RT-PCR, or proximity ligation assay {577,2688,1681, 2870}. Because *NAB2* and *STAT6* are in close proximity on chromosome 12q, it is difficult to detect their fusion by conventional cytogenetic methods, and accounting for the diversity of breakpoints (occurring in both exons and introns) using PCR-based detection assays is challenging. Fortunately, immunohistochemical detection of strong nuclear STAT6 expression is a sensitive and specific surrogate for all fusions {2870}.

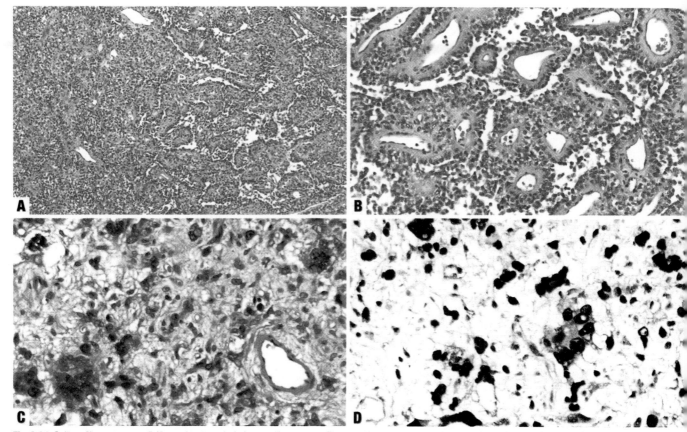

Fig. 8.04 Solitary fibrous tumour. **A** Unusual patterns include a papillary pattern. The transition between a solid and papillary pattern is shown. **B** The unusual papillary architecture is shown at higher power. **C** This tumour shows a markedly pleomorphic pattern with multinucleated tumour giant cells. **D** This markedly pleomorphic tumour with giant cells shows STAT6 nuclear positivity, confirming the diagnosis.

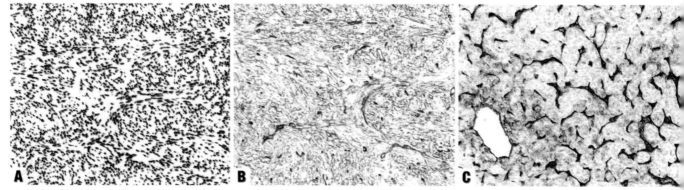

Fig. 8.05 Solitary fibrous tumour. **A** All tumours show nuclear localization of STAT6 by immunohistochemistry. **B** Strong and diffuse positivity for CD34 in a CNS WHO grade 1 tumour. **C** Focal CD34 positivity in a CNS WHO grade 3 tumour.

Essential and desirable diagnostic criteria
See Box 8.01.

Staging
Not relevant

Prognosis and prediction
Two large cohorts of patients with SFTs with confirmed *NAB2::STAT6* gene fusion and/or nuclear overexpression of STAT6 have shown that meningeal SFT has a high propensity for recurrence and metastasis, which sometimes occur decades after the initial diagnosis {1966,988}. In one of these cohorts

Box 8.01 Diagnostic criteria for solitary fibrous tumour

Essential:

Variably cellular tumour composed of spindled to ovoid cells arranged around a branching and hyalinized vasculature

AND

Variable stromal collagen deposition

AND

STAT6 nuclear expression

Desirable (in selected cases):

Demonstration of *NAB2::STAT6* gene fusion

(132 patients) {1966}, recurrent disease occurred in 52 patients after a median period of 36 months (of those cases, 14 recurred after 10 years) and 16 patients died of the disease after a median period of 70 months (range: 22–268 months). In the other cohort (133 patients) {988}, 42 patients experienced at least one adverse event after surgery (local recurrence or metastasis) and 29 died (including 20 of the disease). In both series, several CNS WHO grade 1 tumours recurred over time, reflecting the experience of tertiary referral centres. In one series, 6 (4.5%) of the patients with CNS WHO grade 1 tumours ultimately died, 2 with metastases {1966}. Therefore, long-term follow-up is recommended for the entire meningeal SFT spectrum.

The widely used risk model applied to SFT occurring at other sites is not entirely applicable to meningeal SFT because older age does not correlate with worse outcome {1966,988} and intracranial tumour size is not prognostic {988}. Only mitotic count and presence of necrosis appear to correlate with prognosis, resulting in a histologically based three-tiered grading scheme, as described above. In one series {1966}, progression-free survival (PFS) was associated with grade and extent of surgery, and disease-specific survival was associated with grade as well as its determinants (mitotic count and necrosis). On multivariate analysis, grade, extent of surgery, and mitotic activity remained independent prognostic factors for PFS, while necrosis was an independent prognostic factor for disease-specific survival. The other series {988} compared the 2016 CNS WHO tumour grading scheme to the 2013 WHO soft tissue grading scheme; on univariate analysis, mitotic count, necrosis, CNS WHO grade, and soft tissue grade were associated with PFS but not overall survival. A modified soft tissue grading scheme incorporating necrosis was chosen, which showed a higher correlation with PFS.

Although *NAB2::STAT6* fusion type is associated with phenotype, it is not predictive of outcome {989,3340,988,3561,209, 3104}. *TERT* promoter mutations have not been shown to correlate with worse outcomes {3340}.

Haemangiomas and vascular malformations

Hainfellner JA
Bouvier C
Calonje JE
Sciot R
Thway K

Definition

Haemangiomas are benign neoplastic vascular lesions with multiple tightly packed capillary-sized and cavernous vessels. They may be isolated, multiple, or part of a *PIK3CA*-related overgrowth syndrome.

Cavernous malformations (CMs) are angiographically occult solitary or (rarely) multifocal vascular anomalies. Histologically, they comprise multiple tightly packed sinusoidal vessels with fibrotic walls lacking arterial or venous features, and they contain little or no interposed CNS tissue. Familial and some sporadic CMs are associated with a mutation in *KRIT1* (*CCM1*), *CCM2*, or *PDCD10* (*CCM3*).

Cerebral arteriovenous malformation (AVM) is a fast-flow vascular anomaly consisting of arteriovenous connections through a nidus or fistula of malformed arteries and veins instead of a normal capillary bed. AVMs are typically sporadic; they show intervening brain parenchyma with gliosis between malformed vessels, and they have frequent somatic *KRAS* or *BRAF* mutations.

Capillary telangiectasia is an aggregation of individually dispersed dilated capillary-type vessels with interposed normal brain parenchyma.

ICD-O coding

9121/0 Cavernous haemangioma
9131/0 Capillary haemangioma
9123/0 Arteriovenous malformation

ICD-11 coding

2E81.0Y Other specified neoplastic haemangioma
LA90.3Y Other specified peripheral arteriovenous malformations

Related terminology

Acceptable: cavernous angioma; cerebral cavernous malformation; cavernoma.

Subtype(s)

None

Localization

Haemangiomas arise preferentially in the spine; less frequently in the skull; and exceptionally in the CNS parenchyma, nerve roots, and cauda equina {2944,938,1686,3566}. Spinal haemangiomas favour the thoracic and lumbar vertebrae. They are often multiple, and they may involve vertebral bodies, pedicles, arches, and spinous processes {3159}.

CMs favour supratentorial locations, including the optic nerve or chiasm, pineal gland, and cavernous sinus. Rare locations include the cerebellopontine angle, pons, cerebellum, and spinal cord {3566}. Spinal cord CMs are usually intramedullary.

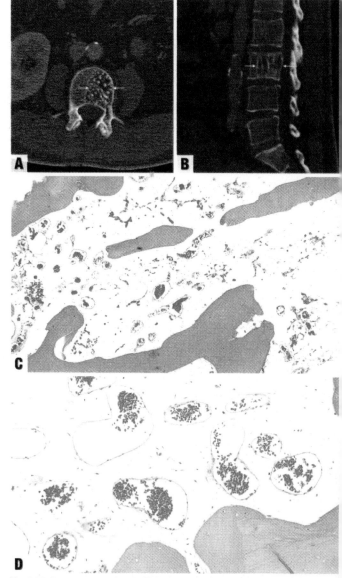

Fig. 8.06 Haemangioma. **A** Axial CT (bone window) of vertebral body L3 showing the polka-dot sign with thickened trabeculae. **B** Sagittal reconstruction of the CT (bone window) showing the corduroy sign in vertebral body L3. **C** Presence of capillary-type and cavernous vessels in the bone marrow space between coarse trabeculae of bone in a calvarial haemangioma. **D** Calvarial haemangioma with cavernous vessels lined by flattened endothelium and separated by loose mesenchymal stroma with fibroblasts.

Cerebral AVMs can involve the meninges, cortical regions, and deep brain (insular region, basal ganglia, thalamus, corpus callosum, brainstem, and cerebellum) {3566}. In the spinal cord, AVMs can be extradural, intradural, or intramedullary, or they can occur in the conus medullaris {2361}.

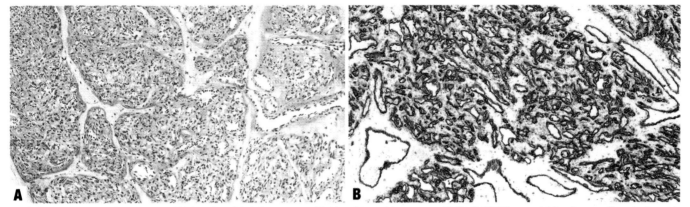

Fig. 8.07 Haemangioma of the conus medullaris region. **A** Lobular pattern and highly cellular, solid appearance (PAS). **B** CD34 immunostaining shows capillary-sized vessels with partly canalized lumina lined by a single layer of plump endothelial cells.

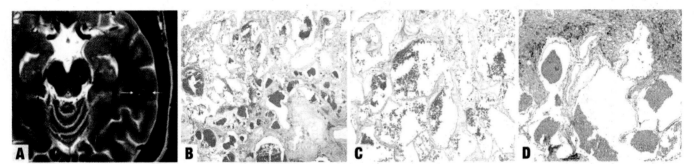

Fig. 8.08 Cavernous malformation. **A** T2-weighted axial MRI of a left temporal cavernous malformation demonstrating the characteristic popcorn-like appearance with a hypointense rim (haemosiderin ring). **B** Sinusoidal vasculature filled with blood. **C** Densely packed sinusoidal vessels with fibrotic walls and no interposed CNS tissue. **D** There is heavy haemosiderin deposition in the perilesional CNS tissue (Prussian blue).

Cerebral capillary telangiectasia shows a predilection for the pons and may extend into the middle cerebellar peduncle. The basal ganglia, cerebral hemispheres, and spinal cord may also be affected {3566}.

Clinical features

Vertebral haemangiomas occur predominantly in male patients. They are usually asymptomatic, but they may also lead to vertebral compression fracture, inducing compressive myelopathy {3159}. Pregnancy may induce progression {3369}.

Patients with cerebral CMs more commonly present with seizures than with acute haemorrhage. The age range is wide. Male patients are affected in the second to third decades of life, and female patients often in the fourth to sixth decades. Intralesional or perilesional haemorrhage may cause acute focal neurological deficits that may improve without neurosurgical intervention {946}. Most CMs remain asymptomatic, and they can be incidental findings on MRI or autopsy {648}.

Patients with spinal CMs may present with pain, myelopathy, or radiculopathy; patients often also have intracranial lesions {1130}.

AVMs can occur at any age, with no sex predilection. Patients with cerebral AVM most frequently present with acute intracerebral, intraventricular, or subarachnoid haemorrhage, typically in the third to fourth decades of life. Other frequent manifestations are seizure, chronic headache, and progressive neurological deficit. AVMs may also be asymptomatic and discovered incidentally on imaging. AVMs most commonly come to clinical attention in the second to fourth decades of life {450,3566}.

Imaging

On CT, vertebral haemangiomas show a typical polka-dot, honeycomb, or corduroy pattern. On MRI, they are hyperintense on T1- and T2-weighted images, and they show postcontrast enhancement {3159}.

On CT, calcifications are frequently visible in CMs. On MRI, T2-weighted images show mixed signal intensities centrally and a surrounding hypointense/low signal rim with blooming (haemosiderin ring). T1-weighted imaging with contrast shows the associated developmental venous anomaly, if present. On angiography, CMs are occult, because they lack feeding arteries and draining veins. CMs are dynamic lesions that may arise de novo and may grow, contract, or remain the same size. In sporadic cases, single isolated lesions with or without associated developmental venous anomaly are seen on MRI; in familial cases, multiple CMs are seen {3567,3566}.

On CT, vessels in AVMs are isodense and strongly enhancing with contrast. Calcifications may be present, and haemorrhage visible, with a nidus in the region. On T2-weighted MRI, AVMs appear as honeycomb flow voids due to rapid signal loss from lesional high flow. T2-weighted and FLAIR images show hyperintensity in surrounding CNS parenchyma because of gliosis due to ischaemia from the vascular steal phenomenon of the AVM shunt. Angiography visualizes AVMs as conglomerates of tortuous vessels with early venous drainage. AVMs are usually solitary, but they may be multiple {3566}.

On MRI with contrast, ectatic capillaries in cerebral capillary telangiectasias show mild to moderate enhancement with an irregular border. T1-weighted postcontrast imaging may show

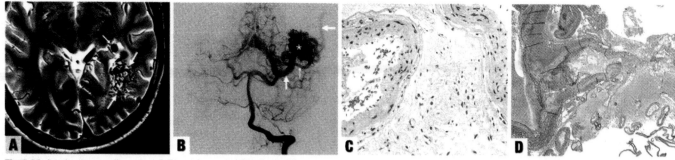

Fig. 8.09 Arteriovenous malformation. **A** T2-weighted axial MRI showing an arteriovenous malformation in the left temporo-occipital region with characteristic flow voids in the nidus area (thick arrows) and dilated draining vein (thin arrows). **B** Digital subtraction angiography via the left vertebral artery (coronal projection). The arteriovenous malformation is visualized as a conglomerate of tortuous vessels; note the large nidus (asterisk), a feeding artery (thin arrow), and the draining veins (thick arrows). **C** CNS tissue with gliosis between two malformed vessels. **D** Variably sized abnormal arteries with a large feeder (left) and interposed CNS tissue (elastica van Gieson).

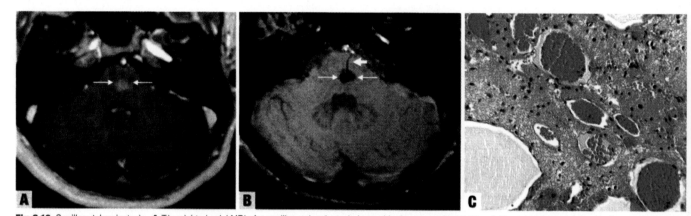

Fig. 8.10 Capillary telangiectasia. **A** T1-weighted axial MRI of a capillary telangiectasia located in the pons, with faint brush-like enhancement (arrows) after contrast administration. **B** Axial susceptibility-weighted MRI demonstrating susceptibility artefacts in the pons due to the capillary telangiectasia (thin arrows). Note the draining vein (thick arrow). **C** Cerebral lesion. Dilated capillary-type vessels with a flattened single-layer endothelium are separated by CNS tissue without gliosis.

a draining vein from the capillary telangiectasia. Susceptibility-weighted imaging shows signal intensity loss due to deoxyhaemoglobin loss in stagnant vessels {3566}.

Epidemiology

Vertebral haemangiomas have a prevalence of 10–12% in the general population {3369}.

For CM, the estimated population-based prevalence ranges from 0.16% to 0.9%. The estimated population prevalence of familial CM ranges from 0.01% to 0.03% {3567}.

For AVM, population-based studies approximate the incidence to be about 1 case per 100 000 person-years {2338}.

The prevalence of capillary telangiectasia is 0.4–0.7% in the general population {3566}.

Etiology

Intraosseous haemangioma can be congenital or can develop de novo (e.g. due to trauma) {2944}. Haemangiomas may also be part of a *PIK3CA*-related overgrowth syndrome (e.g. Klippel–Trénaunay syndrome) {1752}.

Most CM lesions are sporadic, and they can be congenital or acquired. CMs can develop years after brain or spinal irradiation {946}. The molecular basis of inherited CMs (and of a proportion of sporadic CMs) is an autosomal dominant loss-of-function mutation in *KRIT1* (*CCM1*) (common in the Hispanic population), *CCM2* (which encodes malcavernin), or *PDCD10*

(*CCM3*) {3567}. The mutations most commonly result in a truncated protein; rarely, missense mutations lead to protein misfolding {1880}.

Most sporadic AVMs have somatic *KRAS* mutations or, less frequently, a *BRAF* mutation {1149}.

Pathogenesis

The development of CM is thought to be a phenomenon of venous hypertension leading to erythrocyte extravasation and the release of angiogenic growth factors. CMs may also be associated with developmental venous anomalies {3566}.

Familial CMs are associated with a mutation in *KRIT1* (*CCM1*), *CCM2*, or *PDCD10* (*CCM3*). These genes are part of a signalling pathway that regulates cell proliferation, network formation, and endothelial layer growth {3567,160}.

In AVM, dysregulation of angiogenesis, vasculogenesis, and inflammation seems to be involved in pathogenesis {450}. Sporadic AVMs may relate to abnormalities in cerebral vascular autoregulation or in venous architecture. AVMs can also occur in association with hereditary genetic syndromes, such as hereditary haemorrhagic telangiectasia syndrome (Osler–Weber–Rendu disease) {1149}.

Cerebral capillary telangiectasias may be congenital in origin (caused by a failure of capillary involution during development) or acquired due to reactive angiogenesis after insults such as venous hypertension or irradiation {3566}.

Box 8.02 Diagnostic criteria for haemangiomas and vascular malformations

Haemangioma

Essential:

Tightly packed capillary-sized and cavernous vessels with a single layer of benign endothelial cells

AND

Mesenchymal stroma with fibroblasts

AND

Absence of foamy stromal cells

Desirable:

Typical neuroimaging findings

Cavernous malformation

Essential:

Tightly packed sinusoidal vessels with a single-layer attenuated endothelium and fibrotic vessel walls, lacking arterial or venous features

AND

Absence of prominent feeding arteries and draining veins

Desirable:

Deposition of haemosiderin in surrounding CNS tissue

Typical neuroimaging findings

Arteriovenous malformation

Essential:

Aggregates of abnormal arteries and veins of variable diameters with direct connections through a nidus or fistula, instead of a normal capillary bed

Desirable:

Typical neuroimaging findings

Capillary telangiectasia

Essential:

Aggregation of capillary-type dilated vessels lined with a single benign endothelial cell layer

AND

Lack of tissue alterations in the intervening CNS parenchyma

Desirable:

Typical neuroimaging findings

Macroscopic appearance

Macroscopically, haemangiomas are soft, red, and lobular, and they are associated with many small feeder and drainer vessels {1686}.

CMs are macroscopically circumscribed and lobulated, with a reddish-purple raspberry appearance. The surrounding brain tissue contains haemosiderin {946}.

AVMs macroscopically show dilated surface draining veins, a nidus located deep to these, and feeding arteries {2360}.

Cerebral capillary telangiectasias are vascular lesions without mass effect and are usually small (ranging from only a few millimetres up to ~20 mm).

Histopathology

Haemangiomas show a lobular pattern separated by fibrous septa. Each lobule is fed by a separate artery and consists of multiple capillary-sized vessels lined by single layers of bland endothelial cells with very rare mitotic activity. Rare cases with high mitotic activity may be seen. Vessels vary in size from small, poorly canalized channels lined by plump endothelial cells (giving a highly cellular solid appearance) to dilated vessels lined with flattened endothelium. Blood-filled cavernous spaces and fibroendothelial papillae mimicking papillary endothelial hyperplasia may be observed. The stroma displays haemorrhage, haemosiderin, fibroblasts, and oedema, but foamy macrophages are absent. Reticulin stain shows a delicate network of reticulin fibres surrounding vessels. Immunohistochemically, the endothelial cells express ERG, CD31, and CD34. Single SMA-immunostaining cells may be present in the subendothelial layer. VEGF-positive cells are seen in the solid, immature-appearing areas without vessel lumen formation. The Ki-67 (MIB1) index is usually < 10% {7,1686,938}.

CMs are histologically well circumscribed, showing sinusoidal congested vessels (caverns) without intervening arteries, capillaries, or veins. The vessels comprise a single layer of attenuated endothelium and fibrotic walls, without arterial or venous features and without smooth muscle cells. Electron microscopy shows defects in tight junctions between endothelial cells, permitting leakage of blood components. The vessels are arranged back to back with little or no interposed brain tissue. There may be hyalinization, calcification, cholesterol crystals, and microhaemorrhages. The brain parenchyma abutting the lesion shows haemosiderin deposition and gliosis. Macrophages and chronic inflammation may be present {648}.

Histologically, AVMs are composed of variably sized abnormal arteries and veins with direct fistulous connections and without normal intervening capillary beds. Between vessels, there is CNS tissue with gliosis.

Cerebral capillary telangiectasias are localized aggregations of thin-walled, dilated vessels without elastic fibres or smooth muscle cells. They occur within brain parenchyma without adjacent gliosis, calcification, or haemosiderin-laden macrophages.

Cytology
Not clinically relevant

Diagnostic molecular pathology
Not clinically relevant

Essential and desirable diagnostic criteria
See Box 8.02.

Staging
Not relevant

Prognosis and prediction
Haemangiomas of the neuraxis usually do not recur after complete resection {1686}.

In CMs, the annual risk of clinically significant haemorrhage is 1.6–4.6%. Previous haemorrhage and brainstem location are associated with increased risk. Female sex, larger lesion size, and greater number of lesions are also associated with increased risk of haemorrhage {3566}.

In AVM, the risk of haemorrhage is 2–5% per year. In AVM haemorrhage, 5–25% of cases are fatal. Age, hypertension, and previous intracranial haemorrhage are associated with an increased risk of haemorrhage {450}.

Capillary telangiectasia is most often an incidental finding, with only a minor risk of bleeding or progressive course.

Haemangioblastoma

Tihan T
Fanburg-Smith JC
Vortmeyer AO
Zagzag D

Definition

Haemangioblastoma is a highly vascular tumour containing neoplastic stromal cells that have clear to vacuolated cytoplasm and characteristic immunohistochemical features (e.g. inhibin positivity) and molecular findings (e.g. *VHL* alterations) (CNS WHO grade 1).

ICD-O coding

9161/1 Haemangioblastoma

ICD-11 coding

2F7Y & XH6810 Neoplasms of uncertain behaviour of other specified site & Haemangioblastoma

Related terminology

Not recommended: angioblastoma; von Hippel–Lindau disease.

Subtype(s)

None

Localization

Haemangioblastomas typically occur in the cerebellum. Sporadic and multiple tumours are also found in the brainstem, spinal cord, cerebrum, retina, and peripheral nerves. Haemangioblastomas can also occur outside the CNS, such as in bone and soft tissue, liver, lung, pancreas, kidney, intestines, and skin {785,287,2181}.

Clinical features

Haemangioblastomas account for < 2% of all CNS tumours, and they may occur sporadically (most commonly) or in association with von Hippel–Lindau syndrome (VHL) {2244}. Symptoms are generally caused by the mass effect of the lesion through compression of adjacent structures, and/or by the impairment of cerebrospinal fluid flow due to increased intracranial pressure and hydrocephalus. Cerebellar deficits such as dysmetria and ataxia can also occur. Haemangioblastomas produce erythropoietin, and this may cause secondary polycythaemia {1117}. Haemangioblastoma is a frequent manifestation of VHL {1115}. Therefore, genetic counselling and screening for *VHL* germline mutations are critical in the management of patients with haemangioblastoma {1115}.

Imaging

Neuroimaging typically demonstrates contrast-enhancing nodules that are frequently associated with cystic structures. The solid component is usually peripheral in location within the cerebellar hemisphere. Flow voids may be seen within the nodule due to enlarged feeding/draining vessels. Angiography is useful for identifying small lesions, showing a mass with a dense tangle of vessels that may resemble arteriovenous malformation. Spinal tumours can cause pain, hyperaesthesia, or incontinence due to local compression, and they may be associated with a syrinx. Haemorrhage is a rare complication.

Epidemiology

Intracranial haemangioblastoma is estimated to have an annual incidence rate of 0.15 cases per 100 000 population {2244}. Tumours typically occur in adults, with an M:F ratio of 1:1. VHL-associated tumours occur at a younger age than sporadic haemangioblastomas. Symptomatic presentation is usually in people aged 18–30 years, and the disease has 95% penetrance by 60 years, although there is considerable variability.

Etiology

In both sporadic haemangioblastoma and VHL, allelic losses or mutations of the *VHL* gene are found in stromal cells. VHL is autosomal dominant, through a germline inactivating mutation in the *VHL* gene on chromosome 3p25.3 with subsequent inactivation of the second allele in tumours. In the majority of patients

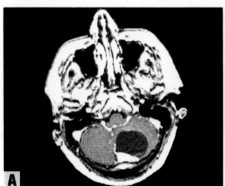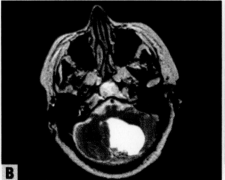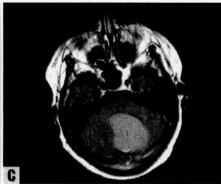

Fig. 8.11 Haemangioblastoma in the posterior fossa in a 52-year-old man, demonstrating typical solid-cystic features. Axial MRI. **A** T1-weighted, contrast-enhanced image. **B** T2-weighted image. **C** FLAIR image.

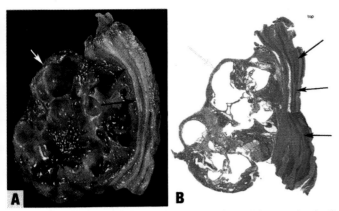

Fig. 8.12 Haemangioblastoma. **A,B** The tumour is multicystic (white arrow) and well demarcated from the surrounding cerebellum (black arrows).

with VHL there is a family history of the syndrome, so only one other disease manifestation is necessary for the diagnosis.

Studies on sporadic tumours (including somatic mutation analyses, assessments of allelic loss, deep-coverage DNA sequencing, and hypermethylation studies) have found a loss or inactivation of the *VHL* gene in as many as 78% of cases {1114A,1837A,2890A}, suggesting that loss of function of *VHL* is a central event in haemangioblastoma formation.

Pathogenesis

The variably lipid-filled stromal cells release angiogenic factors, including vascular endothelial growth factor (VEGF), which leads to the production of the rich vascular network present in the tumour. HIF1, a ubiquitously expressed and highly conserved heterodimeric basic helix–loop–helix PAS transcription factor composed of two subunits, HIF1α and HIF1β, plays an essential role in oxygen homeostasis {2879}. In normoxic conditions, after hydroxylation of HIF1α by the oxygen-dependent prolyl hydroxylases at proline residues 402 and 564 within the oxygen-dependent degradation domain, the protein complex VCB-CUL2 (which includes VHL protein, an E3 ubiquitin ligase) binds HIF1α and polyubiquitinates it, targeting it for proteasomal degradation. In contrast, when VHL protein is inactivated or when cellular oxygen concentration decreases, HIF1α accumulates in the cytoplasm, translocates into the nucleus, and binds to hypoxia-response elements in the promoters of a large battery of genes whose protein products function either to increase oxygen availability or to allow metabolic adaptation to oxygen deprivation {1524}. For example, the inactivation of VHL protein in haemangioblastomas leads to the accumulation of HIF1α in stromal cells {3572} and triggers increased transcription of HIF1α-regulated genes (including those encoding VEGF, erythropoietin, glucose transporters, and glycolytic enzymes).

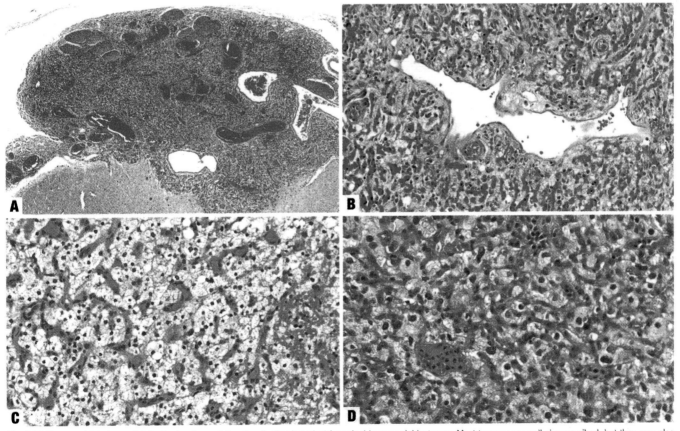

Fig. 8.13 Haemangioblastoma. **A** Intradural, extramedullary localization is typical for spinal haemangioblastomas. Most tumours are well circumscribed, but they may also encroach on the spinal cord parenchyma. **B** Abundant vascularity of haemangioblastoma is often in the form of thin-walled vessels, some of which appear as highly branching staghorn vessels. **C** Neoplastic stromal cells with clear to vacuolated cytoplasm admixed with abundant capillary vessels. **D** The stromal cells show mild nuclear pleomorphism and a rich capillary network.

More than 1000 unique *VHL* mutations (substitutions, deletions, insertions, and duplications) have been described in the Catalogue of Somatic Mutations in Cancer (COSMIC), about 25% of which are pathogenic. Recurrent DNA copy-number losses of chromosomes 6q and 6, somatic gain-of-function *EPAS1* (*HIF2A*) mutations, and loss of SDHB expression have been reported. Various cell signalling mechanisms are upregulated in CNS haemangioblastomas, including EGFR (HER1), TGF-α, FGFR3, PDGFRA, and Notch signalling pathways or receptors. Copy-number variations in various genes, including gain of *EGFR* and microdeletion of *FGFR1*, have been identified in haemangioblastomas. Recent whole-exome sequencing of familial and sporadic CNS haemangioblastomas identified multiple somatic single-nucleotide variations and several copy-number variations associated with angiogenesis. Mutations in *BRCA2* (COSM3753648, COSM5019704) have also been reported.

Macroscopic appearance

Haemangioblastomas are typically well-circumscribed pseudoencapsulated masses that may be cystic with a mural solid nodule or (less commonly) entirely solid {3363}. There is a variegated yellow cut surface due to the high lipid content. Tumours are up to 125 mm in diameter in extraneuraxial locations and generally < 30 mm in the cerebellum {287,785,1373}.

Histopathology

Haemangioblastomas demonstrate two main components: (1) neoplastic stromal cells that are characteristically large and vacuolated but that can show considerable cytological variation, and (2) abundant reactive vascular cells. In many tumours, vascular cells are more abundant than stromal cells; in other tumours, stromal cells are more abundant and may reveal solid epithelioid aggregates that may be associated with extramedullary haematopoiesis {3349A}. The most characteristic and distinguishing morphological feature of the stromal cell is numerous lipid-containing vacuoles. Tumour cell nuclei can vary in size, with occasional atypical and hyperchromatic nuclei. Mitotic figures are rare. In adjacent reactive tissues, particularly in cystic and syrinx walls, astrocytic gliosis and Rosenthal fibres are frequently observed. The tumour edge is generally well demarcated, but infiltration into surrounding neural tissues can be detected. Cellular tumours with clear cell aggregates can resemble metastatic renal cell carcinoma.

The neoplastic stromal cells frequently express α-inhibin {1321A}, D2-40 {2741A}, and brachyury (cytoplasmic expression), which may be helpful for differentiating haemangioblastoma from metastatic renal clear cell carcinoma, particularly in the context of VHL. Identification of stromal cells is further facilitated by positive immunoreactivity for NSE, NCAM1 {314}, S100 {1420}, ezrin {315}, CXCR4 {1885,3570}, aquaporin-1

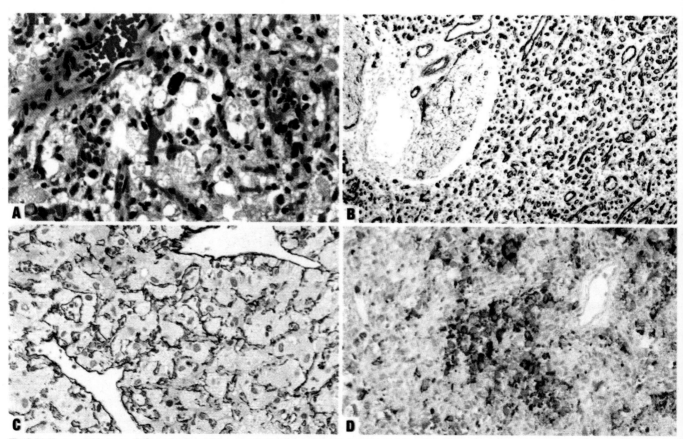

Fig. 8.14 Haemangioblastoma. **A** Stromal cell nuclei may vary in size. Enlarged atypical and hyperchromatic nuclei may be observed occasionally. **B** Immunohistochemical staining with antibodies against endothelial markers highlights the abundant vascular structures that are not considered to be neoplastic. **C** Reticulin surrounds single strips to clusters of stromal cells and highlights small capillary vessels and larger vessels with a staghorn appearance. **D** Inhibin immunohistochemistry is at least focally positive in the characteristic stromal cells, confirming the diagnosis.

{1922}, several carbonic anhydrase isozymes {2577}, occasionally GFAP {1593}, and EGFR {313A}. Positivity of these markers, in addition to negative staining with RCCm, EMA, CD10, and CAM5.2 antibodies, may be helpful for excluding a metastatic renal cell carcinoma. Especially in patients with VHL, staining for these antigens may be helpful in the differentiation of haemangioblastoma from many different tumours, but there is overlap with the immunohistochemical profile of renal cell carcinoma. Stromal cells lack endothelium-associated markers, such as von Willebrand factor (factor VIII–related antigen), CD34, ERG, and CD31 {314,3464A}.

Cytology

Cytological smear preparations often appear as cohesive tissue fragments and yield few individual cells. Stromal cells with spindled morphology and cytoplasmic vacuoles can be identified at the periphery of the tissue fragment. Occasionally, tissue fragments may demonstrate large irregular nuclei. Rare cells with clear cytoplasm can be seen {623}.

Diagnostic molecular pathology

Not clinically relevant

Essential and desirable diagnostic criteria

See Box 8.03.

Staging

No currently accepted staging system is recognized.

Box 8.03 Diagnostic criteria for haemangioblastoma

Essential:

A tumour composed of large, multivacuolated, and lipidized stromal cells with occasional hyperchromatic nuclei, as well as a rich capillary network

AND

> Stromal cells with immunohistochemical positivity for markers such as inhibin (at least focally)
>
> **OR**
>
> Loss or inactivation of the *VHL* gene
>
> **OR**
>
> In a patient with von Hippel–Lindau syndrome

Desirable:

In patients with von Hippel–Lindau syndrome, absence of immunohistochemical staining for markers of renal cell carcinoma

Prognosis and prediction

Haemangioblastoma has excellent prognosis after complete excision. Permanent neurological deficits are rare {631}, and they can be avoided when the haemangioblastoma is treated early {1116}. Sporadic tumours have a better prognosis than VHL-associated tumours because the latter show multiplicity and occur in combination with other VHL-associated neoplasms {2131}. Tumours may persist locally after incomplete excision {785}. Features that affect outcome include age, size, growth pattern, treatment, multifocality, and location (e.g. brainstem vs cerebellum) {1373}.

Rhabdomyosarcoma

Kleinschmidt-DeMasters BK
Bouvier C
Dry SM
Hainfellner JA
Rudzinski ER

Definition

Rhabdomyosarcomas are a family of malignant primitive neoplasms that show at least focal, predominantly skeletal muscle differentiation and are rarely identified as a primary tumour in the CNS.

ICD-O coding

8910/3 Embryonal rhabdomyosarcoma
8920/3 Alveolar rhabdomyosarcoma
8901/3 Rhabdomyosarcoma, pleomorphic-type
8912/3 Spindle cell rhabdomyosarcoma

ICD-11 coding

2B55.Z & XH83G1 Rhabdomyosarcoma & Embryonal rhabdomyosarcoma, NOS
2B55.Z & XH7099 Rhabdomyosarcoma & Alveolar rhabdomyosarcoma
2B55.Z & XH5SX9 Rhabdomyosarcoma, primary site & Pleomorphic rhabdomyosarcoma, NOS
2B55.Z & XH7NM2 Rhabdomyosarcoma, primary site & Spindle cell rhabdomyosarcoma

Related terminology

None

Subtype(s)

None

Localization

There is no stereotypical location for primary intracerebral rhabdomyosarcoma; examples have occurred in the cerebellopontine angle {458,3544,2196} and in meningeal {2379,3494}, pineal {1812,1418}, posterior third ventricular and pineal {1501}, and sellar {803,135,3025} locations. A recent study of 12 examples plus cases published in the literature since 1946 found

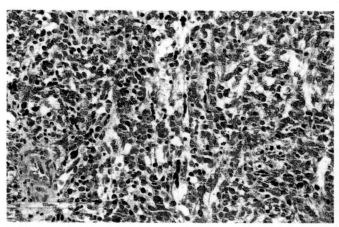

Fig. 8.15 Rhabdomyosarcoma. Tumours occasionally contain elongate strap cells with eosinophilic cytoplasm, as seen here. Note, however, that the majority of tumour cells are poorly differentiated and contain scant cytoplasm.

that infratentorial / skull base sites (66% of cases) predominated over supratentorial locations (34% of cases) {3603}.

Clinical features

Symptoms are referable to tumour location, but many patients present with headache {3603} and mass effects such as nausea and vomiting {1501}. Supratentorial examples may cause hemiparesis {727} or extremity weakness {2379}. Infratentorial / skull base examples are often associated with cranial nerve palsies {3603}, and intrasellar examples have mimicked symptoms seen in pituitary adenomas, such as bitemporal hemianopsia {3025}.

Epidemiology

The majority of rhabdomyosarcomas develop in children, but adults may also be affected {1269,740,2379,1501,135,3025}.

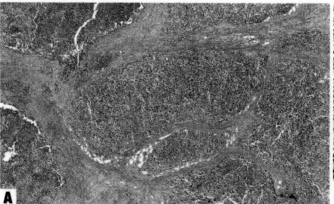
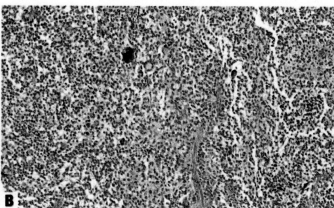

Fig. 8.16 Alveolar rhabdomyosarcoma. **A** A highly cellular tumour composed of primitive round cells with scant cytoplasm and hyperchromatic nuclei. Fibrovascular septa are seen in this example of the solid type of tumour. **B** The alveolar type often contains scattered multinucleated, wreath-like, giant tumour cells, as seen here.

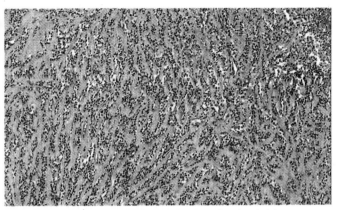

Fig. 8.17 Rhabdomyosarcoma. This example of a sclerosing rhabdomyosarcoma shows abundant collagenized stroma creating cords of tumour cells.

Etiology

The etiology is unknown. Although systemic-site embryonal rhabdomyosarcomas have been seen in patients with naevoid basal cell carcinoma syndrome (Gorlin syndrome) {2564}, that association has yet to be documented for primary intracerebral examples. Patients with neurofibromatosis type 1 have a small risk (< 1%) of developing systemic rhabdomyosarcomas {879}; one intracranial case has been described in association with neurofibromatosis type 1, although the patient had received prior cranial irradiation for bilateral optic nerve glioma {727}. A definite radiation-induced brainstem rhabdomyosarcoma has been reported in a patient with neurofibromatosis type 2 {468}. A meningeal rhabdomyosarcoma was found in a 15-month-old infant with hypomelanosis of Ito {3494}.

Pathogenesis

Sporadic cases of embryonal rhabdomyosarcoma are aneuploid with whole-chromosome gains including polysomy 8, followed in number by cases with extra copies of chromosomes 2, 11, 12, 13, and/or 20. In most embryonal rhabdomyosarcomas, a genomic event such as chromosome loss or deletion, or uniparental disomy, results in the loss of one of the two alleles at many chromosome 11 loci. This loss of heterozygosity involves chromosomal region 11p15, which contains imprinted genes that encode a growth factor (*IGF2*) and growth suppressors (*H19* and *CDKN1C*) {2906}. Genomic studies of embryonal rhabdomyosarcomas have identified somatic driver mutations in genes involved in the RAS pathway (*NRAS, KRAS, HRAS, NF1, FGFR4*), genes encoding effectors of PI3K (*PTEN, PIK3CA*), and genes that control the cell cycle (*FBXW7, CTNNB1*) {2905,2949}.

A t(2;13)(q36;q14) translocation is found in the majority of alveolar rhabdomyosarcomas, and a t(1;13)(p36;q14) translocation is seen in a smaller subset. These translocations juxtapose *PAX3* (at 2q36.1) or *PAX7* (at 1p36.13) with the *FOXO1* gene at 13q14.11, to generate chimeric genes that encode PAX3::FOXO1 and PAX7::FOXO1 fusion proteins {202,693,1024}. PAX3 and PAX7 are transcription factors that play essential roles in myogenesis {400}.

Please refer to the *Soft tissue and bone tumours* volume for additional details of pathogenesis.

Macroscopic appearance

Gross specimens are usually described as being moderately vascular and firm; these characteristics can make it difficult to achieve complete neurosurgical removal without complications {3544}.

Histopathology

The two most common types in systemic sites are embryonal and alveolar rhabdomyosarcomas; recently reported examples of primary intracerebral rhabdomyosarcomas have also been embryonal {1269,135,3025} and alveolar {1501,740} when histologically characterized. Pleomorphic rhabdomyosarcoma is less commonly reported {1501}. No intracerebral cases of spindle cell / sclerosing rhabdomyosarcoma have yet been confirmed; however, spindle cell / sclerosing rhabdomyosarcoma is frequently parameningeal.

Microscopy

Rhabdomyosarcomas manifest varying proportions of undifferentiated small cells and strap cells with cross-striations. Mitotic activity is often brisk.

Typical embryonal rhabdomyosarcomas are composed of variably differentiated rhabdomyoblasts within a loose, myxoid mesenchyme, with alternating areas of dense and loose cellularity. The proportions of myxoid matrix and spindled cells vary greatly between examples. Many tumour cells may be small with scant amphophilic cytoplasm, but differentiating rhabdomyoblasts show larger cytoplasmic volume, more cytoplasmic eosinophilia, and elongation. Terminal differentiation with cross-striations or myotube formation may be evident.

Alveolar rhabdomyosarcomas are highly cellular and composed of primitive round cells with scant cytoplasm and

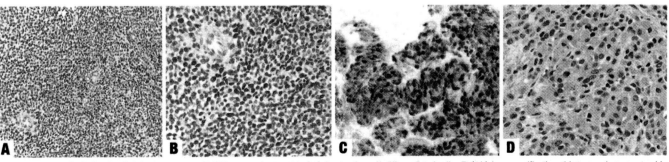

Fig. 8.18 Primary CNS alveolar rhabdomyosarcoma. **A** This tumour is composed of sheets of poorly differentiated cells. **B** At higher magnification, this tumour is monomorphic with round to ovoid nuclei and fine chromatin with inconspicuous nucleoli. **C** Myogenin (MYF4) stains the majority of tumour nuclei in this *PAX3::FOXO1* fusion–positive alveolar rhabdomyosarcoma. **D** After chemotherapy, this tumour showed cytodifferentiation. Differentiated tumour cells have abundant eosinophilic cytoplasm and eccentrically located nuclei with stippled chromatin and small nucleoli.

hyperchromatic nuclei arranged in nests separated by fibrovascular septa. Loss of cellular cohesion centrally may result in irregular alveolar spaces and cystic change; the solid pattern lacks these fibrovascular septa. Multinucleated, wreath-like tumour giant cells are frequent, but overt rhabdomyoblastic differentiation is not typically seen.

Spindle cell / sclerosing rhabdomyosarcoma is heterogeneous. Purely spindle cell forms demonstrate fascicular, whorling, or herringbone architecture with uniform spindled cells in intersecting fascicles. The sclerosing pattern contains round, oval, or (less often) spindled cells within a hyalinized/collagenized stroma typically showing cord-like or nested patterns suggesting vascular or alveolar spaces.

Pleomorphic rhabdomyosarcoma shows sheets of large, pleomorphic rhabdoid, spindled, or polygonal cells, often multinucleated.

Immunophenotype

All rhabdomyosarcomas should show cytoplasmic immunoreactivity for desmin, although the extent of immunoreactivity is variable. The skeletal muscle–specific nuclear regulatory proteins myogenin (MYF4) and MYOD1 are also positive in essentially all cases, although the number of immunopositive nuclei varies. Myogenin is usually diffusely positive in the alveolar type, but the embryonal and spindle cell / sclerosing types may have only scattered positive cells. MSA and SMA immunoreactivity is often present. Aberrant expression of keratins, S100, and NFP has been reported in systemic examples, but few primary intracranial examples have been assessed for these markers.

A potential diagnostic pitfall for primary intracranial alveolar rhabdomyosarcoma is that OLIG2 has been shown in systemic *PAX3::FOXO1* or *PAX7::FOXO1* fusion–positive alveolar rhabdomyosarcomas {2602}. Therefore, OLIG2 immunoreactivity in a primary intracerebral alveolar rhabdomyosarcoma should not be misinterpreted as representing the presence of a glial component. The Ki-67 labelling index is usually high.

Differential diagnosis

CNS metastases from systemic primary tumours must be excluded {699}, as must parameningeal involvement by rhabdomyosarcoma {3520}. Primary intracranial spindle cell sarcoma with rhabdomyosarcoma-like features and *DICER1* mutations (see *Primary intracranial sarcoma, DICER1-mutant*, p. 323) is now considered to be a distinct and separate entity {1677,2788}.

Rhabdomyosarcomas must be differentiated from other brain tumours that predominantly manifest other features but occasionally show focal skeletal muscle differentiation. Examples of primary CNS or peripheral nervous system tumours in which there may be focal rhabdomyosarcomatous differentiation include rare medulloblastomas with myoid elements (medullomyoblastomas), glioblastomas with a sarcomatous element (i.e. gliosarcomas, especially postirradiation examples), malignant peripheral nerve sheath tumours with a myoid component (malignant triton tumours), and even rare meningiomas {1439}. Germ cell tumours with a prominent rhabdomyosarcomatous component may be difficult to distinguish from primary intracerebral rhabdomyosarcoma, especially when located in the pineal gland {1812} and when small amounts of other tissues such as cartilage are present {1418}. Malignant ectomesenchymoma, a mixed tumour composed of ganglion cells or neuroblasts and one or more mesenchymal elements (usually rhabdomyosarcoma), also rarely occurs in the brain {2432}. Benign rhabdomyoma consisting of mature skeletal muscle should be excluded.

Cytology

Cytological preparations of embryonal rhabdomyosarcoma demonstrate primitive round, spindled, and stellate cells with scattered rhabdomyoblasts. Fine-needle biopsies of alveolar rhabdomyosarcoma are highly cellular and consist of uniform round cells with scant cytoplasm and variable rhabdomyoblastic differentiation. Wreath-like multinucleated giant cells may be seen {2393}.

Diagnostic molecular pathology

Most alveolar rhabdomyosarcomas in systemic sites are characterized by the presence of *PAX3::FOXO1* or *PAX7::FOXO1* fusion, with a worse prognosis in those without the fusion. Diverse molecular changes have been reported in spindle cell / sclerosing rhabdomyosarcomas, suggesting that this group may contain several subgroups. Congenital and infantile spindle cell / sclerosing rhabdomyosarcomas usually contain rearrangements of *NCOA2* and *VGLL2*, whereas those arising in older children and adults often show mutations in *MYOD1* {2354}. Embryonal and pleomorphic rhabdomyosarcomas do not show characteristic mutations or rearrangements, although embryonal rhabdomyosarcomas often display whole-chromosome gains, especially of chromosome 8.

Essential and desirable diagnostic criteria

See Box 8.04.

Staging

CNS rhabdomyosarcomas are not currently staged, because of their very limited numbers; however, they almost always show clinically aggressive behaviour.

Prognosis and prediction

Prognosis is usually poor due to local recurrence, with 44% survival at 1 year {1995}; long-term survival > 24 months is exceptional {1418}. Metastasis occurs in < 20% of primary intracranial examples {3603}.

Box 8.04 Diagnostic criteria for rhabdomyosarcoma

Essential:

A malignant primitive tumour with at least focal immunohistochemical demonstration of skeletal muscle lineage

AND

Absence of non-rhabdomyosarcomatous components, as detailed in the text

Desirable:

Confirmation of a *FOXO1* gene fusion in diagnostically difficult cases (other than alveolar rhabdomyosarcoma, in which such confirmation is essential rather than desirable)

Intracranial mesenchymal tumour, FET::CREB fusion–positive

Kleinschmidt-DeMasters BK
Bouvier C
Hainfellner JA
Perry A

Definition

Intracranial mesenchymal tumour with FET::CREB fusion (a provisional entity) is a mesenchymal neoplasm arising intracranially with variable histomorphology and fusion of a FET RNA-binding protein family gene (usually *EWSR1*, rarely *FUS*) with a member of the CREB family of transcription factors (*CREB1*, *ATF1*, or *CREM*).

ICD-O coding

None

ICD-11 coding

2F7C & XH9362 Neoplasms of uncertain behaviour of connective or other soft tissue

Related terminology

Acceptable: intracranial mesenchymal tumour / angiomatoid fibrous histiocytoma.

Not recommended: intracranial myxoid variant of angiomatoid fibrous histiocytoma; intracranial myxoid mesenchymal tumour with *EWSR1*::CREB family gene fusions.

Subtype(s)

None

Localization

These intracranial masses are more commonly located in supratentorial sites than in infratentorial sites. Most are extra-axial, attached to the meninges or dura, or located intraventricularly {2954}.

Clinical features

Tumours produce symptoms referable to mass effect and specific location, including headache, nausea, vomiting, tinnitus, and occasionally seizures {3002} or focal neurological deficits. Patients with anaemia {1230} or haemorrhage {2296} have been reported.

Imaging

Tumours are usually circumscribed extra-axial neoplasms with attachment to the meninges or dura and compression of the subjacent brain parenchyma. Other radiological characteristics include lobulated growth (often with both solid and cystic components), avid enhancement after contrast administration, intratumoural blood products, and substantial peritumoural oedema. Some demonstrate a dural tail or bony involvement of the overlying skull, mimicking meningioma {87,2954}.

Epidemiology

Most cases occur in children or young adults, although cases in adults in their fifties and sixties have been reported {1691,184, 1078,2954}.

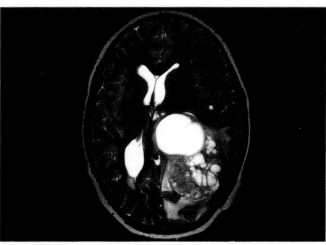

Fig. 8.19 Intracranial mesenchymal tumour, FET::CREB fusion–positive. This 12-year-old boy presented with hemiparesis and headache and was found on neuroimaging to have a bulky left parietal tumour with heterogeneous signal features. The mass, as seen on T2-weighted axial MRI, is supratentorial, as are most examples of this tumour type. On testing, an *EWSR1::ATF1* fusion transcript was identified.

Etiology

The etiology is unknown, but no cases to date have been associated with familial tumour predisposition syndromes.

Pathogenesis

The cell of origin is unknown. These tumours harbour fusion of a FET RNA-binding protein family gene (mostly *EWSR1*) with a member of the CREB family of transcription factors: *CREB1* {3304,181,1552}, *ATF1* {1701,2873,1552,804}, or *CREM* {1701, 1039,181,1552}. One case with *FUS::CREM* fusion has been identified {2954}.

The relationship of these intracranial tumours to extracranial angiomatoid fibrous histiocytoma or to the many different types of extracranial tumours harbouring the same FET::CREB fusions (e.g. clear cell sarcoma of soft tissue, angiomatoid fibrous histiocytoma, primary pulmonary myxoid sarcoma, hyalinizing clear cell carcinoma of the salivary gland, and gastrointestinal clear cell sarcoma) is uncertain.

Macroscopic appearance

Examples have been described as partially encapsulated, focally haemorrhagic, tan brown, and focally gelatinous {804}.

Histopathology

Tumours demonstrate a wide morphological spectrum, usually including a collagenous stroma with dense intercellular matrix highlighted by reticulin staining. Architecture ranges from syncytial or sheet-like growth to reticular cord-like structures, and a subset of tumours contain fibrous septa separating nodules of tumour cells. Not all examples contain a myxoid stroma {2954}.

Chapter 8

Tumour cell morphology varies from epithelioid/rhabdoid cells to stellate/spindle cells to monotonous round cells. Mitotic activity is generally low (typically < 5 mitoses/mm²). Haemangioma-like collections of dilated thin-walled vessels are a frequent finding.

Dense lymphoplasmacytic cuffing at the tumour periphery or along fibrous septa and haemosiderin or haematoidin are often present. Additional morphological features can include meningothelial-like whorls and amianthoid-type fibres {1691,1552}.

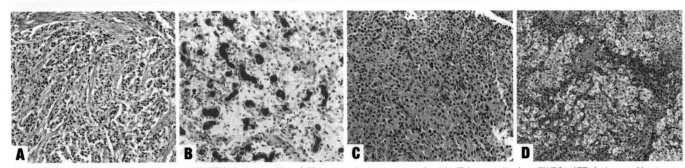

Fig. 8.20 Intracranial mesenchymal tumour, FET::CREB fusion–positive. **A** The morphological spectrum is wide. This example of an *EWRS1::ATF1* fusion–positive tumour shows cords of small, cytologically uniform cells. **B** This example shows very prominent small vessels in an angiomatoid pattern. The tumour harboured an *EWSR1::CREB* fusion, one of several types of characteristic fusions in this tumour type. **C** Architectural patterns in this tumour type include reticular, cord-like, spindled, and sheet-like; this example with an *EWSR1::ATF1* fusion shows sheet-like architecture. **D** These tumours can show a wide range of histological features, making the differential diagnosis broad in some cases. This example with *EWSR1::ATF1* fusion shows numerous clear cells.

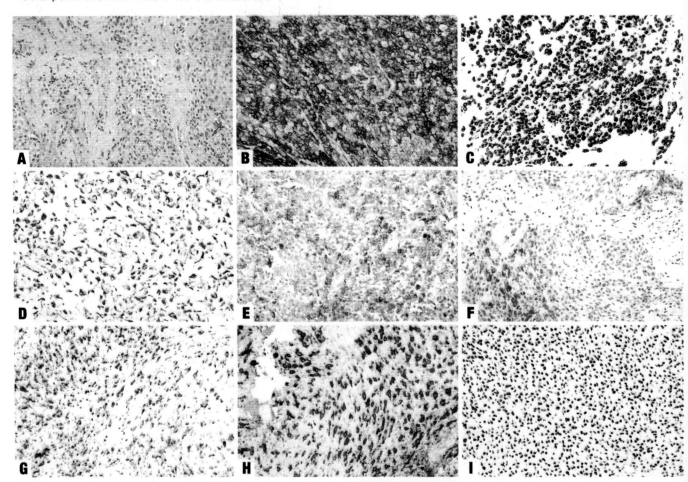

Fig. 8.21 Intracranial mesenchymal tumour, FET::CREB fusion–positive. **A** Alcian blue highlights the myxoid background seen in some intracranial examples. **B** Most examples of this tumour show immunopositivity for CD99. Immunostaining is strong and diffuse in this example, which harboured an *EWSR1::ATF1* fusion. **C** Desmin immunoreactivity is variable in this tumour type, and it can even be negative. In this example with *EWSR1::ATF1* fusion, the cytoplasmic immunostaining is strong and diffuse. **D** Desmin immunoreactivity is strong and diffuse in this example and highlights the slight variation in morphology from one cell to the next. **E** This example shows patchy EMA immunoreactivity, but the immunostaining can be quite variable. **F** Occasional examples may show immunoreactivity for AE1/AE3; there is focal immunostaining in this example. **G** Immunostaining for CD68 is frequently positive. **H** Although the immunohistochemical profile is varied, CD163 immunostaining is often identified. It is strong and diffuse in this example. **I** Some examples of this tumour may prompt diagnostic consideration of an atypical teratoid/rhabdoid tumour, but in this example, nuclear staining for both SMARCB1 (INI1) and SMARCA4 (BRG1) is retained, which excludes atypical teratoid/rhabdoid tumour. SMARCA4 staining is illustrated here.

Tumours with *EWSR1::CREB1* fusions more often have stellate/spindle cell morphology, mucin-rich stroma, and haemangioma-like vasculature, whereas tumours with *EWSR1::ATF1* fusions are more commonly composed of sheets of epithelioid cells with mucin-poor collagenous stroma {2954}.

The immunohistochemical profile is also variable, with the most commonly reported immunoreactivities being for EMA, CD99, and desmin; all three are usually diffusely or focally positive, but in a minority of reports, CD99 or desmin were negative. CD68 {804}, CD163 {87}, and vimentin, when assessed, have been positive. Variable positivity has been reported for synaptophysin, S100, and MUC4 {2954}.

Tumours have been negative for SSTR2A, OLIG2, GFAP, and CAM5.2 {181}; for myogenin, MYOD1, and myoglobin {2296}; and for SMA {1552,1230}, MSA, melan-A, HMB45, MITF, nuclear STAT6, and CD34 {1230}. SMARCB1 (INI1) and SMARCA4 (BRG1) expression is retained {181,1039}. Proliferation (Ki-67 labelling index) is generally low {2954}.

Differential diagnosis
The broad morphological spectrum of these tumours and the fact that their features overlap with those of other tumour entities make diagnosis challenging {1039}. Only documentation of a pathognomonic gene fusion provides diagnostic confidence. The differential diagnosis is usually with sarcomas or meningioma {87,1078}, especially of chordoid, microcystic {181}, or rhabdoid {1230} types.

Cytology
Not relevant

Diagnostic molecular pathology
Diagnostic FET::CREB family gene fusions may be detected using FISH or DNA/RNA sequencing strategies. Demonstrating *EWSR1* rearrangement via break-apart FISH assay is not specific in isolation, and confirmation of a CREB family fusion partner is recommended.

Essential and desirable diagnostic criteria
See Box 8.05.

Staging
Not applicable

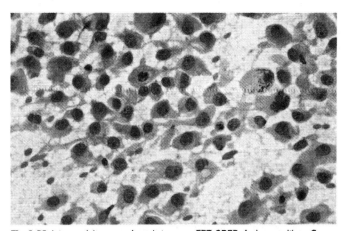

Fig. 8.22 Intracranial mesenchymal tumour, FET::CREB fusion–positive. Smear preparations from some examples may prompt diagnostic consideration of atypical teratoid/rhabdoid tumour due to the rounded cytoplasmic profiles, prominent nucleoli, mitoses, and somewhat eccentrically located nuclei (at least in some cells), as in this example. Fortunately, atypical teratoid/rhabdoid tumour can be excluded at the time of permanent section if there is retention of nuclear immunoreactivity for SMARCB1 (INI1) and SMARCA4 (BRG1).

Box 8.05 Diagnostic criteria for intracranial mesenchymal tumour, FET::CREB fusion–positive

Essential:

Primary intracranial neoplasm

AND

Variable morphological features including spindle cells, mucin-rich stroma, haemangioma-like vasculature, or epithelioid cells in a mucin-poor collagenous stroma

AND

Demonstration of a FET::CREB family fusion

Desirable:

CD99, EMA, and desmin immunoreactivity

Prognosis and prediction
The full spectrum of clinical behaviour is not yet known, but it ranges from slow growth to rapid recurrences {2873,2296,1701, 2954}. Rarely, cerebrospinal fluid dissemination or systemic metastases (including to pulmonary and thoracic lymph nodes) and bony metastases to spine have been seen {2954}.

CIC-rearranged sarcoma

Yip S
Orr BA
Sturm D
von Hoff K
Yoshida A

Definition

CIC-rearranged sarcoma of the neural axis is a high-grade, poorly differentiated sarcoma defined by *CIC* fusion with different gene partners.

ICD-O coding

9367/3 *CIC*-rearranged sarcoma

ICD-11 coding

None

Related terminology

Not recommended: CIC::DUX4, CIC::NUTM1 sarcoma; CNS Ewing sarcoma family tumour with *CIC* alteration.

Subtype(s)

None

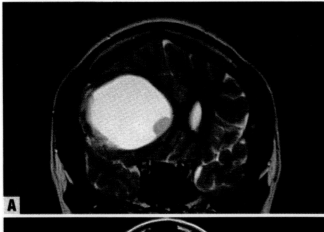
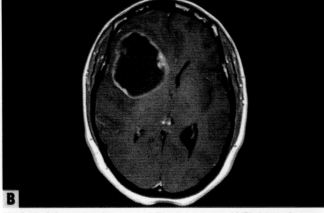

Fig. 8.23 *CIC*-rearranged sarcoma. **A** T2-weighted coronal MRI shows a large cystic tumour with several mural nodules in the right frontal lobe of a 35-year-old woman. **B** The axial postcontrast T1-weighted image shows enhancement of the capsule and demonstration of the solid components. Note the strictly intra-axial localization of the lesion. These tumours may appear as cystic lesions or as solid masses.

Localization

Most occur in the deep soft tissues with about 10% involving the viscera {120,3543,3059}, including the craniospinal intra-axial and extra-axial compartments {3059,1426,774,3507,278}. CNS metastasis may also occur {1286}.

Clinical features

Patients with *CIC*-rearranged sarcoma can present with focal neurological deficits or with globally raised intracranial pressure. The symptoms are location-dependent and due to mass effect.

Epidemiology

In a prospective registry, *CIC*-rearranged sarcoma identified using DNA methylation microarray accounted for 0.44% of all newly diagnosed CNS tumours in patients aged ≤ 21 years. There is a preference for adolescents and young adults, but older patients can be affected {120,1808}.

Etiology

Unknown

Pathogenesis

All *CIC*-rearranged sarcomas, irrespective of location, uniformly contain an oncogenic gene fusion of *CIC* transcriptional repressor with various partners (most often *DUX4*, but also *FOXO4*, *LEUTX*, *NUTM1*, or *NUTM2A*) {1578,1424,1818,3066,3067, 1371}. The t(4;19)(q35;q13) or t(10;19)(q26;q13) translocation that results in *CIC::DUX4* fusion in the majority of peripheral tumours leads to the fusion of the C-terminus of *CIC* to the N-terminus transactivating domain of *DUX4*, and to the subversion of the *CIC* transcriptional repressor function to one that is activating {3003}. A subset of *CIC::DUX4* cases contain a stop codon immediately after the breakpoint, resulting in a chimeric protein without a *DUX4* sequence, suggesting that truncated *CIC* may be sufficient for oncogenesis {1551,3542}. *CIC::DUX4* fusion leads to the pathological upregulation of normal targets of *CIC* inhibition including the PEA3 family genes (e.g. *ETV1*, *ETV4*, *ETV5*), *CCND2*, and *MUC5AC* {3003,1578,1551,3549}. The majority of CNS *CIC*-rearranged sarcoma fusions are associated with *NUTM1* {1818}.

Macroscopic appearance

The tumours are typically well-circumscribed, white or tan, soft masses, with frequent haemorrhage and necrosis.

Histopathology

CNS *CIC*-rearranged sarcomas display similar histological features to those of their extra-CNS counterparts {120}. Tumours are composed of sheets of highly undifferentiated small round cells interposed with foci of necrosis, a variably lobulated growth pattern, and desmoplastic stroma {774,1426,1818,3507}. The

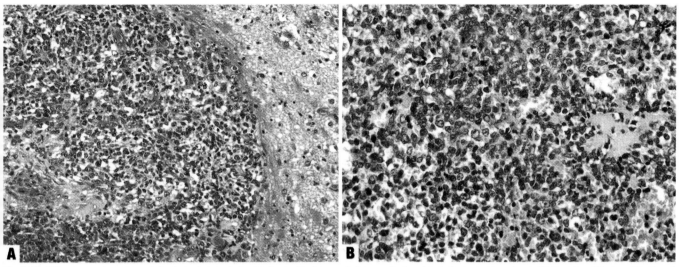

Fig. 8.24 *CIC*-rearranged sarcoma. **A** A primary tumour in the cerebrum showing a well-circumscribed nodule in the brain parenchyma. **B** There is a diffuse proliferation of small round cells with minimally pleomorphic nuclei and variably prominent nucleoli.

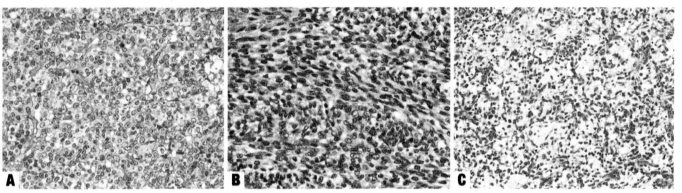

Fig. 8.25 *CIC*-rearranged sarcoma. **A** Some tumours are composed of epithelioid cells, mimicking metastatic carcinoma. **B** A spindle cell component may be present. **C** Some tumours may show prominent myxoid change.

predominant round cell component may be interspersed with epithelioid/spindle cell morphology. Myxoid change is common. Cytological features also include prominent nucleoli and eosinophilic cytoplasm. Tumours with *CIC*::non-*DUX4* fusion variants have similar histology to that of *CIC*::*DUX4* tumours {1818,3066, 3067}.

Grading
CIC-rearranged sarcomas are designated CNS WHO grade 4.

Immunophenotype and differential diagnosis
CNS *CIC*-rearranged sarcomas can express patchy and weak CD99; WT1 and ETV4 are frequently positive and NKX2-2 is typically negative, which distinguishes *CIC*-rearranged sarcoma from Ewing sarcoma. Scattered expression of cytokeratin AE1/AE3, calretinin, α-SMA, and neurofilament has been reported {1426,774,3507}. Sarcomas with *CIC*::*NUTM1* fusion express NUT protein. Nuclear preservation of SMARCB1 and SMARCA4 rules out atypical teratoid/rhabdoid tumour.

Cytology
Not clinically relevant

Diagnostic molecular pathology
Suspected cases require positive confirmation of *CIC* gene fusion events. Break-apart FISH offers a simple approach but does not inform on the binding partner and is affected by

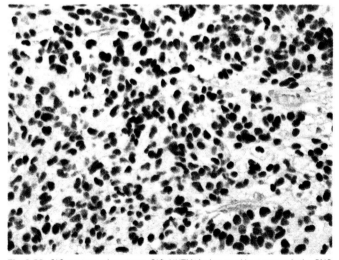

Fig. 8.26 *CIC*-rearranged sarcoma. *CIC*::*NUTM1* fusion–positive tumours in the CNS can be identified by nuclear immunoreactivity for NUT protein.

Chapter 8

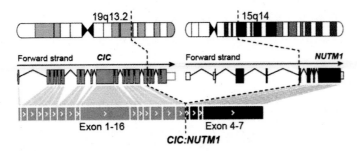

Fig. 8.27 *CIC*-rearranged sarcoma. Schematic of chromosomal location, wildtype RNA transcript, and exon structure resulting from a *CIC::NUTM1* gene fusion.

Box 8.06 Diagnostic criteria for *CIC*-rearranged sarcoma

Essential:

Evidence of a *CIC* gene fusion

AND

Predominant round cell phenotype

AND

Mild nuclear pleomorphism

AND

Variable admixture of epithelioid and/or spindle cells

AND

Variably myxoid stroma

AND

Variable CD99 and frequent ETV4 and WT1 expression

Desirable:

DNA methylation pattern matching that of *CIC*-rearranged sarcoma

false negative results {1424,3542}. Next-generation sequencing of transcriptome (RNA sequencing) or with anchored multiplex PCR are practical yet sensitive approaches {1921, 1794,2005}. Detection of upregulation of ETV1, ETV4, or ETV5 complements FISH and RNA sequencing findings {1551}. The unique methylome {3059} permits the use of DNA methylation microarray profiling {1675}. RNA sequencing and methylation profiling is helpful in ruling out other tumours with overlapping histology {3059}.

Essential and desirable diagnostic criteria
See Box 8.06.

Staging
Radiological survey and cerebrospinal fluid cytology should be undertaken. There is no relevant staging system for *CIC*-rearranged sarcoma in the CNS.

Prognosis and prediction
There is a lack of clinical data specific for CNS *CIC*-rearranged sarcomas; however, peripheral *CIC*-rearranged sarcomas are characterized by a highly aggressive course that is markedly worse than that of Ewing sarcoma {120,3543}, and they have an inferior response to Ewing sarcoma chemotherapy regimens {120}.

Primary intracranial sarcoma, *DICER1*-mutant

Solomon DA
Alexandrescu S
Foulkes WD
Haberler C
Huang A
Kölsche C
Kool M
Orr BA
Pfister SM
Sturm D
von Deimling A
von Hoff K

Definition

Primary intracranial sarcoma, *DICER1*-mutant, is a primary intracranial sarcoma composed of spindled or pleomorphic tumour cells typically displaying eosinophilic cytoplasmic globules, immunophenotypic evidence of myogenic differentiation, and occasionally foci of chondroid differentiation. These tumours are genetically defined by mutations in the *DICER1* gene (either somatic or germline as part of *DICER1* syndrome).

ICD-O coding

9480/3 Primary intracranial sarcoma, *DICER1*-mutant

ICD-11 coding

None

Related terminology

Not recommended: primary intracranial spindle cell sarcoma with rhabdomyosarcoma-like features, *DICER1*-mutant.

Subtype(s)

None

Localization

The characteristic localization of these lesions is intracranial, often in supratentorial forebrain regions, and there is typically leptomeningeal and sometimes dural involvement {1677,1836}.

Clinical features

Presenting symptoms include headaches, seizures, or focal neurological signs representing the typical spectrum of clinical signs for tumours arising in the respective brain regions {1677,1836}.

Epidemiology

The sex distribution has been reported as almost equal, and the median age at diagnosis as 6 years (range: 2–76 years) {1677,

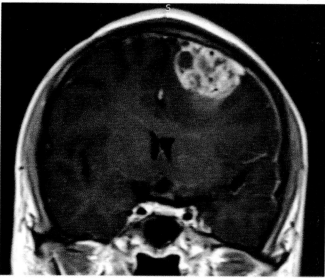

Fig. 8.28 Primary intracranial sarcoma, *DICER1*-mutant. Coronal T1-weighted post-contrast MRI showing a heterogeneously enhancing mass with dural involvement and marked mass effect on the underlying brain parenchyma.

1836,2788,3391,1535}. Clear ethnicity biases have not been reported to date, because of a lack of population-based studies.

Etiology

By definition, at least one pathogenic alteration in the *DICER1* gene located at chromosome 14q32 is present. These *DICER1* mutations can be either somatic or present in the germline as part of *DICER1* syndrome {704,1677}. An association with neurofibromatosis type 1 has also been observed {1836}. Therefore, genetic counselling and germline testing may be warranted in patients with this tumour entity. However, the exact incidence of *DICER1*-mutant primary intracranial sarcoma in DICER1 syndrome and in neurofibromatosis type 1 remains to be elucidated.

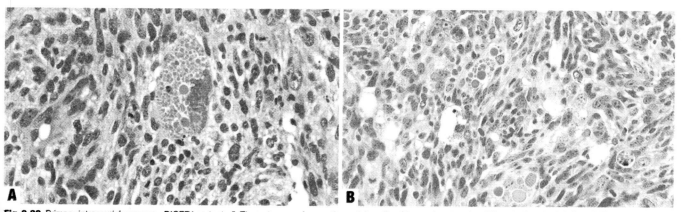

Fig. 8.29 Primary intracranial sarcoma, *DICER1*-mutant. **A** These tumours frequently contain cells with prominent eosinophilic cytoplasmic globules. **B** These tumours are typically composed of pleomorphic spindle cells arranged in fascicles or disorganized sheets. Brisk mitotic activity and eosinophilic cytoplasmic globules are common features.

Chapter 8

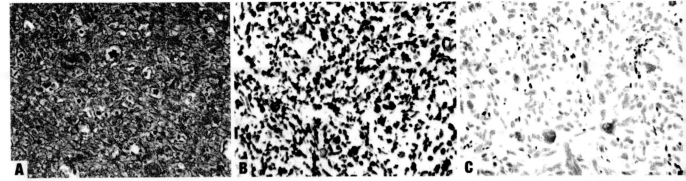

Fig. 8.30 Primary intracranial sarcoma, *DICER1*-mutant. **A** These tumours often feature dense intercellular basement membrane deposition that can be highlighted by reticulin staining. **B** In addition to the defining *DICER1* mutation, these tumours often have accompanying *TP53* mutation resulting in aberrant accumulation of p53 protein that can be visualized by immunohistochemistry. **C** In addition to the defining *DICER1* mutation, these tumours often have genetic inactivation of the *ATRX* gene resulting in loss of *ATRX* protein expression as visualized by immunohistochemistry.

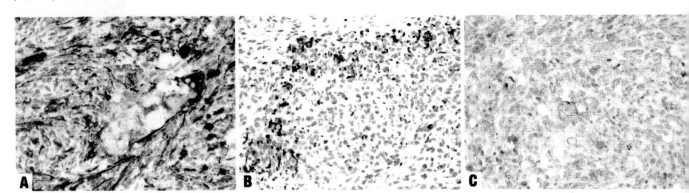

Fig. 8.31 Primary intracranial sarcoma, *DICER1*-mutant. **A** These tumours demonstrate immunophenotypic evidence of myogenic differentiation, most frequently with expression of desmin as shown here. **B** These tumours demonstrate immunophenotypic evidence of myogenic differentiation, but this finding can often be focal rather than diffuse. This example had desmin immunostaining in only a few small clusters of tumour cells. **C** While these tumours demonstrate immunophenotypic evidence of myogenic differentiation with expression of desmin and SMA, they typically have limited or absent expression of myogenin, distinguishing them from rhabdomyosarcoma. This example has complete absence of nuclear staining for myogenin (a skeletal muscle–specific transcription factor), with only nonspecific background staining in the cytoplasmic globules.

Pathogenesis

DICER1-mutant primary intracranial sarcoma is driven by the genetic disruption of the *DICER1* gene, which encodes a microRNA processing enzyme. The typical combination of events is a loss-of-function variant on one allele and one of a few recurrent missense mutations occurring in base pairs coding for metal-ion binding residues in the RNase IIIb domain of *DICER1* on the other allele {969,1677}. In addition to the disruption of microRNA processing, the majority of these tumours have disruption of p53 signalling via inactivating mutations in the *TP53* tumour suppressor gene, *ATRX* mutation or deletion, and activation of the MAPK signalling pathway via mutations in *KRAS*, *NF1*, or *PDGFRA* {1677,1836,1535}. All tumours studied to date have lacked the *NAB2::STAT6* fusion that defines solitary fibrous tumour, the *PAX3::FOXO1* and/or *PAX7::FOXO1* fusions that characterize alveolar rhabdomyosarcoma, and mutations in known genetic drivers of meningioma (*NF2*, *TRAF7*, *KLF4*, *SMO*, *AKT1*, *SMARCB1*). The exact histogenesis and cell of origin are unknown, as is the relationship with extracranial sarcomas of the kidney, uterine cervix, and other sites that harbour *DICER1* mutation {966,3483,2049}.

Macroscopic appearance

DICER1-mutant primary intracranial sarcomas are typically unifocal, relatively circumscribed lesions. They tend to be firm and often feature haemorrhage.

Histopathology

DICER1-mutant primary intracranial sarcomas are malignant pleomorphic or spindle cell neoplasms often with fascicular or patternless growth, which may demonstrate myogenic and/or cartilaginous differentiation {1677,1836,679}. Cytoplasmic eosinophilic globules and myxoid stroma are often present {1836,1535}. These tumours typically have compact growth, usually with involvement of the leptomeninges and dura, but they may also invade into surrounding brain tissue.

Special stains and immunophenotype

As with other sarcomas, there is abundant intercellular basement membrane deposition that can be highlighted with reticulin or collagen IV staining. The eosinophilic cytoplasmic globules stain with PAS. The typical immunophenotype involves positivity for markers of myogenic differentiation (desmin, SMA, and occasionally myogenin), which is often focal or patchy {1677,1836,705}. p53 expression is variable, and loss of ATRX expression occurs in a subset of tumours {1836}. Immunohistochemistry is typically negative for GFAP, OLIG2, cytokeratins, EMA, S100, SOX10, and SOX2. These tumours frequently demonstrate nuclear positivity for TLE1 and loss of H3 p.K28me3 (K27me3) {72}.

Differential diagnosis

Histologically, the resemblance to pleuropulmonary blastoma is striking. Because the brain is a known sanctuary for metastatic

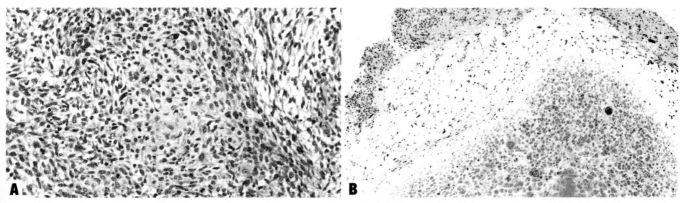

Fig. 8.32 Primary intracranial sarcoma, *DICER1*-mutant. A subset of these tumours display chondroid differentiation, which can range from small foci of chondroid matrix production (**A**) to frank malignant cartilage (**B**).

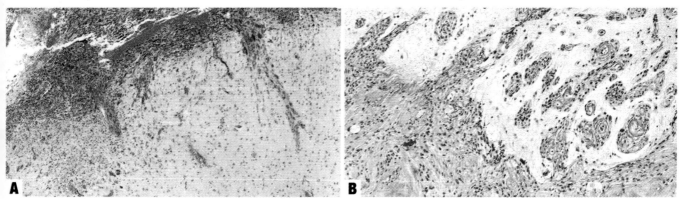

Fig. 8.33 Primary intracranial sarcoma, *DICER1*-mutant. **A** These tumours typically have a solid/compact growth pattern, but this example demonstrates invasion into the underlying brain parenchyma. **B** This tumour was located extra-axially and demonstrated meningioangiomatosis-like invasion through Virchow–Robin spaces into the subjacent brain parenchyma.

pleuropulmonary blastoma {2085}, clinical history and imaging studies are essential for ruling out pleuropulmonary blastoma metastasis. Other tumours in the differential diagnosis based on location or histological features are anaplastic/malignant meningioma, solitary fibrous tumour, gliosarcoma, and other sarcoma subtypes such as rhabdomyosarcoma, fibrosarcoma, and synovial sarcoma.

Cytology
Not relevant

Diagnostic molecular pathology
The *DICER1* mutations in these tumours are most often a hot-spot missense mutation in the RNase IIIb domain on one allele combined with a truncating mutation (frameshift, nonsense, or splice-site) occurring in trans on the other allele. Some tumours harbour a single mutation accompanied by loss of heterozygosity eliminating the remaining wildtype allele. *DICER1*-mutant primary intracranial sarcoma harbours a DNA methylation profile distinct from those of other CNS tumours {1677,1836}; however, the epigenetic overlap with extracranial sarcomas harbouring *DICER1* mutation is unknown.

Essential and desirable diagnostic criteria
See Box 8.07.

Box 8.07 Diagnostic criteria for primary intracranial sarcoma, *DICER1*-mutant

Essential:

Primary intracranial sarcoma

AND

Pathogenic *DICER1* mutation (either germline or somatic)

AND *(for unresolved lesions)*

DNA methylation profile aligned with primary intracranial sarcoma, *DICER1*-mutant

Staging
Staging is not clinically relevant to date, although spinal imaging and cerebrospinal fluid sampling should be considered.

Prognosis and prediction
The prognosis for patients with *DICER1*-mutant primary intracranial sarcoma remains unknown, because only limited clinical data are available so far. In one series of 22 patients, an aggressive clinical course was suspected, but long-term follow-up data were not sufficient for reliable conclusions {1677}. No prognostic or predictive factors have yet been reported, and the prognostic relevance of tumours arising in the setting of germline *DICER1* or *NF1* mutation has not yet been established {704,1677,1836}.

Ewing sarcoma

Perry A
de Álava E
Haberler C
Jacques TS
Kool M

Orr BA
Park SH
Sturm D
Yip S
Yoshida A

Definition

Ewing sarcoma of the nervous system is an extraosseous small round cell sarcoma containing a fusion between one FET family gene (usually *EWSR1*) and one ETS family gene (most often *FLI1*).

ICD-O coding

9364/3 Ewing sarcoma

ICD-11 coding

2B52.3 Ewing sarcoma of soft tissue
2B52.Y Ewing sarcoma of bone and articular cartilage of other specified sites

Related terminology

Not recommended: (peripheral) primitive neuroectodermal tumour.

Subtype(s)

None

Localization

Roughly 12% of Ewing sarcomas are extraosseous tumours, a small subset of which involve the craniospinal axis {1172}. Most of the latter are meningeal (intracranial or spinal), paraspinal, and/or peripheral nerve–associated masses, including those that involve the cauda equina. Direct extension from adjacent bone primaries can also occur.

Clinical features

Signs and symptoms vary with location and are typically due to mass effect. They include localized pain, cranial/radicular neuropathies, bone fractures, and/or fever, the last being more frequent in patients with metastatic disease. Imaging studies are necessary for defining the site of origin, extent of local disease, and metastatic spread, but they do not otherwise show specific diagnostic findings.

Epidemiology

Ewing sarcoma is most commonly encountered in children and young adults, with older patients more commonly presenting with extraosseous disease, including in the nervous system. Presentation beyond 50 years of age is rare {1443}.

Etiology

The majority of Ewing sarcomas are sporadic and idiopathic, although rare examples have been reported in patients with germline *TP53*, *PMS2*, or *RET* mutations; whether these were causal or coincidental is unclear {3596}.

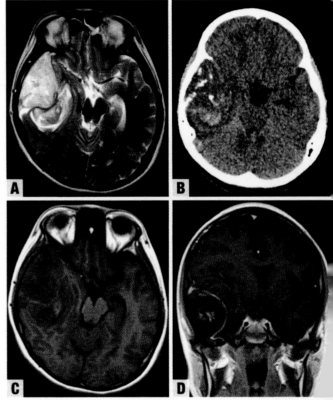

Fig. 8.34 Intracranial Ewing sarcoma. **A** T2-weighted MRI of a dural-based solid mass lesion in the right middle cranial fossa, about 55 × 75 mm in size, showing heterogeneous signal intensity. The mass effect on the right temporal lobe with impending transtentorial (uncal) herniation is observed. Probable extra-axial location extending into the right temporal lobe with dural tear and adjacent parenchymal oedema was suspected. **B** CT image reveals the multifocal calcifications and haemorrhages within the tumour. **C** The mass lesion is mainly hypointense with multifocal hyperintensity on T1-weighted imaging. **D** Contrast-enhanced T1-weighted imaging demonstrates multifocal enhancement within the tumour and the medial displacement and thickening of the right temporal dura.

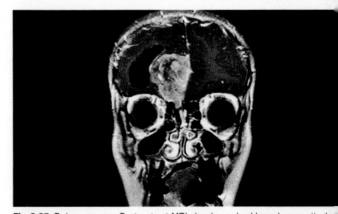

Fig. 8.35 Ewing sarcoma. Postcontrast MRI showing a dural-based mass attached to the falx cerebri.

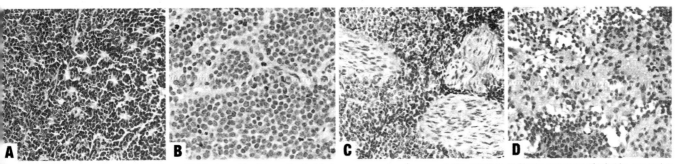

Fig. 8.36 Ewing sarcoma. **A** The focal Homer Wright (neuroblastic) rosettes in this tumour are a sign of neuronal differentiation. **B** Sheets and nests of primitive-appearing small round cells with delicate chromatin, high N:C ratios, and high mitotic count. **C** Cauda equina lesion. Native nerves are entrapped in this small round cell neoplasm. **D** A rare form of neuronal differentiation in Ewing sarcoma is ganglion cell maturation.

Pathogenesis

Ewing sarcomas uniformly contain an oncogenic gene fusion that combines a FET RNA-binding protein family member (mostly *EWSR1* and rarely *FUS*) with an ETS transcription factor family member (*FLI1* > *ERG* >> *ETV1*, *ETV4* [*E1AF*], and *FEV*) {1172}. The t(11;22)(q24;q12) translocation that results in the *EWSR1::FLI1* fusion transcript and protein product accounts for roughly 85% of all cases. Additional *STAG2* (in 15–22% of cases), *CDKN2A* (12%), and/or *TP53* (7%) mutations are occasionally found, and they may be associated with a worse prognosis {382,3201,1172}.

Macroscopic appearance

Ewing sarcoma has a soft, grey, fleshy appearance, often with foci of necrosis and haemorrhage on the cut surface. Nerve roots may be entrapped within the tumour, especially in the cauda equina.

Histopathology

Classic Ewing sarcoma is composed predominantly of monomorphic, primitive-appearing, and mitotically active small round cells arranged in sheets. The chromatin is delicate and there are small amounts of clear to amphophilic cytoplasm, which is often glycogen-rich (PAS-positive and diastase-sensitive). Like other sarcomas, Ewing sarcoma is also reticulin-rich. Evidence of neuronal differentiation most commonly manifests as Homer Wright rosettes with central neuropil (cases previously referred to as "peripheral primitive neuroectodermal tumour"), although rare cases may show ganglion cell differentiation {3413}. Postchemotherapy specimens are often extensively necrotic.

Grading

Ewing sarcoma is considered CNS WHO grade 4.

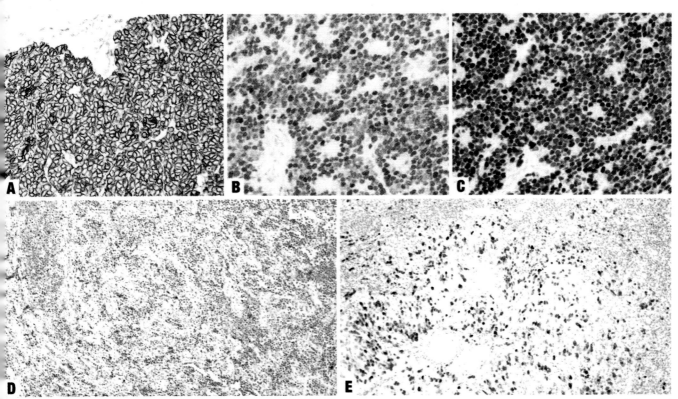

Fig. 8.37 Ewing sarcoma. **A** Diffuse membranous immunostaining with CD99. **B** Most Ewing sarcomas express NKX2-2. **C** Most Ewing sarcomas express PAX7. **D** Scattered synaptophysin-positive cells provide evidence of limited neuronal differentiation. **E** Extensive NeuN positivity in regions of ganglion cell differentiation.

Table 8.01 Useful immunostains for the diagnostic workup of Ewing sarcoma

Immunostain	Sensitivity estimate	Specificity estimate	Notes
CD99 (diffuse membranous pattern)	Nearly 100%	87%	Can be positive in desmoplastic small round cell tumour, alveolar/embryonal rhabdomyosarcoma, and small cell osteosarcoma
PAX7 (nuclear)	Nearly 100%	88%	Can be positive in EWSR1::NFATC2 sarcoma, alveolar rhabdomyosarcoma, poorly differentiated synovial sarcoma, BCOR::CCNB3 sarcoma, small cell osteosarcoma, and desmoplastic small round cell tumour
NKX2-2 (nuclear)	93–100%	85–88%	Can be positive in small cell carcinoma or neuroendocrine tumours, olfactory neuroblastoma, neuroblastoma, mesenchymal chondrosarcoma, CIC::DUX sarcoma, synovial sarcoma, and melanoma

Immunophenotype and differential diagnosis

The three most useful immunostains for differentiating Ewing sarcoma from other round cell sarcomas are summarized in Table 8.01 {1971,1615,3208}. Otherwise, lineage markers are mostly negative, except neuronal markers, which are variably positive depending on the extent of neuronal differentiation. Cytokeratin may be expressed focally. The differential diagnosis for cases with Homer Wright rosettes and/or ganglionic differentiation includes peripheral neuroblastoma, although patients with Ewing sarcoma are typically much older and neuroblastomas are virtually always CD99-negative. In contrast, the diffuse CD99 positivity encountered in mesenchymal chondrosarcoma is an occasional pitfall, but hyaline cartilage is seen only in mesenchymal chondrosarcoma, as is the pathognomonic HEY1::NCOA2 gene fusion. CD99 can also be expressed in other tumour types, including solitary fibrous tumour and atypical teratoid/rhabdoid tumour, as well as other embryonal CNS neoplasms. Solitary fibrous tumour is distinguished by

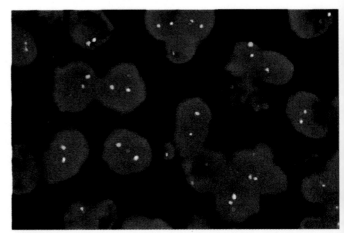

Fig. 8.38 Ewing sarcoma of the dura. Locus-specific identifier (LSI) EWSR1 gene (22q12) dual-colour break-apart FISH shows separated SpectrumOrange and SpectrumGreen signals in addition to a fused signal (normal) in the nuclei of Ewing sarcoma cells.

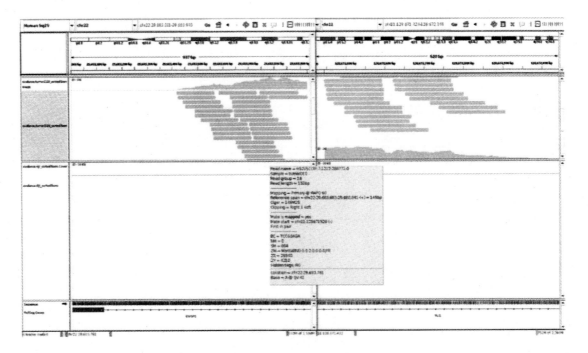

Fig. 8.39 Ewing sarcoma. EWSR1::FLI1 fusion in the Integrative Genomics Viewer (IGV). The red bar on the chromosome track (below 29 683 900 bp of chromosome 22 and below 128 671 400 bp of chromosome 11) represents a breakpoint. The red reads are positive strands, and the blue reads are negative strands. The mated reads exist on a different chromosome (chromosome 11) upon mouseover on chromosome 22 (H52V5CCXY:7:1212:288771:0).

its nuclear STAT6 immunoreactivity, whereas atypical teratoid/ rhabdoid tumour shows a loss of SMARCB1 (INI1) expression or, rarely, of SMARCA4 (BRG1) expression.

Cytology

Not relevant

Diagnostic molecular pathology

Most Ewing sarcomas of the nervous system require molecular confirmation of a FET::ETS–type gene fusion for definitive diagnosis. With classic histopathological features, a positive *EWSR1* break-apart FISH assay may suffice, but potential mimics with other *EWSR1* fusions must be excluded (e.g. desmoplastic small round cell tumour; intracranial mesenchymal tumour, FET::CREB fusion–positive; myoepithelial neoplasms). For example, *CIC::DUX4* fusion is frequently found in *EWSR1* fusion–negative small round cell sarcoma {3003,120}. Also, *EWSR1* fusion has been identified in other intra-axial CNS tumours, including ganglioglioma and ependymoma {2928,3470}. Given the sometimes limited sensitivity of FISH {541} and the diversity of gene fusion partners and junctional breakpoints, next-generation sequencing–based approaches are considered more efficient, comprehensive, and informative for fusion drivers.

Essential and desirable diagnostic criteria

See Box 8.08.

Staging

There is no relevant staging system for Ewing sarcoma in the CNS.

Prognosis and prediction

Patient outcome greatly improves with induction chemotherapy followed by tumour resection and radiation therapy {1172,1615}. Nonetheless, roughly a quarter of cases come to clinical attention with metastatic disease and this is the strongest negative prognostic variable; the estimated 5-year overall survival rate in patients with localized disease is 70–80%, but it decreases to about 30% in those with disseminated disease. In localized disease, complete response to induction chemotherapy (0% viable tumour in the posttherapy specimen) is associated with a favourable prognosis {57}.

Mesenchymal chondrosarcoma

Kleinschmidt-DeMasters BK
Baumhoer D
Bouvier C
Flanagan AM
Hainfellner JA
Inwards CY

Definition

Mesenchymal chondrosarcoma is a rare, biphasic, malignant tumour composed of undifferentiated small, round or oval to spindle-shaped cells and islands of well-differentiated hyaline cartilage. The presence of a *HEY1::NCOA2* gene fusion is characteristic.

ICD-O coding

9240/3 Mesenchymal chondrosarcoma

ICD-11 coding

2B50.Z & XH8X47 Chondrosarcoma of bone and articular cartilage of unspecified sites & Mesenchymal chondrosarcoma

Related terminology

None

Subtype(s)

None

Localization

Intracranial location {1898} is more frequent than intraspinal {535}, and these are followed by frontoparietal and thoracic cord locations. Approximately 60% have a dural attachment {1898}.

Clinical features

Symptoms relate to intracranial mass effect or spinal cord compression {535}.

Epidemiology

Most mesenchymal chondrosarcomas arise in the second and third decades of life, although patients at either end of the age spectrum have been reported {2771,3314,1898}.

Etiology

Unknown

Pathogenesis

Almost all mesenchymal chondrosarcomas show the highly specific *HEY1::NCOA2* fusion transcript.

Macroscopic appearance

Typically, the tumours are lobular, grey-brown, firm masses {1787,2771,3314} with varying amounts of calcification {542}.

Histopathology

Mesenchymal chondrosarcoma shows primitive small round cells intermingled with islands of well-differentiated hyaline cartilage. The absence of the latter in core needle biopsies can render the diagnosis particularly challenging {1898}. CNS examples show more spindling and less necrosis than musculoskeletal tumours {888}. A staghorn, solitary fibrous tumour–like vascular pattern is often (but not invariably) present. Varying amounts of central calcification and/or enchondral ossification of cartilaginous islands with eosinophilic osteoid-like matrix are seen.

Immunohistochemistry

The primitive small round cells can show expression of CD99, EMA, desmin, myogenin, MYOD1 and NKX3-1, whereas they are negative for GFAP, keratins, SMA, and ER {888,953,3545}. SMARCB1 (INI1) is retained and Ki-67 labelling is generally increased. S100 and SOX10 can be positive in both components {889,3406}.

Differential diagnosis

The main differential for mesenchymal chondrosarcoma in the CNS is solitary fibrous tumour. The presence of hyaline cartilage,

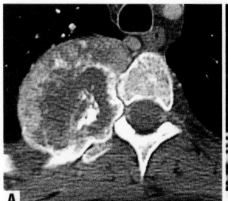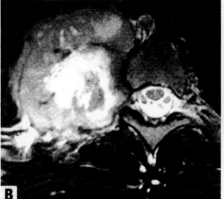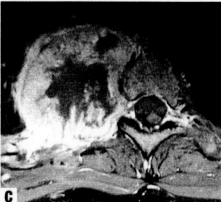

Fig. 8.40 Mesenchymal chondrosarcoma. **A** Axial CT shows a partially calcified right paraspinal soft tissue mass that extends into the adjacent neural foramen. **B** T2-weighted axial MRI shows the mass is hyperintense compared with adjacent paraspinal musculature and contains an irregular, very hyperintense necrotic centre. **C** T1-weighted axial postcontrast MRI shows an intensely enhancing ring of tumour surrounding a central non-enhancing necrotic core.

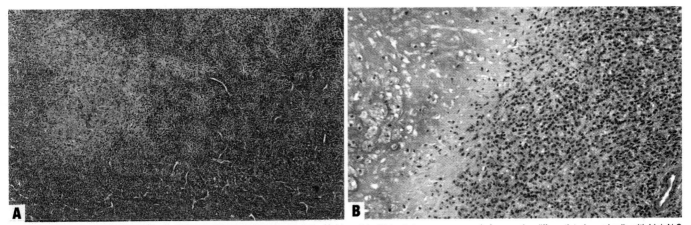

Fig. 8.41 Mesenchymal chondrosarcoma. **A** Mesenchymal chondrosarcoma is a highly cellular biphasic tumour composed of areas of undifferentiated round cells with high N:C ratios, as well as numerous staghorn vessels, and islands of hyaline cartilage. **B** Mesenchymal chondrosarcoma typically shows a biphasic pattern of small malignant cells with scant cytoplasm and islands of hyaline cartilage, both seen here.

SOX9 positivity and *HEY1::NCOA2* fusion in the former versus nuclear STAT6 expression and a *NAB2::STAT6* fusion in the latter usually allows an unequivocal diagnosis. Areas of ossification and/or calcification of the cartilage component in mesenchymal chondrosarcoma can mimic an osteosarcoma (either small cell or chondroblastic). On neuroimaging, dural-based examples most often mimic meningioma {2787}. Histologically, meningioma with metaplastic cartilage is distinguishable by lower-grade features, a meningothelial/fibroblastic architecture, and positive EMA and/ or SSTR2A immunolabelling. Other small round cell tumours, including Ewing sarcoma, monophasic synovial sarcoma, rhabdomyosarcoma, and atypical teratoid/rhabdoid tumour, may enter the differential diagnosis, particularly when there is insufficient hyaline cartilage in a small biopsy {1898,3254}

Cytology

Tumours show oval to spindled cells with high N:C ratios and hyperchromatic nuclei. The cytoplasm may be vacuolated and cells may be associated with myxoid stromal material and/or necrotic debris. Intraoperative smear preparations may feature a prominent perivascular arrangement of cells {3324}.

Diagnostic molecular pathology

Mesenchymal chondrosarcoma typically harbours an underlying *HEY1::NCOA2* gene fusion.

Essential and desirable diagnostic criteria

See Box 8.09.

Staging

Not relevant

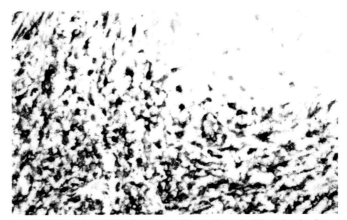

Fig. 8.42 Mesenchymal chondrosarcoma. The small, poorly differentiated cells express diffuse cytoplasmic CD99.

Box 8.09 Diagnostic criteria for mesenchymal chondrosarcoma

Essential:

Poorly differentiated tumour composed of small blue round cells with high N:C ratios and variable amounts of hyaline cartilage

AND *(in cases lacking cartilage)*

Demonstration of the characteristic fusion transcript (*HEY1::NCOA2*)

Prognosis and prediction

Spinal examples show low recurrence rates, and most patients survive for > 2 years after diagnosis {535}; intracranial examples have a high rate of recurrence and (rarely) can show leptomeningeal dissemination {1994} or metastasize outside the cranial vault {2754,1748}.

Chondrosarcoma

Kleinschmidt-DeMasters BK
Bouvier C
Flanagan AM
Hainfellner JA
Inwards CY
Rosenberg AE

Definition

Chondrosarcomas are a family of malignant mesenchymal tumours with cartilaginous differentiation, comprising conventional central, dedifferentiated central, conventional peripheral, dedifferentiated peripheral, and clear cell chondrosarcomas.

ICD-O coding

9220/3 Chondrosarcoma
9243/3 Dedifferentiated chondrosarcoma

ICD-11 coding

2B50.Y Chondrosarcoma of bone or articular cartilage of other specified sites
2B50.Z & XH0FY0 Chondrosarcoma of bone and articular cartilage of unspecified sites & Atypical cartilaginous tumour / chondrosarcoma, grade 1
B50.Z & XH6LT5 Chondrosarcoma of bone and articular cartilage of unspecified sites & Chondrosarcoma, grade 2
2B50.Z & XH0Y34 Chondrosarcoma of bone and articular cartilage of unspecified sites & Chondrosarcoma, grade 3

Related terminology

None

Subtype(s)

None

Localization

Conventional chondrosarcoma is the most common tumour type that arises in the cranial bones. The most common sites are the skull base (spheno-occipital and sphenopetrosal synchondroses), spine, and sacrum. Parafalcine examples are uncommon; parenchymal intracranial, meningeal, and extraosseous examples are rare. Peripheral chondrosarcoma is exceptionally rare at these sites.

Clinical features

Patients with chondrosarcoma present with a painful enlarging mass. Neurological symptoms are site-dependent; skull base examples may produce cranial nerve palsies.

Epidemiology

Intracranial chondrosarcomas comprise approximately 1% of all chondrosarcomas {781}; in this site, they are less frequent than chordoma {1644}. In one study of 200 patients with skull base tumours, the age range was 10–79 years (mean: 39 years), and the M:F ratio was 1:1.3 {2724}.

Etiology

Most chondrosarcomas are sporadic. Individuals with enchondromatosis (Ollier disease, Maffucci syndrome) have an

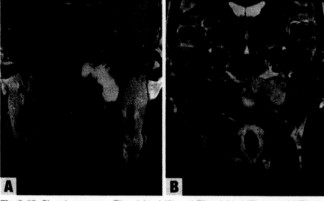

Fig. 8.43 Chondrosarcoma. T1-weighted (**A**) and T2-weighted (**B**) coronal MRI of a 33-year-old man who presented with dysphagia shows a skull base lesion that extensively involves left-sided basilar skull regions (right side of images).

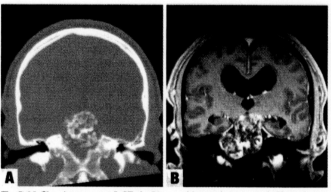

Fig. 8.44 Chondrosarcoma. **A** CT of a 56-year-old man who presented with ataxia and weakness demonstrates a heavily calcified skull base mass near the prepontine and basal cisterns, behind the sella. Preoperative considerations included craniopharyngioma and chondrosarcoma. Biopsy proved that the lesion was a low-grade chondrosarcoma. **B** T1-weighted postcontrast coronal MRI of a 56-year-old man with a skull base low-grade tumour shows the characteristic heterogeneous signal seen within the tumour.

increased risk of developing chondrosarcoma, possibly associated with pre-existing enchondroma. Individuals with multiple osteochondromas arising in association with germline *EXT1* or *EXT2* mutation have a greater propensity to develop a secondary peripheral chondrosarcoma {3312}.

Pathogenesis

Approximately 60% of central cartilaginous tumours harbour an *IDH1* or *IDH2* mutation, the former being considerably more common. When this alteration occurs as an early postzygotic mutation, it causes mosaic disorders including Ollier disease and Maffucci syndrome. The rate of IDH mutations is high in skull base chondrosarcomas, whereas chondrosarcomas of the facial skeleton lack IDH mutations {3118}. The additional genetic alterations in conventional chondrosarcoma are similar to those in IDH-mutant and IDH-wildtype tumours and in central and peripheral chondrosarcoma {3426}.

Macroscopic appearance

Chondrosarcomas are glistening, grey, firm lobular masses that are usually non-haemorrhagic but may have more mucinous areas reflecting myxoid change microscopically; skull base tumours are usually resected piecemeal.

Histopathology

Microscopy

Hyaline-type conventional chondrosarcoma grows with an infiltrative pattern. It is moderately cellular and composed of polyhedral cells residing in lacunar spaces within a solid basophilic matrix. In myxoid conventional chondrosarcoma, the tumour cells are spindle and stellate, and they float in a basophilic, flocculent, mucinous matrix. The tumour cells are small to medium in size. They do not form cohesive nests or aggregates, but elongate cytoplasmic processes of adjacent cells may come into contact with one another and form complex interconnecting networks. In a study of 200 skull base chondrosarcomas (the largest such study to date), > 60% showed mixed hyaline and myxoid features {2724}.

Grading schemes of conventional chondrosarcoma (CNS WHO grades 1–3) are based on the degree of cellularity, cytological atypia, and mitotic activity. Most skull base chondrosarcomas are low-grade (CNS WHO grade 1) {2724}; CNS WHO grade 3 tumours are uncommon at this site {3118}. Dedifferentiated chondrosarcomas often show abrupt transition from a low-grade to a high-grade phenotype, usually with the latter showing features of a pleomorphic spindle cell sarcoma, although osteosarcomatous or other lines of differentiation can occur.

Immunophenotype

Immunoreactivity for S100 and D2-40 (podoplanin) is typical, and immunoreactivity for ERG is possible; keratin and brachyury stains show no positivity. There is a good antibody for IDH1 p.R132H, but this variant represents < 20% of IDH mutations in cartilaginous tumours. Immunostaining can be abrogated by harsh decalcification. Dedifferentiated chondrosarcomas may show loss of H3 p.K28me3 (K27me3), but only in the dedifferentiated areas {1990}.

Proliferation and grading

Proliferative activity is low in grade 1 neoplasms and high in grade 3 and dedifferentiated neoplasms. The grading criteria from the *Soft tissue and bone tumours* volume of this series can be used: for grade 1, nuclei are generally uniform in size, and binucleation is frequently seen, but mitoses are absent; for grade 2, there is increased cellularity, a greater degree of nuclear atypia, hyperchromasia, increased nuclear size, myxoid matrix change, and the presence of mitoses; for grade 3, the tumour is highly cellular and more pleomorphic, mitoses are easily found, and the cells at the periphery of the mostly myxoid tumour lobules are spindled and less differentiated. As noted in this same reference, however, "histological grading is subject to interobserver variability".

Differential diagnosis

Chondrosarcoma can be distinguished from chordoma by the absence of cohesive nests of cells, and the neoplastic chondrocytes are negative for cytokeratin and brachyury; approximately 6% of chondrosarcomas are positive for EMA. SOX9 is common to both notochordal and cartilaginous differentiation and is therefore not useful in the chordoma–chondrosarcoma differential diagnosis {2294}. The presence of osteoid matrix indicates a diagnosis of osteosarcoma, although a diagnosis of a dedifferentiated chondrosarcoma must also be entertained.

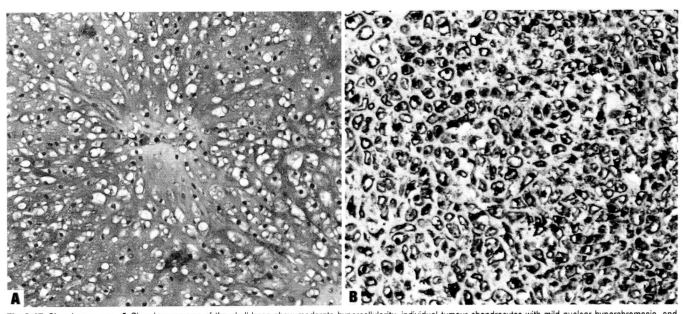

Fig. 8.45 Chondrosarcoma. **A** Chondrosarcomas of the skull base show moderate hypercellularity, individual tumour chondrocytes with mild nuclear hyperchromasia, and absence of mitotic activity. **B** This skull base chondrosarcoma shows the typical strong diffuse immunoreactivity for S100 in tumoural cells, both in cytoplasm and in nuclei. Strong immunostaining for S100 can also be found in chordomas of the skull base; chordoma often is the main tumour type in the differential diagnosis, so S100 immunostaining does not help distinguish these two tumour types.

Box 8.10 Diagnostic criteria for chondrosarcoma

> ***Essential:***
>
> A histologically malignant tumour with cartilaginous differentiation
>
> **AND**
>
> Immunohistochemical profile characteristic of chondrosarcoma

Cytology

Cytology is rarely used because it is difficult to access skull base lesions with a needle, but when it is used, discohesive round to elongate cells in a hyaline or myxoid matrix are seen. The degree of cellularity and atypia varies with grade. In rare instances of high-grade tumours, examples may show necrosis and pleomorphic cells {1841}.

Diagnostic molecular pathology

IDH1 or *IDH2* mutation is present in approximately 60% of central conventional and dedifferentiated chondrosarcomas.

Essential and desirable diagnostic criteria

See Box 8.10.

Staging

Not applicable

Prognosis and prediction

Most skull base chondrosarcomas are primary and low-grade, but they are locally destructive, requiring adjuvant therapy (often proton beam therapy or radiosurgery). Metastases are rare.

Chordoma

Varlet P
Nielsen GP
Righi A
Tanaka S
Tirabosco R

Definition
Chordomas are a family of primary malignant bone neoplasms demonstrating notochordal differentiation, comprising conventional, chondroid, poorly differentiated, and dedifferentiated types.

ICD-O coding
9370/3 Chordoma

ICD-11 coding
2B5Y & XH9GH0 Other specified malignant mesenchymal neoplasms & Chordoma, NOS
2B5Y & XH17D8 Other specified malignant mesenchymal neoplasms & Chondroid chordoma
2B5Y & XH7303 Other specified malignant mesenchymal neoplasms & Dedifferentiated chordoma

Related terminology
None

Subtype(s)
None

Localization
Chordomas almost always arise within the axial skeleton, particularly in the skull base and the sacrococcygeal region. The anatomical distribution varies depending on age {2876} and histopathological type (detailed in Table 8.02). Extra-axial locations are exceptional {2676,3200}.

Clinical features
Patients with chordomas most commonly present with pain and site-related neurological symptoms.

Imaging
Chordomas are lobular, lytic, destructive midline lesions, hypointense on T1-weighted MRI and hyperintense on T2-weighted MRI, with enhancement on postcontrast imaging.

Epidemiology
Chordoma has an incidence of 0.088 cases per 100 000 person-years, representing 0.5% of all primary CNS tumours {680}. Sex and age predominance according to histopathological type are detailed in Table 8.02.

Table 8.02 Characteristics of histopathological types of chordoma

Characteristic	Conventional chordoma	Chondroid chordoma	Dedifferentiated chordoma	Poorly differentiated chordoma, SMARCB1-deficient
Age at diagnosis	Adults (96%) Median: 55 years	Adults (86%) Median: 45 years	Adults (96%) Median: 61 years	Children (86%) Median: 7 years
M:F ratio	1.7	1.1	1.8	0.7
Prior irradiation	No	No	Yes (25%)	No
Localization	Sacrococcygeal region (55%)	Skull base (73%)	Sacrococcygeal region (60%)	Skull base (64%)
Histopathology	Classic	Chondroid	Conventional juxtaposed with sarcomatous (91%) Chondroid juxtaposed with sarcomatous (2%) Conventional chordoma transformed into pure sarcomatous tumour (7%)	Epithelioid No physaliphorous cells
Immunohistochemical profile	SMARCB1 (INI1) preserved Brachyury+ Pancytokeratin+ EMA+ S100+	SMARCB1 (INI1) preserved Brachyury+ Pancytokeratin+ EMA+ S100+	SMARCB1 (INI1) preserved Brachyury+/–[a] Pancytokeratin– EMA– S100–/+	Loss of SMARCB1 (INI1) Brachyury+ Pancytokeratin+ EMA+ S100+/–
Outcome	Metastasis: 13% Local progression: 46% Median PFS: 24 months Death during follow-up: 29% Median OS: 48 months	Metastasis: 9% Local progression: 54% Median PFS: 26.5 months Death during follow-up: 42% Median OS: 43 months	Metastasis: 30% Local progression: 65% Median PFS: 6 months Death during follow-up: 61% Median OS: 15 months	Metastasis: 30% Local progression: 54% Median PFS: 4 months Death during follow-up: 43% Median OS: 13 months

+, immunopositive; –, immunonegative; OS, overall survival; PFS, progression-free survival.
[a]Positive in the conventional or chondroid component, negative in the sarcomatous component.
Note: Data are based on the systematic review of 245 conventional chordomas (main references: {3349,3144}), 210 chondroid chordomas (main references: {2876,3144}), 57 dedifferentiated chordomas (main references: {1581,3144}), and 65 poorly differentiated chordomas (main references: {1258,2912}).

Etiology

The majority of chordomas are sporadic, but rare associations with tuberous sclerosis in children {668} or familial cases with germline duplication of the *TBXT* gene have been reported {1585}.

Pathogenesis

The *TBXT* gene encodes the protein brachyury, a notochord tissue–specific transcription factor critical for notochord development. The notochord undergoes regression and disappears by birth to become the nucleus pulposus of the intervertebral discs. In a subset of the population, notochordal remnants persist, particularly in the odontoid process and the coccyx. The molecular mechanisms of the notochordal tumoural transformation are not completely understood but duplications of *TBXT* gene (27% of cases) and *PIK3CA* signalling mutations (16% of cases) have recently been described {3137,3144,1585}. A *LYST* inactivating mutation (in 10% of cases) may represent a novel cancer gene in chordoma {3137}. Unlike in most atypical teratoid/rhabdoid tumours, loss of SMARCB1 (INI1) expression in chordomas results from a homozygous deletion of the *SMARCB1* gene {1258}.

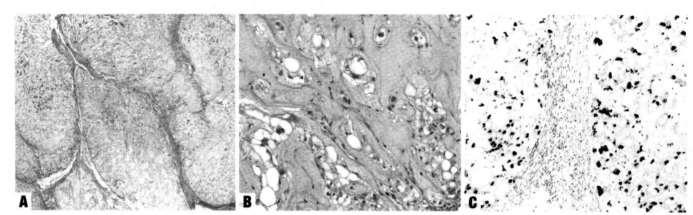

Fig. 8.46 Conventional chordoma. **A** This shows a lobular architecture and abundant myxoid matrix. **B** Nests and cords of cells, sometimes with vacuolated bubbly cytoplasm (physaliphorous cells). **C** Diffuse nuclear expression of brachyury.

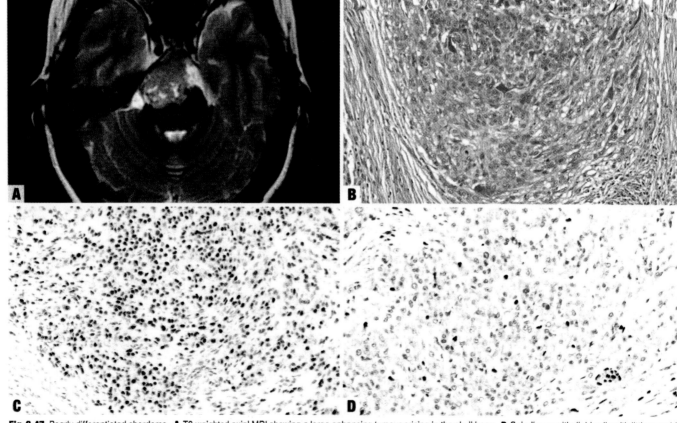

Fig. 8.47 Poorly differentiated chordoma. **A** T2-weighted axial MRI showing a large enhancing tumour arising in the skull base. **B** Spindle or epithelioid cells with little myxoid matrix. **C** The chordoma cells express nuclear brachyury. **D** Loss of SMARCB1 (INI1) expression is essential for this diagnosis.

Macroscopic appearance

Chordomas are lobulated, solid tumours with a gelatinous appearance, destroying bone and extending into surrounding soft tissue.

Histopathology

Conventional chordoma is divided into lobules by fibrous septa. Tumour cells are arranged in cords or ribbons separated by a myxoid matrix. Tumour cells are large with clear to eosinophilic cytoplasm characterized by vacuolated or bubbly cytoplasm (physaliphorous cells). Anisokaryosis and nuclear inclusions may be observed, but prominent nucleoli, mitoses and apoptotic bodies are scarce or absent. Chondroid chordoma is a subtype of conventional chordoma containing extracellular matrix mimicking hyaline cartilage.

Dedifferentiated chordomas are biphasic tumours, composed of conventional chordoma juxtaposed to high-grade sarcoma. Brachyury (nuclear) and cytokeratin expression are preserved in the conventional component but lost in the high-grade sarcomatous component {1379,151}.

Poorly differentiated chordomas are epithelioid and solid, with focal rhabdoid morphology and without physaliphorous cells, and they are characterized by a loss of SMARCB1 (INI1) expression but retained brachyury expression {2912,1258}.

Cytology

Not clinically relevant

Diagnostic molecular pathology

No diagnostic molecular markers have been reported for conventional chordomas, but FISH can be used to identify

Box 8.11 Diagnostic criteria for chordoma

Essential:

Midline axial bone tumour

AND

Lobules of cohesive and physaliphorous cells in a myxoid or chondroid matrix

AND

Brachyury immunopositivity

AND *(in the case of epithelioid/solid forms)*

Loss of SMARCB1 (INI1) expression to confirm the diagnosis of poorly differentiated chordoma

homozygous *SMARCB1* deletions in poorly differentiated chordomas.

Essential and desirable diagnostic criteria

See Box 8.11.

Staging

Union for International Cancer Control (UICC) staging is according to bone sarcoma protocols.

Prognosis and prediction

Outcome data according to type are detailed in Table 8.02 (p. 335). Dedifferentiated and poorly differentiated chordomas appear to have the worst prognosis {3604,228,3144}. In conventional chordomas, the main prognostic factors for worse progression-free and overall survival are age > 60 years, skull base location, regional extension or metastasis at diagnosis, tumour size > 80 mm, and incomplete resection {3604,228,3144,1367}.

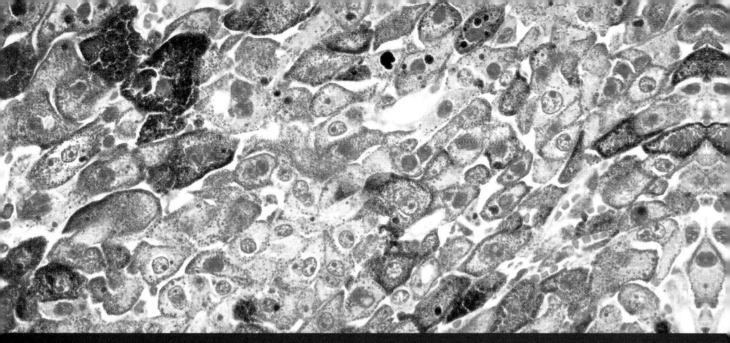

9

Melanocytic tumours

Edited by: Singh R, Wesseling P

Melanocytic tumours: Introduction

Wesseling P

Primary meningeal melanocytic tumours are rare, and they can be circumscribed or diffuse, and benign or malignant. Well-differentiated, circumscribed tumours are called meningeal melanocytomas; their malignant counterparts are meningeal melanomas. Meningeal melanocytomas with increased mitotic activity or invasion of the CNS parenchyma are considered inter-mediate-grade lesions. Diffuse meningeal melanocytic tumours are characterized by the involvement of large expanses of the subarachnoid space, with or without focal nodularity. Based on whether the lesion has a benign or malignant histological phenotype, it is called meningeal melanocytosis or meningeal melanomatosis, respectively {1772}.

Molecular analysis is often very helpful for corroborating the diagnosis of a primary meningeal melanocytic tumour. Analy-sis of GNAQ, GNA11, PLCB4, and CYSLTR2, as well as meth-ylation profiling, is especially useful for recognizing these neo-plasms as primary CNS tumours and discriminating them from other pigmented CNS tumours such as malignant melanotic nerve sheath tumours {1676,637,1774,1164,1007,1772}. The presence of an additional SF3B1, EIF1AX, or BAP1 mutation (BAP1 mutation leading to a loss of BAP1 protein expression on immunohistochemistry); of chromosome 3 monosomy; or of complex copy-number variations indicates aggressive behav-iour consistent with meningeal melanoma {3269}. In children, primary meningeal melanomas and meningeal melanocytosis and melanomatosis are often NRAS-mutant and occasionally BRAF-mutant {2233,1635,1637,2436,2791}.

The lack of large clinical studies with adequate patient follow-up has hindered definitive assessment of the correlation between histology, molecular features, and clinical behaviour. Meningeal melanomas are usually highly aggressive and radioresistant tumours with a poor prognosis, and they may cause extradural metastases. Still, the prognosis may be substantially better for patients with primary meningeal melanoma (particularly if com-plete resection of the primary tumour can be achieved) than for those with CNS metastasis of cutaneous melanoma {1772,983, 1007}. Meningeal melanocytosis may remain asymptomatic for a variable period of time, but once symptoms develop, the prog-nosis is usually poor; currently, the prognosis for NRAS-mutant meningeal melanoma and meningeal melanomatosis in children is very poor {2233,1635,1772}.

Of note, in the fourth edition of the WHO classification of skin tumours (2018), the taxonomy of cutaneous melanocytic neo-plasms is based, where possible, on different underlying evo-lutionary trajectories (pathways) associated with differences in genetics, clinical presentation, and/or histopathological features {830}. Perpendicular to this axis, another axis contains informa-tion on the recognizable progression stages of the respective neoplastic disorder. In this scheme, cutaneous melanocytomas are considered intermediate lesions because they have more pathogenic mutations than their fully benign counterparts, but fewer than the melanomas they can produce. It is not yet pos-sible to follow exactly the same approach for primary meningeal melanocytic tumours because of their rarity and the relative lack of data on their genetic evolution. Therefore, the term "melano-cytoma" as in (intermediate-grade) meningeal melanocytoma has somewhat different connotations from those of cutaneous melanocytomas.

Diffuse meningeal melanocytic neoplasms: Melanocytosis and melanomatosis

Gessi M
Bastian BC
Kölsche C
Küsters-Vandevelde HV
Reyes-Múgica M

Definition

Meningeal melanocytosis is a diffuse or multifocal meningeal proliferation of cytologically bland melanocytic cells that arises from leptomeningeal melanocytes. Meningeal melanomatosis is a diffuse or multifocal meningeal proliferation of melanoma cells that arises from leptomeningeal melanocytes and often shows CNS invasion.

ICD-O coding

8728/0 Meningeal melanocytosis
8728/3 Meningeal melanomatosis

ICD-11 coding

2A01.0Y & XH8974 Other specified meningeal tumours & Meningeal melanocytosis
2A01.0Y & XH1BP7 Other specified meningeal tumours & Meningeal melanomatosis

Related terminology

None

Subtype(s)

None

Localization

Meningeal melanocytosis and melanomatosis involve the leptomeninges, often extending into Virchow–Robin spaces. Meningeal melanomatosis frequently displays invasion of the CNS parenchyma. The lesions generally involve large expanses of the subarachnoid space, with focal or multifocal nodularity occasionally present. The sites of highest frequency include the temporal lobes, cerebellum, pons, medulla, and spinal cord {1523}.

Clinical features

Neurological symptoms associated with meningeal melanocytosis or melanomatosis arise secondarily to either hydrocephalus or local effects on the CNS parenchyma. Neuropsychiatric symptoms, bowel and bladder dysfunction, and sensory and motor disturbances are common. Once malignant transformation occurs, symptoms progress rapidly, with increasing intracranial pressure resulting in irritability, vomiting, lethargy, and seizures. Diffuse meningeal melanocytic tumours frequently occur in the setting of neurocutaneous melanosis, a syndrome that is further characterized by giant or numerous congenital melanocytic naevi of the skin that usually involve the trunk or the head and neck {1523}. About 10–15% of patients with large congenital melanocytic naevi of the skin develop clinical symptoms related to meningeal melanocytosis {720}, and radiological evidence of CNS involvement has been reported in as many as 23% of asymptomatic children with giant congenital naevi {965}. Other features are communicating hydrocephalus, arachnoid

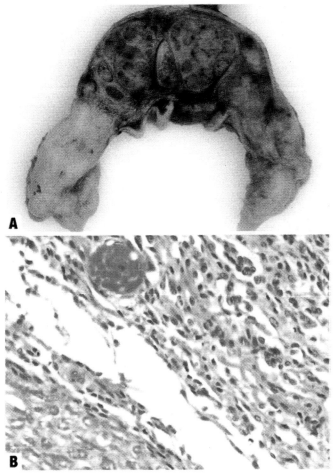

Fig. 9.01 Meningeal melanocytosis. **A** Autopsy findings in a child with meningeal melanocytosis. The meninges of the lower spinal cord appear diffusely packed with tumour tissue. The lesion harboured an *NRAS* p.Q61K mutation. **B** Melanocytic cells with benign features diffusely proliferate within the meninges between the nerve roots of the lower spinal cord.

cysts, syringomyelia, brain tumours (including astrocytoma, choroid plexus papilloma, ependymoma, and germinoma), and structural defects such as Dandy–Walker or Chiari malformations {2611}. The incidence of neurological involvement, melanoma, and death is significantly associated with the projected adult size of the largest congenital melanocytic naevus {1637}.

Imaging

CT and MRI of meningeal melanocytosis and melanomatosis typically show diffuse thickening and enhancement of the leptomeninges, often with focal or multifocal nodularity {2519}. Depending on melanin content, they may have a characteristic appearance on MRI due to the paramagnetic properties of melanin, resulting in an isodense or hyperintense signal on T1-weighted images and a hypointense signal on T2-weighted images {2959}.

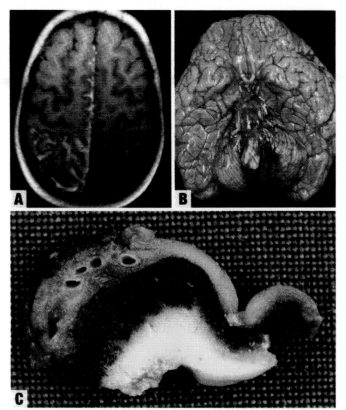

Fig. 9.02 Meningeal melanomatosis. **A** T1-weighted axial MRI revealing a hyperintense, contrast-enhancing lesion outlining the gyri and sulci in the left fronto-parieto-occipital region in a 5-year-old child. **B** Macroscopy of meningeal melanomatosis in a child with neurocutaneous melanosis who succumbed at the age of 17 months due to rapid disease progression. **C** Macroscopic appearance of the cerebral tissue shows brownish discolouration of the thickened leptomeninges and black discolouration of the underlying cerebral cortex.

Epidemiology

Diffuse meningeal melanocytic neoplasms are rare, so a population-based incidence is difficult to estimate. The incidence of neurocutaneous melanosis is reported as 0.5–2 cases per 100 000 person-years. Melanocytosis mainly affects children, mostly in the context of neurocutaneous melanosis, and it rarely occurs without cutaneous melanocytic lesions. Melanomatosis has a bimodal age distribution and may become manifest in children with or without neurocutaneous melanosis, as well as in adults (mostly in the fourth decade of life) {1772}.

Etiology

Diffuse meningeal melanocytic neoplasms associated with neurocutaneous melanosis derive from melanocyte precursor cells that reach the CNS after acquiring postzygotic somatic mutations, mostly of *NRAS* (chromosome 1p13) {1637,2436}. Diffuse melanocytosis may be associated with *BRAF* mutations in a minority of cases {2791}. Copy-number variations found in newly acquired or clinicoradiologically progressive diffuse meningeal melanocytic neoplasms show overlap with those described in cutaneous melanoma, even the in absence of malignant features at the histopathological level {1636,3281}.

Pathogenesis

Meningeal melanomatosis and melanocytosis are mostly associated with postzygotic somatic mutations in *NRAS*, which predispose to oncogenesis as a first hit in a multistep process {1637,2436}. *NRAS* is part of the family of RAS GTPases acting as a molecular switch that regulates the activation of the RAF/MEK/ERK and PI3K/AKT/mTOR pathways. *NRAS* mutations mainly occur at codon 61, the catalytic centre of the GTPase, and cause constitutive activation of *NRAS*, resulting in cell proliferation and growth {1772}. Amplification of the mutated *NRAS* gene has also been described in an aggressive form of neurocutaneous melanosis leading to CNS and widely disseminated congenital melanoma {2790}.

Macroscopic appearance

Dependent on melanin content, diffuse meningeal melanocytic neoplasms appear as dense black replacement of the subarachnoid space or as dusky clouding of the meninges.

Histopathology

The pathological proliferation of leptomeningeal melanocytes and their production of melanin account for the main microscopic findings in meningeal melanocytosis and melanomatosis. The tumour cells may assume a variety of shapes, including

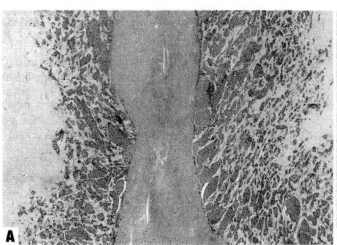
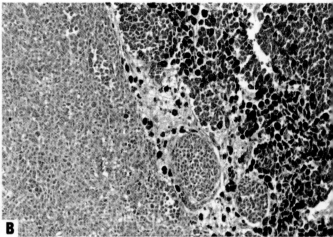

Fig. 9.03 Meningeal melanomatosis. **A** Malignant melanocytic cells diffusely infiltrate the underlying brain parenchyma. The tumour carries an *NRAS* p.Q61R mutation. **B** A subpopulation of melanoma cells are heavily pigmented.

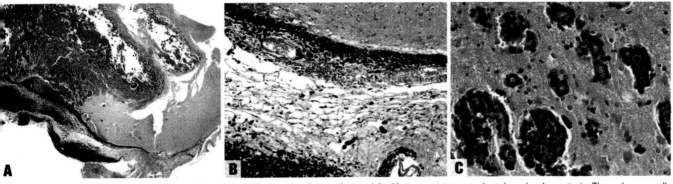

Fig. 9.04 Melanoma arising from meningeal melanocytosis. **A** Meningeal melanoma in an adult with neurocutaneous melanosis and melanocytosis. The melanoma cells infiltrate the surrounding brain tissue. **B** The areas with meningeal melanocytosis are heavily pigmented. **C** The meningeal melanoma infiltrates the brain around the small vessels.

spindled, round, oval, and cuboidal. In meningeal melanocytosis, individual cells are cytologically bland and accumulate within the subarachnoid and Virchow–Robin spaces. Lesions that histologically look like meningeal melanocytosis but show unequivocal invasion of the CNS parenchyma should be considered as meningeal melanomatosis {2959}. The presence of marked cytological atypia, mitotic activity, or necrosis also warrants a diagnosis of meningeal melanomatosis. Distinction from metastasis of cutaneous melanoma may be impossible using microscopy alone; additional molecular testing may help to solve this diagnostic problem {637}.

Cytology
Diagnostic cerebrospinal fluid cytology in patients with meningeal melanomatosis may reveal atypical cells that often have epithelioid features but immunocytochemically express melanocytic markers and may contain melanin pigment {1689}.

Diagnostic molecular pathology
See the *Diagnostic molecular pathology* subsection in *Circumscribed meningeal melanocytic neoplasms: Melanocytoma and melanoma* (p. 347). Mutation and DNA methylation profile analyses often help distinguish metastatic cutaneous melanoma from primary meningeal melanocytic tumours. In children, meningeal melanocytosis and meningeal melanomatosis are often associated with somatic mutations in *NRAS*.

Essential and desirable diagnostic criteria
See Box 9.01.

Box 9.01 Diagnostic criteria for diffuse meningeal melanocytic neoplasms

Essential:

Diffuse or multifocal primary meningeal melanocytic neoplasm

AND

- *For meningeal melanocytosis:* absence of CNS parenchyma invasion, absence of marked cytological atypia, absence of mitotic activity, and absence of necrosis
- *For meningeal melanomatosis:* invasion of the CNS parenchyma and/or marked cytological atypia and/or mitotic activity and/or necrosis

Desirable:

In children, meningeal melanocytosis/melanomatosis is often *NRAS*-mutant and rarely *BRAF*-mutant

Staging
Not relevant

Prognosis and prediction
Melanocytosis may remain asymptomatic for a variable period of time, but once symptoms develop the prognosis is usually poor {1772}. Melanomatosis is usually a very aggressive disease with a dismal prognosis {1635}. A particularly ominous complication in patients with ventriculoperitoneal shunting to relieve hydrocephalus is peritoneal melanomatosis {439}. Distinction of a primary (diffuse) meningeal melanocytic tumour from metastatic spread derived from an extradural (usually cutaneous) melanoma is critical for guiding prognostication and therapy.

Circumscribed meningeal melanocytic neoplasms: Melanocytoma and melanoma

Gessi M
Bastian BC
Kölsche C
Küsters-Vandevelde HV

Definition

Circumscribed meningeal melanocytic neoplasms are tumours that arise from leptomeningeal melanocytes and range histologically from well-differentiated tumours (meningeal melanocytoma) to frankly malignant neoplasms with aggressive growth properties (meningeal melanoma). Tumours with a bland histological appearance but increased mitotic activity or invasion of the CNS parenchyma have been defined as melanocytoma of intermediate grade.

ICD-O coding

8728/1 Meningeal melanocytoma
8720/3 Meningeal melanoma

ICD-11 coding

2A01.0Y & XH3DN1 Other specified meningeal tumours & Melanoma, meningeal

Related terminology

Not recommended: melanocytoma (without site); melanoma (without site).

Subtype(s)

None

Localization

Meningeal melanocytomas occur mostly in the cervical and thoracic spine. They can be dural based or associated with nerve roots or spinal foramina {359,1121}. Less frequently, they arise from the leptomeninges in the posterior fossa or supratentorial compartments. The trigeminal cave and cranial base is a site with a peculiar predilection for primary meningeal melanocytic neoplasms that are associated with ipsilateral naevus of Ota {1761,1129}. Rare cases of intraventricular

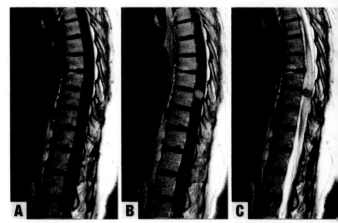

Fig. 9.05 Meningeal melanocytoma. **A** T1-weighted pre-contrast MRI reveals a slightly hyperintense lesion at the T8–T9 level of the spinal cord. **B** The lesion shows strong contrast enhancement (T1-weighted MRI). **C** On T2-weighted MRI, the lesion is hypointense.

or intramedullary localization have been reported {2183,1667}. Meningeal melanomas may occur throughout the neuraxis but, like melanocytomas, they show a predilection for the spinal canal and posterior fossa {1007,359}. A purely intraparenchymal location of a melanoma in the CNS is highly indicative of metastatic disease.

Clinical features

Patients with meningeal melanocytomas and melanomas present mostly with symptoms related to compression of the spinal cord, cerebellum, or cerebrum by an extra-axial mass with focal neurological signs depending on location {359,3516, 1917}. Distant metastasis from meningeal melanocytic tumours, mostly melanomas, are rare; they have been reported in liver, bone, and lungs {1772,1771}.

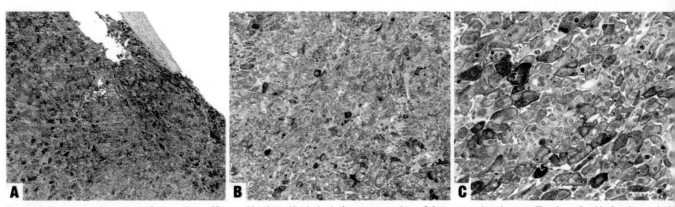

Fig. 9.06 Meningeal melanocytoma. A tumour from a 25-year-old patient with a lesion in the cavernous sinus. **A** Low-power view shows proliferating cells with abundant melanin pigment but no major atypia or necrosis. **B** A higher-power view from the same tumour. **C** High-power view of the same tumour shows an absence of malignant features in the proliferating pigmented cells. The cells have a low N:C ratio, small nuclei, and inconspicuous nucleoli.

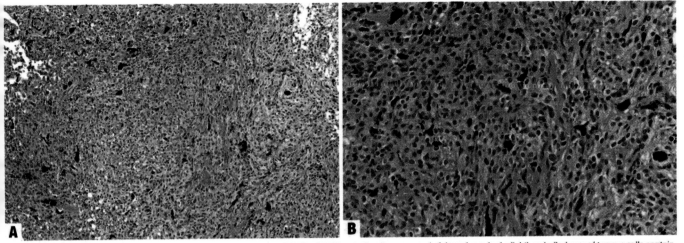

Fig. 9.07 Meningeal melanocytoma. **A** A melanocytoma, harbouring a *GNAQ* p.Q209L mutation, is composed of densely packed, slightly spindled or oval tumour cells containing variable melanin pigment. **B** The tumour does not show marked nuclear polymorphism.

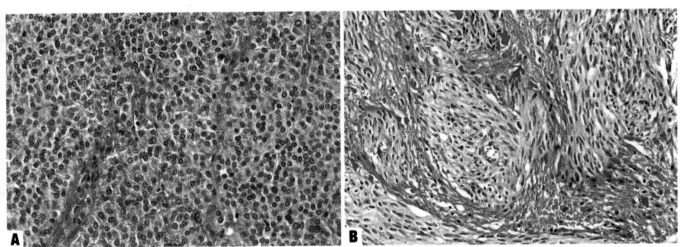

Fig. 9.08 Meningeal melanocytoma, intermediate grade. **A** This tumour, affecting the tentorium, is composed of rounded cells without marked nuclear polymorphism but with increased mitotic activity. The tumour carries *GNA11* and *EIF1AX* mutations. **B** This *GNAQ*-mutant tumour diffusely infiltrates CNS tissue of the filum terminale. The surrounding nervous tissue shows marked gliosis and Rosenthal fibres.

Imaging

Meningeal melanocytomas and melanomas are isoattenuating to hyperattenuating, contrast-enhancing on CT, with an imaging appearance similar to that of meningiomas but usually without hyperostosis or intratumoural calcification {2959}. On MRI, they often show T1 hyperintensity due to the paramagnetic properties of melanin pigment, and they are typically isointense to hypointense on T2-weighted images {2957}, hyperintense on FLAIR images, and they enhance after gadolinium {1917}. CNS structures adjacent to a meningeal melanoma are often T2-hyperintense as a result of vasogenic oedema generated in response to rapid tumour growth, which may be accompanied by invasion by tumour cells into the CNS parenchyma {637}.

Epidemiology

Meningeal melanocytomas and melanomas are rare, accounting for 0.06–0.1% of meningeal tumours. Melanocytomas have an estimated incidence of 1 case per 10 million person-years {2344,1917}. They can occur in patients of any age, but they are most frequent in the fourth and fifth decades of life. In

two relatively large series, the mean patient age at diagnosis of meningeal melanocytoma and melanoma was 45.6 years (range: 23–69 years) and 53.7 years (range: 15–86 years), respectively {1769,1164}. In other studies, the mean age at the time of diagnosis of meningeal melanoma was found to be 48.5 years for adults and 5.4 years (median: 3.0 years) for children {2000,2233}. For meningeal melanomas an annual incidence of 0.005 cases per 100 000 population has been reported {1917}.

Etiology

In most well-differentiated meningeal melanocytomas, copy-number variations are either absent or limited in number; when present, they usually affect a single whole chromosome or large parts of a single chromosome or a limited number of chromosomes {3268,1773}. The chromosomal alterations identified in melanocytoma may include gains of chromosome arms 8q and 6p, loss of chromosome arms 1p and 6q, and monosomy of chromosome 3 – this last alteration found in tumours with intermediate-grade histology {1164,1773}. Such alterations, including monosomy of chromosome 3, can be found in meningeal

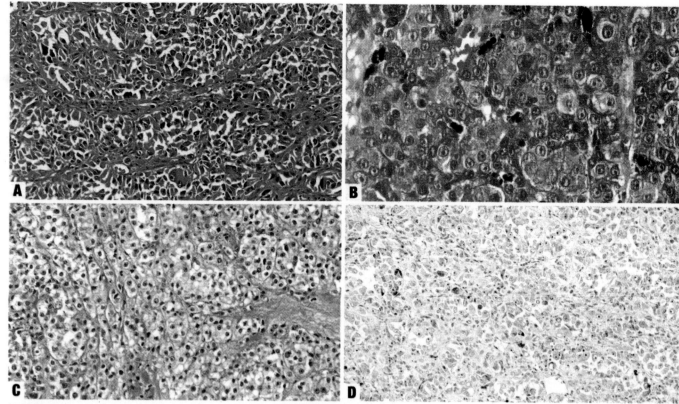

Fig. 9.09 Meningeal melanoma. **A** The tumour is composed of pleomorphic cells arranged in loose nests. **B** This *GNA11*-mutant meningeal melanoma shows a prominent epithelioid cytology and variable melanin content. **C** A nested architecture and epithelioid cytology characterize this spinal tumour. **D** The tumour shows loss of BAP1 expression immunohistochemically, corresponding at the molecular level to a *BAP1* p.Q267 frameshift mutation.

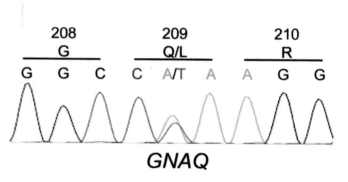

Fig. 9.10 Meningeal melanocytoma. Detection of a *GNAQ* p.Q209L mutation by Sanger sequencing.

melanomas as well, but (like cutaneous and uveal melanomas) meningeal melanomas usually have a more complex copy-number variation profile, with multiple large chromosomal gains and/or losses {1773,1164}.

Meningeal melanocytomas and melanomas harbour mutually exclusive activating hotspot mutations in *GNAQ*, *GNA11*, *PLCB4*, or *CYSLTR2*. *GNAQ* and *GNA11* mutations are most frequent, observed in about 60–70% of cases {1770,2176, 1164,3268,3271}. Usually, meningeal melanocytomas and melanomas do not harbour *HRAS*, *KRAS*, *BRAF*, or *KIT* mutations {1770,1676,3370,1071}. *TERT* promoter mutations are also usually absent {1075}. Meningeal melanocytomas of

intermediate grade and meningeal melanomas may carry an additional *EIF1AX*, *SF3B1*, or *BAP1* mutation, again in a mutually exclusive pattern and with a higher incidence reported in melanomas {1769,1164,3268}. Childhood meningeal melanomas in patients with neurocutaneous melanosis typically harbour *NRAS* mutations {2436,1637}.

Pathogenesis
Mutually exclusive mutations in *GNAQ*, *GNA11*, *PLCB4*, and *CYSLTR2* are considered the first step in oncogenesis of meningeal melanocytic tumours not associated with neurocutaneous melanosis. The glutamine at codon 209 or arginine at codon 183 of *GNAQ* and *GNA11* is essential for GTP hydrolysis, and mutations at these codons impair GTPase activity, leading to constitutive activation of downstream intracellular pathways including the RAF/MEK/ERK and Hippo/YAP1 signalling pathways that regulate cell growth and proliferation {212,1772}. Like in uveal melanomas, mutation in *EIF1AX*, *SF3B1*, or *BAP1* is considered to represent a next step in the oncogenic process {2397,212}. *EIF1AX* and *SF3B1* encode eukaryotic translation initiation factor 1A (EIF1A) and splicing factor 3b subunit 1 (SF3B1), respectively, but their role in the oncogenesis of meningeal melanocytic tumours is not yet fully understood. *BAP1* is a well-characterized tumour suppressor gene. Carriers of germline *BAP1* mutations are at risk of developing cutaneous, uveal, and meningeal melanomas, as well as mesotheliomas, clear cell renal cancer, and various other tumour types {708}. *BAP1* (chromosome 3p21.1) encodes a nuclear ubiquitin hydrolase with multiple nuclear and cytoplasmic substrates, regulating DNA repair, transcription,

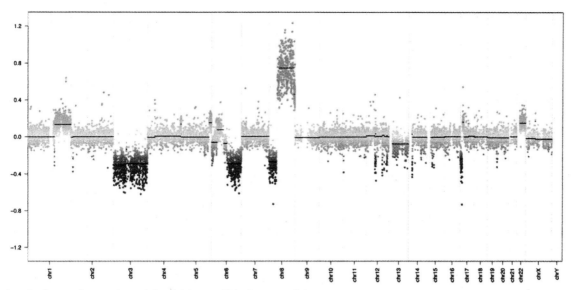

Fig. 9.11 Meningeal melanoma. Copy-number variation plot shows multiple chromosomal changes.

and cell death. Loss-of-function hemizygous mutations combined with chromosome 3 monosomy result in decreased or absent BAP1 protein expression.

Macroscopic appearance
Meningeal melanocytomas and melanomas are circumscribed mass lesions that may be black, reddish-brown, blue, or macroscopically non-pigmented, depending on the melanin content.

Histopathology
Circumscribed meningeal melanocytic tumours show a spectrum of histopathological features, ranging from bland-appearing, low-grade, well-differentiated melanocytomas to overtly malignant melanomas. Usually, all meningeal melanocytic tumours strongly express S100, vimentin, melan-A (MART1), HMB45, and MITF {3516}. Well-differentiated melanocytomas may show variable (sometimes high) cell density and are usually composed of densely packed, slightly spindled or oval tumour cells containing variable (at times abundant) melanin. The tumour cells may form tight nests with a superficial resemblance to the whorls of meningioma. Heavily pigmented tumour cells and intratumoural macrophages are especially seen at the periphery of nests. Other melanocytomas may show storiform, vasocentric, or sheet-like arrangements. Only rare amelanotic melanocytomas have been described. The nuclei are oval or bean-shaped, occasionally showing grooves, with small eosinophilic nucleoli. Cytological atypia, necrosis, and mitoses are generally absent (on average < 0.5 mitoses/mm², equating to < 1 mitosis/10 HPF of 0.5 mm in diameter and 0.2 mm² in area). Melanocytomas generally do not show invasion of CNS parenchyma {359,1772,3370}.

Based on data from a relatively large study, meningeal melanocytic tumours with the histology of melanocytoma but showing CNS invasion or increased mitotic activity (0.5–1.5 mitoses/mm², equating to 1–3 mitoses/10 HPF of 0.5 mm in diameter and 0.2 mm² in area) have been defined as intermediate-grade melanocytic neoplasms {359}.

Melanomas are more pleomorphic and mitotically active, and they may have a high cell density. In addition, meningeal melanomas often demonstrate unequivocal invasion of the CNS parenchyma or coagulative necrosis. They may be composed of pleomorphic spindled or epithelioid cells (arranged in loose nests, fascicles, or sheets) and display variable cytoplasmic melanin {359,1007}. Some meningeal melanomas contain large cells with bizarre nuclei, numerous (typical and atypical) mitotic figures, and large nucleoli; others are highly cellular and less pleomorphic, usually consisting of smaller, tightly packed spindle cells with a high N:C ratio. Meningeal melanomatosis may arise from diffuse spreading of a primary meningeal melanoma through the subarachnoid space.

Cytology
In patients with meningeal melanoma, cytological examination of cerebrospinal fluid may show atypical or frankly malignant cells, often with epithelioid cytology and containing melanin pigment.

Diagnostic molecular pathology
Mutation analysis (including for *GNAQ*, *GNA11*, *PLCB4*, and *CYSLTR2*) and methylation profiling are useful for recognizing meningeal melanocytic tumours as primary CNS tumours and discriminating them from other pigmented CNS tumours such as malignant melanotic nerve sheath tumours {1676,637, 1774}. Primary meningeal melanomas in adults are rare, and when encountered, they raise suspicion of metastatic disease. In adults, the identification *BRAF*, *NRAS*, or *TERT* promoter mutations help differentiate a cutaneous melanoma metastasis from a primary meningeal melanoma. Conversely, the presence of *GNAQ* or *GNA11* mutation in the absence of a uveal melanoma or a blue naevus–like melanoma strongly favours a primary meningeal tumour. Combining mutation, copy-number, and DNA methylation profiles has been described as a method of further distinguishing cutaneous melanoma metastases from other melanocytic tumours {1676,1164,1007}.

Essential and desirable diagnostic criteria

See Box 9.02.

Staging

Not relevant

Prognosis and prediction

The clinical behaviour of circumscribed meningeal melanocytic tumours correlates with histopathological features. However, the lack of large clinical studies with adequate patient follow-up has hindered definitive assessment of the correlation between histology, molecular features, and clinical behaviour, in particular for melanocytomas of intermediate grade. Although melanocytomas lack anaplastic features, in some patients local recurrence or leptomeningeal seeding occurs; intermediate-grade melanocytic tumours seem to be more recurrence prone. Malignant transformation of a melanocytoma and metastatic spread outside the CNS have been reported {2729,1771,1684}. Some meningeal melanocytic tumours (not necessarily associated with worrisome histology) harbour *EIF1AX*, *SF3B1*, and *BAP1* mutations and show aggressive clinical behaviour {1769,3268}. Therefore, the diagnosis of a meningeal melanoma should be considered in the presence of additional *EIF1AX*, *SF3B1*, or *BAP1* mutations (*BAP1* mutations leading to a loss of BAP1 protein expression at the immunohistochemical level); chromosome 3 monosomy; or complex copy-number variations {3269}. Meningeal melanoma is usually a highly aggressive and radioresistant tumour with a poor

prognosis, and it can rarely metastasize to distant organs {1772}. Nevertheless, the prognosis tends to be better for patients with primary meningeal melanoma (particularly if complete resection of the primary tumour can be achieved) than for patients with CNS metastasis of cutaneous melanoma {983,1007}. Currently, the prognosis for *NRAS*-mutant meningeal melanoma in children is very poor {2233,1635}.

Box 9.02 Diagnostic criteria for circumscribed meningeal melanocytic neoplasms

Essential:

Circumscribed/localized primary melanocytic neoplasm in the meninges

AND

- *For melanocytoma:* limited cytological atypia, (almost) no mitoses, no necrosis, and (in cases of evaluable CNS parenchyma) no CNS invasion
- *For intermediate-grade melanocytoma:* mitotic count[a] of 0.5–1.5 mitoses/mm^2 and/or CNS invasion, but limited cytological atypia and no necrosis
- *For melanoma:* mitotic count[a] > 1.5 mitoses/mm^2 and/or necrosis, often accompanied by marked cytological atypia

Desirable:

Demonstration of *GNAQ*, *GNA11*, *PLCB4*, or *CYSLTR2* mutation corroborates the CNS origin of the neoplasm, especially after exclusion of uveal or blue naevus–like melanoma

Additional molecular markers (*SF3B1*, *EIF1AX*, and *BAP1* mutations; chromosome 3 monosomy; complex copy-number variations) indicating aggressive behaviour

[a] 1 mm^2 equates approximately to 5 HPF of 0.5 mm in diameter and 0.2 mm^2 in area.

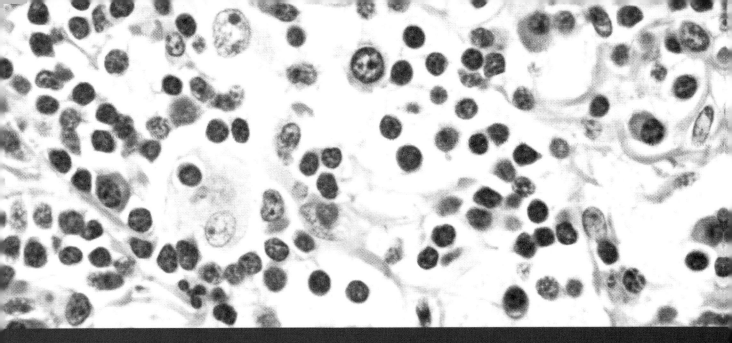

10

Haematolymphoid tumours involving the CNS

Edited by: Chan JKC, Reifenberger G, Soffietti R

Lymphomas
    Primary diffuse large B-cell lymphoma of the CNS
    Immunodeficiency-associated CNS lymphomas
    Lymphomatoid granulomatosis
    Intravascular large B-cell lymphoma
    MALT lymphoma of the dura
    Other low-grade B-cell lymphomas of the CNS
    Anaplastic large cell lymphoma (ALK+/ALK−)
    T-cell and NK/T-cell lymphomas
Histiocytic tumours
    Erdheim–Chester disease
    Rosai–Dorfman disease
    Juvenile xanthogranuloma
    Langerhans cell histiocytosis
    Histiocytic sarcoma

Haematolymphoid tumours involving the CNS: Introduction

Soffietti R

The following sections cover lymphomas and histiocytic tumours that may occur as solitary or multifocal CNS lesions in primary intraparenchymal and meningeal localizations. Virtually all of these tumour types may also manifest in other organs. Therefore, primary CNS manifestation needs to be distinguished from secondary manifestation in the CNS, i.e. metastases from systemic lesions. The way the different tumour types are presented here follows the revised fourth-edition volume of the WHO classification of CNS tumours, with the sections on less common CNS lymphoma types being slightly expanded. Of the primary CNS lymphomas, diffuse large B-cell lymphoma of the CNS (CNS-DLBCL), previously called "primary CNS lymphoma", is the most common tumour type encountered. There has long been only modest insight into the pathogenesis of CNS-DLBCL, mainly because of limited tissue availability (because most patients undergo stereotactic biopsy rather than surgical resection), and a lack of correlations between histological or molecular data and clinical outcomes. Large-scale genomic investigations have characterized the mutation profile and identified relevant genetic drivers in these tumours. In particular, the B-cell receptor, toll-like receptor, and NF-κB pathways are frequently activated by recurrent mutations; in addition, genes involved in chromatin structure and modification, cell-cycle regulation, and immune recognition are commonly altered {2153,2150,2154,2205,349,3298}. Among these various genetic changes, *MYD88* and *CD79B* mutations are of potential clinical interest because they are frequent and may be detected in several body fluids (plasma, cerebrospinal fluid, vitreous fluid). Liquid biopsy–based detection of these mutations may assist disease monitoring under treatment {1305,2149,1306,1265}, although their detection in blood (for non-invasive initial diagnosis) has not been proved to be a reliable approach {2149}. Genetically activated pathways in CNS-DLBCL can be targeted by small molecules such as ibrutinib {1169,1908}, and the immune microenvironment may be modulated by drugs such as lenalidomide and pomalidomide {2146,1406}. An increase in the mutation burden, the presence of translocations involving the *CD274* (*PD-L1*) and *PDCD1LG2* (*PD-L2*) loci in a subset of tumours {53}, and the expression of immune response biomarkers {2350} suggest a potential susceptibility of CNS-DLBCL to immune checkpoint inhibitors, but clinical evidence of this is still limited {2220,1406}.

Other lymphoid neoplasms (including various types of low-grade B-cell lymphomas, as well as T-cell and NK/T-cell lymphomas) rarely arise primarily in the CNS and may therefore pose problems in differential diagnosis. Lymphomatoid granulomatosis is part of a group of EBV-associated B-cell lymphoproliferative disorders that also includes other immunodeficiency-associated lymphomas. Because the histological features may overlap, the clinical context is critical {2064}. Intravascular large B-cell lymphoma {524} may obstruct small and medium-sized vessels in the brain and thereby typically induces progressive neurocognitive deterioration (mimicking dementias) or acute neurological deficits (mimicking cerebrovascular diseases), with a stroke-like appearance on MRI. Primary MALT lymphoma of the dura is a rare lymphoma type that clinically and radiologically may be mistaken for meningioma and has a similarly good outcome after local treatment {1564}.

Despite impressive advances in our understanding of the etiology and pathogenesis of primary CNS lymphomas, in particular for CNS-DLBCL, the mainstay of their diagnostic assessment remains tissue-based classification using histological and immunohistochemical analysis of biopsy specimens. Molecular pathology investigations, such as the demonstration of a clonal proliferation of B cells or (rarely) T cells, are occasionally helpful as adjunct methods, for example to distinguish neoplastic from inflammatory lymphoid infiltrates. In addition, in individual cases, molecular testing may provide helpful information by detecting diagnostically relevant translocations / gene fusions (e.g. by FISH) or an underlying EBV infection (e.g. by in situ hybridization). The importance of avoiding corticosteroid administration before tissue biopsy in the diagnostic assessment of CNS lymphomas has long been recognized. Highly potent corticosteroids like dexamethasone may induce rapid tumour waning, impeding histological diagnosis in as many as 50% of cases {389}.

Histiocytic neoplasms may represent a clinical challenge because of their rarity, broad clinical spectrum (often mimicking non-neoplastic conditions), and varied histology {264}. For instance, Erdheim–Chester disease of the CNS, which preferentially occurs in middle-aged adults, can be clinically mistaken for various other diseases, such as multiple sclerosis, neurosarcoidosis, CNS vasculitis, IgG4-related disease, and others. In addition to focal neurological deficits due to tumour-like masses, a peculiar clinical finding across several histiocytoses (in as many as 30–50% of patients) is cognitive impairment associated with brain and cerebellar atrophy and neurodegenerative lesions, whose pathophysiology is still unknown. Comprehensive histological and immunohistochemical assessment, complemented by molecular characterization such as mutation analysis for *BRAF* p.V600E and other MAPK pathway gene alterations, is therefore of utmost importance for confirming the diagnosis and guiding targeted treatment {753, 755,1155,2707}. In addition to the common types of histiocytic tumours addressed in the individual sections of this chapter, ALK-positive histiocytosis has been identified as a novel type of systemic histiocytic proliferative disorder that predominantly occurs in young children and is driven by *ALK* fusions, most commonly *KIF5B::ALK* {513,520}. Rare cases of ALK-positive histiocytosis with exclusive involvement of the CNS have been reported {1952}, underlining the importance of a thorough molecular workup of CNS histiocytoses for diagnostic purposes and for targeted therapy.

Primary diffuse large B-cell lymphoma of the CNS

Deckert M   Nagane M
Batchelor T   Paulus W
Ferry JA   Weller M
Hoang-Xuan K

Definition
Diffuse large B-cell lymphoma of the CNS (CNS-DLBCL) is a DLBCL confined to the CNS at presentation. Its cytological features, and many of its molecular features, correspond to those of its systemic counterparts.

ICD-O coding
9680/3 Primary diffuse large B-cell lymphoma of the CNS

ICD-11 coding
2A81.5 Primary diffuse large B-cell lymphoma of central nervous system

Related terminology
Acceptable: primary central nervous system lymphoma.

Subtype(s)
None

Localization
Primary CNS-DLBLCs are solitary brain lesions in 65% of cases, with the remaining cases being multifocal lesions. Tumours are mainly located in the cerebral hemispheres (38%), thalamus and basal ganglia (16%), corpus callosum (14%), periventricular region (12%), or cerebellum (9%) {1755, 350}. The leptomeninges may be involved, but exclusive meningeal involvement is unusual. Ocular manifestation (i.e. in the vitreous, retina, or optic nerve) occurs in as many as 20% of patients and may antedate intracranial disease {1444}. Isolated spinal cord involvement occurs in < 1% of cases. Extraneural dissemination is rare. In cases with systemic spread, CNS-DLBCL has a propensity to home to the testis, an immunoprivileged organ {322,1445}.

Clinical features
Patients present with cognitive dysfunction, psychomotor slowing, and focal neurological symptoms more frequently than with headache, seizures, and cranial nerve palsies. Blurred vision and eye floaters are symptoms of ocular involvement {213,1709, 2446}.

MRI is the most sensitive technique for detecting CNS-DLBCL. Lesions are hypointense on T1-weighted images, isointense to hyperintense on T2-weighted images, densely enhancing on postcontrast images, and may manifest restricted diffusion on diffusion-weighted images. Peritumoural oedema is relatively limited, and it is less severe than in malignant gliomas and brain metastases {1709}. Meningeal involvement may manifest as hyperintense enhancement {1755}. With steroid therapy, lesions may vanish within hours {719}.

Biopsy is the gold standard for establishing the diagnosis and classification of CNS-DLBCL. It is important to withhold corticosteroids before biopsy because they induce rapid tumour

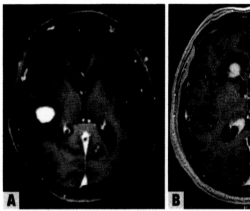

Fig. 10.01 Primary diffuse large B-cell lymphoma of the CNS. **A** Single homogeneously enhancing lesion on postcontrast T1-weighted axial MRI. **B** Multiple enhancing lesions with periventricular and subependymal location on postcontrast T1-weighted axial MRI.

waning. Corticosteroids have been shown to prevent diagnosis in as many as 50% of cases {389}.

Epidemiology
Primary CNS-DLBCL accounts for 2.4–3% of all brain tumours and 4–6% of all extranodal lymphomas {2847}. The overall annual incidence rate is 0.47 cases per 100 000 population {3327}. The incidence in patients aged > 60 years has been reported to have increased over the past two decades {3327}. CNS-DLBCL can affect patients of any age, with a peak incidence during the fifth to seventh decades of life. The median patient age is 66 years, and the M:F ratio is 3:2 {2347}.

Etiology
In immunocompetent individuals, etiological factors are unknown. There is no evidence that viruses such as EBV, HHV6 {2429}, HHV8 {2151}, and the polyomaviruses SV40 and BK virus {2148,2178} play a role.

Genetic susceptibility
In immunocompetent individuals, genetic predispositions to CNS-DLBCL have not been described. About 8% of patients have had a prior extracranial tumour {2652}, most of which arose in the haematopoietic system. In patients with CNS-DLBCL and preceding extraneural lymphoma, comparative molecular analyses of primary and secondary lymphomas may confirm or exclude a common clonal origin of these tumours, distinguishing CNS relapse from an unrelated secondary cerebral lymphoma. In individual patients, associations between CNS-DLBCL and other tumours (e.g. carcinoma, meningioma, and glioma) or hereditary tumour syndromes (e.g. neurofibromatosis type 1) are likely to be coincidental. Folate and methionine metabolism have been proposed to be relevant to CNS-DLBCL

susceptibility. The G allele of the *MTR*:c.2756A>G p.D919G missense polymorphism was found to be underrepresented among patients with CNS-DLBCL, suggesting that this allele has a protective function {1907}.

Pathogenesis

Tumour cells correspond to mature, late germinal-centre exit B cells derived from self-reactive/polyreactive precursor cells, which have escaped elimination, possibly fostered by early acquisition of *MYD88* mutations. During a dysregulated germinal-centre reaction, the tumour cells have increased self-reactivity/polyreactivity, allowing the tumour cell B-cell receptor to bind to multiple CNS antigens {2156}, which may, in part, underlie the affinity and confinement of these lymphoma cells to the CNS microenvironment. Tumour cells carry rearranged and somatically mutated IG genes with evidence of ongoing somatic hypermutation {2152,2445,3189}. Consistent with the ongoing germinal-centre programme, they show persistent BCL6 activity {392,2152,3189,2156}. The process of somatic hypermutation is not confined to its physiological targets (IG genes and *BCL6*) but extends to other genes that have been implicated in tumorigenesis, including *BCL2, MYC, PIM1, PAX5, RHOH, KLHL14, OSBPL10,* and *SUSD2* {393,2157,3298}. These data indicate that aberrant somatic hypermutation has a major impact on the pathogenesis of CNS-DLBCL. The fixed IgM/IgD phenotype of the tumour cells is in part due to miscarried IG class-switch rearrangements during which the Sμ region is deleted {2155}. *PRDM1* mutations also contribute to impaired IG class-switch recombination {645}.

Translocations affect the IG genes (in 38% of cases), *BCL6* (in 17–47%), and *ETV6* {2158,434,394} recurrently, whereas *MYC* translocations are rare and translocations of the *BCL2* gene are absent {392,434,2158}. FISH and genome-wide SNP analyses have shown recurrent gains of genetic material, most frequently affecting 18q21-q23 (in 43% of cases), which includes the *BCL2* and *MALT1* genes; chromosome 12 (in 26%); and 10q23.21 (in 21%) {2872}. Losses of genetic material most frequently involve chromosome bands 6q21 (in 52% of cases), 6p21 (in 37%), 8q12.1-q12.2 (in 32%), and 10q23.21 {2872}. *CDKN2A* gene deletions are recurrent {613,349}. Heterozygous or homozygous loss or partial uniparental disomies of chromosomal region 6p21.32 affect 73% of CNS-DLBCLs; this region harbours the HLA class II–encoding HLA-DRB, HLA-DQA, and HLA-DQB genes {1499,2674,2872}. Correspondingly, 55% and 46% of CNS-DLBCLs show loss of expression of HLA class I and class II gene products, respectively {322}.

Several important pathways (i.e. the B-cell receptor, toll-like receptor, and NF-κB pathways) are frequently activated due to genetic alterations affecting the genes *CD79B* (in 20–83% of cases), *INPP5D* (in 25%), *CBL* (in 4%), *BLNK* (in 4%), *CARD11* (in 16%), *MALT1* (in 43%), *BCL2* (in 43%), and *MYD88* (in > 50%), which may foster proliferation and prevent apoptosis {1136,1732, 2150,2154,2153,2872,2205,2223}. Epigenetic changes may also contribute to pathogenesis, including epigenetic silencing by DNA methylation. DNA hypermethylation of *DAPK1* (in 84% of cases), *CDKN2A* (in 75%), *MGMT* (in 52%), and RFC genes (in 30%) may be of potential therapeutic relevance {594,613, 915,2872}. However, the DNA methylome does not unequivocally distinguish primary CNS-DLBCL from non-CNS DLBCL {3341}.

Macroscopic appearance

CNS-DLBCLs occur as single or multiple masses in the brain parenchyma, most frequently in the cerebral hemispheres. Often, they are deep-seated and adjacent to the ventricular system. The tumours are firm, friable, granular, haemorrhagic, and greyish-tan or yellow, with central necrosis. They can also be virtually indistinguishable from the adjacent neuropil. Demarcation from surrounding parenchyma is variable. Some tumours appear well delineated, like carcinoma metastases. When diffuse borders and architectural effacement are present, the lesions may resemble gliomas. Meningeal involvement may resemble meningitis or meningioma, or it may be inconspicuous macroscopically.

Histopathology

CNS-DLBCLs are highly cellular, diffusely growing, patternless tumours. Centrally, large areas of geographical necrosis are common. Necrotic zones may harbour viable perivascular lymphoma islands. At the periphery, an angiocentric infiltration pattern is frequent. Infiltration of cerebral blood vessels causes splitting of their argyrophilic fibre network. From these perivascular cuffs, tumour cells invade the CNS parenchyma, either with a well-delineated invasion front with small clusters, or with single tumour cells diffusely infiltrating the tissue. Cytologically, CNS-DLBCLs consist of large atypical cells with large round, oval, irregular, or pleomorphic nuclei and distinct nucleoli, corresponding to centroblasts or immunoblasts. Mitotic activity is brisk. Tumour cells are intermingled with reactive inflammatory infiltrates consisting of mature, small T and B lymphocytes. CD3-positive T cells predominantly correspond to CD8-positive cytotoxic T cells {2536,2008}, which characteristically accumulate between tumour cells and vessel walls {2536}. Intermingled with the tumour cells are reactive GFAP-positive astrocytes; prominently activated CD45med (leukocyte common antigen), CD68+, HLA-DR+ microglia; and macrophages.

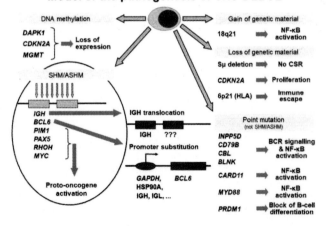

Fig. 10.02 Primary diffuse large B-cell lymphoma of the CNS (CNS-DLBCL). Alterations of specific pathways contributing to the pathogenesis of primary CNS-DLBCL. ASHM, aberrant somatic hypermutation; BCR, B-cell receptor; CSR, class-switch recombination; SHM, somatic hypermutation.

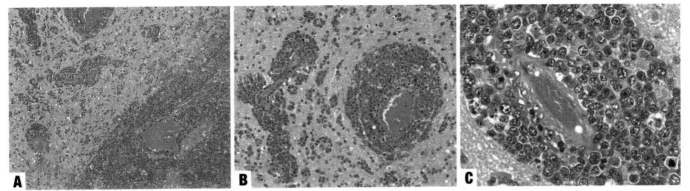

Fig. 10.03 Primary diffuse large B-cell lymphoma of the CNS. **A** The lymphoma cells form dense sheets (right) and show the characteristic perivascular spread (left). **B** The lymphoma cells infiltrate around blood vessels (left) and also into their walls (right). **C** The lymphoma cells are large, with vesicular nuclei, prominent nucleoli, and amphophilic cytoplasm.

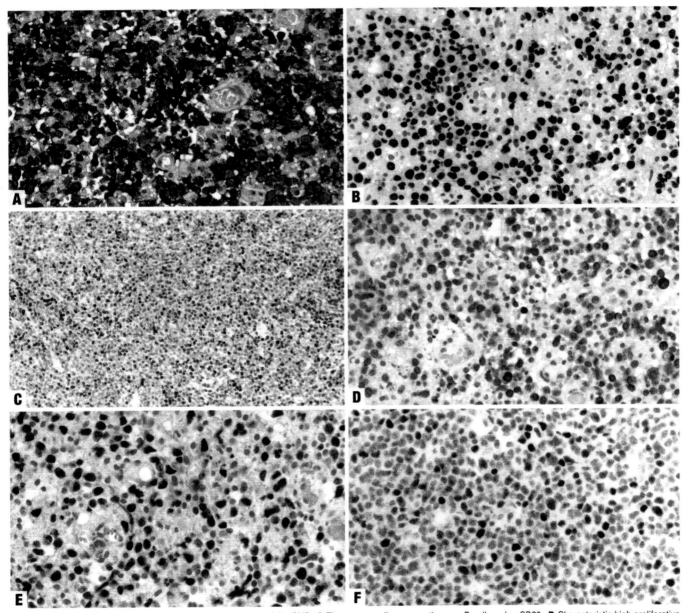

Fig. 10.04 Immunophenotype of diffuse large B-cell lymphoma of the CNS. **A** The tumour cells express the pan–B-cell marker CD20. **B** Characteristic high proliferative activity evidenced by nuclear Ki-67 expression in the majority of tumour cells. **C** Strong nuclear expression of MYC protein in the majority of the tumour cells in the absence of a *MYC* rearrangement. **D** Expression of BCL2. **E** Strong nuclear staining of the tumour cells for IRF4 (MUM1). **F** The majority of the tumour cells show nuclear expression of BCL6.

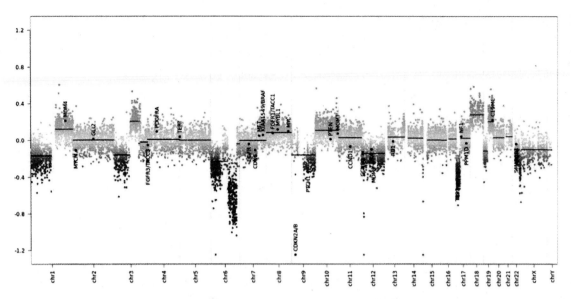

Fig. 10.05 Diffuse large B-cell lymphoma of the CNS. Copy-number profile. Note losses of chromosome arm 6q and homozygous deletion of *CDKN2A* on chromosome arm 9p, among other copy-number variations. The tumour also carried mutations in *MYD88* and *CD79B*, determined by next-generation sequencing (not shown).

Immunophenotype

The tumour cells are mature B cells that are immunohistochemically positive for PAX5, CD19, CD20, CD22, and CD79a. IgM and IgD, but not IgG, are expressed on the surface of tumour cells {2155}, with either kappa or lambda light chain restriction. Most cells express BCL6 (60–80%) and IRF4 (MUM1) (90%), whereas plasma cell markers (e.g. CD38 and CD138) are negative. Fewer than 10% of all CNS-DLBCLs express CD10 {718}, whereas CD10 expression is more frequent in systemic DLBCL; therefore, CD10 positivity in a CNS lymphoma with DLBCL characteristics should prompt a thorough investigation for systemic DLBCL that might have spread to the CNS. HLA-A, HLA-B, HLA-C, and HLA-DR are variably expressed, with approximately 50% of CNS-DLBCLs showing a loss of HLA class I and/or class II expression {322,2675}. BCL2 expression is common: 82% of CNS-DLBCLs have a BCL2high, MYChigh phenotype {392}. The Ki-67 proliferation index is usually > 70% or even > 90% {392}. Apoptotic cells may be frequent. Only isolated cases show evidence of EBV infection {2152}, and the presence of EBV should prompt evaluation for underlying immunodeficiency.

Corticoid-mitigated lymphoma

Because the tumour cells are highly susceptible to steroid-induced apoptosis, CNS-DLBCL may vanish rapidly after corticosteroid treatment. Microscopically, neoplastic B cells may then be present in only small numbers (or they may even be absent), and apoptotic debris may be abundant. Tissue samples may show only nonspecific inflammatory and reactive changes and/or necrosis; foamy macrophages are particularly frequent {389,718}. High numbers of large T cells with Ki-67 expression indicative of prominent activation may dominate, raising the possibility of T-cell lymphoma as a differential diagnosis. In some cases, PCR analysis of the CDR3 region of the IGH gene may reveal a monoclonal B-cell population. However, pseudoclonality due to very low numbers of B cells poses a problem.

Sentinel lesions

In rare cases, CNS-DLBCL has been reported to be preceded (for as long as 2 years) by demyelinating and inflammatory lesions similar to those occurring in multiple sclerosis {63,1386, 1753}.

Cytology

Smear preparations performed in the intraoperative setting show enlarged, highly atypical neoplastic cells that are discohesive and have minimal detectable cytoplasm, which can be useful in distinguishing CNS-DLBCL from metastatic neoplasms and high-grade gliomas. Anaplastic nuclear features, apoptosis, and mitotic activity are typical. Intraoperative smear is a useful technique for increasing diagnostic security in tiny serial stereotactic biopsies to identify blasts {899}. Final diagnosis requires further tumour cell characterization including immunophenotyping.

The diagnostic value of cerebrospinal fluid cytology is limited {1709}. Meningeal dissemination is diagnosed in 15.7% of cases (of which 12.2% are diagnosed by cerebrospinal fluid cytomorphology, 10.5% by PCR, and 4.1% by MRI) {1710}. Pleocytosis is found in 35–60% of cases and correlates with meningeal dissemination {1710}. Cell counts may even be normal. The cerebrospinal fluid harbours neoplastic cells in a minority of patients with leptomeningeal involvement, and their detection may require repeated lumbar puncture. The combination of cytological and immunohistochemical analyses with multiparameter flow cytometry may facilitate the detection of cerebrospinal fluid lymphoma cells {2858}. PCR analysis of the CDR3 region of the IGH gene followed by sequencing of the PCR products may identify a clonal B-cell population in the cerebrospinal fluid, but it does not enable lymphoma classification. Elevated cerebrospinal fluid levels of several microRNAs (miR-21, miR-19, miR-92a, miR-30) {196} and of CXCL13 plus IL-10 {2742} have been reported to distinguish CNS-DLBCL from inflammatory and other CNS disorders

{197}. Cumulative data suggest that pretherapeutic and post-treatment IL-10 levels in the cerebrospinal fluid have prognostic value {2246,2813}.

Diagnostic molecular pathology
PCR demonstrates clonal rearrangement of IG genes with the introduction of somatic mutations.

Essential and desirable diagnostic criteria
See Box 10.01.

Staging
Staging at diagnosis includes CT of thorax and abdomen as well as bone marrow analysis to exclude systemic lymphoma.

Prognosis and prediction
CNS-DLBCL has a worse outcome than does systemic DLBCL. However, a minority of younger patients may be cured. Older patient age (> 65 years) is a major negative prognostic factor and is associated with reduced survival and an increased risk of neurotoxicity {13,1709}. High-dose methotrexate-based polychemotherapy is currently the induction therapy of choice {1709}. The inclusion of consolidative whole-brain irradiation may improve progression-free survival, but it does not improve overall survival (OS) {3172}; moreover, it increases the risk of neurotoxicity resulting in cognitive dysfunction, especially in patients aged > 60 years {13}. In eligible patients with CNS-DLBCL, consolidative high-dose chemotherapy and autologous stem cell transplantation after methotrexate-based polychemotherapy is associated with prolonged survival and with maintenance of or improvement in cognitive outcomes and quality of life. At recurrence, there is no standard approach and prognosis is poor.

Box 10.01 Diagnostic criteria for primary diffuse large B-cell lymphoma of the CNS (CNS-DLBCL)

Essential:

Biopsy-proven mature large B-cell lymphoma confined to the CNS at presentation

AND

Expression of one or more B-cell markers (CD20, CD19, CD22, CD79a, PAX5)

Desirable:

Immunohistochemical phenotype of late germinal-centre exit B cells (IRF4 [MUM1]+, BCL6+/−, CD10−); CD10 expression does not exclude the diagnosis, but it is uncommon and indicates possible systemic DLBCL

Immunohistochemical positivity for BCL2 and MYC

Absence of EBV-associated markers (in > 97% of cases)

Molecular detection of a clonal B-cell population in cases in which histology is not definitive, such as corticoid-mitigated CNS-DLBCL

The transcobalamin missense variant *TCN2*:c.776C>G p.P259R has been associated with shorter survival and neurotoxicity {1906}. Most protocols report a median progression-free survival of about 12 months and an OS of approximately 3 years. In a subgroup of elderly patients with CNS-DLBCL with a methylated *MGMT* promoter, temozolomide monotherapy appeared to be therapeutically effective {1768}.

The presence of reactive perivascular CD3 T-cell infiltrates on biopsy has been associated with improved survival {2536}. LMO2 protein expression by the tumour cells has been associated with prolonged OS {1930}. BCL6 expression has been suggested as a prognostic marker in several studies, although conflicting conclusions as to whether it is a favourable or unfavourable marker have been reported {2144,2570,2619,2990}. In one study, del(6)(q22) was associated with inferior OS {434}.

Chapter 10

Immunodeficiency-associated CNS lymphomas

Deckert M
Batchelor T
Ferry JA
Hoang-Xuan K
Nagane M
Paulus W
Weller M

Definition

Immunodeficiency-associated CNS lymphomas comprise a family of CNS lymphomas arising in patients with inherited or acquired immunodeficiency, including that related to AIDS and iatrogenic disease.

ICD-O coding

None

ICD-11 coding

2B32 Immunodeficiency-associated lymphoproliferative disorders

Related terminology

Acceptable: AIDS-related diffuse large B-cell lymphoma.

Subtype(s)

None

Localization

Immunodeficiency-associated CNS lymphomas typically manifest in the CNS parenchyma.

Clinical features

The clinical presentation and imaging features of immunodeficiency-associated CNS lymphoma may be similar to those of CNS lymphoma in immunocompetent patients. Multiple lesions and areas of necrosis occur more frequently in immunodeficiency-associated CNS lymphoma than in CNS lymphoma of immunocompetent patients {719}.

Epidemiology

Immunodeficiency-associated CNS lymphomas may develop in rare hereditary immunodeficiency syndromes or (more commonly) in acquired immunodeficiency conditions related to infectious, autoimmune, or neoplastic diseases, or to immunosuppressive therapies. AIDS-related primary diffuse large B-cell lymphoma of the CNS (CNS-DLBCL) has become less common with the introduction of highly active antiretroviral therapy (HAART) {3327}. EBV-positive DLBCL of the elderly is related to immunosenescence and occurs in patients aged > 50 years {2356}.

Etiology

Immunodeficiency syndromes underlying immunodeficiency-associated CNS lymphoma include ataxia telangiectasia, Wiskott–Aldrich syndrome, and IgA deficiency. Other underlying conditions include autoimmune disorders (e.g. systemic lupus erythematosus and Sjögren syndrome), neoplastic diseases, and iatrogenic immunosuppression (either for the purpose of organ transplantation or due to treatment with immunosuppressive drugs). Infectious disorders such as HIV and HTLV

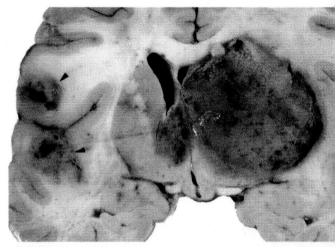

Fig. 10.06 HIV-associated primary diffuse large B-cell lymphoma of the CNS. This case was in an HIV-infected patient. In addition to the large tumour in the basal ganglia, there are further foci in the contralateral insular region (arrowheads).

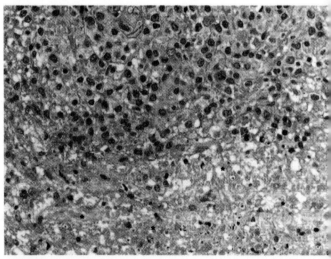

Fig. 10.07 HIV-associated primary diffuse large B-cell lymphoma of the CNS. Tumour in an HIV-infected patient.

infections that lead to immunodeficiency also increase the risk of CNS lymphomas, as does immunosenescence.

Pathogenesis

EBV infection is important because most immunodeficiency-associated lymphomas are EBV-related.

Macroscopic appearance

Multifocal presentation is more frequent than in CNS lymphomas in immunocompetent patients, as is a tendency to contain more and larger areas of necrosis. Tumours may simulate necrotizing cerebral toxoplasmosis, which may occur concomitantly {3032}

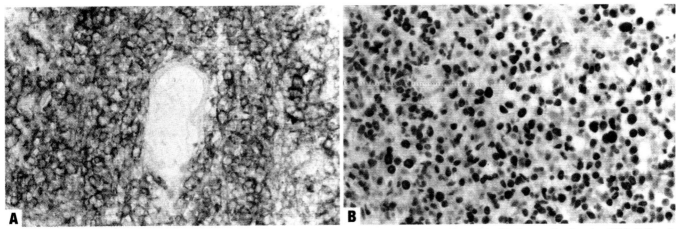

Fig. 10.08 EBV+ diffuse large B-cell lymphoma of the CNS. **A** Large tumour cells clustering around a blood vessel are stained by the pan–B-cell marker CD20. **B** There is strong expression of EBV-encoded small RNA (EBER) in the nuclei of the tumour cells.

Histopathology

Immunodeficiency-associated CNS lymphomas are typically EBV-related, so in addition to B-cell markers such as CD19, CD20, and CD79a, the lymphoma cells express the EBV-associated proteins EBNA1–6, LMP1, and EBV-encoded small RNAs 1 and 2 (EBER1 and EBER2) {1669}.

Otherwise, AIDS-related CNS-DLBCL shares the characteristics of CNS-DLBCL in immunocompetent patients.

Cytology

Cytology is of limited value for immunodeficiency-associated CNS lymphomas.

Diagnostic molecular pathology

Demonstration of a clonal B-cell population may be helpful in diagnostically ambiguous cases.

Essential and desirable diagnostic criteria

See Box 10.02.

Box 10.02 Diagnostic criteria for immunodeficiency-associated CNS lymphoma

> ### Essential:
> A B-cell lymphoma confined to the CNS at presentation, in an immunodeficient patient
>
> ### AND
> EBV positivity of tumour cells demonstrated by immunohistochemistry or in situ hybridization
>
> ### Desirable:
> Demonstration of a clonal B-cell population by PCR (in diagnostically difficult cases)

Staging

Not clinically relevant

Prognosis and prediction

Overall, outcome for immunodeficiency-associated CNS lymphoma is poor {1063}.

Lymphomatoid granulomatosis

Deckert M
Batchelor T
Ferry JA
Hoang-Xuan K
Nagane M
Paulus W
Weller M

Definition

Lymphomatoid granulomatosis is an angiocentric and angiodestructive lymphoproliferative disorder characterized by polymorphous lymphoid infiltrates composed of EBV-positive atypical B cells in a T cell–rich inflammatory background.

ICD-O coding

9766/1 Lymphomatoid granulomatosis
9766/1 Lymphomatoid granulomatosis, grade 1
9766/1 Lymphomatoid granulomatosis, grade 2
9766/3 Lymphomatoid granulomatosis, grade 3

ICD-11 coding

2A81.3 Lymphomatoid granulomatosis

Related terminology

None

Subtype(s)

None

Localization

The brain may show multiple focal intraparenchymal lesions. Leptomeninges and cranial nerves may also be involved {2423}. The spinal cord may also be affected {1620}.

Clinical features

This angiocentric and angiodestructive lymphoproliferative disorder affects the brain in 26% of patients, who may present with focal neurological symptoms and/or headache or cognitive impairment {2423}. Presentation may even be indistinct from that of systemic manifestation {1623,1272}. MRI may reveal mass lesions throughout the CNS {1272}; multiple punctate lesions along perivascular and periventricular spaces have also been reported {1623}.

Epidemiology

This rare disease usually manifests in adults in the fifth and sixth decade; a male predilection has been reported {1570, 2485}.

Etiology

Lymphomatoid granulomatosis is an EBV-driven disease. Immunodeficiency increases the risk of lymphomatoid granulomatosis.

Pathogenesis

Disease is hypothesized to result from defective immunosurveillance of EBV and an abnormal immune response towards EBV {2064}.

Macroscopic appearance

Macroscopically, the lesions may resemble tumour or infarct-like areas of necrosis.

Histopathology

Lesions are characterized by polymorphous lymphoid infiltrates consisting of lymphocytes (including CD4+ and CD8+ T lymphocytes), and plasma cells intermingled with varying numbers of atypical EBV+, CD20+, CD30+/−, CD15− large neoplastic B cells. Grading of lymphomatoid granulomatosis depends on the proportion of EBV-expressing CD20+ B cells (see Table 10.01). Most cases affecting the CNS correspond to grade 3, with large aggregates of EBV+ CD20+ B cells, and they should be classified as EBV+ diffuse large B-cell lymphoma of the CNS. The infiltrates invade blood vessel walls

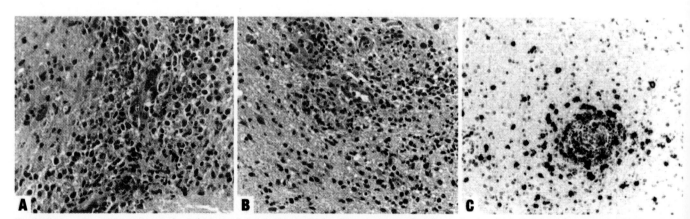

Fig. 10.09 Lymphomatoid granulomatosis. **A** Angiocentric lymphoid lesion harbouring some large cells with prominent nucleoli. **B** Polymorphous lymphoid infiltrate in the CNS parenchyma. Lymphocytes predominate, admixed with histiocytes and some plasma cells. Lymphocytes show some irregularity, with slightly increased nuclear size and increased nuclear basophilia. **C** Enlarged CD20+ B cells as part of a lymphoid infiltrate within a blood vessel wall. Note that some enlarged B cells have also invaded the CNS parenchyma.

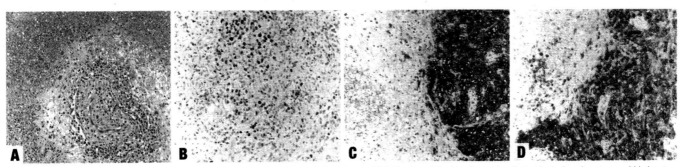

Fig. 10.10 Lymphomatoid granulomatosis, CNS WHO grade 3. **A** An angiotropic lymphoma with infiltration of the blood vessel walls by blasts, lymphocytes, and histiocytes. Blasts also invade the perivascular brain tissue, which is largely necrotic. **B** Note the high number of EBV-encoded small RNA (EBER)-positive cells. **C** Tumour cells express the pan–B-cell marker CD20. **D** Tumour cells express the CD30 antigen.

Table 10.01 Grading of lymphomatoid granulomatosis (adapted from the 2017 *WHO classification of tumours of haematopoietic and lymphoid tissues*)

	Lymphoid cells	Transformed B cells	EBER+ lymphoid cells[a]	Necrosis
Grade 1	Polymorphous background	Rare or absent	< 40 cells/mm² (< 5 cells/HPF)	Focal or absent
Grade 2	Polymorphous background	Single or in small clusters	40–400 cells/mm² (5–50 cells/HPF)	More common
Grade 3	Polymorphous background	Large atypical B cells or aggregates	> 400 cells/mm² (> 50 cells/HPF)	Extensive

EBER, EBV-encoded small RNA.
[a]Originally reported per HPF of 0.16 mm².

Box 10.03 Diagnostic criteria for lymphomatoid granulomatosis

Essential:

Morphology of an intracerebral polymorphous lymphoid infiltrate with atypical EBV+, CD20+, CD30+/−, CD15− large neoplastic B cells of variable numbers

AND

Blood vessel destruction

and may induce infarct-like necrosis of tumour and/or brain tissue. Rarely, CNS WHO grade 2 lesions may occur in the CNS.

Cytology
Not relevant

Diagnostic molecular pathology
Detection of clonal rearrangement of IG genes may be helpful in diagnostically difficult cases.

Essential and desirable diagnostic criteria
See Box 10.03.

Staging
Not relevant

Prognosis and prediction
Lymphomatoid granulomatosis of the CNS usually follows an aggressive course because most CNS biopsies demonstrate EBV-positive diffuse large B-cell lymphoma of the CNS. Current treatments of lymphomatoid granulomatosis are based on its histological grade, although clinical courses and treatment responses are largely unclear {1623}, particularly in cases with CNS involvement. Since most cases of CNS lymphomatoid granulomatosis correspond to diffuse large B-cell lymphoma of the CNS, treatment options include corticosteroids, radiation, or chemotherapy {1272}.

Intravascular large B-cell lymphoma

Deckert M
Batchelor T
Ferry JA
Hoang-Xuan K
Nagane M
Paulus W
Weller M

Definition
Intravascular large B-cell lymphoma is a distinctive type of aggressive B-cell lymphoma characterized by exclusively intravascular growth.

ICD-O coding
9712/3 Intravascular large B-cell lymphoma

ICD-11 coding
2A81.1 Intravascular large B-cell lymphoma

Related terminology
Not recommended: angiotropic large cell lymphoma.

Subtype(s)
None

Localization
The brain is nearly always involved; spinal cord involvement is less common.

Clinical features
Except for the solely cutaneous cases, CNS involvement occurs in 75–85% of cases {251}. The hallmark intravascular growth leads to clinical symptoms mimicking those of cerebral infarction or subacute encephalopathy {954}.

Epidemiology
Intravascular large B-cell lymphoma is rare and usually manifests in adults. The median patient age is 70 years (range: 34–90 years). There is no sex predilection {2538}.

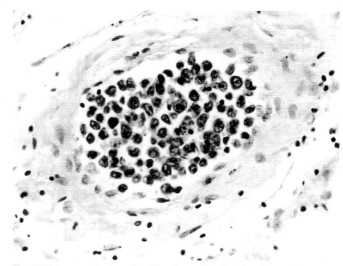

Fig. 10.11 Intravascular large B-cell lymphoma. Neoplastic lymphoma cells are confined to the vessel lumen.

Etiology
Unknown

Pathogenesis
Absence of CD29 and CD54 (ICAM1) expression is thought to underlie the tumour cells' inability to migrate transvascularly {2535}. Expression levels of the chemokine receptors CXCR5, CCR6, and CCR7 are decreased, and MMP2 and MMP9 are not expressed. Thus, the tumour cells express molecules that enable their adhesion to the endothelium but not those involved in extravasation {2538}.

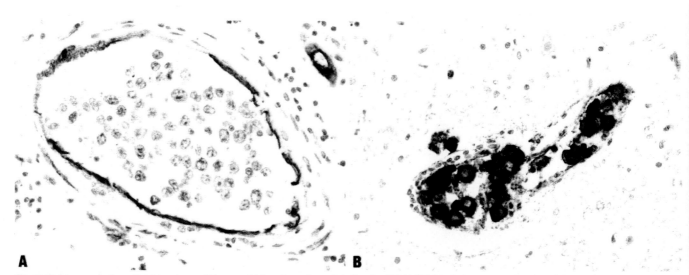

Fig. 10.12 Intravascular large B-cell lymphoma. **A** Immunostaining of vascular endothelium for CD34 highlights the intravascular location of the lymphoma cells. **B** There is intravascular accumulation of CD20+ lymphoma cells.

Macroscopic appearance

Macroscopy reveals infarcts (acute and/or old), necrosis, and/or haemorrhage, although abnormalities may be inconspicuous.

Histopathology

Microscopically, large atypical B cells are present, confined to the lumina of cerebral blood vessels; they may occlude these vessels, but they do not invade into the brain parenchyma, although, exceptionally, a few cells may extravasate. Immunohistochemically, the neoplastic B cells typically show a strong expression of CD20. However, exceptional CD20-negative cases have been reported that require immunostaining for additional B-cell markers (e.g. CD79a and PAX5) {2538}.

Cytology

Not relevant

Diagnostic molecular pathology

Detection of clonal rearrangement of the IG genes may be helpful for the diagnosis.

Box 10.04 Diagnostic criteria for intravascular large B-cell lymphoma

Essential:

Biopsy showing a large B-cell lymphoma with morphological and immunohistochemical confinement of neoplastic B cells to the blood vessel lumen without invasion of the surrounding tissue

Essential and desirable diagnostic criteria

See Box 10.04.

Staging

Staging should determine involvement of other organs because intravascular lymphoma may be widely disseminated.

Prognosis and prediction

The prognosis of intravascular large B-cell lymphoma involving the CNS is poor. Methotrexate-based chemotherapy is beneficial in a subset of patients {1582}.

MALT lymphoma of the dura

Deckert M
Batchelor T
Ferry JA
Hoang-Xuan K
Nagane M
Paulus W
Weller M

Definition
MALT lymphoma of the dura is a distinctive low-grade lymphoma of mucosa-associated lymphoid tissue (MALT) composed of marginal zone B cells, sometimes with plasmacytic differentiation, arising in the dura.

ICD-O coding
9699/3 MALT lymphoma of the dura

ICD-11 coding
2A85.3 Extranodal marginal zone B-cell lymphoma, primary site excluding stomach or skin

Related terminology
Acceptable: extranodal marginal zone lymphoma of mucosa-associated lymphoid tissue.

Subtype(s)
None

Localization
Lymphomas arising in the dura mater are much less frequent than those arising in the brain {1428}. By far the most common dural lymphoma is MALT lymphoma {1759,1847}. MALT lymphoma originating in the dura is much more common than MALT lymphoma originating in the brain {163,3071}. Most MALT lymphomas arise in the cranial dura; a small minority arise in the dura covering the spinal cord {3306,2274}, and these may be associated with spinal cord compression {1536}.

Clinical features
Patients may present with headache, seizures, visual changes, focal neurological defects, and other symptoms {1759,1534,90, 1428,1536,3306,1029,163}.

Epidemiology
Dural MALT lymphoma affects adults, with a median age in the sixth decade {163,3071}. Women are affected more often than men, with an M:F ratio of approximately 1:5–7 {3237,1428,

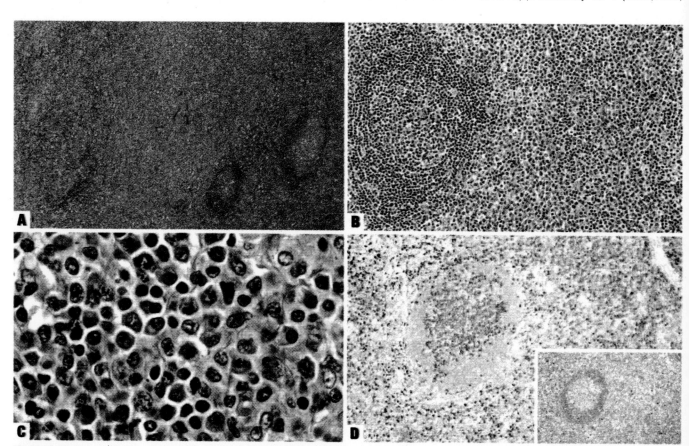

Fig. 10.13 MALT lymphoma. **A** Low-power view of a dense lymphoid infiltrate with residual follicles visible. **B** Lymphoma cells are small or of medium size and have colonized follicles. **C** High-power view of the plasmacytoid infiltrate that may be present in MALT lymphomas. **D** Staining for kappa light chains is positive; inset: staining for lambda light chains is negative.

3306,1029}. No racial or geographical associations have been identified.

Etiology

MALT lymphoma outside the CNS has been attributed to chronic inflammation (of either infectious or autoimmune origin) {3171}. Regarding MALT lymphoma of the dura, it is still unknown whether there is an association with inflammatory disorders. One patient with hepatitis C who developed dural MALT lymphoma has been reported {3328}. One patient with CNS extranodal marginal zone lymphoma had a long history of white matter disease with some features of multiple sclerosis {2834}, and another patient with extranodal marginal zone lymphoma had *Chlamydia psittaci* infection {2537}.

Pathogenesis

Trisomies, most often of chromosome 3, are occasionally detected {3237,3306}. Inactivation of *TNFAIP3* by mutation or loss appears common in cases with plasmacytic differentiation {1029}. Activating *NOTCH2* mutations accompanied by inactivating *TBL1XR1* mutations are common in cases with monocytoid morphology {1029}. Recurrent gains of 6p25.3 and losses at 1p36.32 have been documented. IGH translocation and MALT lymphoma–associated translocations are rare {163, 2274}, but a translocation involving the *MALT1* and IGH genes, consistent with IGH::*MALT1* fusion [t(14;18)(q32;q21)], has been identified in 1 case {263}.

Macroscopic appearance

There is a solitary mass or plaque-like thickening of the dura {1759,3237,1428,1536,3306}, often mimicking a meningioma {163}.

Histopathology

Dural MALT lymphomas share histological and immunohistological features with MALT lymphomas at other sites. They are composed of small lymphocytes and marginal zone cells, often with plasmacytic differentiation, sometimes with remnants of reactive follicles with follicular colonization {1759,1534,3237,1428,3306}. A subset of cases have tumour cells with abundant clear cytoplasm (monocytoid morphology) {1029}. Occasionally, associated amyloid deposition is seen {1847,3237}. Dural MALT lymphomas may arise in association with meningothelium (just as marginal zone lymphomas often arise in association with epithelium in other sites), so entrapped meningothelial cells may be present {1759,1847}. Infrequently, lymphoma cells invade Virchow–Robin spaces and the subjacent brain parenchyma {3306}.

Immunohistochemistry

Neoplastic B cells are CD20+, CD79a+, CD5–, CD10–, BCL6–, CD23–, IRF4 (MUM1)+/–, cyclin D1–, BCL2+, and they have a low proliferation index {1029,163,2274}. A component of clonal plasma cells is often found {1536,3306}. The monotypic plasma cells are often IgG4+ {3306,1029}, but evidence of systemic IgG4-related disease has been absent to date {3306}.

Cytology

The cerebrospinal fluid is occasionally involved {1428}.

Diagnostic molecular pathology

IG genes are clonally rearranged {1759,263}.

Essential and desirable diagnostic criteria

See Box 10.05.

Staging

MALT lymphomas of the dura are typically localized at presentation {1759,3237,1428,3306}. Clinical staging is performed to exclude extracranial manifestations.

Prognosis and prediction

Patients are treated with resection, radiation, and/or chemotherapy, and they typically achieve complete remission {585, 1029,163,2274,3071}. The prognosis is very good. One case series reported 22 complete remissions and 1 partial response in 23 evaluable patients, with a 3-year progression-free survival rate of 89% {709}. Local and systemic relapses are rare {1428,709}.

Other low-grade B-cell lymphomas of the CNS

Deckert M
Batchelor T
Ferry JA
Hoang-Xuan K
Nagane M
Paulus W
Weller M

Definition

Other low-grade B-cell lymphomas of the CNS are those lymphomas confined to the CNS at presentation that histologically correspond to one of the types of systemic low-grade B-cell lymphomas, most commonly extranodal marginal zone lymphoma; other cases have been diagnosed as small lymphocytic lymphoma, lymphoplasmacytic lymphoma, or low-grade B-cell lymphoma NOS.

ICD-O coding

9671/3 Lymphoplasmacytic lymphoma
9690/3 Follicular lymphoma

ICD-11 coding

2A85.Y Further specified mature B-cell neoplasms or lymphoma

Related terminology

None

Subtype(s)

None

Localization

Tumours may occur as a solitary lesion or (infrequently) as multiple discrete lesions, or as diffuse involvement of the white matter of the brain. Lesions are mostly supratentorial (affecting lobes of the cerebral cortex or basal ganglia) {2387,163,1188, 2274}, but the cerebellum and spinal cord also may be affected {2387,3248}. Involvement of the leptomeninges and choroid plexus has been reported {1586,2537,1050,163}.

Clinical features

Male and female patients are roughly equally affected. Patients are almost all adults, with only rare paediatric cases being reported (age range: 5–79 years; median: 49 years) {2387,163, 2274,3071}. Symptoms are variable, and they are occasionally present for months or years before diagnosis {2537,1188}. The most common symptoms and signs include headache, seizures, and speech impairment {2387,165,1188,3071}. The clinical differential diagnosis can include glioma, intravascular lymphoma, and demyelinating disease {163,2274}. Radiographically, lesions may be well defined or infiltrative {2387, 3248,165}.

Epidemiology

Low-grade B-cell lymphomas of the CNS are rare, and epidemiological data are not available.

Etiology

The etiology is unknown.

Pathogenesis

Limited data are available on genetic alterations in low-grade B-cell lymphoma arising in the CNS. Clonal rearrangement of IGH and/or IGK has been reported {2950,1050,2274}. One case with loss of heterozygosity on 6q (including the locus for *TNFAIP3*) and one with *MALT1* rearrangement are on record {2274}. In the few cases tested, *MYD88* p.L265P was absent {2274}, and FISH for translocations of IGH, *BCL2*, and *CCND1* was negative {1586,163}.

Macroscopic appearance

Limited data are available on macroscopy.

Histopathology

Most cases of low-grade B-cell lymphoma of the CNS correspond to extranodal marginal zone lymphoma {3248,2274}; other cases have been diagnosed as small lymphocytic lymphoma {165,1188}, lymphoplasmacytic lymphoma {2950}, or low-grade B-cell lymphoma NOS {1446,2387}.

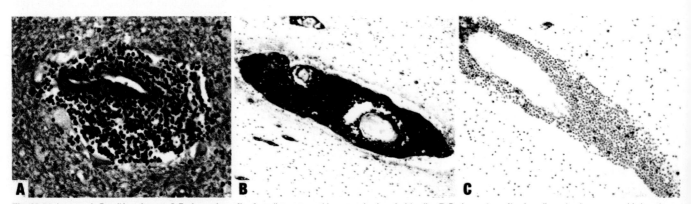

Fig. 10.14 Low-grade B-cell lymphoma. **A** Perivascular cuffs of small, monomorphic-appearing lymphoid cells. **B** Perivascular cuffs of medium-sized, monomorphic lymphoma cells, which express the pan–B-cell marker CD20. **C** Admixed with the lymphoma cells are some reactive CD3 T cells.

Immunophenotype

Neoplastic cells are typically CD20+, CD3–, CD5–, CD10–, CD23–, BCL6–, BCL2+, cyclin D1–, TdT–, EBV-encoded small RNA (EBER)– {2834,3248,2274}. When present, plasma cells (CD138+) often express monotypic light chain. The proliferation index is low (< 10%) {165,1188}.

Cytology

Cerebrospinal fluid is negative in most cases, but occasional cases have cerebrospinal fluid involved by lymphoma, with the diagnosis confirmed by flow cytometry {2834,1050,1188}.

Diagnostic molecular pathology

Clonal rearrangement of IGH and/or IGK genes has been reported {2950,1050,2274}.

Essential and desirable diagnostic criteria

See Box 10.06.

Staging

Extent of disease is established using lumbar puncture for cytology and flow cytometry, complete blood count with differential, bone marrow biopsy with flow cytometry, and imaging to investigate sites of disease outside the CNS.

Prognosis and prediction

Low-grade B-cell lymphomas show a less aggressive course and have a better prognosis than do primary diffuse large B-cell lymphomas of the CNS. Patients have been treated with resection, steroids, radiation, and/or chemotherapy. Most are alive and free of disease or have stable disease on follow-up {3407, 163,2274,3071}. Progression outside the CNS is very rare. A small subset of patients succumb to lymphoma {2274}.

Anaplastic large cell lymphoma (ALK+/ALK−)

Deckert M
Batchelor T
Ferry JA
Hoang-Xuan K
Nagane M
Paulus W
Weller M

Definition

Anaplastic large cell lymphoma (ALCL) is a distinctive CD30-positive peripheral T-cell lymphoma that is rare in the CNS and is separated into two distinct types: ALK-positive (ALK+ ALCL) and ALK-negative (ALK− ALCL).

ICD-O coding

9714/3 Anaplastic large cell lymphoma (ALK+/ALK−)

ICD-11 coding

2A90.A Anaplastic large cell lymphoma, ALK-positive
2A90.B Anaplastic large cell lymphoma, ALK-negative

Related terminology

None

Subtype(s)

None

Localization

ALK+ ALCL occurs as single or multiple supratentorial parenchymal lesions with or without infratentorial involvement, and rarely with spinal cord involvement. Extension to involve the meninges and (rarely) the skull can occur {2751,2398,3447,776}.

ALK− ALCL occurs as single or multiple lesions, usually supratentorial {1057}.

Clinical features

Patients present with headache, seizures, nausea, fever, or a combination of these {251,2275,2398,1760}. They are often initially thought to have an infection {916,2398,1017,776}.

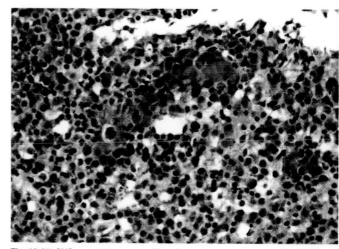

Fig. 10.15 CNS anaplastic large cell lymphoma. There is a polymorphic lymphomatous infiltrate with occasional markedly atypical hallmark cells.

Epidemiology

ALK+ ALCL occurs from early childhood to young adulthood (median age: ~17 years), with a male preponderance. ALK− ALCL affects adults (median age: 65 years), also with a male preponderance {2275}.

Etiology

Unknown

Pathogenesis

ALK+ ALCL is driven by oncogenic *ALK* gene fusions, most commonly with *NPM1* (in > 80% of cases). *ALK* fusions increase ALK expression, leading to aberrant activation of downstream signalling pathways including JAK/STAT3 and others {3420}.

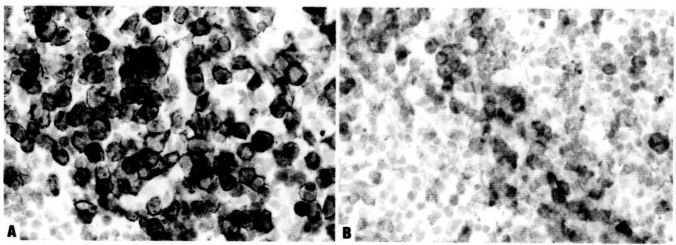

Fig. 10.16 ALK+ anaplastic large cell lymphoma. **A** The lymphoma cells strongly express the CD30 antigen. **B** Neoplastic large tumour cells with round nuclei and prominent nucleoli show cytoplasmic expression of ALK.

ALK− ALCL carries mutations or gene fusions of other receptor tyrosine kinase genes that eventually activate signalling pathways similar to those activated in ALK+ ALCL, including JAK/STAT3 {653}. Clonal rearrangements of T-cell receptor genes are present in the vast majority of cases of ALCL.

Macroscopic appearance

Insufficient data available

Histopathology

ALK+ ALCL shows a diffuse proliferation of large atypical cells with abundant cytoplasm, including hallmark cells with bean-shaped nuclei and an eosinophilic paranuclear area {2081, 1057,2751,1760}. Rare examples of the lymphohistiocytic and small cell patterns have been described {2539,3447}. Tumour cells are CD30+, ALK+, and EMA+, and they may express one or more T-cell antigens.

ALK− ALCL histopathology is similar to that of ALK+ ALCL, but ALK is not expressed {1057}. The differential diagnosis includes classic Hodgkin lymphoma and diffuse large B-cell lymphoma with pleomorphic cells. Hodgkin lymphoma is very rare in the CNS {1064}, typically has more admixed reactive cells, and cells express PAX5 (weakly) and often CD15, in addition to CD30. In contrast to ALCL, diffuse large B-cell lymphoma is typically positive for CD20 and other B-cell antigens.

Cytology

The cerebrospinal fluid may be involved. The large atypical neoplastic cells may have cytoplasmic azurophilic granules {3447,2081}.

Diagnostic molecular pathology

Molecular analysis demonstrates clonally rearranged TR genes in the vast majority of tumours. ALK+ ALCL carries chromosomal translocations involving *ALK*, most commonly a t(2;5)(p23;q35) causing an oncogenic fusion with *NPM1* (*NPM1::ALK* fusion).

Essential and desirable diagnostic criteria

See Box 10.07.

Staging

Staging is required to exclude a systemic primary lymphoma.

Prognosis and prediction

ALK+ ALCL of the CNS has a prognosis similar to or worse than that of systemic ALK+ ALCL, although sustained remission is possible. Treatment failures tend to occur in the CNS and are rarely systemic. ALK− ALCL has a poor prognosis {1057,2275, 3336,2081}.

Chapter 10

T-cell and NK/T-cell lymphomas

Deckert M
Batchelor T
Ferry JA
Hoang-Xuan K
Nagane M
Paulus W
Weller M

Definition
Primary CNS T-cell and NK/T-cell lymphomas are groups of malignant non-Hodgkin lymphomas, including peripheral T-cell lymphoma (PTCL) and NK/T-cell lymphoma (nasal type), with primary manifestation in the CNS.

ICD-O coding
9702/3 T-cell lymphoma
9719/3 NK/T-cell lymphoma

ICD-11 coding
2B2Z Mature T-cell or NK-cell neoplasms, unspecified

Related terminology
None

Subtype(s)
None

Localization
In a series of 45 patients with primary CNS T-cell lymphoma, 19% had positive cerebrospinal fluid cytology, 4% had eye involvement, and 29% had multiple brain lesions {2902,2072}.

Extranodal NK/T-cell lymphoma usually forms a single mass, but it may also occur with multiple lesions {1175,2135}. Involved sites include the frontal and temporal lobes, cerebellum, pituitary {2135,1866}, and (rarely) the leptomeninges {66}.

Clinical features
Patients with primary CNS T-cell lymphoma are adults aged 21–81 years (median: sixth decade), with an M:F ratio of about 1.5:1 {2072}. Patients present with headache, neurological decline, seizures, and abnormalities of sensory and/or motor function {2072,2160}.

Extranodal NK/T-cell lymphoma of the CNS affects patients aged 21–77 years (median: fifth decade), with a male preponderance (M:F ratio: ~2:1) {2135}. Patients present with symptoms that are often rapidly progressive, including dizziness, headache, vomiting {1175}, weakness, paralysis, aphasia {2553}, dysphagia, dysarthria {1866}, and mental deterioration {2303}. Manifestations can mimic a cerebrovascular accident {2303,2553}.

Epidemiology
PTCLs accounted for 2–4% of primary CNS lymphomas in a European series {914}, and as many as 17% of primary CNS lymphomas in an Asian series {583}. Extranodal NK/T-cell lymphoma is rare. Most reported patients were Asian {1175,2303, 2135,1866}; rarely, patients were African-American {2553,2135} or Hispanic {2135}.

Etiology
Rare T-cell lymphomas {1809} and one extranodal NK/T-cell lymphoma {614} of the CNS have been reported in HIV-positive patients, and one CNS NK/T-cell lymphoma has been reported in a transplant recipient {2135}, suggesting that immunodeficiency might play a role in the etiology of the disease in a subset of patients. One patient with a CD4-positive primary CNS T-cell lymphoma was seropositive for HTLV-1 {1931}.

Pathogenesis
Mutations of DNMT3A, TET2, and several JAK/STAT pathway genes have been found in a subset of cases {2072}.

Macroscopic appearance
Necrosis is common in extranodal NK/T-cell lymphomas {1175, 2135} and T-cell lymphomas {2072}.

Histopathology
Most T-cell lymphomas in the CNS are PTCL-NOS {2072,2160}. A minority of tumours (17% in one series) are anaplastic large cell lymphoma (see *Anaplastic large cell lymphoma (ALK+, ALK–)*, p. 366) {2072}. Most tumours in PTCL-NOS are composed of small and/or medium-sized atypical lymphoid cells; a minority are composed of medium-sized to large cells or mainly of large cells {583,1446,802,2072}. PTCL often shows

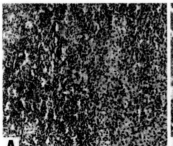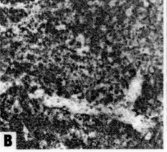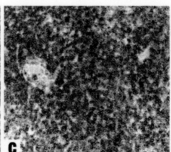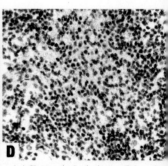

Fig. 10.17 Peripheral T-cell lymphoma. **A** Highly cellular lymphoma of medium-sized to large tumour cells with frequent mitoses diffusely infiltrates the brain tissue. **B** Lymphoblastic and moderately sized lymphoma cells express the pan–T-cell marker CD3. **C** The tumour cells show a sheet-like growth pattern and have invaded the wall of a cerebral blood vessel. They strongly express the CD8 antigen. **D** Many tumour cells express granzyme B, a cytotoxic granule, in their cytoplasm.

a prominent perivascular growth pattern and areas of necrosis {583,1446,2902,802,2072}. Tumours are accompanied by reactive gliosis and a histiocytic reaction, but plasma cells, neutrophils, and eosinophils are usually inconspicuous {802,2072}.

Extranodal NK/T cell lymphomas are composed of medium-sized, medium-sized and large, or large atypical, pleomorphic lymphoid cells with irregular nuclei (featuring dark or coarse chromatin and inconspicuous nucleoli) and a moderate amount of pale cytoplasm {1175,2303,2135}, accompanied by vascular proliferation and histiocytic infiltrates {1866}. Mitotic figures are readily found, and angiocentric growth and extensive necrosis are common {2135}. Necrosis is coagulative and apoptotic bodies are also seen {1866}. A single case of a collision tumour with meningioma has been reported {3515}.

Immunophenotype
Neoplastic cells in CNS PTCL are usually CD3-positive and CD56-negative; CD8 is expressed more often than CD4 {2072}. Most tumours are of αβ T-cell lineage, but γδ lineage has been documented in a few cases {2072,2160}. They typically express one or more cytotoxic granule proteins (TIA1, granzyme B, and/or perforin). CD2, CD5, and CD7 are each lost in subsets of cases {2072}. Proliferation index is usually > 50% {2072}. A case with aberrant coexpression of CD20 and CD79a has been reported {1192}.

Extranodal NK/T-cell lymphoma is usually positive for CD3, CD56, cytotoxic granule protein, and EBV-encoded small RNA (EBER), and negative for CD5 and B-cell antigens {2135}. Occasional cases express CD5 or lack CD56 {2303,2135}. CD30 may be expressed {1866}. A single case showed aberrant CD20 expression {1866}.

Differential diagnosis
The differential diagnosis of T-cell lymphoma often includes a reactive inflammatory process because of the often relatively small size of tumour cells {2072,1192}. Pan–T-cell antigen loss and clonal TR favour a PTCL; a polymorphous infiltrate with admixed inflammatory cells favours a reactive process {802, 2072,1192}.

The differential diagnosis of NK/T-cell lymphoma includes B-cell lymphoma, especially lymphomatoid granulomatosis, because of the angiocentric growth and necrosis. Immunohistochemistry distinguishes the two entities. If the biopsy mainly shows necrosis, an infectious lesion can be considered in the differential diagnosis.

Cytology
Cerebrospinal fluid involvement is reported in extranodal NK/T-cell lymphoma with leptomeningeal disease; involvement can be documented by cytology augmented by flow cytometry {66}.

Diagnostic molecular pathology
Clonal rearrangement of TR genes can be demonstrated in most T-cell lymphomas {2072,1192}. In extranodal NK/T-cell lymphomas, TR genes are usually in germline configuration, but they may be clonally rearranged {1175,2303}.

Box 10.08 Diagnostic criteria for T-cell and NK/T-cell lymphomas

T-cell lymphoma

Essential:

Biopsy-proven lymphoma manifesting in the CNS

AND

Expression of one or more T-cell markers in variable combination (CD2, CD3, CD4, CD8, CD5, CD7)

Desirable:

Abnormal T-cell immunophenotype with loss of one or more pan–T-cell antigens

Demonstration of clonal TR gene rearrangement, if inflammation is considered in the differential diagnosis

NK/T-cell lymphoma

Essential:

Biopsy-proven lymphoma manifesting in the CNS

AND

    NK-cell immunophenotype (typically CD3+, CD2+, CD5−, CD7+, CD56+)

    OR

    Cytotoxic T-cell immunophenotype (typically CD3+, CD8+)

Desirable:

Expression of cytotoxic molecules (perforin, granzyme B)

Absence of clonal TR gene rearrangement in cases of NK-cell lineage

Essential and desirable diagnostic criteria
See Box 10.08.

Staging
Staging is required to exclude a systemic primary; for cases of extranodal NK/T-cell lymphoma in particular, the possibility of an occult primary in the upper respiratory tract should be excluded.

Prognosis and prediction
The outcome for patients with CNS T-cell lymphoma appears similar to that for patients with primary diffuse large B-cell lymphoma of the CNS. T-cell lymphomas with low-grade histological features may be associated with a more favourable outcome than high-grade T-cell lymphomas {1446}. In one series, 20% of patients with PTCL-NOS were alive without lymphoma at last follow-up, whereas 40% were alive with disease and 40% had died of the disease {2072}. Methotrexate-based chemotherapy is the most common treatment regimen used. In a cohort of 45 patients with primary CNS lymphoma of T-cell origin, the median progression-free survival and overall survival were 22 and 25 months, respectively {2902}.

The prognosis of patients with extranodal NK/T-cell lymphoma of the CNS is poor, and most patients experience rapidly progressive disease. Median survival is approximately 6 months (range: 1–18 months) {1175,2553,2135}. Long-term survival is rare {2135}. Because primary CNS NK/T-cell lymphomas are rare, no standard treatment protocol exists. Methotrexate-based chemotherapy may be beneficial {2553}.

Erdheim–Chester disease

Paulus W
Chan JKC
Idbaih A
Perry A
Sahm F

Definition

Erdheim–Chester disease of the CNS or the meninges, with or without systemic lesions, pathologically corresponds to its counterparts occurring elsewhere. It is a clonal histiocytosis with foamy histiocytes, occasional Touton giant cells, chronic inflammation, and variable fibrosis.

ICD-O coding

9749/3 Erdheim–Chester disease

ICD-11 coding

2B31.Y & XH1VJ3 Other specified histiocytic or dendritic cell neoplasms & Erdheim–Chester disease

Related terminology

None

Subtype(s)

None

Localization

All parts of the CNS may be involved, including the dura (in 15–25% of cases), cerebrum (60%), hypothalamus (3%), brainstem and cerebellum (25%), and spinal cord (12%) {1781,2402, 492}. Neurodegenerative lesions are typically located in the posterior fossa, including in the brainstem, cerebellar peduncles, and dentate nuclei.

Clinical features

Tumour-like lesions are characterized by symptoms related to tumour location, including increased intracranial pressure, focal neurological deficits, and seizures. Neurodegenerative lesions may lead to cerebellar symptoms, pyramidal tract signs, pseudobulbar palsy, or cognitive disturbances {1781}. Infiltration of large arteries may induce stroke {892}.

Imaging

On MRI, tumour lesions are isointense or hypointense on T1-weighted images, contrast enhancing, and associated with mass effect and perilesional oedema. Diffuse CNS atrophy may appear over time, even without direct tumour cell infiltration {754}. More than 10% of patients are asymptomatic despite abnormal CNS MRI findings {2402}.

Epidemiology

Neurological complications occur in 30–50% of patients with Erdheim–Chester disease, predominantly in men aged about 50 years {2402,2381}.

Etiology

Unknown

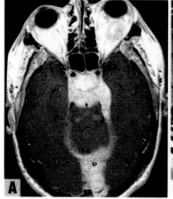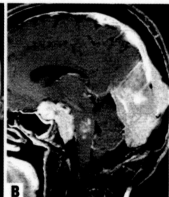

Fig. 10.18 Erdheim–Chester disease. This 39-year-old man presented with headaches and severe proptosis. **A** T1-weighted postcontrast axial MRI shows severe proptosis with intensely enhancing intraconal retrobulbar masses in both orbits. The cavernous sinus and pituitary gland are infiltrated and intensely enhancing. There is an additional enhancing mass along the tentorium and posteroinferior falx. **B** T1-weighted postcontrast sagittal MRI shows a mass infiltrating the pituitary gland and hypothalamus, extending inferiorly along the clivus. Multiple lobulated masses are present along the falx and tentorium. This is an important scan because it shows patchy enhancing lesions in the pons, indicating parenchymal involvement.

Pathogenesis

Common alterations include *BRAF* p.V600E mutations (in as many as 50% of cases) {168,1241,1300,845}, *MAP2K1* mutations (in up to 30% of cases), *KRAS* and/or *NRAS* mutations (in up to 20% of cases) {845,753,2389}, and other genetic alterations pertaining to the MAPK pathway, with single cases exhibiting *ARAF* mutations or *BRAF*, *NTRK1*, *ALK*, or *ETV3* fusions {753,810}. Single cases with *CSF1R* mutations or *RET* fusions have been reported {810}. *PIK3CA* mutations can occur as single events or in combination with other alterations, mostly with *BRAF* p.V600E mutations (in about 11% of all cases) {845}. In general, *EPHB2* (*ERK*) activation and a potentially therapeutically relevant alteration of a MAPK pathway gene can be found in nearly all cases {753}.

Patients with additional haematopoietic tumours may have other mutation profiles. In patients with both Erdheim–Chester disease and Langerhans cell histiocytosis, the frequency of *BRAF* p.V600E mutation is even higher (82% of lesions) according to one study {1300}. In patients with a concomitant myeloid neoplasm, the alterations typical for Erdheim–Chester disease can overlap with mutations frequently found in myeloid tumour cells (e.g. *JAK2* mutations) {2388}.

Macroscopic appearance

Erdheim–Chester disease manifests as widespread infiltrative parenchymal lesions (in 44% of cases), dural thickening to a meningioma-like mass (37%), or a combination of both (19%) {1781}. Nerve root or pituitary stalk lesions also occur {1156}.

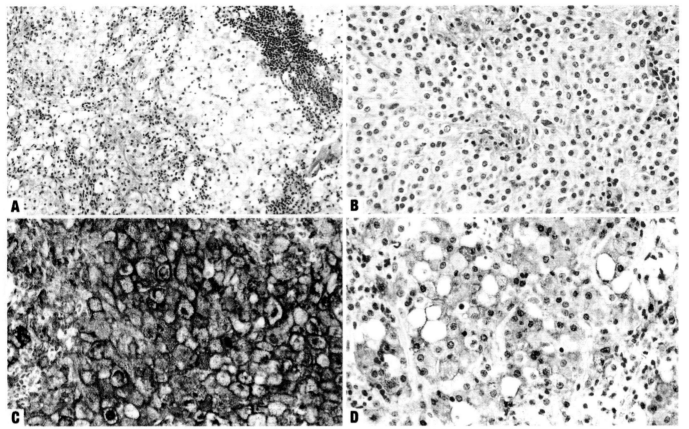

Fig. 10.19 Erdheim–Chester disease. **A** Sheets of large foamy histiocytes are seen, along with a lymphoid infiltrate, but no obvious emperipolesis. **B** Sheets of epithelioid histiocytes. **C** Strong CD163 immunoreactivity. **D** Extensive factor XIIIa positivity.

Histopathology

Like in juvenile xanthogranuloma, infiltrates are composed of foamy to epithelioid histiocytes with small nuclei, Touton-type multinucleated giant cells, scant lymphocytes, rare eosinophils, and variable fibrosis or gliosis that is often rich in Rosenthal fibres (piloid gliosis). This potential mimicry of pilocytic astrocytoma is exacerbated by histiocytes resembling astrocytes when embedded in densely fibrillar CNS parenchyma.

Immunophenotype

The neoplastic histiocytes are positive for CD68, CD163, CD14, and factor XIIIa; variably positive for S100; and negative for CD1a. About half express BRAF p.V600E {2381}.

Cytology

Not clinically relevant

Diagnostic molecular pathology

Testing for potentially mutant genes (*BRAF*, some in combination with *PIK3CA*, *MAP2K1*, and *KRAS* or *NRAS*) should be performed with sensitive assays, reflecting the frequently low proportion of neoplastic cells. If none of these is detected, testing can progress to the fusions of *NTRK1*, *ALK*, or *ETV3*, known from peripheral Erdheim–Chester disease.

Essential and desirable diagnostic criteria

See Box 10.09.

Box 10.09 Diagnostic criteria for Erdheim–Chester disease

Essential:

A population of foamy cells expressing histiocytic antigens

AND

Negativity for Langerhans cell markers (CD1a and/or CD207 [langerin])

Desirable:

Exclusion of other lines of differentiation (glial, epithelial, melanocytic, lymphocytic, etc.)

Exclusion of reactive and demyelinating lesions

BRAF, *MAP2K1*, and *KRAS* or *NRAS* mutation status

Potential systemic manifestations on imaging

Staging

Not applicable

Prognosis and prediction

Therapeutic options include surgery, cladribine, immunomodulators, and molecular targeted therapies including BRAF inhibitors and MEK inhibitors. These therapies yield a significant tumour response rate. In contrast, neurodegenerative lesions are relatively resistant to therapeutic interventions.

Rosai–Dorfman disease

Paulus W
Chan JKC
Idbaih A
Perry A
Sahm F

Definition
Rosai–Dorfman disease of the CNS or the meninges, with or without systemic lesions, pathologically corresponds to its counterparts occurring elsewhere. It is a clonal histiocytic proliferation characterized by large S100-positive histiocytes with variable emperipolesis.

ICD-O coding
9749/3 Rosai–Dorfman disease

ICD-11 coding
EK92 Histiocytoses of uncertain malignant potential

Related terminology
Not recommended: sinus histiocytosis with massive lymphadenopathy.

Subtype(s)
None

Localization
Rosai–Dorfman disease of the CNS forms solitary or multiple dural masses, especially in the cerebral convexity, cranial base, and cavernous sinuses, as well as parasagittal, suprasellar and petroclival regions {3194}. Parenchymal or intrasellar lesions may also occur.

Clinical features
Patients may exhibit signs of increased intracranial pressure or focal neurological deficits. Patients with sellar lesions present with signs of hypopituitarism and diabetes insipidus. The classic systemic signs – cervical lymphadenopathy, fever, and weight

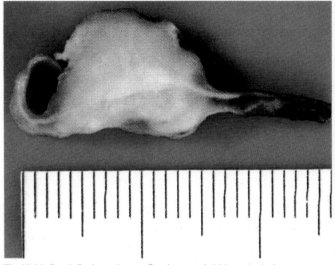

Fig. 10.20 Rosai–Dorfman disease. Dural mass, mimicking a meningioma.

loss – are absent in 70% of patients, and 52% have no associated systemic disease {2582}. On MRI, Rosai–Dorfman disease resembles meningioma. Lesions are isointense or hypointense on T1-weighted images, and they show homogeneous contrast enhancement. Hypointensity on T2-weighted images may help in the differential diagnosis between Rosai–Dorfman disease and classic meningioma.

Epidemiology
The M:F ratio is estimated at 2:1, and the mean age of patients with CNS Rosai–Dorfman disease is approximately 40 years {2799}.

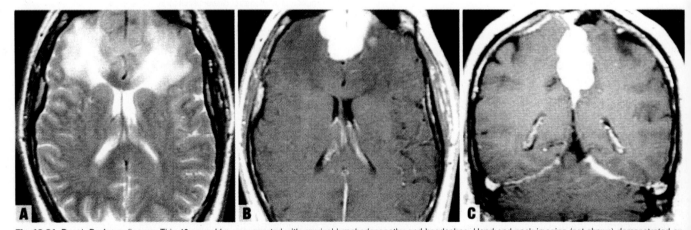

Fig. 10.21 Rosai–Dorfman disease. This 42-year-old man presented with cervical lymphadenopathy and headaches. Head and neck imaging (not shown) demonstrated extensive enhancing, enlarged cervical lymph nodes. **A** This T2-weighted axial MRI shows a lobulated, nearly isointense dural-based mass along the anterior falx cerebri. The adjacent frontal white matter is severely oedematous. **B** T1-weighted, postcontrast axial MRI shows that the dural-based bifrontal lobulated mass enhances intensely and uniformly. **C** Coronal postcontrast T1-weighted image shows another lobulated, intensely enhancing mass along the posterior falx cerebri. Both tentorial leaves are thickened and there is another focal mass along the left tentorium.

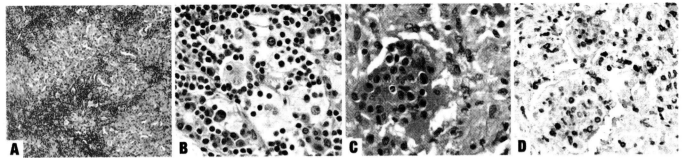

Fig. 10.22 Rosai–Dorfman disease. **A** Multinodular mass composed of a mixed inflammatory infiltrate, including large pale histiocytes, numerous lymphocytes, and plasma cells. **B** This mass involved the dura. Some large histiocytes contain plasma cells or lymphocytes in the cytoplasm (emperipolesis). **C** Emperipolesis with histiocytic engulfment of intact lymphocytes, plasma cells, neutrophils, and eosinophils. **D** CD45 expression by phagocytosed haematopoietic cells.

Etiology
Unknown

Pathogenesis
Two recent studies found *BRAF* p.V600E (in 12.5% of cases) and mutations in *KRAS* or *NRAS* (in 25% and 12.5% of cases, respectively) {810,753}. Single cases with *ARAF, MAP2K1,* and *CSF1R* mutations have been reported {810}. However, the numbers of Rosai–Dorfman cases were limited in these high-throughput sequencing analyses of histiocytic disorders, and Rosai–Dorfman samples were among those types in which no alteration could be detected in a large proportion.

Macroscopic appearance
Rosai–Dorfman disease of the CNS is typically a firm, vaguely lobulated, yellow to greyish-white dural mass.

Histopathology
Rosai–Dorfman disease occurs as a multinodular mass composed of a mixed inflammatory infiltrate including large pale histiocytes, numerous lymphocytes and plasma cells, and variable fibrosis. Emperipolesis with histiocytic engulfment of intact lymphocytes, plasma cells, neutrophils, and occasionally eosinophils is typical, but it may be inconspicuous or absent. Notably, emperipolesis is not pathognomonic of Rosai–Dorfman disease, occasionally being encountered in other neoplastic or non-neoplastic disorders.

Immunophenotype
The neoplastic histiocytes are positive for CD11c, CD68, CD163, fascin, and S100; variably positive for lysozyme; and negative for CD1a and CD207 (langerin). Expression of cyclin D1 (possibly reflecting MAPK activation) can be diagnostically useful {195}, particularly because most cases are negative for BRAF p.V600E.

Cytology
Not applicable

Diagnostic molecular pathology
Testing for potentially mutant genes (*BRAF, ARAF, KRAS* and *NRAS,* and the rare *MAP2K1* and *CSF1R*) should be performed with sensitive assays, reflecting the frequently low proportion of neoplastic cells.

Essential and desirable diagnostic criteria
See Box 10.10.

Staging
Not applicable

Prognosis and prediction
For resectable lesions, surgery is the first therapeutic option. For non-resectable lesions, steroids, radiotherapy, and MAPK signalling pathway inhibitors may be considered. Although little is known about the long-term natural history of Rosai–Dorfman disease of the CNS, the overall prognosis appears to be favourable in most cases.

Chapter 10

Juvenile xanthogranuloma

Paulus W
Chan JKC
Idbaih A
Perry A
Sahm F

Definition

Juvenile xanthogranuloma of the CNS or the meninges, with or without systemic lesions, pathologically corresponds to its cutaneous counterpart. It is a mostly paediatric, non–Langerhans cell histiocytosis characterized by foamy histiocytes, occasional Touton giant cells, and inflammation.

ICD-O coding

9749/1 Juvenile xanthogranuloma

ICD-11 coding

2B31.0 Juvenile xanthogranuloma

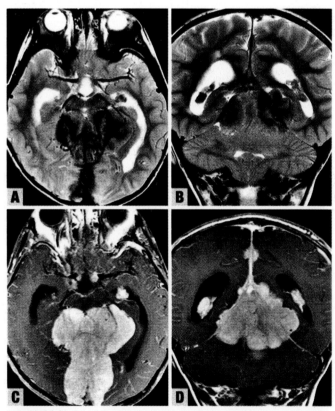

Fig. 10.23 Juvenile xanthogranuloma. A 7-year-old boy with proptosis. **A** T2-weighted axial MRI shows proptosis; both orbits are infiltrated with very hypointense soft tissue masses. There is an extensive, lobulated, hypointense mass involving the tentorium and straight sinus. Moderate obstructive hydrocephalus is present and there is a lesion in the choroid plexus of the left temporal horn. **B** T2-weighted coronal MRI shows symmetrical hypointense masses along the tentorium. The glomus in each choroid plexus is enlarged and hypointense. **C** T1-weighted, contrast-enhanced axial MRI with fat saturation. The orbital masses enhance intensely, as does the mass along the straight sinus and tentorium. **D** T1-weighted postcontrast MRI shows that the dural-based lobulated masses enhance intensely and quite uniformly, as do the masses in the choroid plexuses. There is a smaller dural-based mass along the falx cerebri.

Related terminology

None

Subtype(s)

None

Localization

Juvenile xanthogranuloma of the CNS localizes to the brain (in 53% of cases), intradural extramedullary spine (in 13%), or nerve roots (in 15%), with meningeal involvement also being common {722}.

Clinical features

Tumour lesions induce location-related neurological symptoms, whereas the rare neurodegenerative-like lesions induce more diffuse symptoms including cognitive disturbances {2503}. On MRI, tumour lesions appear isointense to hyperintense on T1-weighted images, with homogeneous contrast enhancement, and neurodegenerative-like lesions include non-enhancing hyperintense T2 signals and atrophy {2503,2371}.

Epidemiology

CNS juvenile xanthogranuloma typically occurs in children and young adults {2503,722,3365}. Neurological involvement is seen in < 5% of patients with cutaneous juvenile xanthogranuloma.

Etiology

Unknown

Pathogenesis

The frequency of *BRAF* p.V600E mutations is currently unclear. *ARAF* mutations occur in 18% of cases. *KRAS* and *NRAS* mutations are also frequent (in as many as 20% of cases) {810,753}. One study found that occasional cases can have combined *NRAS* and *ARAF* mutations {753}.

Macroscopic appearance

Juvenile xanthogranuloma lesions are often received as fragmented, soft, yellow to tan-pink biopsy specimens.

Histopathology

Juvenile xanthogranuloma (overlapping with Erdheim–Chester disease) is composed of rounded to spindled, variably vacuolated histiocytes, scattered Touton and foreign body–type giant cells, lymphocytes, and occasional eosinophils {2503}.

Immunophenotype

The neoplastic histiocytes of juvenile xanthogranuloma are CD1a-negative, CD11c-positive, CD14-positive, CD68-positive, factor XIIIa–positive, lysozyme-negative, and S100-negative. BRAF p.V600E protein is present in mutant cases {2503}.

Cytology

Not relevant

Diagnostic molecular pathology

Testing for potentially mutant genes (*BRAF*, *ARAF*, *KRAS*, and *NRAS*) should be performed with sensitive assays, reflecting the frequently low proportion of neoplastic cells. Mutations of *CSF1R* and fusions involving an NTRK gene have been reported for peripheral juvenile xanthogranuloma, so their assessment may be particularly useful in cases not limited to the CNS. For NTRK fusions, RNA sequencing or in situ hybridization can be applied, depending on the tumour cell density.

Essential and desirable diagnostic criteria

See Box 10.11.

Staging

Not applicable

Prognosis and prediction

Therapy relies on maximally safe surgery when feasible. Cytotoxic chemotherapies, radiotherapy, and molecular targeted therapies including MAPK signalling pathway inhibitors are therapeutic alternatives based on molecular characterization {2503}. Drawing prognostic conclusions about juvenile xanthogranuloma of the CNS is difficult because of its rarity.

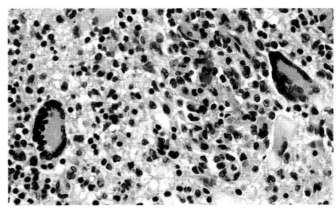

Fig. 10.24 Juvenile xanthogranuloma. Numerous foamy histiocytes and two large multinucleated Touton cells.

Box 10.11 Diagnostic criteria for juvenile xanthogranuloma

Essential:

A histiocytic tumour composed of foamy cells and a mixed inflammatory infiltrate

Desirable:

Exclusion of other lines of differentiation (glial, epithelial, melanocytic, lymphocytic, Langerhans cell, meningothelial, etc.)

BRAF, *ARAF*, *KRAS*, and *NRAS* mutation status

Evidence of cutaneous manifestations

Chapter 10

Langerhans cell histiocytosis

Paulus W
Chan JKC
Idbaih A
Osborn AG
Perry A
Sahm F

Definition

Langerhans cell histiocytosis of the CNS or the meninges is a clonal proliferation of Langerhans-type cells manifesting in the CNS or the meninges, with or without systemic lesions, which pathologically corresponds to its counterparts occurring elsewhere.

ICD-O coding

9751/1 Langerhans cell histiocytosis

ICD-11 coding

2B31.2Y & XH1J18 Other specified Langerhans cell histiocytosis & Langerhans cell histiocytosis, NOS

Related terminology

Not recommended: histiocytosis X; eosinophilic granuloma; Hand–Schüller–Christian disease; Letterer–Siwe disease; Langerhans cell granulomatosis.

Subtype(s)

None

Localization

The most common CNS involvement is via lesions of the craniofacial bone and skull base (seen in 56% of cases), with or without soft tissue extension. Intracranial, extra-axial masses are also common, particularly in the hypothalamic–pituitary region (in 25–50% of patients), meninges (30%), and choroid plexus (6%). A leukoencephalopathy-like pattern, with or without dentate nucleus or basal ganglia neurodegeneration, is seen in 36% of patients with Langerhans cell histiocytosis, and cerebral atrophy occurs in 8%. Rare intraparenchymal CNS masses have also been described {1291,1767,2557}. Langerhans cell sarcoma primarily occurring in the CNS has not been reported.

Clinical features

Patients with circumscribed tumour lesions experience acute or subacute, nonspecific and/or location-dependent neurological symptoms. Patients with neurodegenerative-like lesions present with a chronic and slowly progressing neurological pattern combining cerebellar syndrome, pyramidal tract signs, pseudobulbar palsy, and/or neuropsychiatric symptoms {1291}.

On MRI, tumour-like lesions are characterized by one or multiple masses that appear hypointense on T1-weighted images and contrast-enhanced after gadolinium infusion. On T2-weighted images, lesions and perilesional oedema are hyperintense. Neurodegenerative lesions do not exert mass effect, are not contrast enhancing, and are not surrounded by perilesional oedema. They are mainly located in the posterior fossa with symmetrical T2 hyperintensity of the corpus

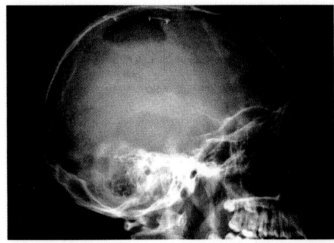

Fig. 10.25 Langerhans cell histiocytosis. X-ray showing bone lucency at site of disease.

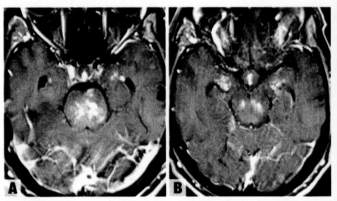

Fig. 10.26 Langerhans cell histiocytosis in a 46-year-old man with multiple cranial nerve palsies. **A** T1-weighted postcontrast axial MRI shows a thickened, enhancing infundibulum with multiple patchy enhancing lesions in the pons and both temporal lobes. **B** More cephalad T1-weighted postcontrast axial MRI shows a thickened, enhancing infundibulum with multiple patchy enhancing lesions in the pons and both temporal lobes.

medullare and symmetrical T1 hyperintensity of the dentate nuclei. Similar lesions are observed in supratentorial areas with nonspecific white matter T2 hyperintensity and symmetrical T1 hyperintensity of the basal ganglia. Over time, diffuse CNS atrophy may appear.

Epidemiology

Most cases of Langerhans cell histiocytosis occur in childhood, with an annual incidence of 0.5 cases per 100 000 individuals aged < 15 years and with an M:F ratio estimated at 1:2 {1203}.

Etiology

Unknown

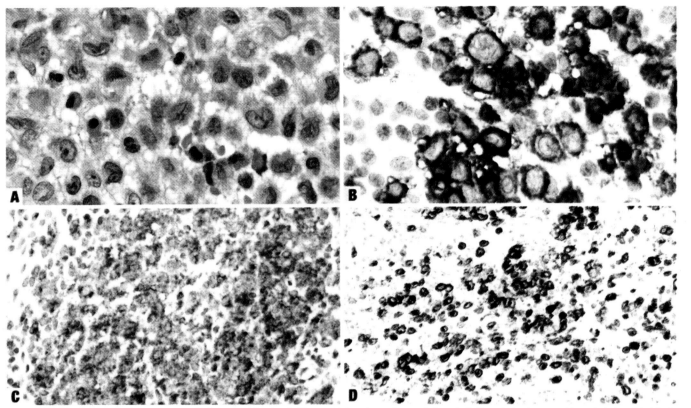

Fig. 10.27 Langerhans cell histiocytosis. **A** In this lesion involving the skull bone and dura, Langerhans cells have typically oval, deeply grooved to contorted nuclei, delicate nuclear membranes, fine chromatin, and ample lightly eosinophilic cytoplasm. There are admixed eosinophils. **B** CD1a expression by neoplastic Langerhans cells. **C** BRAF p.V600E expression in neoplastic Langerhans cells. **D** Langerhans cells are immunoreactive for CD207 (langerin).

Pathogenesis

The most frequent molecular alteration is *BRAF* p.V600E mutation, which occurs in about 50% of cases {169,2711,810}. Single cases of *BRAF* p.V600D or *ARAF* mutations, or *BRAF* fusions, have been reported {1550,2231,810}. Of the *BRAF*-wildtype cases, *MAP2K1* mutations are found in about 25% {753,386}. *NRAS*, *KRAS*, and *PIK3CA* mutations have been reported in single cases {1292,169,2711,810}.

Macroscopic appearance

Intracranial Langerhans cell histiocytosis lesions are often yellow or white and range from discrete dural-based nodules to granular parenchymal infiltrates. CNS lesions may be well delineated or poorly defined.

Histopathology

Infiltrates include neoplastic Langerhans cells and variable reactive macrophages, lymphocytes, plasma cells, and eosinophils. The nuclei of Langerhans cells are typically slightly eccentric, ovoid, and reniform or convoluted, with linear grooves and inconspicuous nucleoli. There is abundant pale to eosinophilic cytoplasm, and Touton giant cells may be seen. Copious collagen deposition is common. In the neurodegenerative lesions of the cerebellum, brainstem, and basal ganglia, there are often no obvious Langerhans cells, but inflammation accompanies severe neuronal and axonal loss, with perivascular BRAF p.V600E–positive cells with monocyte phenotype (CD14+ CD33+ CD163+ P2RY12–) nonetheless

found in some {1168,2047}. Eosinophils may aggregate and undergo necrosis, producing granulomas or abscesses.

Immunophenotype

Neoplastic Langerhans cells consistently express CD1a (surface), CD207 (also known as langerin; granular cytoplasmic), S100 (nuclear and cytoplasmic), and CD68 (Golgi dot-like staining, sometimes weak); about 50–60% express BRAF p.V600E

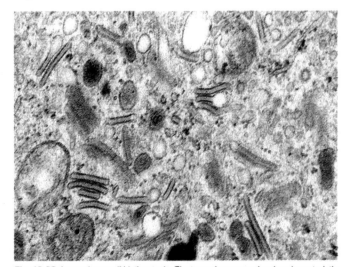

Fig. 10.28 Langerhans cell histiocytosis. Electron microscopy showing characteristic rod-shaped structures (Birbeck granules).

{1156,2778}. The Ki-67 proliferation index is highly variable, but it can reach 50%.

Cytology
Not relevant

Diagnostic molecular pathology
Testing for potentially mutant genes (*BRAF*, *MAP2K1*, *ARAF*, *NRAS*, *KRAS*, *PIK3CA*) should be performed with sensitive assays, reflecting the frequently low proportion of neoplastic cells. BRAF p.V600E can also be detected via immunohistochemistry. Independent of the specific alteration, activation of the MAPK pathway can be inferred from immunohistochemistry for phosphorylated ERK.

Essential and desirable diagnostic criteria
See Box 10.12.

Staging
Not applicable

Prognosis and prediction
Tumour-like lesions are sensitive to conventional anti-tumour treatments including vinblastine or cladribine and, in cases with an actionable target, to molecular targeted therapies (i.e. MAPK signalling pathway inhibitors), allowing a high tumour response rate and a favourable prognosis {2241,2707}. In contrast, neurodegenerative lesions are resistant or poorly sensitive to multiple therapeutic strategies, including radiotherapy, differentiating agents, immunosuppressive drugs, cytotoxic chemotherapies, and molecular targeted drugs. Neurological symptoms tend to worsen slowly over decades {1407}.

Histiocytic sarcoma

Paulus W
Chan JKC
Idbaih A
Perry A
Sahm F

Definition
Histiocytic sarcoma is a malignant proliferation of cells showing morphological and immunophenotypic features of tissue histiocytes and exhibiting no other lines of differentiation.

ICD-O coding
9755/3 Histiocytic sarcoma

ICD-11 coding
2B31.1 Histiocytic sarcoma

Related terminology
None

Subtype(s)
None

Localization
Histiocytic sarcoma can involve any site of the CNS and the meninges.

Clinical features
Neurological symptoms are related to tumour location. Neuroimaging mimics a malignant primary CNS tumour.

Epidemiology
Fewer than 100 cases have been reported, most of them in adults {2045}.

Etiology
Isolated cases of radiation-associated histiocytic sarcoma of the CNS have been reported {505,3484}.

Pathogenesis
A study of 28 histiocytic sarcomas found RAS/MAPK pathway gene alterations in 16 cases (57%; affecting mostly *MAP2K1*,

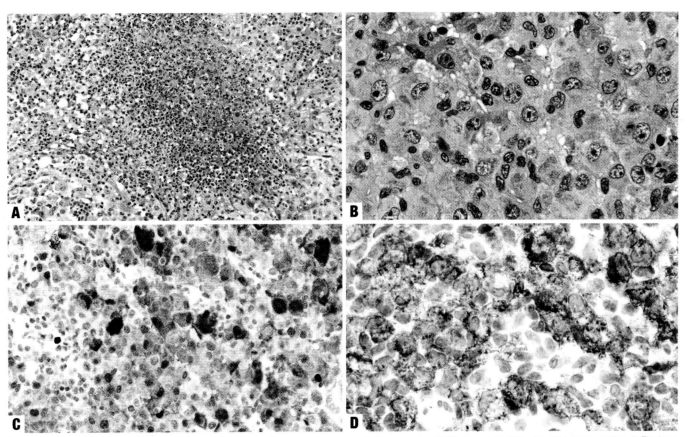

Fig. 10.29 Histiocytic sarcoma of brain. **A** This example of histiocytic sarcoma is accompanied by a prominent infiltrate of neutrophils, with areas of suppuration. **B** The large tumour cells have oval or reniform nuclei and abundant eosinophilic cytoplasm. **C** Positive immunostaining for S100 in a proportion of tumour cells is common. **D** The lineage-specific marker CD163 was diagnostic in this high-grade neoplasm.

KRAS, and *BRAF*, but also *NRAS*, *PTPN11*, *NF1*, and *CBL*) and PI3K/AKT/mTOR pathway gene alterations in 6 cases (21%; in *PTEN*, *MTOR*, *PIK3R1*, and *PIK3CA*) {2892}. Alterations in both pathways were not mutually exclusive. In addition, *CDKN2A* and/or *CDKN2B* was altered in 13 cases (46%), half of which displayed homozygous deletions. Independently, a recent study reported single cases with *KRAS*, *NRAS*, or *CSF1R* mutations, or *BRAF* fusion {810}. A single case is described with concurrent *BRAF* p.F595L and *HRAS* mutation {1707}.

Macroscopic appearance

Histiocytic sarcomas are destructive, soft, fleshy, white masses with occasional yellow necrotic foci.

Histopathology

Histiocytic sarcoma is characterized by highly cellular, non-cohesive infiltrates of large, moderately pleomorphic, mitotically active histiocytes, which have abundant eosinophilic cytoplasm, variably indented to irregular nuclei, and often prominent nucleoli. Occasional multinucleated or spindled forms are also common, as is background reactive inflammation {534,558}.

Immunophenotype

The tumour cells are typically positive for histiocytic markers (e.g. CD68, CD163, lysozyme, CD11c, and CD14); variably positive for CD34; and negative for myeloid antigens, dendritic antigens, CD30, ALK, and other lymphoid markers, as well as for glial, epithelial, and melanocytic antigens. The tumour cells are negative for the follicular dendritic cell antigens CD23 and CD35. However, follicular dendritic cell sarcoma expressing these antigens may primarily arise in the brain and must be differentiated from histiocytic sarcoma {1257}. Although MAPK alterations are common, BRAF p.V600E expression is rare {1630,2892}.

Cytology

Not relevant

Diagnostic molecular pathology

Although the proportion of *BRAF* p.V600E–mutant cases is relatively small, a variety of other MAPK gene alterations have been reported in non-CNS histiocytic sarcoma, so high-throughput sequencing may be advisable. Sequencing should cover all the potentially affected genes of the MAPK pathway (*MAP2K1*, *KRAS*, *NRAS*, *PTPN11*, *NF1*, and *CBL*), the reported altered genes of the mTOR pathway (*PTEN*, *MTOR*, *PIK3R1*, and *PIK3CA*), and *CSF1R* mutations. Rare *BRAF* fusions can be detected via in situ hybridization or RNA sequencing. *CDKN2A* and/or *CDKN2B* alterations often constitute homozygous deletions, which can be detected by in situ hybridization or array-based approaches.

Essential and desirable diagnostic criteria

See Box 10.13.

Staging

Not applicable

Prognosis and prediction

Survival time has been < 12 months after initial presentation in most reported patients.

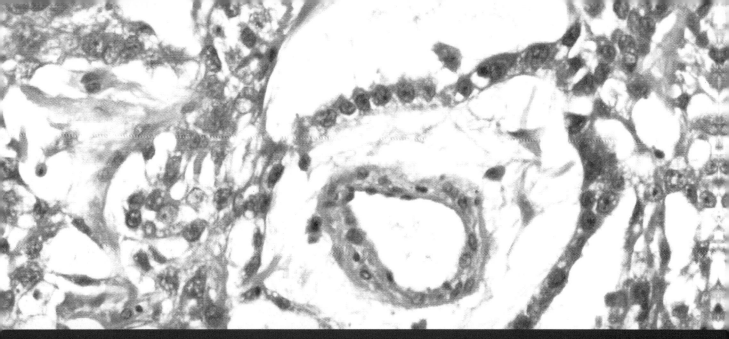

11

Germ cell tumours

Edited by: Ng HK, Srigley JR

Germm cell tumours of the CNS

Rosenblum MK
Ichimura K
Lau CC
Nishikawa R
Pietsch T
Wong TT

Definition
Germ cell tumours of the CNS are a family of morphological and immunophenotypic homologues of gonadal and other extra-neuraxial germ cell neoplasms sharing certain genetic features (see Table 11.01 for definitions of individual types).

ICD-O coding
9080/0 Mature teratoma
9080/3 Immature teratoma
9084/3 Teratoma with somatic-type malignancy
9064/3 Germinoma
9070/3 Embryonal carcinoma
9071/3 Yolk sac tumour
9100/3 Choriocarcinoma
9085/3 Mixed germ cell tumour

ICD-11 coding
2A00.1Y & XH1E13 Other specified embryonal tumours of brain & Germinoma
2A00.1Y & XH8MB9 Other specified embryonal tumours of brain & Embryonal carcinoma, NOS
2A00.1Y & XH09W7 Other specified embryonal tumours of brain & Yolk sac tumour
2A00.1Y & XH83G5 Other specified embryonal tumours of brain & Teratoma, NOS
2A00.1Y & XH8PK7 Other specified embryonal tumours of brain & Choriocarcinoma, NOS
2A00.1Y & XH2PS1 Other specified embryonal tumours of brain & Mixed germ cell tumour

Related terminology
Teratoma with somatic-type malignancy
Not recommended: malignant teratoma; teratoma with secondary malignant component; teratoma with malignant transformation.

Germinoma
Not recommended: seminoma (used for germinoma in the testis); dysgerminoma (used for germinoma in the ovary).

Yolk sac tumour
Not recommended: endodermal sinus tumour.

Choriocarcinoma
Not recommended: chorionepithelioma.

Subtype(s)
None

Localization
Approximately 80–90% of CNS germ cell tumours arise in the midline, most frequently in the pineal region followed by the suprasellar compartment (where they originate in the posterior

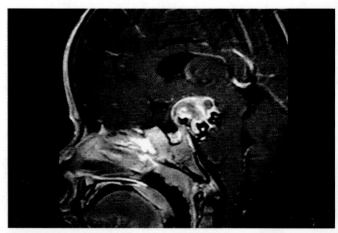

Fig. 11.01 Mature teratoma. T1-weighted, contrast-enhanced sagittal MRI in a 3-year-old boy shows a suprasellar tumour with strong contrast enhancement and teeth in the posterior and inferior parts.

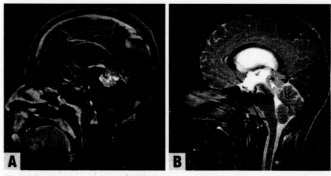

Fig. 11.02 Germinoma. Sagittal MRI of a 21-year-old man who developed headache, nausea, and Parinaud syndrome. **A** T1-weighted image shows a contrast-enhancing tumour of the pineal region. **B** T2-weighted image.

pituitary / infundibular stalk) {3108,3111}. Bifocal and multifocal examples (nearly all germinomas) typically involve these sites, but they may also occur in the basal ganglia, thalami, or other locations {3108}. A basal ganglionic location has been more frequently reported in patients in eastern Asia than in those in the USA, with the reverse being recorded for a bifocal (posterior pituitary and pineal) presentation {3111}. Germinomas can also grow as diffuse periventricular lesions, and they can arise in the cerebrum, cerebellum, posterior fossa structures, spinal cord, and sella. Congenital holocranial examples (typically teratomas) are encountered.

Clinical features
Pineal region tumours compress the cerebral aqueduct, causing hydrocephalus and intracranial hypertension, and they can produce paralysis of upward gaze and convergence (Parinaud syndrome) by compressing or invading the tectal plate. Preserved pupillary accommodation with impaired constriction

Table 11.01 Definitions and diagnostic criteria for germ cell tumours of the CNS

Type	Definition	Essential diagnostic criteria
Mature teratoma	A germ cell tumour composed solely of fully differentiated, adult-type somatic tissue components that recapitulate the differentiating potential of the ectoderm, endoderm, and mesoderm	• A germ cell tumour with components exhibiting differentiation along at least two of the three somatic tissue lines (ectoderm, endoderm, mesoderm) • Fully differentiated, adult-type histology (absence of fetal-type elements) • Absence of other germ cell tumour components
Immature teratoma	A germ cell tumour containing incompletely differentiated, fetal-like somatic tissue components that recapitulate the differentiating potential of the ectoderm, endoderm, and mesoderm; mature elements may be admixed	• Identification of incompletely differentiated elements exhibiting differentiation along at least two of the three somatic tissue lines (ectoderm, endoderm, mesoderm) in a teratoma, or the identification of any such elements within a tumour otherwise qualifying as a mature teratoma • Absence of other germ cell tumour components
Teratoma with somatic-type malignancy	A germ cell tumour of mature or immature teratomatous type that develops a distinct secondary component resembling a somatic-type malignant neoplasm (e.g. sarcoma or carcinoma) as seen in other organs and tissues	• Identification of a distinct histological component that has the cytological features, architecture, mitotic activity, and disorderly growth pattern expected of a sarcoma, carcinoma, or other defined type of somatic cancer in a mature or immature teratoma
Germinoma	A malignant germ cell tumour composed of cells resembling primordial germ cells	• A germ cell tumour containing large tumour cells with typical cytological characteristics • Nuclear OCT4 and widespread membranous KIT (or podoplanin [D2-40]) immunoreactivity, or absence of 5-methylcytosine expression • Absence of CD30 expression • Absence of AFP expression • hCG immunoreactivity in syncytiotrophoblastic giant cells (for the specific diagnosis of germinoma with syncytiotrophoblastic elements) • Absence of other germ cell tumour components (except syncytiotrophoblastic giant cells for the specific diagnosis of germinoma with syncytiotrophoblastic giant cells)
Embryonal carcinoma	A malignant germ cell tumour composed of large epithelioid cells resembling those of the embryonic germ disc	• A germ cell tumour with large epithelioid cells as described in the *Histopathology* subsection • CD30 and OCT4 expression • Absent or only focal, non-membranous KIT expression • Absence of hCG expression • Absence of AFP expression • Absence of other germ cell tumour components • Cytokeratin expression is desirable
Yolk sac tumour	A malignant germ cell tumour that differentiates to resemble extraembryonic structures, including the yolk sac, allantois, and extraembryonic mesenchyme	• A germ cell tumour with epithelioid cells arranged in any of the patterns described in the *Histopathology* subsection, with or without mesenchymal components • Absence of other germ cell tumour components • AFP expression • Absent or only focal, non-membranous KIT expression • Absent or only focal CD30 expression • Absence of β-hCG expression
Choriocarcinoma	A malignant germ cell tumour that differentiates to resemble the trophoblastic cells of the extraembryonic chorion, including syncytiotrophoblastic and cytotrophoblastic elements	• A germ cell tumour with both syncytiotrophoblastic and cytotrophoblastic elements but no other germ cell tumour components • β-hCG expression • Absence of KIT (or podoplanin [D2-40]) expression • Absence of AFP expression • Absence of OCT4 expression
Mixed germ cell tumours	Malignant germ cell tumours harbouring at least two germ cell tumour subtypes in any combination	• A germ cell tumour with at least two distinct germ cell tumour subtypes

(Argyll Robertson pupil) is also frequent. Posterior pituitary / suprasellar lesions produce visual disturbances by impinging on the optic chiasm, and they often cause diabetes insipidus, delayed growth, and delayed sexual maturation by disrupting the hypothalamic–pituitary axis. Germ cell tumours producing hCG can cause precocious puberty in boys and (rarely) in girls {2325,3020}.

Imaging
Teratomas excepted, germ cell tumours are usually solid and contrast enhancing on CT/MRI {995,1884}. Intratumoural cysts, calcification, and regions of low signal attenuation characteristic of fat suggest teratoma, whereas haemorrhage is commonly associated with choriocarcinomatous elements.

Epidemiology
CNS germ cell tumours principally affect children, and they are more prevalent in eastern Asia than in Europe and the USA. Age-adjusted annual incidence rates of 0.45 cases per 100 000 population aged < 15 years and 0.49 cases per 100 000 population aged < 19 years have been reported from Japan {1989} and the Republic of Korea {1546}, respectively; these rates (the highest recorded) are more than triple those in Germany {1520} and the USA {2344}. CNS germ cell tumours account for 2–3% of

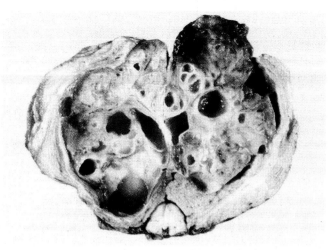

Fig. 11.03 Teratoma. Large immature teratoma of the cerebellum in a 4-week-old infant, with characteristic cysts and chondroid nodules.

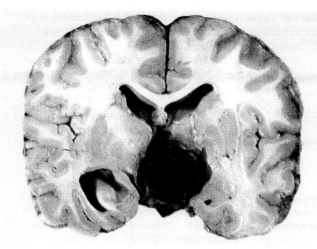

Fig. 11.04 Germinoma. Suprasellar tumour from a 7-year-old girl.

all primary intracranial neoplasms and for 8–15% of paediatric examples in series from Japan {350}; Taiwan, China {1321}; and the Republic of Korea {1546}. In contrast, these tumours account for only 0.3–0.6% of primary intracranial tumours in adults, and 3–4% of those affecting children, in series from India {1527}, Europe {656}, England {715}, and North America {1326,290}. Incidence peaks in patients aged 10–14 years, and a clear majority of all histological types involve male patients {290,1321,2817,1989,1546}. More than 90% of pineal examples affect male patients, but there is no sex predilection in posterior pituitary / suprasellar cases {2042,3110}. Cases involving members of the same family are rare {1160}. Pure germinomas outnumber other types, with mixed lesions and teratomas being next most common; embryonal carcinomas, yolk sac tumours, and choriocarcinomas occur uncommonly in pure form {1321, 290,2042,3111}.

Etiology

Germline variants of the *JMJD1C* gene, which encodes a jumonji domain–containing histone demethylase, have been associated with a heightened risk of CNS germ cell tumours in Japanese people {1762}. An increased risk of CNS germ cell tumours in the setting of Klinefelter syndrome (47,XXY) {1526, 3450,2362} implicates X chromosome–associated genes that presumably escape normal inactivation. An excess of CNS germ cell tumours appears to occur in Down syndrome (trisomy 21) {2133}.

Genetic observations argue against a shared etiology (or pathogenesis) for all CNS germ cell tumours. Whereas intracranial teratomas of infancy resemble teratomas of the infant testis in their generally diploid status and chromosomal integrity {2666}, CNS germ cell tumours arising after early childhood, irrespective of histological composition, share with their testicular counterparts in young men frequent aneuploidy with complex chromosomal anomalies and overlapping copy-number alterations {2851,3166,1005,3374,2861}. Particularly common are gains on chromosomes 12p, 21q, 8q, 1q, 2p, and X, and losses of 11q, 13q, 5q, 9q, and 10q. The weight of evidence, however, indicates that fewer CNS tumours exhibit isochromosome 12p, a signature abnormality of testicular (and mediastinal) primaries {2316,3068,3166,1005}. Regions of particular gain have been

reported to encompass *KRAS*, *CCND2*, and *PRDM14* (this last gene being a regulator of primordial germ cell specification), and losses of the *RB1* locus could implicate the cyclin/CDK/RB1/E2F pathway {3166,2861}.

As regards genetic drivers, gain-of-function mutations involving genes encoding MAPK pathway components (*KIT*, RAS family members) and (less frequently) PI3K/AKT/mTOR pathway components (*MTOR*, *PTEN*, and PIK3 family members) are the most common gene abnormalities identified in CNS germ cell tumours occurring beyond infancy and early childhood {1005,3374,1397,2861}. These occur across all subtypes, but they are variably represented. Germinomas exhibit a particularly high frequency of MAPK pathway–activating *KIT* (exons 11, 13, and 17) and RAS gene family mutations (found in ~60% of cases) as well as frequent coactivation of the RAS/ERK and AKT pathways, with associated severe chromosomal instability and global DNA hypomethylation signatures similar to those of primordial germ cells (and generally foreign to other CNS germ cell tumours) {1005,2861,1006}. *KIT* alterations have predominated in germinomas derived from Japanese patients {1005,1397,1006}, but they were outnumbered by RAS lesions in a cohort reported from Germany {2861}. Copy-number gains and amplifications of *KIT* and RAS genes have been documented, as have loss-of-function mutations in the tumour-suppressing *BCORL1* and *CBL* genes (the latter a negative regulator of MAPK signalling) {3374,1397}. Specific microRNAs (e.g. miR-302, miR-335, miR-371-3, and miR-654-3p) appear to be upregulated in CNS germ cell tumours {3371,2377}.

Pathogenesis

CNS germ cell tumours arising beyond infancy and early childhood may share a unifying pathogenesis and cytogenesis despite their morphological variety and epigenetic differences. This is suggested by overlapping genetic alterations leading to the activation of the MAPK and/or AKT/mTOR pathways (albeit with strikingly different mutation frequencies of *KIT* and other individual genes) {1397,2861} and by the detection of identical *MTOR* mutations in both the globally hypomethylated germinomatous component and the highly methylated non-germinomatous component of mixed lesions {1006}. The similarity of

CNS and gonadal germ cell tumours in appearance and immunophenotype, as well as in their chromosomal, genetic, and epigenetic landscapes, accords with the view that CNS germ cell tumours derive from primordial germ cells that migrate to the CNS during development. Germinomas express a panoply of primordial germ cell–associated antigens {1324} and closely resemble migratory primordial germ cells at the E10.5 stage in their widespread DNA hypomethylation and in the differentially methylated status of their imprinted genes {1006}. Mutations of *KIT* leading to ligand-independent activation could save primordial germ cells in the CNS from the apoptotic death that follows physiological suppression of *KIT* signalling in primordial germ cells that fail to migrate properly from the midline {2750}. Such cells could then spawn pure germinomas or, via epigenetic reprogramming, other germ cell tumour types. The ability of murine primordial germ cells to dedifferentiate into pluripotent stem cells and to generate teratomas in vivo has been documented {2786}, but primordial germ cells have never been identified in the human CNS {901}, and alternative theories of cytogenesis implicate other pluripotent ancestors {2327}. These include embryonic stem cells and neural stem cells, which can generate teratomas after activation of the *POU5F1* (*OCT4*) pluripotency gene {3122}, although why these stem cells would be reprogrammed to the germ cell differentiation pathway remains unexplained. The genetically distinct infantile CNS teratomas could derive, alternatively, from non-germinal stem cell elements. Whether the characteristically pure and mature teratomas of the spinal cord represent germ cell neoplasms {85} or complex malformations {1683} is debated.

Subsequent genetic events occurring within the differentiated tissue components of teratomas are presumed to drive the development of somatic cancers in these lesions; one enteric-type adenocarcinoma arising from a mature teratoma exhibiting an acquired *KRAS* mutation has been reported {1619}.

Macroscopic appearance

Mature teratomas typically have both solid components and cysts of varying diameter that may contain mucinous material. Areas of calcification and chondroid nodules may be appreciable. Haemorrhage and necrosis are typically absent.

Immature teratomas may contain cysts, regions of calcification, and chondroid nodules, but they generally have soft, fleshy components reflecting the high cellularity of immature elements.

Teratomas with somatic-type malignancy may resemble mature or immature teratomas but are more likely to exhibit regional necrosis. Overgrowth by sarcomatous components may impart a fleshy appearance, whereas mucoid/gelatinous regions may reflect the presence of mucin-producing adenocarcinoma.

Germinomas are usually solid, tan-white, soft, and friable. Focal cystic change can occur, but haemorrhage and necrosis are rare.

Embryonal carcinomas are solid, grey-white, friable masses that may exhibit regional haemorrhage and necrosis.

Yolk sac tumours are solid, grey-tan, and friable or gelatinous (due to myxoid alterations). Focal haemorrhage may be seen.

Choriocarcinomas are typically solid, haemorrhagic, and often extensively necrotic masses containing foci of grey-tan tumour tissue.

The appearances of mixed germ cell tumours reflect the macroscopic features of the constituent germ cell tumour components, as described for these tumours in pure form.

Histopathology

Mature teratoma

Mature teratomas harbour only fully differentiated, adult-type tissue elements that exhibit little if any mitotic activity. Ectodermal components commonly include epidermis and skin adnexa, central nervous tissue, choroid plexus, and salivary gland acini. Smooth and striated muscle, cartilage, bone, and adipose tissue are typical mesodermal representatives. Glands that are lined by respiratory or enteric-type epithelia and are often cystically dilated are the usual endodermal participants, but hepatic and pancreatic tissue may be encountered. Gut- and bronchus-like structures replete with mucosa and muscular coats or with cartilaginous rings, respectively, can be formed. Exceptional intracranial teratomas contain remarkably organized, fetus-like bodies {2218}.

Re-resection specimens deriving from germ cell tumours displaying progressive enlargement in the course of adjuvant

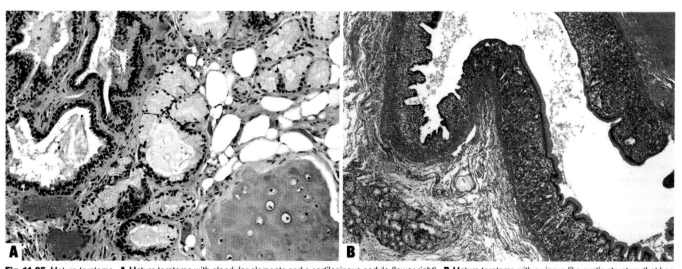

Fig. 11.05 Mature teratoma. **A** Mature teratoma with glandular elements and a cartilaginous nodule (lower right). **B** Mature teratoma with a viscus-like cystic structure that has a mucosa that is partly of gastric type, with muscularis mucosa and submucosal glands.

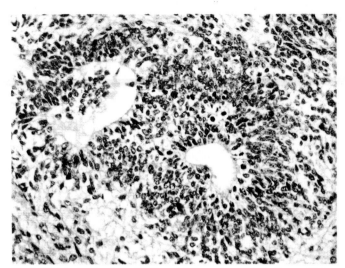

Fig. 11.06 Immature teratoma. Undifferentiated neural component with neural tube–like formations in an immature teratoma.

therapy or recurrence after initially complete response to treatment may be composed solely of mature teratomatous elements, a seemingly paradoxical scenario termed "growing teratoma syndrome" {2355,3236}. Although the simple expansion of cystic components can play a role in this phenomenon, Ki-67 immunohistochemistry may reveal surprisingly elevated labelling activity within their ostensibly differentiated tissues {2355}.

Immature teratoma

The identification of even minor tissue components having incompletely differentiated, fetal-like appearances mandates the classification of a teratoma as immature. Commonly represented are hypercellular and mitotically active stromal elements resembling embryonic mesenchyme, glands lined by crowded columnar cells with clear subnuclear and apical cytoplasm (in mimicry of fetal gut and respiratory mucosa), and primitive central neuroepithelial elements that may form multilayered rosettes or canalicular arrays of neural tube–like appearance. Abortive retinal differentiation is reflected in the presence of clefts lined by melanotic neuroepithelium.

The components of immature teratomas exhibit the immunohistochemical profiles expected of their somatic tissue counterparts. Retained expression of SMARCB1 (INI1), a general feature of CNS germ cell tumours {1208}, may assist in distinguishing teratomas with multilayered neuroepithelial rosettes from atypical teratoid/rhabdoid tumours containing similar structures {3373}. For the distinction of immature teratomas and C19MC-altered embryonal tumours with multilayered rosettes, see the *Diagnostic molecular pathology* subsection, below.

Teratoma with somatic-type malignancy

The somatic-type cancers most commonly encountered in teratomas with somatic-type malignancy are rhabdomyosarcomas and undifferentiated sarcomas {290,2042,2746}, followed by enteric-type adenocarcinomas {982,1619} and squamous carcinomas {2042}. The possibility of a teratomatous derivation must also be kept in mind in the evaluation of primitive-appearing neuroepithelial neoplasms arising in the age groups and locations favoured by CNS germ cell tumours {3252}. Erythroleukaemia {1285} and leiomyosarcoma {2951} have been described as secondary malignant components, as has a carcinoid tumour associated with an intradural spinal teratoma {1416}. The pathogenesis of a composite intrasellar tumour containing elements of Burkitt-like B-cell lymphoma and germinoma is unclear {3262}. Yolk sac tumour components have been the speculated progenitors of enteric-type adenocarcinomas encountered in selected cases {982}. Cytological atypia alone, even when pronounced, should not prompt the diagnosis of somatic-type malignant transformation, this being a feature of some otherwise mature teratomas (especially after adjuvant therapy).

Germinoma

Germinomas are composed of large, undifferentiated-looking cells that have round, vesicular, and centrally positioned nuclei with prominent nucleoli, and abundant cytoplasm that is often clear due to glycogen accumulation. An example exhibiting rhabdoid features has been described {3106}. Tumour cells are disposed in sheets, lobules, or (in cases manifesting desmoplasia) regimented cords and trabeculae. Mitotic activity is variable, necrosis uncommon. Delicate fibrovascular septa infiltrated by small lymphocytes are typical, with tumour cells occasionally being obscured by florid lymphoplasmacytic and histiocytic infiltrates {3579} or an intense granulomatous reaction mimicking sarcoidosis or tuberculosis {1698}.

Consistent cell membrane and Golgi region immunoreactivity for KIT and membranous labelling for D2-40 distinguish germinomas from solid variants of yolk sac tumour, embryonal carcinomas, and other germ cell neoplasms {1399,1034}. Complete loss of nuclear 5-methylcytosine immunoreactivity by tumour cells is also unique to germinomas, reflecting a global DNA hypomethylation foreign to other germ cell tumour types {2861}. Germinomas share nuclear OCT4 expression with embryonal carcinomas {1399}. Inconsistent and nonspecific is PLAP expression {290,1321}, and similarly non-discriminating is reactivity for LIN28A {457} as well as nuclear labelling for the transcription factors NANOG {2804}, HESRG {3388}, UTF1 {2383}, and SALL4 {1399}. CD30 and AFP expression is typically absent. Labelling of a minority of germinomas by the CAM5.2 and AE1/AE3 cytokeratin antibodies (in dot-like or more diffuse cytoplasmic fashion) may signal early differentiation along epithelial/carcinomatous lines but is without demonstrated clinical significance {2118}. Germinoma cell subsets may express β-hCG, and syncytiotrophoblastic elements expressing hPL and β-hCG may be found in otherwise pure germinomas and should not prompt a diagnosis of choriocarcinoma. Tumours having such components must be reported as germinoma with syncytiotrophoblastic giant cells.

Immunohistochemical and other studies have shown that the reactive infiltrates within germinomas include T cells (both CD4+ and CD8+ elements being represented), B cells, plasma cells, and histiocytes, in varying proportions {3452,3579,3109}. PD1-immunoreactive lymphocytes are commonly present but variable in number {3579,3445}. One RNA sequencing / in situ hybridization study {3109} and an immunohistochemical analysis using the SP142 antibody {3445} reported PDL1 expression by germinoma cells, but this was restricted to activated macrophages in a series using the EIL3N antibody {3579}.

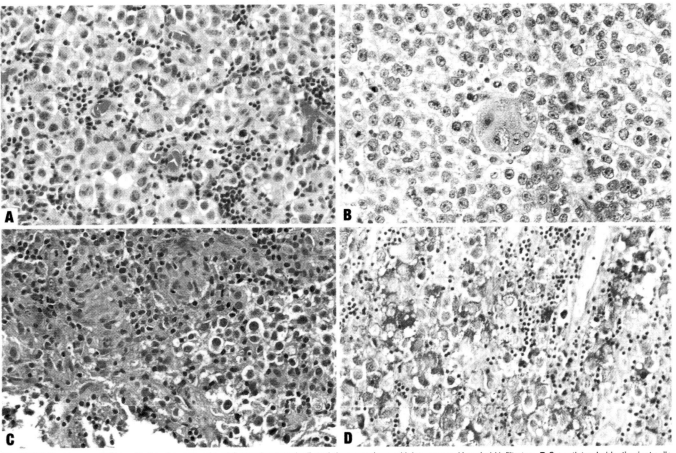

Fig. 11.07 Germinoma. **A** The cells show large round nuclei, prominent nucleoli, and clear cytoplasm with interspersed lymphoid infiltrates. **B** Syncytiotrophoblastic giant cells are sometimes present. **C** This tumour shows granulomatous inflammation. **D** There is granular cytoplasmic PAS positivity.

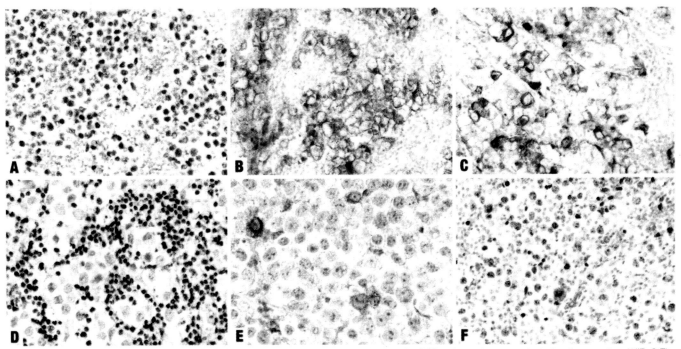

Fig. 11.08 Germinoma. **A** Immunohistochemistry for OCT4 shows nuclear expression in germinoma cells. **B** There is membranous and cytoplasmic expression of KIT. **C** The cells show PLAP expression. **D** Immunohistochemistry for 5-methylcytosine. In contrast to inflammatory cells, germinoma cells show unmethylated chromatin. **E** Germinoma cells can express β-hCG. **F** Ki-67 immunohistochemistry shows that most germinoma cells are proliferating.

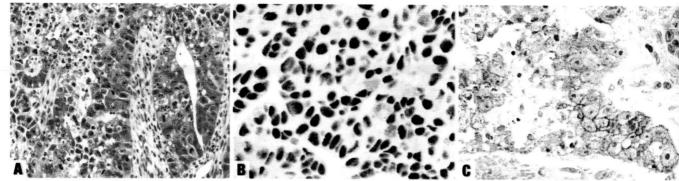

Fig. 11.09 Embryonal carcinoma. **A** The tumour is composed of pleomorphic epithelioid cells with large nuclei containing prominent nucleoli. **B** There is nuclear OCT4 expression. **C** There is CD30 expression on the cell membrane.

Embryonal carcinoma

Embryonal carcinomas are composed of large epithelioid cells with vesicular nuclei, macronucleoli, and clear to violet-hued cytoplasm. These can form nests and sheets, line gland-like spaces, and be disposed in abortive or true papillae. Embryoid bodies replete with germ discs and miniature amniotic cavities may be encountered (rarely). Conspicuous mitotic activity and zones of necrosis are common.

Cell membrane immunoreactivity for CD30, although potentially shared by the epithelial and mesenchymal components of teratomas, distinguishes embryonal carcinomas from other germ cell tumours {1399}. Consistently displaying strong cytokeratin expression, with nuclear OCT4 and SALL4 labelling {1399}, and often being PLAP-positive and LIN28A-reactive {457}, embryonal carcinomas also manifest nuclear expression of HESRG {3388}, UTF1 {2383}, and SOX2 {2805}. Focal and

non-membranous KIT expression may be seen {1399}, but AFP, β-hCG, and hPL are typically not expressed {290,1321}.

Yolk sac tumour

The neoplasm is composed of primitive-looking epithelial cells that may be associated with loose, variably cellular, and frequently myxoid stromal components resembling extraembryonic mesoblast. Epithelial elements may form solid sheets but are more commonly punctuated by irregular tissue spaces (reticular pattern) or aligned in cuboid profile along sinusoidal channels, in some cases draping fibrovascular projections to form papillae known as Schiller–Duval bodies. Flattened epithelial elements may line eccentrically constricted cysts (polyvesicular vitelline pattern), some examples containing enteric-type glands with goblet cells or exhibiting hepatocellular differentiation (hepatoid pattern). Diagnostically useful, but inconstantly

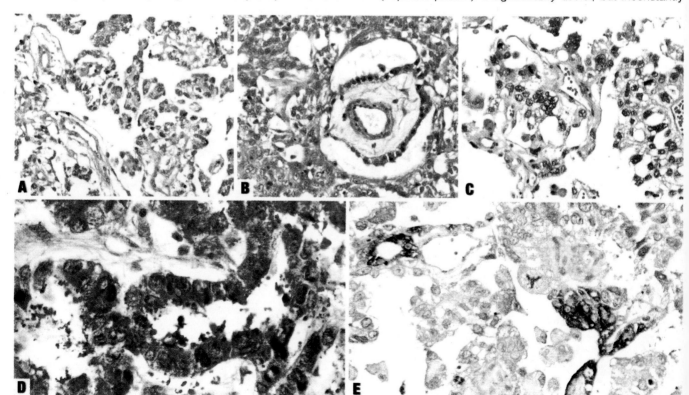

Fig. 11.10 Yolk sac tumour. **A** The characteristic growth pattern with loose histoarchitecture is shown. **B** A Schiller–Duval body. **C** Epithelioid tumour cells show trabecular and sinusoidal patterns, with increased mitotic activity. **D** There is strong, often globular PAS positivity. **E** There is focal AFP expression.

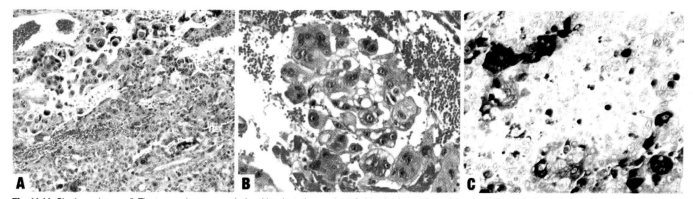

Fig. 11.11 Choriocarcinoma. **A** The tumour is composed of multinucleated syncytiotrophoblastic giant cells and cytotrophoblasts. **B** Extensive haemorrhage surrounds the tumour cells. **C** Expression of β-hCG.

present, are brightly eosinophilic, PAS-positive, diastase-resistant globules clustered in the cytoplasm of epithelial cells or extracellular spaces.

Cytoplasmic immunoreactivity for AFP, although potentially shared by the enteric glandular and hepatocellular components of teratomas, distinguishes yolk sac tumours from other germ cell neoplasms {290,1321,1034}. Hyaline globules are also reactive for AFP. Epithelial components consistently label for cytokeratins, show intense nuclear expression of SALL4, often express glypican-3 (GPC3), and may be PLAP-positive {2062}. Yolk sac tumours also express LIN28A {457} but not β-hCG or hPL. OCT4 expression is most exceptional, and KIT reactivity (rare) is focal, non-membranous, and without Golgi area accentuation when present {1399}.

Choriocarcinoma

Syncytiotrophoblastic elements are represented by giant cells containing multiple hyperchromatic or vesicular nuclei, which are often clustered in knot-like fashion within a large expanse of basophilic or violaceous cytoplasm. Such cells surround or partially drape cytotrophoblastic components, which consist of cohesive sheets of large mononucleated cells with vesicular nuclei and clear or lightly eosinophilic cytoplasm. Ectatic vascular channels, blood lakes, and haemorrhagic necrosis are characteristic. Syncytiotrophoblastic cells exhibit diffuse cytoplasmic immunoreactivity for β-hCG and hPL {290,1321,1034}. Cytokeratin expression is the rule, with some choriocarcinomas also expressing PLAP, but KIT and OCT4 labelling is not seen {1399,1034}.

Mixed germ cell tumours

Any combination of germ cell tumour subtypes can be encountered in mixed germ cell tumours. Pathologists reporting such lesions should specify the subtypes present and the relative proportions of each. The individual components display the same immunophenotypes as the subtypes in pure form (see Table 11.02).

Cytology

The cytological appearances of teratomas reflect their somatic-type tissue components. In smear and squash preparations, germinomas display large tumour cells with delicate, vacuolated cytoplasm and prominent nucleoli admixed with small lymphocytes {2239,1477}. A tigroid extracellular background may be appreciated in material stained by the Giemsa method or related methods {1477}. A pseudopapillary structuring of tumour cells can be encountered in squash preparations {156}. Embryonal carcinomas show cohesive clusters of large epithelioid tumour cells with prominent nucleoli and abundant cytoplasm in squash and smear preparations. Yolk sac tumours show cohesive clusters of epithelioid cells with distinct nucleoli in smear and squash preparations, which may also contain spindled mesenchymal elements and myxoid material. The presence of syncytiotrophoblastic giant cells in squash or smear preparations should raise the question of choriocarcinoma, particularly in a haemorrhagic and necrotic background. In mixed germ cell tumours, cytological appearances reflect the germ cell tumour components present, as described in pure form.

Table 11.02 Expression patterns of germ cell tumour markers in individual germ cell tumour components

Germ cell tumour component	OCT4	5mC	PLAP	KIT	SALL4	CD30	AFP	β-hCG	LMWCK
Germinoma	+	–	+	+	+	–	–	–/+[a]	–/+[b]
Embryonal carcinoma	+	+	+	–	+	+	–	–	+
Yolk sac tumour	–	+	+/–	–	+	–	+	–	+
Choriocarcinoma	–	+	+/–	–	+	–	–	+	+
Teratoma	–	+	–	+/–[c]	+	–	+/–[d]	–	+[e]

5mC, 5-methylcytosine; LMWCK, low-molecular-weight cytokeratin.

[a]β-hCG can be expressed in a proportion of typical germinoma cells and in syncytiotrophic giant cells in otherwise pure germinomas. [b]Cytokeratin can be expressed in a proportion of typical germinoma cells, often in a dot-like pattern. [c]KIT can be found in mesenchymal or epithelioid components (e.g. melanocytes). [d]AFP can be expressed by enteric or hepatic components. [e]Cytokeratin is expressed in the epithelial components of teratoma.

Diagnostic molecular pathology

Molecular diagnostic methods currently play only a minor role in the diagnosis and subclassification of CNS germ cell tumours, which generally rest on histopathological and immunophenotypic features. Some of the microRNAs upregulated in these lesions may be detected in the cerebrospinal fluid (CSF) or blood, making liquid biopsy potentially feasible {3371,2377}.

Immature teratomas harbouring multilayered neuroepithelial rosettes and developing neuroectodermal tissues do not demonstrate chromosome 19q13.42 amplification {2270}, a feature that distinguishes them from C19MC-altered embryonal tumours with multilayered rosettes. Genome-wide copy-number analysis may help in distinguishing immature teratomas from other tumour types, the former generally having balanced genomes.

Essential and desirable diagnostic criteria

See Table 11.01 (p. 383).

Staging

Extent of disease is established by craniospinal MRI and CSF cytology. Current pretreatment recommendations also include the examination of serum and CSF levels of AFP and hCG (see *Prognosis and prediction*, below) {2179}. Highly elevated AFP and hCG levels suggest the presence of aggressive yolk sac tumour and choriocarcinoma components, respectively, although the correlation between marker elevation and histology is imperfect (particularly in cases of limited biopsy or subtotal resection).

Prognosis and prediction

CNS germ cell tumours occurring as congenital lesions (usually immature teratomas and often immense on discovery) are associated with a high mortality rate. A literature survey of 90 fetal intracranial teratomas identified only 7 survivors after resection {1417}. The prognosis of tumours arising beyond early childhood varies by histology. The best outcomes attach to pure and fully mature teratomas (curable by surgical means alone), pure germinomas (curable by irradiation or chemoradiotherapy), and mixed tumours combining only these elements; 10-year survival rates approach or exceed 90% in these cases {2042,33,441, 3108}. Comparable rates of control have been achieved with appropriate radiation dosing {2910,2301} and radiochemotherapy {441} of germinomas that harbour syncytiotrophoblastic elements or that are associated with elevated hCG levels in the serum and/or CSF. Select series have found atypical (e.g. basal ganglionic / thalamic) locations {3108}, evidence of chromosomal instability {3108}, and high intratumoural levels of

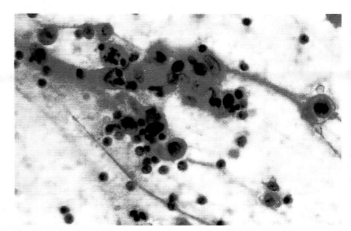

Fig. 11.12 Germinoma. Cytological touch preparation showing large pleomorphic tumour cells with clear cytoplasm admixed with inflammatory cells.

macrophage-derived NOS2 {3109} to be negative prognostic indicators, whereas conspicuous immune cell infiltration and high-level CD4 expression may carry positive implications {3109}.

Historically, dismal outcomes have characterized intracranial yolk sac tumours, embryonal carcinomas, and choriocarcinomas in pure form, as well as mixed tumours in which these were prominently represented {2042,2817,2041}. An analysis of 153 patients treated from 1963 through 1994 found that the 3-year survival rates of patients with these pure and mixed tumour types were 27% and 9.3%, respectively {2042}. Mixed tumours in which these aggressive elements were only minor components, immature teratomas, and teratomas with somatic malignant change were associated with a 3-year survival rate of 70% in this series. Regimens combining irradiation and chemotherapy have now pushed overall 5- and 10-year survival rates for patients with aggressive lesions to 75–80% {440,3108}. Logarithmic decreases of serum AFP and hCG in response to chemotherapy are favourable predictive indicators {1577}, whereas CSF or serum AFP levels > 1000 ng/ml and residual disease on completion of treatment carry negative connotations {440}. An important exception to the latter is the scenario in which a tumour that is persistent or enlarging after therapy is found to consist entirely of mature teratoma (growing teratoma syndrome), because in such cases radical resection may effect disease control {1617}. Unfortunately, long-term survivors of both germinoma and non-germinomatous tumours remain at risk of premature death due to treatment-associated malignant neoplasms, stroke, and other unwanted effects of therapy {14}.

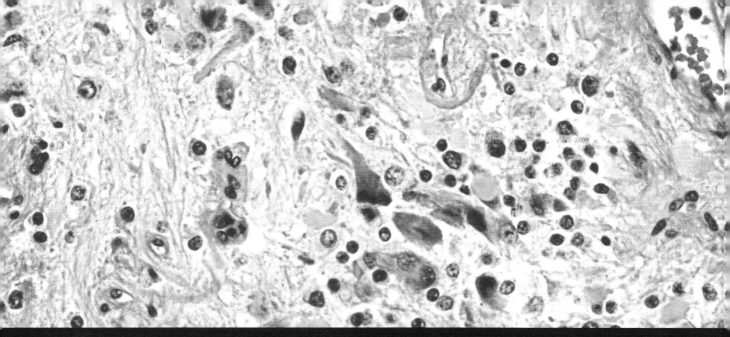

12

Tumours of the sellar region

Edited by: Brat DJ, Gill AJ, Wesseling P

Adamantinomatous craniopharyngioma
Papillary craniopharyngioma
Pituicytoma, granular cell tumour of the sellar region, and spindle cell oncocytoma
Pituitary adenoma / pituitary neuroendocrine tumour
Pituitary blastoma

Tumours of the sellar region: Introduction

Lopes MBS

Tumours of the sellar region include a diverse set of paediatric and adult neoplasms that arise in the region extending from the sella turcica inferiorly to the floor of the third ventricle superiorly. Based on current understanding of the clinical, molecular, and morphological features of these neoplasms, there have been additions of new tumour types and modifications of existing tumour types in the fifth-edition WHO classification of CNS tumours.

In past editions, adamantinomatous and papillary craniopharyngiomas were considered to be histological subtypes of craniopharyngioma. In the current edition, adamantinomatous craniopharyngioma and papillary craniopharyngioma are classified as distinct tumour types, each discussed in their own section. Although these tumours arise in the same general location and both display squamous differentiation, it is now clear that they should be classified separately, because they have distinct clinical demographics, radiological features, histopathological findings, genetic alterations, and methylation profiles {2173,1335}.

Pituicytoma, granular cell tumour of the sellar region, and spindle cell oncocytoma, which constitute a highly related family of tumour types, are discussed together in a single section {2094}. These neoplasms are all circumscribed and low-grade and arise along the posterior pituitary or infundibulum. Because of their shared immunoreactivity for thyroid transcription factor 1 (TTF1) and close clustering on methylation profiling, they are all thought to have a shared histogenesis from pituicytes, the primary glial cell of the posterior pituitary. Although these tumours may in fact represent morphological variations of the same entity, their patient demographics and clinical outcomes differ, and they are still classified separately in the current edition {832}.

Pituitary adenomas / pituitary neuroendocrine tumours (PitNETs) have been included in this fifth-edition volume because they are typically resected by neurosurgeons and diagnosed by neuropathologists. We have followed the guidelines set forth in the fourth-edition classification of endocrine tumours {1919},

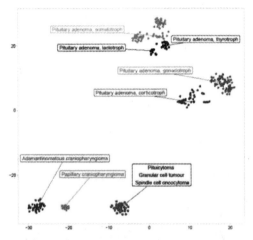

Fig. 12.01 Tumours of the sellar region. Methylation profiling of tumours of the sellar region demonstrates distinct clusters for adamantinomatous craniopharyngioma, papillary craniopharyngioma, and subtypes of pituitary adenoma / pituitary neuroendocrine tumour (PitNET). Pituicytoma, granular cell tumour, and spindle cell oncocytoma cluster together.

including the concept of classifying tumours by their anterior pituitary cell lineage according to combined immunohistochemical expression of pituitary hormones and transcription factors, as well as the definition of new subtypes, and modifications in histological grading. This chapter also introduces the new nomenclature for PitNETs proposed by the WHO Classification of Tumours' endocrine group, which will be further discussed in the fifth-edition classification of endocrine tumours {2678}.

Pituitary blastoma, a rare embryonal neoplasm of infancy composed of primitive blastemal cells, neuroendocrine cells, and Rathke pouch epithelium, has been added as a tumour type to this fifth-edition volume on CNS tumours. These tumours are strongly associated with underlying germline variation in *DICER1* {707}.

Adamantinomatous craniopharyngioma

Santagata S
Kleinschmidt-DeMasters BK
Komori T
Müller HL
Pietsch T

Definition

Adamantinomatous craniopharyngioma is a mixed solid and cystic squamous epithelial tumour with stellate reticulum and wet keratin, usually localized to the hypothalamic–pituitary axis and characterized by activating *CTNNB1* mutations.

ICD-O coding

9351/1 Adamantinomatous craniopharyngioma

ICD-11 coding

2F7A.Y & XH15X9 Other specified neoplasms of uncertain behaviour of endocrine glands & Craniopharyngioma, adamantinomatous

Related terminology

None

Subtype(s)

None

Localization

Adamantinomatous craniopharyngiomas arise anywhere along the craniopharyngeal canal, but most occur in the sellar and infundibulotuberal region {2173}. The majority (~95%) have a suprasellar component (purely suprasellar, 20–41% of cases; both suprasellar and intrasellar, 53–75%), whereas purely intrasellar craniopharyngiomas are less common (~5%) {1558}. Occasionally, a tumour extends into the anterior (9%), middle (8%), or posterior (12%) fossa. Very rare examples occur in the cerebellopontine angle and other ectopic sites {1019}.

Clinical features

Craniopharyngiomas are rarely detected incidentally (in < 2% of cases) {311}. The diagnosis is often made years after initial manifestation of nonspecific symptoms related to increased intracranial pressure, such as headache {1330,2171}. Primary manifestations include visual impairment (62–84%) {2575} and endocrine deficits (52–87%) affecting growth hormone (75%), LH or FSH (40%), TSH (25%), ACTH (25%), and antidiuretic hormone (17–27% of patients have central diabetes insipidus at diagnosis) {1558,2173}. Reduced growth rates before diagnosis may occur in patients aged as young as 12 months {2171}. Weight gain, predictive of hypothalamic obesity, tends to occur as a later manifestation, shortly before diagnosis and during the first year after diagnosis {2170}. Almost half of patients develop hypothalamic syndrome from disease- or treatment-related hypothalamic involvement or damage {2170, 2171,2172,313,843}; the hypothalamic syndrome is associated with morbid obesity, cognitive impairment, personality changes, and psychiatric symptoms {2363,2407}.

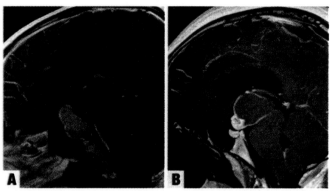

Fig. 12.02 Adamantinomatous craniopharyngioma. **A** T1-weighted postcontrast MRI showing a 34 mm sellar mass with suprasellar extension stretching the optic nerves and optic chiasm in a 22-year-old man with a 1-year history of excessive thirst and urination, fatigue, and hair loss. **B** T1-weighted postcontrast MRI showing a 37 mm predominantly cystic mass with a thin rim of enhancement extending into the third ventricle. In prior imaging there was a 16 mm region of nodular enhancement inferiorly. The 18-year-old man had a 2-month history of headache that had become acutely worse, with new onset of nausea and vomiting. The mass demonstrated peripheral calcification on CT.

Imaging

On MRI and CT images, adamantinomatous craniopharyngiomas are intrasellar and parasellar tumours with solid and cystic components {3389}. Imaging features follow a 90% rule: about 90% are predominantly cystic, about 90% have prominent calcifications, and about 90% take up contrast media in cyst walls {1486,2173}.

Spread

Local invasion of hypothalamic, visual tract, and vascular structures (including encasement of the internal carotid arteries) is common (occurring in ~25% of cases) {3556,2173}. Subarachnoid dissemination or implantation along the spinal cord, the surgical track, or the path of needle aspiration is rare {1331, 1708,2848,437}.

Epidemiology

Craniopharyngiomas constitute 1.2–4.6% of all intracranial tumours, with an incidence of 0.5–2.5 cases per 1 million person-years {409,2253,3562,2323}. Adamantinomatous craniopharyngiomas are the most common non-neuroepithelial intracerebral neoplasms in children (accounting for 5–11% of intracranial tumours in this age group) {2323,2722}. They account for nearly all craniopharyngioma diagnoses in children and about 80% of craniopharyngioma diagnoses in adults {2438,3562,2380}.

There is a bimodal age distribution {2253,3562}, with incidence peaks in children (5–15 years) and adults (45–60 years). Rare neonatal/fetal cases occur {2174,555,1525}. There is no sex predilection {409,3562,2323}.

Chapter 12

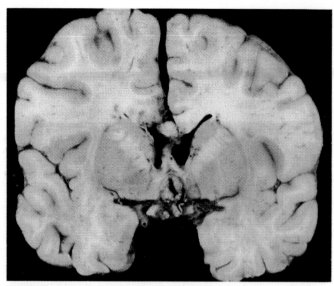

Fig. 12.03 Adamantinomatous craniopharyngioma. Solid and cystic mass with calcification, first diagnosed 4 years earlier.

Etiology

The etiology is unknown. Occasional familial adenomatous polyposis 1–associated cases of adamantinomatous cranio-pharyngioma that lack *CTNNB1* mutation and instead harbour germline *APC* mutation with somatic loss of heterozygosity have been reported {2413}.

Pathogenesis

Craniopharyngiomas are proposed to arise from cellular elements related to the Rathke pouch (craniopharyngeal duct), which is integral to pituitary development {2173}. Expression of oncogenic β-catenin in early embryonic precursors and in stem cell populations of the pituitary drive the formation of tumours resembling adamantinomatous craniopharyngioma {1047,110}. SOX2-positive progenitors may also underlie the formation of papillary craniopharyngiomas {1263} and Rathke cleft cysts {376}. Similar stem cell populations for adamantinomatous and papillary craniopharyngiomas {1037} may explain shared patterns of cytokeratin expression {1763,3143,3491,1815}; scattered cells expressing pituitary hormones {3093}, chromogranin A {3504}, and hCG {3101}; and the occasional presence of mixed transitional tumour and cyst phenotypes {2815,1128,935, 2845,2001}. In adamantinomatous craniopharyngioma, SOX2-positive stem cells may contribute to the formation of epithelial whorls with nuclear localized β-catenin. The whorls are quiescent and secrete numerous factors including sonic hedgehog, FGF, TGF-β, BMPs, and proinflammatory mediators {425,109, 649,1138,651,127,376}. These signalling centres are analogous to the enamel knot that controls tooth morphogenesis {127,376}, and they implicate paracrine signalling in tumour formation and signal transduction via primary cilia {649}. Histological and molecular parallels with odontogenic tumours suggest similar cells of origin and similar mechanisms of pathogenesis {254, 2433}, and they explain the occasional presence of teeth in adamantinomatous craniopharyngioma {225}.

Adamantinomatous craniopharyngiomas are characterized by mutations in exon 3 of *CTNNB1*, the gene that encodes the WNT signalling pathway regulator β-catenin {2877,1567, 426,355,1335,1993,1147,1234,129}. These are activating mutations, as evidenced by overexpression of β-catenin targets such as *AXIN2* and *LEF1* {1334}. Many publications report *CTNNB1* mutations in about 60–75% of samples {426,1567, 2877}, and more sensitive sequencing methods and analytical approaches identify *CTNNB1* mutations in as many as 100% of samples {355,129} by more reliably identifying low allelic fraction mutations in samples with small amounts of tumour epithelium. *CTNNB1* mutations are clonal driver events {355, 128,129}, but nuclear localization of β-catenin is observed in only some tumour cells. Additional recurrent mutations have not been reported. However, in a familial case of adamantinomatous craniopharyngioma with wildtype *CTNNB1*, germline and somatic inactivating mutations were identified in *APC* {1142}, suggesting that mutations in other components of the WNT signalling pathway may rarely contribute to the pathogenesis of craniopharyngioma. Consistent with the distinct histology and driver mutations in adamantinomatous craniopharyngioma and papillary craniopharyngioma, the tumours also display distinct methylation and transcriptional profiles {1335}. Recurrent focal deletions of Xp28 have been described in a subset of samples from male patients, and other recurrent gains have also been described {1147}.

Macroscopic appearance

Craniopharyngiomas are solid and cystic. The cyst fluid is dark greenish-brown, resembling machinery oil. Secondary changes are common, such as fibrosis, gliosis, calcifications, and cholesterol deposition. The lobulated masses have irregular surfaces that strongly adhere to surrounding structures.

Histopathology

The well-differentiated tumour epithelium forms cords, lobules, ribbons, nodular whorls, and irregular trabeculae. Peripheral crowding and palisading are prominent. Degenerative features such as fibrosis, calcification, and nodules/whorls of anucleate remnants of ghost-like squamous cells (termed "wet keratin") are common. Loose microcystic areas of stellate reticulum often intermingle between the wet keratin and more densely arranged areas of tumour epithelium. Cysts are often lined by an attenuated, flattened epithelium. Finger-like tumour protrusions extend into surrounding gliotic brain tissue with numerous Rosenthal fibres. A secondary degenerative feature is xanthogranulomatous reaction to ruptured cyst material, which is characterized by cholesterol clefts, haemosiderin deposits, xanthoma cells, multinucleated giant cells, and lymphoplasmacytic infiltrates. This extensive reaction can constitute a substantial (sometimes near-total) component of the surgically excised material, necessitating a careful search for residual, identifiable epithelium and wet keratin, as xanthogranulomas of the sellar region are associated with a ruptured/haemorrhagic Rathke cleft cyst.

Histological malignant progression in adamantinomatous craniopharyngioma is exceedingly rare, and it generally only develops after multiple recurrences and radiation therapy, often decades after first diagnosis {2701,2980,2211,3367}. Histopathological features range from squamous cell carcinoma to ameloblastic or odontogenic ghost cell carcinoma, but a large percentage lack specific histological features {2701,2102}.

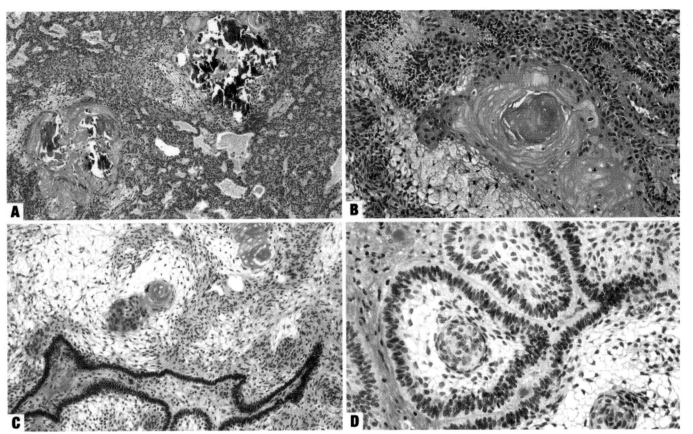

Fig. 12.04 Adamantinomatous craniopharyngioma. **A** This adamantinomatous craniopharyngioma in an adult is composed of cords and trabeculae of cells punctuated by irregularly distributed clumps of wet keratin with superimposed calcification. **B** A characteristic feature of adamantinomatous craniopharyngioma but not papillary craniopharyngioma is the presence of wet keratin, which is composed of anucleate ghost cells. A second characteristic feature limited to this type is a concentration of cells at the perimeter of the epithelial trabeculae, i.e. tumour palisading. **C** Basal palisading of tumour cells along the tumour–brain interface, epithelial whorls, stellate reticulum, and wet keratin. **D** High-power view of the interface of adamantinomatous craniopharyngioma and brain tissue; Rosenthal fibres are present in the reactive piloid gliosis.

Immunophenotype

p63 is expressed in all epithelial layers of adamantinomatous craniopharyngiomas {2142}; high–molecular weight cytokeratins (34βE12 [K903], CK5/6) and low- to intermediate-molecular-weight cytokeratins (CK7, CK17, and CK19) are also expressed {3491}. In contrast to Rathke cleft cysts, craniopharyngiomas in some studies lack CK8 and CK20 expression except in rare cells; the value of cytokeratin expression for distinguishing these two lesions is unclear {3491,1815}. PDL1 is expressed in the cyst-lining epithelium of adamantinomatous craniopharyngioma {651}. SOX2 is present in a small proportion of cells and SOX9 is widely expressed {3175}.

Adamantinomatous craniopharyngiomas have activating mutations in *CTNNB1*, which encodes the β-catenin protein. The mutation is clonal and present across the tumour epithelium {355,1147,129}; however, nuclear accumulation of β-catenin is spatially restricted and found in only a small percentage of cells, most pronounced within small epithelial whorls {426,425, 651,129}. Nuclear β-catenin is observed even when *CTNNB1* mutations are not detected {1147}.

Proliferation

Ki-67 is generally confined to palisading regions and absent in epithelial whorls. The Ki-67 proliferation index varies widely between cases and provides no prognostic information {2600, 808,1929,354}.

Grading

Adamantinomatous craniopharyngioma is regarded as CNS WHO grade 1.

Differential diagnosis

The differential diagnosis includes papillary craniopharyngioma, xanthogranuloma, Rathke cleft cyst, epidermoid and dermoid cysts, and pilocytic astrocytoma. Xanthogranuloma of the sellar region is a reactive lesion resulting from leakage, rupture, or haemorrhage of a Rathke cleft cyst, indicated by strips of columnar or ciliated columnar epithelium in the resected material {2427,94,1657,793}. They comprise cholesterol clefts, multinucleated giant cells, macrophages (xanthoma cells), lymphoplasmacytic inflammation, fibrosis, eosinophilic granular necrotic debris, and haemosiderin deposits. Epidermoid cysts are distinguished by the presence of a single cavity lined by keratinizing squamous epithelium and filled with flaky, dry keratin. Dermoid cysts additionally have adnexal structures. Rathke cleft cysts have a wall lined by simple columnar or cuboidal epithelium, which often is ciliated, with mucinous goblet cells. Myxoid/mucoid cyst contents are common. Rosenthal fibres and dense piloid gliosis adjacent to adamantinomatous craniopharyngioma can mimic pilocytic astrocytoma, but the dense cellularity and biphasic nature characteristic of pilocytic astrocytoma are absent.

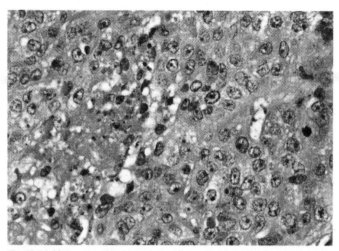

Fig. 12.05 Malignant craniopharyngioma. High-power view of malignant craniopharyngioma emerging 19 years after resection and radiation treatment of previously grade 1 craniopharyngioma. Sheets of poorly differentiated cells show severe cytological atypia, large vesicular nuclei, prominent nucleoli, mitotic activity, and necrosis.

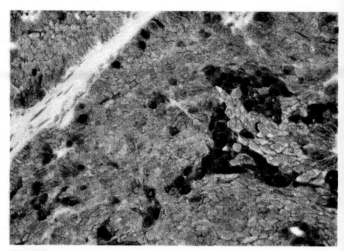

Fig. 12.06 Adamantinomatous craniopharyngioma. Even though mutations in exon 3 of the *CTNNB1* gene, which encodes β-catenin, are clonal and present across the neoplastic epithelium, β-catenin protein only accumulates in the nucleus in a subset of cells such as those scattered individually and in small clusters.

Box 12.01 Diagnostic criteria for adamantinomatous craniopharyngioma

Essential:

Tumour in the sellar region

AND

Squamous non-keratinizing epithelium, benign

AND

Stellate reticulum and/or wet keratin

Desirable:

Nuclear immunoreactivity for β-catenin

Mutation in *CTNNB1*

Absence of *BRAF* p.V600E mutation

Cytology

Not relevant

Diagnostic molecular pathology

Demonstration of *CTNNB1* mutation, as well as an absence of *BRAF* p.V600E, may be helpful in selected cases.

Essential and desirable diagnostic criteria

See Box 12.01.

Staging

Not relevant

Prognosis and prediction

Current treatment strategies for craniopharyngioma are debated; they range from gross total resection to the extended transsphenoidal endoscopic endonasal approach, through to limited surgical approaches focused on the preservation of hypothalamic and visual integrity and quality of life {959,1304,130,1979,688}. Safe total resection remains the goal when feasible (i.e. when hypothalamic integrity can be preserved). Gross total resection is associated with better recurrence-free survival than subtotal resection, but many studies do not support an advantage of gross total resection over subtotal resection followed by adjuvant radiation {800,3033,3126,673,3368,2328,2772}. Other radiotherapeutic approaches and techniques such as proton beam therapy are often considered {46,2762}.

Overall survival rates that have been described in paediatric series are 83–96% at 5 years, 65–100% at 10 years, and 62% at 20 years {1899,618}. In mixed cohorts including adults and children, reported overall survival rates are 54–96% at 5 years, 40–93% at 10 years, and 66–85% at 20 years {3290,2455, 2448}. Because overall survival rates are high, quality of life is an essential consideration. Disease- and/or treatment-related hypothalamic damage results in morbid obesity, metabolic syndrome, circadian rhythm disturbances, memory deficits, and neuropsychological impairments {843,3033,880,942,2169, 3282,313}. Although craniopharyngioma corresponds biologically to CNS WHO grade 1, the prognosis is often worse because of the large percentage of tumours that invade adjacent structures, often precluding safe gross total resection. A novel MRI-based grading system of presurgical hypothalamic involvement and surgical hypothalamic lesions shows that posterior hypothalamic involvement has a major negative impact on hypothalamic morbidity and quality of life {3033,313,880}. Accordingly, hypothalamus-sparing surgical and radiotherapeutic treatment strategies are recommended. Late mortality without tumour progression results from type 2 diabetes, cerebral and myocardial infarction, fracture, and severe infection {3335,2323}. Malignant transformation of craniopharyngioma is rare and associated with a poor prognosis {2701,2980,2211, 3367}. Although there are few studies of molecular features predictive of worse outcome, tumours with *CTNNB1* p.T41 mutations or focal deletions of Xp28 may be associated with a worse outcome {1147}.

Papillary craniopharyngioma

Santagata S
Kleinschmidt-DeMasters BK
Komori T
Müller HL
Pietsch T

Definition
Papillary craniopharyngioma is a solid or partially cystic, non-keratinizing squamous epithelial tumour that develops in the infundibulotuberal region of the third ventricle floor, most often in adults, and is characterized by *BRAF* p.V600E mutations.

ICD-O coding
9352/1 Papillary craniopharyngioma

ICD-11 coding
2F7A.Y & XH2BF0 Other specified neoplasms of uncertain behaviour of endocrine glands & Craniopharyngioma, papillary

Related terminology
None

Subtype(s)
None

Localization
Papillary craniopharyngiomas arise anywhere along the hypothalamic–pituitary axis, but there is a strong predilection for intrinsic localization within the infundibulum and tuber cinereum of the third ventricle floor. They can expand into the third ventricle cavity, and they can be located entirely within the ventricle above an intact ventricular floor. Intrasellar involvement is not common {2408,2380,3556,996,2574}.

Clinical features
Primary manifestations include headache (in 70% of cases) and visual deficits (in 63%), the latter resulting from compression of the optic chiasm, which often stabilizes or improves after surgery. Nearly all patients have some evidence of hypopituitarism (either partial hypopituitarism or panhypopituitarism, in a 70:30 ratio) manifesting as hypothyroidism (80%), hypogonadotropic hypogonadism (56%), hypocortisolaemia (50%), and growth hormone deficiency (20%). Hyperprolactinaemia is also seen due to stalk effect (in 30% of cases). Diabetes insipidus is a primary manifestation in 25% of patients, and in 70% of those patients it develops anew after surgery. Hydrocephalus is common, occurring in 30% of cases. Preoperative hypothalamic disturbances (in 63% of cases) include weight gain and psychiatric and cognitive disturbances {1777, 2407} as well as alterations in core body temperature and sleep–wake cycles {3618}.

Imaging
Papillary craniopharyngiomas are often solid, but some tumours are mixed solid/cystic or predominantly cystic. They are generally spherical (not lobulated or irregular) and calcification is infrequently seen {2812,1831,1777,996}. T1-weighted postcontrast

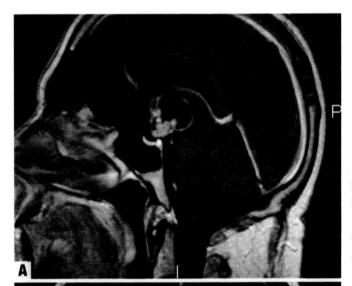
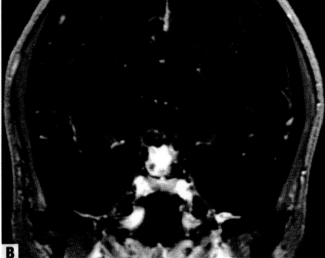

Fig. 12.07 Papillary craniopharyngioma. **A** T1-weighted postcontrast MRI showing a cystic and solid mass with peripheral and central enhancement, which proved on biopsy to be a papillary craniopharyngioma. Although the cyst and papillary mural nodule pattern is archetypal for this tumour on imaging, other examples of papillary craniopharyngioma can be predominantly solid or cystic. **B** T1-weighted postcontrast coronal MRI of a 28 mm complex cystic mass with nodular enhancement in the infundibulotuberal region and cystic components extending up into the third ventricle. The mass involved the pituitary stalk, was predominantly posterior to the optic chiasm, and abutted and displaced the hypothalamus superiorly. The 31-year-old woman presented with visual loss, headache, and mild endocrine disturbance.

MRI most often shows homogeneous enhancement, with only a small proportion of cases showing heterogeneous enhancement. The pituitary stalk is often visible and thickened, and the hypothalamus is often below the tumour {3556,2574}. Cystic lesions often have a solid, cauliflower-like nodule. Cysts are hypointense on T1-weighted non-contrast images {2812}.

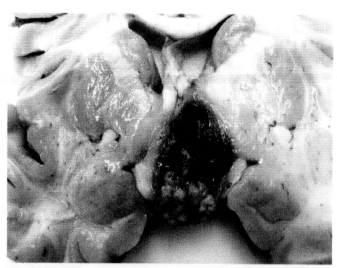

Fig. 12.08 Papillary craniopharyngioma. Fixed coronal section of papillary craniopharyngioma showing a solid and cystic mass involving the infundibulotuberal region and third ventricle in an adult patient without prior surgical intervention. The tumour mass has a cauliflower-like configuration. Calcifications are absent.

Spread

Local recurrence occurs in about 25% of patients who have involvement of the hypothalamus and other vital neural and vascular structures {2380,2173}. Ectopic recurrence is a rare complication that occurs along the surgical track or at other sites in the CNS via cerebrospinal fluid spread in the subarachnoid space {3525,437}.

Epidemiology

Incidence

Papillary craniopharyngiomas constitute 1.2–4.6% of all intracranial tumours, with an incidence of 0.5–2.5 cases per 1 million person-years {409,2253,3562,2323}. They account for about 10% of all craniopharyngioma diagnoses and 12–33% of those arising in adults {800,19,2438,2380,1777,2772}.

Age and sex distribution

Papillary craniopharyngioma is principally a disease of adults (peak incidence in patients aged 30–59 years), with tumours arising in paediatric patients only rarely {657,2438,3562,329}. There is no reported sex predilection {657,3562}.

Etiology

Unknown

Pathogenesis

Craniopharyngiomas have been proposed to arise from cellular elements related to the Rathke pouch / craniopharyngeal duct, which is integral to pituitary development {2173}. SOX2-positive progenitors may underlie the formation of papillary craniopharyngiomas {1263} and Rathke cleft cysts {376}. The development of papillary and adamantinomatous types of craniopharyngioma from similar stem cell populations {1037} may explain shared patterns of cytokeratin expression {1763, 3143,3491,1815}; scattered cells expressing pituitary hormones {3093}, chromogranin A {3504}, and hCG {3101}; as well as the occasional presence of mixed transitional tumour and cyst phenotypes {2815,1128,935,2845,2001}.

Almost all papillary craniopharyngiomas have *BRAF* p.V600E mutations {355,1803,2869,1147,1335,1993,1234} leading to activation of the MAPK/ERK pathway. No other recurrent mutations have been reported. Only a relatively low number of non-synonymous somatic mutations are present in papillary craniopharyngiomas compared with other tumour types in large cohorts {355}. Consistent with the distinct histology and driver mutations in papillary craniopharyngioma (*BRAF* p.V600E mutations) and adamantinomatous craniopharyngioma (*CTNNB1* mutations) the tumours also display distinct methylation and transcriptional profiles {1335}. Papillary craniopharyngiomas show stable genomic copy-number profiles without recurrent chromosomal gains or losses {2665,1147}.

Macroscopic appearance

Papillary craniopharyngiomas tend to be predominantly solid or mixed solid/cystic, but a small proportion can also be mostly cystic; the cystic tumours generally have a cauliflower-like solid nodule. The cyst contents are typically described as viscous and yellow {657}. Calcifications are generally absent. The tumours are generally circumscribed, spherical, and not widely adherent to surrounding brain tissue. The surface can have a papillary pattern.

Histopathology

Papillary craniopharyngiomas have non-keratinizing mature squamous epithelium covering fibrovascular cores or a cyst wall. Stellate reticulum and flaky and wet keratin are absent {19,657}. Calcifications are rare. Crowding is present in the basal cell layer but pronounced palisading is absent. Epithelial whorls and collagenous whorls are present, but they are distinct from those of adamantinomatous craniopharyngioma. Mitoses are infrequent. The tumour–brain interface is well demarcated and invasive protrusions are absent {19}. Tumour-infiltrating neutrophils are common; T cells and macrophages are also present throughout the fibrovascular cores and tumour epithelium. In as many as one third of cases, there are single or small groups of PAS-positive goblet cells within the squamous epithelium, and in a small number of cases there are regions of ciliated epithelium. These histological features overlap those of Rathke cleft cysts with extensive squamous metaplasia.

Histological malignant progression in craniopharyngioma is exceedingly rare; it generally develops after multiple recurrences of adamantinomatous craniopharyngioma and receipt of radiation therapy, often decades after initial diagnosis {2701, 2980,2211,3367}. Malignant progression of papillary craniopharyngioma has been reported {1032,3367}, but none of those cases were tested for *BRAF* p.V600E mutations.

Immunophenotype

p63 is expressed in all epithelial layers {2142}. High-molecular-weight cytokeratins (34βE12 [K903] and CK5/6) and low- to intermediate-molecular-weight cytokeratins (CK7, CK17, and CK19) are expressed {3491}. CK7 expression is confined to the superficial epithelial layer {1763}. Some studies indicate that craniopharyngiomas lack CK8 and CK20 expression except in rare cells, in contrast to Rathke cleft cysts; the value of cytokeratin expression for distinguishing these two lesions is unclear {3491,1815}. Primary cilia are present in the basally

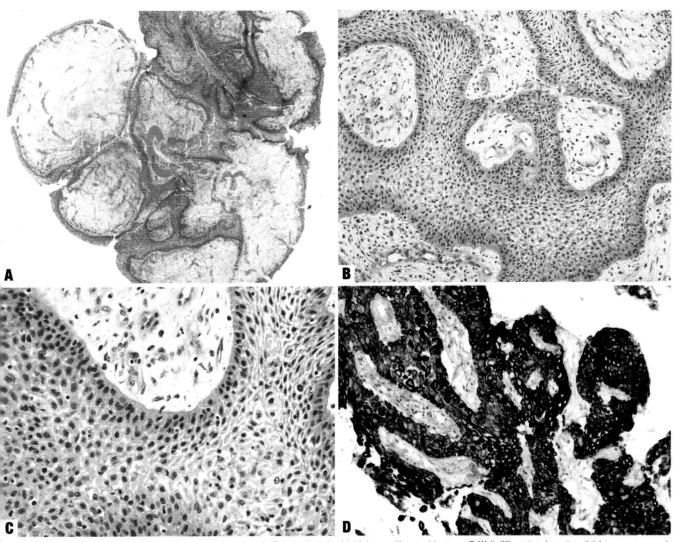

Fig. 12.09 Papillary craniopharyngioma. **A** Low-power view of an H&E-stained section highlights papillary architecture. **B** Well-differentiated non-keratinizing squamous epithelium covering fibrovascular cores that contain a low density of fibroblasts and immune cells including lymphocytes, macrophages, and neutrophils. **C** Well-differentiated non-keratinizing squamous epithelium with intercellular bridges and abundant tumour-infiltrating neutrophils, which are common in these tumours. **D** Immunohistochemistry for CK5/6 (an antibody against the intermediate-weight keratins CK5 [58 kDa] and CK6 [56 kDa]) is positive throughout all layers. Staining for CK19 is also positive. Another marker commonly used to assess squamous cell carcinomas of all types, p63, is also immunoreactive in almost all papillary and adamantinomatous craniopharyngiomas.

oriented tumour cells near the fibrovascular stroma {649}. PDL1 is expressed in multiple layers of tumour cells circumferentially surrounding the fibrovascular stroma {651}. SOX9 is variably expressed, and the expression of SOX2 requires further assessment {1263,3175}.

Nearly all papillary craniopharyngiomas have *BRAF* p.V600E mutations {355}, which can be identified across the tumour epithelium using mutation-specific antibodies, thereby distinguishing papillary craniopharyngioma from adamantinomatous craniopharyngioma and Rathke cleft cyst {1498,2869,1622}; Rathke cleft cyst displays antibody cross-reactivity in motile cilia {1498}. In papillary craniopharyngioma, β-catenin is confined to the cytoplasmic membrane {355}.

Grading

Papillary craniopharyngioma is regarded as CNS WHO grade 1.

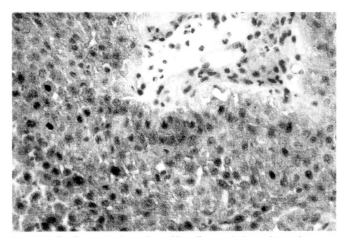

Fig. 12.10 Papillary craniopharyngioma. All papillary craniopharyngiomas show cytoplasmic immunoreactivity for BRAF p.V600E.

Proliferation

Ki-67 is generally confined to the basal layers {354,1263}. The proliferation index varies widely between cases and provides no prognostic information {808,1929}.

Differential diagnosis

The differential diagnosis of papillary craniopharyngioma includes adamantinomatous craniopharyngioma, xanthogranuloma, Rathke cleft cyst, epidermoid and dermoid cysts, and pilocytic astrocytoma. When accompanied by extensive squamous metaplasia, Rathke cleft cyst can be difficult to discriminate from papillary craniopharyngioma because the latter can also contain ciliated columnar cells and goblet cells. Importantly, Rathke cleft cysts lack *BRAF* p.V600E mutations {1498,2869}.

Cytology

Not clinically relevant

Diagnostic molecular pathology

Demonstration of *BRAF* mutation confirms the diagnosis, whereas *CTNNB1* mutation suggests adamantinomatous craniopharyngioma {1234}.

Essential and desirable diagnostic criteria

See Box 12.02.

Staging

Not relevant

Prognosis and prediction

Studies often report outcome measures that include patients with adamantinomatous and papillary craniopharyngioma, with papillary craniopharyngioma often making up only 10–20% of the total. Therefore, information about prognosis and complications specifically for patients with papillary craniopharyngioma is limited. It has been proposed that papillary

Box 12.02 Diagnostic criteria for papillary craniopharyngioma

Essential:

Tumour in the sellar region

AND

Non-keratinizing mature squamous epithelium covering fibrovascular cores or a cyst wall

Desirable:

Immunoreactivity for BRAF p.V600E

Presence of *BRAF* p.V600E mutation

Absence of nuclear β-catenin immunoreactivity

Absence of *CTNNB1* mutation

craniopharyngioma has a better prognosis, in part because of its well-demarcated spherical shape and fewer points of adhesion, which facilitate complete resection {3149,19}, but other studies have shown no significant difference in prognosis between adamantinomatous and papillary craniopharyngioma {657,3410,800,2380}. Extent of resection is > 95% in 80% of patients {1777}. Recurrence for papillary craniopharyngioma occurs in 20–35% of patients {1777,2380}. For craniopharyngioma as a whole, a higher recurrence-free survival rate is achieved with gross total resection than with subtotal resection, but many studies do not support the notion that gross total resection has an advantage over subtotal resection followed by adjuvant radiation therapy in terms of progression-free survival {800,673,2328,2772}. In mixed cohorts including adults and children, overall survival rates are 54–96% at 5 years, 40–93% at 10 years, and 66–85% at 20 years {3290,2455,2448}. Rapid and dramatic tumour responses have been reported in patients with *BRAF* p.V600E–mutant papillary craniopharyngioma treated with BRAF and/or MEK inhibitors {354,1515}; a multicentre phase II clinical trial is ongoing to evaluate targeted treatment {610}.

Pituicytoma, granular cell tumour of the sellar region, and spindle cell oncocytoma

Lopes MBS
Kleinschmidt-DeMasters BK
Mete O
Roncaroli FR
Shibuya M

Definition

Pituicytoma, granular cell tumour of the sellar region, and spindle cell oncocytoma constitute a distinct family of low-grade neoplasms that arise from pituicytes of the posterior pituitary or infundibulum, most likely representing a spectrum of a single nosological entity, all showing expression of thyroid transcription factor 1 (TTF1).

ICD-O coding

9432/1 Pituicytoma
9582/0 Granular cell tumour of the sellar region
8290/0 Spindle cell oncocytoma

ICD-11 coding

2F7A.Y & XH59V4 Other specified neoplasms of uncertain behaviour of endocrine glands & Pituicytoma
2F7A.Y & XH2XW8 Other specified neoplasms of uncertain behaviour of endocrine glands & Granular cell tumour of the sellar region
2F7A.Y & XH26P7 Other specified neoplasms of uncertain behaviour of endocrine glands & Spindle cell oncocytoma

Related terminology

Pituicytoma
Not recommended: pilocytic astrocytoma of the posterior pituitary; posterior pituitary astrocytoma; infundibuloma.

Granular cell tumour of the sellar region
Not recommended: Abrikossoff tumour; choristoma; granular cell myoblastoma; granular cell neuroma; granular cell schwannoma.

Spindle cell oncocytoma
Not recommended: spindle cell oncocytoma of the adenohypophysis.

Subtype(s)

None

Localization

Pituicytomas, granular cell tumours, and spindle cell oncocytomas arise along the length of the posterior pituitary and infundibulum, forming suprasellar or sellar/suprasellar masses. Spindle cell oncocytomas occasionally extend into the cavernous sinus and invade the sellar floor {2911}.

Clinical features

Symptoms are indistinguishable from those of other regional lesions and include headaches, visual field defects, and hypopituitarism {2911}. Diabetes insipidus is uncommon {647}. Pituicytomas and granular cell tumours have been reported in association with synchronous functional corticotroph and somatotroph adenomas/tumours {1402,2749,444}. A small number of patients with pituicytomas and granular cell tumours have presented with hypercortisolism or acromegaly without demonstration of a synchronous pituitary adenoma / pituitary neuroendocrine tumour (PitNET) {1402}. Massive intraoperative bleeding or spontaneous haemorrhage can occur in spindle cell oncocytomas, possibly owing to their hypervascularity {1658}.

Imaging

No specific features have been identified to distinguish these three lesions from clinically non-functioning pituitary tumours. They are isointense on T1-weighted MRI and show either homogeneous or heterogeneous enhancement. T2-weighted MRI reveals various intensities {647,2911}.

Epidemiology

Pituicytoma, granular cell tumour, and spindle cell oncocytoma are rare; there are no epidemiological data available at present. A recent meta-analysis of literature published in either English or Spanish identified about 270 cases of the entire group {1180}. The majority of these tumours occurred in adults in the fifth and sixth decades of life (median: 48 ± 21.8 years) {1180}; patients with spindle cell oncocytoma were older (mean age: 61.6 years) {2718}. Sex distribution varies in the literature; a slight male predominance is reported for pituicytoma {647,2792} and a slight female predominance has been reported for spindle cell oncocytoma {647} and granular cell tumour {647,3600}.

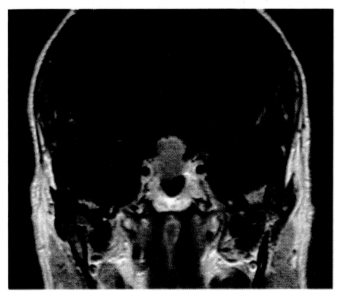

Fig. 12.11 Pituicytoma. This 55-year-old man presented with symptoms identical to those of a non-functioning pituitary adenoma, and his preoperative neuroimaging studies were similarly thought to be non-functioning pituitary adenoma based on the presence of a homogeneous, well-demarcated sellar/suprasellar mass, as seen here. However, biopsy proved this to be a pituicytoma.

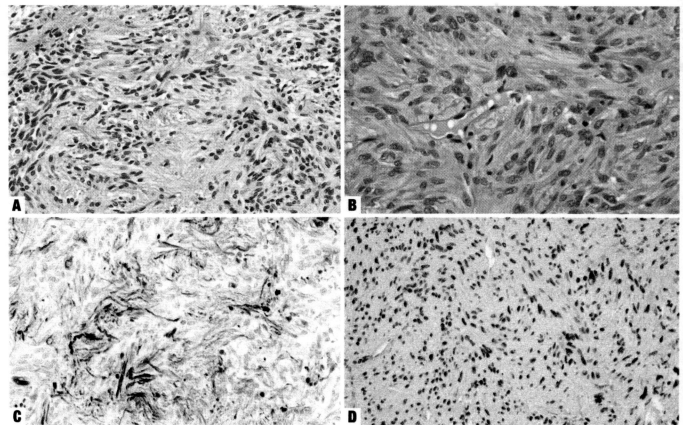

Fig. 12.12 Pituicytoma. **A** Tumours are composed of fibrillary cells that have elongated nuclei and are arranged in fascicles. **B** Tumour cells are cytologically bland, with oval nuclei, minimal hyperchromatism, and eosinophilic cytoplasm. **C** Pituicytomas show variable immunoreactivity for GFAP (shown), and they are also immunoreactive for vimentin. **D** Diffuse nuclear immunoreactivity for thyroid transcription factor 1 (TTF1) is typical of pituicytoma and confidently distinguishes it from schwannoma, meningioma, or pituitary adenoma / pituitary neuroendocrine tumour (PitNET), all of which are TTF1-immunonegative.

Etiology

The etiology of these neoplasms is unknown. No germline susceptibility has been identified. DNA methylation classification demonstrates close clustering between the three tumour types, with assignment to a single methylation class {460}.

Pathogenesis

Ubiquitous nuclear TTF1 expression indicates a common derivation of pituicytoma, granular cell tumour, and spindle cell oncocytoma from the pituitary infundibulum / forebrain ganglionic eminence (ventral neuroectoderm) rather than from endocrine cells of the anterior pituitary or from folliculostellate cells {1829}. Similarities between these tumours and the normal light, dark, granular, and oncocytic pituicyte subtypes are consistent with an origin from the posterior pituitary {3115,1829,2094}.

Genetic profile

The pathogenesis of these tumours has yet to be fully elucidated. Methylation-based classification studies show close clustering, suggesting they may be a single tumour type with a shared histogenesis but distinctive morphology {460}. *IDH1* p.R132H mutation and *KIAA1549::BRAF* oncogene fusion are absent {2094}. A limited number of case series reported variable somatic alterations with some evidence supporting MAPK pathway activation in pituicytoma and spindle cell oncocytoma {2114,3323}. Whole-exome sequencing identified

several mutations, including in the *HRAS*, *SND1*, and *FAT1* genes in 4 spindle cell oncocytomas from 3 patients {2114}. The *HRAS*-mutant case also had a *MEN1* frameshift mutation {2114}. Similarly, constitutive MAPK activation was found in 10 of 11 pituicytomas including *HRAS* somatic mutations as well as pathogenic *BRAF* p.V600E, *NF1*, and *TSC1* sequence variants {3323}. An additional case of a spindle cell oncocytoma with *BRAF* p.V600E mutation has been shown to respond to targeted inhibition of the MAPK/ERK signalling pathway {2986}. A recent study provided the first whole-microRNA signature of spindle cell oncocytomas, with distinct microRNA profiles distinguishing primary tumours from recurrent tumours {1741}. The same study also linked these tumours to an altered metabolic phenotype related to lipid metabolism and the Krebs cycle {1741}.

Macroscopic appearance

The three types of tumours cannot be distinguished by their gross features. Their texture reportedly ranges from similar to that of normal brain to firm and vascular, and their colour from grey to yellow {2167}. Pituicytoma and spindle cell oncocytoma can occasionally be associated with haemorrhage {324,1180}.

Histopathology

Pituicytomas

Pituicytomas are composed of elongate bipolar spindle cells often arranged in solid sheets and short fascicles, which can have a storiform pattern {365,2094,2093,1658,1919}. Tumour cells tend to show distinct cell borders. These tumours lack eosinophilic granular bodies, Rosenthal fibres, cytoplasmic eosinophilic coarse granularity, cytoplasmic vacuolization, and hyalinized blood vessels {1658}. Like in spindle cell oncocytomas, inflammatory infiltrates can sometimes be present {1658, 1829}. Some pituicytomas can display regions with ependymal and oncocytic change {2773,3548}. These observations have raised the possibility of morphological continuity among pituicyte-related tumours of the posterior lobe {2773,2911,2093}. Pituicytomas may be distinguished from normal posterior pituitary by the identification of Herring bodies and the presence of axons (NFP expression) in non-tumorous posterior lobe.

Although pituicytomas typically show a low mitotic activity and low Ki-67 labelling index (often < 3%) {1215,3323}, rare examples with atypical features characterized by increased cellularity, pleomorphism, mitotic activity, and elevated Ki-67 labelling index (> 5%) have been reported {3323,1215}.

Unlike granular cell tumours, pituicytomas lack the PAS-positive and diastase-resistant intracytoplasmic granules {1658}. Unlike schwannomas, reticulin histochemistry shows no pericellular staining {1658}.

By immunohistochemistry, pituicytomas invariably express TTF1, and they are negative for cytokeratins, pituitary hormones and transcription factors, chromogranin A, synaptophysin, and neurofilaments. They show strong reactivity for vimentin and S100, but variable GFAP immunostaining. The tumours also express variable EMA, CD56, galectin-3, CD68, and BCL2 {2094,1098}. Staining patterns for α1-antitrypsin and antimitochondrial antibody can also assist in the distinction of

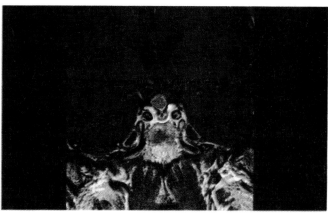

Fig. 12.13 Granular cell tumour. Postcontrast coronal MRI shows homogeneous mild enhancement within the mass and a relatively normal calibre of the more caudal stalk.

pituicytomas from granular cell tumours and spindle cell oncocytomas, respectively {2715,1658}.

Pituicytomas show ultrastructural characteristics of light and dark pituicytes – two of five ultrastructural subtypes of non-tumorous pituicytes {3115} that are enriched in intermediate filaments {2094}.

Granular cell tumour of the sellar region

Granular cell tumours consist of densely packed polygonal cells with granular eosinophilic cytoplasm. The architecture is typically nodular; sheets and/or spindled/fascicular patterns can also be seen. PAS staining of cytoplasmic granules is resistant to diastase digestion. The tumour cell nuclei are small, with inconspicuous

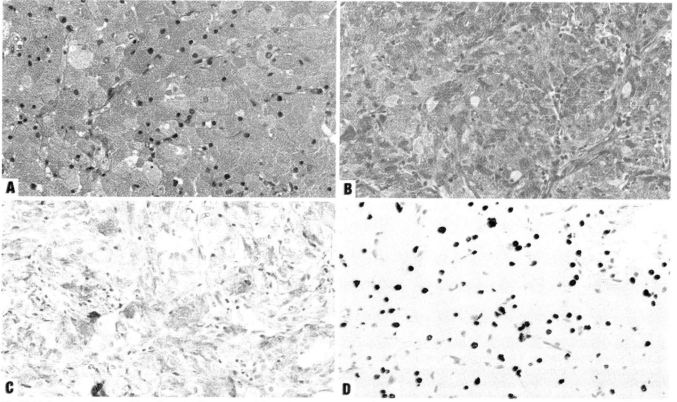

Fig. 12.14 Granular cell tumour of the sellar region. Tumours are characterized by eosinophilic polygonal cells with abundant granular eosinophilic cytoplasm (**A**). The cells show marked PAS positivity (**B**), strong EMA expression (**C**), and nuclear expression of thyroid transcription factor 1 (TTF1) (**D**).

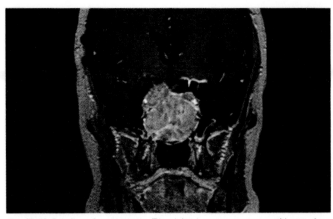

Fig. 12.15 Spindle cell oncocytoma. T1-weighted, postcontrast coronal image demonstrates a large, expansile, heterogeneously enhancing sellar mass with parasellar extension and invasion of the clivus.

nucleoli and evenly distributed chromatin. Perivascular lymphocytic aggregates are common. Mitotic activity is usually inconspicuous, and proliferative activity is usually very low.

Granular cell tumours show nuclear staining for TTF1 {1829, 2094}. The tumours are variably immunoreactive for S100 and vimentin, but only occasionally immunoreactive for GFAP and EMA {2094,1658}. The tumours are also positive for CD68, α1-antitrypsin, α1-antichymotrypsin, and cathepsin B, and they

are negative for NFPs, cytokeratins, chromogranin A, synaptophysin, desmin, SMA, and the pituitary hormones and transcription factors {2094,1658}.

Ultrastructural analysis highlights the abundant cytoplasmic lysosomal population of the tumour cells that confers the granular aspect of the cytoplasm seen on light microscopy. Neurosecretory granules are absent.

Spindle cell oncocytoma

Spindle cell oncocytomas are typically composed of interlacing fascicles and poorly defined lobules of spindle to epithelioid cells with eosinophilic, variably granular cytoplasm. Oncocytic changes can be focal to widespread. Whorls, myxoid changes, clear cells, osteoclastic-like giant cells, and follicle-like structures can also be features of these tumours {2733,3261,3548}. Mild to moderate nuclear atypia and (less commonly) marked pleomorphism can be observed. Focal infiltrates of mature lymphocytes are common.

Their immunoprofile includes TTF1, vimentin, S100, EMA, ANXA1, and galectin-3 expression. EMA expression varies from diffuse to limited to a few tumour cells. Focal GFAP expression can be present. MU213-UC, an antibody against a non-glycosylated 60-kDa mitochondrial protein, can help identify oncocytic features {2715}. Chromogranin A is absent, but synaptophysin {619} and faint and focal CD56 immunoreactivity have been described in some cases {2094,2004,1181}. Pituitary

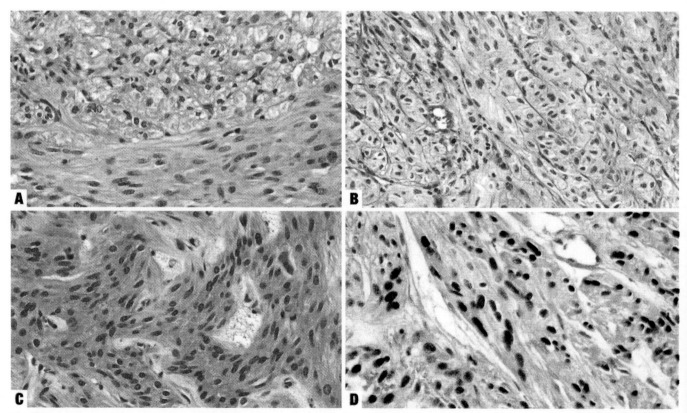

Fig. 12.16 Spindle cell oncocytoma. **A** Intersecting fascicles of tumour cells show the plump eosinophilic cytoplasm typical of this tumour. Increased cytoplasmic volume is due to increased mitochondrial content. **B** The clear cell appearance of the tumour cells can be seen, here with cells arranged in a nested pattern. **C** Tumour cells generally show more oval nuclei than do those in schwannoma (which usually contain tapering nuclei with pointed ends). Note the absence of nuclear pseudoinclusions, as can be seen in some meningiomas. Note also the uniformity of nuclear features and absence of mitotic activity. **D** There is diffuse nuclear immunoreactivity for thyroid transcription factor 1 (TTF1) in spindle cell oncocytomas, but it is also in pituicytomas, in granular cell tumours of the posterior pituitary, and even in normal posterior pituitary gland, so this immunostain does not distinguish these types of lesions from each other.

Box 12.03 Diagnostic criteria for pituicytoma, granular cell tumour of the sellar region, and spindle cell oncocytoma

Pituicytoma	Granular cell tumour	Spindle cell oncocytoma
Essential:	**Essential:**	**Essential:**
Bipolar spindle cell neoplasm in sheets and short fascicles	Neoplasm composed of polygonal cells with granular cytoplasm	Spindled or epithelioid tumour with eosinophilic, granular cytoplasm
AND	AND	AND
Sellar or suprasellar location	Sellar or suprasellar location	Sellar or suprasellar location
AND	AND	AND
Nuclear TTF1 expression	Nuclear TTF1 expression	Nuclear TTF1 expression
AND	AND	AND
Absence of pituitary hormone and transcription factor expression	Absence of pituitary hormone and transcription factor expression	Absence of pituitary hormone and transcription factor expression
AND	AND	AND
Absence of neuronal and neuroendocrine marker expression	Absence of neuronal and neuroendocrine marker expression	Absence of neuronal and neuroendocrine marker expression
Desirable:	**Desirable:**	**Desirable:**
Absence of interspersed reticulin fibres	Absence of interspersed reticulin fibres	Absence of interspersed reticulin fibres
	PAS-positive/diastase-resistant	Antimitochondrial antigen immunoreactivity
	CD68 or α1-antitrypsin immunoreactivity	

TTF1, thyroid transcription factor 1.

hormones and transcription factors are absent. Other positive markers include BCL2, CD44, nestin, and αB-crystallin {2094, 70}. Cytokeratins, CD34, and markers of skeletal and smooth muscle differentiation are absent. Phosphorylated ERK, AKT, and S6 expression has been reported {70,2114}. Expression of SSTRs and DRD2 has also been documented {2995,1881}.

Spindle cell oncocytomas usually show low proliferation. Mitotic activity is rarely reported in studies; when documented, mitoses are usually limited to a few. The reported Ki-67 labelling index ranges from < 1% to 17%, although reports of values > 5% are few {1098}.

Hallmark ultrastructural features include an increased number of often abnormal mitochondria, intermediate filaments, and cell-to-cell junctions including well-formed desmosomes and intermediate-type junctions {2718,1174}. A few cases may show sparse small neurosecretory granules {667,2094,619,998}. Follicular structures {619} and intracytoplasmic lumina with microvillous projections are reported {3261,2167}.

Cytology

In cytological preparations, pituicytomas can display fibrillary to fine and wispy cytoplasm with occasional spindled cell morphology, sharing glial and meningioma-like features {3322}. Granular cell tumour cytological preparations are characterized by the uniform appearance of the polygonal cells, which have round to ovoid nuclei and abundant eosinophilic granular cytoplasm dispersed in a granular background {2530}.

Diagnostic molecular pathology

No specific molecular test results are used in the diagnosis.

Essential and desirable diagnostic criteria

See Box 12.03.

Staging

Not applicable

Prognosis and prediction

Pituicytoma, granular cell tumour, and spindle cell oncocytoma are typically benign, slow-growing tumours, curable by gross total surgical excision. However, there seems to be a higher frequency of recurrence in spindle cell oncocytomas than in the other tumours {1663,2004,324,1098,503,1658}. Malignant transformation and distant metastases have not been reported.

Pituitary adenoma / pituitary neuroendocrine tumour

Lopes MBS
Asa SL
Kleinschmidt-DeMasters BK
Mete O
Osamura RY
Villa C

Definition

Pituitary adenoma / pituitary neuroendocrine tumour (PitNET) is a clonal neoplastic proliferation of anterior pituitary hormone–producing cells.

ICD-O coding

8272/3 Pituitary adenoma / pituitary neuroendocrine tumour (PitNET)

ICD-11 coding

2F37.Y & XH94U0 Other specified benign neoplasm of endocrine glands & Pituitary adenoma, NOS

2F9A & XH94U0 Neoplasms of unknown behaviour of endocrine glands & Pituitary adenoma, NOS

Related terminology

Acceptable: PitNET; pituitary adenoma.

Subtype(s)

The types and subtypes of pituitary adenomas / PitNETs are described in Table 12.01.

Localization

These tumours are usually identified in the sellar region, often with suprasellar extension, but ectopic locations include the sphenoid sinus, and rare clival and suprasellar tumours have also been described {28}. Rarely, pituitary adenomas / PitNETs may arise in teratomas {56,161,3305}.

Clinical features

Pituitary adenomas / PitNETs have a spectrum of clinical features. They may be small, slow-growing, and found incidentally, or they may give rise to hormone excess syndromes, including hyperprolactinaemia, acromegaly/gigantism, Cushing disease, or hyperthyroidism {2089,1133}. Large tumours may cause symptoms of an intracranial mass (e.g. headache, visual field disturbances) and cause hypopituitarism {2089}. Some tumours invade downwards and appear as a nasal or paranasal mass {1392}. Occasional examples undergo acute haemorrhagic necrosis, resulting in rapid expansion and causing a clinical presentation termed "pituitary apoplexy" {1543}, characterized by severe headache, lethargy, and signs of increased intracranial pressure.

Imaging

MRI with and without gadolinium is used to identify the sellar/suprasellar mass and to characterize size, optic chiasm compression, cavernous sinus and/or sphenoid sinus invasion, haemorrhage, or cystic changes. Most lesions are hypointense on T1-weighted images and show variable gadolinium enhancement {771}. On T2-weighted images, densely granulated

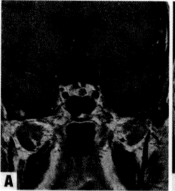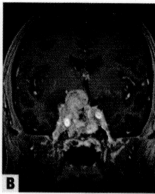

Fig. 12.17 Pituitary adenoma / pituitary neuroendocrine tumour (PitNET). **A** Corticotroph adenoma/tumour. T1-weighted postcontrast coronal MRI demonstrates the classic appearance of a homogeneously hypoenhancing pituitary lesion compatible with corticotroph microadenoma. **B** Invasive adenoma/tumour. T1-weighted postcontrast coronal MRI demonstrates a very large heterogeneously enhancing tumour centred in the sellar region with suprasellar and parasellar extension and invasion of the sphenoid sinus and clivus. Both internal carotid arteries are completely encased.

tumours tend to be hypointense, whereas sparsely granulated tumours are hyperintense {1278,2545}.

Epidemiology

Pituitary adenomas / PitNETs are identified incidentally in up to 20% of the population {882}. Clinically diagnosed tumours were once considered rare; however, recent population studies report a prevalence of 78–116 cases per 100 000 population {671,909, 36,955}. The Central Brain Tumor Registry of the United States (CBTRUS) reports that pituitary adenomas / PitNETs account for 16.5% of brain tumours, with an incidence of 3.94 cases per 100 000 person-years {2347}; however, this database reports surgically resected tumours and does not include those treated with medical therapy alone.

The incidence of pituitary adenoma / PitNET increases with age. Approximately 5% of patients are diagnosed before the age of 20 years {1541,2168}. Pituitary adenomas / PitNETs occur equally in both sexes, although some studies show an overall female predominance of certain subtypes {36,2347, 2090}. Cushing disease and prolactin-secreting tumours are more common in female patients {909}, whereas non-functioning {909} and lactotroph tumours are more often surgically resected in male patients {2090}.

Etiology

Risk factors

Risk factors for pituitary adenoma / PitNET related to exposure or lifestyle have not been definitively identified. Preliminary studies showed that environmental pollutants influence the biological behaviour of somatotroph adenomas/tumours in vivo and induce proliferation in normal pituitary cells after long-term incubation in vitro {1814,1141,2480,454,3624,3135, 963,453,2599}.

Established carcinogenic agents like X- and γ-radiation do not seem to play a role in pituitary tumorigenesis {617}. Use of oral contraceptives or menopausal hormone therapy is not significantly associated with an increase in the risk of tumours {242, 643}.

Genetic factors
Pituitary adenomas / PitNETs are monoclonal proliferations, and the great majority occur sporadically {1293}. The most common recurrent somatic mutations that drive tumorigenesis affect *GNAS* in as many as 40% of somatotroph adenomas/ tumours and lead to hormone hypersecretion via upregulation of the cAMP/PKA pathway {1800,3000,2501}. *USP8* and *USP48* mutations rescue the EGFR (HER1) and CRH/SHH pathways resulting in aberrant ACTH synthesis in approximately 50% of corticotroph adenomas/tumours {2642,1964, 2457,1270,897,2458,55}. Novel mutations associated with sporadic tumours include *USP48* {2819,538}, *NR3C1* {2819, 1375,121}, *CABLES1* {1294,2736} in corticotroph adenomas/ tumours, and *TP53* {3133} in pituitary carcinomas. Apart from these rare events, recurrent molecular alterations have

Table 12.01 Classification of pituitary neuroendocrine tumours (PitNETs) in the upcoming WHO Classification of Tumours volume *Endocrine and neuroendocrine tumours* {3425A}

Tumour type[a]	Transcription factor(s)	Hormone(s)	Keratin (CAM5.2 or CK18)	Tumour subtypes (if applicable)	Hormone excess syndrome[b]
PIT1-lineage tumours					
Somatotroph tumours	PIT1	GH, α-subunit	Perinuclear	Densely granulated somatotroph tumour	Florid acromegaly
		GH	Fibrous bodies (> 70%)	Sparsely granulated somatotroph tumour	Subtle acromegaly
Lactotroph tumours	PIT1, ERα	PRL (paranuclear)	Weak or negative	Sparsely granulated lactotroph tumour	Hyperprolactinaemia[c]
		PRL (diffuse cytoplasmic)	Weak or negative	Densely granulated lactotroph tumour	Hyperprolactinaemia[c]
Mammosomatotroph tumour	PIT1, ERα	GH (often predominant), PRL, α-subunit	Perinuclear		Acromegaly and hyperprolactinaemia[c]
Thyrotroph tumour	PIT1, GATA2/3[d]	α-subunit, TSH-β	Weak or negative		Hyperthyroidism
Mature PIT1-lineage tumour	PIT1, ERα, GATA2/3[d]	GH (often predominant), PRL, α-subunit, TSH-β	Perinuclear		Acromegaly, hyperprolactinaemia[c], and hyperthyroidism
Acidophil stem cell tumour	PIT1, ERα	PRL (predominant), GH (focal/variable)	Scattered fibrous bodies		Hyperprolactinaemia[c] and subclinical acromegaly
Immature PIT1-lineage tumour	PIT1, ERα, GATA2/3[d]	GH, PRL, α-subunit, TSH-β	Focal/variable		Acromegaly, hyperprolactinaemia[c], and hyperthyroidism
TPIT-lineage tumours					
			Strong	Densely granulated corticotroph tumour	Florid Cushing, often microtumour
Corticotroph tumours	TPIT (TBX19), NeuroD1 (β2)	ACTH and other POMC derivatives	Variable	Sparsely granulated corticotroph tumour	Subtle Cushing, often macrotumour
			Intense ring-like perinuclear	Crooke cell tumour	Variable, Cushing
SF1-lineage tumours					
Gonadotroph tumour	SF1, ERα, GATA2/3[d]	α-subunit, FSH-β, LH-β	Variable		Hypogonadism (virtually all) or hypergonadism (exceptional)
Tumours without distinct cell lineage					
Unclassified plurihormonal tumours	Multiple combinations	Multiple combinations	Variable		Variable
Null cell tumour	None	None	Variable		None

α-subunit, glycoprotein hormones alpha subunit; GH, growth hormone; PRL, prolactin.
[a]Mixed tumours also occur and can constitute any combination of tumours shown; the most common is mixed somatotroph–lactotroph tumour. [b]Any tumour type can be clinically non-functioning. [c]Moderate hyperprolactinaemia can occur with any sellar mass that has suprasellar extension, interrupting hypothalamic tonic dopaminergic inhibition; however, the PRL level rarely exceeds 150 ng/mL; lactotroph tumours usually show a characteristic correlation between tumour size and PRL levels, whereas other PRL-secreting tumours do not. [d]GATA2 and GATA3 are paralogues and show cross-reactivity with some available antisera.

not been identified in sporadic tumours. Instead, epigenetic alterations may be relevant to tumorigenesis in the majority of sporadic cases {3141,883,268,1267,884,3613}. Chromosomal alterations are common, which is unusual for tumours with largely indolent behaviour {267}.

A minority of tumours are associated with known familial predisposition syndromes, implicating specific germline mutations in the development of pituitary adenomas / PitNETs (see Table 12.02) {3038,3013,3289}.

Pathogenesis

Cell of origin

Pituitary adenomas / PitNETs are considered to represent a clonal neoplastic proliferation of hormone-producing neuroendocrine anterior pituitary cells.

Somatic genetic alterations

See *Genetic factors* in the *Etiology* subsection, above.

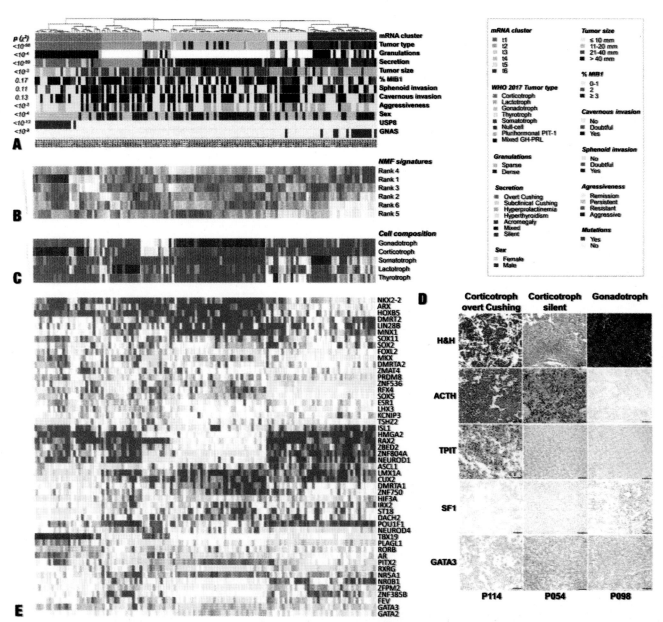

Fig. 12.18 Transcriptome of pituitary neuroendocrine tumours (PitNETs). **A** Unsupervised classification of PitNETs identifies six main groups, corresponding to corticotroph with overt Cushing (t1), lactotroph (t2), silent corticotroph (t3), gonadotroph (t4), thyrotroph (t5), and somatotroph (t6) PitNETs. Pathological and clinical annotations are provided. The association with transcriptome groups is detailed (p (χ^2): chi-squared *P* values). **B** Heat map of the six non-negative matrix factorization (NMF) ranks used for generating the unsupervised classification. **C** Proportion of gonadotroph, corticotroph, somatotroph, lactotroph, and thyrotroph canonical signatures in each PitNET. **D** Magnification (20×) of H&E staining and immunohistochemistry for the corticotroph-related markers ACTH and TPIT and the gonadotroph-related markers SF1 and GATA3 performed on tissue sections of corticotroph of overt Cushing (P114), silent corticotroph (P054), and gonadotroph (P098) PitNETs. Scale bars represent 100 mm. **E** Expression profiles related to the top 50 most significantly differentially expressed transcription factors among the six transcriptome groups.

Table 12.02 Inherited genetic susceptibility to pituitary tumours

Disease	Gene(s)	Pituitary lesions (in order of frequency)
Isolated pituitary tumours		
Familial isolated pituitary adenoma	*AIP* or unknown	Somatotroph, lactotroph, mammosomatotroph, corticotroph, and other tumours Rarely, somatotroph hyperplasia
X-linked acrogigantism	*GPR101*[a]	Mammosomatotroph adenomas and/or hyperplasia
Syndromes associated with pituitary tumours		
Multiple endocrine neoplasia type 1	*MEN1*	Lactotroph, non-functioning, somatotroph, and corticotroph tumours Multiple or plurihormonal tumours Somatotroph or mammosomatotroph hyperplasia
Multiple endocrine neoplasia type 4	*CDKN1B*	Somatotroph, non-functioning, and corticotroph tumours
Carney complex	*PRKAR1A*	Somatotroph, lactotroph, and corticotroph tumours Mammosomatotroph or somatotroph hyperplasia
McCune–Albright syndrome	*GNAS* (mosaic)[a]	Mammosomatotroph and somatotroph tumours Mammosomatotroph or somatotroph hyperplasia
Familial paraganglioma, phaeochromocytoma, pituitary adenoma syndrome	*SDHA, SDHB, SDHC, SDHD*	Lactotroph, somatotroph, gonadotroph, and (rarely) corticotroph tumours
DICER1 syndrome	*DICER1*	Pituitary blastoma (majority ACTH-secreting; rarely, growth hormone–secreting and prolactin-secreting)
Neurofibromatosis type 1	*NF1*	Corticotroph and somatotroph adenomas Pituitary duplication
Lynch syndrome	*MSH2, MSH6, MLH1, PMS2*	Corticotroph and lactotroph tumours
USP8-related syndrome	*USP8*[a]	Corticotroph tumours
Tuberous sclerosis	*TSC1, TSC2*	Corticotroph tumours

[a]Mutation can also be somatic.

Gene expression

A recent transcriptome-based classification identified distinct molecular subtypes of pituitary tumours, each associated with specific secretion phenotypes, genetic alterations, and epigenetic profiles {2232}. In this classification, clinically aggressive tumours did not appear as a distinct molecular entity.

Protein expression

A limited number of transcription factors currently bridge the differing types of pituitary tumours and lineages. However, recent multiomics and protein expression profiling studies have shown less rigid pituitary lineage {2232,2670,635}. For instance, silent corticotroph tumours display both corticotroph and gonadotroph signatures, suggesting a transdifferentiation state {2232,2092,635,2670}. In addition, SF1 is expressed in a subset of somatotroph tumours (mainly *GNAS*-wildtype tumours) {2232}.

Macroscopic appearance

At autopsy, pituitary adenomas / PitNETs range from small pale nodules within the gland to large cohesive hyperaemic masses with pushing borders. Variable extension into the suprasellar space and invasion into the sphenoid and/or cavernous sinus are frequent; dura mater and bone invasion may be seen. Tumours with apoplexy may show haemorrhagic necrosis.

Histopathology

Pituitary adenomas / PitNETs are generally monomorphic, with cells arranged in a variety of histological patterns, including diffuse, papillary, and trabecular arrangements. Cytologically, tumour cells may be acidophilic, basophilic, or chromophobic; however, these tinctorial characteristics are nonspecific. Cells may show densely or sparsely granulated cytoplasm according to the tumour subtype (see *Histopathological subtypes*, below). Nuclei tend to be bland with regularly distributed chromatin. Mitotic activity is generally low. The presence of extensive cellular pleomorphism, brisk mitotic activity, and necrosis is not typical and should prompt consideration of alternative diagnoses. Calcification or ossification is rare, except in lactotroph and thyrotroph subtypes.

Histopathological subtypes

Pituitary adenomas / PitNETs reflect their derivation from six cell types (see Fig. 12.19, p. 410), with each lineage differentiating into multiple subtypes. Some are composed of less differentiated cells.

TPIT-lineage corticotroph adenomas/tumours

The subtypes within this group reflect their hormonal activity. They can be clinically functioning or silent, the silent ones probably arising due to failure of enzymatic cleavage of the POMC precursor into the active hormone. All tumours variably express nuclear TPIT (TBX19) {2090,481,2262,2089}. Silent corticotroph tumours can be any of the subtypes below.

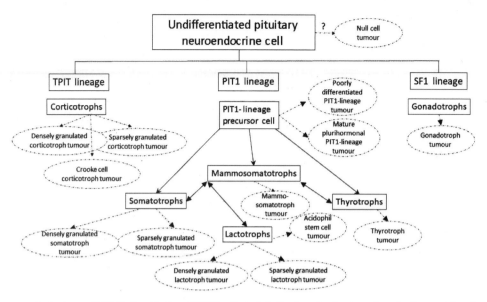

Fig. 12.19 Pituitary neuroendocrine tumour (PitNET). Classification of PitNETs reflects derivation from six adenohypophyseal cell types of three lineages, with multiple subtypes of some cell types and some tumours showing incomplete differentiation.

Densely granulated corticotroph adenomas/tumours are strongly basophilic and PAS-positive, and they have intense cytoplasmic ACTH and cytokeratin reactivity. They are usually small and associated with florid Cushing disease, and they tend to harbour *USP8* mutations {1270}.

Sparsely granulated corticotroph adenomas/tumours are chromophobic or weakly basophilic, with faint or focal PAS positivity and weak cytoplasmic ACTH reactivity but intense cytokeratin reactivity {2090}. They are usually large {770} with subtle clinical features of Cushing disease {52,2625}.

Crooke cell adenomas/tumours show Crooke hyaline change (required in > 50% of tumour cells for the diagnosis), consisting of abundant cytoplasmic accumulation of pale acidophilic hyaline material with focal basophilia, PAS and ACTH positivity

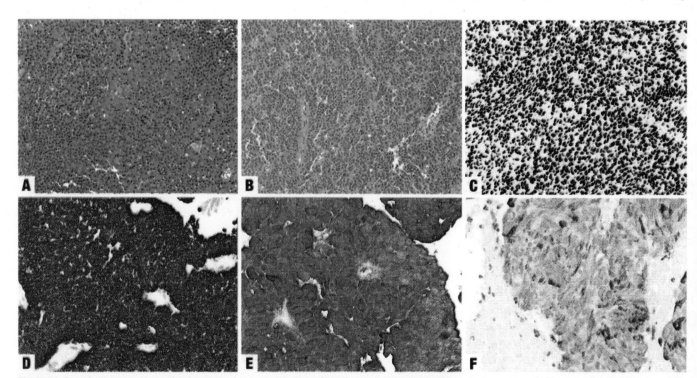

Fig. 12.20 Densely and sparsely granulated corticotroph adenomas/tumours. Densely granulated corticotroph tumours are composed of tumour cells with dense basophilic granular cytoplasm (**A**), whereas sparsely granulated corticotroph tumours display a lightly basophilic appearance (**B**). Irrespective of their subtypes, these tumours are positive for TPIT (**C**), and they tend to display diffuse cytoplasmic reactivity for low-molecular-weight cytokeratin (CAM5.2) (**D**). Consistent with their cytoplasmic granularity pattern, densely granulated tumours are diffusely positive for ACTH (**E**), whereas sparsely granulated tumours are variably and weakly positive (**F**). The same pattern of reactivity can be identified when using PAS histochemistry (not shown).

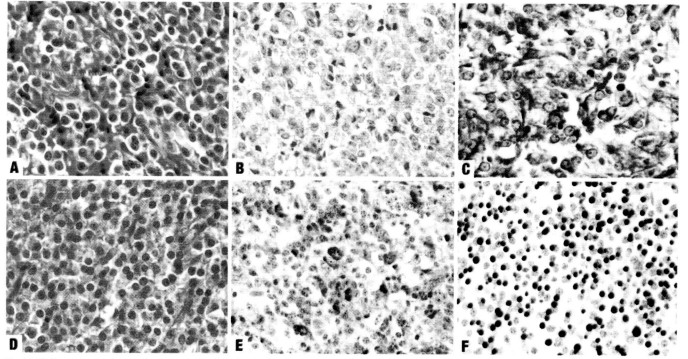

Fig. 12.21 Somatotroph adenomas/tumours. **A–C** A densely granulated somatotroph tumour showing eosinophilic, granular cytoplasm and a central nucleus with a prominent nucleolus (**A**), as well as intense and diffuse growth hormone expression (**B**); cytokeratin (CAM5.2) staining reveals perinuclear deposition with very few fibrous bodies (**C**). **D–F** A sparsely granulated somatotroph tumour with slightly eosinophilic cytoplasm and showing paranuclear fibrous bodies (**D**), as well as focal growth hormone expression in the cytoplasm (**E**); cytokeratin (CAM5.2) staining highlights a large proportion (> 70%) of fibrous bodies (**F**).

in juxtanuclear or perimembranous distributions, and intense cytokeratin staining in a concentric pattern {1058,749,2089}. These are usually large, invasive tumours and about 76% occur with Cushing disease {749}.

SF1 gonadotroph adenomas/tumours

These show a spectrum of morphologies and degrees of differentiation, from trabecular proliferations of elongated cells with basal nuclei and prominent pseudorosettes to solid sheets of round cells. They can show prominent oncocytic change. They have a range of gonadotropin hormone expression: most often focal FSH, with scant LH and variable α-subunit immunoreactivity. About 40% are negative for cytokeratins {2090}. They are characterized by variable nuclear expression of SF1 {142}, GATA3 {2092,3243}, and focal ER {3568,2924}. Hormone-negative gonadotroph tumours with SF1 and GATA3 positivity alone are the least differentiated and must be distinguished from null cell tumours {2262,83,185,1210}.

PIT1-lineage adenomas/tumours

This is the most complex group. It comprises a range of tumours, from those composed of a single cell population with the ability to secrete one or more of the PIT1-lineage hormones (growth hormone [GH], prolactin, and TSH) to tumours consisting of two types of cells with bihormonal or plurihormonal secretory abilities {147,985}.

Somatotroph adenomas/tumours that usually cause acromegaly or gigantism are characterized as densely or sparsely granulated based on GH immunoexpression and cytokeratin pattern {3505}. The presence of a predominant (> 70%) fibrous body pattern is the hallmark of the sparsely granulated subtype, whereas the densely granulated subtype has perinuclear cytokeratin and may have focal fibrous bodies {2295}. The distinction is clinically critical because the two subtypes have different treatment responses {145,49}. Densely granulated adenomas/tumours occur in about 30–50% of patients with acromegaly, whereas sparsely granulated adenomas/tumours account for about 15–35% of acromegaly cases {2295,49,1736}.

Densely granulated somatotroph adenomas/tumours are acidophilic, with strong GH staining dispersed diffusely throughout the entire tumour; glycoprotein hormones α-subunit is typically expressed {2090}.

Sparsely granulated somatotroph adenomas/tumours are less acidophilic than their densely granulated counterparts. They often show cytoplasmic clearing due to fibrous bodies, and eccentric nuclei that are often bilobed or contorted around the fibrous body. GH expression is focal in the cytoplasm, and α-subunit expression is negative {2803,2090}.

Lactotroph adenomas/tumours are generally sparsely granulated with juxtanuclear hormone positivity in the Golgi complex; rare densely granulated lactotroph tumours have diffuse cytoplasmic hormone staining {2090}. The tumours often show intense nuclear ER staining {3568,986} and absence of α-subunit. Sparsely granulated lactotroph tumours often show hyperprolactinaemia that is proportional to their tumour size.

Thyrotroph adenomas/tumours are usually large and composed of relatively monomorphic, polygonal cells with some degree of nuclear pleomorphism. The tumours express TSH and α-subunit, and coexpress PIT1 and GATA3 {3506,2089}. They may have intense stromal fibrosis {3506} and calcification.

Plurihormonal tumours of PIT1 lineage

This is a complex family, characterized as follows:

Mammosomatotroph adenomas/tumours are composed of a monomorphic cell population with eosinophilic cell cytoplasm {902,1348} that coexpresses GH, α-subunit, prolactin, and ER. They often cause acromegaly/gigantism and hyperprolactinaemia, and they are more common in the paediatric age group and younger adults than in older populations.

Mixed somatotroph–lactotroph adenomas/tumours are composed of two discrete tumour cell populations, typically with one expressing GH and the other expressing prolactin (see Table 12.01, p. 407). Many combinations of sparsely and/or densely granulated somatotroph and lactotroph cells have been described {2090}. Patients may present with acromegaly/gigantism or with hyperprolactinaemia.

Acidophilic stem cell adenomas/tumours are rare; they most closely resemble lactotrophs but may express scant GH and be associated with fugitive acromegaly {1349,1350}. They are usually oncocytic, but they may have abundant clear to vacuolated cytoplasm due to mitochondrial dilatation {1350}. Tumours predominantly express prolactin with variable intensity, and they often express focal to variable GH {1350,1349,2090}. Staining for cytokeratin highlights small, scattered fibrous bodies in about two thirds of these tumours {2090}.

GH-producing plurihormonal adenomas/tumours are also rare; they may arise in the setting of acromegaly/gigantism, hyperprolactinaemia, and in some cases synchronous hyperthyroidism. These are monomorphic eosinophilic tumours that express variable amounts of TSH in addition to GH, prolactin, and α-subunit {2090}. GATA3 expression correlates with the TSH staining pattern {2092}. Intense acidophilia and abundant GH and prolactin immunoexpression distinguish these tumours from the immature PIT1-lineage pituitary adenomas / PitNETs that may be plurihormonal {2091}.

Immature PIT1-lineage adenomas/tumours were formerly known as "silent subtype 3 adenoma" and are referred to in the 2017 WHO classification of endocrine tumours as "plurihormonal PIT1-positive adenoma/tumour". These tumours are composed of cells that do not show terminal differentiation to one of the well-known PIT1 lineage anterior pituitary cells. They are usually chromophobic, rather than acidophilic like more differentiated tumours. They always express nuclear PIT1 {2091}, and they may express focal ER and/or GATA3 {2092}. They may be immunonegative for hormones, but more often they are focally positive for one or more of GH, prolactin, TSH, and α-subunit {855,2091,2090}. Cytokeratin patterns are variable and there may be occasional fibrous bodies {2091,2090}. These tumours are frequently clinically silent, but they may be associated with acromegaly/gigantism, hyperprolactinaemia, and/or hyperthyroidism {2091,855,1351}. They tend to be aggressive and invasive, with an increased risk of recurrence {2091,855}.

Unclassified plurihormonal adenomas/tumours

These are extremely rare, with only individual case reports published. Tumours show differentiation across more than one lineage, expressing several combinations of hormones (e.g. GH/ACTH, prolactin/ACTH, and LH/ACTH) and corresponding transcription factors (e.g. PIT1/TPIT, PIT1/SF1, TPIT/SF1) {1987, 2802,2621,3217,2456}. Multiple synchronous tumours of distinct lineages should not be confused for plurihormonal tumours {2088}.

Null cell adenomas/tumours

These are anterior pituitary tumours that show no immunohistochemical expression of biomarkers of known anterior pituitary cell lineages. They are usually positive for chromogranin A and cytokeratins but must be negative for pituitary transcription factors and hormones. Recently, some cases expressing focal

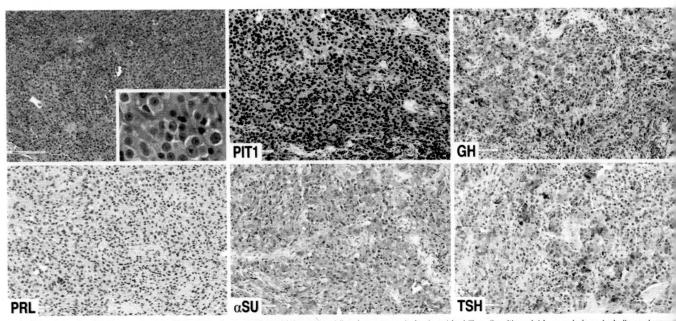

Fig. 12.22 Immature PIT1-lineage tumour. This tumour from a patient with hyperthyroidism is composed of pale acidophilic cells with variable morphology, including polygonal cells that resemble thyrotrophs. They have prominent nuclear inclusions that resemble irregular nucleoli (inset); these have been called spheridia. This tumour expressed nuclear PIT1 with variable growth hormone (GH) and TSH but no prolactin (PRL); there is diffuse α-subunit (αSU) positivity. Tumours of this lineage have variable positivity for the three PIT1-lineage hormones.

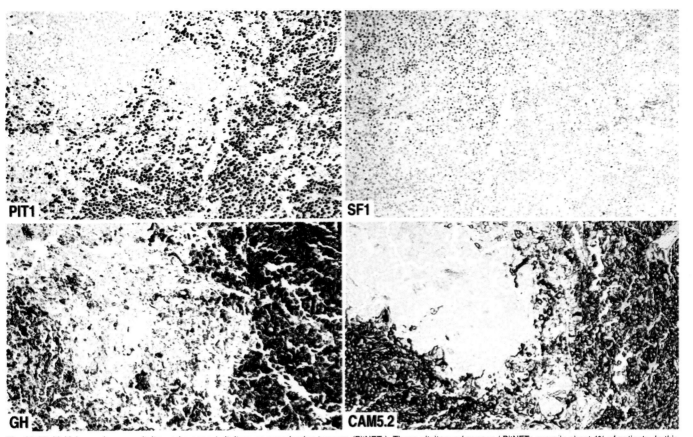

Fig. 12.23 Multiple synchronous pituitary adenomas / pituitary neuroendocrine tumours (PitNETs). These pituitary adenomas / PitNETs occur in about 1% of patients. In this example, a densely granulated somatotroph tumour stains for PIT1 and growth hormone (GH) and shows diffuse cytoplasmic CAM5.2 reactivity. It traps a small gonadotroph tumour that stains for SF1 and is negative for the other biomarkers examined. Tumours like this one and the common occurrence of trapped non-tumorous tissue may explain why SF1 expression is detected in some tumours causing acromegaly.

glycoprotein hormones α-subunit have been reported {2090}. They represent < 5% of surgically resected pituitary tumours {2090,2262,83,185,1210}, and they may have a high incidence of recurrence and cavernous sinus invasion {83,1210,185,2262}.

Grading
There is no formal grading system.

Invasion
Pituitary tumours may invade the surrounding tissues, including the sphenoid and cavernous sinus, dura mater, and bone. Invasion of the cavernous sinus prevents gross total tumour surgical resection. MRI evaluation using the Knosp scale and its modifications may predict the degree of invasion {1668,2107}. Tumour invasion is closely related to tumour size, with about 55% of tumours > 10 mm showing histological dural invasion, compared with about 24% of tumours < 10 mm {2063}. Nonfunctioning tumours have a higher incidence of invasion than functioning tumours {2063,3229}.

Differential diagnosis
Tumour metastases to the sellar region, such as carcinomas (especially breast and lung) and neuroendocrine tumours, can mimic pituitary adenomas / PitNETs. Metastases are immunonegative for pituitary transcription factors, with the exception of ER, GATA3, and SF1, which can be expressed in some

metastatic carcinomas {2092}. Primary sellar paragangliomas {1238,144} are distinguished from cytokeratin-negative pituitary adenomas / PitNETs by their positivity for GATA3 (without SF1

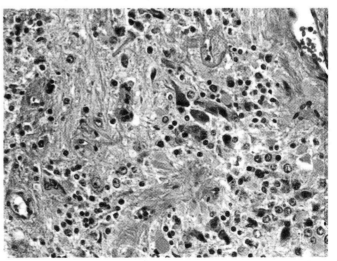

Fig. 12.24 Mixed gangliocytoma–somatotroph adenoma/tumour. A minority of patients with acromegaly may have a mixed gangliocytoma–somatotroph adenoma/tumour. The two cellular elements can be seen intermixed or in isolated areas. Ganglionic cells vary in shape and size, some with dense Nissl substance, and they are commonly embedded in a neuropil-like matrix.

and PIT1) and tyrosine hydroxylase {144}. Sinonasal neuroendocrine tumour and olfactory neuroblastoma can also involve the sellar region; these do not express pituitary hormones or transcription factors. Spindle cell oncocytoma should be excluded in the differential diagnosis of pituitary adenoma / PitNET with oncocytic features; the former uniformly stain for thyroid transcription factor 1 (TTF1) {1829,2094}. The rare sellar neurocytomas are negative for cytokeratins but express neurofilaments, TTF1, and hypothalamic hormones {143,146}. Pituitary hyperplasia should be distinguished using reticulin staining; reticulin shows complete breakdown in tumours, whereas in hyperplasia the acini are expanded but intact.

Cytology

At low magnification, pituitary adenomas / PitNETs are distinguished from normal anterior pituitary gland in cytological preparations by their hypercellularity and homogeneous appearance. Because pituitary adenomas / PitNETs have less stroma than normal tissue, their cells do not aggregate in large numbers; rather, they are seen predominantly as individual cells and small clusters. Tumour cells tend to have enlarged, pleomorphic, or atypical nuclei with variable amounts of cytoplasm and embedded in a granular background. Papillary formations are easily recognized on cytological touch or smear preparations.

Diagnostic molecular pathology

Pituitary adenomas / PitNETs do not yet have specific molecular characteristics that are applied to routine diagnostic algorithms (see *Prognosis and prediction*, below, for prognostic biomarkers).

Essential and desirable diagnostic criteria

See Box 12.04.

Staging

Craniospinal spread may be observed at progression/transformation of pituitary adenomas / PitNETs {2300,1248}; by definition, cerebrospinal fluid spread is indicative of pituitary carcinoma. Cerebrospinal fluid cytology may be helpful for the detection of meningeal spread {1248}. For monitoring progression, structural (MRI and CT) and/or functional (FDG PET and/or SSTR PET) imaging has been recommended {2623}.

Prognosis and prediction

The 2017 WHO classification of tumours of endocrine organs categorized pituitary neuroendocrine tumours as "pituitary adenomas and carcinomas" {1919}. Notably, the term "atypical adenoma" (defined in the 2004 WHO classification) was abandoned, because a definite correlation between histological diagnosis and clinical behaviour could not be established. The 2017 volume did not introduce a new tumour grading system, but it emphasized the identification of high-risk adenomas by recognizing (1) tumours with increased proliferation (evaluated by mitotic count and Ki-67 labelling index), which most likely relates to tumour recurrence {2050,3228}; and (2) the following five tumour subtypes that have an increased propensity for early recurrence and resistance to treatment: sparsely granulated somatotroph adenomas/tumours, silent corticotroph adenomas/tumours, Crooke cell adenomas/tumours, plurihormonal PIT1-positive adenomas/tumours, and lactotroph adenomas/tumours in men {1919}.

Pituitary carcinomas correspond to 0.12–0.4% of all tumours {2775,86}. They are characterized by craniospinal dissemination and/or systemic metastases. The most common subtypes are lactotroph and corticotroph carcinomas {2598,2461,1275}. However, predictive markers of malignant progression are not well established and no single histopathological marker has been shown to reliably predict pituitary tumour behaviour.

Many pituitary adenomas / PitNETs are non-invasive and may exhibit expansive growth in the sellar region and surrounding tissue. A substantial subset (30–65% {2063,3220,3229,2483}) are invasive, with corresponding residual tumour {2063,3565} and regrowth after surgery {3120}. Therefore, a considerable number of patients with pituitary adenoma / PitNET require clinical surveillance and/or adjuvant treatment.

A subset of pituitary adenomas / PitNETs may display aggressive clinical behaviour and rapid growth, with early and multiple recurrences despite multimodal therapy {2624}. The prevalence of these clinically aggressive pituitary adenomas / PitNETs is unknown, probably because they are inconsistently defined {2624,3573,526,750,723}. Pituitary tumour proliferation alone does not always correlate with clinical behaviour {1167}; however, the correlation of proliferation and radiological evidence of invasive growth appears to have prognostic value, and it identifies tumours with aggressive potential {3229,150,1854,2623,3228,545}.

Tumour biomarkers may be relevant for guiding treatment of pituitary adenomas / PitNETs. SSTR expression level may predict the response to treatment with somatostatin analogues {2140,3230,1393,1640}, and a low expression of ER in lactotroph tumours may predict resistance to dopamine agonists {729}. DRD2 expression in gonadotroph tumours and in *GNAS*-mutant somatotroph tumours suggests potentially new indications for dopamine treatment {2521,3583}. MGMT protein expression appears to be negatively correlated with response to temozolomide {2623,2050}. In distinction from IDH-wildtype glioblastoma, MGMT promoter methylation status in pituitary adenomas / PitNET is not related to tumour response {424}. Finally, losses of MSH2 and MSH6 expression have been linked to temozolomide resistance {239}.

Pituitary blastoma

Jarzembowski JA
de Kock L
Mete O
Rotondo F
Schultz KAP

Definition

Pituitary blastoma is an embryonal neoplasm of the sellar region, composed of primitive blastemal cells, neuroendocrine cells, and Rathke pouch epithelium.

ICD-O coding

8273/3 Pituitary blastoma

ICD-11 coding

2D12.Y & XH5QV8 Other specified malignant neoplasms of other endocrine glands or related structures & Pituitary blastoma

Related terminology

Not recommended: pituitary embryoma.

Subtype(s)

None

Localization

Pituitary blastoma originates within the sellar region and frequently extends into the suprasellar region and invades the cavernous sinus {2828}.

Clinical features

Cushing syndrome is one of the most common presenting symptoms; the elevated and non-suppressible serum ACTH level is due to its overexpression by tumour cells {707,2828}. Other hormones may also be overexpressed {562}. Ophthalmoplegia frequently occurs due to extension of the tumour in the suprasellar and parasellar region {2828}.

Epidemiology

Pituitary blastoma is an exceptionally rare tumour, with fewer than 20 published cases. It usually occurs in children aged < 2 years, with a median age of 9 months and a slight female predominance {707,2828}. Patients may present with or subsequently develop other *DICER1*-related tumours {707}.

Etiology

Pituitary blastoma is linked to underlying germline and somatic variation in *DICER1*, a critical gene in microRNA processing {707}.

Pathogenesis

Pituitary blastoma appears to arise because of a genetic alteration in *DICER1*, which encodes an enzyme involved in microRNA

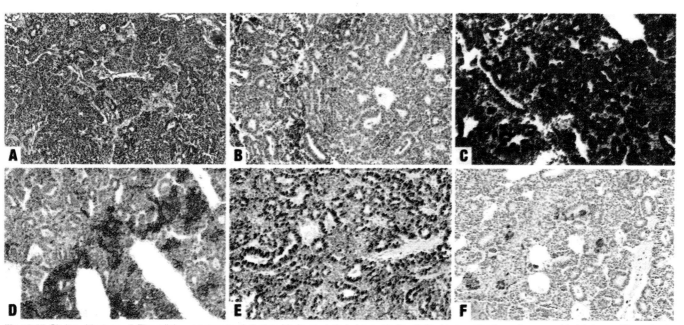

Fig. 12.25 Pituitary blastoma. **A** The cellular components of pituitary blastomas include large anterior pituitary neuroendocrine cells arranged in lobules or diffuse sheets, cuboidal primitive Rathke pouch epithelium with rosette or gland/follicle formation, and scattered small undifferentiated blastemal cells. **B** The anterior pituitary neuroendocrine tumour cells are arranged in diffuse sheets or lobules, and they are variably positive for ACTH. In contrast, rosette- or follicle-forming cuboidal or columnar primitive Rathke pouch epithelium and blastemal undifferentiated cells are negative for ACTH. **C** CAM5.2 stains almost all cellular components in pituitary blastomas. **D** Strong membranous CD56 expression distinguishes areas of neuroendocrine cells, whereas other cellular elements show less intense staining for CD56. **E** Proliferative heterogeneity of various cellular components is illustrated in this photomicrograph. The follicle-forming cuboidal or columnar primitive Rathke pouch epithelium shows a higher Ki-67 proliferation index than do the other cellular elements. **F** S100 stains scattered folliculostellate cells.

processing; mature microRNAs in turn regulate the translation of mRNA. Virtually all tumours (15 of 15 tested cases) harbour at least one *DICER1* alteration, typically a germline loss-of-function pathogenic variant coupled with a somatic RNase IIIb hotspot missense mutation {2776,707}. In a minority of cases, the second somatic alteration may be loss of the wildtype allele {707}.

Macroscopic appearance
Descriptions of the macroscopic details of pituitary blastomas are limited. Focal cystic or haemorrhagic changes and partial necrosis can be seen {2829}.

Histopathology
Pituitary blastomas are composed of three cellular components: (1) large, anterior pituitary neuroendocrine cells arranged in lobules or diffuse sheets; (2) cuboidal or columnar primitive Rathke pouch epithelium with rosette or gland/follicle formation; and (3) small undifferentiated blastemal cells {2829,2828,707}.

Ultrastructurally, pituitary blastomas resemble fetal pituitary gland of 10–12 weeks, but they are distinguished by (1) a marked complex cellular proliferation of mature TPIT-lineage corticotroph cells (some with Crooke hyaline change), (2) PIT1-lineage somatotrophs with a background of anterior pituitary cells with small secretory granules that simulate null cells, and (3) other elements including undifferentiated Rathke pouch epithelial cells and folliculostellate cells {2829,2828}.

Neuroendocrine cells variably express pro-opiomelanocortin derivatives including ACTH, β-endorphin, and MSH, and to a lesser extent growth hormone {2829}. Rare LH-β {2829} and/or FSH-β {2829,2776} staining has also been reported. Unlike neuroendocrine cells, blastemal and Rathke pouch cells rarely show pituitary transcription factor expression {2828}. EMA and keratins are expressed in various components, with stronger staining in the Rathke pouch epithelium {2829}. Galectin-3 variably stains cellular components {2829}. Proliferative heterogeneity varies between cases and between tumour components {2829,2828}. A high Ki-67 labelling index (up to 60%) and p53 expression are more frequent in the Rathke pouch epithelium {2829,2828,707}. Necrosis can occur {2828}.

The differential diagnosis includes sellar teratoma, germ cell tumours, and pituitary adenomas / pituitary neuroendocrine tumours (PitNETs) with synchronous Rathke cleft cyst {2774, 694}.

Cytology
Details of intraoperative cytological preparations have not been described.

Diagnostic molecular pathology
DICER1 variants may be considered a diagnostic molecular marker of pituitary blastoma. Germline and tumour sequencing should be performed.

Essential and desirable diagnostic criteria
See Box 12.05.

Staging
Staging should include brain and spine MRI with and without contrast, endocrine evaluation (including ACTH level), and ophthalmological evaluation. The role of cerebrospinal fluid cytology is uncertain, and its use in individual situations may depend on the safety of lumbar puncture in the clinical setting.

Prognosis and prediction
Because of the rarity of this tumour, prognostic factors are not yet fully understood. In the largest series of 13 patients with pituitary blastoma, 5 children (38%) died: 4 from early or late treatment-related complications and 1 from progression {707}.

Box 12.05 Diagnostic criteria for pituitary blastoma

Essential:

Rathke pouch epithelial glands, primitive blastomatous cells, and secretory and folliculostellate anterior pituitary cells

AND

DICER1 alterations

Desirable:

Diagnosed in children aged < 2 years

Cushing syndrome

Personal or family history of *DICER1* syndrome

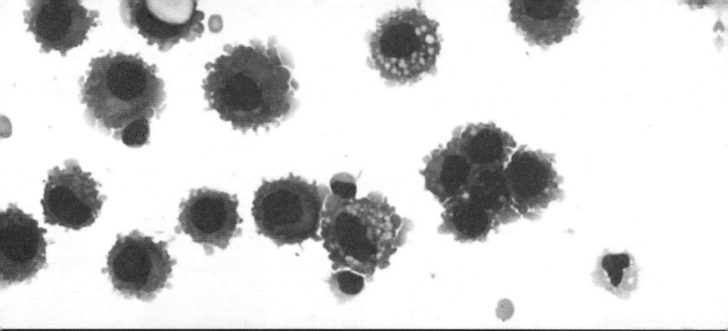

13

Metastases to the CNS

Edited by: Soffietti R, Wesseling P

Metastases to the brain and spinal cord parenchyma
Metastases to the meninges

Metastases to the brain and spinal cord parenchyma

Mittelbronn MGA
Ahluwalia MS
Brastianos PK
Preusser WM
Rosenblum MK
Tanaka S
Winkler FA

Definition

Metastases to the brain and spinal cord parenchyma are tumours originating outside the CNS and spreading into the brain and spinal cord parenchyma via a haematogenous route or (less frequently) directly from adjacent anatomical structures.

ICD-O coding

None

ICD-11 coding

2D50 Malignant neoplasm metastasis in brain, with extension code for primary tumour type

Related terminology

None

Subtype(s)

None

Localization

Approximately 80% of all brain metastases are located in the cerebral hemispheres, particularly in arterial border zones and at the junction of the cerebral cortex and white matter; 15% occur in the cerebellum and 5% occur in the brainstem. Fewer than 50% occur as a single brain metastasis and very few as the only (solitary) metastasis in the body {1049,2439}. Occasionally, CNS metastases seed along ventricular walls or are located in the pituitary gland or choroid plexus.

Non-parenchymal, non-diffuse meningeal metastases

In addition to having diffusely or multifocally disseminated leptomeningeal metastases (see *Metastases to the meninges*, p. 421), 8–9% of patients with advanced cancer may also present with circumscribed dural metastases {1791}. The distinction between diffuse and circumscribed meningeal metastases is clinically important because the latter has a slightly better prognosis and patients can usually undergo local treatment strategies {1822}. Metastases to the dura and leptomeninges are most frequently linked to extension from or to other CNS compartments, with the vast majority affecting the spinal cord via expansion from vertebral or paravertebral tissues into the epidural space {1791,2219,2182}. Dural metastases are relatively common in cancers of the prostate, breast, and lung, and in haematological malignancies {1791,2219}. Spinal epidural metastases are most common in cancers of the prostate, breast, lung, and kidney, as well as in non-Hodgkin lymphoma and multiple myeloma. Intramedullary spinal cord metastases are most common in small cell lung carcinoma {2182}.

Clinical features

Neurological symptoms of intracranial metastases are generally caused by increased intracranial pressure and local tumour

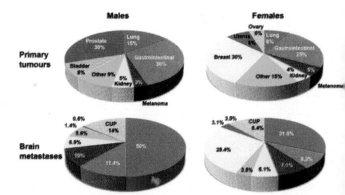

Fig. 13.01 Relative frequencies of primary tumours and of brain metastases derived from them. Tumours with a high propensity to metastasize to the brain are lung cancer, breast cancer, renal cell carcinoma, and melanoma. In this series of brain metastases, about 14% of cases in male patients and 8% of cases in female patients were diagnosed as carcinoma of unknown primary (CUP) {459,2568}. Data are based on the histology of archival tissue samples: 874 cases collected in 1990–2011 at the Institute of Neurology (Neuropathology), Medical University of Vienna. Metastases for which surgery was not performed are not represented. The relative frequencies of brain metastases may differ substantially in other regions of the world.

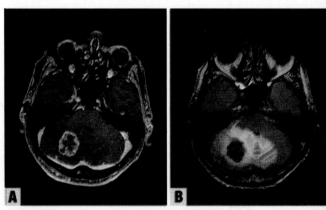

Fig. 13.02 Single brain metastasis from colorectal cancer. **A** Ring-enhancing lesion in the cerebellum on T1-weighted, postcontrast axial MRI. **B** FLAIR MRI showing great extent of vasogenic oedema.

effects on the adjacent brain tissue. The symptoms may progress gradually and include headache, altered mental status, paresis, ataxia, visual changes, nausea, and sensory disturbances. Some patients present with seizure, infarct, or haemorrhage {1830}. The interval between diagnosis of the primary tumour and the CNS metastasis is frequently < 1 year for lung carcinoma, but it can be many years for breast cancer and melanoma {248}.

Imaging

On MRI, intraparenchymal metastases are generally circumscribed and show mild T1 hypointensity, T2 hyperintensity, and diffuse or ring-like contrast enhancement with a surrounding zone of parenchymal oedema. Haemorrhagic metastases and metastatic melanomas containing melanin pigment may demonstrate hyperintensity on non-contrast MRI or CT {3551}.

Epidemiology

The incidence rates reported in the literature probably underestimate the true incidence of brain metastases because of underdiagnosis and inaccurate reporting {972,3099}. In a large population-based study in Sweden, the incidence of patients admitted to hospital with brain metastases doubled to 14 cases per 100 000 person-years between 1987 and 2006. More efficient control of disease spread outside the CNS and the use of more advanced neuroimaging techniques may have contributed to this increase {2956,2353,3099}. Autopsy studies have shown that CNS metastases occur in about 25% of patients who die of cancer {1049}.

Age and sex distribution

CNS metastases are the most common CNS neoplasms in adults, but metastases account for only about 2% of all paediatric CNS tumours. As many as 30% of adults and 6–10% of children with cancer develop brain metastases. The relative proportions of various primary tumours are different between the two sexes, but for most tumour types, sex has no significant independent effect on the occurrence of CNS metastasis {201,972,3437}. The incidence of brain metastases has been reported to be highest among patients diagnosed with primary lung cancer at the age of 40–49 years; with primary melanoma, renal cancer, or colorectal cancer at the age of 50–59 years; and with breast cancer at the age of 20–39 years {3099}.

Etiology

The most common source of brain metastasis in adults is lung cancer (especially adenocarcinoma and small cell carcinoma), followed by breast cancer, melanoma, renal cell carcinoma, and colorectal cancer {459,2252,2568}. Tumours and their molecular subtypes vary in their propensity to metastasize to the CNS {201,661,248}. In as many as 10% of patients with brain metastases, no primary tumour is found at presentation {2568}. In children, the most common sources of CNS metastases are leukaemias and lymphomas, followed by non-haematopoietic CNS neoplasms such as germ cell tumours, osteosarcoma, neuroblastoma, Ewing sarcoma, and rhabdomyosarcoma {661, 3437}. Occasionally, primary neoplasms in the head and neck region extend intracranially by direct invasion, sometimes along cranial nerves, and manifest as intracranial tumours {2882}.

Pathogenesis

Before they manifest as haematogenous metastases in the CNS, tumour cells must successfully complete a series of steps: escape from the primary tumour, enter into and survive in the blood stream, get arrested in brain capillaries, extravasate into the CNS, and colonize the perivascular niche that allows survival and subsequent growth in the CNS microenvironment. This process occurs via interactions with various cell types, including neurons, and with the extracellular matrix {1609,2568, 3586}. An alternative, direct route to the brain using bridging vessels from the bone marrow has only been described for leukaemia cells so far {3527}. The molecular basis of CNS spread

in the various tumour types is still incompletely understood and requires further study. Local spread of CNS tumours may also occur by direct extension from primary tumours in adjacent anatomical structures (e.g. paranasal sinuses and bone) {2882}. Such tumours are not formally considered metastases because they remain in continuity with the primary neoplasm.

Macroscopic appearance

Metastases in the brain and spinal cord parenchyma often form grossly circumscribed and rounded greyish-white or tan masses with variable central necrosis and peritumoural oedema. Metastases of adenocarcinomas may contain collections of mucoid material. Haemorrhage is relatively frequent in metastases of choriocarcinoma, hepatocellular carcinoma, melanoma, and clear cell renal cell carcinoma. Melanoma metastases with abundant melanin pigment are brown to black in colour. Primary neoplasms in the head and neck region that extend intracranially by direct invasion generally cause marked destruction of the skull bones. However, in some cases, the skull is penetrated by relatively subtle perivascular or perineural invasion, without major bone destruction {2882}.

Histopathology

The histological and immunohistochemical features of CNS metastases are as diverse as those of the primary tumours from which they arise. Most brain metastases are fairly well demarcated, with variable perivascular growth (vascular cooption) in the adjacent CNS tissue {247}. On occasion, small cell carcinomas and lymphomas may show more diffuse infiltration (pseudogliomatous growth) in the adjacent brain parenchyma {219, 2237}. Tumour necrosis may be extensive, leaving recognizable tumour tissue only at the periphery of the lesion and around blood vessels {2439}.

Proliferation

Metastatic CNS tumours show variable and often marked mitotic activity. The Ki-67 proliferation index may be significantly higher than that of the primary neoplasm {246}.

Immunophenotype

The immunohistochemical characteristics of CNS metastases are generally similar to those of the tumours from which they originate. Immunohistochemical analysis is often very helpful for distinguishing between primary CNS tumours and metastases and for assessing the exact nature and origin of the metastatic neoplasm (particularly in cases with an unknown primary tumour) {229,2439} (see Table 13.01, p. 420).

Cytology

Cytological features depend mainly on the type of primary tumour.

Diagnostic molecular pathology

The use of molecular markers for CNS metastases is becoming increasingly important because the molecular profiles of primary tumour brain metastases can vary and treatment has to be adapted accordingly {245,3009}. In addition, some markers such as PDL1 are evaluable by immunohistochemistry and are already used in a broad spectrum of entities {691}, but shortcomings of this approach (e.g. intratumoural heterogeneity, multiple

Table 13.01 Diagnostic and theragnostic markers for CNS metastases

Primary tumour	Diagnostic markers	Predictive diagnostic markers
Melanoma	Melan-A, HMB45, SOX10, BRAF p.V600E	*BRAF, NRAS, KIT*, PDL1
Non-small cell lung carcinoma	CK7, TTF1, napsin A	*EGFR, ALK, KRAS, BRAF, ERBB2* (HER2), *MET, ROS1*, PDL1
Small cell lung carcinoma	CK7, CD56, TTF1	None
Breast adenocarcinoma	CK7, GCDFP-15, GATA3, mammaglobin	ER, PR, ERBB2 (HER2), PDL1, gene expression panels
Ovarian carcinoma	CK7, WT1, PAX8	*BRCA1, BRCA2, CHEK2, PALB2, RAD51C* and/or *RAD51D*
Squamous cell carcinoma	CK5/6, p63, p40	None
Renal cell carcinoma	PAX8, CD10, RCCm	None
Urothelial carcinoma	CK5/6, CK7, CK20	PDL1
Colorectal carcinoma	CK20, CDX2	*KRAS, BRAF, NRAS*, microsatellite instability (MLH1), mismatch repair immunohistochemistry (e.g. MSH2, MSH6, MLH1, PMS2)
Gastric adenocarcinoma	CK7, CK20	ERBB2 (HER2), PDL1
Prostate adenocarcinoma	Pancytokeratin, PSA, PSAP, NKX3-1	None
Thyroid carcinoma	TTF1, thyroglobulin, PAX8	None
B-cell lymphoma	CD45, CD20, CD79a	B-cell clonality (IG genes)
T-cell lymphoma	CD45, CD3, CD4, CD8	T-cell clonality (TR genes)

TTF1, thyroid transcription factor 1.

different antibodies for distinct entities or treatment schemes, entity-specific evaluation algorithms) are associated with poor interobserver reproducibility {2677}. In addition, there is increasing evidence that tumour cell expression of PDL1 might be induced by infiltrating immune cells, and it may therefore (at least partly) be considered an indirect effect, thus potentially being of lower predictive value than the immune cell infiltration itself {1951}. Molecular alterations that are frequently found, and that are of high clinical importance because of the availability of targeted drugs with activity against brain metastases, include *EGFR* mutations and *ALK* fusions in lung cancer {1902}, *BRAF* mutations in melanoma {2884}, and ERBB2 overexpression in breast cancer {3265}. For other treatable molecular alterations that are found at low frequencies in various cancers (e.g. NTRK fusions, involving various oncogenic fusion partners), broad immunohistochemical screening might be useful in the future {2989}.

Essential and desirable diagnostic criteria

See Box 13.01.

Staging

Despite the high incidence of brain metastases, in certain cancers like metastatic melanoma, lung adenocarcinoma, and ERBB2 (HER2)-positive and triple-negative breast cancer, brain imaging is not an established part of primary staging, but it should be considered whenever clinically meaningful (at the latest when neurological symptoms develop in patients with known cancer). MRI is recommended over CT when available, because of its much higher sensitivity and the opportunity it provides to exclude differential diagnoses {446,68}. If the primary tumour is not known, a skin examination, gynaecological examination, and

Box 13.01 Diagnostic criteria for metastases to the brain and spinal cord parenchyma

Essential:

Detection of malignant non-primary cells within the brain or spinal cord parenchyma

Desirable:

Fulfilment of specific diagnostic criteria for the primary tumour type

CT of the chest +/– abdomen is typically performed. FDG PET may be of additional value in cases of unknown primary tumour {2982}. After treatment of brain metastases, regular follow-up imaging is recommended, normally every 3 months.

Prognosis and prediction

The main established prognostic factors for patients with brain metastases are patient age, Karnofsky performance status, number of brain metastases, and status of extracranial disease. Several prognostic scores taking these parameters into account have been described, but they require validation in independent and prospective studies {1696,3006}. Other factors of prognostic significance include the specific tumour type and the molecular drivers involved (e.g. ERBB2 [HER2] in breast cancer) {3010,3007,3008}. Neuroradiological parameters such as peritumoural brain oedema may also provide prognostic information {3001}. In more recent studies, the reported improvement in the overall survival of patients with CNS metastases may be attributable to improvements in focal surgical removal for single lesions, stereotactic radiosurgery, and systemic therapies, in combination with earlier detection of such metastases {2252,2982}.

Metastases to the meninges

Mittelbronn MGA   Rosenblum MK
Ahluwalia MS   Tanaka S
Brastianos PK   Winkler FA
Preusser WM

Definition

Metastases to the meninges are tumours originating outside the CNS with diffuse and/or multifocal spread within the leptomeninges and the subarachnoid space.

ICD-O coding

None

ICD-11 coding

2D51 Malignant neoplasm metastasis in meninges

Related terminology

Not recommended: leptomeningeal cancer; neoplastic meningitis; (lepto)meningeal carcinomatosis.

Subtype(s)

None

Localization

Meninges. For non-diffuse meningeal metastases, see *Metastases to the brain and spinal cord parenchyma* (p. 418).

Clinical features

Many patients with leptomeningeal metastasis (LM) have multiple and varied neurological symptoms at presentation, including headache, mental alteration, ataxia, cranial nerve dysfunction, and radiculopathy. Clinical diagnosis can be made according to current diagnostic criteria {1822}. Cytological examination reveals malignant cells in the initial cerebrospinal fluid (CSF) sample in about 50% of such patients; this proportion may increase to ≥ 80% when CSF sampling is repeated and adequate volumes (≥ 10 mL) are available for cytological analysis {506,1830}. Spinal metastases generally result in compression of the spinal cord or nerve roots, and they may cause back pain, weakness of the extremities, sensory disturbances, and incontinence over the course of hours, days, or weeks {1830}.

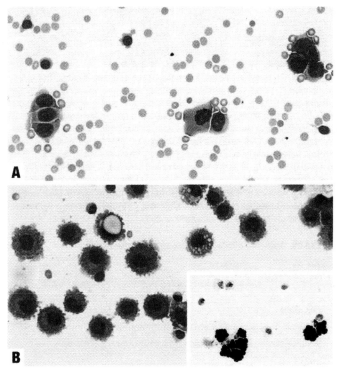

Fig. 13.03 Metastases to the meninges. Cytological preparations showing metastatic cells within the cerebrospinal fluid. **A** Lobular breast carcinoma, showing single-file–like group and mitosis. **B** Melanoma metastasis; **inset:** S100 immunochemistry.

Imaging

In patients with LM, MRI can show focal or diffuse leptomeningeal thickening and contrast enhancement (sometimes with dispersed tumour nodules in the subarachnoid space). Enhancement and enlargement of the cranial nerves and communicating hydrocephalus may also be found {1119}.

Epidemiology

LM occurs in 4–15% of patients with solid tumours {506,3105}; however, this number might be underestimated due to lack of specific symptoms. In cases of already existing brain metastasis, rates of LM may increase to 33–54% in breast cancer, 56–82% in lung cancer, and 87–96% in melanoma {1822}. The highest incidence rates of LM have been reported in metastatic melanoma (23%) and lung cancer (9–25%) followed by breast carcinoma (5%) {3170}.

Etiology

Metastatic spread is usually haematogenous and from non-CNS malignant neoplasms.

Pathogenesis

Once in contact with the CSF compartment via direct invasion from the brain or spinal cord or indirectly via the blood stream,

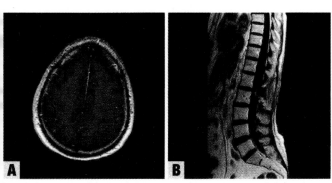

Fig. 13.04 Leptomeningeal metastases from breast carcinoma. **A** Diffuse enhancement of cortical sulci on T1-weighted, postcontrast axial MRI. **B** Linear enhancement of the spinal leptomeninges on T1-weighted, postcontrast sagittal MRI.

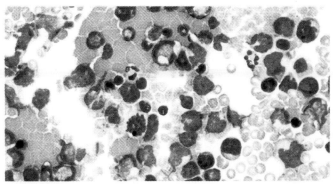

Fig. 13.05 Cerebrospinal fluid (CSF) metastasis of B-cell lymphoma. The cellular component of normal CSF consists almost exclusively of cytologically atypical lymphocytes (60–70% of the cells) with round nuclei and sparse cytoplasm, mainly of the CD4+ memory phenotype, and monocytes with a bean-shaped nucleus (30–40% of the cells), without associated haemorrhage (red blood cell) as in the present case; neutrophils in the CSF indicate a barrier disturbance. When there is leptomeningeal spread, tumour cells are primarily recognized by their large nuclei (here 4–5 times larger than the nuclei of normal lymphocytes and monocytes), which are often irregular and hyperchromatic. Frequently, the neoplastic cells display prominent nucleoli, a cytological feature that is absent in cells of the normal CSF. Abnormal binucleated or multinucleated cells are also observed. Mitoses are a frequent finding in leptomeningeal spread of tumour cells. (Pappenheim stain)

Box 13.02 Diagnostic criteria for metastases to the meninges

Essential:

Unequivocal clinical and/or radiological evidence of leptomeningeal metastasis

Desirable:

Presence of malignant cells within the cerebrospinal fluid

Immunohistochemical demonstration of the origin of the metastatic cells

metastatic tumour cells may disseminate (seed) diffusely along the leptomeninges.

Macroscopic appearance
LM may produce diffuse opacification of the membranes or manifest as multiple nodules {2439}.

Histopathology
In LM, the tumour cells are dispersed in the subarachnoid (including Virchow–Robin) space and may invade the adjacent CNS parenchyma and nerve roots {3105}.

Cytology
More than 90% of patients with LM show at least one of the following non-diagnostic pathological features in the CSF: increased opening pressure (> 200 mm H2O), increased leukocyte count (> 4/µL), elevated protein (> 50 mg/dL) and lactate (> 2.4 mmol/L), and decreased glucose levels (< 60 mg/dL) {762,1822}. However, the final proof of LM is still provided by the highly specific detection of malignant cells in CSF samples by cytology. Normal CSF samples almost exclusively consist of lymphocytes (60–70%) and monocytes (30–40%), whereas > 50% of all patients with LM also show elevated numbers of granulocytes indicating a barrier disturbance {762}. Neoplastic cells within the CSF are typically recognized by increased nuclear and total cell size, irregular cytoplasmic and nuclear shape, and prominent nucleoli. Furthermore, mitoses and

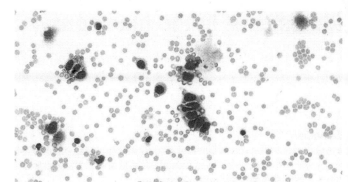

Fig. 13.06 Diffuse meningeal metastasis. Cerebrospinal fluid showing the presence of numerous metastatic breast adenocarcinoma cells. Note the clustering and large size of the carcinoma cells in relation to the small lymphocytes.

apoptotic nuclei can be present. Finally, immunocytochemical assessment for lineage-specific or even therapeutic markers can be an asset to the diagnostic procedure. The unequivocal detection of malignant cells in the CSF should be reported as "positive", the detection of suspicious or atypical cells as "equivocal", and the absence of malignant or equivocal cells as "negative" {1822}.

Diagnostic molecular pathology
Novel liquid biopsy approaches hold promise for more accurate detection of, for example, circulating tumour cells and cell-free tumour DNA, so they may help improve diagnostic precision, therapeutic management, and treatment monitoring. There is increasing evidence that such liquid biopsies of CSF constitute a reliable additional diagnostic tool, especially in cases that are highly suspicious for LM but that have negative or equivocal results in classic cytological assessments of the CSF {316}.

Essential and desirable diagnostic criteria
See Box 13.02.

Staging
Central staging methods are MRI of the brain and spine, and CSF diagnostics (cytology, as well as measurement of opening pressure, protein, glucose, and lactate). The highly variable clinical presentation – with many possible combinations of solid meningeal manifestation in various places throughout the CNS, and/ or the presence of non-adherent (fluid) tumour cells in the CSF – has complicated the development of generally accepted criteria for diagnosis, response assessment, and follow-up {1820}.

Union for International Cancer Control (UICC) staging should be performed according to the criteria for the specific primary tumour, when known.

Prognosis and prediction
The prognosis is dismal for patients with LM, so pragmatic treatment approaches primarily focus on life prolongation with an acceptable quality of life {1822}. Besides standard intravenous or intra-CSF pharmacotherapy, focal radiotherapy can be used for circumscribed, symptomatic lesions, whereas whole-brain irradiation might be preferential for extensively disseminated LM. The increasing availability of targeted treatments and liquid biopsy approaches allow for more individualized therapy according to molecular cancer profiles.

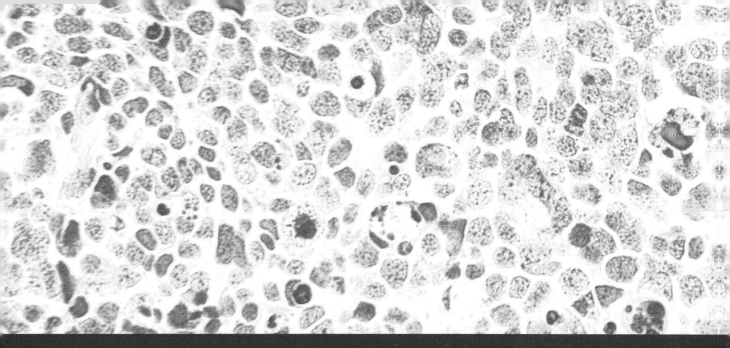

14

Genetic tumour syndromes involving the CNS

Edited by: Lax SF, Lazar AJ, Perry A

Neurofibromatosis type 1
Neurofibromatosis type 2
Schwannomatosis
Von Hippel–Lindau syndrome
Tuberous sclerosis
Li–Fraumeni syndrome
Cowden syndrome
Constitutional mismatch repair deficiency syndrome
Familial adenomatous polyposis 1
Naevoid basal cell carcinoma syndrome
Rhabdoid tumour predisposition syndrome
Carney complex
DICER1 syndrome
Familial paraganglioma syndromes
Melanoma-astrocytoma syndrome
Familial retinoblastoma
BAP1 tumour predisposition syndrome
Fanconi anaemia
ELP1-medulloblastoma syndrome

The central and peripheral nervous systems are frequently implicated in a wide range of genetic tumour predisposition syndromes. These disorders are often highly complex, and patients are typically best served in specialized centres with broad multidisciplinary expertise. Traditionally, most of these patients' diagnoses have been based purely on clinical features and family histories. However, more and more often, a heritable pathogenic variant is first detected as part of a genomic screening assay, such as next-generation sequencing of tumour and/ or germline DNA. Not uncommonly though, the pathologist encounters the first clue, so it is critically important to be aware of when to raise the possibility of genetic tumour syndromes to the patient's clinical team for further workup. Some of the common relationships between syndromes and tumours have long been appreciated; for instance, most pathologists know of the tight associations between multiple and/or plexiform neurofibromas (sometimes with transformation to malignant peripheral nerve sheath tumour) and neurofibromatosis type 1, between bilateral vestibular schwannomas and neurofibromatosis type 2, between haemangioblastomas and von Hippel–Lindau

Table 14.01 Tumour scenarios that should prompt a pathologist to consider a potential underlying genetic tumour syndrome

Tumour scenario	Genetic tumour syndrome(s)
Bilateral vestibular schwannomas	NF2
Choroid plexus carcinoma	Li–Fraumeni syndrome
Dysplastic cerebellar gangliocytoma (Lhermitte–Duclos disease)	Cowden syndrome
Embryonal tumour with multilayered rosettes lacking C19MC alteration	DICER1 syndrome
Haemangioblastoma	Von Hippel–Lindau syndrome
Hybrid neurofibroma/schwannoma	NF1, NF2, and schwannomatosis
IDH- and H3-wildtype, p53-positive glioblastoma in a child	Li–Fraumeni syndrome
IDH-wildtype giant cell glioblastoma in a young patient	Constitutional mismatch repair deficiency, Lynch syndrome, and Li–Fraumeni syndrome
IDH1 p.R132C/S–mutant astrocytoma in an adult	Li–Fraumeni syndrome
Malignant melanotic nerve sheath tumour	Carney complex
Malignant peripheral nerve sheath tumour arising from a neurofibroma	NF1
Meningioma in a child	NF2
Multiple meningiomas	NF2
Multiple neurofibromas, a plexiform neurofibroma, or a massive soft tissue neurofibroma	NF1
Multiple schwannomas or one with mosaic SMARCB1 (INI1) expression	NF2 and schwannomatosis
Paraganglioma with loss of SDHB expression	Familial paraganglioma syndromes (see Table 14.06, p. 465)
Pineoblastoma	DICER1 syndrome and familial retinoblastoma syndrome
Pituitary blastoma	DICER1 syndrome
Primary intracranial sarcoma, DICER1-mutant	DICER1 syndrome
Rhabdoid and/or papillary meningioma	BAP1 tumour predisposition syndrome
Rhabdoid tumour(s) in an infant	Rhabdoid tumour predisposition syndrome
SHH-activated medulloblastoma	Naevoid basal cell carcinoma (Gorlin) syndrome, ELP1-medulloblastoma syndrome, and GPR161 (Gorlin-like) syndrome
SHH-activated, TP53-mutant medulloblastoma (often the large cell / anaplastic histological type)	Li–Fraumeni syndrome and Fanconi anaemia
Subependymal giant cell astrocytoma	Tuberous sclerosis
WNT-activated medulloblastoma, CTNNB1-wildtype	Familial adenomatous polyposis

NF1, neurofibromatosis type 1; NF2, neurofibromatosis type 2; SHH, sonic hedgehog.

syndrome, and between subependymal giant cell astrocytomas and tuberous sclerosis. However, many pathologists are less aware of many of the other syndromic associations highlighted in Table 14.01. The combination of colonic polyposis and brain tumours was historically designated as Turcot syndrome, but this designation is no longer appropriate, because it is now clear that this outdated eponym in fact comprises multiple now well-defined cancer predisposition syndromes, each with a different pathogenesis.

Our understanding of genetic tumour syndromes has evolved rapidly since the 2016 WHO classification of CNS tumours, such that eight additional disorders are now covered in this new edition: Carney complex, *DICER1* syndrome, familial paraganglioma syndrome, melanoma-astrocytoma syndrome, familial retinoblastoma, *BAP1* tumour predisposition syndrome, Fanconi anaemia, and ELP1-medulloblastoma syndrome. Several of the 19 syndromes covered here are additionally described in other volumes of the WHO classification. Nonetheless, there is naturally a greater focus on nervous system findings in this volume. For some of these syndromes, the clinical guidelines for diagnosis have also evolved; therefore, the newest or most widely used iterations are emphasized, often in table format. Practical diagnostic approaches utilizing surrogate immunostains are also highlighted when appropriate, along with the more traditional molecular diagnostic techniques that may be requisite for a definitive diagnosis. In most cases, the macroscopy, histopathology, and cytology descriptions of individual tumour types seen within a genetic syndrome are covered entirely or in greater detail within the earlier sections dedicated to the sporadic counterparts of those distinct entities. In contrast, the clinical spectrum, pathogenesis, and molecular genetics of the syndromes are covered in greater detail here.

Neurofibromatosis type 1

Legius E
Fisher MJ
Gutmann DH
Reuss DE
Rodriguez FJ

Definition

Neurofibromatosis type 1 (NF1) is an autosomal dominant disorder caused by sequence variation in the *NF1* gene, diagnosed clinically when at least two of the following are present: multiple café-au-lait macules, skinfold freckling, iris hamartomas (Lisch nodules), optic pathway glioma / pilocytic astrocytoma (OPG), multiple neurofibromas or one plexiform neurofibroma, specific osseous lesions, and an affected first-degree relative.

MIM numbering

162200 Neurofibromatosis, type I; NF1

ICD-11 coding

LD2D.10 Neurofibromatosis type 1

Related terminology

Not recommended: von Recklinghausen disease; peripheral neurofibromatosis.

Subtype(s)

Mosaic neurofibromatosis type 1, including segmental neurofibromatosis type 1; spinal neurofibromatosis; neurofibromatosis–Noonan syndrome; 17q11.2 microdeletion syndrome

Localization

NF1 affects many different cell types and tissues in the body, including both the central and peripheral nervous systems.

Clinical features

Multiple café-au-lait macules are usually present at birth, and they increase in number during the first 2 years of life. Skinfold freckling in the axillary, inguinal, and submammary regions occurs in > 80% of adults with NF1. Lisch nodules (asymptomatic iris hamartomas), present in > 90% of adults with NF1, are best detected by slit-lamp examination. Lisch nodules and skinfold freckling both usually develop before puberty. Cutaneous neurofibromas, present in > 85% of adults with NF1 {1199}, typically develop during puberty. In contrast, plexiform neurofibromas are probably congenital lesions, arising in 30–50% of children with NF1 {1199}. Individual plexiform neurofibromas have variable growth rates, which can be relatively constant for long periods of time, but they exhibit the highest growth potential during infancy and childhood. A subset of plexiform neurofibromas transform into atypical neurofibroma / atypical neurofibromatous neoplasm of uncertain biological potential (ANNUBP), which can be a premalignant lesion with increased risk to progress to high-grade malignant peripheral nerve sheath tumour (MPNST) {2109,231}. Possible transformation to ANNUBP or MPNST should be considered in patients with growing nodular plexiform neurofibromas, plexiform neurofibromas in which an isolated portion exhibits disproportionate

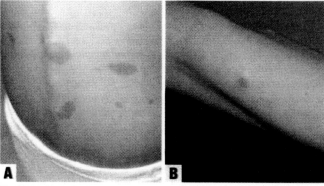

Fig. 14.01 Neurofibromatosis type 1 (NF1). **A** Multiple café-au-lait spots on the back in a child with NF1. **B** Cutaneous neurofibromas on the left arm of an adult with NF1.

growth relative to the rest of the tumour, or continued growth of a plexiform neurofibroma into adulthood.

Specific bone abnormalities can be present in individuals with NF1. These include severe scoliosis, sphenoid wing dysplasia, non-ossifying fibromas, and congenital tibial bowing. Progressive tibial bowing can result in pathological fracture, with the development of a pseudarthrosis {2840}.

Many children with NF1 exhibit learning disabilities, attention deficit hyperactivity disorder, and problems with reciprocal social interactions {2165}. MRI brain morphometry reveals a large grey matter volume and large corpus callosum, both features associated with learning disabilities {2161}.

About 15% of children with NF1 will develop an OPG, which can cause progressive vision loss in ≥ 50% of affected individuals {1912}. The second most common location for a glioma is the brainstem {1986}; however, gliomas can develop in other locations {1985}. Young adults with NF1 are also prone to malignant gliomas {2364}. In children, T2-weighted brain MRI shows focal areas of high signal intensity that tend to disappear with age and are sometimes difficult to differentiate from low-grade gliomas {1166}.

Epilepsy is more common in individuals with NF1 than in the general population, and drug-resistant epilepsy requiring surgery is often associated with dysembryoplastic neuroepithelial tumours {2340}. Sleep disturbances are also more common in people with NF1 {1890}.

Other neoplasms observed at increased frequency are juvenile myelomonocytic leukaemia, rhabdomyosarcoma, glomus tumours of the digits, gastrointestinal stromal tumours, phaeochromocytoma, female breast cancer, and duodenal neuroendocrine tumours (somatostatinomas) {369}.

Epidemiology

NF1 is a common autosomal dominant disorder, with a birth incidence of 1 case per 3000 live births {3260}.

Etiology

NF1 is caused by heterozygous pathogenic variants in the *NF1* gene, which encodes neurofibromin {3360,493,3334}. Half of the individuals with NF1 have unaffected parents; those cases of NF1 represent de novo mutations.

Pathogenesis

Neurofibromin primarily functions as a GAP for the RAS family of oncogenes {1846}. The EVH1 domain of SPRED1 (the protein implicated in Legius syndrome) binds to neurofibromin on both sides of the GAP-related domain and recruits neurofibromin to the membrane where it can accelerate RAS inactivation {3047, 1313,807}.

Most clinical features of NF1, including café-au-lait macules, bony abnormalities, and benign tumours, result from a complete loss of neurofibromin function (biallelic *NF1* inactivation), leading to increased RAS and RAS effector (MEK/ERK or AKT/mTOR) signalling. Atypical neurofibromas / ANNUBPs harbour additional genetic alterations, including loss of the *CDKN2A*, *CDKN2B*, and *SMARCA2* regions on chromosome 9p {231, 2449,3518}. MPNSTs have a highly rearranged karyotype, and they frequently show additional aberrations in the PRC2 complex and, to a lesser extent, *TP53* genes {712,1842,3598}. Low-grade gliomas in NF1 are typically characterized by biallelic *NF1* loss alone, although other mutations are occasionally seen. Alterations in *CDKN2A*, *CDKN2B*, and/or *ATRX* have been detected in some low-grade gliomas in NF1, where they are often associated with worrisome histological features (anaplasia and increased proliferation) and more aggressive tumour behaviour. In the absence of a low-grade precursor such as pilocytic astrocytoma, high-grade gliomas in NF1 are also characterized by frequent *TP53* mutations, as well as *CDKN2A*, *CDKN2B*, and *ATRX* mutations {675}.

In neurofibromas and OPGs, murine studies have revealed that non-neoplastic (stromal) cells with a heterozygous *Nf1* mutation, including mast cells, macrophages, neurons, T cells, and microglia, are critical for tumorigenesis and continued growth.

Macroscopic appearance

Macroscopic appearances of nerve sheath neoplasms affecting people with NF1 include small sessile or pedunculated growths of the skin (cutaneous neurofibromas), plaque-like thickening of the skin (diffuse neurofibroma), fusiform segmental expansions of individual peripheral nerve fascicles (intraneural neurofibromas), and multinodular/multifascicular nerve expansions, described as a "bag of worms" (plexiform neurofibromas). Massive soft tissue neurofibromas occur exclusively in individuals with NF1 and are characterized by large neurofibromatous involvement of anatomical segments, even of entire limbs, with infiltration of soft tissue and skeletal muscle. Fleshy masses and areas of necrosis and haemorrhage characterize MPNST.

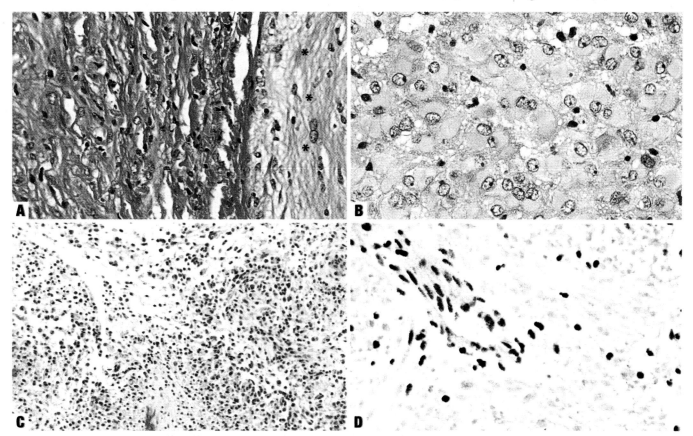

Fig. 14.02 Neurofibromatosis type 1 (NF1). **A** Pilocytic astrocytoma. The most common brain tumour in patients with NF1 is pilocytic astrocytoma, which is frequently located in the optic nerve (asterisks). **B** Low-grade astrocytoma with subependymal giant cell astrocytoma (SEGA)-like morphology. A variety of gliomas may also affect patients with NF1, including low-grade astrocytomas that are difficult to classify, occasionally demonstrating SEGA-like morphology. **C** High-grade glioma tumours usually afflict adult patients and may show infiltration, mitotic activity, and palisading necrosis, similar to glioblastoma. **D** Loss of ATRX staining in an NF1-associated high-grade glioma. *ATRX* mutations lead to protein loss shown by immunohistochemistry, with preservation in blood vessels and other non-neoplastic cells.

Histopathology

Nerve sheath tumours in NF1 are predominantly neurofibromas, which resemble their sporadic counterparts. Cells of the haematopoietic lineage (including histiocytes and mast cells) are also encountered, which contribute to the tumour microenvironment {1560}.

Recently proposed criteria for ANNUBPs are used to describe premalignant or worrisome changes in neurofibromas, and they include at least two of the following: cytological atypia, hypercellularity, loss of neurofibroma architecture, and a mitotic count of > 0.2 mitoses/mm^2 and < 1.5 mitoses/mm^2 (equating to > 1 mitosis/50 HPF and < 3 mitoses/10 HPF of 0.51 mm in diameter and 0.2 mm^2 in area) {2109}. These changes may be present in clinically designated atypical neurofibromas, which, in a subset of cases, later transform into MPNST {1307}.

Most MPNSTs in individuals with NF1 are high-grade malignant spindle cell neoplasms with brisk mitotic activity and necrosis, which either develop in a pre-existing plexiform neurofibroma or arise de novo. A wide spectrum of heterologous differentiation (cartilaginous, osseous, rhabdomyoblastic, glandular) may be present.

Immunohistochemical analyses frequently demonstrate p16 and H3 p.K28me3 (K27me3) loss {608}, as well as decreased or absent expression of Schwann cell markers (S100, SOX10).

Individuals with NF1 are also predisposed to a variety of glial neoplasms, with pilocytic astrocytomas being the predominant histological subtype. Difficult-to-classify gliomas with ambiguous features may also be encountered, as well as low-grade gliomas with morphological similarities to subependymal giant cell astrocytomas {2378}. High-grade astrocytomas in NF1 tend to affect young adults, and their aggressiveness is similar to that of their sporadic counterparts. High-grade astrocytomas in NF1 frequently have loss of ATRX expression, resulting in an alternative-lengthening-of-telomeres phenotype {2694,675}.

Cytology

Not clinically relevant

Diagnostic molecular pathology

Although no mutation hotspots have been identified, a pathogenic *NF1* variant is detected in 95% of people with NF1 {2084}. Nonsense, frameshift, and splice-site mutations, as well as small insertions, small deletions, or small duplications, all result in *NF1* inactivation. In 5–10% of cases a 17q11.2 microdeletion is identified, in which multiple genes are codeleted along with the *NF1* gene. One of these deleted genes, *SUZ12*, a component of the polycomb complex PRC2, has been implicated in MPNST development {712,1842,3598}.

To date, the most striking genotype–phenotype correlations have involved individuals with a specific 3 bp deletion (c.2970_2972del) or with a missense mutation affecting codon

Box 14.01 Diagnostic criteria for neurofibromatosis type 1 (NF1)

Essential:

A clinical diagnosis of NF1 requires the presence of at least two of the following features:

- Six or more café-au-lait macules (diameter > 5 mm in children, > 15 mm in adults)
- Two or more cutaneous or subcutaneous neurofibromas or one plexiform neurofibroma
- Axillary/inguinal freckling
- Optic pathway glioma / pilocytic astrocytoma
- Two or more iris hamartomas (Lisch nodules)
- Distinctive bony abnormality (tibial dysplasia, pseudarthrosis, orbital dysplasia)
- First-degree relative with NF1 (by the above criteria)

In the future, these criteria may be revised to include genetic testing and other common newly recognized clinical features. In young children, multiple café-au-lait macules are usually the only clinical sign of NF1, such that in the absence of an affected parent, a diagnosis of NF1 cannot be rendered. Multiple café-au-lait spots with or without skinfold freckling can be seen in other conditions, including Legius syndrome (MIM number: 611431). Multiple neurofibromas can also be associated with certain forms of Noonan syndrome, making molecular analysis of the *NF1* gene increasingly more important for diagnostic purposes {2083,2409,625}. In children with multiple café-au-lait spots and malignant tumours (e.g. leukaemia), constitutive mismatch repair deficiency should also be considered {3062}.

p.R1809: these individuals do not develop neurofibromas or OPGs {1672,2710,2516,3257}. In addition, patients with missense mutations involving codons 844–848 appear to exhibit more severe disease symptomatology, including a higher incidence of externally visible plexiform neurofibromas, symptomatic spinal nerve root neurofibromas, OPG, and MPNST {1673}.

Essential and desirable diagnostic criteria

See Box 14.01.

Staging

Not relevant

Prognosis and prediction

NF1 is an autosomal dominant disorder, where affected parents harbour a 50% risk of disease transmission with each pregnancy. Individuals often have a shortened lifespan, mainly due to malignant disease and stroke {3260,875,2620}. The standard mortality ratio for many complications is higher in women aged < 50 years {3260}. Genetic counselling is recommended and includes the possibility of prenatal and/or preimplantation genetic testing.

MEK inhibitors are approved for use in children (aged 2–18 years) with NF1 who have symptomatic, inoperable plexiform neurofibromas, and they are currently being evaluated for use in adults with plexiform neurofibromas as well as in children with low-grade glioma {1170,2462,1660}.

Neurofibromatosis type 2

Stemmer-Rachamimov AO
Kratz CP
Louis DN
Schuhmann MU

Definition

Neurofibromatosis type 2 (NF2) is an autosomal dominant disease caused by a pathological sequence variant of the *NF2* gene, characterized by multiple benign tumours and dysplastic/hamartomatous lesions in the nervous system, including multiple schwannomas (particularly bilateral vestibular schwannomas), meningiomas, and spinal ependymomas.

MIM numbering

101000 Neurofibromatosis, type II; NF2

ICD-11 coding

LD2D.11 Neurofibromatosis type 2

Related terminology

Acceptable: bilateral acoustic neurofibromatosis; central neurofibromatosis.
Not recommended: von Recklinghausen disease.

Subtype(s)

Wishart phenotype (severe); Gardner phenotype (mild)

Localization

Tumours and hamartomas associated with NF2 affect all locations of the central and peripheral nervous system, with predilections for cranial, paraspinal, and peripheral nerves, as well as the meninges and the spinal cord.

Clinical features

Patients with NF2 often present in early adulthood, although the disease can manifest in childhood. The most common presentation in adults is with symptoms referable to a vestibular schwannoma (hearing loss, tinnitus, or imbalance). Presentation with vestibular schwannomas is uncommon in children (15%) whereas cutaneous schwannomas (NF2 plaques) and ocular abnormalities are more frequent {865}. NF2 mosaics, in which a somatic mutation occurs during embryogenesis, have variable phenotypes depending on the cell lineages involved. They may be challenging to diagnose and have clinical symptoms overlapping with schwannomatosis {2524}.

Clinical diagnostic criteria

The original clinical diagnostic criteria for NF2 were established at the US National Institutes of Health (NIH) Consensus Development Conference on neurofibromatosis in 1987 {2217}. Several revisions of these criteria have since been proposed, including the 1991 NIH criteria, the Manchester criteria (see Box 14.02, p. 432), the National Neurofibromatosis Foundation (NNFF) criteria, the Baser criteria, and the Smith criteria. Each of these revisions expanded the original criteria, aiming to also identify patients with multiple NF2 features who do not present

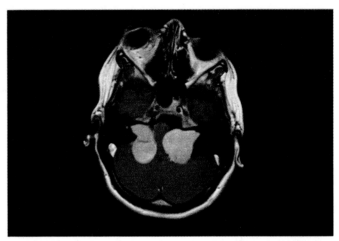

Fig. 14.03 Neurofibromatosis type 2 (NF2) schwannomas. Postcontrast T1-weighted MRI of bilateral vestibular schwannomas, the hallmark of NF2. When large, vestibular schwannomas may compress the brainstem.

with bilateral vestibular schwannomas and have no family history {210,871,1197}.

Because of the wide variability of symptoms and time of onset, it may be challenging to diagnose NF2 on the basis of clinical features alone. Particularly difficult to diagnose are genetic mosaics (accounting for 30% of sporadic cases), in which segmental involvement or milder disease may occur {1665}, and paediatric cases in which the full manifestations of the disease have not yet developed. The distinction from other forms is difficult in some cases. There is clinical phenotypic overlap between NF2 mosaic, early NF2, and schwannomatosis; some cases that fulfil the clinical diagnostic criteria for schwannomatosis are later proved to be NF2 {2524}. Molecular analysis of *LZTR1* and *SMARCB1* mutations (the two schwannomatosis genes) as well as *NF2* mutations is helpful when a patient does not meet the clinical criteria for a definite diagnosis and or has overlapping features of NF2 and schwannomatosis.

Schwannomas

NF2-associated schwannomas differ from sporadic tumours in several ways. They occur in younger patients (in the third decade of life, versus the sixth decade for sporadic tumours), and many patients develop bilateral vestibular schwannomas by their fourth decade of life {871,2025}. Recent studies with high-resolution MRI showed that in many cases patients have multiple discrete tumour nodules along both the superior and inferior vestibular nerve branches, as well as along the cochlear and facial nerves {3039}. This finding refutes the previous hypothesis of schwannoma originating at the junction of central and peripheral myelination in the internal auditory meatus proposed by Harvey Cushing. In some cases, tumours are a coalescence of multiple nodules/tumours, each with its own somatic *NF2*

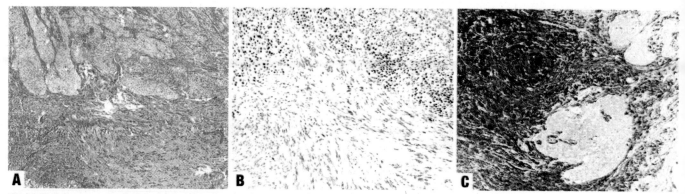

Fig. 14.04 Schwannoma/meningioma. **A** A collision tumour of schwannoma (lower half) and meningioma (upper half) is characteristic of neurofibromatosis type 2. **B** The meningioma component is highlighted with PR immunostaining. **C** The schwannoma component is highlighted with S100 immunostaining.

mutation or deletion {744}. This explains the characteristic gross and microscopic feature of multinodularity {2979} as well as the observed lower rates of surgical efficacy and higher rates of surgical complications than in cases of sporadic vestibular schwannoma {584,864}. In addition to the eighth cranial nerve, other sensory nerves may be affected, including the fifth cranial nerve and spinal dorsal roots. However, motor nerves such as the twelfth cranial nerve may also be involved {871,1941}. In addition to having larger schwannomas, patients with NF2 may have numerous small Schwann cell tumourlets on peripheral nerves and spinal nerves, which despite their small size show biallelic *NF2* inactivation suggestive of precursor neoplastic lesions {3030}. Plexiform schwannomas are common and may involve large plexuses (brachial, sacral), skin, or subcutaneous tissues. Cutaneous plexiform schwannomas are common in paediatric patients and are characteristically associated with a pigmented, plaque-like lesion {871,2025,486}.

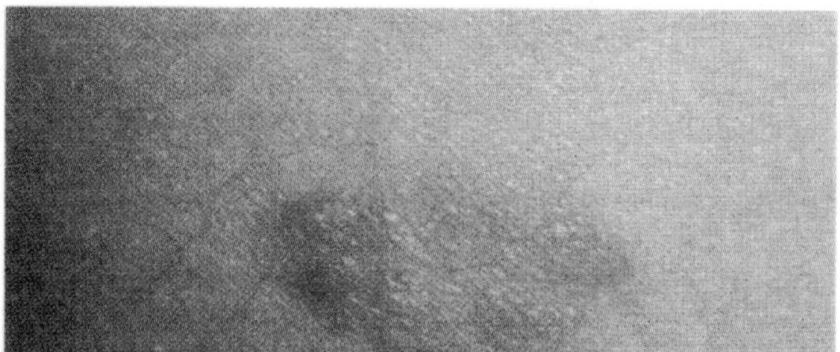

Meningiomas
Multiple meningiomas are the second hallmark of NF2, afflicting half of all patients {1941}. NF2-associated meningiomas can occur throughout the meninges, but they are more common in intracranial compartments (including along the falx cerebri) than in spinal compartments {448,652}, and they may affect sites such as the cerebral ventricles. NF2-associated meningiomas occur earlier in life than sporadic meningiomas {2404} and may be the presenting feature, especially in paediatric patients {865, 871,2025}.

Gliomas
Ependymomas account for most of the histologically diagnosed gliomas in NF2, and for almost all spinal gliomas {2705, 2759}. In most cases, NF2 spinal ependymomas are multiple, intramedullary, slow-growing, asymptomatic masses {2705, 2759}. Most (70–80%) occur in the cervicomedullary junction or cervical spine; a minority occur in the thoracic spine {2422, 2044}. Diffuse and pilocytic astrocytomas have been reported in NF2, but they probably constitute misdiagnosed tanycytic ependymomas {1216}.

Meningioangiomatosis
Meningioangiomatosis is a cortical lesion characterized by a plaque-like proliferation of perivascular meningothelial and fibroblast-like cells. It occurs both sporadically and in NF2. Sporadic meningioangiomatosis is a single lesion that usually occurs in young adults or children, who present with seizures or persistent headaches. In contrast, NF2-associated meningioangiomatosis may be multifocal and often asymptomatic, diagnosed only at autopsy {3029}. Meningioangiomatosis may be predominantly vascular (resembling a vascular malformation) or predominantly meningothelial, sometimes with an associated meningioma, although most cases of the latter probably

Fig. 14.05 Schwannoma. **A** Cutaneous schwannoma is a common manifestation in children with neurofibromatosis type 2 (NF2), and it is often associated with a raised pigmented lesion of the skin (plaque). **B** S100 immunostaining highlights a cutaneous plexiform schwannoma. **C** NF2 schwannoma. A mosaic pattern of SMARCB1 (INI1) staining is common in syndromic (NF2 and schwannomatosis) schwannomas.

represent meningiomas with perivascular spread along Virchow–Robin spaces instead {2469}.

Glial hamartias (also called microhamartomas)

These are circumscribed cellular clusters of the neocortex with medium to large atypical nuclei. They are scattered throughout the cortex and basal ganglia, and they show strong S100 immunoreactivity but only focal GFAP positivity. Glial hamartias are common in and pathognomonic of NF2 {2743,3440}, and they are not associated with mental retardation or gliomas. The hamartias are usually intracortical, with a predilection for the molecular and deeper cortical layers, but they have also been observed in the basal ganglia, thalamus, cerebellum, and spinal cord {3440}. The fact that merlin (NF2) expression is retained in glial hamartias suggests the possibility that haploinsufficiency during development underlies these malformations {3028}.

Peripheral neuropathies

Neuropathies not related to tumour masses are increasingly recognized as a common feature of NF2 {641,1941}. Mononeuropathies may be the presenting symptom in children {865}, whereas progressive polyneuropathies are more common in adults. Sural nerve biopsies from patients with NF2 suggest that NF2 neuropathies are mostly axonal and may be due to focal nerve compression by Schwann cell tumourlets, or that they may be onion-bulb–like Schwann cell or perineurial cell proliferations without associated axons {3011,3186}.

Ophthalmological manifestations

Posterior lens opacities are common in children (juvenile posterior cataract) and highly characteristic of NF2. A variety of retinal abnormalities, including hamartomas, tufts, dysplasias, and epiretinal membranes, may also be found {509,1185}.

Neurofibromas

Cutaneous neurofibromas have been reported in patients with NF2. However, on histological review, many such neurofibromas prove to be schwannomas, including plexiform schwannomas and hybrid schwannomas/neurofibromas. Café-au-lait spots may be present in patients with NF2, but they are fewer in number than in NF1 and not associated with freckling.

Epidemiology

NF2 affects 2.5–4 individuals per 100 000 population {874}. There is no evidence of racial or sex preference.

Etiology

NF2 is an autosomal dominant disease caused by inactivation of the NF2 gene. About half of all NF2 cases are sporadic, occurring in individuals with no family history and caused by newly acquired germline mutations. More than 50% of de novo cases are somatic mosaics, where the pathogenic variant is present only in some of the individual's cells {868,1665,3227}.

Pathogenesis

The NF2 gene

The NF2 gene maps to chromosome 22 {2734,3227}, spans 110 kb, and consists of 17 exons. NF2 mRNA transcripts encode at least two protein forms generated by alternative splicing at

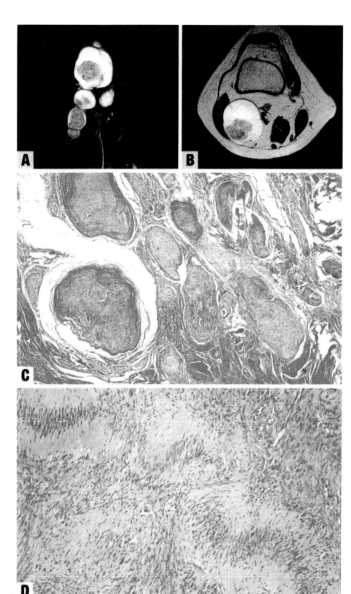

Fig. 14.06 Plexiform schwannoma. **A,B** MRI showing a large plexiform schwannoma in a patient with neurofibromatosis type 2. **C** Multiple nerve fascicles are expanded and replaced by tumour, a pattern similar to that of a plexiform neurofibroma. **D** High-power view shows the typical histological features of a schwannoma, including Verocay bodies.

the C-terminus. The predominant gene product, merlin (NF2), encoded by exons 1–15 and 17, is a cytoskeletal protein with intramolecular interactions similar to those of the ERM proteins (ezrin, radixin, and moesin) {1194,3496}.

Gene mutations

Numerous germline and somatic NF2 mutations have been detected in neoplasms, supporting the hypothesis that NF2 functions as a tumour suppressor gene {1195,1941}. Germline NF2 mutations differ somewhat from the somatic mutations identified in sporadic schwannomas and meningiomas. The most frequent germline mutations are point mutations that alter splice junctions or create new stop codons {341,1941,1968, 2077,2734,2784,3227}. Germline mutations occur preferentially in exons 1–8 {2077}.

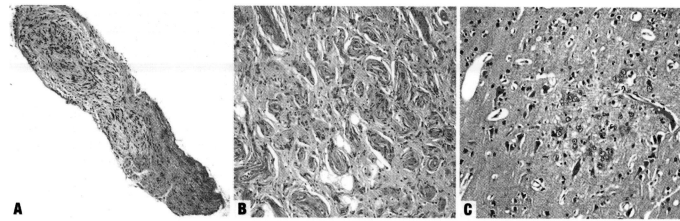

Fig. 14.07 Other lesions in neurofibromatosis type 2. **A** Schwann cell tumourlet embedded in a peripheral nerve. **B** Meningioangiomatosis histologically consists of an intracortical proliferation of small capillaries with a cuff of perivascular meningothelial cells separated by brain parenchyma. In neurofibromatosis type 2, most cases are asymptomatic. **C** Small clusters of atypical large cells, known as glial microhamartomas, are asymptomatic and pathognomonic of neurofibromatosis type 2.

Box 14.02 Clinical diagnostic criteria for neurofibromatosis type 2 (revised Manchester criteria) {872}

1. Bilateral vestibular schwannomas

OR

2. Family history of neurofibromatosis type 2 **AND**

    a. Unilateral vestibular schwannoma **OR**

    b. Any two of: meningioma, ependymoma, schwannoma, posterior subcapsular opacities

OR

3. Unilateral vestibular schwannoma **AND**

    • Any two of: meningioma, ependymoma, schwannoma, posterior subcapsular opacities

OR

4. Multiple meningiomas **AND**

    a. Unilateral vestibular schwannoma **OR**

    b. Any two of: ependymoma, schwannoma, posterior subcapsular opacities

Gene expression

The *NF2* gene is expressed in most normal human tissues, including brain {2734,3227}. The structural similarity of merlin to the ERM proteins suggests that merlin links membrane-associated proteins and the actin cytoskeleton, thus regulating signal transmission from the extracellular environment to the cell {2048} and influencing multiple downstream pathways, including the MAPK, FAK/SRC, PI3K/AKT, RAC/PAK/JNK, mTOR, and WNT/β-catenin pathways. Many merlin binding partners have been identified, including integrins and tyrosine receptor kinases {1642,2180}. In addition to its tumour suppressor function at the cell membrane, merlin translocates to the nucleus where it suppresses the E3 ubiquitin ligase IL-17RB, which is involved in transcription activity {1879}.

Macroscopic appearance

NF2 schwannomas may have a multilobular (bunch-of-grapes) appearance on both gross and microscopic examination {3425}. Multiple Schwann cell tumourlets may develop along individual nerves, particularly on spinal roots and the cauda equina {1941,3030}. The gross appearance of meningiomas

and ependymomas in NF2 is similar to that of non-syndromic tumours.

Histopathology

NF2 schwannomas may have a multilobular appearance on microscopic examination {3425}, which may reflect a multicentric origin. NF2 vestibular schwannomas may entrap seventh cranial nerve fibres {1431} and have higher proliferative activity than sporadic schwannomas {117}, although these features do not necessarily connote more aggressive behaviour. A mosaic pattern of immunostaining for SMARCB1 expression (indicating patchy loss) has been reported in most syndrome-associated schwannomas, including in both NF2 and schwannomatosis {2421}. Hybrid schwannoma/neurofibroma tumours are common in NF2 (accounting for 30% of NF2 schwannomas) {1237, 2159}.

All major subtypes of meningioma can occur in patients with NF2, but the most common subtype is fibrous {116,1941}. Although many NF2-associated meningiomas are CNS WHO grade 1 tumours, a wide spectrum of tumours are encountered, including aggressive subtypes {116,2467}. Some reports have characterized their growth as saltatory {760}. Collision tumours of meningioma and schwannoma are characteristic of NF2.

Cytology

Not relevant

Diagnostic molecular pathology

A pathogenic variant of the *NF2* gene is detected in 70–90% of patients with NF2 (and in 60% of patients with de novo NF2, most likely because of somatic mosaicism) {3359,877}. The risk of transmission to offspring in familial cases is 50%. Risk of transmission in individuals with mosaicism is unknown. Prenatal diagnosis by mutation analysis and testing of children of patients with NF2 is possible when the mutation is known.

Essential and desirable diagnostic criteria

See Box 14.02 and Box 14.03.

Staging

Not relevant

Box 14.03 Diagnostic criteria for neurofibromatosis type 2

Essential:

Clinical criteria as outlined in Box 14.02

OR

A demonstrable germline pathological variant of the *NF2* gene in addition to one of the clinical criteria

Prognosis and prediction

The clinical course in patients with NF2 varies widely between and (to a lesser extent) within families {871,2025}. Some families feature early-onset disease with diverse tumours and high tumour load (Wishart phenotype), whereas others present later, with only vestibular schwannomas (Gardner phenotype). An effect of maternal inheritance on severity has been noted, as have families with genetic anticipation. Genotype–phenotype correlations have been identified wherein truncating mutations are associated with a more severe phenotype, whereas missense mutations, large deletions, and somatic mosaicism have been associated with milder disease {211,878,1666,2077}. In addition to mutation type, the position of the mutation within the gene also affects the phenotype: splice-site mutations upstream from exon 7 have more severe phenotypes {1664} and mutations towards the 5′ end of the gene are associated with a higher risk of intracranial meningiomas {2965}. The life expectancy of people with NF2 is shortened when compared with lifespan in a White control population (69 years vs 80 years, respectively) {3446}.

Schwannomatosis

Stemmer-Rachamimov AO
Hulsebos TJM
Wesseling P

Definition

Schwannomatosis is a disorder caused by pathogenic variants in *SMARCB1* or *LZTR1* (both on chromosome 22q11) and associated with inactivation of the *NF2* gene in the tumours but not in the germline; it is characterized by multiple schwannomas (spinal, cutaneous, and cranial) and, less commonly, meningiomas (cranial and spinal).

MIM numbering

162091 Schwannomatosis 1; SWNTS1
615670 Schwannomatosis 2; SWNTS2

ICD-11 coding

LD2D.1Y Other specified neurofibromatoses

Related terminology

Not recommended: neurilemomatosis.

Subtype(s)

SMARCB1 schwannomatosis 1; *LZTR1* schwannomatosis 2

Localization

Tumours associated with schwannomatosis affect the central and peripheral nervous systems, with predilections for paraspinal and peripheral nerves, as well as (less commonly) the meninges.

Clinical features

Schwannomas

Patients with schwannomatosis typically have multiple schwannomas that may develop in spinal nerve roots, and less

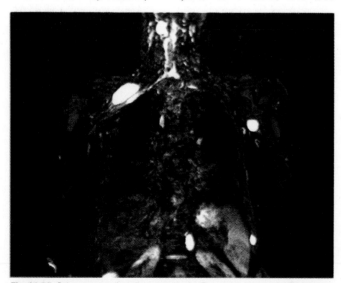

Fig. 14.08 Schwannomas in schwannomatosis. T1-weighted coronal MRI showing multiple bright, discrete peripheral tumours in a patient with schwannomatosis.

commonly in cranial nerves, including unilaterally in the vestibular nerve (in patients with *LZTR1* mutations, schwannomatosis 2). The tumours have a segmental distribution in about 30% of patients, presumed to be the result of genetic mosaicism {1967,2080,2966,2967}. Unlike in neurofibromatosis type 2 (NF2), severe chronic pain associated with the tumours is characteristic of the disease, and neurological deficits and polyneuropathy are uncommon {2080}. Patients with schwannomatosis most often develop symptoms of pain, a mass, or both, in the second or third decade of life, but a formal diagnosis is usually delayed for years {2526}.

Meningiomas

Various studies have shown that *SMARCB1* germline mutations also predispose individuals to the development of multiple meningiomas, with the falx cerebri being a preferential location for cranial meningiomas {167,592,3278}. The reported proportion of patients with schwannomatosis who develop a meningioma is 5% {2962}. Occasionally, patients present with multiple meningiomas.

Other tumours

Other tumours associated with schwannomatosis are rare. The occurrence of malignant peripheral nerve sheath tumours has been reported {1212,476,827}. Also, patients with *SMARCB1*-related schwannomatosis have been described who developed a leiomyoma, a leiomyosarcoma, or a renal cell carcinoma with a molecular profile similar to that of the schwannomas, as well as the corresponding mosaic staining for the SMARCB1 protein {1377,827,2367,1376}.

Epidemiology

Schwannomatosis was found to be almost as common as NF2, with an estimated annual incidence of 1.25–2.5 cases per 100 000 population {118,2881}.

Etiology

Schwannomatosis is often caused by mutations in *SMARCB1* or *LZTR1*, both located on chromosome 22q11. The great majority of schwannomatosis cases are sporadic, with only about 15% of patients having a positive family history {1970,2881}. In the familial form, the disease displays an autosomal dominant pattern of inheritance, with incomplete penetrance {1969}. In 2007, the *SMARCB1* gene on chromosome arm 22q11 was identified as a familial schwannomatosis-predisposing gene {1378}. In 2014, the *LZTR1* gene was identified as a second causative gene in schwannomatosis {2518}. In 2020, the *DGCR8* gene (which maps very close to *LZTR1* on chromosome 22q11) was identified as the predisposing gene in a family with multinodular goitre and schwannomatosis {2681}.

Pathogenesis

According to the tumour suppressor gene model, both copies of the *SMARCB1* or *LZTR1* gene are inactivated in the tumours of patients with schwannomatosis. In addition, there is inactivation of both copies (by mutation and deletion) of the *NF2* gene, located distal to *SMARCB1* and *LZTR1* in chromosome region 22q12.2 {345,1212,2883,1213,1388,2366,2518,2966}. A four-hit, three-step model of tumorigenesis has been proposed for schwannomatosis: first, an (inherited) *SMARCB1* (or *LZTR1*) germline mutation occurs (hit 1); next, loss of the other chromosome 22 follows, with the wildtype copy of *SMARCB1* (and *LZTR1*) and one copy of *NF2* (hits 2 and 3); finally, a somatic mutation of the remaining copy of the *NF2* gene occurs (hit 4) {2524,2883}.

The SMARCB1 gene

SMARCB1 is located in chromosome region 22q11.23 and contains nine exons spanning 50 kb of genomic DNA {3318}. The SMARCB1 protein is a core subunit of mammalian SWI/SNF chromatin remodelling complexes. These act as master regulators of transcription, using ATP for sliding the nucleosomes along the DNA helix {3453}. In schwannomatosis 1, most germline mutations in *SMARCB1* are hypomorphic, non-truncating mutations, which are predicted to result in the synthesis of an altered SMARCB1 protein with modified activity {2969}. The mosaic staining pattern seen in many schwannomatosis-associated schwannomas suggests the absence of SMARCB1 protein in part of the tumour cells {2421}. In contrast to schwannomatosis, in malignant rhabdoid tumours of the kidney and atypical teratoid/rhabdoid tumours of the CNS, the two copies of the *SMARCB1* gene are inactivated by a truncating mutation and deletion of the wildtype gene, resulting in total loss of SMARCB1 expression in tumour cells. Because children with a rhabdoid tumour usually die before the age of 3 years, familial inheritance of the predisposition is extremely rare, and most cases are sporadic {2885,3151}. A few families have been reported in which the affected individuals inherited a *SMARCB1* mutation and developed schwannomatosis or a rhabdoid tumour {476,816,3092}. However, the schwannomas in these families (as well as the rhabdoid tumours) displayed total loss of SMARCB1 protein expression {476,3092}.

The LZTR1 gene

The *LZTR1* gene is situated proximal to *SMARCB1* in chromosome region 22q11.21 and contains 21 exons, spanning 17 kb

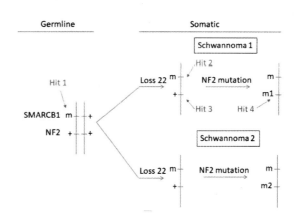

Fig. 14.09 The four-hit mechanism for the formation of tumours in schwannomatosis. Schwannomatosis tumour pathogenesis involves three steps in which two genes (*SMARCB2* and *NF2*) are lost as a result of three different hits. Different tumours will have a different *NF2* mutation (somatic), but they will share the same *SMARCB1* mutation (germline).

of genomic DNA {2518}. It was suggested that LZTR1 may function as a substrate adaptor in cullin-3 ubiquitin ligase complexes, binding to cullin-3 and targeting substrates for ubiquitination {981}, and it may function as a negative modulator of RAS activity {3027,2166}. The reported *LZTR1* germline mutations in schwannomatosis include non-truncating as well as truncating mutations, and they are found along the entire coding sequence of the gene, affecting the functionally important domains of the LZTR1 protein {1388,2366,2518,2966}. Immunostaining of *LZTR1*-associated schwannomas with an LZTR1-specific antibody demonstrates absent or reduced expression of the protein, consistent with its function as a tumour suppressor {2366}. Germline *LZTR1* mutations (but no germline *NF2* mutations) were found in patients with schwannomatosis who had a unilateral vestibular schwannoma {2966,2964}. Because these patients phenotypically resemble patients with mosaic NF2, this causes the misdiagnosis with NF2 in a small number of cases (1–2%) {866}.

Macroscopic appearance

Schwannomas in schwannomatosis are identical to their non-schwannomatosis counterparts.

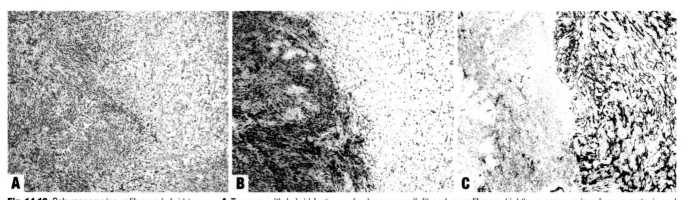

Fig. 14.10 Schwannoma/neurofibroma hybrid tumour. **A** Tumours with hybrid features of schwannoma (left) and neurofibroma (right) are common in schwannomatosis and neurofibromatosis type 2. **B** SOX10 is diffusely positive in the schwannoma component of the tumour and shows patchy positivity in the neurofibroma component. **C** This CD34 immunostain highlights a lattice-like pattern in the neurofibroma component but not the schwannoma component.

Histopathology

The histopathology of schwannomatosis-related tumours largely overlaps with that of their non-schwannomatosis counterparts. Most (70%) of the schwannomas associated with schwannomatosis are hybrid schwannoma/neurofibroma tumours with prominent myxoid stroma, and they may sometimes be misdiagnosed as neurofibromas or malignant peripheral nerve sheath tumours {2080}. Cutaneous schwannomas may be plexiform.

Immunohistochemically, almost all schwannomas of patients with familial schwannomatosis show a mosaic pattern of staining for SMARCB1 (with considerable intertumoural and intratumoural heterogeneity; < 10% to > 50% immunonegative nuclei) {2421}. This mosaic staining is also frequently seen in the schwannomas of patients with sporadic schwannomatosis (55–100% of cases) and in most (non-vestibular) schwannomas of patients with NF2, but it is rare in solitary, sporadic schwannomas {1378,2421,443}. What causes this absence of SMARCB1 staining in part of the tumour cells is unknown at present; the synthesis of a mutant SMARCB1 protein is not a prerequisite because mosaic expression was found in the schwannomas of patients with schwannomatosis with a germline LZTR1 mutation (and no SMARCB1 mutation) and in those of patients lacking germline mutations in both genes {443}.

Cytology

Not relevant

Diagnostic molecular pathology

In patients with schwannomatosis, SMARCB1 appears to be involved as a causative gene in about 50% of familial cases but in < 10% of sporadic cases {345,1212,2735,2969}. In patients without SMARCB1 germline mutations, LZTR1 mutations were found in about 40% of familial cases and 25% of sporadic cases {1388,2366,2966}. The fact that most schwannomatosis cases cannot be explained by the involvement of SMARCB1 or LZTR1 suggests the existence of additional causative genes {1388}. Indeed, the DGCR8 gene was recently identified as the predisposing gene in a family with multinodular goitre and schwannomatosis {2681}. Patients with schwannomatosis typically have somatically acquired NF2 mutations in their schwannomas, but no germline NF2 mutations {1436,1572,1969}.

Essential and desirable diagnostic criteria

See Box 14.04.

Staging

Not applicable

Prognosis and prediction

Life expectancy in schwannomatosis is near normal (76.9 years); it is higher than the mean life expectancy of patients with NF2 (66.2 years) {866}.

Box 14.04 Diagnostic criteria for schwannomatosis

Essential:

Two or more schwannomas (non-intradermal and pathologically confirmed)
    AND No bilateral vestibular schwannomas on high-quality MRI

OR

One schwannoma or meningioma
    AND One affected first-degree relative

Desirable:

Loss of heterozygosity / deletion of chromosome 22 and two different NF2 mutations

Germline SMARCB1 or LZTR1 mutation

Clinical history of pain, hybrid neurofibroma/schwannoma histology, multiple peripheral schwannomas

Von Hippel–Lindau syndrome

Plate KH
Aldape KD
Neumann HPH
Vortmeyer AO
Zagzag D

Definition

Von Hippel–Lindau syndrome (VHL) is an autosomal dominant disorder caused by pathogenic germline variants of the *VHL* tumour suppressor gene (located on chromosome 3p25.3) and characterized by the development of haemangioblastoma of the CNS and retina, clear cell renal cell carcinoma (RCC), phaeochromocytoma, pancreatic neuroendocrine tumours, and endolymphatic sac tumours (ELSTs).

MIM numbering

193300 Von Hippel–Lindau syndrome; VHLS

ICD-11 coding

None

Related terminology

None

Subtype(s)

Von Hippel–Lindau syndrome types 1, 2A, 2B, and 2C

Localization

Haemangioblastomas most often involve the retina, cerebellum, and spinal cord (especially paraspinal nerve roots), but they can occur anywhere along the craniospinal axis, including

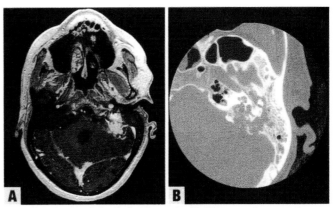

Fig. 14.11 Endolymphatic sac tumour in a patient with von Hippel–Lindau syndrome. **A** This contrast-enhancing tumour (T1-weighted postcontrast MRI) occurred in the cerebellopontine angle and was therefore resected by a neurosurgeon. **B** A CT of this same tumour shows destruction of the temporal bone, essentially excluding the diagnostic consideration of choroid plexus papilloma.

peripheral nerves and even tissues outside the nervous system {3352,3351,102,785,287,2181}. ELSTs arise from the vestibular aqueduct and may invade through the temporal bone and into the cerebellopontine angle {1118,789}.

The sites of involvement in VHL are summarized in Table 14.02 (p. 438).

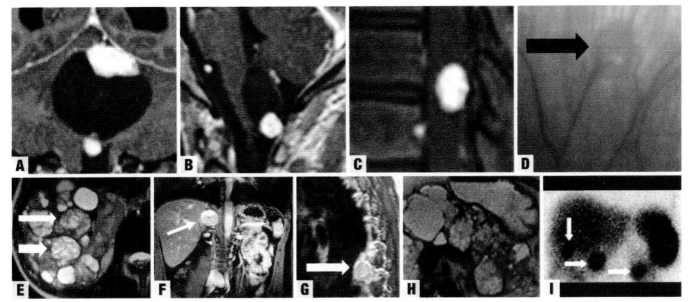

Fig. 14.12 Von Hippel-Lindau syndrome. **A** Transverse MRI of a cystic cerebellar haemangioblastoma; solid tumour shows contrast enhancement. **B** Sagittal MRI of a cystic brain stem haemangioblastoma; solid tumour shows contrast enhancement. **C** Contrast-enhanced MRI of a spinal haemangioblastoma. **D** Retinal haemangioblastoma. Angiography shows the tumour (arrow) with a pair of feeder vessels. **E** Contrast-enhanced MRI showing multiple renal cell carcinomas (arrows) and renal cysts, after contralateral nephrectomy. **F** Contrast-enhanced MRI showing right adrenal phaeochromocytoma (arrow). **G** Contrast-enhanced MRI showing thoracic phaeochromocytoma (paraganglioma) (arrow). **H** Multiple pancreatic cysts on MRI. **I** Two pancreatic neuroendocrine tumours (horizontal arrows); vertical arrow denotes the gall bladder. Somatostatin receptor scintigraphy, planar anterior projection.

Table 14.02 Organ/tissue distribution and pathology of lesions in von Hippel–Lindau syndrome

Organ/tissue	Tumour(s)	Non-neoplastic lesions
CNS	Haemangioblastoma	
Eye (retina)	Haemangioblastoma	
Kidney	Clear cell renal cell carcinoma	Cysts
Adrenal gland	Phaeochromocytoma	
Pancreas	Neuroendocrine islet cell tumours	Cysts
Inner ear	Endolymphatic sac tumour	
Epididymis	Papillary cystadenoma	

Clinical features

Retinal haemangioblastomas manifest at a mean age of 25 years (earlier than RCC) and thus offer the possibility of an early diagnosis {1813}. CNS haemangioblastomas develop mainly in young adults (mean age: 29 years). They are predominantly located in the cerebellum and next most commonly in the brainstem or spinal cord {782}. Approximately 25% of all cases of CNS haemangioblastoma are associated with hereditary VHL. Key clinical characteristics of VHL-associated versus sporadic haemangioblastoma are presented in Table 14.03.

Renal cysts and clear cell RCCs are typically multifocal and bilateral. The mean patient age at presentation is 37 years (vs 61 years for sporadic clear cell RCC), with a patient age at onset of 16–67 years. Patients with VHL have a 70% chance of developing clear cell RCC by the age of 70 years. Metastatic RCC is the leading cause of death from VHL.

Adrenal phaeochromocytomas arise in 20% of patients with VHL; the mean age at onset is 30 years.

Pancreatic manifestations are predominantly multiple cysts but also neuroendocrine tumours {1735}.

Other VHL-associated tumours include ELSTs (associated with hearing loss, tinnitus, and vertigo) and epididymal and broad ligament cystadenomas.

VHL type 1 is characterized by haemangioblastomas and RCCs (phaeochromocytomas are rare or absent), and it is typically caused by *VHL* deletions, truncations, and missense mutations. Type 2A is characterized by haemangioblastomas and phaeochromocytomas (RCCs are rare), and it is caused by missense mutations. Type 2B is characterized by a high frequency of haemangioblastomas, RCCs, and phaeochromocytomas, and it is mainly caused by missense mutations. Type 2C is characterized by phaeochromocytomas (haemangioblastomas and RCCs are absent), and it is mainly caused by missense mutations.

Epidemiology

VHL is estimated to have an annual incidence rate of 2.8 cases per 100 000 population.

Etiology

VHL is caused by heterozygous germline pathogenic sequence variants of the *VHL* gene on chromosome 3p25.3; these are spread over the three exons. Missense mutations are most common, but nonsense mutations, microdeletions/insertions, splice-site mutations, and large deletions also occur. In total,

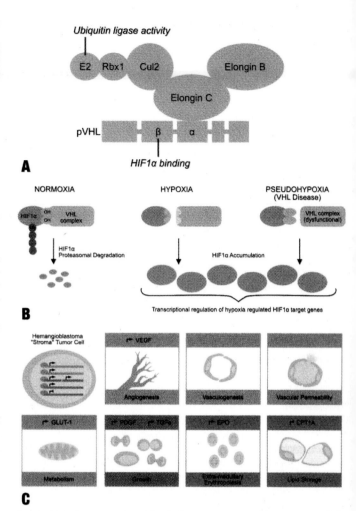

Fig. 14.13 Pathogenesis of von Hippel–Lindau syndrome. **A** The β domain of VHL protein interacts with HIF1α, whereas the α domain interacts with other partners of the VHL protein complex. In von Hippel–Lindau syndrome, alterations in the α domain prevent the formation of a functional VHL protein complex. **B** In normoxia, the VHL complex binds to HIF1α and promotes ubiquitination and proteasomal degradation in an oxygen-dependent manner. In hypoxia, binding of VHL protein to HIF1α is impaired, resulting in the accumulation of HIF1α and increased activation of target genes. In von Hippel–Lindau syndrome, HIF1α accumulation results from failed binding of HIF1α to the dysfunctional VHL protein complex. **C** HIF accumulation in haemangioblastoma stromal tumour cells leads to altered gene expression of HIF-responsive genes and results in increased vascularization due to angiogenesis and vasculogenesis; cyst formation due to increased vascular permeability; and metabolic adaptation, growth stimulation, extramedullary haematopoiesis, and lipid deposition (clear cell phenotype).

> 1000 mutations have been described in the *VHL* gene. The heterogeneous clinical manifestations of VHL are a reflection of the diversity of germline mutations.

Pathogenesis

Mutational inactivation of the *VHL* tumour suppressor gene in affected family members is responsible for their genetic susceptibility to tumour development at various organ sites, but the mechanisms by which the inactivation or loss of the suppressor gene product (VHL protein) causes neoplastic transformation are only partly understood {1150}. The cell of origin (haemangioblast, stromal cell) is not well defined, but current evidence points to a developmentally arrested haemangioblast precursor {3350}. In accordance with the function of *VHL* as a tumour

Table 14.03 Clinical characteristics of sporadic versus von Hippel–Lindau syndrome (VHL)-associated haemangioblastoma

Characteristic	Sporadic	VHL-associated
Female sex	41%	56%
Median patient age	44 years (range: 7–82 years)	23 years (range: 7–64 years)
Intracranial location	79%	73%
Spinal location	11%	75%
Multiple haemangioblastomas	5%	65%

suppressor gene, mutations are also common in sporadic haemangioblastomas (occurring in as many as 78% of cases) and ubiquitous in clear cell RCCs.

The VHL protein has many different functions, and it is critically involved in protein degradation. The α domain of the VHL protein forms a complex with elongin B (transcription elongation factor B, also known as TCEB2), elongin C (TCEB1), cullin-2, and RBX1; this is called VCB-CUL2, and it has ubiquitin ligase activity, thereby targeting cellular proteins for ubiquitination and proteasome-mediated degradation. The α domain of the gene involved in the binding to elongin B is frequently mutated in neoplasms associated with VHL.

VHL protein plays a key role in cellular oxygen sensing, by polyubiquitination and proteasomal degradation of hypoxia-inducible factors (HIF1α and HIF2α) {3572,943}, which mediate cellular responses to hypoxia. This leads to a loss of function of VHL protein with a pseudohypoxic state characterized by altered expression of genes that drive vascularization, cyst formation, lipid storage, metabolic adaptation, and extramedullary erythropoiesis. The β domain of VHL protein interacts with HIF1α. Binding of the hydroxylated subunit of the VHL protein causes polyubiquitination and thereby targets HIF1α for proteasomal degradation. In the absence of functional VHL protein, HIF1α accumulates and activates the transcription of several hypoxia-inducible genes, including *VEGFA*, *PDGFB*, *TGFA*, and *EPO* by binding to the respective hypoxia-responsive elements in the promoter region (leading to pseudohypoxia).

Constitutive overexpression of VEGF-A {3464,3051} explains the extraordinary vascularization of neoplasms associated with VHL due to increased angiogenesis/vasculogenesis, as well as the formation of cysts due to increased vascular permeability (VEGF-A has also been denominated "vascular permeability factor [VPF]") {1972}. Increased erythropoietin expression is common in haemangioblastomas {1737} and is responsible for intratumoural (extramedullary) haematopoiesis and for the paraneoplastic erythrocytosis syndrome that can occur in patients with VHL. HIF-dependent downregulation of carnitine palmitoyltransferase 1A leads to enhanced lipid storage, a characteristic of VHL-dependent tumours {2732}.

Macroscopic appearance

The macroscopic appearance of VHL-associated tumours is similar to that of their sporadic counterparts.

Histopathology

The histopathology of VHL-associated tumours is similar to that of their sporadic counterparts. Notably, however, ELSTs occurring in the cerebellopontine angle may closely mimic choroid plexus papilloma; neuroimaging is helpful in this differential because only ELSTs invade and destroy temporal bone.

Cytology

The cytology of VHL-associated tumours is similar to that of their sporadic counterparts.

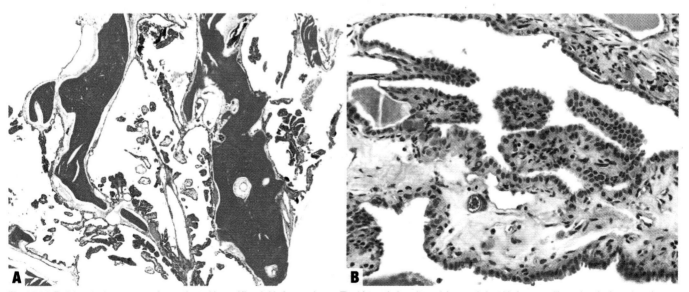

Fig. 14.14 Endolymphatic sac tumour in a patient with von Hippel–Lindau syndrome. The histopathology is reminiscent of choroid plexus papilloma, but the bone invasion essentially excludes that diagnosis. **A** Low-power view. **B** High-power view.

Diagnostic molecular pathology

Demonstration of a *VHL* germline sequence variant is desirable to confirm the diagnosis.

Essential and desirable diagnostic criteria

See Box 14.05.

Staging

Not relevant

Prognosis and prediction

The median life expectancy of patients with VHL is 49 years. Clinical surveillance guidance has been published {285,2631}.

Tuberous sclerosis

Lopes MBS
Rodriguez FJ
Santosh V
Sharma MC
Stemmer-Rachamimov AO

Definition

Tuberous sclerosis is a group of autosomal dominant disorders caused by a pathogenic variant of *TSC1* on 9q or *TSC2* on 16p and characterized by hamartomas and benign neoplastic lesions that affect the CNS and various non-neural tissues.

MIM numbering

191100 Tuberous sclerosis 1; TSC1
613254 Tuberous sclerosis 2; TSC2

ICD-11 coding

LD2D.2 Tuberous sclerosis

Related terminology

None

Subtype(s)

Tuberous sclerosis 1; tuberous sclerosis 2

Localization

Major CNS manifestations of tuberous sclerosis include cortical dysplasias (tubers and white matter glioneuronal hamartomas), subependymal nodules, and subependymal giant cell astrocytomas (SEGAs). Major extraneural manifestations include cutaneous angiofibromas, shagreen patches, subungual fibromas, cardiac rhabdomyomas, pulmonary lymphangioleiomyomatosis, and renal angiomyolipomas.

Clinical features

Diagnostic criteria

The diagnosis of tuberous sclerosis is based primarily on clinical features, and it may be challenging due to the considerable variability in phenotype, patient age at symptom onset, and penetrance among mutation carriers. The diagnostic criteria for tuberous sclerosis were revised in 2012 at the International Tuberous Sclerosis Complex Consensus Conference and are based on genetic testing and/or clinical manifestations {2286}. Clinical manifestations are categorized as either major or minor. The diagnostic categories, which are based on the number of major/minor manifestations present in a given individual, define disease likelihood as being definite or possible {2286} (Box 14.06, p. 444). Most patients have manifestations of tuberous sclerosis before the age of 10 years, although some cases may manifest much later in life {37}. Confirmatory testing for *TSC1* or *TSC2* mutations may be helpful when a patient does not meet the clinical criteria for a definite diagnosis but the phenotype is compelling. Antenatal diagnosis by mutation analysis is possible when parents or other family members are known to be affected {348}.

Clinical features

Cardiac rhabdomyomas are often a presenting feature of tuberous sclerosis in newborns and infants aged < 2 years,

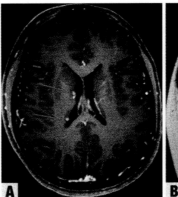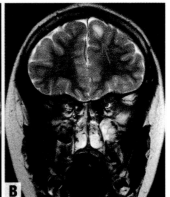

Fig. 14.15 Tuberous sclerosis. **A** T1-weighted postcontrast axial MRI demonstrates two small enhancing subependymal nodules along the right caudate nucleus (arrows). **B** T2-weighted coronal MRI demonstrates a minimally expansile hyperintense lesion in the left frontal white matter compatible with a cortical/subcortical tuber (arrow).

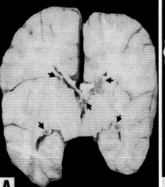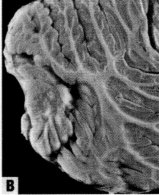

Fig. 14.16 Tuberous sclerosis. **A** Gross autopsy section from a patient with tuberous sclerosis illustrates axially cut cerebral hemispheric parenchyma with multiple subependymal nodules in the lateral and third ventricles (arrows). **B** Gross image of a brain from a 57-year-old man showing an unusual tuber in the cerebellar hemisphere with extensive calcification.

and more than half of cardiac rhabdomyomas are associated with tuberous sclerosis {2683}. Cutaneous manifestations include hypomelanotic nodules, facial angiofibromas, and shagreen patches. Ungual (or subungual) fibromas often develop in childhood. Renal angiomyolipomas develop by the age of 10 years in as many as 80% of people with tuberous sclerosis. Renal cysts are present in as many as 20% of affected individuals, but polycystic kidney disease only occurs in 3–5%. Lymphangioleiomyomatosis severely impairs lung function and may be fatal; it is present in as many as 40% of women with tuberous sclerosis. All the phenotypic features of tuberous sclerosis can also occur sporadically in individuals without the genetic condition {2683}. About 50% of patients with lymphangioleiomyomatosis do not have tuberous sclerosis. Sporadic angiomyolipomas are typically solitary, whereas tuberous sclerosis–associated angiomyolipomas are often multiple or bilateral.

Neurological symptoms are among the most frequently observed and serious (sometimes life-threatening) manifestations of tuberous sclerosis {654,3173}. The most common initial signs of tuberous sclerosis are intractable epilepsy, including infantile spasms (in 80–90% of cases); cognitive impairment (in 50%); and a combination of neurobehavioral disorders known as tuberous sclerosis–associated neuropsychiatric disorders (TAND; in > 60%), including autism spectrum disorder (in as many as 40%) {1132,3173,2285}. Cortical tubers and white matter glioneuronal hamartomas (see *CNS manifestations*, below) are both commonly associated with intractable epilepsy and learning difficulties in tuberous sclerosis {2286}, although meticulous autopsy studies on small numbers of patients have also suggested that there may be more subtle degrees of cortical and white matter disorganization {2010}.

CNS manifestations

CNS lesions in tuberous sclerosis include cerebral cortical tubers, white matter glioneuronal heterotopia, subependymal hamartomatous nodules, and SEGAs. Schizencephaly, agenesis of the corpus callosum, and cerebellar dysplasia are rare abnormalities. Cortical tubers can involve the cortex, subcortical white matter, or both. They are both detected by CT or MRI, although MRI is considered the reference method for defining CNS involvement in tuberous sclerosis {2760}. Diffusion tensor imaging and metabolic brain studies using AMT PET or FDG PET {2904,2760} in addition to intraoperative electrocorticography can identify epileptogenic tubers, facilitating tuberectomy as a reasonable surgical approach to treating intractable seizures in these patients. Tubers resemble sporadic cortical dysplasias of the cortex not associated with tuberous sclerosis, classified as focal cortical dysplasia type 2b by the classification proposed by the International League Against Epilepsy (ILAE) {305}.

Epidemiology

The variability of the clinical manifestations of tuberous sclerosis previously led to underdiagnosis. Recent data indicate that the disorder affects as many as 25 000–40 000 individuals in the USA and about 1–2 million individuals worldwide, with an estimated incidence of 1 case per 6000–10 000 live births and a population prevalence of about 1 in 20 000 {2286}.

Etiology

Tuberous sclerosis is caused by a pathogenic variant of *TSC1* on chromosome 9q or *TSC2* on 16p.

The TSC1 gene

The *TSC1* gene maps to chromosome 9q34 {626} and contains 23 exons {3285}, 21 of which carry coding information (exons 3–23).

Gene expression: The *TSC1*-encoded protein, hamartin, has a molecular weight of 130 kDa. Hamartin is strongly expressed in brain, kidney, and heart, all of which are tissues frequently affected in tuberous sclerosis {2522}. Its pattern of expression overlaps with that of tuberin, the product of the *TSC2* gene.

Gene mutations: Mutation analysis of large cohorts {530,3286} showed that the most common mutations in the *TSC1* gene are small deletions and nonsense mutations (each accounting for about 30% of all mutations in the gene). Virtually all mutations result in a truncated gene product, and more than half of the changes affect exons 15 and 17 {3286}. Large deletions of the *TSC1* gene are rare.

The TSC2 gene

The *TSC2* gene maps to chromosome 16p13.3 {1538} and contains 42 exons, with exons 2–42 encoding the functional protein. *Gene expression:* *TSC2* encodes a large transcript of 5.5 kb, which shows widespread expression in many tissues, including the brain and other organs affected in tuberous sclerosis. Alternatively spliced mRNAs have been reported {3488}. A portion of the 180 kDa protein product tuberin has substantial homology with the catalytic domain of RAP1GAP, a member of the RAS family.

Gene mutations: The mutation spectrum of *TSC2* is wider than that of *TSC1*; it includes large deletions and missense mutations, and (less frequently) splice-junction mutations {76,662, 1492}. Exons 16, 33, and 40 have the highest number of mutations. Large deletions in the *TSC2* gene may extend into the adjacent *PKD1* gene, with a resulting phenotype of tuberous sclerosis and polycystic kidney disease {310,3286}. Multiple studies of genotype–phenotype correlations have demonstrated that *TSC2* mutations are associated with a more severe phenotype overall, with earlier seizure onset, a higher number of tubers, and a lower cognition index. However, within that spectrum, *TSC2* missense mutations are associated with milder phenotypes {159,2798}.

Like in other tumour suppressor gene syndromes, somatic inactivation of the wildtype allele (i.e. loss of heterozygosity for the *TSC1* or *TSC2* locus) has been reported in kidney and cardiac lesions associated with tuberous sclerosis, as well as in SEGAs {512}. However, there is conflicting evidence of whether a so-called second hit is required for cortical tuber formation, raising the possibility that some lesions in tuberous sclerosis may be due to haploinsufficiency {2256,3455}. Recent studies have predominantly found activating mTOR mutations in focal cortical dysplasias, but rarely *TSC1* and *TSC2* mutations as well {179,1894}. In recent studies, loss of *TSC1* in periventricular zone neuronal stem cells was sufficient to cause aberrant migration and giant cell phenotype, supportive of the two-hit hypothesis for tuber formation {900,3606}.

Most of the cases in which no mutation is identified (15% of patients with tuberous sclerosis) {662,1492} were found to be somatic mosaics when newer sequencing methods were used {3246}. Mosaicism occurs when the pathogenic variant occurs in embryogenesis, resulting in only some of the fetal cell lines carrying the pathogenic variants while other cell lines have two wildtype alleles. Clinical features of tuberous sclerosis are milder in individuals with mosaicism and may have limited distribution (e.g. they may involve only one organ).

Inheritance and genetic heterogeneity

Most tuberous sclerosis cases (~60%) are sporadic, with no family history, indicating a high rate of de novo mutations {2796}. Familial cases are inherited in an autosomal dominant fashion. In affected kindreds, the disease follows an autosomal dominant pattern of inheritance, with high penetrance but considerable phenotypic variability {2921}.

Pathogenesis

The impact of *TSC1* and *TSC2* sequence variants is mediated by effects on signalling pathways involving tuberin and hamartin. Tuberin, hamartin, and TBC1D7 form a heteromeric protein complex (known as TSC) that functions as a signalling node that integrates growth factor and stress signals from the upstream PI3K/AKT pathway and transmits signals downstream to coordinate multiple cellular processes, including cell proliferation and cell size {2586,626,1538,2523}. The complex negatively regulates the mTOR pathway {155,1033,3158}. Disruption of TSC causes upregulation of the mTOR pathway and increases proliferation and cell growth through two effector molecules: 4E-BP1 and S6K1 {155,3158}. The understanding of the basic mechanism of mTOR pathway activation in tuberous sclerosis lesions has led to the use of mTOR inhibitors in the treatment of manifestations of tuberous sclerosis. Several tuberous sclerosis–associated tumours (e.g. renal angiomyolipomas, SEGAs, and lymphangioleiomyomas) show a marked size reduction in response to treatment with mTOR inhibitors (e.g. everolimus), and they regrow when treatment is stopped. mTOR inhibitors were also shown to be effective in reducing seizure frequency in children with refractory epilepsy {660,659}.

Macroscopic appearance

See individual tumour types within the classification.

Histopathology

Microscopically, CNS tubers consist of a disorganized cortex with disrupted cortical lamination and containing dysmorphic, markedly enlarged neurons; balloon cells (also designated by some authors as "giant cells" {2138,2010}); dense fibrillary gliosis; calcification of blood vessel walls and/or parenchyma; and myelin loss. The surrounding cortex, which usually appears normal in cytoarchitecture, shows changes on more detailed immunohistochemical and morphometric investigations {1387,2010}. Dysmorphic neurons and balloon cells may be seen in all cortical layers and in the underlying white matter. The dysmorphic neurons show altered radial orientation in the cortex, aberrant dendritic arborization, and accumulation of perikaryal fibrils. The perikaryal fibrils can be highlighted using silver impregnation techniques, which show many neurons with neurofibrillary tangle–like morphology. Although the dysmorphic neurons express neuronal-associated proteins, they display cytoarchitectural features of immature or poorly differentiated neurons, such as reduced axonal projections

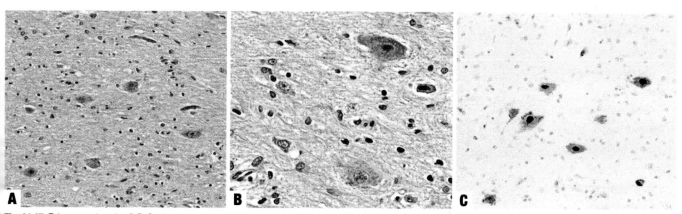

Fig. 14.17 Tuberous sclerosis. **A,B** Cortical tuber with dysmorphic enlarged neurons embedded in a densely fibrillary background. **C** Cortical tuber with large neuronal cells highlighted by NeuN.

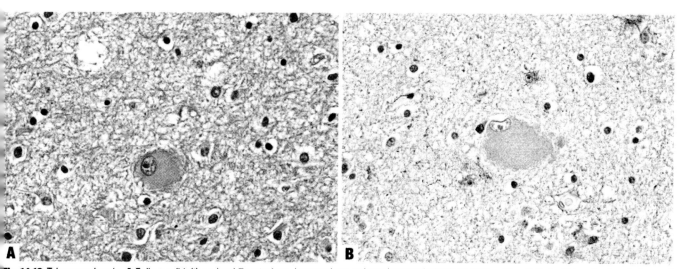

Fig. 14.18 Tuberous sclerosis. **A** Balloon cell (with eosinophilic cytoplasm, large nucleus, and prominent nucleolus) in the white matter. **B** Cortical tuber showing a balloon cell with a ganglion-like nucleus and strong immunoreactivity for S100.

Table 14.04 Major manifestations of tuberous sclerosis {2286}

Manifestation	Frequency
CNS	
Cortical dysplasias (tubers and white matter heterotopias)	~90%
Subependymal nodule	80%
Subependymal giant cell astrocytoma	5–15%
Skin	
Facial angiofibroma	75%
Hypomelanotic macule	90%
Shagreen patch	50%
Forehead plaque	25%
Confetti skin (hypopigmented macules)	58%
Subungual fibroma	20%
Eye	
Retinal hamartoma	30–50%
Retinal giant cell astrocytoma	20–30%
Retinal achromic patch	40%
Kidney	
Angiomyolipoma[a]	80%
Isolated renal cyst	10–20%
Polycystic kidney cysts	2–3%
Heart	
Cardiac rhabdomyoma	50%
Digestive system	
Liver angiomyolipomas	10–15%
Lung	
Lymphangioleiomyomatosis	30–40% (female patients)
Pulmonary cysts	10–12% (male patients)
Micronodular pulmonary pneumocyte hyperplasia	40–58%
Other	
Intraoral fibroma	20–50%
Dental enamel pits	Variable (up to 100%)
Bone cyst	40%
Non-renal hamartomas	Rare

[a]May occur in other locations besides kidneys.

Box 14.06 Diagnostic criteria for tuberous sclerosis (2012) {2286}

Essential:

A. Genetic diagnostic criteria

Identification of either a *TSC1* or a *TSC2* pathogenic mutation in DNA from normal tissue is sufficient to make a definitive diagnosis of tuberous sclerosis according to strict criteria {1849,1850}.

B. Clinical diagnostic criteria

Major features:

1. Hypomelanotic macules (≥ 3, at least 5 mm in diameter)
2. Angiofibromas (≥ 3) or fibrous cephalic plaque
3. Ungual fibromas (≥ 2)
4. Shagreen patch
5. Multiple retinal hamartomas
6. Cortical dysplasias (including tubers and cerebral white matter migration lines)
7. Subependymal nodules
8. Subependymal giant cell astrocytoma
9. Cardiac rhabdomyoma
10. Lymphangioleiomyomatosis[a]
11. Angiomyolipomas (≥ 2)[a]

Minor features:

1. Confetti-like skin lesions
2. Dental enamel pits (≥ 3)
3. Intraoral fibromas (≥ 2)
4. Retinal achromic patch
5. Multiple renal cysts
6. Non-renal hamartomas

Definite diagnosis: Two major features[a] **OR** one major feature with at least two minor features

Possible diagnosis: One major feature **OR** at least two minor features

[a]A combination of the two major clinical features lymphangioleiomyomatosis and angiomyolipomas without other features does not meet the criteria for a definite diagnosis.

---

identical morphological phenotype express neuronal markers including connexin 26, connexin 32, neurofilaments, class III β-tubulin, MAP2, and α-internexin {655,1317,3511}. However formation of well-defined synapses between balloon cells and adjacent neurons is not a consistent finding. As previously mentioned, cortical dysplasias morphologically indistinguishable from tubers may occur in chronic focal epilepsies without clinical or genetic evidence of an underlying tuberous sclerosis condition {301,305}. The pathogenesis of these sporadic lesions is unclear.

White matter glioneuronal heterotopias and radial migration lines are linear or flame-shaped bands radiating from the periventricular zone to the subcortical white matter. They are composed of dysplastic glioneuronal cells, and they can extend from the cortex down to the periventricular region. Subependymal glial nodules are elevated, often calcified nodules. They are composed of enlarged glioneuronal cells indistinguishable from those found in SEGAs, but they are smaller than those in cortical tubers.

The proteins tuberin and hamartin are identifiable by immunohistochemistry and western blotting in many organs and tissues throughout the body {1489}; both proteins are widely expressed throughout the CNS of the normal developing brain

and spine density {1317,1387}. The other frequently observed element in tubers and adjacent cortex and white matter is the characteristic balloon cell {1983,1317,1387}. Balloon cells may resemble gemistocytic astrocytes with glassy eosinophilic cytoplasm and eccentric, often multinucleated nuclei; however, immunohistochemical markers characteristic of glial and neuronal phenotypes suggest a mixed glioneuronal origin of these cells. Many balloon cells express nestin mRNA and protein {655}. Some balloon cells demonstrate immunoreactivity for vimentin and GFAP {1317}, while others with an

{1488,3333}. Immunostaining a given tuber with anti-hamartin or anti-tuberin antibodies does not provide evidence of which mutation is present in a given subject, and therefore is not of diagnostic value.

Extraneural manifestations
The extraneural manifestations of tuberous sclerosis and the frequencies at which they occur are summarized in Table 14.04.

Cytology
Not relevant

Diagnostic molecular pathology
In the revised diagnostic criteria, demonstration of a pathogenic variant of *TSC1* or *TSC2* in DNA from normal tissue is an independent diagnostic criterion and is sufficient for a definitive diagnosis of tuberous sclerosis {1745}. Therefore, genetic testing is recommended when tuberous sclerosis is suspected but cannot be clinically confirmed. On molecular testing, 75–90% of patients with tuberous sclerosis are found to be positive for a pathogenic genetic variant, so a negative result does not rule out the diagnosis {1745}. Genetic testing is recommended for family members of an affected patient, especially in babies, and may be offered as a preimplantation or prenatal test.

Essential and desirable diagnostic criteria
Clinical and genetic diagnostic criteria are summarized in Box 14.06.

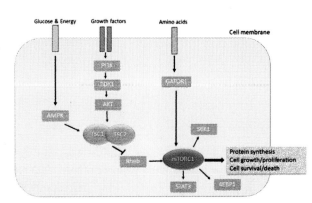

Fig. 14.19 The mTOR molecular signalling pathway. The TSC genes are integral members of the mTOR pathway, the inactivation of which leads to cell growth and survival. mTOR is modulated by the TSC1-TSC2 complex and regulated upstream by several protein kinases, such as PI3K, PDK1, AKT, and AMPK.

Staging
Not relevant

Prognosis and prediction
Tuberous sclerosis tends to shorten lifespan slightly (as compared with lifespan in a White control population) {2903}. The most common causes of death in the second decade of life are brain tumours and status epilepticus, followed by renal abnormalities {2286,99}. In patients aged > 40 years, mortality is most commonly associated with renal abnormalities (i.e. cystic disease or neoplasm) or lymphangioleiomyomatosis.

Li–Fraumeni syndrome

Orr BA
Hawkins CE
Kratz CP
Malkin D
Solomon DA

Definition

Li–Fraumeni syndrome (LFS) is an autosomal dominant disorder caused by pathogenic sequence variants of the *TP53* tumour suppressor gene on chromosome 17p13.1 and characterized by multiple primary neoplasms in children and adults, with a predominance of soft tissue sarcomas, osteosarcomas, breast cancer, brain tumours, and adrenocortical carcinoma.

MIM numbering

151623 Li–Fraumeni syndrome; LFS

ICD-11 coding

None

Related terminology

Not recommended: Li–Fraumeni syndrome, p53-associated.

Subtype(s)

None

Localization

Cancers of the breast, soft tissue, CNS, adrenal glands, and bone are the most frequent manifestations of LFS, accounting for about 80% of all tumours. The most common CNS tumour manifestations of LFS are choroid plexus carcinoma, medulloblastoma, and diffuse astrocytic gliomas.

Clinical features

LFS is characterized by the early onset of a broad spectrum of cancers and a high lifetime risk for cancer. Breast cancer is the most common tumour in *TP53* mutation carriers (24–31.2% {2028}, followed by soft tissue sarcomas (11.6–17.8%), brain tumours (3.5–14%), osteosarcomas (12.6–13.4%), and adrenocortical tumours (6.5–9.9%) {2251,3199,336}. However, almost all cancer types have been reported in *TP53* mutation carriers, and tumour patterns and penetrance demonstrate distinct phases by age {93}.

Candidates for *TP53* germline testing are identified based on fulfilment of the classic LFS criteria, the Birch or Eeles criteria for LFS-like syndrome {286,826}, or the 2015 Chompret criteria {1869,336} (Table 14.05). The classic clinical criteria used to identify individuals potentially harbouring pathogenic *TP53* germline mutations or structural variants and thus affected by LFS are: (1) occurrence of sarcoma before the age of 45 years, (2) at least one first-degree relative with any tumour before the age of 45 years, and (3) a first- or second-degree relative with cancer before the age of 45 years or a sarcoma at any age {1869}.

In general, tumours associated with a *TP53* germline mutation develop earlier than their sporadic counterparts, but there are marked organ-specific differences {3607}. For example, adrenocortical carcinoma associated with a *TP53* germline mutation develops almost exclusively in children, in contrast to sporadic

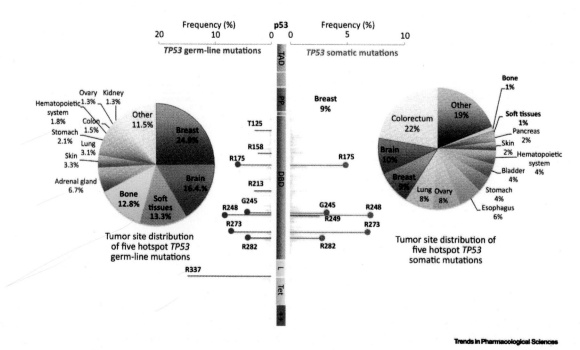

Fig. 14.20 Li–Fraumeni syndrome. Mutation landscape of *TP53* germline and somatic mutations in human cancer. ++, lysine-rich basic C-terminal domain; DBD, sequence-specific core DNA-binding domain; L, linker region; PP, proline domain; TAD, transcriptional activation domain; Tet, tetramerization domain.

Table 14.05 Clinical criteria for recommending *TP53* germline testing

Clinical criteria for recommending *TP53* germline testing		Reference(s)
Classic LFS criteria	A proband with: • a sarcoma diagnosed before the age of 45 years **AND** • a first-degree relative with any cancer before the age of 45 years **AND** • a first- or second-degree relative with any cancer before the age of 45 years or a sarcoma at any age	{1869}
LFS-like syndrome criteria	*Birch criteria* A proband with: • any childhood cancer or with a sarcoma, brain tumour, or adrenocortical carcinoma diagnosed before the age of 45 years **AND** • a first- or second-degree relative with a typical LFS cancer (sarcoma, breast cancer, brain tumour, adrenocortical carcinoma, or leukaemia) at any age **AND** • a first- or second-degree relative with any cancer before the age of 60 years	{286,826}
	Eeles criteria Two first- or second-degree relatives with LFS-related malignancies at any age	
Chompret criteria	1. A proband with: • a tumour belonging to the LFS tumour spectrum (soft tissue sarcoma, osteosarcoma, premenopausal breast cancer, brain tumour, adrenocortical carcinoma, leukaemia, or bronchoalveolar lung cancer) before the age of 46 years **AND** • at least one first- or second-degree relative with an LFS tumour (except breast cancer if the proband has breast cancer) before the age of 56 years or with multiple tumours **OR** 2. A proband with multiple tumours (except multiple breast tumours), two of which belong to the LFS tumour spectrum and the first of which occurred before the age of 46 years **OR** 3. A proband diagnosed with adrenocortical carcinoma or choroid plexus tumour, or anaplastic rhabdomyosarcoma of embryonal subtype, irrespective of family history **OR** 4. Breast cancer before the age of 31 years	{587,337,3199}

LFS, Li–Fraumeni syndrome.

adrenocortical carcinoma, which has a broad age distribution with peak incidence in patients aged > 40 years {894}. Furthermore, sonic hedgehog (SHH)-activated medulloblastoma and acute lymphoblastic leukaemia tend to occur at older ages than do their sporadic counterparts.

Nervous system neoplasms

In the 1245 individuals carrying a *TP53* germline mutation who were included in the IARC *TP53* Database as of July 2019, a total of 2591 tumours were reported; 289 (11.15%) of these were located in the nervous system. The M:F ratio of patients with brain tumours associated with *TP53* germline mutation is 1.5:1 {1394}. As with sporadic brain tumours, the age of patients with nervous system neoplasms associated with *TP53* germline mutations shows a bimodal distribution. The first incidence peak is in children (mainly SHH-activated medulloblastomas, IDH-wildtype high-grade gliomas, and choroid plexus carcinomas), and the second is in the third and fourth decades of life (mainly IDH-mutant diffuse astrocytic gliomas).

Epidemiology

TP53 germline variants have been estimated to occur at a rate of about 1 in 500 to 1 in 5000 live births, and they account for as many as 17% of all familial cancer cases {1134,2302,333, 697,696}. There is a variant-dependent gradient of phenotype severity, with the most functionally severe mutations associated with early tumour onset {695}. Tumour patterns are generally stable regardless of geographical or population demographics, with the only notable exceptions being an excess of gastric cancers in south-eastern Asia, an excess of soft tissue sarcomas in the western Pacific {695}, and an excess of a low-penetrance mutation at codon 334 in patients of Ashkenazi Jewish descent {2549}.

Etiology

LFS is caused by heterozygous germline alterations (mutation, rearrangement, or partial/complete deletion) in the *TP53* gene on chromosome 17p13.

Pathogenesis

The p53 protein is a multifunctional transcription factor involved in a wide range of biological processes {1860}. Its best-characterized functions are in the control of cell-cycle progression, DNA integrity, and the survival of cells exposed to DNA-damaging agents. Evidence indicates that p53 also regulates other important processes, such as cell oxidative metabolism, the cellular response to nutrient deprivation, fertility, ferroptosis, and stem cell maintenance. The extent and consequences of the biological response elicited by p53 vary according to stress and cell type {1566}. The functions of p53 rely mainly on its transcriptional activity, but it can also act via interactions with various proteins {2007,1727}.

In most human cancers, *TP53* is inactivated through gene alterations that confer loss of the protein's tumour suppressor function. Mutant p53 isoforms differ from each other in the extent to which they have lost suppressor function and in their capacity to inhibit wildtype p53 in a dominant negative manner {1568,2482}. In addition, some p53 mutants seem to exert oncogenic activity, but the molecular basis of this gain-of-function phenotype is still unclear {1082}.

Macroscopic appearance
The macroscopic appearance of tumours in LFS is similar to that of their sporadic counterparts.

Histopathology
The most common brain tumours occurring in the setting of LFS are choroid plexus carcinomas, medulloblastomas, and diffuse astrocytic gliomas. Their histopathology is similar to that of their sporadic counterparts, although the large cell / anaplastic pattern is observed more frequently in LFS-associated medulloblastomas than in sporadic medulloblastomas {2622}.

Immunophenotype
Immunohistochemistry can be used, albeit imperfectly, as a surrogate marker of *TP53* mutation, although somatic versus germline mutations cannot be distinguished. The typical pattern of a missense *TP53* mutation is strong, diffuse nuclear immunolabelling for p53 protein. Truncating mutations (nonsense, frameshift, or splice-site) are associated with an absence of nuclear staining in tumour cells.

Cytology
Not relevant

Diagnostic molecular pathology
The *TP53* gene on chromosome 17p13 has 11 exons spanning 20 kb. Exon 1 is non-coding, and exons 5–8 are highly conserved among vertebrates.

Distribution of TP53 germline mutations: Most germline *TP53* mutations are spread over exons 5–8, with major hotspots at codons 133, 175, 245, 248, 273 (all within the DNA-binding domain), and 337 (within the tetramerization domain). Missense mutations are most common – accounting for > 85% of all germline *TP53* pathogenic variants – but nonsense mutations, deletions/insertions, and splice-site mutations also occur. Structural variants with breakpoints located in intron 1 have also been identified in families fulfilling clinical criteria for LFS but lacking *TP53* point mutations {2661}. Mutations observed at hotspot codons consist of missense mutations that result in mutant proteins with complete loss of function, dominant negative phenotypes, and oncogenic (gain-of-function) activities.

Genotype/phenotype: Among 139 families with at least 1 case of brain tumour, the mean number of CNS tumours per family

Box 14.07 Diagnostic criteria for Li–Fraumeni syndrome

Essential:

Pathogenic germline alteration (mutation, rearrangement, or partial/complete deletion) in the *TP53* gene

was 1.55 {2331}. Several reported families showed a remarkable clustering of brain tumours {3398,1629}, suggesting potential for organ-specific or cell-specific risk.

An analysis of the IARC *TP53* Database {1394} of germline mutations showed an association between brain tumours and missense mutations located in the p53 DNA-binding surface that make contact with the minor groove of DNA {2320}. The type of mutation was also associated with the patient age at onset of brain tumours: truncating mutations were associated with early-onset brain tumours {2320,336}. Familial clustering may also be due to gene–environment interactions; for example, exposure of families to similar environmental carcinogens or lifestyle factors has been suggested in stomach and breast cancer {466}.

Molecular features of CNS tumours in LFS
(1) Medulloblastoma: Medulloblastomas associated with LFS demonstrate near uniform large cell / anaplastic morphology and belong to the sonic hedgehog (SHH)-activated, *TP53*-mutant molecular subtype. These tumours are characterized by chromothripsis and often have amplification of oncogenes including *MYCN* and *GLI2* {2622}.

(2) Diffuse astrocytic gliomas: Astrocytomas associated with LFS demonstrate distinct age-dependent molecular patterns. In the paediatric population, patients tend to present with IDH-wildtype glioblastomas throughout the neuraxis characterized by frequent *NF1* mutations, *MYCN* amplification, and cell-cycle pathway gene alterations {2955}. In young adults, lower-grade diffuse astrocytic gliomas with *IDH1* mutations located within the cerebral hemispheres are most common. These are enriched for non-*IDH1* p.R132H variants, including p.R132C and p.R132S, along with concurrent *ATRX* mutation or deletion {3398,3070,2955}.

(3) Choroid plexus carcinoma: Choroid plexus carcinomas associated with LFS are not molecularly distinct from the subset of sporadic choroid plexus carcinomas harbouring somatic *TP53* mutations. They are characterized by genomic instability and cluster with the high-risk paediatric, type B methylation class {2507,3182}.

Essential and desirable diagnostic criteria
See Box 14.07.

Staging
Not clinically relevant

Prognosis and prediction
Medulloblastomas arising in the setting of LFS are associated with a dismal prognosis {3392}. Choroid plexus carcinomas harbouring *TP53* mutations, typically occurring in the germline as part of LFS, are associated with a worse prognosis than are choroid plexus carcinomas without *TP53* mutation {3097,1157,2079}. IDH-wildtype high-grade gliomas that arise during childhood in the setting of LFS are associated with a poor prognosis, whereas the IDH-mutant diffuse astrocytic gliomas arising in teenagers and young adults in the setting of LFS are associated with more favourable survival, similar to that associated with their sporadic IDH-mutant astrocytoma counterparts {2955}. Clinical surveillance has been associated with early tumour detection and improved survival in patients with LFS {3326,1733}.

Cowden syndrome

Eberhart CG
Eng CE

Definition

Cowden syndrome is an autosomal dominant disorder caused mainly by germline pathogenic variants of *PTEN*, characterized by multiple hamartomas involving tissues derived from all three germ cell layers and a high risk of breast, thyroid, endometrial, renal, and colon cancers. Adult-onset dysplastic cerebellar gangliocytoma (Lhermitte–Duclos disease) is also considered to be pathognomonic.

MIM numbering

158350 Cowden syndrome 1; CWS1

ICD-11 coding

LD2D.Y Other specified phakomatoses or hamartoneoplastic syndromes

Related terminology

Acceptable: Cowden disease; *PTEN* hamartoma tumour syndrome.
Not recommended: multiple hamartoma syndrome.

Subtype(s)

Bannayan–Riley–Ruvalcaba syndrome; Proteus syndrome

Localization

Dysplastic cerebellar gangliocytoma affects the cerebellum, and macrocephaly the cerebral hemispheres.

Clinical features

Dysplastic cerebellar gangliocytoma (Lhermitte–Duclos disease)

Adult-onset dysplastic cerebellar gangliocytoma, even in the absence of other features or family history, is highly predictive of a germline pathogenic variant in *PTEN* {3609}, and dysplastic cerebellar gangliocytoma is now considered pathognomonic of Cowden syndrome. For further details, see *Dysplastic cerebellar gangliocytoma (Lhermitte–Duclos disease)* (p. 146).

Intestinal hamartomatous polyps and colorectal cancer

Several varieties of hamartomatous polyps are seen in this syndrome, including hamartomas most similar to juvenile polyps composed of a mixture of connective tissues normally present in the mucosa, lipomatous and ganglioneuromatous lesions, and lymphoid hyperplasia {467,3401}. These polyps are found in the stomach, duodenum, small bowel, and colon. The presence of some ganglion tissue is not unusual in the juvenile-like polyps. Lesions in which autonomic nerves are predominant (resulting in a ganglioneuroma-like appearance) have also been described, but these seem to be exceptional {1805}. A prospective study of a large series of patients with germline *PTEN* pathogenic variants found that ≥ 90% of adults undergoing colonoscopy had polyps with various histological features and even mixed

polyposis {1274}. In that series, 9 of 127 patients were found to have colorectal cancer, all before the age of 50 years, with a standardized incidence ratio of 224 (*P* < 0.0001). Because of this prospective study, the National Comprehensive Cancer Network (NCCN) practice guidelines have advocated starting routine colon surveillance for patients when they are in their thirties. In an unselected series of 4 children with juvenile polyposis of infancy, germline 10q23 deletion also involved *BMPR1A*, upstream of *PTEN*. Subsequently, germline deletion involving both *PTEN* and *BMPR1A* was shown to characterize at least a subset of juvenile polyposis of infancy {730}.

Breast and thyroid cancer

The two most commonly occurring cancers in Cowden syndrome are carcinomas of the breast and thyroid {3019,3584}. In the general population, the lifetime risks of breast and thyroid cancers are approximately 11% (among women) and 1% (among both sexes), respectively. In women with Cowden syndrome, a prospective series revealed lifetime breast cancer risks of 85% with an elevated standardized incidence ratio of 25.4 {3125}. The mean patient age at diagnosis is about 10 years younger than that for breast cancer occurring in the general population {1924,3019}. Although Rachel Cowden died of breast cancer at 31 years of age {388,1918} and the youngest reported patient was aged 14 years at diagnosis {3019}, the great majority of breast cancers are diagnosed in patients aged > 30 years (range: 14–65 years) {1924,3125}. The predominant histology is ductal adenocarcinoma. Most breast carcinomas in Cowden syndrome occur in a background of ductal carcinoma in situ, atypical ductal hyperplasia, adenosis, and sclerosis {2856}.

The lifetime risk of epithelial thyroid cancer can be as high as 35% in patients with Cowden syndrome {3125}. The youngest patient reported was 8 years old at diagnosis. Based on this and two other studies, routine thyroid surveillance should begin at about 7 years of age. Histologically, follicular carcinoma predominates, although papillary histology has also been rarely observed {1232,1997,3019,3584}. Medullary thyroid carcinoma has not been reported.

Other tumour types

A prospective series of individuals with Cowden syndrome with *PTEN* pathogenic variants revealed lifetime risks of endometrial (28%), renal cell (30%), and colorectal (9%) carcinomas, as well as melanoma (6%) {3125}.

The most important benign tumours in Cowden syndrome are trichilemmomas and papillomatous papules of the skin. Benign tumours and disorders of the breast and thyroid are the next most common, and probably constitute true component features of the syndrome. Fibroadenomas and fibrocystic disease of the breast are common signs of Cowden syndrome, as are follicular adenomas and multinodular goitre of the thyroid.

Chronic lymphocytic thyroiditis is a common finding accompanying thyroid pathology in Cowden syndrome with *PTEN* mutations.

Other malignancies and benign tumours have also been reported in patients or families with Cowden syndrome. It remains to be determined whether these (e.g. sarcomas, lymphomas, leukaemias, and meningiomas) are true components of the syndrome.

Epidemiology

Before the identification of *PTEN*, the incidence of Cowden syndrome was estimated to be 1 case per 1 million person-years {3019}. After the gene was identified {1889}, a molecular-based estimate of prevalence in the same population was 1 case per 200 000 population {2227}. Because of difficulties in recognizing this syndrome, prevalence figures are likely to be underestimates. One recent study estimated de novo *PTEN* mutation frequency to be about 11% at minimum and 48% at maximum in tested probands {2087}.

Etiology

Approximately 85% of Cowden syndrome cases, as strictly defined by the International Cowden Consortium (ICC) criteria, have a germline pathogenic variant in *PTEN*, including intragenic mutations, promoter mutations, and large deletions/rearrangements {1889,2018,3610}. If the diagnostic criteria are relaxed, this mutation frequency drops to 10–50% {1961,2229, 3232}. A formal study that ascertained 64 unrelated Cowden syndrome–like cases found a mutation frequency of 2% if the criteria were not met, even if the diagnosis was made short of only one criterion {2019}. However, this study only looked at the nine exons of *PTEN*; presumably, further mutations would have been identified in the promoter or in *SDHB* or *SDHD*. A single-centre study involving 37 unrelated families affected by Cowden syndrome (as strictly defined by the ICC criteria) found a pathogenic variant frequency of 80% {2018}. Exploratory genotype–phenotype analyses showed that the presence of a germline pathogenic variant was associated with a familial risk of developing breast cancer {2018}. Additionally, missense mutations and/or mutations of the phosphatase core motif seem to be associated with a surrogate for disease severity (multiorgan involvement). A small study of 13 families with 8 *PTEN* mutation–positive members did not show any genotype–phenotype associations {2227}, but this may be due to the small sample size.

Recently, other Cowden syndrome predisposition genes have also been identified: the SDH genes, *PIK3CA*, *KLLN*, and *WWP1*.

Pathogenesis

PTEN, on 10q23, consists of 9 exons spanning 120–150 kb of genomic distance, and it encodes a 1.2 kb transcript and a 403 amino acid and lipid dual-specificity phosphatase (dephosphorylating both protein and lipid substrates), which is homologous to the focal adhesion molecules tensin and auxilin {1872,2018,3023}. The amino acid sequence that is homologous to tensin and auxilin is encoded by exons 1–6. A classic phosphatase core motif is encoded within exon 5, which is the largest exon, constituting 20% of the coding region {1868, 1872,3023}. A longer isoform of *PTEN* has also been described,

which apparently interacts with the mitochondrion, but its clinical impact is still unclear {2581}.

PTEN is virtually ubiquitously expressed {3023}. Detailed studies of expression in human development have not been performed, and only a single study has examined PTEN expression during human embryogenesis using a monoclonal antibody against the terminal 100 amino acids of PTEN {1110}. The study revealed high levels of expression of PTEN protein in the skin, thyroid, and CNS – organs that are affected by the component neoplasms of Cowden syndrome. It also revealed prominent expression in the developing autonomic nervous system and gastrointestinal tract. Early embryonic death in *Pten*[-/-] mice also implies a crucial role for PTEN in early development {748,2527, 3081}. PTEN is a tumour suppressor and a dual-specificity lipid phosphatase that plays multiple roles in the cell cycle, apoptosis, cell polarity, cell migration, and even genomic stability {2185,2901,3584}. The major substrate of PTEN is PIP3, which is part of the PI3K pathway {665,1013,1871,1980,3015}. When PTEN is ample and functional, PIP3 is converted to PIP2, which results in hypophosphorylated AKT, a known cell-survival factor. Hypophosphorylated AKT is apoptotic. When PTEN is in the cytoplasm, it predominantly signals via its lipid phosphatase activity down the PI3K/AKT pathway {2120}. In contrast, when PTEN is in the nucleus, it predominantly signals via protein phosphatase activity down the cyclin D1 / MAPK pathway, eliciting G1 arrest at least in breast and glial cells {1013,1014,1871, 2120}. It is also thought that PTEN can dephosphorylate FAK and inhibit integrin and MAPK signalling {1173,3121}.

Bannayan–Riley–Ruvalcaba syndrome, which is characterized by macrocephaly, lipomatosis, haemangiomatosis, and speckled penis, was previously thought to be clinically distinct, but it is now considered a likely allelic variant of Cowden syndrome {2020}. In a combined cohort of 16 sporadic and 27 familial cases, approximately 60% of the patients carried a germline pathogenic variant in *PTEN* {2021}. Of the 27 familial cases studied, 11 were classified as exhibiting true overlap of Cowden syndrome and Bannayan–Riley–Ruvalcaba syndrome, and 10 of those 11 had a *PTEN* mutation. Another 10% of patients with Bannayan–Riley–Ruvalcaba syndrome were subsequently found to harbour large germline deletions of *PTEN* {3610}. The overlapping mutation spectrum, the existence of true overlap between familial cases, and genotype–phenotype associations suggest that a germline *PTEN* pathogenic variant is associated with cancer, and they strongly suggest that these two syndromes are allelic and part of a single spectrum at the molecular level. The aggregate term "*PTEN* hamartoma tumour syndrome" was first proposed in 1999 {2021} and has since become even more apt, now that germline *PTEN* pathogenic variants have been identified in autism spectrum disorder with macrocephaly, in Proteus syndrome, and in VATER/VACTERL association (the co-occurrence of several birth defects) with macrocephaly {427,2629,3608}. In one case, the identification of a germline intragenic *PTEN* mutation in a patient thought to have juvenile polyposis {2321} was subsequently considered to exclude that specific clinical diagnosis; the finding instead suggests a molecular designation of *PTEN* hamartoma tumour syndrome {850,1358,1359,1764,2022,2329}. This conclusion has been further supported by the identification of germline *PTEN* pathogenic variants in individuals with juvenile polyps, and of large deletions involving both *PTEN* and *BMPR1A* in juvenile polyposis of infancy {730,3090}. An important finding of the polyp ascertainment study was that the reasons for referral listed in the original pathology reports were often incorrect, suggesting that a re-review of all polyp histology by gastrointestinal pathologists based in major academic medical centres is a vital step for determining correct genetic etiology {3090}.

Macroscopic appearance
Dysplastic cerebellar gangliocytomas, the main CNS lesions associated with Cowden syndrome, are discrete lesions characterized by hypertrophy of cerebellar gyri.

Histopathology
Dysplastic cerebellar gangliocytoma shows diffuse enlargement of the molecular and internal granular layers by ganglionic cells of various size, with relative preservation of the overall cerebellar architecture {11}.

Cytology
The cytology varies by tumour type.

Diagnostic molecular pathology
Cowden syndrome is an autosomal dominant disorder, with age-related penetrance and variable expression {849,2255, 3125}. The major Cowden syndrome susceptibility gene, *PTEN*, is located on 10q23.3 {1872,1889,2228}. Other predisposition genes in non-*PTEN* Cowden syndrome include the SDH genes as well as *PIK3CA*, *AKT1*, *KLLN*, *USF3*, *SEC23B*, and *WWP1* {241,2248,2250,2330,2249,3534,1843}.

Essential and desirable diagnostic criteria
Pathognomonic and major diagnostic criteria are listed in Box 14.08.

Staging
Staging varies by tumour type.

Box 14.08 International Cowden Consortium (ICC) and National Comprehensive Cancer Network (NCCN) operational criteria for Cowden syndrome without known family history of *PTEN* mutation

Pathognomonic criteria:
Adult dysplastic cerebellar gangliocytoma (cerebellar tumours)

Mucocutaneous lesions[a]

- Facial trichilemmomas, any number[a] (at least two biopsy-proven trichilemmomas[b])
- Acral keratoses
- Papillomatous papules

Mucosal lesions (especially hamartomatous gastrointestinal polyps)

Autism spectrum disorder and macrocephaly[b]

Major criteria:
Breast cancer

Thyroid cancer (non-medullary)

Macrocephaly (megalocephaly; i.e. 97th percentile and above)

Endometrial cancer

Mucocutaneous lesions[b]

- One biopsy-proven trichilemmoma
- Multiple palmoplantar keratoses
- Multifocal cutaneous facial papules
- Macular pigmentation of the glans penis

Multiple gastrointestinal hamartomas or ganglioneuromas[b]

[a]ICC criteria only, [b]NCCN 2010 criteria only (modified from {3124}).
Note: In 1996, the ICC {2228} compiled operational diagnostic criteria for Cowden syndrome on the basis of the published literature and their own clinical experience {848,3584}. NCCN has also established a set of operational clinical diagnostic criteria for identifying individuals with possible Cowden syndrome {2216}.

Prognosis and prediction
There have been no systematic studies to indicate whether the prognosis for patients with Cowden syndrome and cancer is different from that of non-syndromic patients with the same cancer types.

Constitutional mismatch repair deficiency syndrome

Tabori U
Abedalthagafi MS
Legius E
Solomon DA

Definition

Constitutional mismatch repair deficiency syndrome (CMMRD) is an autosomal recessive cancer predisposition syndrome caused by biallelic germline mutations in one of four mismatch repair genes (*MLH1*, *PMS2*, *MSH2*, and *MSH6*). Individuals with CMMRD develop ultrahypermutated malignant gliomas, CNS embryonal tumours, and a variety of other cancers during childhood and early adulthood.

MIM numbering

276300 Mismatch repair cancer syndrome 1; MMRCS1

ICD-11 coding

None

Related terminology

Not recommended: mismatch repair cancer syndrome; Turcot syndrome; brain tumour polyposis syndrome type 1.
Acceptable: biallelic mismatch repair deficiency syndrome.

Subtype(s)

None

Localization

The glioblastomas arising in the setting of CMMRD, Lynch syndrome, and polymerase proofreading deficiency can occur both in the cerebral hemispheres and in the posterior fossa, including a gliomatosis-like dissemination pattern in a subset of cases. Medulloblastomas centred in the posterior fossa, and other embryonal CNS tumours, have also been reported {178}.

Clinical features

The combination of café-au-lait skin macules, consanguinity, and specific brain, haematological, and gastrointestinal cancers arising during childhood should raise suspicion for CMMRD. A scoring system has been developed for determining those patients in whom genetic testing for CMMRD should be performed {3457}. Importantly, family history of cancer is often uninformative, especially for those children with biallelic *PMS2* mutations, because of the substantially lower cancer risk associated with heterozygous mutations in this gene compared with the other mismatch repair genes.

Nervous system neoplasms

Brain tumours, most commonly gliomas, occur in the first two decades of life and account for 25–40% of all CMMRD-associated cancers {178,3457}. Medulloblastoma and CNS embryonal tumours have also been described in patients with CMMRD {1183}. Molecularly, all brain tumours arising in the setting of CMMRD have a unique ultrahypermutation genotype, which distinguishes them from the typically low somatic mutation burdens in their sporadic paediatric counterparts {335,447}.

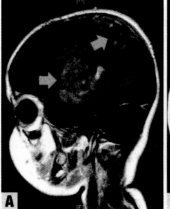
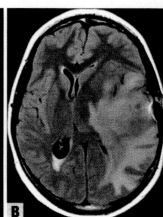

Fig. 14.21 Representative imaging of replication repair–deficient glioblastomas. **A** T1-weighted postcontrast MRI of a patient with constitutional mismatch repair deficiency syndrome with a homozygous *MSH2* pathogenic germline variant. Note two synchronous tumours (arrows). Both tumours had secondary somatic mutations and ultrahypermutation, one involving *POLE* and one involving *POLD1*. **B** A FLAIR sequence of a patient with Lynch syndrome and *MLH1* heterozygous pathogenic germline variant. This gliomatosis-like pattern is typical for somatic mutation in *IDH1* and hypermutation.

Other CNS manifestations

Agenesis of the corpus callosum and venous anomalies have been reported in children with CMMRD. Developmental venous anomalies are extremely common and may point towards the possibility of CMMRD {2917}.

Extraneural manifestations

More than 90% of patients with CMMRD have café-au-lait macules and other dermatological abnormalities such as hyperpigmented or hypopigmented areas {178}. These café-au-lait macules can mimic those found in patients with neurofibromatosis type 1. However, patients with CMMRD typically lack other stigmata of neurofibromatosis type 1, such as axillary and groin freckling, cutaneous neurofibromas, and Lisch nodules {3457,813}. Haematological malignancies, predominantly T-cell leukaemia/lymphoma, occur in as many as 30% of patients, mostly in the first two decades of life, whereas gastrointestinal polyposis and cancers are present in virtually all patients by the second decade of life. Other cancers (e.g. urinary tract cancers and sarcomas) have also been reported {178,3457}. Multiple pilomatrixomas appear to be frequent and might suggest CMMRD when present in combination with another feature of the condition {576}. An increased frequency of paediatric systemic lupus erythematosus has been reported in patients with CMMRD {3210}; all 5 patients with CMMRD and paediatric systemic lupus erythematosus were girls, and 4 of them had biallelic *MSH6* mutations.

Differential diagnosis

CMMRD should not be confused with Lynch syndrome (also known as hereditary nonpolyposis colorectal cancer syndrome). Whereas CMMRD is an autosomal recessive syndrome resulting from biallelic germline mutation in one of the mismatch repair genes, Lynch syndrome is an autosomal dominant syndrome resulting from a heterozygous germline mutation. It results in a different cancer spectrum and different age of onset (mostly colorectal, genitourinary, and sebaceous carcinomas during adulthood). Hypermutant cancers including glioblastomas, accompanied by some of the features of CMMRD including café-au-lait macules, can also occur with germline mutations in the *POLE* gene encoding DNA polymerase E, which has been termed "polymerase proofreading deficiency" {3267,114}.

Epidemiology

More than 200 kindreds with CMMRD have been reported {178, 3457}. However, this syndrome is probably underdiagnosed and highly prevalent in populations where consanguinity is high {96,811}. In countries with a low level of consanguinity, the prevalence of this condition has been estimated at 1 case per 1 million children.

Etiology

CMMRD is caused by biallelic germline inactivation of one of the four main mismatch repair genes: *MLH1* at chromosome 3p22.2, *MSH2* at 2p21-p16.3, *MSH6* at 2p16, and *PMS2* at 7p22. This can be the result either of two different mutations present in trans (compound heterozygous) or of the same mutation present on both alleles (homozygous), the latter being common in consanguinity.

Pathogenesis

The genetic defect underlying CMMRD is the inability to recognize and repair DNA mismatches during replication. Recognition and repair of base-pair mismatches in human DNA is mediated by heterodimers of MSH2 and MSH6, which form a sliding clamp on DNA. The C-terminus of PMS2 interacts with MLH1, and this complex binds to MSH2/MSH6 heterodimers to form a functional strand-specific mismatch recognition complex {2946}. Cells that are deficient in any of the above genes are defective in the repair of mismatched bases and insertions/deletions of single nucleotides, resulting in high mutation rates and microsatellite instability. Unlike in heterozygous carriers with Lynch syndrome (in whom microsatellite instability is robustly observed in the resultant endometrial and colorectal cancers), glioblastomas arising in patients with CMMRD often lack classic microsatellite instability and are characterized instead by extremely high rates of single-nucleotide mutations with a significantly smaller component of small insertions/deletions {178, 2920}. CMMRD-associated glioblastomas commonly acquire mutations in *POLE* or *POLD1* to create complete replication deficiency and ultrahypermutation {178,2920}. These tumours almost invariably inactivate tumour suppressor genes such as *TP53*.

Genotype/phenotype

In CMMRD, the genotype/phenotype correlation is difficult to ascertain due to the syndrome's rarity. Whereas germline *MLH1*

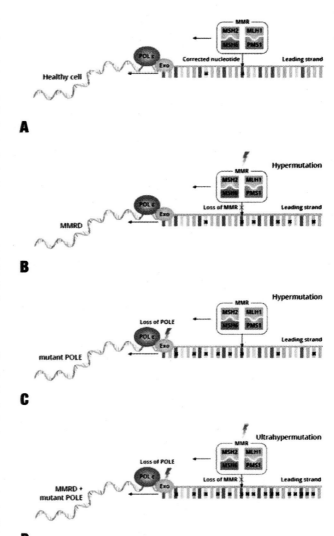

Fig. 14.22 A model of replication repair deficiency and the consequent mutation accumulation. **A** Replication repair in normal cells. **B** Mismatch repair deficiency from mutation in one on the four mismatch repair genes leads to hypermutation. **C** Mutations in the proofreading domain of the DNA polymerases *POLE* or *POLD1* overwhelm the mismatch repair system and result in hypermutation. **D** Combined mismatch repair deficiency and polymerase mutations result in ultrahypermutation.

and *MSH2* mutations are most prevalent in Lynch syndrome, *PMS2* and *MSH6* mutations predominate in CMMRD. Heterozygous *PMS2* mutation carrier parents are usually unaffected due to the substantially lower cancer risks. The *MLH1* and *MSH2* group tends to have a younger age of first malignancy diagnosis and a more severe overall cancer phenotype {3457}.

All tumour types are observed among specific CMMRD mutation carriers. Some studies suggest that brain tumours are more frequent in patients with biallelic *PMS2* than in those with *MLH1* or *MSH2* mutations, with the *MLH1* and *MSH2* group more frequently having haematological malignancies {3457}.

Macroscopic appearance

The macroscopic appearance of tumours in CMMRD is as described for the individual tumour types.

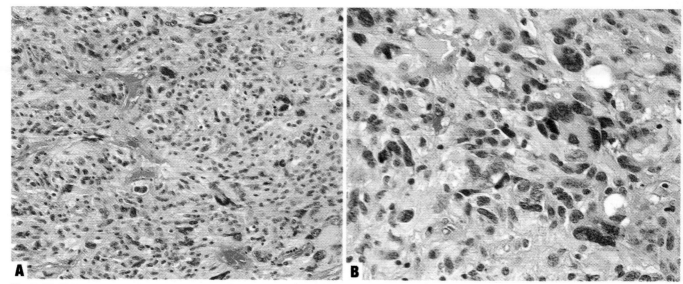

Fig. 14.23 Glioblastoma arising in the setting of constitutional mismatch repair deficiency syndrome. **A,B** Glioblastomas arising in this setting often demonstrate severe nuclear pleomorphism with bizarre and multinucleated giant cells.

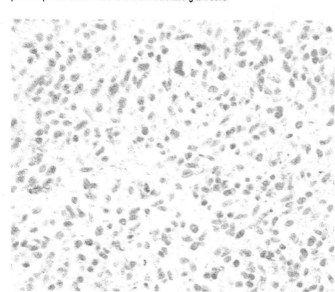

Fig. 14.24 Glioblastoma arising in the setting of constitutional mismatch repair deficiency syndrome (CMMRD). This glioblastoma in the cerebral hemispheres of a child with CMMRD demonstrates a complete absence of PMS2 protein both in tumour cells and in normal cells, resulting from biallelic inactivation of the *PMS2* mismatch repair gene in the germline of this patient.

Box 14.09 Diagnostic criteria for constitutional mismatch repair deficiency syndrome

Essential:

Biallelic pathogenic germline mutation/deletion in one of the four main mismatch repair genes (*MSH2, MSH6, PMS2, MLH1*)

OR

A combination of the presence of two clinical criteria and positive results in two functional assays (see text)

Desirable:

Genomic profiling of the index brain tumour demonstrating an ultrahypermutated genotype with mutation signature characteristic of mismatch repair deficiency

Absence of expression of mismatch repair proteins in both tumour cells and normal cells on immunohistochemistry

Histopathology

The glioblastomas arising in the setting of CMMRD often have severe nuclear pleomorphism and/or bizarre multinucleated giant cells {1183}. Other brain tumours in CMMRD appear morphologically as sheets of primitive small blue cells, raising the differential diagnosis of a CNS embryonal tumour or medulloblastoma depending on the location {178,1183}. Whether all the brain tumours that arise in the setting of CMMRD are in fact glioblastomas or whether true medulloblastomas, pleomorphic xanthoastrocytomas, and other tumour types can occur in this syndrome remains to be determined.

The finding of a paediatric high-grade glioma or glioblastoma with severe pleomorphism or giant cell features should raise suspicion for possible CMMRD and prompt immunohistochemical testing for the mismatch repair proteins.

Cytology

Not relevant

Diagnostic molecular pathology

Detection of biallelic germline mutation (either homozygous or compound heterozygous) in one of the four main mismatch repair genes is required for the diagnosis of CMMRD. The abundance of variants of unknown significance and the technical problems with sequencing *PMS2*, which has multiple pseudogenes, has led to the development of several functional assays that can aid in the rapid detection of CMMRD. Microsatellite instability testing on glioblastomas is not a reliable test because they typically demonstrate only a low level of microsatellite instability despite being mismatch repair–deficient and ultrahypermutated. Immunohistochemistry demonstrates loss of expression of the inactivated mismatch repair protein (and when appropriate, its heterodimer) in both tumour and normal tissue in > 90% of CMMRD-associated cancers {178}. In vitro cell-based assays on normal fibroblasts and lymphoblasts can detect microsatellite instability, resistance to several compounds, and failure to repair G–T mismatches {2920,308}. Recently, screening tests based on microsatellite instability using next-generation sequencing of normal tissue reported successful identification of patients with CMMRD {1026,1135}.

Essential and desirable diagnostic criteria
See Box 14.09.

Staging
Not applicable

Prognosis and prediction
Patients with CMMRD and their family members benefit from genetic counselling, because surveillance protocols exist and early detection may result in increased survival for both biallelic and heterozygous carriers {812,3294}. The inherent resistance of mismatch repair–deficient cells to several common chemotherapies, including temozolomide, makes them ineffective in the management of gliomas in the setting of CMMRD. In contrast, the ultrahypermutation phenotype of CMMRD-associated cancers results in a greater neoantigen burden on cancer cells, which can be therapeutically exploited by immune checkpoint blockade {2920,1816}. Because the prognosis for children with glioblastomas arising in the setting of CMMRD is unfavourable, immunotherapeutic approaches and prevention strategies are now being tested {335,8,1183}.

Familial adenomatous polyposis 1

Varlet P
Abedalthagafi MS
Ellison DW
Hawkins CE
Legius E

Pfister SM
Pietsch T
Solomon DA
Tabori U

Definition

Familial adenomatous polyposis 1 (FAP1) is an autosomal dominant cancer syndrome caused by an inactivating germline pathogenic sequence variant in the tumour suppressor gene *APC*. In FAP1, gastrointestinal neoplasms predominate. A subset of patients with FAP1 develop a primary brain tumour, which is also referred to as brain tumour polyposis syndrome 2 (BTP2). The principal brain tumour in BTP2 is medulloblastoma with WNT activation.

MIM numbering

175100 Familial adenomatous polyposis 1; FAP1

ICD-11 coding

2B90.Y & XH1CV4 Other specified malignant neoplasms of colon & Adenomatous polyposis coli

Related terminology

Not recommended: Turcot syndrome.

Subtype(s)

None

Localization

For WNT-activated medulloblastoma arising in the setting of BTP2, no differences in location (cerebellar midline / cerebellopontine angle) have been found from that of their sporadic counterparts with somatic *CTNNB1* mutations {3076}.

Clinical features

FAP1 is a common gastrointestinal polyposis syndrome and is characterized by the development of multiple adenomas in the colon and rectum, predisposing to colorectal carcinoma. More than 70% of patients also develop multiple extracolonic manifestations, including gastric and duodenal adenomas,

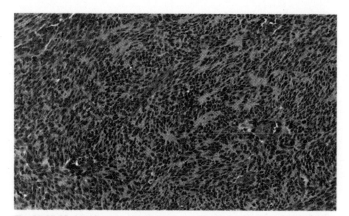

Fig. 14.25 Medulloblastoma in brain tumour polyposis syndrome 2. Classic medulloblastoma with Homer Wright rosettes.

congenital retinal pigment epithelial hypertrophy, epidermal cysts, dental abnormalities, and a high risk of developing extracolonic tumours such as osteomas (50–90%), desmoid tumours (10–15%), thyroid cancers (2–3%), and hepatoblastoma (1%) {1855}. Therefore, FAP1 is a multiorgan cancer predisposition syndrome. Timely diagnosis and awareness will help in early detection of other cancers and appropriate interventions.

Medulloblastoma represents the only primary brain tumour clearly associated with BTP2 {3392,1616}. No difference in age at diagnosis has been found between patients with a syndromic medulloblastoma due to germline *APC* mutations and sporadic medulloblastoma with somatic *CTNNB1* mutations {3076,3392}. Colonic symptoms may be mild or even absent and medulloblastoma can be the initial tumour, predating manifestations of the polyposis syndrome. In this setting, family history can be suggestive of FAP1. The recommendation is therefore to carefully investigate family history and offer genetic counselling for patients with *CTNNB1* wildtype WNT-activated medulloblastomas.

Occasional FAP1-associated cases of adamantinomatous craniopharyngioma that lack *CTNNB1* mutation and instead harbour germline *APC* mutation with somatic loss of heterozygosity have been reported {2413}.

Epidemiology

Only a small proportion of WNT-activated medulloblastomas are familial (approximately 5% of cases), and these are so far exclusively due to germline *APC* pathogenic variants. Medulloblastomas are a rare manifestation of FAP1, accounting for only 1% of all malignancies in FAP1 patients {1855}. FAP1 occurs in 1–3 per 10 000 births, with an almost 100% penetrance. In 20–30% of cases, the disease is caused by a de novo mutation, with no clinical or genetic evidence of FAP1 in the parents or family {1391}.

The lifetime risk of developing a medulloblastoma in the context of FAP1 is about 1%, which is 92 times as high as that in the general population {158}.

Etiology

FAP1 results from a heterozygous pathogenic variant in the *APC* tumour suppressor gene, located on chromosome band 5q22.2. A second hit (additional somatic mutation or deletion/ loss of heterozygosity) in the *APC* gene is required for tumour formation {1225}.

Pathogenesis

APC acts as a negative regulator of the WNT signalling pathway, playing an important role in ubiquitination and degradation of β-catenin. APC loss leads to a nuclear translocation of β-catenin that impacts proliferation, differentiation, and migration {1855}. The activation of the WNT signalling pathway by APC loss is similar to that caused by common mutant oncogenic β-catenin proteins occurring in sporadic WNT-activated medulloblastomas.

Box 14.10 Diagnostic criteria for a familial adenomatous polyposis 1–associated brain tumour

Essential:

Occurrence of a brain tumour, typically WNT-activated medulloblastoma, in a patient with familial adenomatous polyposis 1

OR

Identification of a pathogenic germline mutation in the *APC* gene in a child with WNT-activated medulloblastoma lacking *CTNNB1* mutation

Macroscopic appearance

Not relevant

Histopathology

In a series of 12 medulloblastomas in patients with BTP2, all had a classic histology, including frequent Homer Wright rosettes and nuclear β-catenin accumulation {3076}.

Cytology

Not relevant

Diagnostic molecular pathology

WNT-activated medulloblastomas without *CTNNB1* mutation should be tested for *APC* pathogenic variants. These patients and their families should be offered genetic counselling and tested for germline pathogenic variants because the frequency of germline *APC* mutations is very high in this setting {3392}.

Essential and desirable diagnostic criteria

See Box 14.10.

Staging

Staging involves cerebrospinal fluid cytology, cranial and spinal MRI to exclude metastasis, and postoperative imaging to evaluate gross residual disease.

Prognosis and prediction

The overall and progression-free survival of patients with FAP1 with WNT-activated medulloblastoma is excellent (similar to that reported for sporadic WNT-activated medulloblastomas) {841, 3076,3392}. Given the relatively low prevalence of CNS tumours in patients with FAP1, imaging-based screening is not recommended for children of these families. However, identification of a germline *APC* pathogenic variant is key in initiating early surveillance for gastrointestinal and other FAP1-related neoplasms. The guidelines are well established and include surveillance during childhood {1391}.

Naevoid basal cell carcinoma syndrome

Pietsch T
Eberhart CG
Ellison DW
Evans DGR
Pajtler KW

Definition

Naevoid basal cell carcinoma syndrome (NBCCS), also known as Gorlin syndrome, is a complex syndrome involving multiple organ systems. It is caused by germline mutations in genes involved in the hedgehog signalling pathway (most commonly *PTCH1*). The most common CNS finding is medulloblastoma of the desmoplastic/nodular subtype.

MIM numbering

109400 Basal cell naevus syndrome; BCNS

ICD-11 coding

LD2D.4 Gorlin syndrome

Related terminology

Acceptable: Gorlin syndrome; Gorlin–Goltz syndrome.
Not recommended: basal cell naevus syndrome; fifth phakomatosis.

Subtype(s)

None

Localization

Manifestations of NBCCS occur in the skin (basal cell carcinomas, sebaceous cysts), jaw (keratocysts), bone (congenital anomalies), and brain (macrocephaly, falx calcification, medulloblastoma), as well as in the eyelid, mouth (cleft lip/palate), and ovary (fibromas).

Clinical features

The most frequent manifestations of NBCCS are multiple basal cell carcinomas, as well as odontogenic keratocysts of the jaw. In one study, basal cell carcinomas and odontogenic keratocysts were found together in > 90% of affected individuals by the age of 40 years {873}. Other frequent manifestations include calcification of the falx cerebri, palmar and plantar pits, and bifid or fused ribs {1631,2891}. These findings (apart from rib anomalies) are considered major diagnostic criteria (see Box 14.11). Minor criteria include medulloblastoma {100}, ovarian fibroma, macrocephaly, congenital facial abnormalities (e.g. cleft lip or palate), skeletal abnormalities (e.g. digit polydactyly), and radiological bone abnormalities (e.g. bridging of the sella turcica) {100,1631}. The clinical features manifest at different points in life. Macrocephaly and rib anomalies can be detected at birth, and medulloblastomas typically develop within the first 3 years of life. Jaw cysts do not usually become evident before the age of about 8 years, and basal cell carcinomas are usually found 10 years later {993}. Radiation treatment of patients with NBCCS (e.g. craniospinal irradiation for the treatment of cerebellar medulloblastoma) induces multiple basal cell carcinomas of the skin as well as various other tumour types (e.g. meningioma) within the radiation field {511,2324,3021}.

NBCCS-associated medulloblastoma

In a review of 33 reported medulloblastoma cases associated with NBCCS, all but 1 tumour had developed in children aged < 5 years, and 22 cases (66%) had arisen in patients aged < 2 years {100}. Medulloblastomas associated with NBCCS seem to be exclusively the extensively nodular or desmoplastic/nodular types {100,1042,2855,2963}. It has been proposed that nodular/desmoplastic medulloblastomas in young children should serve as a major criterion for the diagnosis of NBCCS {100,1042}.

Epidemiology

A UK prevalence of 3.2 cases per 100 000 individuals and a birth incidence of 5.3 cases per 100 000 births have been reported {869}, although lower prevalence rates have been reported from Italy (0.39 cases per 100 000 population) {3317}, Japan (0.42 cases per 100 000 population) {993}, and Australia (0.61 cases per 100 000 population) {2891}. Of 131 children with medulloblastomas, 6% had germline *SUFU* mutations {391}. About 1–2% of patients with NBCCS with germline *PTCH1* pathogenic variants develop medulloblastoma, compared with about 20% of patients with germline *SUFU* pathogenic variants {2963}.

Etiology

NBCCS results from inactivating germline mutations in the human homologue of the *Drosophila* segment polarity patched gene (*PTCH1*) on 9q22 {1217,1491}, its paralog *PTCH2* on 1p34 in rare cases {887,994}, or *SUFU* on 10q24 {2963}.

Numerous different *PTCH1* germline pathogenic variants associated with NBCCS have been reported {993,1904}, although pathogenic variants are only detected in about 50–60% of cases {2017}. However, the detection rate of specific pathogenic variants has increased significantly (with as many as 93% of cases found positive in one study in recent years) because of the development of improved methods of detection {993}. The (mostly truncating) mutations are distributed over the entire *PTCH1* coding region, with no mutation hotspots {3433}. Missense mutations cluster in a highly conserved region (the sterol-sensing domain), and particularly in transmembrane domain 4. *SUFU* pathogenic variants are only detected in approximately 5–6% of tested probands, and they are mostly truncating {2963}.

The rate of new *PTCH1* pathogenic variants has not been precisely determined. It has been estimated that a high proportion (14–81%) of cases are the result of new pathogenic variants {873,1144,2891,3432}. In 4 of 6 cases of NBCCS with a germline *SUFU* pathogenic variant, the mutation was inherited from an unaffected, healthy parent. In the other 2 cases, the mutation was new {2963}.

Pathogenesis

The *PTCH1* gene encodes a 12-transmembrane protein expressed on many progenitor cell types. It functions as a

Box 14.11 Diagnostic criteria for naevoid basal cell carcinoma syndrome

Major criteria:

Lamellar (sheet-like) calcification of the falx

Jaw keratocyst

Palmar or plantar pits (≥ 2)

Multiple basal cell carcinomas (> 5 in a lifetime) or a basal cell carcinoma in a patient aged < 30 years

First-degree relative with naevoid basal cell carcinoma syndrome

Minor criteria:

Childhood medulloblastoma[a]

Lymphomesenteric or pleural cysts

Macrocephaly (occipitofrontal circumference > 97th percentile)

Cleft lip or palate

Vertebral or rib anomalies

Preaxial or postaxial polydactyly

Bifid or fused ribs

Ovarian or cardiac fibromas

Ocular anomalies

Requirements for diagnosis:

Two major diagnostic criteria and one minor diagnostic criterion

OR

One major and three minor diagnostic criteria

OR

Identification of a heterozygous germline *PTCH1* or *SUFU* pathogenic variant on molecular genetic testing and supporting clinical criteria

[a]Medulloblastoma with sonic hedgehog activation, mostly desmoplastic/nodular or extensive nodular types.

---

receptor for members of the hedgehog protein family of secreted signalling molecules (sonic hedgehog, IHH, and DHH) {2014, 3043}. PTCH1 controls another transmembrane protein, SMO {61,3043}. In the absence of its ligand, PTCH1 inhibits the activity of SMO {61,3043}. Hedgehog signalling takes place in the primary cilium {157}. Binding of hedgehog proteins to PTCH1 can relieve its inhibition of SMO, allowing its translocation to the tip of the primary cilium, which results in the activation and translocation of GLI transcription factors into the cell nucleus and the transcription of a set of specific target genes controlling the survival, differentiation, and proliferation of progenitor cells. In vertebrates, this pathway is critically involved in the development of various tissues and organ systems, such as limbs, gonads, bone, and the CNS {1140,1412}. SUFU is located downstream in the hedgehog pathway. SUFU has been found to directly interact with GLI proteins, and it is a negative regulator of hedgehog signalling {3044}. *PTCH1* and *SUFU* are classic tumour suppressor genes; the second allele of the mutant gene is lost in most NBCCS-related tumours. Inactivation of *PTCH1* or *SUFU* leads to the pathological activation of the sonic hedgehog signalling pathway. In cases where *PTCH1* and *SUFU* are wildtype, a much less common source of a Gorlin-like syndrome to consider is that caused by pathogenic germline *GPR161* variants {232}.

Macroscopic appearance
Not relevant

Histopathology
Practically all medulloblastomas associated with NBCCS have the morphological features of desmoplastic tumours, including the desmoplastic/nodular medulloblastoma and the medulloblastoma with extensive nodularity {2855,100,1042,391,2963}.

Cytology
Not relevant

Diagnostic molecular pathology
A comprehensive mutation analysis of the *PTCH1* and *SUFU* genes by DNA sequencing along with a search for deletions/duplications by appropriate methods (e.g. multiplex ligation-dependent probe amplification, targeted array-based analysis) can identify most NBCCS-related germline pathogenic variants {867}. To detect more complex alterations, additional analysis on the transcript level may be necessary in some cases. The detection rate of specific pathogenic variants has increased significantly thanks to improved methods of detection {993}. Still, in 15–27% of index cases, neither *PTCH1* nor *SUFU* pathogenic variants can be identified {876}.

Because germline pathogenic variants are frequent in children younger than 5 years with extensive nodular or desmoplastic/nodular medulloblastomas, human genetic counselling should be offered to the families, and early pathogenic variant analysis of *PTCH1* and *SUFU* should be performed with appropriate methods. The detection of a germline condition is important for planning appropriate treatment that avoids radiation therapy {1042,391,2963,1182,3392}.

Essential and desirable diagnostic criteria
The major and minor diagnostic criteria are listed in Box 14.11.

Staging
Not relevant

Prognosis and prediction
The prognosis of NBCCS-associated medulloblastomas seems to be better than that of sporadic cases, and it has been suggested that therapy protocols be adjusted in patients aged < 5 years with NBCCS, to prevent the formation of radiation-induced secondary tumours {100,3021}. A recent retrospective review of patients with medulloblastoma with a *SUFU* germline pathogenic variant, however, indicated a worse prognosis {1182}. In another retrospective series, no difference in survival was found between patients with medulloblastoma carrying a *PTCH1* pathogenic variant versus those carrying a *SUFU* pathogenic variant {3392}.

Surveillance guidelines are well established and include surveillance during childhood {968}. For carriers of the *SUFU* pathogenic variant, these include a recommendation for repeated brain MRI screening for medulloblastoma development within the first 5 years of life {968}.

Rhabdoid tumour predisposition syndrome

Judkins AR
Biegel JA
Eberhart CG
Huang A
Kool M
Wesseling P

Definition

Rhabdoid tumour predisposition syndrome (RTPS) is a disorder characterized by a markedly increased risk of developing malignant rhabdoid tumours (MRTs), including atypical teratoid/rhabdoid tumours (AT/RTs), due to constitutional loss or inactivation of *SMARCB1* (in the syndrome subtype RTPS1), or rarely *SMARCA4* (in RTPS2).

MIM numbering

609322 Rhabdoid tumour predisposition syndrome 1; RTPS1
613325 Rhabdoid tumour predisposition syndrome 2; RTPS2

ICD-11 coding

None

Related terminology

Not recommended: rhabdoid predisposition syndrome; familial posterior fossa brain tumour syndrome of infancy.

Subtype(s)

Rhabdoid tumour predisposition syndrome 1; rhabdoid tumour predisposition syndrome 2

Localization

Both the nervous system and extraneural organs/tissues can be involved.

Clinical features

The median age at tumour onset is younger in patients with RTPS than in patients with sporadic tumours. To date, no other clinical features have been identified that distinguish RTPS-associated tumours from sporadic rhabdoid tumours.

Nervous system

Individuals with RTPS1 often present with isolated AT/RTs or an AT/RT with a synchronous renal or extrarenal MRT {1832}.

In the past, a variety of other CNS tumours have been reported to be associated with RTPS, including choroid plexus carcinoma {1069}, medulloblastoma, and supratentorial primitive neuroectodermal tumours {2885}. However, because these tumours may be hard to distinguish from AT/RTs, and because some AT/RTs lack well-developed rhabdoid cells, whether such tumours occur in RTPS is controversial {1208,1509,1511,3255}.

Extraneural manifestations

By far the most common extraneural manifestation is MRT of the kidney. Bilateral renal MRTs are almost always associated with a germline *SMARCB1* mutation, but infants with an isolated MRT may carry germline mutations as well. MRTs have been reported to originate in the head and neck region, paraspinal soft tissues, heart, mediastinum, and liver {3424}. Children surviving a primary MRT can develop a second primary in a different location {961}. *SMARCB1* mutations may occasionally underlie the oncogenesis of other neoplasms, such as the proximal type of epithelioid sarcoma {2139}, but to date, these sarcomas have not been described in RTPS. Germline and somatic mutations in *SMARCA4* also give rise to small cell carcinoma of the ovary, hypercalcaemic type – a rare and highly aggressive tumour in adolescents and young adults {967,3203}. The incidence of germline mutations is high in hypercalcaemic type small cell carcinoma of the ovary, and in one family with a *SMARCA4* germline mutation, AT/RT and ovarian cancer were diagnosed in a newborn and his mother, respectively {3461}.

Epidemiology

AT/RTs generally occur in early childhood, but they are occasionally found in adults {2605}. RTPS is found in 25–35% of all patients with AT/RT {273,816}; these patients are more likely to present in their first year of life. Second primary tumours may arise as late as 8 years after the primary diagnosis {265}, suggesting that lifetime surveillance is required.

Etiology

RTPS1 and RTPS2 are caused by germline *SMARCB1* and *SMARCA4* mutations, respectively. De novo germline mutations can occur during oogenesis/spermatogenesis, or postzygotically during the early stages of embryogenesis (mosaic) {816,1254,1453,2885}. Tumours in rare families with multiple affected children and no parental *SMARCB1* mutation are probably due to gonadal mosaicism. In some families, apparently unaffected carriers develop schwannomas in the fourth or fifth decade.

SMARCB1 has also been identified as a predisposing gene in familial schwannomatosis, germline mutations in *SMARCA4* as predisposing in hypercalcaemic type small cell carcinoma of the ovary, and germline mutations in both *SMARCB1* and *SMARCA4* have been identified to contribute to syndromes, such as Coffin–Siris syndrome, associated with dysmorphic features and intellectual disability.

Pathogenesis

The SMARCB1 gene

The *SMARCB1* gene was the first subunit of the SWI/SNF complex found to be mutated in cancer. This gene is located in chromosome region 22q11.23 and contains nine exons spanning 50 kb of genomic DNA {3318}. Alternative splicing of exon 2 results in two transcripts and two proteins with lengths of 385 and 376 amino acid residues, respectively. The SNF5 homology domain in the second half of the protein harbours highly conserved structural motifs through which SMARCB1 interacts with other proteins {3042}. The SMARCB1 protein is a core subunit of mammalian SWI/SNF chromatin remodelling complexes, and it regulates gene expression via ATP-mediated nucleosomal remodelling {3453}. The SMARCB1 protein functions as a tumour suppressor via repression of *CCND1* gene expression, induction of the *CDKN2A* gene, and hypophosphorylation of retinoblastoma protein, resulting in G0/G1 cell-cycle arrest {262,2685}. Loss of SMARCB1 leads to activation of EZH2, a histone lysine methyltransferase and catalytic component of the PRC2 complex, resulting in increased H3 p K28me3 (K27me3) marks associated with repression of polycomb gene targets. The Hippo signalling pathway is involved in the detrimental effects of SMARCB1 deficiency, and its main effector (YAP1) is overexpressed in AT/RTs {1462,3454}.

SMARCB1 is a classic tumour suppressor requiring biallelic loss of function, with the second event typically being loss of heterozygosity / deletion. The types of *SMARCB1* mutations observed in sporadic MRTs are similar to those observed in the germline mutations in RTPS. However, single base deletions in exon 9 occur most often in sporadic AT/RTs {273,816,3092}. The second inactivating event is most frequently a deletion of the wildtype allele, often due to monosomy 22. Schwannomatosis mutations are significantly more likely than sporadic mutations to occur at either end of the gene and to be non-truncating {2969}.

Germline *SMARCB1* mutations may predispose individuals to the development of rhabdoid tumours or schwannomatosis. In rhabdoid tumours, the two copies of the *SMARCB1* gene are inactivated by a truncating mutation and deletion of the wildtype gene, resulting in the total loss of SMARCB1 expression in tumour cells. This is in contrast to the non-truncating *SMARCB1* mutations and mosaic SMARCB1 expression in schwannomas in patients with schwannomatosis {2969}. Because of the high mortality and morbidity associated with rhabdoid tumours, familial inheritance of RTPS is extremely rare {2885,3151}. It has been reported that as many as 35% of patients with a rhabdoid tumour carry a germline *SMARCB1* alteration as the first hit {338,816}. However, a recent study demonstrated a lower incidence, suggesting that prior studies may have been biased by the inclusion of patients with multiple primary tumours, virtually all of whom have a germline *SMARCB1* alteration {2630}. A few families have been reported wherein affected individuals inherited a *SMARCB1* mutation and developed either schwannomatosis or a rhabdoid tumour {476,816,3092}. In these families, both the rhabdoid tumours and schwannomas displayed total SMARCB1 loss {476,3092}. Recently, a patient with co-occurrence of a rhabdoid tumour and schwannomas was reported {1584}.

The SMARCA4 gene

The *SMARCA4* gene, located on chromosome 19p13.2 and encoding a catalytic subunit of the SWI/SNF complex, was the second member of this complex reported in a cancer predisposition syndrome {274,2853}. More recently, other SWI/SNF subunit genes have also been implicated in cancers. Collectively, 20% of all human cancers contain a SWI/SNF mutation, and because most of these tumours are not classic MRTs, the definition of RTPS may need adjustment in the future {1624}.

Box 14.12 Diagnostic criteria for rhabdoid tumour predisposition syndrome

Essential:

Demonstration of a germline *SMARCB1* or *SMARCA4* mutation in a patient with malignant rhabdoid tumour (MRT) or atypical teratoid/rhabdoid tumour (AT/RT)

Desirable:

Multiple MRTs or AT/RTs

Siblings or other relatives with MRT or AT/RT

Macroscopic appearance

The macroscopic appearance of tumours in RTPS is similar to that of their sporadic counterparts.

Histopathology

The histopathology of tumours in RTPS is similar to that of their sporadic counterparts.

Cytology

The cytology of tumours in RTPS is similar to that of their sporadic counterparts.

Diagnostic molecular pathology

Loss of immunohistochemical staining for SMARCB1 (INI1) or SMARCA4 (BRG1) expression allows for the identification of MRTs and AT/RTs associated with RTPS1 and RTPS2, respectively. However, molecular genetic testing of the patient is needed to confirm a suspected germline alteration.

Essential and desirable diagnostic criteria

See Box 14.12.

Staging

Not relevant

Prognosis and prediction

Transcriptome and DNA methylation profiling separate AT/RTs into three molecular groups, which by consensus have been designated "AT/RT-TYR", "AT/RT-SHH", and "AT/RT-MYC" {1320}. Although these subgroups show differences in patient age and in localization, no pattern of germline predisposition by subgroup has been confirmed to date.

Because only a relatively small number of patients with RTPS have been reported in prospective therapeutic studies, the impact of germline alterations on patient outcome remains unclear. Although earlier data suggested a poorer outcome for patients with *SMARCB1* germline alterations, an increasing number of AT/RT survivors with germline *SMARCB1* alterations are being seen, suggesting that other variables such as intensity or type of therapy, as well as specific *SMARCB1* genotypes, may influence outcome.

Carney complex

Legius E
Folpe AL
Jo VY
Reuss DE

Definition
Carney complex (CNC) is an autosomal dominant syndrome characterized by myxomas, endocrinopathy, and pigmented skin lesions; the main nervous system manifestation is malignant melanotic nerve sheath tumour. In > 70% of patients a heterozygous inactivating pathogenic variant is detected in the *PRKAR1A* gene coding for the type 1α regulatory (R1α) subunit of PKA.

MIM numbering
160980 Carney complex, type 1; CNC1
605244 Carney complex, type 2; CNC2

ICD-11 coding
2F7A.0 Multiple polyglandular tumours

Related terminology
Not recommended: LAMB syndrome (lentigines, atrial myxoma, mucocutaneous myoma, blue naevus); NAME syndrome (naevi, atrial myxomas, myxoid neurofibromas, and ephelides); myxoma, spotty pigmentation, and endocrine overactivity.

Subtype(s)
Isolated primary pigmented nodular adrenocortical disease caused by a specific splice mutation; severe Carney complex caused by a chromosomal microdeletion

Localization
Manifestations of CNC arise in the skin, endocrine organs (adrenal cortex, thyroid, pituitary, testis, ovaries), peripheral and central nervous systems, heart, bone, breast, and (to a lesser extent) pancreas.

Clinical features
CNC was reported for the first time in 1985 as a complex of myxomas, spotty pigmentation, and endocrine overactivity {471}. Multiple lentigines might be present at birth {3049} but the typical appearance usually develops around puberty. Lentigines are predominantly localized on the lips, conjunctiva, eyelids, ears, and external genitalia. Other pigmentation abnormalities such as hypopigmented macules, blue naevi, epithelioid blue naevi, and café-au-lait spots develop in early childhood. Skin and mucosal myxomas are seen in 10–30% of patients {2034,256,859}. Myxomas of the breast are often bilateral and are seen in as many as 25% of women with CNC {256,3049,859}. Cardiac myxomas can occur in childhood. The prevalence of cardiac myxomas in different cohorts ranges from 22% to 53% {3049,256,859}. Recurrence after surgery was observed in 62% in one study {859}. Patients with cardiac myxomas present with symptoms of systemic embolism, heart failure, or intracardiac obstruction of blood flow. Myxomas can affect any chamber of the heart, and continued surveillance is advocated. Osteochondromyxoma is a

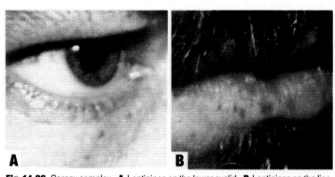

Fig. 14.26 Carney complex. **A** Lentigines on the lower eyelid. **B** Lentigines on the lips.

rare form of myxoma found in bone. A recent study showed vertebral nodular lesions on MRI in 31.6% of patients {859}.

Malignant melanotic nerve sheath tumour is a rare but potentially lethal complication occurring in 8–10% of adults {3049, 256,859}. Gastrointestinal tract and the paraspinal sympathetic chain are most frequently involved.

Endocrine neoplasms are characteristic for CNC. The most frequent endocrine tumour is primary pigmented nodular adrenocortical disease (PPNAD), which frequently results in an ACTH-independent hypercortisolism (Cushing syndrome). PPNAD is reported in 26–58% of patients in cohorts with CNC {256,3049, 859}. A recent study diagnosed PPNAD in 57% of patients, and in an additional 11.4% there was possible PPNAD {859}. Another study of 353 individuals found PPNAD in 58% of patients with a proven *PRKAR1A* pathogenic variant. The frequency was higher in female patients (71%; median age at onset: 30 years) than in male patients (29%; median age at onset: 46 years) {256}. Multiple thyroid nodules were seen in 5–28% of patients {256,3049, 859}. Sometimes a thyroid papillary or follicular carcinoma is present. A somatotroph pituitary adenoma / pituitary neuroendocrine tumour (PitNET) is diagnosed in 10–18% of adults {256, 3049,859}. Large cell calcifying Sertoli cell tumours are reported in 33–49% of male patients; they can be hormone-producing and are mostly benign {256,3049,859}. They are more frequent in male patients with a proven *PRKAR1A* pathogenic variant {256} than in those with CNC without a pathogenic variant.

Conditions associated with Carney complex are listed in Box 14.13.

Epidemiology
CNC is a rare autosomal dominant disease known to affect > 700 individuals worldwide {3050}.

Etiology
CNC is caused by heterozygous inactivating pathogenic variants in the *PRKAR1A* gene in an estimated 70% of patients fulfilling diagnostic criteria {3049,1639,256,2793}. The penetrance of CNC caused by *PRKAR1A* pathogenic variants is estimated to be virtually 100% {3049}.

Pathogenesis

PRKAR1A codes for the R1α subunit of PKA. PKA is a hetero-tetramer with two regulatory and two catalytic subunits. There are four isoforms of the regulatory subunits (R1α, R1β, R2α, R2β) and of the catalytic subunits (Cα, Cβ, Cγ, PRKX) {3156}. G-protein coupled receptors bound to a ligand will activate adenylyl cyclase and the synthesis of cAMP, which binds to the regulatory subunits of PKA. This allows the catalytic subunits to dissociate and phosphorylate downstream targets. Inactivating pathogenic variants of *PRKAR1A* will result in an overactivation of the cAMP/PKA pathway. This pathway is essential in many endocrine cell types. Inactivation of the wildtype allele in CNC-associated tumours has been demonstrated, reflecting the tumour-suppressor function of the R1α protein {1639}. Some mutations are not associated with nonsense-mediated RNA decay, and it has been suggested that a specific splice variant leading to skipping of exon 6 might have a dominant negative effect and that this is sufficient for tumorigenesis in CNC-affected tissues {1171}, but the evidence for this is incomplete.

Macroscopic appearance

The macroscopic appearance of CNC-associated tumours is similar to that of their sporadic counterparts.

Histopathology

The histopathology of CNC-associated tumours is similar to that of their sporadic counterparts.

Cytology

The cytology of CNC-associated tumours is similar to that of their sporadic counterparts.

Diagnostic molecular pathology

A mutation in the *PRKAR1A* gene is identified in 70% of patients fulfilling diagnostic criteria for CNC {3049,1639,256,2793, 3321}. Many types of mutations have been found, such as missense, nonsense, splice, indels, and small and large deletions in the *PRKAR1A* gene {1639,256,2793}. Genetic heterogeneity is likely. Initial linkage studies in 1996 suggested a locus on chromosome 2 but a gene has never been identified in this region {3048}. There are a number of genotype–phenotype correlations reported. Lentigines, cardiac myxomas, and thyroid tumours are more frequent in patients with the hotspot pathogenic variant *PRKAR1A* c.491_492del, and isolated PPNAD is frequently associated with splice variant *PRKAR1A* c.709-7_709-2del {256}. CNC patients without a detectable *PRKAR1A* pathogenic variant usually represent sporadic cases that occur later in life with a milder phenotype {256}. Large gene deletions might be associated with developmental delay and other features not typically seen in CNC {2793}.

Certain pathogenic variants affecting the 3′ end of the gene result in the synthesis of a mutant R1α protein unable to bind cAMP. The resulting PKA tetramer cannot be activated by cAMP and results in impaired signalling through the cAMP/PKA pathway {1905}. These variants do not cause CNC or tumours but an autosomal dominant form of acrodysostosis with hormone resistance.

Essential and desirable diagnostic criteria

See Box 14.14.

Staging

Not relevant

Prognosis and prediction

CNC is an autosomal dominant disorder; affected parents harbour a 50% risk of disease transmission with each pregnancy. Genetic counselling is recommended, and it includes the possibility of prenatal and/or preimplantation genetic testing.

The average life expectancy is 50 years because of excess mortality related to cardiac myxoma, malignant melanotic nerve sheath tumour, postoperative complications, and a variety of carcinomas {3049,3050}.

Box 14.13 Conditions associated with Carney complex {3049}

Intense freckling

Blue naevus

Café-au-lait spots

Elevated IGF1 levels, abnormal oral glucose tolerance test, or paradoxical growth hormone responses to TRH testing in the absence of clinical acromegaly

Cardiomyopathy

Pilonidal sinus

Cushing syndrome

Acromegaly

Sudden death in extended family

Multiple skin tags

Lipomas

Colonic polyps

Hyperprolactinaemia

Thyroid nodule

Family history of carcinoma (especially of the thyroid, colon, pancreas, or ovary)

Box 14.14 Diagnostic criteria for Carney complex; diagnosis of Carney complex requires two major criteria or one major criterion plus one supplemental criterion {3049}

Major diagnostic criteria:

Spotty skin pigmentation with typical distribution (lips, conjunctiva, inner or outer canthi, vaginal or penile mucosa)

Cardiac myxoma[a]

Myxoma (cutaneous and mucosal)[a]

Breast myxomatosis[a] or fat-suppressed MRI findings suggestive of this diagnosis

Primary pigmented nodular adrenocortical disease[a] or paradoxical positive response of urinary glucocorticoid excretion to dexamethasone administration during the Liddle test

Acromegaly due to growth hormone (GH)-producing pituitary adenoma / pituitary neuroendocrine tumour (PitNET)[a]

Large cell calcifying Sertoli cell tumour[a] or characteristic calcification on testicular ultrasound

Thyroid follicular adenoma or carcinoma[a] or multiple, hypoechoic nodules on thyroid ultrasound in a young patient

Malignant melanotic nerve sheath tumour[a]

Blue naevus, epithelioid blue naevus (multiple)[a]

Breast ductal adenoma (multiple)[a]

Osteochondromyxoma[a]

Supplemental criteria:

Affected first-degree relative

Inactivating mutation of the *PRKAR1A* gene

[a]These tumours all require histological confirmation.

DICER1 syndrome

Hill DA
Alexandrescu S
Kölsche C
Korshunov A
Solomon DA

Definition

DICER1 syndrome is an autosomal dominant tumour predisposition syndrome caused by heterozygous germline pathogenic sequence variants in the DICER1 gene, which encodes a micro-RNA-processing enzyme. It is characterized by increased incidence of benign and malignant neoplasms involving multiple organ systems. The CNS tumour manifestations associated with DICER1 syndrome are metastatic pleuropulmonary blastoma; pineoblastoma; embryonal tumour with multilayered rosettes; pituitary blastoma; and primary intracranial sarcoma, DICER1-mutant.

MIM numbering

606241 DICER 1, ribonuclease III; DICER1

ICD-11 coding

None

Related terminology

Acceptable: pleuropulmonary blastoma familial tumour and dysplasia syndrome.

Subtype(s)

None

Localization

The most commonly involved organs are the lungs, kidneys, thyroid, ovaries, uterine cervix, eyes, and brain.

Clinical features

The clinical features are listed in Table 14.06.

CNS manifestations

The most common CNS manifestation of DICER1 syndrome is metastasis of pleuropulmonary blastoma to the cerebrum {2571}. The CNS is the most frequent site of distant pleuropulmonary blastoma metastasis, with CNS metastasis occurring in 11% of patients with advanced pleuropulmonary blastoma. The International Pleuropulmonary Blastoma/DICER1 Registry recommends brain MRI surveillance every 3 months until 36 months after a diagnosis of type II or type III pleuropulmonary blastoma {3280,2862}. The primary CNS tumour manifestations of DICER1 syndrome are pineoblastoma, pituitary blastoma, embryonal tumour with multilayered rosettes, and DICER1-mutant primary intracranial sarcoma. Pituitary blastoma virtually always occurs in the setting of DICER1 syndrome, arises in young children typically aged < 2 years, and often occurs with Cushing syndrome and diabetes insipidus {2776,707}. The clinical features of pineoblastoma, embryonal tumour with multilayered rosettes, and DICER1-mutant primary intracranial sarcoma that are associated with germline DICER1 mutations

are indistinguishable from those encountered in their sporadic counterparts {2769,706,1677,3259,1836,705,1797,1913,1865}.

Extracranial manifestations

These include pleuropulmonary blastoma, pulmonary cysts, thyroid gland neoplasia, ovarian sex-cord stromal tumours, cystic nephroma, renal anaplastic sarcoma, ciliary medulloepithelioma, nasal chondromesenchymal hamartoma, and embryonal rhabdomyosarcoma of the uterine cervix {2572,1309,175,2952, 3035,969,3483,3280}.

Epidemiology

Pathogenic germline variants in DICER1 are estimated to occur in about 10 in 100 000 individuals {1621}. DICER1 syndrome has variable penetrance. Benign thyroid nodules and lung cysts are the most common phenotypic manifestations, occurring in a large subset of individuals with pathogenic germline variants {1601}. The exact incidence of specific neoplasms in individuals carrying germline DICER1 mutations remains uncertain. Pituitary blastoma is pathognomonic of DICER1 syndrome, with all reported cases to date arising in the setting of this syndrome.

Etiology

DICER1 syndrome is caused by heterozygous germline loss-of-function variants in the DICER1 gene on chromosome 14q32.13 {1309}. Mutations are most often transmitted in a familial manner, although approximately 13% of affected individuals with pleuropulmonary blastoma harbour de novo mutations {372}. Additionally, a subset of affected individuals acquire DICER1 mutations during postzygotic development and have a mosaic phenotype. Individuals with somatic mosaicism for a DICER1 RNase IIIb hotspot mutation show an increased tumour incidence and are younger at presentation than individuals with germline loss-of-function truncating variants {372}.

Pathogenesis

In addition to the germline DICER1 loss-of-function pathogenic variant, DICER1 syndrome–related tumours typically harbour an additional somatically acquired missense mutation in exon 24 or 25 encoding the RNase IIIb cleavage domain, involving one of the following codons: p.E1705, p.D1709, p.G1809, p.D1810, or p.E1813. This leads to a unique combination of two hits, but in contrast to the classic Knudson hypothesis, the second hit does not fully abrogate the function of the DICER1 gene {969}. Some sporadic tumour counterparts harbour somatic biallelic DICER1 alterations. These patients are not considered syndromic, although the possibility of unrecognized mosaicism should be entertained {588,372}. However, the pathogenesis of DICER1 syndrome–associated pineoblastoma diverges from the mechanism described above, with the somatic event being loss of heterozygosity of the DICER1 allele {969,724}.

Table 14.06 Key clinical phenotypes associated with germline *DICER1* pathogenic variants

Phenotype and relative frequency	Approximate ages of clinical diagnosis, range (peak)	Malignant (M) or benign (B)	Deaths associated with *DICER1*-mutated cases?
Most frequent phenotypes			
Pleuropulmonary blastoma (PPB)			
Type I (cystic) PPB	0–24 months (8 months)	M	Yes, if it progresses to type II or III
Type II (cystic/solid) PPB	12–60 months (31 months)	M	Yes, ~40%
Type III (solid) PPB	18–72 months (44 months)	M	Yes, ~60%
Type Ir (cystic) PPB	Any age	B or M	None observed
Multinodular goitre[a]	5–40 years (10–20 years)	B	No
Cystic nephroma	0–48 months (undetermined)	B	No (see anaplastic sarcoma of the kidney below)
Sertoli–Leydig cell tumour of the ovary	2–45 years (10–25 years)	M	Yes, < 5%
Moderate-frequency phenotypes			
Embryonal rhabdomyosarcoma of the cervix	4–45 years (10–20 years)	M	None observed
Rare phenotypes			
Differentiated thyroid carcinoma[b]	5–40 years (10–20 years)	M	None observed
Wilms tumour[b]	3–13 years (undetermined)	M	None observed
Juvenile hamartomatous intestinal polyps[b]	0–4 years (undetermined)	B	No
Ciliary body medulloepithelioma	3–10 years (undetermined)	B or M	None observed
Nasal chondromesenchymal hamartoma	6–18 years (undetermined)	B	No
Pituitary blastoma	0–24 months (undetermined)	Undetermined	Yes, ~50%
Pineoblastoma	2–25 years (undetermined)	M	Yes
Very rare phenotypes			
Anaplastic sarcoma of the kidney	Estimated 2–20 years	M	Yes
Embryonal tumour with multilayered rosettes[b]	Undetermined	M	Unknown
Primary intracranial sarcoma, *DICER1*-mutant	Median 6 years	M	Unknown
Embryonal rhabdomyosarcoma of the bladder	Estimated < 5 years	M	None observed
Embryonal rhabdomyosarcoma of the ovary	Undetermined	M	None observed
Neuroblastoma[b]	Estimated < 5 years	M	Yes
Congenital phthisis bulbi[b]	Birth	B	No
Juvenile granulosa cell tumour[b]	Undetermined	M	None observed
Gynandroblastoma	Undetermined	M	None observed

[a]Multinodular goitre occurring in patients aged < 18 years may warrant *DICER1* testing, even if it occurs in the absence of other syndromic features in the patient or their family.
[b]These phenotypes may not be sufficiently associated with *DICER1* mutations to warrant testing in the absence of other personal or family history suggestive of *DICER1* syndrome.

In general, the *DICER1* alterations in benign and malignant syndrome-associated tumours are identical, and it is hypothesized that the variable malignant potential is due to the presence of additional oncogenic alterations, such as *TP53* and *NRAS* RAF mutations {2580,1913,1865}. The mutations in *DICER1* are thought to promote tumorigenesis via the disruption of microRNA regulation of gene expression, permitting aberrant oncofetal transcriptional programmes to persist beyond fetal development {969}.

Macroscopic appearance

The macroscopic appearance of tumours in *DICER1* syndrome is similar to that of their sporadic counterparts.

Histopathology

The histopathology of tumours in *DICER1* syndrome is similar to that of their sporadic counterparts.

Cytology

The cytology of tumours in *DICER1* syndrome is similar to that of their sporadic counterparts.

Diagnostic molecular pathology

Most germline pathogenic variants are nonsense mutations, small insertion/deletions, or splice-site substitutions resulting in truncation of the protein. Larger deletions and pathogenic missense variants make up a small percentage of causative variants.

There are no well-established clinical algorithms for the diagnosis of *DICER1* syndrome beyond germline testing. The identification of a heterozygous germline *DICER1* pathogenic variant that is known or suspected to cause loss of function establishes the diagnosis. The hallmark manifestation of *DICER1* syndrome is pleuropulmonary blastoma, although any of the other manifestations can appear first. In the presence of pleuropulmonary blastoma or any other condition that has been described in the setting of *DICER1* syndrome, there should be a low threshold for germline testing.

Essential and desirable diagnostic criteria

See Box 14.15.

Staging

Not relevant

Box 14.15 Diagnostic criteria for *DICER1* syndrome

Essential:

Pathogenic germline variant in the *DICER1* gene

Desirable:

Genomic tumour testing demonstrating loss of heterozygosity or a somatic mutation involving the remaining *DICER1* allele, often a hotspot missense mutation in the RNase IIIb domain

Prognosis and prediction

No difference in clinical outcomes has been observed for *DICER1* syndrome–associated versus sporadic pineoblastoma, embryonal tumour with multilayered rosettes, or *DICER1*-mutant primary intracranial sarcoma.

Familial paraganglioma syndromes

Asa SL
Brandner S
Lloyd RV

Definition
Familial paraganglioma syndromes are a group of inherited cancer syndromes characterized by the presence of paragangliomas (including phaeochromocytoma).

MIM numbering
See Table 14.07 (p. 468).

ICD-11 coding
None

Related terminology
Acceptable: familial paraganglioma-phaeochromocytoma syndromes; hereditary paraganglioma-phaeochromocytoma syndromes; hereditary phaeochromocytoma-paraganglioma.

Subtype(s)
Familial paraganglioma syndromes are shown in Table 14.07 (p. 468).

Localization
Sympathetic-derived paragangliomas are usually intra-adrenal (phaeochromocytoma) or they may be retroperitoneal, occurring alongside the aorta and the inferior mesenteric artery, and above the aortic bifurcation. Parasympathetic-derived paragangliomas commonly arise in the head-and-neck region, including the carotid body and cervical branches of the glossopharyngeal and vagus nerves {2923}. Familial paragangliomas may be multifocal; they occur anywhere in the body with the exception of bone, brain, and lymph nodes {144}. Spinal paragangliomas are usually non-familial, but one study identified an *SDHD* germline mutation in one patient with recurrent spinal paraganglioma and cerebellar metastasis {2033}.

Clinical features
Clinical manifestations may be due to catecholamine excess and/or mass effects.

Symptoms of adrenaline/noradrenaline excess include sweating, palpitation, and anxiety; signs include hypertension and tachycardia. These are generally associated with sympathetic paragangliomas. Some parasympathetic paragangliomas may secrete dopamine with minimal clinical manifestations, whereas others, mainly those of the head and neck and the cauda equina, are non-secretory. There is strong genotype–phenotype correlation in catecholamine profile. Cluster 1 tumours are those with pseudohypoxic pathogenesis, and they tend to be clinically silent and non-secretory or dopamine-secreting; cluster 2 comprises tumours with kinase signalling and rare phaeochromocytomas with WNT-pathway activation that are usually functional.

Cluster 1 tumours express SSTRs, and they are well visualized with 68Ga-DOTATATE PET-CT or the less sensitive

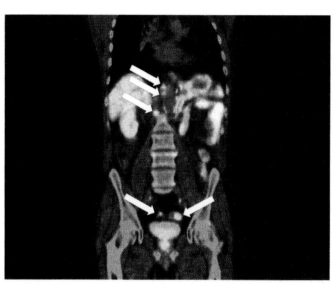

Fig. 14.27 Paragangliomas in familial paraganglioma syndrome. Multiple para-aortic and pelvic paragangliomas are identified with 68Ga-DOTATATE PET-CT in a patient with a pathogenic germline *SDHB* mutation.

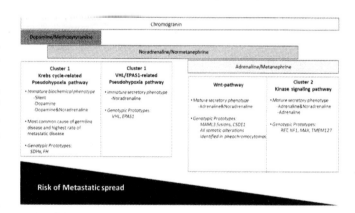

Fig. 14.28 Familial paraganglioma syndromes. Biochemical and genetic clusters of paragangliomas {144}.

indium-labelled somatostatin PET. Cluster 2 tumours can be imaged with 18F-DOPA PET-CT or iobenguane (metaiodobenzylguanidine; 123I-MIBG) PET.

Epidemiology
Overall, 30–40% of paragangliomas in adults are hereditary; cascade testing of index patients facilitates risk reduction strategies across entire kindreds {309,2024}. Younger age at presentation, multiple tumours, and extra-adrenal tumours are significantly associated with the presence of a germline mutation {2234}. In contrast, cauda equina paragangliomas are sporadic and exceptionally rare in the familial setting.

Table 14.07 Familial paraganglioma syndromes

Gene	Chromosomal location	Syndrome	Commonest locations	Associated lesions	MIM numbers
RET	10q11.2	MEN2	Adrenal	Medullary thyroid carcinoma Parathyroid proliferations Mucocutaneous ganglioneuromas	171400, 162300, 164761
VHL	3p25.3	VHL	Adrenal, EA-PGL	Clear cell renal cell carcinoma Haemangioblastomas Neuroendocrine tumours Pancreatic serous cystadenomas	193300, 608537
NF1	17q11.2	NF1	Adrenal, EA-PGL	Neurofibroma and MPNST Ocular manifestations Duodenal neuroendocrine tumour	162200
SDHA	5p15.33	PGL5	EA-PGL, adrenal	Renal cell carcinoma Gastrointestinal stromal tumour Pituitary tumour	614165, 600857
SDHB	1p36.13	PGL4	EA-PGL, A&T, H&N	Renal cell carcinoma Gastrointestinal stromal tumour Pituitary tumour	606864[a], 115310, 185470
SDHC	1q23.3	PGL3	EA-PGL, H&N	Renal cell carcinoma Gastrointestinal stromal tumour	605373, 602413
SDHD	11q23	PGL1	EA-PGL, adrenal	Renal cell carcinoma Gastrointestinal stromal tumour Pituitary tumour	168000, 602690
SDHAF2	11q12.2	PGL2	EA-PGL, H&N	Insufficient data	601650, 613019
TMEM127	2q11.2	Unknown	Adrenal, EA-PGL	Renal cell carcinoma	171300, 613403
MAX	14q23.3	Unknown	Adrenal, EA-PGL	Insufficient data	171300, 154950
FH	1q43	HLRCC	Adrenal, EA-PGL	Cutaneous and uterine leiomyomas Renal cell carcinoma	150800
EPAS1	2p21	PZS	Adrenal, EA-PGL, A&T	Duodenal neuroendocrine tumour Polycythaemia Ocular manifestations	611783
EGLN1	1q42.2	Unknown	Adrenal, EA-PGL, A&T	Polycythaemia	609070, 609820
EGLN2	19q13.2	Unknown	Adrenal, EA-PGL, A&T	Polycythaemia	606424
MDH2	7q11.23	Unknown	EA-PGL, A&T	Insufficient data	617339
KIF1B	1p36.22	Unknown	Insufficient data	Ganglioneuroma/neuroblastoma Leiomyosarcoma Lung adenocarcinoma	605995
MEN1	11q13	Unknown	Adrenal, EA-PGL, H&N	Parathyroid proliferations Pituitary tumour Neuroendocrine tumours	131100, 613733

A&T, abdomen and thorax; EA-PGL, extra-adrenal paraganglioma; H&N, head and neck; HLRCC, hereditary leiomyomatosis and renal cell carcinoma; MEN2, multiple endocrine neoplasia type 2; MIM number, Mendelian Inheritance in Man number; MPNST, malignant peripheral nerve sheath tumour; NF1, neurofibromatosis type 1; PGL1–5, hereditary paragangliomas 1–5; PZS, Pacak–Zhuang syndrome; VHL, von Hippel–Lindau syndrome.
[a]Paraganglioma and gastric stromal sarcoma, also known as Carney–Stratakis syndrome.

Etiology

Familial paragangliomas are caused by germline pathogenic variants (Table 14.07) that predispose to tumour development {939,3241}.

Pathogenesis

See Table 14.07.

Macroscopic appearance

Familial paragangliomas are often multifocal. Adrenal disease in patients with multiple endocrine neoplasia type 2 is often bilateral and grossly multinodular.

Histopathology

Some SDH-associated tumours have a distinct pseudorosette pattern {1632}. SDH-related paragangliomas from the head and neck usually have small cells with clear cytoplasm. Other unique features include a prominent nested architecture with well-formed, almost circular nests and monotonous cells with

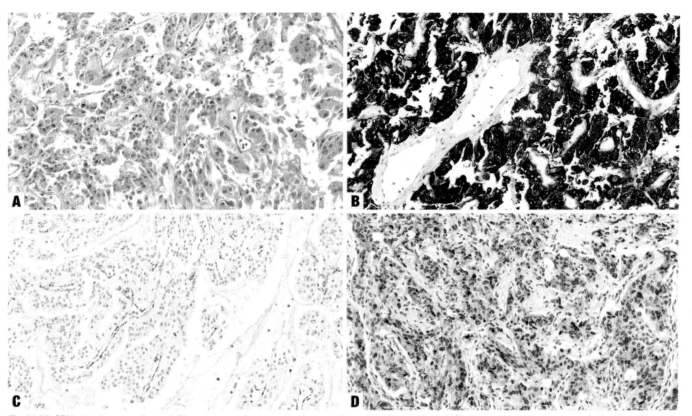

Fig. 14.29 SDH-related paraganglioma. **A** These tumours often have abundant granular eosinophilic cytoplasm. **B** They express cytoplasmic tyrosine hydroxylase. **C** Lack of cytoplasmic SDHB with intact stromal positivity indicates SDH-related disease. **D** Tumours associated with a pseudohypoxia pathway alteration also express inhibin.

vacuolated eosinophilic cytoplasm {3242}. Unlike sporadic paragangliomas, they are rarely associated with a spindled morphology or densely granular cytoplasm {3242}. VHL-associated tumours may have clear cells with vacuolated cytoplasm and stromal oedema {2617,1671}.

Immunohistochemistry localizes neuroendocrine markers such as nuclear INSM1 {2723} and cytoplasmic synaptophysin and chromogranin. S100 highlights sustentacular cells. Paragangliomas express nuclear GATA3 {2978} and cytoplasmic tyrosine hydroxylase {144}. With the exception of cauda equina tumours, most paragangliomas are immunonegative for cytokeratins {739}. Loss of SDHB immunoreactivity in tumour cells with granular cytoplasmic staining of stromal cells supports the diagnosis of SDH-associated disease {1107,3283}; in tumours that lack SDHB immunoreactivity, loss of SDHA staining identifies patients with *SDHA* mutations {1712}. VHL-associated tumours have membranous CAIX positivity {2515} and express inhibin. *FH* mutations can also be screened by immunohistochemistry {487}.

Cytology
The cytological diagnosis of paragangliomas is challenging, but immunohistochemistry may assist in the diagnosis and in determination of familial disease {941}.

Diagnostic molecular pathology
Not relevant

Essential and desirable diagnostic criteria
See Box 14.16.

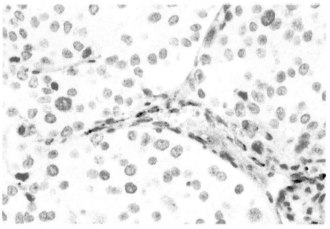

Fig. 14.30 SDH disease. Succinate dehydrogenase (SDH) staining in SDH disease. Familial head and neck paraganglioma immunostained for SDHB showing an SDH-deficient paraganglioma with granular cytoplasmic staining of endothelial cells and completely negative tumour cells.

Box 14.16 Diagnostic criteria for familial paraganglioma syndromes

Essential:

Manifestation in multiple locations

AND

Germline mutation in a susceptibility gene

Desirable:

Loss of SDHB immunoreactivity has a high predictive value for *SDHB, SDHC,* or *SDHD* mutations

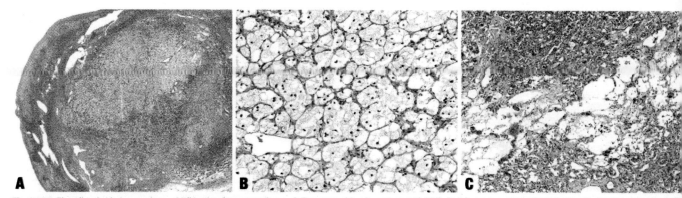

Fig. 14.31 Von Hippel–Lindau syndrome (VHL)-related paraganglioma. **A** Tumours arising in patients with VHL (in this case, a phaeochromocytoma) often have tumour cells with abundant clear cytoplasm (top) and stromal oedema (bottom). They express CAIX and have intact SDHB staining but also express inhibin (not shown). **B** Higher power of area with clear cytoplasm. **C** Higher power of area with stromal oedema.

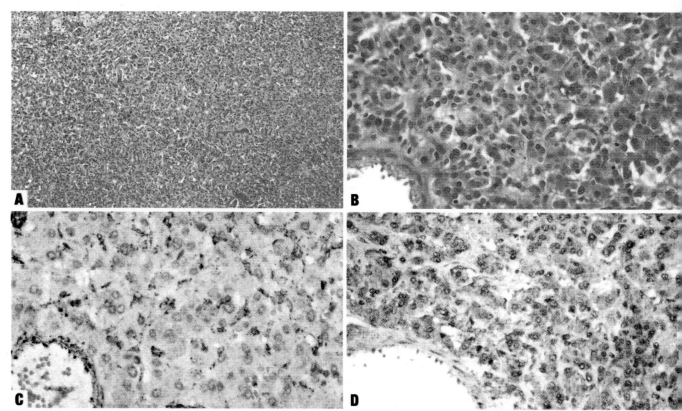

Fig. 14.32 Fumarate hydratase–deficient phaeochromocytoma arising in a patient with confirmed germline *FH* mutation. Although there are no diagnostic morphological features of fumarate hydratase deficiency on H&E (**A,B**), staining for fumarate hydratase (**C**) shows loss of reactivity in the cytoplasm with staining in stromal elements, and there is intact staining for 2-succinocysteine (**D**).

Staging

Staging is available using the Union for International Cancer Control (UICC) eighth edition staging system.

Prognosis and prediction

Most paragangliomas can be surgically resected; however, large tumours and some extra-adrenal tumour locations may preclude complete excision. Familial lesions are often multifocal; the presentations may be asynchronous, mimicking metastasis. Catecholamine profile and *SDHB* mutation increase risk of metastasis. Aggressiveness in sporadic phaeochromocytoma is associated with *MAML3* fusions and with *ATRX* and *CSDE1* mutations but these are not reported in familial tumours. Five-year overall survival rates in patients with metastatic paraganglioma range from 50% to 70% {162, 148,940,1223}.

Melanoma-astrocytoma syndrome

Solomon DA
Reuss DE

Definition

Melanoma-astrocytoma syndrome is an autosomal dominant tumour predisposition syndrome caused by germline pathogenic variants of the *CDKN2A* tumour suppressor gene encoding the p16INK4a and p14ARF cell-cycle regulators. The syndrome is characterized by an increased risk of multiple neoplasms including cutaneous melanoma, astrocytomas, nerve sheath tumours, pancreatic cancer, and squamous cell carcinoma of the oropharynx.

MIM numbering

155755 Melanoma-astrocytoma syndrome

ICD-11 coding

None

Related terminology

Acceptable (depending on the tumour spectrum present in the kindred): melanoma and neural system tumour syndrome; melanoma–pancreatic cancer syndrome; familial atypical mole–melanoma (FAMM) syndrome; susceptibility to cutaneous melanoma type 2 (CM2).

Subtype(s)

None

Localization

The dysplastic naevi and melanomas arising in the setting of melanoma-astrocytoma syndrome are usually cutaneous and not mucosal, acral, or uveal. The astrocytomas are usually located in the cerebral hemispheres or cerebellum.

Clinical features

Melanoma-astrocytoma syndrome is characterized by multiple cutaneous dysplastic naevi and an increased risk of melanoma, astrocytomas, nerve sheath tumours, pancreatic cancer, and squamous cell carcinoma of the oropharynx {1571,166,174, 3553,2874,430,3291,987,2809,507}. Nerve sheath tumours including both paraspinal schwannoma-like neoplasms involving spinal nerve roots and cutaneous neurofibroma-like neoplasms have been reported {174,3291,2809,507}. It is currently unknown why some kindreds exclusively develop dysplastic naevi and melanoma while others also develop astrocytomas, pancreatic cancer, and other neoplasms.

Epidemiology

Melanoma-astrocytoma syndrome is rare, with < 100 genetically confirmed kindreds reported to date. The exact incidence is unknown, but this syndrome probably accounts for < 0.1% of astrocytomas and nerve sheath tumours.

Etiology

Melanoma-astrocytoma syndrome is an autosomal dominant tumour predisposition syndrome caused by heterozygous germline mutation or deletion of the *CDKN2A* tumour suppressor gene on chromosome 9p21.3 {1532,173}.

Pathogenesis

Melanoma-astrocytoma syndrome is caused by genetic disruption of the *CDKN2A* tumour suppressor gene, which encodes the p16INK4a and p14ARF cell-cycle regulators {1532,173}. The p16INK4a protein binds and inhibits cyclin-dependent kinases 4 and 6 to maintain cells in the resting G1 phase of the cell cycle. The structurally unrelated p14ARF protein is produced from an alternative reading frame and acts by antagonizing the p53 regulatory protein MDM2. The neoplasms that arise in the setting of melanoma-astrocytoma syndrome are thought to be due to abnormal proliferation of melanocytes, astrocytes, and other cells after somatic inactivation of the remaining *CDKN2A* allele, typically via loss of heterozygosity {2809,507}.

Macroscopic appearance

The macroscopic appearance of tumours in melanoma-astrocytoma syndrome is as described for the individual tumour types.

Histopathology

The astrocytomas arising in the setting of melanoma-astrocytoma syndrome include both pleomorphic xanthoastrocytoma and diffuse astrocytic gliomas ranging from low-grade (diffuse astrocytoma) to high-grade (glioblastoma) {507}. No histopathological features distinguishing these syndrome-associated astrocytomas from their sporadic counterparts have been identified to date. The nerve sheath tumours have been reported to histologically resemble either schwannoma or neurofibroma {3291,2809}.

Cytology

Not relevant

Diagnostic molecular pathology

Sequencing analysis of the *CDKN2A* gene in a constitutional DNA sample assessing for pathogenic mutations or deletions is required for the diagnosis of melanoma-astrocytoma syndrome. Genomic analysis of astrocytomas and other tumours arising in the setting of melanoma-astrocytoma syndrome demonstrates somatic inactivation of the remaining *CDKN2A* allele via loss of heterozygosity or an acquired second mutation/deletion {507}. One study of a syndromic pleomorphic xanthoastrocytoma revealed *CDKN2A* homozygous deletion and *BRAF* p.V600E mutation, and a separate diffuse astrocytoma in this patient was IDH- and histone H3-wildtype with *CDKN2A* homozygous deletion and *PTPN11*, *NF1*, and *ATRX* mutations {507}. The molecular pathogenesis of nerve sheath tumours arising in the setting of melanoma-astrocytoma syndrome has not been investigated to date, but *CDKN2A* deletion is not characteristic of either sporadic schwannomas or typical neurofibromas, suggesting that their pathogenesis is distinct from that of their sporadic counterparts. Nevertheless, it is seen in atypical neurofibroma / atypical neurofibromatous neoplasm of uncertain biological potential and in malignant peripheral nerve sheath tumour {231,2449}.

Essential and desirable diagnostic criteria
See Box 14.17.

Staging
Not relevant

Prognosis and prediction
Clinical outcomes for the astrocytomas and nerve sheath tumours arising in the setting of melanoma-astrocytoma syndrome relative to their sporadic counterparts have not been well described to date. Surveillance protocols have not yet been established but should include regular dermatological examinations and perhaps also brain imaging.

Familial retinoblastoma

Eagle RC Jr
Jones DTW

Definition

Retinoblastoma is a malignant paediatric retinal neoplasm. Familial cases are caused by germline *RB1* pathogenic variants.

ICD-O coding

9510/3 Retinoblastoma

MIM numbering

180200 Retinoblastoma; RB1

ICD-11 coding

2D02.2 Retinoblastoma

Related terminology

Acceptable: trilateral retinoblastoma.
Not recommended: glioma retinae.

Subtype(s)

None

Localization

Retinoblastoma is an intraocular tumour of the retina. In familial retinoblastoma syndrome, synchronous or metachronous malignant intracranial tumours (pineal or suprasellar) may develop.

Clinical features

Leukocoria (a white pupillary reflex) and strabismus caused by visual loss are characteristic presenting manifestations. Eventually, tumour progression leads to extraocular extension and involvement of adnexal structures. About 60% of patients who have germline *RB1* pathogenic variants develop bilateral tumours. Familial tumours tend to arise at an earlier age (~12 months) than do sporadic counterparts (~24 months). Germline carriers are at significant risk for secondary non-ocular neoplasms including sarcomas and pineoblastoma; the combination of intraocular retinoblastoma and a histologically similar brain tumour, most commonly in the pineal gland, is called trilateral retinoblastoma {2011,3616,1646,703}. For intracranial tumours, a maximal safe surgical resection is encouraged at diagnosis, followed by craniospinal irradiation and high-dose chemotherapy {4}.

Epidemiology

Retinoblastoma is the most common primary intraocular tumour in infants and the most common primary intraocular tumour worldwide {1645}. It has a reported incidence of 5.6–6.3 cases per 100 000 live births {422,3329,378,1645}. There is no racial or sex predilection. The large majority (80%) of cases are diagnosed before 3 years of age, and the mean age at diagnosis is 18 months (typically younger for bilateral retinoblastoma) {3163, 131}. Patients with heritable retinoblastoma account for about

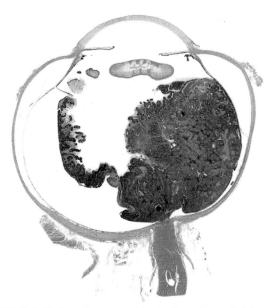

Fig 14.33 Retinoblastoma. Low-power view showing replacement of the retina by retinoblastoma.

45% of cases, with an approximate 5% risk of developing trilateral retinoblastoma {703}.

Etiology

Familial retinoblastoma is caused by germline pathogenic sequence variants in the *RB1* gene.

Pathogenesis

Most retinoblastomas are caused by germline or somatic mutations in the *RB1* tumour suppressor gene on chromosome 13 (13q14.2) {788,58,352}. About 40% have de novo or inherited germline pathogenic variants that are transmissible as an autosomal dominant trait. Amplification of the *MYCN* oncogene causes rare cases of the non-hereditary form without *RB1* mutations (accounting for 2% of all cases of retinoblastoma) {2757}.

Macroscopic appearance

Retinoblastoma arises from and destroys the retina. The tumour has a white or encephaloid appearance with lighter calcific flecks. Endophytic and exophytic tumours arise from the inner and outer layers of the retina causing vitreous invasion and retinal detachment, respectively. Rare diffuse infiltrative retinoblastomas (1.5% of cases) lack calcification and a discrete mass. They occur in older children (mean age: 6–7 years) and contribute to misdiagnosis. Patients with limited access to medical care frequently present with ocular destruction, extraocular extension, and an orbital mass.

Histopathology

Retinoblastoma is a mitotically active small blue cell tumour composed of primitive neuroblastic cells. Perivascular cuffs of viable cells, tumour necrosis, and dystrophic calcification are common {422}. Flexner–Wintersteiner rosettes are a characteristic feature of retinoblastoma, but they may occur in other neoplasms such as pineoblastoma and medulloepithelioma. They represent early retinal differentiation and have a central lumen {3231}. Rosettes are more common in very young infants {815}. Photoreceptor differentiation is found in 15–20% of retinoblastomas {2097,815,757}, and it is characterized by aggregates of neoplastic photoreceptors called fleurettes. Massive posterior uveal invasion (defined as > 3 mm in largest diameter) and retrolaminar optic nerve invasion are high-risk histopathological markers that are indications for adjuvant chemotherapy {2814, 561}. Involvement of anterior segment structures and severe tumour anaplasia are thought to increase metastatic risk {2069}. The histological features of the intracranial tumour/pineoblastoma in trilateral retinoblastoma are essentially identical to those in retinoblastoma.

Cytology

Cytology shows small blue cells, singly or in aggregates, mixed with necrotic tumour. Rosettes are found occasionally {529}. Fine-needle aspiration biopsy is discouraged due to concern about needle track contamination and extraocular spread.

Diagnostic molecular pathology

Retinoblastoma syndrome is defined by a constitutional genetic alteration in the *RB1* gene leading to a high risk for (often bilateral and sometimes trilateral) retinoblastoma. Genetic counselling should therefore be considered for patients with combined ocular disease (particularly bilateral retinoblastoma) and pineal disease (pineoblastoma/retinoblastoma). Genetic testing is used to determine if patients have germline or somatic *RB1* mutations {2590}. Intracranial pineoblastomas/retinoblastomas, whether sporadic or germline, have a distinct DNA methylation profile from that of other pineal tumours and share common copy-number features with ocular retinoblastoma (e.g. chromosome 16 loss and 1q gain) {1865,2490}.

Essential and desirable diagnostic criteria

See Box 14.18.

Staging

Retinoblastoma is staged according to the Union for International Cancer Control (UICC) TNM classification, eighth edition. In bilateral cases, each eye should be staged separately.

Prognosis and prediction

Untreated retinoblastomas are fatal. In developed countries, the survival rate of treated cases approaches 95%. Worldwide, the survival rate is only 50% {2985,1645,456}. In a prospective study of > 300 enucleated eyes, the most significant predictive factors for recurrence and death were extensive retrolaminar optic nerve invasion concomitant with massive (> 3 mm) choroidal invasion {561}.

In patients with retinoblastoma syndrome, the prognosis depends on the stage at which the different tumours are diagnosed and treated: the earlier the diagnosis, the better the prognosis. It is important to screen survivors of hereditary retinoblastoma for second malignancies, including osteosarcomas (typically in the first and second decade of life) and soft tissue sarcomas (10–50 years after retinoblastoma diagnosis). Other epithelial tumours of the bladder, lung, and breast, or melanoma, may arise after the second decade of life. Patients with retinoblastoma syndrome may have more than one second primary malignancy, and screening should continue throughout the patient's life.

BAP1 tumour predisposition syndrome

Santagata S
Wesseling P

Definition

BAP1 tumour predisposition syndrome is an autosomal dominant disorder caused by pathogenic germline variants in the *BAP1* tumour suppressor gene. The syndrome is characterized by a predisposition to various tumours including uveal melanoma, mesothelioma, cutaneous melanoma, and renal cell carcinoma, with less frequently occurring tumours including meningioma, basal cell carcinoma, and cholangiocarcinoma.

MIM numbering

614327 Tumour predisposition syndrome; TPDS

ICD-11 coding

None

Related terminology

None

Subtype(s)

None

Localization

Multiple sites and organ systems are involved, including the eye {1235,6,1442}, pleura, peritoneum {3169}, skin {3438, 3353}, kidney {2540}, liver {2514}, and meninges {6,559,3353, 2888,3361}.

Clinical features

The median age of tumour onset is younger in people with *BAP1* tumour predisposition syndrome than in the general population. Affected individuals can have multiple types of primary cancers {3361}. Mesotheliomas have substantially different clinical features when arising in *BAP1* tumour predisposition syndrome: they arise 20 years earlier, lack male

predominance, and are frequently peritoneal rather than pleural {218,2308,2414}. Histologically distinctive *BAP1*-inactivated naevi/melanocytomas occur in three quarters of germline carriers {1266,3486}, yet they are not specific for the syndrome {431}. An association between meningioma formation and *BAP1* germline pathogenic variants was first reported in three affected families {6,559,3353} and subsequently linked to meningiomas with rhabdoid and papillary morphology {2888, 2890,3449}.

Criteria for genetic counselling and testing include: (1) a medical history of at least two *BAP1* tumour predisposition syndrome-associated tumours, (2) one *BAP1* tumour predisposition syndrome-associated tumour and a first- or second-degree relative with at least one *BAP1* tumour predisposition syndrome-associated tumour(s), and/or (3) young age of tumour onset {2604,3361,527}. In the context of these criteria, loss of BAP1 on immunohistochemistry or detection of *BAP1* variants in relevant tumours further supports a need for germline testing {1266, 3361}. To identify tumours at early stages, screening includes eye and skin examinations and ultrasound or MRI {2604,3018, 3361,527}. *BAP1*-inactivated naevi/melanocytomas often precede the onset of other tumours; their recognition facilitates early syndrome detection.

Epidemiology

More than 180 families have been described, with 140 unique pathogenic germline *BAP1* variants, of which 104 are null variants and 9 are missense variants in the UCH domain {3361}. The carrier frequency of germline pathogenic variants is about 1 in 50 000 in people without cancer and about 1 in 1900 among cancer patients, suggesting that the syndrome prevalence is underestimated {2030}. The most prevalent founder variant is *BAP1* p.L573Wfs*2 {3361}. The lifetime risk of developing cancer is reported to be as high as 80–100%, with many carriers

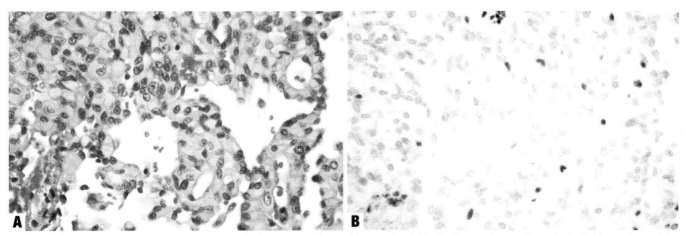

Fig. 14.34 *BAP1* meningioma. A recurrent meningioma arising in a 59-year-old man with a germline *BAP1* p.Y173X truncating mutation and a family history of mesothelioma. **A** The tumour has mixed rhabdoid and papillary features. **B** BAP1 expression is lost in neoplastic cells and retained in associated non-neoplastic cells.

Table 14.08 Frequency of germline and somatic (sporadic) *BAP1* mutations in tumours and occurrence of tumours in probands with null variants in *BAP1*

Tumour type	Prevalence of germline *BAP1* mutations	Prevalence of somatic *BAP1* mutations	Occurrence of tumours in *BAP1*-TPDS probands with null *BAP1* variants
Uveal melanoma	1–2%	40–45%	36.2%
Mesothelioma	1–2%	23–64%	24.8%
Cutaneous melanoma	< 1%	2–3%	23.4%
Renal cell carcinoma	< 1%	10–15%	5.7%
Basal cell carcinoma	< 1%	1–3%	< 10%
Intrahepatic cholangiocarcinoma	1–2%	15–25%	1.4%
Meningioma (all histologies)	< 1%	< 1%	8.5%

BAP1-TPDS, *BAP1* tumour predisposition syndrome.

developing multiple cancers; most families have at least two types of tumours in first- or second-degree relatives {2604, 3361}. Null variants predispose to earlier tumour formation than do missense variants {3361}.

BAP1 is the most frequently mutated gene in sporadic mesothelioma {406} and in metastatic uveal melanoma {1235, 6,1442}, but < 1–4% of these *BAP1*-mutant tumours arise in germline carriers {3169,2752,2890,2653}. This may contrast with meningioma, where half of *BAP1*-mutant meningiomas in a small series arose in germline carriers {2888,2890}. *BAP1*-mutant meningiomas account for < 1% of all meningiomas.

The frequency of germline and somatic *BAP1* mutations in various tumour types and the occurrence of those tumours in probands with null variants in *BAP1* are listed in Table 14.08.

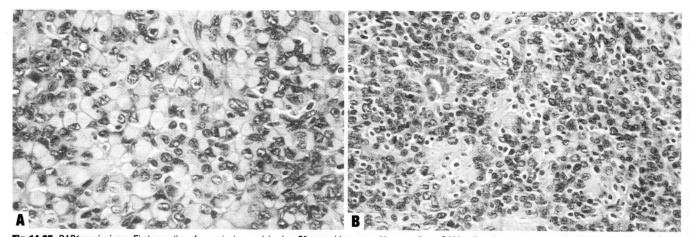

Fig. 14.35 *BAP1* meningioma. First resection of a meningioma arising in a 59-year-old woman with a germline p.G220 splice-site mutation and a family history of mesothelioma and cutaneous melanoma. The tumour had a heterogeneous appearance, with rhabdoid features (**A**) and poorly differentiated regions (**B**).

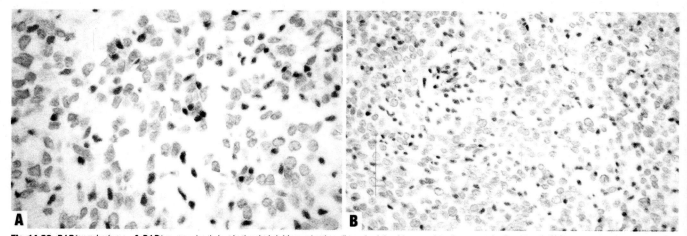

Fig. 14.36 *BAP1* meningioma. **A** BAP1 expression is lost in the rhabdoid neoplastic cells and retained in associated non-neoplastic cells. **B** BAP1 expression is also lost in the poorly differentiated tumour cells and retained in associated non-neoplastic cells.

Box 14.19 Diagnostic criteria for *BAP1* tumour predisposition syndrome

Essential:

Demonstration of a germline pathogenic variant in *BAP1*

Etiology

BAP1 tumour predisposition syndrome is caused by pathogenic germline variants in the *BAP1* tumour suppressor gene on chromosome 3p21.1. More data are required to evaluate the effect of environmental mutagens (e.g. asbestos, UV radiation) on modulating the penetrance of germline mutations. De novo *BAP1* germline mutations are uncommon {3361,527}.

Pathogenesis

The *BAP1* gene on chromosome 3p21.1 comprises 17 exons encoding a protein with ubiquitin carboxyl hydrolase activity first identified as interacting with BRCA1 {1468}. BAP1 interactors include ASXL1, ASXL2, FOXK1, FOXK2, HCFC1, and YY1, consistent with roles in DNA damage response, transcriptional regulation, cell-cycle regulation, metabolism, inflammatory responses, and lineage differentiation {2890,560,3361,1775}. Nuclear localization and deubiquitination activity are both necessary for BAP1-mediated tumour suppression {3310}.

Macroscopic appearance

The macroscopic appearance of tumours in *BAP1* tumour predisposition syndrome is similar to that of sporadic tumours.

Histopathology

The histopathology of *BAP1* tumour predisposition syndrome-associated tumours is similar to that of their sporadic counterparts. Many *BAP1*-mutant meningiomas have overt rhabdoid cytomorphology, but the histology can be diverse, including epithelioid-type cells and papillary growth {2888,2890}.

Cytology

The cytology of tumours in *BAP1* tumour predisposition syndrome is similar to that of sporadic tumours.

Diagnostic molecular pathology

Loss of BAP1 immunoreactivity in tumour cell nuclei readily identifies deficient tumours. Concordance between immunohistochemistry and genotyping is high but incomplete {332,1704, 2215,3270}. In sequencing data, appraising pathogenicity is straightforward for indels and frameshift, nonsense, and splice-site mutations; guidelines for interpreting sequence variants can assist in the classification of missense mutations {2662,1877}.

Essential and desirable diagnostic criteria

See Box 14.19.

Staging

Not relevant

Prognosis and prediction

Sporadic *BAP1*-mutant tumours are often more aggressive than corresponding tumours lacking such mutations {1220,282}. The prognosis of germline carriers with tumours is incompletely characterized because most studies of single tumour histology contain few patients with *BAP1* tumour predisposition syndrome. Uveal melanomas arising in *BAP1* tumour predisposition syndrome have an increased risk of metastasis {2265,1191}. *BAP1*-mutant meningiomas display aggressive behaviour with frequent recurrences {2888,2890}, although it is unclear whether meningiomas arising in *BAP1* tumour predisposition syndrome have a different prognosis than sporadic *BAP1*-mutant meningiomas. In contrast, patients with germline *BAP1*-related mesothelioma have a better 5-year survival rate (47%) than those with sporadic mesotheliomas (6.7%) {218,2308,2414}.

Fanconi anaemia

Solomon DA
Kratz CP

Definition

Fanconi anaemia (FA) is a clinically and genetically heterogeneous disorder caused by underlying genomic instability. Characteristic clinical features include developmental abnormalities in major organ systems, early-onset bone marrow failure, and a high predisposition to cancer. The predominant CNS tumour manifestation is medulloblastoma, resulting from biallelic pathogenic germline variants in either *BRCA2* or *PALB2*.

MIM numbering

605724 Fanconi anaemia, complementation group D1; FANCD1
610832 Fanconi anaemia, complementation group N; FANCN

ICD-11 coding

3A70.0 Congenital aplastic anaemia

Related terminology

None

Subtype(s)

None

Localization

Manifestations of FA may develop in all organs and tissues. The predominant CNS tumour arising in the setting of FA is medulloblastoma.

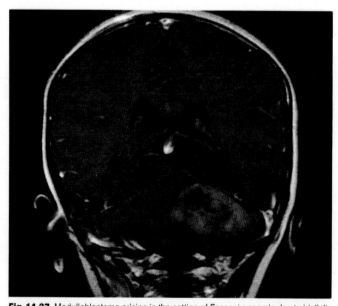

Fig. 14.37 Medulloblastoma arising in the setting of Fanconi anaemia due to biallelic germline *BRCA2* mutations. T1-weighted postcontrast coronal MRI demonstrating a medulloblastoma in the cerebellar hemisphere of a young child with Fanconi anaemia due to biallelic germline *BRCA2* mutations.

Clinical features

FA is characterized by a range of physical abnormalities, progressive bone marrow failure, and an increased cancer risk. Classic features include abnormal thumbs, absent radii, short stature, skin hyperpigmentation, abnormal facies (triangular face, microcephaly), abnormal kidneys, and decreased fertility {717}, although the absence of these features does not exclude FA. The most common neoplasms associated with FA are myelodysplastic syndrome and myeloid leukaemia, squamous cell carcinoma of the head and neck, Wilms tumour, and medulloblastoma.

CNS tumours

Patients with FA due to biallelic germline mutation in *BRCA2* or *PALB2* have a dramatically increased risk of malignancies during childhood, with the predominant CNS tumour manifestation being medulloblastoma {717,2297,1319,3204,89,2633,2810, 2682,2108,3085,1662,3392}. Rare examples of patients with FA with other CNS embryonal tumours or glioblastoma have also been reported {745,769}. Children with medulloblastoma and other childhood cancers that arise in the setting of FA may have a family history of breast, ovarian, and pancreatic cancer in the maternal and/or paternal lineages, caused by heterozygous carrier status for *BRCA2* or *PALB2* pathogenic variants.

Epidemiology

FA is most often an autosomal recessive disorder resulting from homozygous or compound heterozygous germline mutations in the 22 different FANC genes. The two exceptions are complementation group B (*FANCB*), which is X-linked, and complementation group R (*RAD51*), which is autosomal dominant. The estimated carrier frequency for FA is 1:100–200 persons, while the approximate syndrome incidence is 1 case per 130 000 births {2725}.

Etiology

FA is a heritable syndrome caused by germline transmission of deleterious mutations or deletions in the various FANC genes. FA can be caused by disruptions in 22 different genes, which result in a mostly similar clinical phenotype but with some differences, including variable tumour predisposition. Depending on the specific causative gene, FA is differentiated into complementation groups A through W (e.g. complementation group A is caused by biallelic germline mutation in the *FANCA* gene). To date, only two complementation groups have been associated with an increased risk of CNS tumours: D1 and N, which result from biallelic germline mutations in the *BRCA2* and *PALB2* genes, respectively. Complementation group D1 is caused by homozygous or compound heterozygous germline mutations in the *BRCA2* gene on chromosome 13q13.1 {1319}. Complementation group N is caused by homozygous or compound

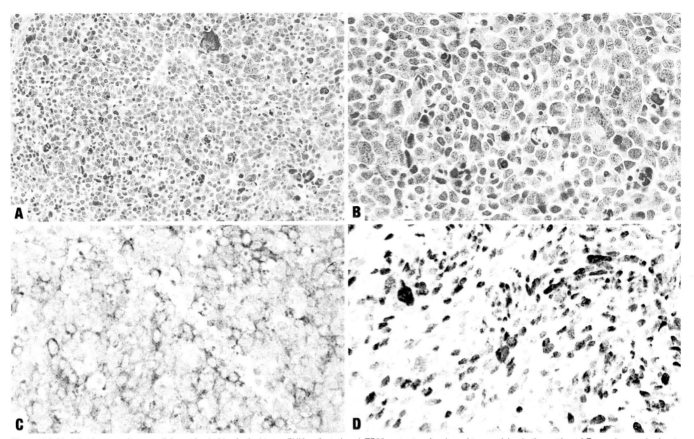

Fig. 14.38 Medulloblastoma. Large cell / anaplastic histological type, SHH-activated and *TP53*-mutant molecular subtype, arising in the setting of Fanconi anaemia due to biallelic germline *BRCA2* mutations. **A** This medulloblastoma in a young child with Fanconi anaemia due to biallelic germline *BRCA2* mutations demonstrates severe anaplasia. **B** High power demonstrates the large cells with severe anaplasia. **C** This medulloblastoma demonstrates immunopositivity for GAB1, indicative of SHH pathway activation. **D** This medulloblastoma also demonstrates strong nuclear staining for p53 protein in the majority of tumour cells, corresponding with the somatic *TP53* mutation that is present.

heterozygous germline mutations in the *PALB2* gene on chromosome 16p12.2 {2633}.

Pathogenesis

The FANC genes encode proteins involved in the homologous recombination of DNA double-strand breaks and in the repair of DNA crosslinks. The deleterious mutations in the FANC genes

causative of FA result in impaired homologous recombination and crosslink repair, which drives chromosomal aberrations such as amplifications, deletions, and translocations that promote tumorigenesis {979}.

Macroscopic appearance

Not relevant

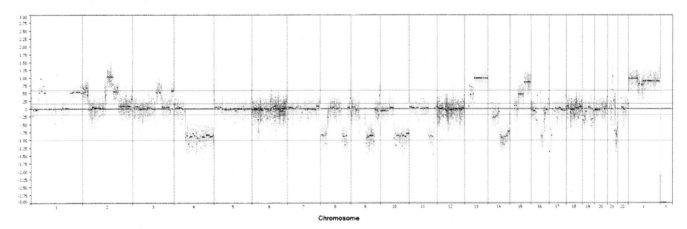

Fig. 14.39 Medulloblastoma, SHH-activated and *TP53*-mutant, arising in the setting of Fanconi anaemia due to biallelic germline *BRCA2* mutations. Genome-wide copy plot showing the aneuploid genome, with most chromosomes in the genome harbouring multiple intrachromosomal copy-number breakpoints, reflective of the defect in double-strand DNA break repair caused by the *BRCA2* biallelic inactivation.

Histopathology

Medulloblastomas arising in the setting of FA are usually of the large cell / anaplastic histological type, or they can have desmoplastic/nodular histology with superimposed anaplasia {3392}.

Cytology

Not relevant

Diagnostic molecular pathology

Diagnosis of FA has traditionally employed chromosomal breakage analysis performed on patient-derived cultures of either leukocytes from a peripheral blood sample or dermal fibroblasts from a skin biopsy after treatment with an agent that induces DNA interstrand crosslinks, such as diepoxybutane. Mutation analysis of a constitutional DNA sample to assess for pathogenic mutations or deletions in the FANC genes is a complementary diagnostic methodology that can identify the causative gene abnormality.

Medulloblastomas and other cancers arising in the setting of FA are genomically characterized by a large number of intrachromosomal breaks, which can be visualized by copy-number analysis as several chromosomes having multiple segmental gains and losses {1662,3392}. A distinct mutation signature has also been observed in medulloblastomas arising in the setting of FA, featuring elevated numbers of large (> 3 bp) insertions and deletions with overlapping microhomology at breakpoint junctions characteristic of BRCA-deficient breast and ovarian cancers {3392}. The medulloblastomas that arise in the setting of FA often belong to the SHH-activated molecular subtype, and they are frequently also *TP53*-mutant {2108,3392}. Notably, medulloblastomas can also arise in the setting of heterozygous germline mutation in either *BRCA2* or *PALB2* (i.e. FA carrier status only); these medulloblastomas have somatic/acquired inactivation of the remaining wildtype allele (often via loss of heterozygosity), and they can belong to the sonic hedgehog–activated, group 3, or group 4 molecular subtypes {1662,3392}.

Essential and desirable diagnostic criteria

See Box 14.20.

Staging

Not relevant

Prognosis and prediction

Medulloblastomas arising in the setting of FA due to biallelic germline *BRCA2* or *PALB2* mutation have a dismal prognosis {3392}. This is probably a reflection of both the aggressive biology of these tumours and the fact that patients with FA cannot tolerate high doses of certain genotoxic chemotherapies. In addition, patients with FA have a dramatically increased risk of developing metastases after therapy.

ELP1-medulloblastoma syndrome

Pfister SM
Waszak SM

Definition

ELP1-medulloblastoma syndrome is an autosomal dominant disorder caused by pathogenic germline variants in the *ELP1* gene and characterized by an increased risk of sonic hedgehog (SHH)-activated medulloblastoma during childhood.

MIM numbering

155255 Medulloblastoma; MDB

ICD-11 coding

None

Related terminology

Acceptable: ELP1-associated medulloblastoma.

Subtype(s)

None

Localization

Tumours arise in the cerebellum.

Clinical features

ELP1-medulloblastoma syndrome is characterized by SHH-activated *TP53*-wildtype medulloblastoma during childhood. The median patient age at diagnosis of medulloblastoma is 6 years (reported range: 2–19 years). Patients with *ELP1*-associated medulloblastoma can have a family history of medulloblastoma {3393}.

Epidemiology

Pathogenic germline *ELP1* variants are estimated to affect 1 in 1000 people worldwide {3393}. ELP1-medulloblastoma syndrome accounts for 1 in 7 cases of SHH-activated medulloblastoma in children and 1 in 3 cases of SHH subgroup 3 medulloblastoma {491,2865,3083,3393}.

Etiology

ELP1-medulloblastoma syndrome is caused by a heterozygous pathogenic germline sequence variant in the *ELP1* gene, located on chromosome 9 at position 9q31.3.

Pathogenesis

ELP1-associated medulloblastomas are characterized by biallelic inactivation of *ELP1* due to somatic loss of chromosome arm 9q (100% of reported cases to date). The majority (84% of reported cases) of *ELP1*-associated medulloblastomas acquire an additional sequence variant or focal deletion in the tumour suppressor gene *PTCH1*, located on chromosome 9 at position 9q22.3, and they are thus predisposed to constitutive activation of SHH signalling during tumour development. A three-step model of tumorigenesis has been proposed for *ELP1*-associated medulloblastomas {3393}: step 1, heterozygous

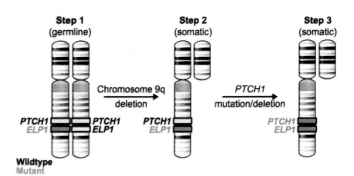

Fig. 14.40 Proposed three-step model of tumorigenesis in ELP1-medulloblastoma syndrome. Step 1: germline variant results in monoallelic inactivation of *ELP1*. Step 2: somatic deletion of chromosome 9q results in biallelic inactivation of *ELP1* and concurrent monoallelic inactivation of *PTCH1*. Step 3: somatic *PTCH1* mutation or focal deletion on 9q22.32 results in biallelic inactivation of *PTCH1*.

pathogenic germline *ELP1* variant; step 2, biallelic inactivation of *ELP1* with concurrent monoallelic inactivation of *PTCH1* due to an acquired deletion of chromosome arm 9q; step 3, biallelic inactivation of *PTCH1* due to an acquired mutation or focal deletion. *ELP1*-associated medulloblastomas also exhibit somatic alterations that converge on the p53 pathway and include amplification of the *PPM1D* (31%) and *MDM4* (10%) genes, yet are mutually exclusive with somatic and germline *TP53* mutations. ELP1 is the largest subunit of the highly conserved eukaryotic Elongator complex {682}, which catalyses translational elongation through transfer RNA (tRNA) modifications at wobble position 34 {1363,2391,2878,3238}. *ELP1*-associated medulloblastomas are characterized by a destabilized Elongator complex, loss of Elongator-dependent tRNA modifications, codon-dependent dysregulation of protein expression, and an unfolded protein response {3393}, consistent with Elongator studies in model systems {1126,1788,2225}.

Macroscopic appearance

ELP1-associated medulloblastomas are similar in appearance to sporadic medulloblastomas.

Histopathology

Patients with ELP1-medulloblastoma syndrome are primarily diagnosed with desmoplastic/nodular medulloblastoma (76%) and less commonly with classic (18%) or large cell / anaplastic (6%) medulloblastoma {3393}.

Cytology

Evaluation of cerebrospinal fluid cytology is required for staging.

Diagnostic molecular pathology

Two dozen rare pathogenic germline variants in the *ELP1* gene are known and include frameshift, nonsense, and canonical

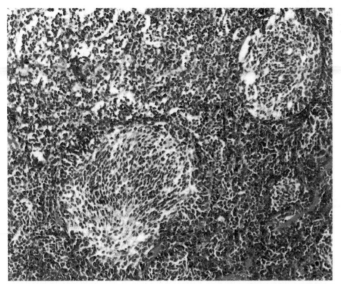

Fig. 14.41 Histopathology of *ELP1*-associated medulloblastoma. Desmoplastic/nodular pattern characterized by nodular, reticulin-free zones and intervening densely packed, poorly differentiated cells that produce an intercellular network of reticulin-positive collagen fibres.

Box 14.21 Diagnostic criteria for ELP1-medulloblastoma syndrome

Essential:

Heterozygous pathogenic germline variant in the *ELP1* gene in the context of a sonic hedgehog (SHH)-activated, *TP53*-wildtype medulloblastoma

Desirable:

Loss of heterozygosity of the *ELP1* gene in resected tumour material and a methylation profile consistent with SHH-activated medulloblastoma subgroup 3 {3393}

splice-site variants {3393}. Pathogenic missense variants and structural variants are identified in 10% of cases. Absence of *ELP1* gene and protein expression in resected tumour material allows for the identification of patients with ELP1-medulloblastoma syndrome. Patients with ELP1-medulloblastoma syndrome show loss of chromosome arm 9q and typically a somatic *PTCH1* mutation in their SHH-activated medulloblastoma, yet no germline *PTCH1* mutation.

Essential and desirable diagnostic criteria
See Box 14.21.

Staging
Clinical staging procedures include MRI examinations of the CNS with contrast agent. This is complemented by cerebrospinal fluid cytology at the time of diagnosis. The postoperative staging system developed by Chang and others in 1969 {519}, which defines the following degrees of metastatic spread, is still being used:

M0 No evidence of gross subarachnoid or haematogenous metastasis
M1 Microscopic tumour cells found in the cerebrospinal fluid
M2 Gross nodular seeding demonstrated in the cerebellar/cerebral subarachnoid space or in the third or lateral ventricles
M3 Gross nodular seeding in the spinal subarachnoid space
M4 Metastasis outside the cerebrospinal axis

Prognosis and prediction
Preliminary data indicates that *ELP1*-associated medulloblastoma is associated with a favourable clinical outcome (5-year overall survival rate: 92%) {3393}.

Contributors

ABEDALTHAGAFI, Malak S.
King Abdulaziz City for Science and
Technology (KACST) and
King Fahad Medical City (KFMC)
King Abdullah Road, Al Raed
Riyadh 11442

AHLUWALIA, Manmeet S.*
Cleveland Clinic
9500 Euclid Avenue, CA5
Cleveland OH 44145

ALDAPE, Kenneth D.
National Cancer Institute
9000 Rockville Pike
Bethesda MD 20892

ALEXANDRESCU, Sanda
Boston Children's Hospital
Harvard Medical School
300 Longwood Avenue, Bader 104
Boston MA 02115

ASA, Sylvia L.*
Case Western Reserve University
11100 Euclid Avenue
Cleveland OH 44106

BAKER, Suzanne J.
St. Jude Children's Research Hospital
262 Danny Thomas Place
Memphis TN 38105

BANDOPADHAYAY, Pratiti*
Dana-Farber/Boston Children's
Cancer and Blood Disorders Center
450 Brookline Avenue, Mayer 658
Dana-Farber Cancer Institute
Boston MA 02215

BASTIAN, Boris C.*
University of California, San Francisco
1450 Third Street, #281
San Francisco CA 94143-3118

BATCHELOR, Tracy*
Brigham and Women's Hospital
60 Fenwood Road, Hale Building, 4th Floor
Boston MA 02115

BAUMHOER, Daniel
University Hospital Basel
Schönbeinstrasse 40
4031 Basel

BIEGEL, Jaclyn A.
Children's Hospital Los Angeles
Department of Pathology
4650 Sunset Boulevard, MS 173
Los Angeles CA 90027

BLÜMCKE, Ingmar
University Hospitals Erlangen
Schwabachanlage 6
91054 Erlangen

BOUVIER, Corinne
Hôpital de la Timone 2
265 Rue Saint-Pierre
13385 Marseille Cedex 05

BRANDNER, Sebastian
UCL Queen Square Institute of Neurology and
National Hospital for Neurology and
Neurosurgery, University College London
Hospitals NHS Foundation Trust
Queen Square
London WC1N 3BG

BRASTIANOS, Priscilla Kaliopi*
Massachusetts General Hospital and
Harvard Medical School
55 Fruit Street, Yawkey 9E
Boston MA 02114

BRAT, Daniel J.
Northwestern University
Feinberg School of Medicine
303 East Chicago Avenue
Ward Building, 3-140
Chicago IL 60611

CAHILL, Daniel Patrick*
Massachusetts General Hospital
55 Fruit Street, Yawkey 9E
Boston MA 02114

CAIRNCROSS, John Gregory*
University of Calgary
3280 Hospital Drive North-West, HRIC 2AA-20
Calgary AB T2N 4Z6

CALONJE, Jaime E.
St John's Institute of Dermatology
St Thomas' Hospital
Westminster Bridge Road
London SE1 7EH

CAPPER, David*
Charité – Universitätsmedizin Berlin
Charitéplatz 1
10117 Berlin

CARNEIRO, Fátima
Ipatimup/i3S
Rua Júlio Amaral de Carvalho, 45
4200-135 Porto

CHAN, John K.C.
Queen Elizabeth Hospital
30 Gascoigne Road
Kowloon, Hong Kong SAR

CHEUNG, Annie Nga-Yin
University of Hong Kong
Queen Mary Hospital
Pok Fu Lam Road
Hong Kong SAR

CHIMELLI, Leila
State Institute of Brain
Rua do Resende 156
Rio de Janeiro RJ 20231-092

CIMINO, Patrick J.
University of Washington
325 Ninth Avenue, Box 359791
98104 Seattle WA

CLAUS, Elizabeth B.
Yale School of Medicine
60 College Street, Box 208034
New Haven CT 06520-8034

CLIFFORD, Steven C.
Newcastle University Centre for Cancer
Herschel Building
Newcastle upon Tyne NE1 7RU

COTTER, Jennifer A.
Children's Hospital Los Angeles and
Keck School of Medicine of USC
4650 Sunset Boulevard, Mail Stop #43
Los Angeles CA 90027

CREE, Ian A.
International Agency for Research on Cancer
150 Cours Albert Thomas
69372 Lyon

DE ÁLAVA, Enrique*
Hospital Universitario Virgen del Rocío-IBiS
University of Seville
Manuel Siurot s/n
41013 Seville

DE KOCK, Leanne
Children's Hospital of Eastern Ontario
Research Institute
401 Smyth Road
Ottawa ON K1H 5B2

* Indicates disclosure of interests (see p. 489).

DECKERT, Martina
Faculty of Medicine and
University Hospital of Cologne
University of Cologne
Kerpener Straße 62
50924 Cologne

DEMICCO, Elizabeth G.
University of Toronto
Mount Sinai Hospital, 600 University Avenue
Toronto ON M5G 1X5

DRY, Sarah M.
University of California, Los Angeles (UCLA)
13-222 CHS, 10833 Le Conte Avenue
Los Angeles CA 90095

EAGLE, Ralph C. Jr
Wills Eye Hospital
840 Walnut Street, Suite 1410
Philadelphia PA 19107

EBERHART, Charles G.
Johns Hopkins University
720 Rutland Avenue, Ross Building 558
Baltimore MD 21205

ELLISON, David W.
St. Jude Children's Research Hospital
262 Danny Thomas Place
Memphis TN 38105

ENG, Charis E.
Cleveland Clinic
9500 Euclid Avenue, NE-50
Cleveland OH 44195

EVANS, D. Gareth R.
University of Manchester
Oxford Road
Manchester M13 9WL

FANBURG-SMITH, Julie C.
Penn State Health
Milton S. Hershey Medical Center
Pathology, Pediatrics, Orthopedics
500 University Drive, C7714
Hershey PA 17033

FERRY, Judith A.
Massachusetts General Hospital
55 Fruit Street
Boston MA 02114

FIELD, Andrew S.
University of NSW and
University of Notre Dame Medical Schools,
Department of Anatomical Pathology
St Vincent's Hospital Sydney
Victoria Street
Darlinghurst NSW 2021

FIGARELLA-BRANGER, Dominique
Assistance Publique des Hôpitaux de
Marseille
264 Rue Saint-Pierre
13005 Marseille

FISHER, Michael J.
Children's Hospital of Philadelphia
3501 Civic Center Boulevard
Philadelphia PA 19104

FLANAGAN, Adrienne Margaret
Royal National Orthopaedic Hospital
Brockley Hill
Stanmore, Middlesex HA7 4LP

FOLPE, Andrew L.
Mayo Clinic
200 First Street South-West
Rochester MN 55905

FOULKES, William D.
McGill University
Research Institute
McGill University Health Centre
1001 Décarie Boulevard
Montréal QC H4A 3J1

FRITCHIE, Karen J.
Cleveland Clinic
9500 Euclid Avenue
Cleveland OH 44195

FULLER, Gregory N.
University of Texas
MD Anderson Cancer Center
1515 Holcombe Boulevard, Unit 85
Houston TX 77030

GESSI, Marco
Fondazione Policlinico Universitario
"Agostino Gemelli" IRCCS
Università Cattolica del Sacro Cuore
Largo Agostino Gemelli 8
00168 Rome RM

GIANGASPERO, Felice
Policlinico Umberto I, Sapienza University
and IRCCS Neuromed (Pozzilli)
Viale Regina Elena 324
00161 Rome RM

GIANNINI, Caterina
Mayo Clinic
(and Alma Mater Studiorum -
University of Bologna)
200 First Street South-West
Rochester MN 55905

GILBERTSON, Richard James*
University of Cambridge
Li Ka Shing Centre, Robinson Way
Cambridge CB2 0RE

GILL, Anthony J.
Royal North Shore Hospital
Pacific Highway
St Leonards NSW 2065

GUPTA, Kirti
Postgraduate Institute of Medical Education
and Research
5th Floor, A Block (Research)
PGIMER, Sector 12
Chandigarh 160012

GUTMANN, David H.
Washington University School of Medicine
660 South Euclid Avenue, Box 8111
St. Louis MO 63110

HABERLER, Christine
Medical University of Vienna
Währinger Gürtel 18–20
1090 Vienna

HAINFELLNER, Johannes A.*
Medical University of Vienna
Währinger Gürtel 18–20
1090 Vienna

HARTMANN, Christian*
Institute of Pathology
Hannover Medical School
Carl-Neuberg-Straße 1
30625 Hannover

HASSELBLATT, Martin
University Hospital Münster
Pottkamp 2
48149 Münster

HAWKINS, Cynthia E.
Hospital for Sick Children
555 University Avenue
Toronto ON M5G 1X8

HILL, D. Ashley*
Children's National Hospital
111 Michigan Avenue North-West
Washington DC 20010

HIROSE, Takanori
Kobe University Graduate School of Medicine
7-5-2 Kusunoki-cho, Chuo-ku, Hyogo
Prefecture
Kobe City 650-0017

HOANG-XUAN, Khe
Hôpital Universitaire Pitié Salpêtrière
Division Mazarin, 47 Boulevard de l'Hôpital
75013 Paris

HONAVAR, Mrinalini
Pedro Hispano Hospital
Rua de Alfredo Cunha 365
4464-513 Matosinhos

---

* Indicates disclosure of interests (see p. 489).

HORBINSKI, Craig Michael
Northwestern University
303 East Superior Street
Chicago IL 60611

HUANG, Annie
Hospital for Sick Children
555 University Avenue
Toronto ON M5G 1X8

HULSEBOS, Theo J.M.
Amsterdam UMC
Meibergdreef 9
1105 AZ Amsterdam

HUSE, Jason T.
University of Texas
MD Anderson Cancer Center
2130 West Holcombe Boulevard
LSP9.4009, Unit 2951
Houston TX 77005

ICHIMURA, Koichi
National Cancer Center Research Institute
5-1-1 Tsukiji, Chuo-ku
Tokyo 104-0045

IDBAIH, Ahmed*
Sorbonne Université, AP-HP, Institut du
Cerveau - Paris Brain Institute - ICM, Inserm,
CNRS, Hôpital de la Pitié Salpêtrière
DMU Neurosciences, Service de Neurologie 2
47-83 Boulevard de l'Hôpital
75013 Paris

INWARDS, Carrie Y.
Mayo Clinic
200 First Street South-West
Rochester MN 55905

JABADO, Nada
McGill University
1001 Décarie Boulevard
Montréal QC H4A 3J1

JACQUES, Thomas S.*
UCL GOS Institute of Child Health
30 Guilford Street
London WC1N 1EH

JARZEMBOWSKI, Jason A.
Medical College of Wisconsin
8701 West Watertown Plank Road
Milwaukee WI 53226

JO, Vickie Y.*
Brigham and Women's Hospital and
Harvard Medical School
75 Francis Street
Boston MA 02115

JONES, Chris*
Institute of Cancer Research
15 Cotswold Road
Suton SM2 5NG

JONES, David T.W.*
Hopp Children's Cancer Center Heidelberg
(KiTZ) and German Cancer Research Center
(DKFZ)
Im Neuenheimer Feld 280
69120 Heidelberg

JUDKINS, Alexander R.*
Children's Hospital Los Angeles and
Keck School of Medicine of USC
4650 Sunset Boulevard, Mail Stop #43
Los Angeles CA 90027

KAUR, Kavneet
All India Institute of Medical Sciences
Ansari Nagar
New Delhi 110029

KLEINSCHMIDT-DeMASTERS, Bette K.
University of Colorado
Health Sciences Center
12605 East 16th Avenue, Room 3.003
Aurora CO 80045

KÖLSCHE, Christian
Institute of Pathology
University Hospital Heidelberg
Im Neuenheimer Feld 224
69115 Heidelberg

KOMORI, Takashi
Neuropathology
Tokyo Metropolitan Neurological Hospital
2-6-1 Musashidai, Fuchu
Tokyo 183-0042

KOOL, Marcel*
Hopp Children's Cancer Center Heidelberg
(KiTZ)
Im Neuenheimer Feld 280
69120 Heidelberg

KORSHUNOV, Andrey
German Cancer Research Center (DKFZ)
Im Neuenheimer Feld 280
69115 Heidelberg

KRATZ, Christian P.
Hannover Medical School
Carl-Neuberg-Straße 1
30625 Hannover

KROS, Johan Marinus
Erasmus Medical Center
Dokter Molewaterplein 40
3015 GD Rotterdam

KÜSTERS-VANDEVELDE, Heidi V.
Canisius Wilhelmina Hospital
Weg door Jonkerbos 100
6532 SZ Nijmegen

LAKHANI, Sunil R.*
University of Queensland and
Pathology Queensland
Royal Brisbane and Women's Hospital
Herston QLD 4029

LAU, Ching C.
Connecticut Children's Medical Center
282 Washington Street
Hartford CT 06106-3322

LAX, Sigurd F.
General Hospital Graz II
Medical University of Graz
Goestingerstrasse 22
8020 Graz

LAZAR, Alexander J.
University of Texas
MD Anderson Cancer Center
1515 Holcombe Boulevard, Unit 85
Houston TX 77030

LEGIUS, Eric
University of Leuven
Herestraat 49
3000 Leuven

LESKE, Henning
Department of Pathology
Rikshospitalet (OUS)
Sognsvannsveien 20
0372 Oslo

LIGON, Keith Lloyd*
Dana-Farber Cancer Institute
Harvard Medical School
450 Brookline Avenue, JF215
Boston MA 02215

LLOYD, Ricardo V.
University of Wisconsin
School of Medicine and Public Health
600 Highland Avenue
53792 Madison WI

LOKUHETTY, Dilani
University of Colombo
25 Kynsey Road
Colombo 00800

LOPES, M. Beatriz S.
University of Virginia
Health System Box 800214 - HSC
Charlottesville VA 22908-0214

---

* Indicates disclosure of interests (see p. 489).

LOUIS, David N.
Massachusetts General Hospital and
Harvard Medical School
55 Fruit Street, Warren 225
Boston MA 02114

MACAGNO, Nicolas
Timone University Hospital
Rue Saint-Pierre
13005 Marseille

MALKIN, David
Hospital for Sick Children
University of Toronto
555 University Avenue
Toronto ON M5G 1X8

MAWRIN, Christian
Otto von Guericke University
Leipziger Straße 44
39120 Magdeburg

METE, Ozgur
University Health Network and
University of Toronto
200 Elizabeth Street, 11th Floor
Toronto General Hospital
Toronto ON M5G 2C4

MITTELBRONN, Michel Guy André
Laboratoire National de Santé (LNS)
1 Rue Louis Rech
3555 Dudelange

MOCH, Holger
University of Zurich and
University Hospital Zurich
Schmelzbergstrasse 12
8091 Zurich

MÜLLER, Hermann L.
University Children's Hospital
Klinikum Oldenburg AöR
Rahel-Straus-Straße 10
26133 Oldenburg

NAGANE, Motoo*
Kyorin University Faculty of Medicine
6-20-2 Shinkawa, Mitaka
Tokyo 181-8611

NAJM, Imad
Cleveland Clinic
9500 Euclid Avenue
Cleveland OH 44195

NEUMANN, Hartmut P.H.
Albert Ludwig University of Freiburg
Hugstetter Straße 55
79106 Freiburg

NG, Ho-Keung
Chinese University of Hong Kong
Prince of Wales Hospital
Shatin
Hong Kong SAR

NIELSEN, G. Petur
Massachusetts General Hospital
55 Fruit Street
Boston MA 02114-2696

NISHIKAWA, Ryo
Saitama Medical University
International Medical Center
1397-1 Yamane, Hidaka-shi
Saitama-ken 350-1298

NORTHCOTT, Paul A.
St. Jude Children's Research Hospital
262 Danny Thomas Place, MS325
Memphis TN 38105-3678

OCHIAI, Atsushi
National Cancer Center
6-5-1 Kashiwanoha
Kashiwa 277-8577

OLIVA, Esther
Massachusetts General Hospital
55 Fruit Street
Boston MA 02114

ORR, Brent A.
St. Jude Children's Research Hospital
262 Danny Thomas Place
Memphis TN 38105

OSAMURA, Robert Y.
Nippon Koukan Hospital and
Keio University School of Medicine
1-2-1 Koukan-dori, Kawasaki-ku, Kawasaki-shi
Kanagawa 210-0852

OSBORN, Anne Gregory
University of Utah
30 North 1900 East, #1A71
Salt Lake City UT 84132

PAJTLER, Kristian W.
Hopp Children's Cancer Center Heidelberg
(KiTZ), German Cancer Research Center
(DKFZ), and Heidelberg University Hospital
Im Neuenheimer Feld 280
69120 Heidelberg

PARK, Sung-Hye
Seoul National University College of Medicine
Seoul National University Hospital
101 Daehak-ro, Jongno-gu
Seoul 03080

PAULUS, Werner
University Hospital Münster
Pottkamp 2
48149 Münster

PEFEROEN, Laura A.N.
Amsterdam University Medical Center
De Boelelaan 1117
1081 HV Amsterdam

PEKMEZCI, Melike
University of California, San Francisco
505 Parnassus Avenue, M551
San Francisco CA 94143

PERRY, Arie
University of California, San Francisco
505 Parnassus Avenue, M551
San Francisco CA 94143-0102

PFISTER, Stefan M.*
Hopp Children's Cancer Center Heidelberg
(KiTZ), German Cancer Research Center
(DKFZ), and Heidelberg University Hospital
Im Neuenheimer Feld 280
69120 Heidelberg

PIETSCH, Torsten
University of Bonn Medical Center
Venusberg-Campus 1
53127 Bonn

PLATE, Karl H.
Frankfurt University Hospital
Theodor-Stern-Kai 7
60590 Frankfurt am Main

PREUSSER, W. Matthias*
Medical University of Vienna
Währinger Gürtel 18–20
1097 Vienna

PUNGAVKAR, Sona A.
Global Hospitals
Dr Ernest Borges Road, Parel
Mumbai 400012

RAMASWAMY, Vijay
Hospital for Sick Children and
University of Toronto
555 University Avenue
Toronto ON M5G 1X8

REIFENBERGER, Guido*
Heinrich Heine University Düsseldorf
Moorenstraße 5
40225 Düsseldorf

REUSS, David Emanuel*
Heidelberg University and
German Cancer Research Center (DKFZ)
Im Neuenheimer Feld 224
69120 Heidelberg

---

* Indicates disclosure of interests (see p. 489).

REYES-MÚGICA, Miguel
University of Pittsburgh Medical Center
4401 Penn Avenue, Main Hospital B260
One Children's Hospital Drive
Pittsburgh PA 15224

RIGHI, Alberto
IRCCS, Istituto Ortopedico Rizzoli
Via di Barbiano 1/10
40136 Bologna BO

RODRIGUEZ, Fausto J.
Johns Hopkins University
Sheikh Zayed Tower, Room M2101
1800 Orleans Street
Baltimore MD 21231

RONCAROLI, Federico R.
University of Manchester
Oxford Road
Manchester M13 9PT

ROSENBERG, Andrew E.
Miller School of Medicine
University of Miami
1400 North-West 12th Avenue
Miami FL 33136

ROSENBLUM, Marc K.
Memorial Sloan Kettering Cancer Center
1275 York Avenue
New York NY 10021

ROTONDO, Fabio
St. Michael's Hospital
30 Bond Street
Toronto ON M5B 1W8

ROUS, Brian
Public Health England
Victoria House, Capital Park
Fulbourn, Cambridge CB21 5XA

RUDÀ, Roberta
University of Turin and
City of Health and Science Hospital, Turin
Via Cherasco 15
10126 Turin TO

RUDZINSKI, Erin R.
Seattle Children's Hospital
4800 Sandpoint Way North-East
Seattle WA 98105

SAHM, Felix
Heidelberg University and
German Cancer Research Center (DKFZ)
Im Neuenheimer Feld 224
69120 Heidelberg

SANSON, Marc
Pitié-Salpêtrière Hospital – Sorbonne Université
47-83 Boulevard de l'Hôpital
75013 Paris

SANTAGATA, Sandro
Brigham and Women's Hospital
60 Fenwood Road, Hale 8002P
Boston MA 02115

SANTOSH, Vani
National Institute of
Mental Health and Neurosciences
Hosur Road
Bengaluru 560029

SARKAR, Chitra
All India Institute of Medical Sciences
Ansari Nagar
New Delhi 110029

SCHUHMANN, Martin Ulrich
University Hospital Tübingen
Hoppe-Seyler-Straße 3
72076 Tübingen

SCHÜLLER, Ulrich
University of Hamburg
Martinistraße 52
20246 Hamburg

SCHULTZ, Kris Ann P.
International PPB/DICER1 Registry
Cancer and Blood Disorders
Children's Minnesota
2530 Chicago Avenue South
Minneapolis MN 55404

SCIOT, Raf
Department of Pathology
University Hospital KULeuven
Herestraat 49
3000 Leuven

SHARMA, Mehar C.
All India Institute of Medical Sciences
Ansari Nagar
New Delhi 110029

SHIBUYA, Makoto
Tokyo Medical University
Hachioji Medical Center
1163 Tatemachi
Hachioji City 193-0998

SIEVERS, Philipp
Heidelberg University and
German Cancer Research Center (DKFZ)
Im Neuenheimer Feld 224
69120 Heidelberg

SINGH, Rajendra
Northwell Health
1991 Marcus Avenue, Suite 300
Lake Success NY 11042

SNUDERL, Matija
NYU Langone Health
240 East 38th Street, 22nd Floor
New York NY 10016

SOARES, Fernando Augusto
Rede D'Or Hospitals
Rua das Perobas 266
São Paulo SP 04321-120

SOFFIETTI, Riccardo
University of Turin and
City of Health and Science Hospital, Turin
Via Cherasco 15
10126 Turin TO

SOLOMON, David A.
University of California, San Francisco
513 Parnassus Avenue, HSW 451
San Francisco CA 94143

SRIGLEY, John R.
Trillium Health Partners
Credit Valley Hospital Site
2200 Eglinton Avenue West
Mississauga ON L5M 2N1

STEMMER-RACHAMIMOV, Anat Olga
Massachusetts General Hospital
55 Fruit Street
Boston MA 02114

STURM, Dominik
Hopp Children's Cancer Center Heidelberg
(KiTZ), German Cancer Research Center
(DKFZ), and Heidelberg University Hospital
Im Neuenheimer Feld 280
69120 Heidelberg

SUVÀ, Mario L.
Massachusetts General Hospital
149 13th Street, Office 6.010
Boston MA 02129

TABORI, Uri
Hospital for Sick Children
555 University Avenue
Toronto ON M5G 1X8

TAN, Puay Hoon
Division of Pathology
Singapore General Hospital
20 College Road, Academia, Level 7
Diagnostics Tower
Singapore 169856

TANAKA, Shinya
Hokkaido University
Graduate School of Medicine
N15 W7
Sapporo 060-8638

* Indicates disclosure of interests (see p. 489).

TAYLOR, Michael D.
University of Toronto
555 University Avenue, Suite 1503
Toronto ON M5G 1X8

THOMPSON, Lester D.R.
Head and Neck Pathology Consultations
21867 Ambar Drive
Woodland Hills CA 91364

THWAY, Khin
Royal Marsden Hospital /
Institute of Cancer Research
203 Fulham Road
London SW3 6JJ

TIHAN, Tarik
University of California, San Francisco
Neuropathology Division
505 Parnassus Avenue, M551
San Francisco CA 94143

TIRABOSCO, Roberto
Royal National Orthopaedic Hospital
Brockley Hill
Stanmore, London HA7 4LP

TSAO, Ming Sound
University Health Network
200 Elizabeth Street, 11th Floor
Toronto ON M5G 2C4

TSUZUKI, Toyonori
Aichi Medical University Hospital
1-1 Yazakokarimata
Nagakute 480-1195

VAN DEN BENT, Martin Jacques
Erasmus MC Cancer Institute
Dokter Molewaterplein 40
3015 GD Rotterdam

VARLET, Pascale
GHU Paris, Site Hôpital Sainte-Anne
1 Rue Cabanis
75014 Paris

VASILJEVIC, Alexandre
Groupement Hospitalier Est
59 Boulevard Pinel
69677 Bron Cedex

VENNETI, Sriram
University of Michigan
1150 West Medical Center Drive
3520E MSRB 1
Ann Arbor MI 48109

VILLA, Chiara
Institut Cochin
24 Rue du Faubourg Saint-Jacques
75014 Paris

VON DEIMLING, Andreas*
Heidelberg University and
German Cancer Research Center (DKFZ)
Im Neuenheimer Feld 224
69120 Heidelberg

VON HOFF, Katja
Charité – Universitätsmedizin Berlin
Augustenburger Platz 1
13353 Berlin

VORTMEYER, Alexander Oliver
Indiana University–Purdue University
Indianapolis
350 West 11th Street
Indianapolis IN 46202

WARREN, Katherine E.*
Dana-Farber/Boston Children's
Cancer and Blood Disorders Center
450 Brookline Avenue, DANA 3154
Boston MA 02215

WASHINGTON, Mary K.
Vanderbilt University Medical Center
C-3321 MCN
Nashville TN 37232

WASZAK, Sebastian M.
Centre for Molecular Medicine Norway
University of Oslo and Oslo University Hospital
Box 1137 Blindern
0318 Oslo

WELLER, Michael*
University Hospital Zurich and
University of Zurich
Frauenklinikstrasse 26
8091 Zurich

WESSELING, Pieter
Princess Máxima Center for Pediatric
Oncology, Utrecht, and
Amsterdam University Medical Centers/VUmc
De Boelelaan 1117
1081 HV Amsterdam

WHITE, Valerie A.
International Agency for Research on Cancer
150 Cours Albert Thomas
69372 Lyon

WICK, Wolfgang*
Heidelberg University Hospital and
German Cancer Research Center (DKFZ)
Im Neuenheimer Feld 400
69120 Heidelberg

WINKLER, Frank A.*
Heidelberg University Hospital and
German Cancer Research Center (DKFZ)
Im Neuenheimer Feld 400
69120 Heidelberg

WONG, Tai-Tong
Taipei Medical University Hospital
Taipei Medical University
250 Wu-Hsing Street
Taipei City 110

YIP, Stephen
University of British Columbia and
Vancouver General Hospital
855 West 12th Avenue
Vancouver BC V5Z 1M9

YOKOO, Hideaki
Gunma University
Graduate School of Medicine
3-39-22 Showa
Maebashi 371-8511

YOSHIDA, Akihiko
National Cancer Center Hospital
5-1-1 Tsukiji, Chuo-ku
Tokyo 104-0045

ZAGZAG, David
NYU Langone Health and
NYU Grossman School of Medicine
550 First Avenue
New York NY 10016

ZARKA, Matthew A.
Mayo Clinic Arizona
13400 East Shea Boulevard
Scottsdale AZ 85259

Declaration of interests

Dr Ahluwalia reports holding stocks in MimiVax and Doctible, that his unit at Cleveland Clinic benefits from research funding from several private pharmaceutical companies, and receiving personal consultancy fees from several private companies.

Dr Asa reports receiving personal consultancy fees, in her capacity as a medical advisory board member, from Leica Biosystems, Ibex Medical Analytics, and PathAI.

Dr Bandopadhayay reports that her unit at Dana-Farber Cancer Institute benefits from research funding from the Novartis Institutes for BioMedical Research, and holds a patent on "Compositions and methods for screening pediatric gliomas and methods of treatment thereof".

Dr Bastian reports having received personal consultancy fees from Lilly in connection with expert testimony in relation to litigation, and that his unit at University of California, San Francisco, holds a patent on GNAQ mutations.

Dr Batchelor reports receiving consultancy fees from GenomiCare (in his capacity as a scientific advisory board member), Merck, Champions Biotechnology, Oxford University Press, and NX Development Corp. (NXDC), and honoraria from Oakstone Publishing. He reports receiving royalties from UpToDate and the American Academy of Neurology, and providing expert opinion in medical malpractice suits.

Dr Brastianos reports having received personal consultancy fees from Angiochem, Dantari, SK Life Science, Genentech/Roche, Voyager Therapeutics, ElevateBio, Merck, Pfizer (Array), Pfizer, and Eli Lilly, and that her unit at Massachusetts General Hospital / Harvard Medical School benefits from research funding from Lilly, Bristol Myers Squibb, Mirati Therapeutics, and Merck.

Dr Cahill reports having received personal consultancy fees from Lilly, GlaxoSmithKline, and Boston Pharmaceuticals, and that he is on the advisory board of Pyramid Biosciences.

Dr Cairncross reports receiving personal consultancy fees from IQVIA in his capacity as a data safety monitoring board member.

Dr Capper reports that he holds a patent on DNA methylation–based tumour classification and patents for IDH1-R132H antibody (clone H09) and for BRAF-V600E antibody (clone VE1).

Dr de Álava reports that his unit at Hospital Universitario Virgen del Rocío-IBiS benefits from research funding from Pfizer, Astra, Bristol Myers Squibb, and Roche, and benefited from research funding from PharmaMar.

Dr Gilbertson reports holding patent PCT/EP2020/063096 licensed to Cancer Research Technology Limited and MedImmune Limited.

Dr Hainfellner reports that his unit at the Medical University of Vienna benefits from research funding from Novocure.

Dr Hartmann reports that his unit at the Hannover Medical School's Institute of Pathology holds a patent on "Methods for the diagnosis and the prognosis of a brain tumor".

Dr Hill reports holding equity interest in ResourcePath in her capacity as co-founder and medical director.

Dr Idbaih reports that his unit at Sorbonne Université benefits from research funding from Nutritheragene, Air Liquide, Transgene, Carthera, and Sanofi, and having provided expert opinion on behalf of Novocure to a public regulatory agency.

Dr Jacques reports holding shares and providing expert witness work to courts in his capacity as director of Hepath Ltd and Neuropath Ltd, and being editor-in-chief of the journal Neuropathology and Applied Neurobiology.

Dr Jo reports that her spouse benefits from restricted Merck stock units.

Dr C. Jones reports that his unit at the Institute of Cancer Research benefited from research funding from Hoffmann-La Roche.

Dr D.T.W. Jones reports holding a patent on DNA methylation–based tumour classification.

Dr Judkins reports that his unit at Children's Hospital Los Angeles and the Keck School of Medicine of USC benefits from research funding from Epizyme.

Dr Kool reports that his unit at the Hopp Children's Cancer Center Heidelberg (KiTZ) benefits from research funding from Bayer, Pfizer, and Lilly.

Dr Lakhani reports receiving personal consultancy fees from Sullivan Nicolaides Pathology.

Dr Ligon reports receiving personal consultancy fees from Bristol Myers Squibb, IntegraGen, RareCyte, BroadCast; that his unit at Dana-Farber Cancer Institute benefits from research funding from Bristol Myers Squibb, Lilly, Amgen, and Deciphera and holds patents for diagnostics devices and methods; and that he holds stocks in Travera in his capacity as a founding scientific advisor.

Dr Nagane reports having benefited and benefiting from personal consultancy fees from, or serving in an advisory role for, several pharmaceutical companies. He also reports that his unit at Kyorin University benefits from research funding from several pharmaceutical companies and holds a patent assigned to Toray.

Dr Pfister reports that his unit at the German Cancer Research Center (DKFZ) benefits from research funding from the Innovative Medicines Initiative 2 (IMI2) and holds a patent on DNA methylation–based tumour classification.

Dr Preusser reports receiving honoraria for lectures, consultation, or advisory board participation from a number of private pharmaceutical companies, and that his unit at the Medical University of Vienna benefits from research funding from a number of private pharmaceutical companies.

Dr Reifenberger reports that his unit at the University Hospital of Düsseldorf benefited from research funding from Merck.

Dr Reuss reports that his unit at Heidelberg University and the German Cancer Research Center (DKFZ) holds a patent on NF1 antibody clone NFC.

Dr von Deimling reports that his unit at the German Cancer Research Center (DKFZ) benefits from research funding from Illumina, and that he holds patents for IDH-R132H antibody (clone H09) and for BRAF-V600E antibody (clone VE1).

Dr Warren reports holding intellectual property rights on CRADA support for clinical trials in children with diffuse intrinsic pontine glioma, licensed to Celgene.

Dr Weller reports that his unit at University Hospital Zurich benefited from research funding from Quercis Pharma.

Dr Wick reports that his unit at the Neurology Clinic of Heidelberg University Hospital benefits from research funding from Pfizer, Roche, and Apogenix.

Dr Winkler reports receiving personal consultancy fees from Divide & Conquer (DC Europa Ltd) in his capacity as head of the scientific advisory board; holding a patent application on "Agents for use in the treatment of glioma"; and that his unit at Heidelberg University Hospital and the German Cancer Research Center (DKFZ) benefits from research funding from Roche, Genentech, Boehringer, and Divide & Conquer.

IARC/WHO Committee for the International Classification of Diseases for Oncology (ICD-O)

BRAY, Freddie
International Agency for Research on Cancer
150 Cours Albert Thomas
69372 Lyon

CREE, Ian A.
International Agency for Research on Cancer
150 Cours Albert Thomas
69372 Lyon

FERLAY, Jacques
International Agency for Research on Cancer
150 Cours Albert Thomas
69372 Lyon

JAKOB, Robert
Classification and Terminology
World Health Organization (WHO)
20 Avenue Appia
1211 Geneva

LOKUHETTY, Dilani
University of Colombo
25 Kynsey Road
Colombo 00800

ROUS, Brian
Public Health England
Victoria House, Capital Park
Fulbourn, Cambridge CB21 5XA

WATANABE, Reiko
National Cancer Center Hospital East
6-5-1 Kashiwanoha, Kashiwa-shi
Chiba 277-8577

WHITE, Valerie A.
International Agency for Research on Cancer
150 Cours Albert Thomas
69372 Lyon

ZNAOR, Ariana
International Agency for Research on Cancer
150 Cours Albert Thomas
69372 Lyon

Sources

Note: For any figure, table, or box not listed below, the original source is this volume; the suggested source citation is

WHO Classification of Tumours Editorial Board. Central nervous system tumours. Lyon (France): International Agency for Research on Cancer; 2021. (WHO classification of tumours series, 5th ed.; vol. 6). https://publications.iarc.fr/601.

Figures

2.01	Martin Sill, Hopp Children's Cancer Center Heidelberg (KiTZ) and German Cancer Research Center (DKFZ), Heidelberg, and Pfister SM, von Deimling A
2.02	Martin Sill, Hopp Children's Cancer Center Heidelberg (KiTZ) and German Cancer Research Center (DKFZ), Heidelberg, and Pfister SM, von Deimling A
2.03	Martin Sill, Hopp Children's Cancer Center Heidelberg (KiTZ) and German Cancer Research Center (DKFZ), Heidelberg, and Pfister SM, von Deimling A
2.04	Martin Sill, Hopp Children's Cancer Center Heidelberg (KiTZ) and German Cancer Research Center (DKFZ), Heidelberg, and Pfister SM, von Deimling A
2.05	Martin Sill, Hopp Children's Cancer Center Heidelberg (KiTZ) and German Cancer Research Center (DKFZ), Heidelberg, and Pfister SM, von Deimling A
2.06	Martin Sill, Hopp Children's Cancer Center Heidelberg (KiTZ) and German Cancer Research Center (DKFZ), Heidelberg, and Pfister SM, von Deimling A
2.07A,B	Kleinschmidt-DeMasters BK
2.08A,B	Kleinschmidt-DeMasters BK
2.08C,D	Cimino PJ
2.09A,B,E,G,H	Brat DJ
2.09C,D	Kleinschmidt-DeMasters BK
2.09F	Cimino PJ
2.10A	Cimino PJ
2.10B–D	Kleinschmidt-DeMasters BK
2.11A–D	Perry A
2.12A–C	Perry A
2.13	Perry A
2.14A,B	Cimino PJ
2.15A–D	Van Den Bent MJ

2.16	Reifenberger G
2.17	Adapted, with permission, from: Suvà ML, Tirosh I. The glioma stem cell model in the era of single-cell genomics. Cancer Cell. 2020 May 11;37(5):630–6. PMID:32396858
2.18A,B	Brat DJ
2.19A–C	Yip S
2.20A	Brat DJ
2.20B,E	Reifenberger G
2.20C	© Yoichi Nakazato Louis DN, Ohgaki H, Wiestler OD, et al., editors. WHO classification of tumours of the central nervous system. Lyon (France): International Agency for Research on Cancer; 2016. (WHO classification of tumours series, 4th rev. ed.; vol. 1). https://publications.iarc.fr/543.
2.20D	© Scott R. VandenBerg Louis DN, Ohgaki H, Wiestler OD, et al., editors. WHO classification of tumours of the central nervous system. Lyon (France): International Agency for Research on Cancer; 2016. (WHO classification of tumours series, 4th rev. ed.; vol. 1). https://publications.iarc.fr/543.
2.21A	Reifenberger G
2.21B–D	© Yoichi Nakazato Louis DN, Ohgaki H, Wiestler OD, et al., editors. WHO classification of tumours of the central nervous system. Lyon (France): International Agency for Research on Cancer; 2016. (WHO classification of tumours series, 4th rev. ed.; vol. 1). https://publications.iarc.fr/543.
2.22A–C	Yip S
2.23	Yip S
2.24A,B	Yip S
2.25	Van Den Bent MJ
2.26A,B	Perry A
2.27A–C	Soffietti R
2.28	Julie Laffy, Weizmann Institute of Science, Rehovot, and

	Suvà ML
2.29	Capper D
2.30	Louis DN, Ohgaki H, Wiestler OD, et al., editors. WHO classification of tumours of the central nervous system. Lyon (France): International Agency for Research on Cancer; 2016. (WHO classification of tumours series, 4th rev. ed.; vol. 1). https://publications.iarc.fr/543. and Suvà ML, Riggi N, Bernstein BE. Epigenetic reprogramming in cancer. Science. 2013 Mar 29;339(6127):1567–70. PMID:23539597
2.31A,B	© Paul Kleihues Louis DN, Ohgaki H, Wiestler OD, et al., editors. WHO classification of tumours of the central nervous system. Lyon (France): International Agency for Research on Cancer; 2016. (WHO classification of tumours series, 4th rev. ed.; vol. 1). https://publications.iarc.fr/543.
2.32A–C	Perry A
2.32D,E	Horbinski CM
2.33A–D	Perry A
2.34A–D	Perry A
2.35A,B	Perry A
2.36A–E	Perry A
2.37A–C	Perry A
2.38A–E	Perry A
2.39A–D	Perry A
2.40	Perry A
2.41	Capper D
2.42A,B	Blümcke I
2.42C,D	Perry A
2.43A–D	Perry A
2.44	Perry A
2.45A–C	Ellison DW
2.46A,C,D	Perry A
2.46B	Ellison DW
2.47	Rosenblum MK
2.48A–C,E	Rosenblum MK
2.48D	Perry A
2.49A,C	Perry A
2.49B	Rosenblum MK
2.50A–C	Giannini C

2.51A–D Giannini C
2.52A,B Ellison DW
2.53A–C Giannini C
2.54A–D Varlet P
2.55A,C–E Varlet P
2.55B Leske H
2.56A–D Varlet P
2.57A–E Solomon DA
2.58 Leske H
2.59A,B Leske H
2.60A,B Leske H
2.61 Varlet P
2.62A–D Varlet P
2.63 Capper D
2.64 Capper D
2.65 Capper D
2.66A,B Hawkins CE
2.67A–C Hawkins CE
2.68A,B Tihan T
2.69A–C,E,F Tihan T
2.69D Perry A
2.70A–C Tihan T
2.71A,B Perry A
2.72A,B Tihan T
2.73A Perry A
2.73B Tihan T
2.74A–D Perry A
2.75 Varlet P
2.76A Georg Bohner, Institute of Neuroradiology, on behalf of Charité – Universitätsmedizin Berlin, Berlin
2.76B Winfried Brenner, Department of Nuclear Medicine, on behalf of Charité – Universitätsmedizin Berlin, Berlin
2.77A–D Capper D
2.78A–D Capper D
2.79 Capper D
2.80 Philipp Jurmeister, Institute of Pathology, Ludwig-Maximilians-Universität München, Munich
2.81 Giannini C
2.82A–C Giannini C
2.83A–D Giannini C
2.84A–C Giannini C
2.85A–C Giannini C
2.86A–C Giannini C
2.87A–E Giannini C
2.88 Giannini C
2.89 Rachael A. Vaubel, Department of Laboratory Medicine and Pathology, Mayo Clinic, Rochester MN
2.90A,B © David A. Ornan
Louis DN, Ohgaki H, Wiestler OD, et al., editors. WHO classification of tumours of the central nervous system. Lyon (France): International Agency for Research on Cancer; 2016. (WHO classification of tumours series, 4th rev. ed.; vol. 1). https://publications.iarc.fr/543.
2.91A,B Rodriguez FJ
2.92A–C Perry A
2.93A,B,D Rodriguez FJ
2.93C Lopes MBS
2.94A,B Kleinschmidt-DeMasters BK
2.95A,E Perry A
2.95B–D,F Solomon DA

2.96A Kleinschmidt-DeMasters BK
2.96B Perry A
2.96C Solomon DA
2.97A,B Perry A
2.98A,B,D Rosenblum MK
2.98C,E Perry A
2.99A,B Perry A
2.100A Rosenblum MK
2.100B,C Perry A
2.101 Blümcke I
2.102A–C Solomon DA
2.103A © Paul Kleihues
Louis DN, Ohgaki H, Wiestler OD, et al., editors. WHO classification of tumours of the central nervous system. Lyon (France): International Agency for Research on Cancer; 2016. (WHO classification of tumours series, 4th rev. ed.; vol. 1). https://publications.iarc.fr/543.
2.103B Blümcke I
2.104A–H Solomon DA
2.105A–D Solomon DA
2.106A–C Giannini C
2.107A,B Giannini C
2.108A,B Giannini C
2.109A–F Simona Gaudino, Radiology and Neuroradiology Unit, Fondazione Policlinico Universitario "Agostino Gemelli" IRCCS, Università Cattolica del Sacro Cuore, Rome
2.110A,B Figarella-Branger D
2.111A–C Figarella-Branger D
2.112A–D Figarella-Branger D
2.113 Varlet P
2.114A,B László Solymosi, Department of Neuroradiology, University Hospital Bonn, Venusberg-Campus, Bonn
2.115A,B Varlet P
2.115C Pietsch T
2.116A,B Pietsch T
2.117A–C Sahm F
2.117D,E Adapted, with permission, from: Deng MY, Sill M, Sturm D, et al. Diffuse glioneuronal tumour with oligodendroglioma-like features and nuclear clusters (DGONC) - a molecularly defined glioneuronal CNS tumour class displaying recurrent monosomy 14. Neuropathol Appl Neurobiol. 2020 Aug;46(5):422–30. PMID:31867747
2.118A–C Sahm F
2.119 Reprinted, with permission, from: Deng MY, Sill M, Sturm D, et al. Diffuse glioneuronal tumour with oligodendroglioma-like features and nuclear clusters (DGONC) - a molecularly defined glioneuronal CNS tumour class displaying recurrent monosomy 14. Neuropathol Appl Neurobiol. 2020 Aug;46(5):422–30. PMID:31867747

2.120A,B Komori T
2.121A–C Rosenblum MK
2.122A,B Rosenblum MK
2.123 Varlet P
2.124A–C Maria T. Schmook, Department of Biomedical Imaging and Image-Guided Therapy, Division of Neuroradiology and Musculoskeletal Radiology, Medical University of Vienna / Vienna General Hospital, Vienna
2.125A–C Hainfellner JA
2.126A,C Rosenblum MK
2.126B Hainfellner JA
2.127A Adapted, with permission, from: Lucas CG, Villanueva-Meyer JE, Whipple N, et al. Myxoid glioneuronal tumor, PDGFRA p.K385-mutant: clinical, radiologic, and histopathologic features. Brain Pathol. 2020 May;30(3):479–94. PMID:31609499
2.127B Solomon DA
2.128A,B Solomon DA
2.129 Adapted, with permission, from: Lucas CG, Villanueva-Meyer JE, Whipple N, et al. Myxoid glioneuronal tumor, PDGFRA p.K385-mutant: clinical, radiologic, and histopathologic features. Brain Pathol. 2020 May;30(3):479–94. PMID:31609499
2.130A,B Perry A
2.131A–D Perry A
2.132A,B Perry A
2.133 Perry A
2.134 Perry A
2.135 Rosenblum MK
2.136A Rosenblum MK
2.136B,C Komori T
2.137A,B Rosenblum MK
2.138A–D Rosenblum MK
2.139A–D Park SH
2.140A,B Park SH
2.141A,B Park SH
2.142A–F Park SH
2.143A–D Park SH
2.144A–D Park SH
2.145A–D Park SH
2.146A–D Sievers P
2.147A,B Sievers P
2.148A–C Timothy J. Kaufmann, Department of Radiology, Mayo Clinic, Rochester MN
2.149A–D Rosenblum MK
2.150 Sievers P
2.151 Ellison DW
2.152 Ellison DW
2.153A Ellison DW
2.153B Rudà R
2.154A–D Ellison DW
2.155A–D Ellison DW
2.156A,B Rudà R
2.157A,B Pietsch T
2.158A Ellison DW
2.158B Pietsch T
2.159 Pajtler KW
2.160A,B Pietsch T
2.161A,B Pietsch T
2.162 Perry A

2.163 Rosenblum MK
2.164A,C–F Perry A
2.164B Rosenblum MK
2.165A Ellison DW
2.165B Rosenblum MK
2.165C,D Perry A
2.166 Ramaswamy V
2.167A,B Ellison DW
2.168A Rosenblum MK
2.168B Venneti S
2.169 Venneti S
2.170A Ellison DW
2.170B Venneti S
2.171 László Solymosi, Department of Neuroradiology, University Hospital Bonn, Venusberg-Campus, Bonn
2.172 Pietsch T
2.173A,B Pietsch T
2.174 Giannini C
2.175A,B Giannini C
2.176A Reuss DE
2.176B–D Giannini C
2.177 Robert B. Jenkins, Department of Laboratory Medicine and Pathology, Mayo Clinic, Rochester MN
2.178 Rosenblum MK
2.179A,B Rosenblum MK
2.180 Rosenblum MK
2.181 Rosenblum MK
2.182 Rosenblum MK
2.183A–C Rosenblum MK

3.01A Neuroradiological Reference Center for the pediatric brain tumor (HIT) studies of the German Society of Pediatric Oncology and Hematology, Faculty of Medicine, University Augsburg, Augsburg; Annika Stock, Department of Neuroradiology, University Hospital Würzburg, Würzburg; Brigitte Bison, Department of Diagnostic and Interventional Neuroradiology, Faculty of Medicine, University Augsburg, Augsburg
3.01B László Solymosi, Department of Neuroradiology, University Hospital Bonn, Venusberg-Campus, Bonn
3.01C Martina Messing-Jünger, Department of Pediatric Neurosurgery, Asklepios Children's Hospital, Sankt Augustin
3.02A,C,D Pietsch T
3.02B Paulus W
3.03 Paulus W
3.04A,B Pietsch T
3.05A,B László Solymosi, Department of Neuroradiology, University Hospital Bonn, Venusberg-Campus, Bonn
3.06 Louis DN
3.07A,B,D Pietsch T
3.07C © Paul Kleihues
Louis DN, Ohgaki H, Wiestler OD, et al., editors. WHO classification of tumours of the central nervous system. Lyon

(France): International Agency for Research on Cancer; 2016. (WHO classification of tumours series, 4th rev. ed.; vol. 1). https://publications.iarc.fr/543.
3.08A–C Pietsch T
3.09 Pietsch T

4.01 Pfister SM
4.02 Ellison DW
4.03 Ellison DW
4.04 Zoltán Patay, Diagnostic Imaging Department, St. Jude Children's Research Hospital, Memphis TN
4.05A–C Ellison DW
4.06 Hawkins CE
4.07 Hawkins CE
4.08A,B © Monika Warmuth-Metz
Louis DN, Ohgaki H, Wiestler OD, et al., editors. WHO classification of tumours of the central nervous system. Lyon (France): International Agency for Research on Cancer; 2016. (WHO classification of tumours series, 4th rev. ed.; vol. 1). https://publications.iarc.fr/543.
4.08C Perry A
4.09A,B © François Doz
Louis DN, Ohgaki H, Wiestler OD, et al., editors. WHO classification of tumours of the central nervous system. Lyon (France): International Agency for Research on Cancer; 2016. (WHO classification of tumours series, 4th rev. ed.; vol. 1). https://publications.iarc.fr/543.
4.09C © Maria Luisa Garrè
Louis DN, Ohgaki H, Wiestler OD, et al., editors. WHO classification of tumours of the central nervous system. Lyon (France): International Agency for Research on Cancer; 2016. (WHO classification of tumours series, 4th rev. ed.; vol. 1). https://publications.iarc.fr/543.
4.10A,B Giangaspero F
4.10C © Paul Kleihues
Louis DN, Ohgaki H, Wiestler OD, et al., editors. WHO classification of tumours of the central nervous system. Lyon (France): International Agency for Research on Cancer; 2016. (WHO classification of tumours series, 4th rev. ed.; vol. 1). https://publications.iarc.fr/543.
4.11A,B © Paul Kleihues
Louis DN, Ohgaki H, Wiestler OD, et al., editors. WHO classification of tumours of the central nervous system. Lyon (France): International Agency for Research on Cancer; 2016. (WHO classification of tumours series, 4th rev. ed.; vol. 1). https://publications.iarc.fr/543.
4.11C © Lucy Balian Rorke-Adams
Louis DN, Ohgaki H, Wiestler OD, et al., editors. WHO

classification of tumours of the central nervous system. Lyon (France): International Agency for Research on Cancer; 2016. (WHO classification of tumours series, 4th rev. ed.; vol. 1). https://publications.iarc.fr/543.
4.12A,B Ellison DW
4.13A–D Pietsch T
4.13E Perry A
4.13F Giangaspero F
4.14A,B Giangaspero F
4.14C,D Ellison DW
4.15A,B Ellison DW
4.16 Wesseling P
4.17 Adapted, with permission from Oxford University Press, from: Ho B, Johann PD, Grabovska Y, et al. Molecular subgrouping of atypical teratoid/rhabdoid tumors-a reinvestigation and current consensus. Neuro Oncol. 2020 May 15;22(5):613–24. PMID:31889194
4.18A,B Gregor Kasprian, Department of Biomedical Imaging and Image-Guided Therapy, Medical University of Vienna, Vienna
4.19 Judkins AR
4.20A–D Haberler C
4.21A,C,D Haberler C
4.21B Hasselblatt M
4.22 Haberler C
4.23 Hasselblatt M
4.24A,B Hasselblatt M
4.25A–D Korshunov A
4.26 Korshunov A
4.27 Korshunov A
4.28A–C Korshunov A
4.29A,B Anna Tietze, Department of Radiation Oncology, on behalf of Charité – Universitätsmedizin Berlin, Berlin
4.30A Pietsch T
4.30B Perry A
4.31A–D Pietsch T
4.32A,B Solomon DA
4.33A Haberler C
4.33B–F Solomon DA
4.34A Haberler C
4.34B–D Solomon DA
4.35 Wesseling P
4.36A,B Wesseling P

5.01 Anthony Pak Yin Liu, Department of Paediatrics & Adolescent Medicine, Queen Mary Hospital, Hong Kong SAR
5.02 Anthony Pak Yin Liu, Department of Paediatrics & Adolescent Medicine, Queen Mary Hospital, Hong Kong SAR
5.03 Vasiljevic A
5.04A–C Vasiljevic A
5.05A–C Vasiljevic A
5.06 Vasiljevic A
5.07A–D Vasiljevic A
5.08A,B Vasiljevic A

5.09A,B	Vasiljevic A
5.10A–C	Vasiljevic A
5.11A,B	© Michelle Fèvre-Montange Louis DN, Ohgaki H, Wiestler OD, et al., editors. WHO classification of tumours of the central nervous system. Lyon (France): International Agency for Research on Cancer; 2016. (WHO classification of tumours series, 4th rev. ed.; vol. 1). https://publications.iarc.fr/543.
5.12A–C	Figarella-Branger D
5.13A–D	Vasiljevic A
5.14	Vasiljevic A
5.15A,B	Hasselblatt M
5.16	Hasselblatt M
6.01A,B	Perry A
6.02A,B	Perry A
6.03A–D	Perry A
6.04	Perry A
6.05A,B	Jo VY
6.06	Perry A
6.07A,B	Rodriguez FJ
6.08A,B	Rodriguez FJ
6.09A–C	Rodriguez FJ
6.10A,B	Rodriguez FJ
6.11A,B	Rodriguez FJ
6.12A–C	Perry A
6.13A–C	Perry A
6.14A–C	Jason L. Hornick, Department of Pathology, Brigham and Women's Hospital, Harvard Medical School, Boston MA
6.15A,B	Reuss DE
6.16	Reuss DE
6.17A–C	Reuss DE
6.18A,B	Jo VY
6.18C,D	Reuss DE
6.19A,B	Hirose T
6.20A–C	Hirose T
6.21A–C	Jo VY
6.22	Hirose T
6.23	Kleinschmidt-DeMasters BK
6.24A,B	Francesco Carletti, Lysholm Department of Neuroradiology, National Hospital for Neurology and Neurosurgery, London
6.25A–D	Brandner S
6.26A,B	Brandner S
7.01A,B	Perry A
7.02A,B	Perry A
7.03	Claus EB; Figure prepared courtesy of the Central Brain Tumor Registry of the United States (CBTRUS)
7.04A–C	Perry A
7.05	Perry A
7.06	Perry A
7.07A,B	Perry A
7.08A,B	Perry A
7.09	Perry A
7.10A,B	Perry A
7.11A,B	Perry A
7.12A,B	Perry A
7.13A,B	Perry A
7.14	Perry A
7.15	Perry A
7.16A,B	Perry A
7.17A–D	Perry A

7.18A–C	Perry A
7.19A,B	Perry A
7.20A–E	Perry A
7.21A,B	Perry A
7.22A–E	Perry A
7.23A	Sahm F
7.23B	Perry A
7.24	Mawrin C; Adapted, with permission, from: Louis DN, Ohgaki H, Wiestler OD, et al., editors. WHO classification of tumours of the central nervous system. Lyon (France): International Agency for Research on Cancer; 2016. (WHO classification of tumours series, 4th rev. ed.; vol. 1). https://publications.iarc.fr/543. and Mawrin C, Kalamarides M. Meningiomas. In: Karajannis M, Zagzag D, editors. Molecular pathology of nervous system tumors. New York (NY): Springer; 2015. (Molecular pathology library; vol. 8). https://doi.org/10.1007/978-1-4939-1830-0_17
8.01A–C	Giannini C
8.02A–D	Giannini C
8.03A–D	Giannini C
8.04A,B	Giannini C
8.04C,D	Perry A
8.05A–C	Giannini C
8.06A,B	Maria T. Schmook, Department of Biomedical Imaging and Image-Guided Therapy, Division of Neuroradiology and Musculoskeletal Radiology, Medical University of Vienna / Vienna General Hospital, Vienna
8.06C,D	Hainfellner JA
8.07A,B	Hainfellner JA
8.08A	Maria T. Schmook, Department of Biomedical Imaging and Image-Guided Therapy, Division of Neuroradiology and Musculoskeletal Radiology, Medical University of Vienna / Vienna General Hospital, Vienna
8.08B–D	Hainfellner JA
8.09A	Maria T. Schmook, Department of Biomedical Imaging and Image-Guided Therapy, Division of Neuroradiology and Musculoskeletal Radiology, Medical University of Vienna / Vienna General Hospital, Vienna
8.09B–D	Hainfellner JA
8.10A,B	Maria T. Schmook, Department of Biomedical Imaging and Image-Guided Therapy, Division of Neuroradiology and Musculoskeletal Radiology, Medical University of Vienna / Vienna General Hospital, Vienna

8.10C	Hainfellner JA
8.11A–C	Tihan T
8.12A,B	Zagzag D
8.13A,B	Tihan T
8.13C,D	Fanburg-Smith JC
8.14A,B	Tihan T
8.14C,D	Fanburg-Smith JC
8.15	Dry SM
8.16A,B	Dry SM
8.17	Dry SM
8.18A–D	Rudzinski ER
8.19	Kleinschmidt-DeMasters BK
8.20A–D	Perry A
8.21A–I	Perry A
8.22	Perry A
8.23A,B	Anna Tietze, Department of Radiation Oncology, on behalf of Charité – Universitätsmedizin Berlin, Berlin
8.24A,B	Yoshida A
8.25A–C	Yoshida A
8.26	Orr BA
8.27	Sturm D, Orr BA, Toprak UH, et al. New brain tumor entities emerge from molecular classification of CNS-PNETs. Cell. 2016 Feb 25;164(5):1060–72. PMID:26919435. Copyright 2016, with permission from Elsevier.
8.28	Solomon DA
8.29A	Julieann C. Lee, University of California, San Francisco (UCSF), San Francisco CA
8.29B	Solomon DA
8.30A–C	Solomon DA
8.31A–C	Solomon DA
8.32A,B	Solomon DA
8.33A,B	Solomon DA
8.34A–D	Seung Hong Choi, Department of Radiology, Seoul National University Hospital, Seoul
8.35	Perry A
8.36A–D	Perry A
8.37A,D,E	Perry A
8.37B,C	Yoshida A
8.38	Park SH
8.39	Park SH
8.40A–C	Osborn AG
8.41A	Bouvier C
8.41B	Pekmezci M
8.42	Pekmezci M
8.43A,B	Thomas Borges, Department of Radiology, University of Colorado Anschutz Medical Campus, Aurora CO
8.44A,B	Thomas Borges, Department of Radiology, University of Colorado Anschutz Medical Campus, Aurora CO
8.45A,B	Kleinschmidt-DeMasters BK
8.46A,C	Tirabosco R
8.46B	Varlet P
8.47A,D	Nielsen GP
8.47B,C	Varlet P
9.01A,B	Küsters-Vandevelde HV
9.02A,C	Adapted and reprinted, with permission from the American Association for Cancer Research, from:

Pedersen M, Küsters-Vandevelde HVN, Viros A, et al. Primary melanoma of the CNS in children is driven by congenital expression of oncogenic NRAS in melanocytes. Cancer Discov. 2013 Apr;3(4):458–69. PMID:23303902

9.02B — Reyes-Múgica M
9.03A,B — Küsters-Vandevelde HV
9.04A–C — Wesseling P
9.05A–C — Küsters-Vandevelde HV
9.06A–C — Clayton A. Wiley & Geoffrey Murdoch, Division of Neuropathology, UPMC Presbyterian, Pittsburgh PA, and Reyes-Múgica M
9.07A,B — Kölsche C
9.08A,B — Küsters-Vandevelde HV
9.09A,D — Kölsche C
9.09B — Gessi M
9.09C — Küsters-Vandevelde HV
9.10 — Kölsche C
9.11 — Kölsche C

10.01A,B — Soffietti R
10.02 — Deckert M
10.03A–C — Chan JKC
10.04A–F — Deckert M
10.05 — Reifenberger G
10.06 — © Paul Kleihues
Louis DN, Ohgaki H, Wiestler OD, et al., editors. WHO classification of tumours of the central nervous system. Lyon (France): International Agency for Research on Cancer; 2016. (WHO classification of tumours series, 4th rev. ed.; vol. 1). https://publications.iarc.fr/543.
10.07 — Deckert M
10.08A,B — Deckert M
10.09A–C — Deckert M
10.10A–D — Deckert M
10.11 — Perry A
10.12A,B — Perry A
10.13A–D — Ferry JA
10.14A–C — Ferry JA
10.15 — Ferry JA
10.16A,B — Ferry JA
10.17A–D — Deckert M
10.18A,B — Osborn AG
10.19A–D — Perry A
10.20 — Perry A
10.21A–C — Osborn AG
10.22A,C,D — Perry A
10.22B — Chan JKC
10.23A–D — Osborn AG
10.24 — Perry A
10.25 — Perry A
10.26A,B — Osborn AG
10.27A,D — Chan JKC
10.27B — Perry A
10.27C — Solomon DA
10.28 — Perry A
10.29A–C — Chan JKC
10.29D — Perry A

11.01 — Neuroradiological Reference Center for the pediatric brain tumor (HIT) studies of the German Society of Pediatric Oncology and Hematology, Faculty of Medicine, University Augsburg, Augsburg; Annika Stock, Department of Neuroradiology, University Hospital Würzburg, Würzburg; Brigitte Bison, Department of Diagnostic and Interventional Neuroradiology, Faculty of Medicine, University Augsburg, Augsburg
11.02A,B — László Solymosi, Department of Neuroradiology, University Hospital Bonn, Venusberg-Campus, Bonn
11.03 — Juan E. Olvera-Rabiela (deceased), and Rosenblum MK
11.04 — © Yoichi Nakazato
Louis DN, Ohgaki H, Wiestler OD, et al., editors. WHO classification of tumours of the central nervous system. Lyon (France): International Agency for Research on Cancer; 2016. (WHO classification of tumours series, 4th rev. ed.; vol. 1). https://publications.iarc.fr/543.
11.05A,B — Rosenblum MK
11.06 — Pietsch T
11.07A,B,D — Pietsch T
11.07C — Rosenblum MK
11.08A–F — Pietsch T
11.09A–C — Pietsch T
11.10A–E — Pietsch T
11.11A–C — Pietsch T
11.12 — Pietsch T

12.01 — Pfister SM
12.02A,B — Santagata S
12.03 — Santagata S
12.04A,B — Kleinschmidt-DeMasters BK
12.04C,D — Santagata S
12.05 — Kleinschmidt-DeMasters BK
12.06 — Kleinschmidt-DeMasters BK
12.07A — Kleinschmidt-DeMasters BK
12.07B — Santagata S
12.08 — Solomon DA
12.09A–C — Santagata S
12.09D — Kleinschmidt-DeMasters BK
12.10 — Santagata S
12.11 — Kleinschmidt-DeMasters BK
12.12A,C — Lopes MBS
12.12B,D — Kleinschmidt-DeMasters BK
12.13 — David A. Ornan, Department of Radiology, University of Virginia, Charlottesville VA
12.14A,B,D — Shibuya M
12.14C — Lopes MBS
12.15 — David A. Ornan, Department of Radiology, University of Virginia, Charlottesville VA
12.16A,C,D — Kleinschmidt-DeMasters BK
12.16B — Lopes MBS
12.17A,B — David A. Ornan, Department of Radiology, University of Virginia, Charlottesville VA
12.18A–E — Reprinted, with permission from Elsevier, from: Neou M, Villa C, Armignacco R, et al. Pangenomic classification of pituitary neuroendocrine tumors. Cancer Cell. 2020 Jan 13;37(1):123–34.e5. PMID:31883967. Copyright 2020.
12.19 — Adapted, with permission from Springer Nature, from: Asa SL, Mete O, Cusimano MD, et al. Pituitary neuroendocrine tumors: a model for neuroendocrine tumor classification. Mod Pathol. 2021 Sep;34(9):1634–50. PMID:34017065. Copyright 2021.
12.20A–F — Mete O
12.21A–F — Lopes MBS
12.22 — Asa SL
12.23 — Asa SL
12.24 — Lopes MBS
12.25A–F — Mete O

13.01 — Wesseling P
13.02A,B — Soffietti R
13.03A,B — Mirthe de Boer, Department of Pathology, University Medical Center Utrecht, Utrecht
13.04A,B — Soffietti R
13.05 — Mittelbronn MGA
13.06 — Mirthe de Boer, Department of Pathology, University Medical Center Utrecht, Utrecht

14.01A,B — Legius E
14.02A–D — Rodriguez FJ
14.03 — Schuhmann MU
14.04A–C — Perry A
14.05A — Schuhmann MU
14.05B,C — Stemmer-Rachamimov AO
14.06A,B — Schuhmann MU
14.06C,D — Perry A
14.07A,B — Stemmer-Rachamimov AO
14.07C — Perry A
14.08 — © Hamid Salamipour
Louis DN, Ohgaki H, Wiestler OD, et al., editors. WHO classification of tumours of the central nervous system. Lyon (France): International Agency for Research on Cancer; 2016. (WHO classification of tumours series, 4th rev. ed.; vol. 1). https://publications.iarc.fr/543.
14.09 — Rodriguez FJ
14.10A–C — Perry A
14.11A,B — Perry A
14.12A — Sven Gläsker, Aram Bani, and colleagues, Praxis für Neurochirurgie, Singen
14.12B — Jan-Helge Klingler, Department of Neurosurgery, Medical Center – University of Freiburg, Freiburg
14.12C — Christian A. Taschner, Department of Neuroradiology, Medical Center – University of Freiburg, Freiburg
14.12D — Hansjürgen Agostini, Retinology Section, Department of Ophthalmology, Medical Center – University of Freiburg, Freiburg
14.12E — Cordula A. Jilg, Department of Urology, Medical Center –

	University of Freiburg, Freiburg
14.12F,H	Tobias Krauß, Department of Radiology, Medical Center – University of Freiburg, Freiburg
14.12G	Martin K. Walz, Department of Surgery, Kliniken Essen-Mitte, Essen
14.12I	Juri Ruf, Department of Nuclear Medicine, Medical Center – University of Freiburg, Freiburg
14.13A–C	Plate KH, and Susanne Berger, graphical-abstracts.com
14.14A,B	Perry A
14.15A,B	David A. Ornan, Department of Radiology, University of Virginia, Charlottesville VA
14.16A	Santosh V
14.16B	Giannini C
14.17A–C	Lopes MBS
14.18A–B	Lopes MBS
14.19	Lopes MBS
14.20	Reprinted, with permission from Elsevier, from: Zhou R, Xu A, Gingold J, et al. Li-Fraumeni syndrome disease model: a platform to develop precision cancer therapy targeting oncogenic p53. Trends Pharmacol Sci. 2017 Oct;38(10):908–27. PMID:28818333. Copyright 2017.
14.21A,B	Tabori U
14.22A–D	Abedalthagafi MS
14.23A,B	Solomon DA
14.24	Solomon DA
14.25	Varlet P
14.26A,B	Legius E
14.27	Shereen Ezzat, Princess Margaret Cancer Centre, Toronto ON
14.28	Reprinted from: Asa SL, Ezzat S, Mete O. The diagnosis and clinical significance of paragangliomas in unusual locations. J Clin Med. 2018 Sep 13;7(9):280. PMID:30217041
14.29A–D	Asa SL
14.30	Lloyd RV
14.31A–C	Asa SL
14.32A–D	Gill AJ
14.33	Eagle RC Jr
14.34A,B	Santagata S
14.35A,B	Adapted, with permission from Oxford University Press, from: Shankar GM, Santagata S. BAP1 mutations in high-grade meningioma: implications for patient care. Neuro Oncol. 2017 Oct 19;19(11):1447–56. PMID:28482042
14.36A,B	Adapted, with permission from Oxford University Press, from: Shankar GM, Santagata S. BAP1 mutations in high-grade meningioma: implications for patient care. Neuro Oncol. 2017 Oct 19;19(11):1447–56. PMID:28482042
14.37	Solomon DA
14.38A–D	Solomon DA
14.39	Solomon DA
14.40	Waszak SM
14.41	Korshunov A

Tables

1.01	Louis DN
1.02	Adapted from: WHO Classification of Tumours Editorial Board. Breast tumours. Lyon (France): International Agency for Research on Cancer; 2019. (WHO classification of tumours series, 5th ed.; vol. 2). https://publications.iarc.fr/581.
2.01	Peferoen LAN
2.02	Capper D
2.03	Louis DN, Ohgaki H, Wiestler OD, et al., editors. WHO classification of tumours of the central nervous system. Lyon (France): International Agency for Research on Cancer; 2016. (WHO classification of tumours series, 4th rev. ed.; vol. 1). https://publications.iarc.fr/543. and Adapted from: Collins VP, Jones DT, Giannini C. Pilocytic astrocytoma: pathology, molecular mechanisms and markers. Acta Neuropathol. 2015 Jun;129(6):775–88. PMID:25792358
2.04	Capper D
2.05	Blümcke I
4.01	Ellison DW
5.01	White VA
6.01	Adapted, with permission from Elsevier, from: Miettinen MM, Antonescu CR, Fletcher CDM, et al. Histopathologic evaluation of atypical neurofibromatous tumors and their transformation into malignant peripheral nerve sheath tumor in patients with neurofibromatosis 1-a consensus overview. Hum Pathol. 2017 Sep;67:1–10. PMID:28551330
8.01	Perry A
8.02	Varlet P
10.01	Deckert M
11.01	White VA
11.02	Pietsch T
12.01	Asa SL WHO Classification of Tumours Editorial Board. Endocrine and neuroendocrine tumours. Lyon (France): International Agency for Research on Cancer; forthcoming. (WHO classification of tumours series, 5th ed.). https://publications.iarc.fr/.
12.02	Lopes MBS

13.01	Mittelbronn MGA
14.01	Perry A
14.02	Reprinted from: Louis DN, Ohgaki H, Wiestler OD, et al., editors. WHO classification of tumours of the central nervous system. Lyon (France): International Agency for Research on Cancer; 2016. (WHO classification of tumours series, 4th rev. ed.; vol. 1). https://publications.iarc.fr/543.
14.03	Reprinted from: Louis DN, Ohgaki H, Wiestler OD, et al., editors. WHO classification of tumours of the central nervous system. Lyon (France): International Agency for Research on Cancer; 2016. (WHO classification of tumours series, 4th rev. ed.; vol. 1). https://publications.iarc.fr/543.
14.05	Orr BA
14.06	WHO Classification of Tumours Editorial Board. Female genital tumours. Lyon (France): International Agency for Research on Cancer; 2020. (WHO classification of tumours series, 5th ed.; vol. 4). https://publications.iarc.fr/592. and Adapted, with permission from Springer Nature, from Nature Reviews Cancer: Foulkes WD, Priest JR, Duchaine TF. DICER1: mutations, microRNAs and mechanisms. Nat Rev Cancer. 2014 Oct;14(10):662–72. PMID:25176334. Copyright 2014.
14.07	Asa SL
14.08	Santagata S

Boxes

1.01	Louis DN and Ellison DW
1.02	Louis DN
1.03	Louis DN
7.01	Louis DN
7.02	Louis DN
14.02	Stemmer-Rachamimov AO
14.06	Adapted, with permission from Elsevier, from: Northrup H, Krueger DA; International Tuberous Sclerosis Complex Consensus Group. Tuberous sclerosis complex diagnostic criteria update: recommendations of the 2012 International Tuberous Sclerosis Complex Consensus Conference. Pediatr Neurol. 2013 Oct;49(4):243–54. PMID:24053982
14.08	Eberhart CG
14.13	WHO Classification of Tumours Editorial Board. Thoracic tumours. Lyon (France): International Agency for Research on Cancer; 2021.

(WHO classification of tumours series, 5th ed.; vol. 5). https://publications.iarc.fr/595.
and
Stratakis CA, Kirschner LS, Carney JA. Clinical and molecular features of the Carney complex: diagnostic criteria and recommendations for patient evaluation. J Clin Endocrinol Metab. 2001 Sep;86(9):4041–6. PMID:11549623. By permission of Oxford University Press.

14.14   WHO Classification of Tumours Editorial Board. Thoracic tumours. Lyon (France): International Agency for Research on Cancer; 2021. (WHO classification of tumours series, 5th ed.; vol. 5). https://publications.iarc.fr/595.
and
Travis WD, Brambilla E, Burke AP, et al., editors. WHO classification of tumours of the lung, pleura, thymus and heart. Lyon (France): International Agency for Research on Cancer; 2015. (WHO classification of tumours series, 4th ed.; vol. 7). https://publications.iarc.fr/17.
and
Adapted, with permission from Oxford University Press, from: Stratakis CA, Kirschner LS, Carney JA. Clinical and molecular features of the Carney complex: diagnostic criteria and recommendations for patient evaluation. J Clin Endocrinol Metab. 2001 Sep;86(9):4041–6. PMID:11549623

Images on the cover

Top left	Fig. 4.08A: © Monika Warmuth-Metz Louis DN, Ohgaki H, Wiestler OD, et al., editors. WHO classification of tumours of the central nervous system. Lyon (France): International Agency for Research on Cancer; 2016. (WHO classification of tumours series, 4th rev. ed.; vol. 1). https://publications.iarc.fr/543.
Middle left	Fig. 2.32E: Horbinski CM
Bottom left	Fig. 2.28: Julie Laffy, Weizmann Institute of Science, Rehovot, and Suvà ML
Top centre	Fig. 3.06: Louis DN
Middle centre	Fig. 5.05C: Vasiljevic A
Bottom centre	Fig. 2.24A: Yip S
Top right	Fig. 5.12C: Figarella-Branger D
Middle right	Fig. 2.14A: Cimino PJ
Bottom right	Fig. 2.15I: Ellison DW

Images on the chapter title pages

Chapter 1	Fig. 4.03: Ellison DW
Chapter 2	Fig. 2.23: Yip S
Chapter 3	Fig. 3.04B: Pietsch T
Chapter 4	Fig. 4.30A: Pietsch T
Chapter 5	Fig. 5.04A: Vasiljevic A
Chapter 6	Fig. 6.08B: Rodriguez FJ
Chapter 7	Fig. 7.22C: Perry A
Chapter 8	Fig. 8.07A: Hainfellner JA
Chapter 9	Fig. 9.06C: Clayton A. Wiley & Geoffrey Murdoch, Division of Neuropathology, UPMC Presbyterian, Pittsburgh PA, and Reyes-Múgica M
Chapter 10	Fig. 10.22B: Chan JKC
Chapter 11	Fig. 11.10B: Pietsch T
Chapter 12	Fig. 12.24: Lopes MBS
Chapter 13	Fig. 13.03B: Mirthe de Boer, Department of Pathology, University Medical Center Utrecht, Utrecht
Chapter 14	Fig. 14.38B: Solomon DA

References

1. AACR Project GENIE Consortium. AACR Project GENIE: powering precision medicine through an international consortium. Cancer Discov. 2017 Aug;7(8):818–31. PMID:28572459

2. Aavikko M, Li SP, Saarinen S, et al. Loss of SUFU function in familial multiple meningioma. Am J Hum Genet. 2012 Sep 7;91(3):520–6. PMID:22958902

3. Abdallah A, Emel E, Gündüz HB, et al. Long-term surgical resection outcomes of pediatric myxopapillary ependymoma: experience of two centers and brief literature review. World Neurosurg. 2020 Apr;136:e245–61. PMID:31899399

4. Abdelbaki MS, Abu-Arja MH, Davidson TB, et al. Pineoblastoma in children less than six years of age: the Head Start I, II, and III experience. Pediatr Blood Cancer. 2020 Jun;67(6):e28252. PMID:32187454

5. AbdelBaki MS, Boué DR, Finlay JL, et al. Desmoplastic nodular medulloblastoma in young children: a management dilemma. Neuro Oncol. 2018 Jul 5;20(8):1026–33. PMID:29156007

6. Abdel-Rahman MH, Pilarski R, Cebulla CM, et al. Germline BAP1 mutation predisposes to uveal melanoma, lung adenocarcinoma, meningioma, and other cancers. J Med Genet. 2011 Dec;48(12):856–9. PMID:21941004

7. Abe M, Misago N, Tanaka S, et al. Capillary hemangioma of the central nervous system: a comparative study with lobular capillary hemangioma of the skin. Acta Neuropathol. 2005 Feb;109(2):151–8. PMID:15365728

8. Abedalthagafi M. Constitutional mismatch repair-deficiency: current problems and emerging therapeutic strategies. Oncotarget. 2018 Oct 23;9(83):35458–69. PMID:30459937

9. Abedalthagafi M, Bi WL, Aizer AA, et al. Oncogenic PI3K mutations are as common as AKT1 and SMO mutations in meningioma. Neuro Oncol. 2016 May;18(5):649–55. PMID:26826201

10. Abedalthagafi MS, Merrill PH, Bi WL, et al. Angiomatous meningiomas have a distinct genetic profile with multiple chromosomal polysomies including polysomy of chromosome 5. Oncotarget. 2014 Nov 15;5(21):10596–606. PMID:25347344

11. Abel TW, Baker SJ, Fraser MM, et al. Lhermitte-Duclos disease: a report of 31 cases with immunohistochemical analysis of the PTEN/AKT/mTOR pathway. J Neuropathol Exp Neurol. 2005 Apr;64(4):341–9. PMID:15835270

12. Abou-El-Ardat K, Seifert M, Becker K, et al. Comprehensive molecular characterization of multifocal glioblastoma proves its monoclonal origin and reveals novel insights into clonal evolution and heterogeneity of glioblastomas. Neuro Oncol. 2017 Apr 1;19(4):546–57. PMID:28201779

13. Abrey LE, DeAngelis LM, Yahalom J. Long-term survival in primary CNS lymphoma. J Clin Oncol. 1998 Mar;16(3):859–63. PMID:9508166

14. Acharya S, DeWees T, Shinohara ET, et al. Long-term outcomes and late effects for childhood and young adulthood intracranial germinomas. Neuro Oncol. 2015 May;17(5):741–6. PMID:25422317

15. Achey RL, Khanna V, Ostrom QT, et al. Incidence and survival trends in oligodendrogliomas and anaplastic oligodendrogliomas in the United States from 2000 to 2013: a CBTRUS report. J Neurooncol. 2017 May;133(1):17–25. PMID:28397028

16. Acquaye AA, Vera E, Gilbert MR, et al. Clinical presentation and outcomes for adult ependymoma patients. Cancer. 2017 Feb 1;123(3):494–501. PMID:27679985

17. Actor B, Cobbers JM, Büschges R, et al. Comprehensive analysis of genomic alterations in gliosarcoma and its two tissue components. Genes Chromosomes Cancer. 2002 Aug;34(4):416–27. PMID:12112531

18. Adam C, Polivka M, Carpentier A, et al. Papillary glioneuronal tumor: not always a benign tumor? Clin Neuropathol. 2007 May-Jun;26(3):119–24. PMID:19157003

19. Adamson TE, Wiestler OD, Kleihues P, et al. Correlation of clinical and pathological features in surgically treated craniopharyngiomas. J Neurosurg. 1990 Jul;73(1):12–7. PMID:2352012

20. Adeleye AO, Okolo CA, Akang EE, et al. Cerebral pleomorphic xanthoastrocytoma associated with NF1: an updated review with a rare atypical case from Africa. Neurosurg Rev. 2012 Jul;35(3):313–9. PMID:22020543

21. Adriani KS, Stenvers DJ, Imanse JG. Pearls & oy-sters: Lumbar paraganglioma: can you see it in the eyes? Neurology. 2012 Jan 24;78(4):e27–8. PMID:22271522

22. Aerts I, Pacquement H, Doz F, et al. Outcome of second malignancies after retinoblastoma: a retrospective analysis of 25 patients treated at the Institut Curie. Eur J Cancer. 2004 Jul;40(10):1522–9. PMID:15196536

23. Agaimy A. Microscopic intraneural perineurial cell proliferations in patients with neurofibromatosis type 1. Ann Diagn Pathol. 2014 Apr;18(2):95–8. PMID:24461704

24. Agamanolis DP, Katsetos CD, Klonk CJ, et al. An unusual form of superficially disseminated glioma in children: report of 3 cases. J Child Neurol. 2012 Jun;27(6):727–33. PMID:22596013

25. Agaram NP, Prakash S, Antonescu CR. Deep-seated plexiform schwannoma: a pathologic study of 16 cases and comparative analysis with the superficial variety. Am J Surg Pathol. 2005 Aug;29(8):1042–8. PMID:16006798

26. Agarwal S, Sharma MC, Sarkar C, et al. Extraventricular neurocytomas: a morphological and histogenetic consideration. A study of six cases. Pathology. 2011 Jun;43(4):327–34. PMID:21532524

27. Agarwal SK, Munjal M, Rai D, et al. Malignant transformation of vagal nerve schwannoma into angiosarcoma: a rare event. J Surg Tech Case Rep. 2015 Jan-Jun;7(1):17–9. PMID:27512546

28. Agely A, Okromelidze L, Vilanilam GK, et al. Ectopic pituitary adenomas: common presentations of a rare entity. Pituitary. 2019 Aug;22(4):339–43. PMID:30895500

29. Aghajan Y, Levy ML, Malicki DM, et al. Novel PPP1CB-ALK fusion protein in a high-grade glioma of infancy. BMJ Case Rep. 2016 Aug 16;2016:bcr2016217189. PMID:27530886

30. Aghi MK, Carter BS, Cosgrove GR, et al. Long-term recurrence rates of atypical meningiomas after gross total resection with or without postoperative adjuvant radiation. Neurosurgery. 2009 Jan;64(1):56–60. PMID:19145156

31. Agnihotri S, Jalali S, Wilson MR, et al. The genomic landscape of schwannoma. Nat Genet. 2016 Nov;48(11):1339–48. PMID:27723760

32. Agrawal D, Singhal A, Hendson G, et al. Gyriform differentiation in medulloblastoma - a radiological predictor of histology. Pediatr Neurosurg. 2007;43(2):142–5. PMID:17337929

33. Agrawal M, Uppin MS, Patibandla MR, et al. Teratomas in central nervous system: a clinico-morphological study with review of literature. Neurol India. 2010 Nov-Dec;58(6):841–6. PMID:21150046

34. Aguilera D, Flamini R, Mazewski C, et al. Response to subependymal giant cell astrocytoma with spinal cord metastasis to everolimus. J Pediatr Hematol Oncol. 2014 Oct;36(7):e448–51. PMID:24276039

35. Aguilera D, Janss A, Mazewski C, et al. Successful retreatment of a child with a refractory brainstem ganglioglioma with vemurafenib. Pediatr Blood Cancer. 2016 Mar;63(3):541–3. PMID:26579623

36. Agustsson TT, Baldvinsdottir T, Jonasson JG. The epidemiology of pituitary adenomas in Iceland, 1955-2012: a nationwide population-based study. Eur J Endocrinol. 2015 Nov;173(5):655–64. PMID:26423473

37. Ahlsén G, Gillberg IC, Lindblom R, et al. Tuberous sclerosis in Western Sweden. A population study of cases with early childhood onset. Arch Neurol. 1994 Jan;51(1):76–81. PMID:8274113

38. Ahmad ST, Rogers AD, Chen MJ, et al. Capicua regulates neural stem cell proliferation and lineage specification through control of Ets factors. Nat Commun. 2019 May 1;10(1):2000. PMID:31043608

39. Ahmed AK, Dawood HY, Gerard J, et al. Surgical resection and cellular proliferation index predict prognosis for patients with papillary glioneuronal tumor: systematic review and pooled analysis. World Neurosurg. 2017 Nov;107:534–41. PMID:28823671

40. Ahn D, Lee GJ, Sohn JH, et al. Fine-needle aspiration cytology versus core-needle biopsy for the diagnosis of extracranial head and neck schwannoma. Head Neck. 2018 Dec;40(12):2695–700. PMID:3045/183

41. Ahuja A, Iyer VK, Mathur S. Fine needle aspiration cytology and immunocytochemistry of myxopapillary ependymoma. Cytopathology. 2013 Apr;24(2):134–6. PMID:22175883

42. Ahuja A, Sharma MC, Suri V, et al. Pineal anlage tumour - a rare entity with divergent histology. J Clin Neurosci. 2011 Jun;18(6):811–3. PMID:21435885

43. Aicardi J. Aicardi syndrome. Brain Dev. 2005 Apr;27(3):164–71. PMID:15737696

44. Aihara K, Mukasa A, Nagae G, et al. Genetic and epigenetic stability of oligodendrogliomas at recurrence. Acta Neuropathol Commun. 2017 Mar 7;5(1):18. PMID:28270234

45. Aizer AA, Bi WL, Kandola MS, et al. Extent of resection and overall survival for patients with atypical and malignant meningioma. Cancer. 2015 Dec 15;121(24):4376–81. PMID:26308667

46. Ajithkumar T, Mazhari AL, Stickan-Verfürth M, et al. Proton therapy for craniopharyngioma - an early report from a single European centre. Clin Oncol (R Coll Radiol). 2018 May;30(5):307–16. PMID:29459099

47. Aker FV, Ozkara S, Eren P, et al. Cerebellar liponeurocytoma/lipidized medulloblastoma. J Neurooncol. 2005 Jan;71(1):53–9. PMID:15719276

48. Akhaddar A, Zrara I, Gazzaz M, et al. Cerebellar liponeurocytoma (lipomatous medulloblastoma). J Neuroradiol. 2003 Mar;30(2):121–6. PMID:12717299

49. Akirov A, Asa SL, Amer L, et al. The clinicopathological spectrum of acromegaly. J Clin Med. 2019 Nov 13;8(11):E1962. PMID:31766255

50. Al Krinawe Y, Esmaeilzadeh M, Hartmann C, et al. Pediatric rosette-forming glioneuronal tumor of the septum pellucidum. Childs Nerv Syst. 2020 Nov;36(11):2867–70. PMID:32219524

51. Al-Adnani M. Soft tissue perineurioma in a child with neurofibromatosis type 1: a case report and review of the literature. Pediatr Dev Pathol. 2017 Sep-Oct;20(5):444–8. PMID:28812461

52. Alahmadi H, Lee D, Wilson JR, et al. Clinical features of silent corticotroph adenomas. Acta Neurochir (Wien). 2012 Aug;154(8):1493–8. PMID:22619024

53. Alame M, Pirel M, Costes-Martineau V, et al. Characterisation of tumour microenvironment and immune checkpoints in primary central nervous system diffuse large B cell lymphomas. Virchows Arch. 2020 Jun;476(6):891–902. PMID:31811434

54. Alameda F, Velarde JM, Carrato C, et al. Prognostic value of stem cell markers in glioblastoma. Biomarkers. 2019 Nov;24(7):677–83. PMID:31496301

55. Albani A, Pérez-Rivas LG, Dimopoulou C, et al. The USP8 mutational status may predict long-term remission in patients with Cushing's disease. Clin Endocrinol (Oxf). 2018 Jun 29. PMID:29957855

56. Al-Bazzaz S, Karamchandani J, Mocarski E, et al. Ectopic prolactin-producing pituitary adenoma in a benign ovarian cystic teratoma. Endocr Pathol. 2014 Sep;25(3):321–3. PMID:24584638

57. Albergo JI, Gaston CL, Laitinen M, et al. Ewing's sarcoma: only patients with 100% of necrosis after chemotherapy should be classified as having a good response. Bone Joint J. 2016 Aug;98-B(8):1138–44. PMID:27482030

58. Albert DM, Dryja TP. Recent studies of the retinoblastoma gene. What it means to the ophthalmologist. Arch Ophthalmol. 1988 Feb;106(2):181–2. PMID:3422555

59. Albrecht S, Rouah E, Becker LE, et al. Transthyretin immunoreactivity in choroid plexus neoplasms and brain metastases. Mod Pathol. 1991 Sep;4(5):610–4. PMID:1758873

60. Alcantara Llaguno S, Sun D, Pedraza AM, et al. Cell-of-origin susceptibility to glioblastoma formation declines with neural lineage restriction. Nat Neurosci. 2019 Apr;22(4):545–55. PMID:30778149

61. Alcedo J, Noll M. Hedgehog and its patched-smoothened receptor complex: a novel signalling mechanism at the cell surface. Biol Chem. 1997 Jul;378(7):583–90. PMID:9278137

62. Aldape K, Nejad R, Louis DN, et al. Integrating molecular markers into the World Health Organization classification of CNS tumors: a survey of the neuro-oncology community.

Neuro Oncol. 2017 Mar 1;19(3):336–44. PMID:27688263

63. Alderson L, Fetell MR, Sisti M, et al. Sentinel lesions of primary CNS lymphoma. J Neurol Neurosurg Psychiatry. 1996 Jan;60(1):102–5. PMID:8558135

64. Alentorn A, Dehais C, Ducray F, et al. Allelic loss of 9p21.3 is a prognostic factor in 1p/19q codeleted anaplastic gliomas. Neurology. 2015 Oct 13;85(15):1325–31. PMID:26385879

65. Alentorn A, Marie Y, Carpentier C, et al. Prevalence, clinico-pathological value, and co-occurrence of PDGFRA abnormalities in diffuse gliomas. Neuro Oncol. 2012 Nov;14(11):1393–403. PMID:23074200

66. Alessandro L, Carpani F, Arakaki N, et al. Primary central nervous system natural killer/T-cell lymphoma: an atypical case of chronic meningitis. J Neuroradiol. 2017 Jun;44(3):228–30. PMID:28222909

67. Alexander BM, Ba S, Berger MS, et al. Adaptive Global Innovative Learning Environment for Glioblastoma: GBM AGILE. Clin Cancer Res. 2018 Feb 15;24(4):737–43. PMID:28814435

68. Alexander BM, Brown PD, Ahluwalia MS, et al. Clinical trial design for local therapies for brain metastases: a guideline by the Response Assessment in Neuro-Oncology Brain Metastases working group. Lancet Oncol. 2018 Jan;19(1):e33–42. PMID:29304360

69. Alexander RT, McLendon RE, Cummings TJ. Meningioma with eosinophilic granular inclusions. Clin Neuropathol. 2004 Nov-Dec;23(6):292–7. PMID:15584214

70. Alexandrescu S, Brown RE, Tandon N, et al. Neuron precursor features of spindle cell oncocytoma of adenohypophysis. Ann Clin Lab Sci. 2012 Spring;42(2):123–9. PMID:22585606

71. Alexandrescu S, Korshunov A, Lai SH, et al. Epithelioid glioblastomas and anaplastic epithelioid pleomorphic xanthoastrocytomas–same entity or first cousins? Brain Pathol. 2016 Mar;26(2):215–23. PMID:26238627

72. Alexandrescu S, Meredith DM, Lidov HG, et al. Loss of histone H3 trimethylation on lysine 27 and nuclear expression of transducin-like enhancer 1 in primary intracranial sarcoma, DICER1-mutant. Histopathology. 2021 Jan;78(2):265–75. PMID:32692439

73. Alghamri MS, Thalla R, Avvari RP, et al. Tumor mutational burden predicts survival in patients with low-grade gliomas expressing mutated IDH1. Neurooncol Adv. 2020 Mar 27;2(1):a042. PMID:32642696

74. Al-Hajri A, Al-Mughairi S, Somani A, et al. Pathology-MRI correlations in diffuse low-grade epilepsy associated tumors. J Neuropathol Exp Neurol. 2017 Dec 1;76(12):1023–33. PMID:29040640

75. Al-Hussaini M, Abuirmeileh N, Swaidan M, et al. Embryonal tumor with abundant neuropil and true rosettes: a report of three cases of a rare tumor, with an unusual case showing rhabdomyoblastic and melanocytic differentiation. Neuropathology. 2011 Dec;31(6):620–5. PMID:22103481

76. Ali JB, Sepp T, Ward S, et al. Mutations in the TSC1 gene account for a minority of patients with tuberous sclerosis. J Med Genet. 1998 Dec;35(12):969–72. PMID:9863590

77. Alkadhi H, Keller M, Brandner S, et al. Neuroimaging of cerebellar liponeurocytoma. Case report. J Neurosurg. 2001 Aug;95(2):324–31. PMID:11780904

78. Alkhaili J, Cambon-Binder A, Belkheyar Z. Intraneural perineurioma: a retrospective study of 19 patients. Pan Afr Med J. 2018 Aug 14;30:275. PMID:30637060

79. Alkonyi B, Nowak J, Gnekow AK, et al. Differential imaging characteristics and dissemination potential of pilomyxoid astrocytomas versus pilocytic astrocytomas. Neuroradiology. 2015 Jun;57(6):625–38. PMID:25666233

80. Allen JC, Judkins AR, Rosenblum MK, et al. Atypical teratoid/rhabdoid tumor evolving from an optic pathway ganglioglioma: case study. Neuro Oncol. 2006 Jan;8(1):79–82. PMID:16443951

81. Allinson KS, O'Donovan DG, Jena R, et al. Rosette-forming glioneuronal tumor with dissemination throughout the ventricular system: a case report. Clin Neuropathol. 2015 Mar-Apr;34(2):64–9. PMID:25373141

82. Almefty R, Webber BL, Arnautovic KI. Intraneural perineurioma of the third cranial nerve: occurrence and identification. Case report. J Neurosurg. 2006 May;104(5):824–7. PMID:16703891

83. Almeida JP, Stephens CC, Eschbacher JM, et al. Clinical, pathologic, and imaging characteristics of pituitary null cell adenomas as defined according to the 2017 World Health Organization criteria: a case series from two pituitary centers. Pituitary. 2019 Oct;22(5):514–9. PMID:31401793

84. al Moutaery K, Aabed MY, Ojeda VJ. Cerebral and spinal cord myxopapillary ependymomas: a case report. Pathology. 1996 Nov;28(4):373–6. PMID:9007962

85. al-Sarraj ST, Parmar D, Dean AF, et al. Clinicopathological study of seven cases of spinal cord teratoma: a possible germ cell origin. Histopathology. 1998 Jan;32(1):51–6. PMID:9522216

86. Alshaikh OM, Asa SL, Mete O, et al. An institutional experience of tumor progression to pituitary carcinoma in a 15-year cohort of 1055 consecutive pituitary neuroendocrine tumors. Endocr Pathol. 2019 Jun;30(2):118–27. PMID:30706322

87. Alshareef MA, Almadidy Z, Baker T, et al. Intracranial angiomatoid fibrous histiocytoma: case report and literature review. World Neurosurg. 2016 Dec;96:403–9. PMID:27667574

88. Alsufayan R, Alcaide-Leon P, de Tilly LN, et al. Natural history of lesions with the MR imaging appearance of multinodular and vacuolating neuronal tumor. Neuroradiology. 2017 Sep;59(9):873–83. PMID:28752311

89. Alter BP, Rosenberg PS, Brody LC. Clinical and molecular features associated with biallelic mutations in FANCD1/BRCA2. J Med Genet. 2007 Jan;44(1):1–9. PMID:16825431

90. Altundag MK, Ozişik Y, Yalcin S, et al. Primary low grade B-cell lymphoma of the dura in an immunocompetent patient. J Exp Clin Cancer Res. 2000 Jun;19(2):249–51. PMID:10965827

91. Alturkustani M, Ang LC. Rosette-forming glioneuronal tumour of the 4th ventricle in a NF1 patient. Can J Neurol Sci. 2012 Jan;39(1):95–6. PMID:22384505

92. Alver BH, Kim KH, Lu P, et al. The SWI/SNF chromatin remodelling complex is required for maintenance of lineage specific enhancers. Nat Commun. 2017 Mar 6;8:14648. PMID:28262751

93. Amadou A, Achatz MIW, Hainaut P. Revisiting tumor patterns and penetrance in germline TP53 mutation carriers: temporal phases of Li-Fraumeni syndrome. Curr Opin Oncol. 2018 Jan;30(1):23–9. PMID:29076966

94. Amano K, Kubo O, Komori T, et al. Clinicopathological features of sellar region xanthogranuloma: correlation with Rathke's cleft cyst. Brain Tumor Pathol. 2013 Oct;30(4):233–41. PMID:23322180

95. Amary MF, Damato S, Halai D, et al. Ollier disease and Maffucci syndrome are caused by somatic mosaic mutations of IDH1 and IDH2. Nat Genet. 2011 Nov 6;43(12):1262–5. PMID:22057236

96. Amayiri N, Tabori U, Campbell B, et al. High frequency of mismatch repair deficiency among pediatric high grade gliomas in Jordan. Int J Cancer. 2016 Jan 15;138(2):380–5. PMID:26293621

97. Amemiya S, Shibahara J, Aoki S, et al. Recently established entities of central nervous system tumors: review of radiological findings. J Comput Assist Tomogr. 2008 Mar-Apr;32(2):279–85. PMID:18379318

98. Amin MB, Edge S, Greene F, et al., editors. AJCC cancer staging manual. 8th ed. New York (NY): Springer; 2017.

99. Amin S, Lux A, Calder N, et al. Causes of mortality in individuals with tuberous sclerosis complex. Dev Med Child Neurol. 2017 Jun;59(6):612–7. PMID:27935023

100. Amlashi SF, Riffaud L, Brassier G, et al. Nevoid basal cell carcinoma syndrome: relation with desmoplastic medulloblastoma in infancy. A population-based study and review of the literature. Cancer. 2003 Aug 1;98(3):618–24. PMID:12879481

101. Ammerlaan AC, Ararou A, Houben MP, et al. Long-term survival and transmission of INI1-mutation via nonpenetrant males in a family with rhabdoid tumour predisposition syndrome. Br J Cancer. 2008 Jan 29;98(2):474–9. PMID:18087273

102. Ammerman JM, Lonser RR, Dambrosia J, et al. Long-term natural history of hemangioblastomas in patients with von Hippel-Lindau disease: implications for treatment. J Neurosurg. 2006 Aug;105(2):248–55. PMID:17219830

103. Ampie L, Choy W, DiDomenico JD, et al. Clinical attributes and surgical outcomes of angiocentric gliomas. J Clin Neurosci. 2016 Jun;28:117–22. PMID:26778052

104. Ampie L, Choy W, Lamano JB, et al. Prognostic factors for recurrence and complications in the surgical management of primary chordoid gliomas: a systematic review of literature. Clin Neurol Neurosurg. 2015 Nov;138:129–36. PMID:26342205

105. Anan M, Inoue R, Ishii K, et al. A rosette-forming glioneuronal tumor of the spinal cord: the first case of a rosette-forming glioneuronal tumor originating from the spinal cord. Hum Pathol. 2009 Jun;40(6):898–901. PMID:19269010

106. Andersen BM, Miranda C, Hatzoglou V, et al. Leptomeningeal metastases in glioma: the Memorial Sloan Kettering Cancer Center experience. Neurology. 2019 May 21;92(21):e2483–91. PMID:31019097

107. Andersen ZJ, Pedersen M, Weinmayr G, et al. Long-term exposure to ambient air pollution and incidence of brain tumor: the European Study of Cohorts for Air Pollution Effects (ESCAPE). Neuro Oncol. 2018 Feb 19;20(3):420–32. PMID:29016987

108. Anderson KJ, Tan AC, Parkinson J, et al. Molecular and clonal evolution in recurrent metastatic gliosarcoma. Cold Spring Harb Mol Case Stud. 2020 Feb 3;6(1):a004671. PMID:31896544

109. Andoniadou CL, Gaston-Massuet C, Reddy R, et al. Identification of novel pathways involved in the pathogenesis of human adamantinomatous craniopharyngioma. Acta Neuropathol. 2012 Aug;124(2):259–71. PMID:22349813

110. Andoniadou CL, Matsushima D, Mousavy Gharavy SN, et al. Sox2(+) stem/progenitor cells in the adult mouse pituitary support organ homeostasis and have tumor-inducing potential. Cell Stem Cell. 2013 Oct 3;13(4):433–45. PMID:24094324

111. Andreiuolo F, Lisner T, Zlocha J, et al. H3F3A-G34R mutant high grade neuroepithelial neoplasms with glial and dysplastic ganglion cell components. Acta Neuropathol Commun. 2019 May 20;7(1):78. PMID:31109382

112. Andreiuolo F, Mazeraud A, Chrétien F, et al. A global view on the availability of methods and information in the neuropathological diagnostics of CNS tumors: results of an international survey among neuropathological units. Brain Pathol. 2016 Jul;26(4):551–4. PMID:27062283

113. Andreiuolo F, Varlet P, Tauziède-Espariat A, et al. Childhood supratentorial ependymomas with YAP1-MAMLD1 fusion: an entity with characteristic clinical, radiological, cytogenetic and histopathological features. Brain Pathol. 2019 Mar;29(2):205–16. PMID:30246434

114. Andrianova MA, Chetan GK, Sibin MK, et al. Germline PMS2 and somatic POLE exonuclease mutations cause hypermutability of the leading DNA strand in biallelic mismatch repair deficiency syndrome brain tumours. J Pathol. 2017 Nov;243(3):331–41. PMID:28805995

115. Anghileri E, Eoli M, Paterra R, et al. FABP4 is a candidate marker of cerebellar liponeurocytomas. J Neurooncol. 2012 Jul;108(3):513–9. PMID:22476608

116. Antinheimo J, Haapasalo H, Haltia M, et al. Proliferation potential and histological features in neurofibromatosis 2-associated and sporadic meningiomas. J Neurosurg. 1997 Oct;87(4):610–4. PMID:9322850

117. Antinheimo J, Haapasalo H, Seppälä M, et al. Proliferative potential of sporadic and neurofibromatosis 2-associated schwannomas as studied by MIB-1 (Ki-67) and PCNA labeling. J Neuropathol Exp Neurol. 1995 Nov;54(6):776–82. PMID:7595650

118. Antinheimo J, Sankila R, Carpén O, et al. Population-based analysis of sporadic and type 2 neurofibromatosis-associated meningiomas and schwannomas. Neurology. 2000 Jan 11;54(1):71–6. PMID:10636128

119. Antonelli M, Korshunov A, Mastronuzzi A, et al. Long-term survival in a case of ETANTR with histological features of neuronal maturation after therapy. Virchows Arch. 2015 May;466(5):603–7. PMID:25697539

120. Antonescu CR, Owosho AA, Zhang L, et al. Sarcomas with CIC-rearrangements are a distinct pathologic entity with aggressive outcome: a clinicopathologic and molecular study of 115 cases. Am J Surg Pathol. 2017 Jul;41(7):941–9. PMID:28346326

121. Antonini SR, Latronico AC, Elias LL, et al. Glucocorticoid receptor gene polymorphisms in ACTH-secreting pituitary tumours. Clin Endocrinol (Oxf). 2002 Nov;57(5):657–62. PMID:12390341

122. Aoki K, Nakamura H, Suzuki H, et al. Prognostic relevance of genetic alterations in diffuse lower-grade gliomas. Neuro Oncol. 2018 Jan 10;20(1):66–77. PMID:29016839

123. Appay R, Dehais C, Maurage CA, et al. CDKN2A homozygous deletion is a strong adverse prognosis factor in diffuse malignant IDH-mutant gliomas. Neuro Oncol. 2019 Dec 17;21(12):1519–28. PMID:31832685

124. Appay R, Macagno N, Padovani L, et al. HGNET-BCOR tumors of the cerebellum: clinicopathologic and molecular characterization of 3 cases. Am J Surg Pathol. 2017 Sep;41(9):1254–60. PMID:28704208

125. Appay R, Pages M, Colin C, et al. Diffuse leptomeningeal glioneuronal tumor: a double misnomer? A report of two cases. Acta Neuropathol Commun. 2020 Jun 30;8(1):95. PMID:32605662

126. Appay R, Tabouret E, Macagno N, et al. IDH2 mutations are commonly associated with 1p/19q codeletion in diffuse adult gliomas. Neuro Oncol. 2018 Apr 9;20(5):716–8. PMID:29522183

127. Apps JR, Carreno G, Gonzalez-Meljem JM, et al. Tumour compartment transcriptomics

demonstrates the activation of inflammatory and odontogenic programmes in human adamantinomatous craniopharyngioma and identifies the MAPK/ERK pathway as a novel therapeutic target. Acta Neuropathol. 2018 May;135(5):757–77. PMID:29541918
128. Apps JR, Martinez-Barbera JP. Genetically engineered mouse models of craniopharyngioma: an opportunity for therapy development and understanding of tumor biology. Brain Pathol. 2017 May;27(3):364–9. PMID:28414891
129. Apps JR, Stache C, Gonzalez-Meljem JM, et al. CTNNB1 mutations are clonal in adamantinomatous craniopharyngioma. Neuropathol Appl Neurobiol. 2020 Aug;46(5):510–4. PMID:32125720
130. Apra C, Enachescu C, Lapras V, et al. Is gross total resection reasonable in adults with craniopharyngiomas with hypothalamic involvement? World Neurosurg. 2019 Sep;129:e803–11. PMID:31203080
131. Apushkin MA, Apushkin MA, Shapiro MJ, et al. Retinoblastoma and simulating lesions: role of imaging. Neuroimaging Clin N Am. 2005 Feb;15(1):49–67. PMID:15927860
132. Arai H, Ikota H, Sugawara K, et al. Nestin expression in brain tumors: its utility for pathological diagnosis and correlation with the prognosis of high-grade gliomas. Brain Tumor Pathol. 2012 Jul;29(3):160–7. PMID:22350668
133. Ardon H, Plets C, Sciot R, et al. Paraganglioma of the cauda equina region: a report of three cases. Surg Neurol Int. 2011;2:96. PMID:21811702
134. Arita H, Narita Y, Fukushima S, et al. Upregulating mutations in the TERT promoter commonly occur in adult malignant gliomas and are strongly associated with total 1p19q loss. Acta Neuropathol. 2013 Aug;126(2):267–76. PMID:23764841
135. Arita K, Sugiyama K, Tominaga A, et al. Intrasellar rhabdomyosarcoma: case report. Neurosurgery. 2001 Mar;48(3):677–80. PMID:11270561
136. Arita N, Taneda M, Hayakawa T. Leptomeningeal dissemination of malignant gliomas. Incidence, diagnosis and outcome. Acta Neurochir (Wien). 1994;126(2-4):84–92. PMID:8042560
137. Arivazhagan A, Anandh B, Santosh V, et al. Pineal parenchymal tumors–utility of immunohistochemical markers in prognostication. Clin Neuropathol. 2008 Sep-Oct;27(5):325–33. PMID:18808064
138. Armocida D, Pesce A, Frati A, et al. EGFR amplification is a real independent prognostic impact factor between young adults and adults over 45yo with wild-type glioblastoma? J Neurooncol. 2020 Jan;146(2):275–84. PMID:31889239
139. Arnold MA, Stallings-Archer K, Marlin E, et al. Cribriform neuroepithelial tumor arising in the lateral ventricle. Pediatr Dev Pathol. 2013 Jul-Aug;16(4):301–7. PMID:23495723
140. Aronica E, Leenstra S, van Veelen CW, et al. Glioneuronal tumors and medically intractable epilepsy: a clinical study with long-term follow-up of seizure outcome after surgery. Epilepsy Res. 2001 Mar;43(3):179–91. PMID:11248530
141. Artzi M, Bressler I, Ben Bashat D. Differentiation between glioblastoma, brain metastasis and subtypes using radiomics analysis. J Magn Reson Imaging. 2019 Aug;50(2):519–28. PMID:30635952
142. Asa SL, Bamberger AM, Cao B, et al. The transcription activator steroidogenic factor-1 is preferentially expressed in the human pituitary gonadotroph. J Clin Endocrinol Metab. 1996 Jun;81(6):2165–70. PMID:8964846
143. Asa SL, Ezzat S, Kelly DF, et al. Hypothalamic vasopressin-producing tumors: often inappropriate diuresis but occasionally Cushing disease. Am J Surg Pathol. 2019 Feb;43(2):251–60. PMID:30379651
144. Asa SL, Ezzat S, Mete O. The diagnosis and clinical significance of paragangliomas in unusual locations. J Clin Med. 2018 Sep 13;7(9):E280. PMID:30217041
145. Asa SL, Kucharczyk W, Ezzat S. Pituitary acromegaly: not one disease. Endocr Relat Cancer. 2017 Mar;24(3):C1–4. PMID:28122798
146. Asa SL, Mete O. Hypothalamic endocrine tumors: an update. J Clin Med. 2019 Oct 20;8(10):E1741. PMID:31635149
147. Asa SL, Puy LA, Lew AM, et al. Cell type-specific expression of the pituitary transcription activator pit-1 in the human pituitary and pituitary adenomas. J Clin Endocrinol Metab. 1993 Nov;77(5):1275–80. PMID:8077321
148. Asai S, Katabami T, Tsuiki M, et al. Controlling tumor progression with cyclophosphamide, vincristine, and dacarbazine treatment improves survival in patients with metastatic and unresectable malignant pheochromocytomas/paragangliomas. Horm Cancer. 2017 Apr;8(2):108–18. PMID:28108930
149. Asencio-Cortés C, de Quintana-Schmidt C, Clavel-Laria P, et al. [Spinal cord metastasis from gliosarcoma. Case report and review of the literature]. Neurocirugia (Astur). 2014 May-Jun;25(3):132–5. Spanish. PMID:24183327
150. Asioli S, Righi A, Iommi M, et al. Validation of a clinicopathological score for the prediction of post-surgical evolution of pituitary adenoma: retrospective analysis on 566 patients from a tertiary care centre. Eur J Endocrinol. 2019 Feb 1;180(2):127–34. PMID:30481158
151. Asioli S, Zoli M, Guaraldi F, et al. Peculiar pathological, radiological and clinical features of skull-base de-differentiated chordomas. Results from a referral centre case-series and literature review. Histopathology. 2020 Apr;76(5):731–9. PMID:31652338
152. Askaner G, Lei U, Bertelsen B, et al. Novel SUFU frameshift variant leading to meningioma in three generations in a family with Gorlin syndrome. Case Rep Genet. 2019 Jul 28;2019:9650184. PMID:31485359
153. Asthagiri AR, Parry DM, Butman JA, et al. Neurofibromatosis type 2. Lancet. 2009 Jun 6;373(9679):1974–86. PMID:19476995
154. Astigarraga S, Grossman R, Díaz-Delfín J, et al. A MAPK docking site is critical for downregulation of Capicua by Torso and EGFR RTK signaling. EMBO J. 2007 Feb 7;26(3):668–77. PMID:17255944
155. Astrinidis A, Henske EP. Tuberous sclerosis complex: linking growth and energy signaling pathways with human disease. Oncogene. 2005 Nov 14;24(50):7475–81. PMID:16288294
156. Ates D, Kosemehmetoglu K, Onder S, et al. Pseudopapillary pattern in intra-operative squash smear preparations of central nervous system germinomas. Cytopathology. 2014 Feb;25(1):45–50. PMID:23551548
157. Athar M, Li C, Kim AL, et al. Sonic hedgehog signaling in basal cell nevus syndrome. Cancer Res. 2014 Sep 15;74(18):4967–75. PMID:25172843
158. Attard TM, Giglio P, Koppula S, et al. Brain tumors in individuals with familial adenomatous polyposis: a cancer registry experience and pooled case report analysis. Cancer. 2007 Feb 15;109(4):761–6. PMID:17238184
159. Au KS, Williams AT, Roach ES, et al. Genotype/phenotype correlation in 325 individuals referred for a diagnosis of tuberous sclerosis complex in the United States. Genet Med. 2007 Feb;9(2):88–100. PMID:17304050
160. Awad IA, Polster SP. Cavernous angiomas: deconstructing a neurosurgical disease. J Neurosurg. 2019 Jul 1;131(1):1–13. PMID:31261134
161. Axiotis CA, Lippes HA, Merino MJ, et al. Corticotroph cell pituitary adenoma within an ovarian teratoma. A new cause of Cushing's syndrome. Am J Surg Pathol. 1987 Mar;11(3):218–24. PMID:3548446
162. Ayala-Ramirez M, Feng L, Johnson MM, et al. Clinical risk factors for malignancy and overall survival in patients with pheochromocytomas and sympathetic paragangliomas: primary tumor size and primary tumor location as prognostic indicators. J Clin Endocrinol Metab. 2011 Mar;96(3):717–25. PMID:21190975
163. Ayanambakkam A, Ibrahimi S, Bilal K, et al. Extranodal marginal zone lymphoma of the central nervous system. Clin Lymphoma Myeloma Leuk. 2018 Jan;18(1):34–37.e8. PMID:29103980
164. Aydin F, Ghatak NR, Salvant J, et al. Desmoplastic cerebral astrocytoma of infancy. A case report with immunohistochemical, ultrastructural and proliferation studies. Acta Neuropathol. 1993;86(6):666–70. PMID:7906073
165. Aziz M, Chaurasia JK, Khan R, et al. Primary low-grade diffuse small lymphocytic lymphoma of the central nervous system. BMJ Case Rep. 2014 Apr 12;2014:bcr2013202051. PMID:24729110
166. Azizi E, Friedman J, Pavlotsky F, et al. Familial cutaneous malignant melanoma and tumors of the nervous system. A hereditary cancer syndrome. Cancer. 1995 Nov 1;76(9):1571–8. PMID:8635060
167. Bacci C, Sestini R, Provenzano A, et al. Schwannomatosis associated with multiple meningiomas due to a familial SMARCB1 mutation. Neurogenetics. 2010 Feb;11(1):73–80. PMID:19582488
168. Badalian-Very G. A common progenitor cell in LCH and ECD. Blood. 2014 Aug 14;124(7):991–2. PMID:25124781
169. Badalian-Very G, Vergilio JA, Degar BA, et al. Recurrent BRAF mutations in Langerhans cell histiocytosis. Blood. 2010 Sep 16;116(11):1919–23. PMID:20519626
170. Bader A, Heran M, Dunham C, et al. Radiological features of infantile glioblastoma and desmoplastic infantile tumors: British Columbia's Children's Hospital experience. J Neurosurg Pediatr. 2015 Aug;16(2):119–25. PMID:25955808
171. Badiali M, Gleize V, Paris S, et al. KIAA1549-BRAF fusions and IDH mutations can coexist in diffuse gliomas of adults. Brain Pathol. 2012 Nov;22(6):841–7. PMID:22591444
172. Bady P, Sciuscio D, Diserens AC, et al. MGMT methylation analysis of glioblastoma on the Infinium methylation BeadChip identifies two distinct CpG regions associated with gene silencing and outcome, yielding a prediction model for comparisons across datasets, tumor grades, and CIMP-status. Acta Neuropathol. 2012 Oct;124(4):547–60. PMID:22810491
173. Bahuau M, Vidaud D, Jenkins RB, et al. Germ-line deletion involving the INK4 locus in familial proneness to melanoma and nervous system tumors. Cancer Res. 1998 Jun 1;58(11):2298–303. PMID:9622062
174. Bahuau M, Vidaud D, Kujas M, et al. Familial aggregation of malignant melanoma/dysplastic naevi and tumours of the nervous system: an original syndrome of tumour proneness. Ann Genet. 1997;40(2):78–91. PMID:9259954
175. Bahubeshi A, Bal N, Rio Frio T, et al. Germline DICER1 mutations and familial cystic nephroma. J Med Genet. 2010 Dec;47(12):863–6. PMID:21036787
176. Bainbridge MN, Armstrong GN, Gramatges MM, et al. Germline mutations in shelterin complex genes are associated with familial glioma. J Natl Cancer Inst. 2014 Dec 7;107(1):384. PMID:25482530
177. Baisden BL, Brat DJ, Melhem ER, et al. Dysembryoplastic neuroepithelial tumor-like neoplasm of the septum pellucidum: a lesion often misdiagnosed as glioma: report of 10 cases. Am J Surg Pathol. 2001 Apr;25(4):494–9. PMID:11257624
178. Bakry D, Aronson M, Durno C, et al. Genetic and clinical determinants of constitutional mismatch repair deficiency syndrome: report from the constitutional mismatch repair deficiency consortium. Eur J Cancer. 2014 Mar;50(5):987–96. PMID:24440087
179. Baldassari S, Ribierre T, Marsan E, et al. Dissecting the genetic basis of focal cortical dysplasia: a large cohort study. Acta Neuropathol. 2019 Dec;138(6):885–900. PMID:31444548
180. Bale TA. FGFR- gene family alterations in low-grade neuroepithelial tumors. Acta Neuropathol Commun. 2020 Feb 21;8(1):21. PMID:32085805
181. Bale TA, Oviedo A, Kozakewich H, et al. Intracranial myxoid mesenchymal tumors with EWSR1-CREB family gene fusions: myxoid variant of angiomatoid fibrous histiocytoma or novel entity? Brain Pathol. 2018 Mar;28(2):183–91. PMID:28281318
182. Bale TA, Sait SF, Benhamida J, et al. Malignant transformation of a polymorphous low grade neuroepithelial tumor of the young (PLNTY). Acta Neuropathol. 2021 Jan;141(1):123–5. PMID:33226472
183. Ballester LY, Dunbar E, Guha-Thakurta N, et al. Primary leptomeningeal oligodendroglioma, IDH-mutant, 1p/19q-codeleted. Front Neurol. 2018 Aug 27;9:700. PMID:30210430
184. Ballester LY, Meis JM, Lazar AJ, et al. Intracranial myxoid mesenchymal tumor with EWSR1-ATF1 fusion. J Neuropathol Exp Neurol. 2020 Mar 1;79(3):347–51. PMID:32016322
185. Balogun JA, Monsalves E, Juraschka K, et al. Null cell adenomas of the pituitary gland: an institutional review of their clinical imaging and behavioral characteristics. Endocr Pathol. 2015 Mar;26(1):63–70. PMID:25403448
186. Balss J, Meyer J, Mueller W, et al. Analysis of the IDH1 codon 132 mutation in brain tumors. Acta Neuropathol. 2008 Dec;116(6):597–602. PMID:18985363
187. Banan R, Stichel D, Bleck A, et al. Infratentorial IDH-mutant astrocytoma is a distinct subtype. Acta Neuropathol. 2020 Oct;140(4):569–81. PMID:32776277
188. Bandopadhayay P, Ramkissoon LA, Jain P, et al. MYB-QKI rearrangements in angiocentric glioma drive tumorigenicity through a tripartite mechanism. Nat Genet. 2016 Mar;48(3):273–82. PMID:26829751
189. Bandopadhayay P, Silvera VM, Ciarlini PDSC, et al. Myxopapillary ependymomas in children: imaging, treatment and outcomes. J Neurooncol. 2016 Jan;126(1):165–74. PMID:26468139
190. Banerjee AK, Sharma BS, Kak VK, et al. Gliosarcoma with cartilage formation. Cancer. 1989 Feb 1;63(3):518–23. PMID:2643455
191. Bannykh S, Strugar J, Baehring J. Paraganglioma of the lumbar spinal canal. J Neurooncol. 2005 Nov;75(2):119. PMID:16283440
192. Bannykh SI, Stolt CC, Kim J, et al. Oligodendroglial-specific transcriptional factor SOX10 is ubiquitously expressed in human gliomas. J Neurooncol. 2006 Jan;76(2):115–27. PMID:16205963
193. Bao ZS, Chen HM, Yang MY, et al. RNA-seq of 272 gliomas revealed a novel, recurrent PTPRZ1-MET fusion transcript in secondary glioblastomas. Genome Res. 2014 Nov;24(11):1765–73. PMID:25135958
194. Bar EE, Lin A, Tihan T, et al. Frequent

gains at chromosome 7q34 involving BRAF in pilocytic astrocytoma. J Neuropathol Exp Neurol. 2008 Sep;67(9):878–87. PMID:18716556
195. Baraban E, Sadigh S, Rosenbaum J, et al. Cyclin D1 expression and novel mutational findings in Rosai-Dorfman disease. Br J Haematol. 2019 Sep;186(6):837–44. PMID:31172509
196. Baraniskin A, Chomiak M, Ahle G, et al. MicroRNA-30c as a novel diagnostic biomarker for primary and secondary B-cell lymphoma of the CNS. J Neurooncol. 2018 May;137(3):463–8. PMID:29327175
197. Baraniskin A, Kuhnhenn J, Schlegel U, et al. Identification of microRNAs in the cerebrospinal fluid as marker for primary diffuse large B-cell lymphoma of the central nervous system. Blood. 2011 Mar 17;117(11):3140–6. PMID:21200023
198. Barba C, Jacques T, Kahane P, et al. Epilepsy surgery in neurofibromatosis type 1. Epilepsy Res. 2013 Aug;105(3):384–95. PMID:23597854
199. Barker FG 2nd, Davis RL, Chang SM, et al. Necrosis as a prognostic factor in glioblastoma multiforme. Cancer. 1996 Mar 15;77(6):1161–6. PMID:8635139
200. Barkovich AJ, Guerrini R, Kuzniecky RI, et al. A developmental and genetic classification for malformations of cortical development: update 2012. Brain. 2012 May;135(Pt 5):1348–69. PMID:22427329
201. Barnholtz-Sloan JS, Sloan AE, Davis FG, et al. Incidence proportions of brain metastases in patients diagnosed (1973 to 2001) in the Metropolitan Detroit Cancer Surveillance System. J Clin Oncol. 2004 Jul 15;22(14):2865–72. PMID:15254054
202. Barr FG, Galili N, Holick J, et al. Rearrangement of the PAX3 paired box gene in the paediatric solid tumour alveolar rhabdomyosarcoma. Nat Genet. 1993 Feb;3(2):113–7. PMID:8098985
203. Barresi V, Eccher A, Simbolo M, et al. Diffuse gliomas in patients aged 55 years or over: a suggestion for IDH mutation testing. Neuropathology. 2020 Feb;40(1):68–74. PMID:31758617
204. Barresi V, Lionti S, Valori L, et al. Dual-genotype diffuse low-grade glioma: is it really time to abandon oligoastrocytoma as a distinct entity? J Neuropathol Exp Neurol. 2017 May 1;76(5):342–6. PMID:28419269
205. Barresi V, Simbolo M, Mafficini A, et al. Ultra-mutation in IDH wild-type glioblastomas of patients younger than 55 years is associated with defective mismatch repair, microsatellite instability, and giant cell enrichment. Cancers (Basel). 2019 Aug 30;11(9):E1279. PMID:31480372
206. Barrett OC, Hackney JR, McDonald AM, et al. Pathologic predictors of local recurrence in atypical meningiomas following gross total resection. Int J Radiat Oncol Biol Phys. 2019 Feb 1;103(2):453–9. PMID:30253235
207. Bartek J Jr, Dhawan S, Thurin E, et al. Short-term outcome following surgery for rare brain tumor entities in adults: a Swedish nation-wide registry-based study and comparison with SEER database. J Neurooncol. 2020 Jun;148(2):281–90. PMID:32424575
208. Barthel FP, Johnson KC, Varn FS, et al. Longitudinal molecular trajectories of diffuse glioma in adults. Nature. 2019 Dec;576(7785):112–20. PMID:31748746
209. Barthelmeß S, Geddert H, Boltze C, et al. Solitary fibrous tumors/hemangiopericytomas with different variants of the NAB2-STAT6 gene fusion are characterized by specific histomorphology and distinct clinicopathological features. Am J Pathol. 2014 Apr;184(4):1209–18. PMID:24513261
210. Baser ME, Friedman JM, Joe H, et al. Empirical development of improved diagnostic criteria for neurofibromatosis 2. Genet Med. 2011 Jun;13(6):576–81. PMID:21451418
211. Baser ME, Kuramoto L, Joe H, et al. Genotype-phenotype correlations for nervous system tumors in neurofibromatosis 2: a population-based study. Am J Hum Genet. 2004 Aug;75(2):231–9. PMID:15190457
212. Bastian BC. The molecular pathology of melanoma: an integrated taxonomy of melanocytic neoplasia. Annu Rev Pathol. 2014;9:239–71. PMID:24460190
213. Batchelor T, Loeffler JS. Primary CNS lymphoma. J Clin Oncol. 2006 Mar 10;24(8):1281–8. PMID:16525183
214. Bates JE, Choi G, Milano MT. Myxopapillary ependymoma: a SEER analysis of epidemiology and outcomes. J Neurooncol. 2016 Sep;129(2):251–8. PMID:27306443
215. Bates JE, Peterson CR, Dhakal S, et al. Malignant peripheral nerve sheath tumors (MPNST): a SEER analysis of incidence across the age spectrum and therapeutic interventions in the pediatric population. Pediatr Blood Cancer. 2014 Nov;61(11):1955–60. PMID:25130403
216. Batzdorf U, Malamud N. The problem of multicentric gliomas. J Neurosurg. 1963 Feb;20:122–36. PMID:14192080
217. Baude A, Lindroth AM, Plass C. PRC2 loss amplifies Ras signaling in cancer. Nat Genet. 2014 Nov;46(11):1154–5. PMID:25352098
218. Baumann F, Flores E, Napolitano A, et al. Mesothelioma patients with germline BAP1 mutations have 7-fold improved long-term survival. Carcinogenesis. 2015 Jan;36(1):76–81. PMID:25380601
219. Baumert BG, Rutten I, Dehing-Oberije C, et al. A pathology-based substrate for target definition in radiosurgery of brain metastases. Int J Radiat Oncol Biol Phys. 2006 Sep 1;66(1):187–94. PMID:16814946
220. Baumgarten P, Gessler F, Schittenhelm J, et al. Brain invasion in otherwise benign meningiomas does not predict tumor recurrence. Acta Neuropathol. 2016 Sep;132(3):479–81. PMID:27464983
221. Baumgarten P, Harter PN, Tönjes M, et al. Loss of FUBP1 expression in gliomas predicts FUBP1 mutation and is associated with oligodendroglial differentiation, IDH1 mutation and 1p/19q loss of heterozygosity. Neuropathol Appl Neurobiol. 2014 Feb;40(2):205–16. PMID:24117486
222. Baumgarten P, Michaelis M, Rothweiler F, et al. Human cytomegalovirus infection in tumor cells of the nervous system is not detectable with standardized pathologico-virological diagnostics. Neuro Oncol. 2014 Nov;16(11):1469–77. PMID:25155358
223. Bayliss J, Mukherjee P, Lu C, et al. Lowered H3K27me3 and DNA hypomethylation define poorly prognostic pediatric posterior fossa ependymomas. Sci Transl Med. 2016 Nov 23;8(366):366ra161. PMID:27881822
224. Baysal BE. Hereditary paraganglioma targets diverse paraganglia. J Med Genet. 2002 Sep;39(9):617–22. PMID:12205103
225. Beaty NB, Ahn E. Images in clinical medicine. Adamantinomatous craniopharyngioma containing teeth. N Engl J Med. 2014 Feb 27;370(9):860. PMID:24571758
226. Beaumont TL, Godzik J, Dahiya S, et al. Subependymal giant cell astrocytoma in the absence of tuberous sclerosis complex: case report. J Neurosurg Pediatr. 2015 Aug;16(2):134–7. PMID:25978531
227. Beaumont TL, Kupsky WJ, Barger GR, et al. Gliosarcoma with multiple extracranial metastases: case report and review of the literature. J Neurooncol. 2007 May;83(1):39–46. PMID:17171442
228. Beccaria K, Tauziède-Espariat A, Monnien F, et al. Pediatric chordomas: results of a multicentric study of 40 children and proposal for a histopathological prognostic grading system and new therapeutic strategies. J Neuropathol Exp Neurol. 2018 Mar 1;77(3):207–15. PMID:29361006
229. Becher MW, Abel TW, Thompson RC, et al. Immunohistochemical analysis of metastatic neoplasms of the central nervous system. J Neuropathol Exp Neurol. 2006 Oct;65(10):935–44. PMID:17021398
230. Becker RL, Becker AD, Sobel DF. Adult medulloblastoma: review of 13 cases with emphasis on MRI. Neuroradiology. 1995 Feb;37(2):104–8. PMID:7760992
231. Beert E, Brems H, Daniëls B, et al. Atypical neurofibromas in neurofibromatosis type 1 are premalignant tumors. Genes Chromosomes Cancer. 2011 Dec;50(12):1021–32. PMID:21987445
232. Begemann M, Waszak SM, Robinson GW, et al. Germline GPR161 mutations predispose to pediatric medulloblastoma. J Clin Oncol. 2020 Jan 1;38(1):43–50. PMID:31609649
233. Behdad A, Perry A. Central nervous system primitive neuroectodermal tumors: a clinicopathologic and genetic study of 33 cases. Brain Pathol. 2010 Mar;20(2):441–50. PMID:19725831
234. Beiko J, Suki D, Hess KR, et al. IDH1 mutant malignant astrocytomas are more amenable to surgical resection and have a survival benefit associated with maximal surgical resection. Neuro Oncol. 2014 Jan;16(1):81–91. PMID:24305719
235. Bellail AC, Hunter SB, Brat DJ, et al. Microregional extracellular matrix heterogeneity in brain modulates glioma cell invasion. Int J Biochem Cell Biol. 2004 Jun;36(6):1046–69. PMID:15094120
236. Beltran H. The N-myc oncogene: maximizing its targets, regulation, and therapeutic potential. Mol Cancer Res. 2014 Jun;12(6):815–22. PMID:24589438
237. Bender S, Tang Y, Lindroth AM, et al. Reduced H3K27me3 and DNA hypomethylation are major drivers of gene expression in K27M mutant pediatric high-grade gliomas. Cancer Cell. 2013 Nov 11;24(5):660–72. PMID:24183680
238. Benesch M, Frappaz D, Massimino M. Spinal cord ependymomas in children and adolescents. Childs Nerv Syst. 2012 Dec;28(12):2017–28. PMID:22961356
239. Bengtsson D, Schrøder HD, Andersen M, et al. Long-term outcome and MGMT as a predictive marker in 24 patients with atypical pituitary adenomas and pituitary carcinomas given treatment with temozolomide. J Clin Endocrinol Metab. 2015 Apr;100(4):1689–98. PMID:25646794
240. Bennett JT, Tan TY, Alcantara D, et al. Mosaic activating mutations in FGFR1 cause encephalocraniocutaneous lipomatosis. Am J Hum Genet. 2016 Mar 3;98(3):579–87. PMID:26942290
241. Bennett KL, Mester J, Eng C. Germline epigenetic regulation of KILLIN in Cowden and Cowden-like syndrome. JAMA. 2010 Dec 22;304(24):2724–31. PMID:21177507
242. Benson VS, Kirichek O, Beral V, et al. Menopausal hormone therapy and central nervous system tumor risk: large UK prospective study and meta-analysis. Int J Cancer. 2015 May 15;136(10):2369–77. PMID:25335165
243. Benzagmout M, Karachi C, Mokhtari K, et al. Hemorrhagic papillary glioneuronal tumor mimicking cavernoma: two case reports. Clin Neurol Neurosurg. 2013 Feb;115(2):200–3. PMID:22717600
244. Berg JC, Scheithauer BW, Spinner RJ, et al. Plexiform schwannoma: a clinicopathologic overview with emphasis on the head and neck region. Hum Pathol. 2008 May;39(5):633–40. PMID:18439936
245. Berghoff AS, Bartsch R, Wöhrer A, et al. Predictive molecular markers in metastases to the central nervous system: recent advances and future avenues. Acta Neuropathol. 2014 Dec;128(6):879–91. PMID:25287912
246. Berghoff AS, Ilhan-Mutlu A, Dinhof C, et al. Differential role of angiogenesis and tumour cell proliferation in brain metastases according to primary tumour type: analysis of 639 cases. Neuropathol Appl Neurobiol. 2015 Feb;41(2):e41–55. PMID:25256708
247. Berghoff AS, Rajky O, Winkler F, et al. Invasion patterns in brain metastases of solid cancers. Neuro Oncol. 2013 Dec;15(12):1664–72. PMID:24084410
248. Berghoff AS, Schur S, Füreder LM, et al. Descriptive statistical analysis of a real life cohort of 2419 patients with brain metastases of solid cancers. ESMO Open. 2016 Mar 16;1(2):e000024. PMID:27843591
249. Bergmann N, Delbridge C, Gempt J, et al. The intratumoral heterogeneity reflects the intertumoral subtypes of glioblastoma multiforme: a regional immunohistochemistry analysis. Front Oncol. 2020 Apr 24;10:494. PMID:32391260
250. Berho M, Suster S. Mucinous meningioma. Report of an unusual variant of meningioma that may mimic metastatic mucin-producing carcinoma. Am J Surg Pathol. 1994 Jan;18(1):100–6. PMID:8279622
251. Beristain X, Azzarelli B. The neurological masquerade of intravascular lymphomatosis. Arch Neurol. 2002 Mar;59(3):439–43. PMID:11890850
252. Berkman RA, Clark WC, Saxena A, et al. Clonal composition of glioblastoma multiforme. J Neurosurg. 1992 Sep;77(3):432–7. PMID:1324297
253. Berns S, Pearl G. Review of pineal anlage tumor with divergent histology. Arch Pathol Lab Med. 2006 Aug;130(8):1233–5. PMID:16879032
254. Bernstein ML, Buchino JJ. The histologic similarity between craniopharyngioma and odontogenic lesions: a reappraisal. Oral Surg Oral Med Oral Pathol. 1983 Nov;56(5):502–11. PMID:6196702
255. Bernthal NM, Putnam A, Jones KB, et al. The effect of surgical margins on outcomes for low grade MPNSTs and atypical neurofibroma. J Surg Oncol. 2014 Dec;110(7):813–6. PMID:25111615
256. Bertherat J, Horvath A, Groussin L, et al. Mutations in regulatory subunit type 1A of cyclic adenosine 5'-monophosphate-dependent protein kinase (PRKAR1A): phenotype analysis in 353 patients and 80 different genotypes. J Clin Endocrinol Metab. 2009 Jun;94(6):2085–91. PMID:19293268
257. Bertrand A, Rondenet C, Masliah-Planchon J, et al. Rhabdoid component emerging as a subclonal evolution of paediatric glioneuronal tumours. Neuropathol Appl Neurobiol. 2018 Feb;44(2):224–8. PMID:28054381
258. Beschorner R, Pantazis G, Jeibmann A, et al. Expression of EAAT-1 distinguishes choroid plexus tumors from normal and reactive choroid plexus epithelium. Acta Neuropathol. 2009 Jun;117(6):667–75. PMID:19283393
259. Bettegowda C, Adogwa O, Mehta V, et al. Treatment of choroid plexus tumors: a 20-year single institutional experience. J Neurosurg Pediatr. 2012 Nov;10(5):398–405. PMID:22938081
260. Bettegowda C, Agrawal N, Jiao Y, et al. Exomic sequencing of four rare central nervous system tumor types. Oncotarget. 2013

Apr;4(4):572–83. PMID:23592488
261. Bettegowda C, Agrawal N, Jiao Y, et al. Mutations in CIC and FUBP1 contribute to human oligodendroglioma. Science. 2011 Sep 9;333(6048):1453–5. PMID:21817013
262. Betz BL, Strobeck MW, Reisman DN, et al. Re-expression of hSNF5/INI1/BAF47 in pediatric tumor cells leads to G1 arrest associated with induction of p16ink4a and activation of RB. Oncogene. 2002 Aug 8;21(34):5193–203. PMID:12149641
263. Bhagavathi S, Greiner TC, Kazmi SA, et al. Extranodal marginal zone lymphoma of the dura mater with IgH/MALT1 translocation and review of literature. J Hematop. 2008 Sep;1(2):131–7. PMID:19669212
264. Bhatia A, Hatzoglou V, Ulaner G, et al. Neurologic and oncologic features of Erdheim-Chester disease: a 30-patient series. Neuro Oncol. 2020 Jul 7;22(7):979–92. PMID:31950179
265. Bhatt MD, Al-Karmi S, Druker H, et al. Second rhabdoid tumor 8 years after treatment of atypical teratoid/rhabdoid tumor in a child with germline SMARCB1 mutation. Pediatr Blood Cancer. 2019 Mar;66(3):e27546. PMID:30393974
266. Bi WL, Greenwald NF, Abedalthagafi M, et al. Genomic landscape of high-grade meningiomas. NPJ Genom Med. 2017;2:15. PMID:28713588
267. Bi WL, Greenwald NF, Ramkissoon SH, et al. Clinical identification of oncogenic drivers and copy-number alterations in pituitary tumors. Endocrinology. 2017 Jul 1;158(7):2284–91. PMID:28486603
268. Bi WL, Larsen AG, Dunn IF. Genomic alterations in sporadic pituitary tumors. Curr Neurol Neurosci Rep. 2018 Feb 2;18(1):4. PMID:29396598
269. Bi Z, Ren X, Zhang J, et al. Clinical, radiological, and pathological features in 43 cases of intracranial subependymoma. J Neurosurg. 2015 Jan;122(1):49–60. PMID:25361493
270. Bianchi E, Roncarati P, Hougrand O, et al. Human cytomegalovirus and primary intracranial tumours: frequency of tumour infection and lack of correlation with systemic immune anti-viral responses. Neuropathol Appl Neurobiol. 2015 Feb;41(2):e29–40. PMID:25041908
271. Bianchi F, Tamburrini G, Massimi L, et al. Supratentorial tumors typical of the infantile age: desmoplastic infantile ganglioglioma (DIG) and astrocytoma (DIA). A review. Childs Nerv Syst. 2016 Oct;32(10):1833–8. PMID:27659826
272. Biczok A, Jungk C, Egensperger R, et al. Microscopic brain invasion in meningiomas previously classified as WHO grade I is not associated with patient outcome. J Neurooncol. 2019 Dec;145(3):469–77. PMID:31713016
273. Biegel JA. Molecular genetics of atypical teratoid/rhabdoid tumor. Neurosurg Focus. 2006 Jan 15;20(1):E11. PMID:16459991
274. Biegel JA, Busse TM, Weissman BE. SWI/SNF chromatin remodeling complexes and cancer. Am J Med Genet C Semin Med Genet. 2014 Sep;166C(3):350–66. PMID:25169151
275. Biegel JA, Zhou JY, Rorke LB, et al. Germline and acquired mutations of INI1 in atypical teratoid and rhabdoid tumors. Cancer Res. 1999 Jan 1;59(1):74–9. PMID:9892189
276. Bielle F, Di Stefano AL, Meyronet D, et al. Diffuse gliomas with FGFR3-TACC3 fusion have characteristic histopathological and molecular features. Brain Pathol. 2018 Sep;28(5):674–83. PMID:28976058
277. Bielle F, Villa C, Giry M, et al. Chordoid gliomas of the third ventricle share TTF-1 expression with organum vasculosum of the lamina terminalis. Am J Surg Pathol. 2015 Jul;39(7):948–56. PMID:25786084
278. Bielle F, Zanello M, Guillemot D, et al. Unusual primary cerebral localization of a CIC-DUX4 translocation tumor of the Ewing sarcoma family. Acta Neuropathol. 2014 Aug;128(2):309–11. PMID:24980961
279. Bieńkowski M, Wöhrer A, Moser P, et al. Molecular diagnostic testing of diffuse gliomas in the real-life setting: a practical approach. Clin Neuropathol. 2018 Jul/Aug;37(4):166–77. PMID:29923492
280. Biernat W, Aguzzi A, Sure U, et al. Identical mutations of the p53 tumor suppressor gene in the gliomatous and the sarcomatous components of gliosarcomas suggest a common origin from glial cells. J Neuropathol Exp Neurol. 1995 Sep;54(5):651–6. PMID:7666053
281. Bigner SH, Mark J, Burger PC, et al. Specific chromosomal abnormalities in malignant human gliomas. Cancer Res. 1988 Jan 15;48(2):405–11. PMID:3335011
282. Bihr S, Ohashi R, Moore AL, et al. Expression and mutation patterns of PBRM1, BAP1 and SETD2 mirror specific evolutionary subtypes in clear cell renal cell carcinoma. Neoplasia. 2019 Feb;21(2):247–56. PMID:30660076
283. Bilzer T, Reifenberger G, Wechsler W. Chemical induction of brain tumors in rats by nitrosoureas: molecular biology and neuropathology. Neurotoxicol Teratol. 1989 Nov-Dec;11(6):551–6. PMID:2696875
284. Bin Abdulrahman AK, Bin Abdulrahman KA, Bukhari YR, et al. Association between giant cell glioblastoma and glioblastoma multiforme in the United States: a retrospective cohort study. Brain Behav. 2019 Oct;9(10):e01402. PMID:31464386
285. Binderup ML, Bisgaard ML, Harbud V, et al. Von Hippel-Lindau disease (vHL). National clinical guideline for diagnosis and surveillance in Denmark. 3rd edition. Dan Med J. 2013 Dec;60(12):B4763. PMID:24355456
286. Birch JM, Hartley AL, Tricker KJ, et al. Prevalence and diversity of constitutional mutations in the p53 gene among 21 Li-Fraumeni families. Cancer Res. 1994 Mar 1;54(5):1298–304. PMID:8118819
287. Bisceglia M, Muscarella LA, Galliani CA, et al. Extraneuraxial hemangioblastoma: clinicopathologic features and review of the literature. Adv Anat Pathol. 2018 May;25(3):197–215. PMID:29189208
288. Bitar M, Danish SF, Rosenblum MK. A newly diagnosed case of polymorphous low-grade neuroepithelial tumor of the young. Clin Neuropathol. 2018 Jul/Aug;37(4):178–81. PMID:29701169
289. Bjerke L, Mackay A, Nandhabalan M, et al. Histone H3.3. mutations drive pediatric glioblastoma through upregulation of MYCN. Cancer Discov. 2013 May;3(5):512–9. PMID:23539269
290. Bjornsson J, Scheithauer BW, Okazaki H, et al. Intracranial germ cell tumors: pathobiological and immunohistochemical aspects of 70 cases. J Neuropathol Exp Neurol. 1985 Jan;44(1):32–46. PMID:4038412
291. Blades DA, Hardy RW, Cohen M. Cervical paraganglioma with subsequent intracranial and intraspinal metastases. Case report. J Neurosurg. 1991 Aug;75(2):320–3. PMID:2072174
292. Blakeley JO, Plotkin SR. Therapeutic advances for the tumors associated with neurofibromatosis type 1, type 2, and schwannomatosis. Neuro Oncol. 2016 May;18(5):624–38. PMID:26851632
293. Blaser SI, Harwood-Nash DC. Neuroradiology of pediatric posterior fossa medulloblastoma. J Neurooncol. 1996 Jul;29(1):23–34. PMID:8817413
294. Blessing MM, Blackburn PR, Balcom JR, et al. Novel BRAF alteration in desmoplastic infantile ganglioglioma with response to targeted therapy. Acta Neuropathol Commun. 2018 Nov 5;6(1):118. PMID:30396366
295. Blessing MM, Blackburn PR, Krishnan C, et al. Desmoplastic infantile ganglioglioma: a MAPK pathway-driven and microglia/macrophage-rich neuroepithelial tumor. J Neuropathol Exp Neurol. 2019 Nov 1;78(11):1011–21. PMID:31562743
296. Blümcke I, Aronica E, Becker A, et al. Low-grade epilepsy-associated neuroepithelial tumours - the 2016 WHO classification. Nat Rev Neurol. 2016 Dec;12(12):732–40. PMID:27857123
297. Blumcke I, Aronica E, Urbach H, et al. A neuropathology-based approach to epilepsy surgery in brain tumors and proposal for a new terminology use for long-term epilepsy-associated brain tumors. Acta Neuropathol. 2014 Jul;128(1):39–54. PMID:24858213
298. Blümcke I, Becker AJ, Normann S, et al. Distinct expression pattern of microtubule-associated protein-2 in human oligodendrogliomas and glial precursor cells. J Neuropathol Exp Neurol. 2001 Oct;60(10):984–93. PMID:11589429
299. Blümcke I, Coras R, Wefers AK, et al. Review: challenges in the histopathological classification of ganglioglioma and DNT: microscopic agreement studies and a preliminary genotype-phenotype analysis. Neuropathol Appl Neurobiol. 2019 Feb;45(2):95–107. PMID:30326153
300. Blümcke I, Giencke K, Wardelmann E, et al. The CD34 epitope is expressed in neoplastic and malformative lesions associated with chronic, focal epilepsies. Acta Neuropathol. 1999 May;97(5):481–90. PMID:10334485
301. Blümcke I, Löbach M, Wolf HK, et al. Evidence for developmental precursor lesions in epilepsy-associated glioneuronal tumors. Microsc Res Tech. 1999 Jul 1;46(1):53–8. PMID:10402272
302. Blümcke I, Luyken C, Urbach H, et al. An isomorphic subtype of long-term epilepsy-associated astrocytomas associated with benign prognosis. Acta Neuropathol. 2004 May;107(5):381–8. PMID:15034726
303. Blümcke I, Müller S, Buslei R, et al. Microtubule-associated protein-2 immunoreactivity: a useful tool in the differential diagnosis of low-grade neuroepithelial tumors. Acta Neuropathol. 2004 Aug;108(2):89–96. PMID:15146346
304. Blumcke I, Spreafico R, Haaker G, et al. Histopathological findings in brain tissue obtained during epilepsy surgery. N Engl J Med. 2017 Oct 26;377(17):1648–56. PMID:29069555
305. Blümcke I, Thom M, Aronica E, et al. The clinicopathologic spectrum of focal cortical dysplasias: a consensus classification proposed by an ad hoc Task Force of the ILAE Diagnostic Methods Commission. Epilepsia. 2011 Jan;52(1):158–74. PMID:21219302
306. Blümcke I, Wiestler OD. Gangliogliomas: an intriguing tumor entity associated with focal epilepsies. J Neuropathol Exp Neurol. 2002 Jul;61(7):575–84. PMID:12125736
306A. Bockmayr M, Körner M, Schweizer L, et al. Cauda equina paragangliomas express HOXB13. Neuropathol Appl Neurobiol. 2021 Oct;47(6):889–90. PMID:33768604
307. Bodi I, Curran O, Selway R, et al. Two cases of multinodular and vacuolating neuronal tumour. Acta Neuropathol Commun. 2014 Jan 20;2:7. PMID:24444358
308. Bodo S, Colas C, Buhard O, et al. Diagnosis of constitutional mismatch repair-deficiency syndrome based on microsatellite instability and lymphocyte tolerance to methylating agents. Gastroenterology. 2015 Oct;149(4):1017–29.e3. PMID:26116798
309. Boedeker CC, Hensen EF, Neumann HP, et al. Genetics of hereditary head and neck paragangliomas. Head Neck. 2014 Jun;36(6):907–16. PMID:23913591
310. Boehm D, Bacher J, Neumann HP. Gross genomic rearrangement involving the TSC2-PKD1 contiguous deletion syndrome: characterization of the deletion event by quantitative polymerase chain reaction deletion assay. Am J Kidney Dis. 2007 Jan;49(1):e11–21. PMID:17185137
311. Boekhoff S, Bison B, Eveslage M, et al. Craniopharyngiomas presenting as incidentalomas: results of KRANIOPHARYNGEOM 2007. Pituitary. 2019 Oct;22(5):532–41. PMID:31440945
312. Boerman RH, Anderl K, Herath J, et al. The glial and mesenchymal elements of gliosarcomas share similar genetic alterations. J Neuropathol Exp Neurol. 1996 Sep;55(9):973–81. PMID:8800093
313. Bogusz A, Boekhoff S, Warmuth-Metz M, et al. Posterior hypothalamus-sparing surgery improves outcome after childhood craniopharyngioma. Endocr Connect. 2019 May 1;8(5):481–92. PMID:30925462
313A. Böhling T, Hatva E, Kujala M, et al. Expression of growth factors and growth factor receptors in capillary hemangioblastoma. J Neuropathol Exp Neurol. 1996 May;55(5):522–7. PMID:8627342
314. Böhling T, Mäenpää A, Timonen T, et al. Different expression of adhesion molecules on stromal cells and endothelial cells of capillary hemangioblastoma. Acta Neuropathol. 1996 Nov;92(5):461–6. PMID:8922057
315. Böhling T, Turunen O, Jääskeläinen J, et al. Ezrin expression in stromal cells of capillary hemangioblastoma. An immunohistochemical survey of brain tumors. Am J Pathol. 1996 Feb;148(2):367–73. PMID:8579099
316. Boire A, Brandsma D, Brastianos PK, et al. Liquid biopsy in central nervous system metastases: a RANO review and proposals for clinical applications. Neuro Oncol. 2019 May 6;21(5):571–84. PMID:30668804
317. Boisseau W, Euskirchen P, Mokhtari K, et al. Molecular profiling reclassifies adult astroblastoma into known and clinically distinct tumor entities with frequent mitogen-activated protein kinase pathway alterations. Oncologist. 2019 Dec;24(12):1584–92. PMID:31346129
318. Boisselier B, Dugay F, Belaud-Rotureau MA, et al. Whole genome duplication is an early event leading to aneuploidy in IDH-wild type glioblastoma. Oncotarget. 2018 Nov 13;9(89):36017–28. PMID:30542515
319. Bongaarts A, Giannikou K, Reinten RJ, et al. Subependymal giant cell astrocytomas in tuberous sclerosis complex have consistent TSC1/TSC2 biallelic inactivation, and no BRAF mutations. Oncotarget. 2017 Sep 8;8(56):95516–29. PMID:29221145
320. Bonnet C, Thomas L, Psimaras D, et al. Characteristics of gliomas in patients with somatic IDH mosaicism. Acta Neuropathol Commun. 2016 Mar 31;4:31. PMID:27036230
321. Bonnin JM, Rubinstein LJ. Astroblastomas: a pathological study of 23 tumors, with a postoperative follow-up in 13 patients. Neurosurgery. 1989 Jul;25(1):6–13. PMID:2755581
322. Booman M, Douwes J, Glas AM, et al. Mechanisms and effects of loss of human leukocyte antigen class II expression in immune-privileged site-associated B-cell lymphoma. Clin Cancer Res. 2006 May 1;12(9):2698–705. PMID:16675561
323. Boonyawat B, Charoenpitakchai M, Suwanpakdee P. A first case report of subependymoma in PTPN11 mutation-associated Noonan syndrome. Case Rep Neurol Med. 2019 Sep 16;2019:6091059. PMID:31637070
324. Borges MT, Lillehei KO,

Kleinschmidt-DeMasters BK. Spindle cell oncocytoma with late recurrence and unique neuroimaging characteristics due to recurrent subclinical intratumoral bleeding. J Neurooncol. 2011 Jan;101(1):145–54. PMID:20495848
325. Borit A, Blackwood W, Mair WG. The separation of pineocytoma from pineoblastoma. Cancer. 1980 Mar 15;45(6):1408–18. PMID:6986979
326. Borit A, Richardson EP Jr. The biological and clinical behaviour of pilocytic astrocytomas of the optic pathways. Brain. 1982 Mar;105(Pt 1):161–87. PMID:7066671
327. Borkowska J, Schwartz RA, Kotulska K, et al. Tuberous sclerosis complex: tumors and tumorigenesis. Int J Dermatol. 2011 Jan;50(1):13–20. PMID:21182496
328. Borni M, Kammoun B, Kolsi F, et al. The Lhermitte-Duclos disease: a rare bilateral cerebellar location of a rare pathology. Pan Afr Med J. 2019 Jun 14;33:118. PMID:31489096
329. Borrill R, Cheesman E, Stivaros S, et al. Papillary craniopharyngioma in a 4-year-old girl with BRAF V600E mutation: a case report and review of the literature. Childs Nerv Syst. 2019 Jan;35(1):169–73. PMID:30069716
330. Boström A, von Lehe M, Hartmann W, et al. Surgery for spinal cord ependymomas: outcome and prognostic factors. Neurosurgery. 2011 Feb;68(2):302–8. PMID:21135741
331. Boström J, Meyer-Puttlitz B, Wolter M, et al. Alterations of the tumor suppressor genes CDKN2A (p16(INK4a)), p14(ARF), CDKN2B (p15(INK4b)), and CDKN2C (p18(INK4c)) in atypical and anaplastic meningiomas. Am J Pathol. 2001 Aug;159(2):661–9. PMID:11485924
332. Bott M, Brevet M, Taylor BS, et al. The nuclear deubiquitinase BAP1 is commonly inactivated by somatic mutations and 3p21.1 losses in malignant pleural mesothelioma. Nat Genet. 2011 Jun 5;43(7):668–72. PMID:21642991
333. Bouaoun L, Sonkin D, Ardin M, et al. TP53 variations in human cancers: new lessons from the IARC TP53 Database and genomics data. Hum Mutat. 2016 Sep;37(9):865–76. PMID:27328919
334. Bouchart C, Trépant AL, Hein M, et al. Prognostic impact of glioblastoma stem cell markers OLIG2 and CCND2. Cancer Med. 2020 Feb;9(3):1069–78. PMID:31568682
335. Bouffet E, Larouche V, Campbell BB, et al. Immune checkpoint inhibition for hypermutant glioblastoma multiforme resulting from germline biallelic mismatch repair deficiency. J Clin Oncol. 2016 Jul 1;34(19):2206–11. PMID:27001570
336. Bougeard G, Renaux-Petel M, Flaman JM, et al. Revisiting Li-Fraumeni Syndrome From TP53 Mutation Carriers. J Clin Oncol. 2015 Jul 20;33(21):2345–52. PMID:26014290
337. Bougeard G, Sesboüé R, Baert-Desurmont S, et al. Molecular basis of the Li-Fraumeni syndrome: an update from the French LFS families. J Med Genet. 2008 Aug;45(8):535–8. PMID:18511570
338. Bourdeaut F, Lequin D, Brugières L, et al. Frequent hSNF5/INI1 germline mutations in patients with rhabdoid tumor. Clin Cancer Res. 2011 Jan 1;17(1):31–8. PMID:21208904
339. Bourdeaut F, Miquel C, Richer W, et al. Rubinstein-Taybi syndrome predisposing to non-WNT, non-SHH, group 3 medulloblastoma. Pediatr Blood Cancer. 2014 Feb;61(2):383–6. PMID:24115570
340. Bourekas EC, Bell SD, Ladwig NR, et al. Anaplastic papillary glioneuronal tumor with extraneural metastases. J Neuropathol Exp Neurol. 2014 May;73(5):474–6. PMID:24709681
341. Bourn D, Carter SA, Mason S, et al. Germline mutations in the neurofibromatosis type 2 tumour suppressor gene. Hum Mol Genet. 1994 May;3(5):813–6. PMID:8081368
342. Bourne TD, Mandell JW, Matsumoto JA, et al. Primary disseminated leptomeningeal oligodendroglioma with 1p deletion. Case report. J Neurosurg. 2006 Dec;105(6 Suppl):465–9. PMID:17184079
343. Bouvier C, Bertucci F, Métellus P, et al. ALDH1 is an immunohistochemical diagnostic marker for solitary fibrous tumours and haemangiopericytomas of the meninges emerging from gene profiling study. Acta Neuropathol Commun. 2013 May 9;1:10. PMID:24252471
344. Bouwmeester T, Bauch A, Ruffner H, et al. A physical and functional map of the human TNF-alpha/NF-kappa B signal transduction pathway. Nat Cell Biol. 2004 Feb;6(2):97–105. PMID:14743216
345. Boyd C, Smith MJ, Kluwe L, et al. Alterations in the SMARCB1 (INI1) tumor suppressor gene in familial schwannomatosis. Clin Genet. 2008 Oct;74(4):358–66. PMID:18647326
346. Boykin FC, Cowen D, Iannucci CA, et al. Subependymal glomerate astrocytomas. J Neuropathol Exp Neurol. 1954 Jan;13(1):30–49. PMID:13118373
347. Bozzai B, Hasselblatt M, Turányi E, et al. Atypical teratoid/rhabdoid tumor arising in a malignant glioma. Pediatr Blood Cancer. 2017 Jan;64(1):96–9. PMID:27472468
348. Brabbing-Goldstein D, Ben-Shachar S. Ante-natal counseling in phacomatoses. Childs Nerv Syst. 2020 Oct;36(10):2269–77. PMID:32623496
349. Braggio E, Van Wier S, Ojha J, et al. Genome-wide analysis uncovers novel recurrent alterations in primary central nervous system lymphomas. Clin Cancer Res. 2015 Sep 1;21(17):3986–94. PMID:25991819
350. Brain Tumor Registry of Japan. Report of Brain Tumor Registry of Japan (2005-2008), 14th edition. Neurol Med Chir (Tokyo). 2017;57(Suppl 1):9–102. PMID:28420810
351. Brandner S, von Deimling A. Diagnostic, prognostic and predictive relevance of molecular markers in gliomas. Neuropathol Appl Neurobiol. 2015 Oct;41(6):694–720. PMID:25944653
352. Brantley MA Jr, Harbour JW. The molecular biology of retinoblastoma. Ocul Immunol Inflamm. 2001 Mar;9(1):1–8. PMID:11262663
353. Brastianos PK, Horowitz PM, Santagata S, et al. Genomic sequencing of meningiomas identifies oncogenic SMO and AKT1 mutations. Nat Genet. 2013 Mar;45(3):285–9. PMID:23334667
354. Brastianos PK, Shankar GM, Gill CM, et al. Dramatic response of BRAF V600E mutant papillary craniopharyngioma to targeted therapy. J Natl Cancer Inst. 2015 Oct 23;108(2):djv310. PMID:26498373
355. Brastianos PK, Taylor-Weiner A, Manley PE, et al. Exome sequencing identifies BRAF mutations in papillary craniopharyngiomas. Nat Genet. 2014 Feb;46(2):161–5. PMID:24413733
356. Brat DJ, Aldape K, Colman H, et al. cIMPACT-NOW update 3: recommended diagnostic criteria for "Diffuse astrocytic glioma, IDH-wildtype, with molecular features of glioblastoma, WHO grade IV". Acta Neuropathol. 2018 Nov;136(5):805–10. PMID:30259105
357. Brat DJ, Aldape K, Colman H, et al. cIMPACT-NOW update 5: recommended grading criteria and terminologies for IDH-mutant astrocytomas. Acta Neuropathol. 2020 Mar;139(3):603–8. PMID:31996992
358. Brat DJ, Castellano-Sanchez AA, Hunter SB, et al. Pseudopalisades in glioblastoma are hypoxic, express extracellular matrix proteases, and are formed by an actively migrating cell population. Cancer Res. 2004 Feb 1;64(3):920–7. PMID:14871821
359. Brat DJ, Giannini C, Scheithauer BW, et al. Primary melanocytic neoplasms of the central nervous systems. Am J Surg Pathol. 1999 Jul;23(7):745–54. PMID:10403296
360. Brat DJ, Hirose Y, Cohen KJ, et al. Astroblastoma: clinicopathologic features and chromosomal abnormalities defined by comparative genomic hybridization. Brain Pathol. 2000 Jul;10(3):342–52. PMID:10885653
361. Brat DJ, Kaur B, Van Meir EG. Genetic modulation of hypoxia induced gene expression and angiogenesis: relevance to brain tumors. Front Biosci. 2003 Jan 1;8:d100–16. PMID:12456339
362. Brat DJ, Prayson RA, Ryken TC, et al. Diagnosis of malignant glioma: role of neuropathology. J Neurooncol. 2008 Sep;89(3):287–311. PMID:18712282
363. Brat DJ, Scheithauer BW, Eberhart CG, et al. Extraventricular neurocytomas: pathologic features and clinical outcome. Am J Surg Pathol. 2001 Oct;25(10):1252–60. PMID:11688459
364. Brat DJ, Scheithauer BW, Medina-Flores R, et al. Infiltrative astrocytomas with granular cell features (granular cell astrocytomas): a study of histopathologic features, grading, and outcome. Am J Surg Pathol. 2002 Jun;26(6):750–7. PMID:12023579
365. Brat DJ, Scheithauer BW, Staugaitis SM, et al. Pituicytoma: a distinctive low-grade glioma of the neurohypophysis. Am J Surg Pathol. 2000 Mar;24(3):362–8. PMID:10716149
366. Brat DJ, Scheithauer BW, Staugaitis SM, et al. Third ventricular chordoid glioma: a distinct clinicopathologic entity. J Neuropathol Exp Neurol. 1998 Mar;57(3):283–90. PMID:9600220
367. Brayer KJ, Frerich CA, Kang H, et al. Recurrent fusions in MYB and MYBL1 define a common, transcription factor-driven oncogenic pathway in salivary gland adenoid cystic carcinoma. Cancer Discov. 2016 Feb;6(2):176–87. PMID:26631070
368. Bremer J, Kottke R, Johann PD, et al. A single supratentorial high-grade neuroepithelial tumor with two distinct BCOR mutations, exceptionally long complete remission and survival. Pediatr Blood Cancer. 2020 Jul;67(7):e28384. PMID:32383815
369. Brems H, Beert E, de Ravel T, et al. Mechanisms in the pathogenesis of malignant tumours in neurofibromatosis type 1. Lancet Oncol. 2009 May;10(5):508–15. PMID:19410195
370. Brennan CW, Verhaak RG, McKenna A, et al. The somatic genomic landscape of glioblastoma. Cell. 2013 Oct 10;155(2):462–77. PMID:24120142
371. Brennan MF, Antonescu CR, Moraco N, et al. Lessons learned from the study of 10,000 patients with soft tissue sarcoma. Ann Surg. 2014 Sep;260(3):416–21. PMID:25115417
372. Brenneman M, Field A, Yang J, et al. Temporal order of RNase IIIb and loss-of-function mutations during development determines phenotype in pleuropulmonary blastoma / DICER1 syndrome: a unique variant of the two-hit tumor suppression model. F1000Res. 2015 Jul 10;4:214. PMID:26925222
373. Bridge JA, Liu XQ, Sumegi J, et al. Identification of a novel, recurrent SLC44A1-PRKCA fusion in papillary glioneuronal tumor. Brain Pathol. 2013 Mar;23(2):121–8. PMID:22725730
374. Brierley JD, Gospodarowicz MK, Wittekind C, editors. TNM classification of malignant tumours. 8th ed. Oxford (UK): Wiley-Blackwell; 2017.
375. Brinkman M, Jentjens S, Boone K, et al. Evaluation of the most commonly used (semi-)quantitative parameters of 18F-FDG PET/CT to detect malignant transformation of neurofibromas in neurofibromatosis type 1. Nucl Med Commun. 2018 Nov;39(11):961–8. PMID:30106798
376. Brinkmeier ML, Bando H, Camarano AC, et al. Rathke's cleft-like cysts arise from Isl1 deletion in murine pituitary progenitors. J Clin Invest. 2020 Aug 3;130(8):4501–15. PMID:32453714
377. Brito C, Azevedo A, Esteves S, et al. Clinical insights gained by refining the 2016 WHO classification of diffuse gliomas with: EGFR amplification, TERT mutations, PTEN deletion and MGMT methylation. BMC Cancer. 2019 Oct 17;19(1):968. PMID:31623593
378. Broaddus E, Topham A, Singh AD. Incidence of retinoblastoma in the USA: 1975-2004. Br J Ophthalmol. 2009 Jan;93(1):21–3. PMID:18621794
379. Brock JE, Perez-Atayde AR, Kozakewich HP, et al. Cytogenetic aberrations in perineurioma: variation with subtype. Am J Surg Pathol. 2005 Sep;29(9):1164–9. PMID:16096405
380. Broderick DK, Di C, Parrett TJ, et al. Mutations of PIK3CA in anaplastic oligodendrogliomas, high-grade astrocytomas, and medulloblastomas. Cancer Res. 2004 Aug 1;64(15):5048–50. PMID:15289301
381. Brohl AS, Kahen E, Yoder SJ, et al. The genomic landscape of malignant peripheral nerve sheath tumors: diverse drivers of Ras pathway activation. Sci Rep. 2017 Nov 8;7(1):14992. PMID:29118384
382. Brohl AS, Solomon DA, Chang W, et al. The genomic landscape of the Ewing sarcoma family of tumors reveals recurrent STAG2 mutation. PLoS Genet. 2014 Jul 10;10(7):e1004475. PMID:25010205
383. Broniscer A, Hwang SN, Chamdine O, et al. Bithalamic gliomas may be molecularly distinct from their unilateral high-grade counterparts. Brain Pathol. 2018 Jan;28(1):112–20. PMID:28032389
384. Broniscer A, Tatevossian RG, Sabin ND, et al. Clinical, radiological, histological and molecular characteristics of paediatric epithelioid glioblastoma. Neuropathol Appl Neurobiol. 2014 Apr;40(3):327–36. PMID:24127995
385. Brown AE, Leibundgut K, Niggli FK, et al. Cytogenetics of pineoblastoma: four new cases and a literature review. Cancer Genet Cytogenet. 2006 Oct 15;170(2):175–9. PMID:17011992
386. Brown NA, Furtado LV, Betz BL, et al. High prevalence of somatic MAP2K1 mutations in BRAF V600E-negative Langerhans cell histiocytosis. Blood. 2014 Sep 4;124(10):1655–8. PMID:24982505
387. Brown R, Zlatescu M, Sijben A, et al. The use of magnetic resonance imaging to noninvasively detect genetic signatures in oligodendroglioma. Clin Cancer Res. 2008 Apr 15;14(8):2357–62. PMID:18413825
388. Brownstein MH, Wolf M, Bikowski JB. Cowden's disease: a cutaneous marker of breast cancer. Cancer. 1978 Jun;41(6):2393–8. PMID:657103
389. Brück W, Brunn A, Klapper W, et al. [Differential diagnosis of lymphoid infiltrates in the central nervous system: experience of the Network Lymphomas and Lymphomatoid Lesions in the Nervous System]. Pathologe. 2013 May;34(3):186–97. German. PMID:23471726
390. Bruford EA, Braschi B, Denny P, et al. Guidelines for human gene nomenclature. Nat Genet. 2020 Aug;52(8):754–8. PMID:32747822
391. Brugières L, Remenieras A, Pierron G, et al. High frequency of germline SUFU mutations in children with desmoplastic/nodular medulloblastoma younger than 3 years of age. J Clin Oncol. 2012 Jun 10;30(17):2087–93. PMID:22508808
392. Brunn A, Nagel I, Montesinos-Rongen M, et al. Frequent triple-hit expression of MYC,

BCL2, and BCL6 in primary lymphoma of the central nervous system and absence of a favorable MYC(low)BCL2 (low) subgroup may underlie the inferior prognosis as compared to systemic diffuse large B cell lymphomas. Acta Neuropathol. 2013 Oct;126(4):603–5. PMID:24061549

393. Bruno A, Boisselier B, Labreche K, et al. Mutational analysis of primary central nervous system lymphoma. Oncotarget. 2014 Jul 15;5(13):5065–75. PMID:24970810

394. Bruno A, Labreche K, Daniau M, et al. Identification of novel recurrent ETV6-IgH fusions in primary central nervous system lymphoma. Neuro Oncol. 2018 Jul 5;20(8):1092–100. PMID:29432597

395. Buccoliero AM, Bacci S, Mennonna P, et al. Pathologic quiz case: infratentorial tumor in a middle-aged woman. Oncocytic variant of choroid plexus papilloma. Arch Pathol Lab Med. 2004 Dec;128(12):1448–50. PMID:15578895

396. Buccoliero AM, Castiglione F, Degl'Innocenti DR, et al. Angiocentric glioma: clinical, morphological, immunohistochemical and molecular features in three pediatric cases. Clin Neuropathol. 2013 Mar-Apr;32(2):107–13. PMID:23073165

397. Buccoliero AM, Castiglione F, Rossi Degl'Innocenti D, et al. Embryonal tumor with abundant neuropil and true rosettes: morphological, immunohistochemical, ultrastructural and molecular study of a case showing features of medulloepithelioma and areas of mesenchymal and epithelial differentiation. Neuropathology. 2010 Feb 1;30(1):84–91. PMID:19563506

398. Buccoliero AM, Franchi A, Castiglione F, et al. Subependymal giant cell astrocytoma (SEGA): is it an astrocytoma? Morphological, immunohistochemical and ultrastructural study. Neuropathology. 2009 Feb;29(1):25–30. PMID:18564101

399. Buccoliero AM, Giordano F, Mussa F, et al. Papillary glioneuronal tumor radiologically mimicking a cavernous hemangioma with hemorrhagic onset. Neuropathology. 2006 Jun;26(3):206–11. PMID:16771176

400. Buckingham M, Relaix F. PAX3 and PAX7 as upstream regulators of myogenesis. Semin Cell Dev Biol. 2015 Aug;44:115–25. PMID:26424495

401. Buckner J, Giannini C, Eckel-Passow J, et al. Management of diffuse low-grade gliomas in adults - use of molecular diagnostics. Nat Rev Neurol. 2017 Jun;13(6):340–51. PMID:28497806

402. Buckner JC, Shaw EG, Pugh SL, et al. Radiation plus procarbazine, CCNU, and vincristine in low-grade glioma. N Engl J Med. 2016 Apr 7;374(14):1344–55. PMID:27050206

403. Buczkowicz P, Bartels U, Bouffet E, et al. Histopathological spectrum of paediatric diffuse intrinsic pontine glioma: diagnostic and therapeutic implications. Acta Neuropathol. 2014 Oct;128(4):573–81. PMID:25047029

404. Buczkowicz P, Hoeman C, Rakopoulos P, et al. Genomic analysis of diffuse intrinsic pontine gliomas identifies three molecular subgroups and recurrent activating ACVR1 mutations. Nat Genet. 2014 May;46(5):451–6. PMID:24705254

405. Budohoski KP, Clerkin J, Millward CP, et al. Predictors of early progression of surgically treated atypical meningiomas. Acta Neurochir (Wien). 2018 Sep;160(9):1813–22. PMID:29961125

406. Bueno R, Stawiski EW, Goldstein LD, et al. Comprehensive genomic analysis of malignant pleural mesothelioma identifies recurrent mutations, gene fusions and splicing alterations. Nat Genet. 2016 Apr;48(4):407–16. PMID:26928227

407. Bühren J, Christoph AH, Buslei R, et al. Expression of the neurotrophin receptor p75NTR in medulloblastomas is correlated with distinct histological and clinical features: evidence for a medulloblastoma subtype derived from the external granule cell layer. J Neuropathol Exp Neurol. 2000 Mar;59(3):229–40. PMID:10744061

408. Bullock N, Simpkin A, Fowler S, et al. Pathological upgrading in prostate cancer treated with surgery in the United Kingdom: trends and risk factors from the British Association of Urological Surgeons Radical Prostatectomy Registry. BMC Urol. 2019 Oct 17;19(1):94. PMID:31623595

409. Bunin GR, Surawicz TS, Witman PA, et al. The descriptive epidemiology of craniopharyngioma. J Neurosurg. 1998 Oct;89(4):547–51. PMID:9761047

410. Burel-Vandenbos F, Pierron G, Thomas C, et al. A polyphenotypic malignant paediatric brain tumour presenting a MN1-PATZ1 fusion, no epigenetic similarities with CNS high-grade neuroepithelial tumour with MN1 alteration (CNS HGNET-MN1) and related to PATZ1-fused sarcomas. Neuropathol Appl Neurobiol. 2020 Aug;46(5):506–9. PMID:32397004

411. Burford A, Mackay A, Popov S, et al. The ten-year evolutionary trajectory of a highly recurrent paediatric high grade neuroepithelial tumour with MN1:BEND2 fusion. Sci Rep. 2018 Jan 18;8(1):1032. PMID:29348602

412. Burger PC, Green SB. Patient age, histologic features, and length of survival in patients with glioblastoma multiforme. Cancer. 1987 May 1;59(9):1617–25. PMID:3030531

413. Burger PC, Heinz ER, Shibata T, et al. Topographic anatomy and CT correlations in the untreated glioblastoma multiforme. J Neurosurg. 1988 May;68(5):698–704. PMID:2833587

414. Burger PC, Kleihues P. Cytologic composition of the untreated glioblastoma with implications for evaluation of needle biopsies. Cancer. 1989 May 15;63(10):2014–23. PMID:2539242

415. Burger PC, Pearl DK, Aldape K, et al. Small cell architecture—a histological equivalent of EGFR amplification in glioblastoma multiforme? J Neuropathol Exp Neurol. 2001 Nov;60(11):1099–104. PMID:11706939

416. Burger PC, Scheithauer BW. Tumors of the central nervous system. Washington, DC: Armed Forces Institute of Pathology; 1994. (AFIP atlas of tumor pathology, series 3; fascicle 10).

417. Burger PC, Vogel FS, Green SB, et al. Glioblastoma multiforme and anaplastic astrocytoma. Pathologic criteria and prognostic implications. Cancer. 1985 Sep 1;56(5):1106–11. PMID:2990664

418. Burger PC, Vollmer RT. Histologic factors of prognostic significance in the glioblastoma multiforme. Cancer. 1980 Sep 1;46(5):1170–86. PMID:6260329

419. Burger PC, Yu IT, Tihan T, et al. Atypical teratoid/rhabdoid tumor of the central nervous system: a highly malignant tumor of infancy and childhood frequently mistaken for medulloblastoma: a Pediatric Oncology Group study. Am J Surg Pathol. 1998 Sep;22(9):1083–92. PMID:9737241

420. Burgy M, Chenard MP, Noël G, et al. Bone metastases from a 1p/19q codeleted and IDH1-mutant anaplastic oligodendroglioma: a case report. J Med Case Rep. 2019 Jun 28;13(1):202. PMID:31248444

421. Burkhard C, Di Patre PL, Schüler D, et al. A population-based study of the incidence and survival rates in patients with pilocytic astrocytoma. J Neurosurg. 2003 Jun;98(6):1170–4. PMID:12816259

422. Burnier MN, McLean IW, Zimmerman LE, et al. Retinoblastoma. The relationship of proliferating cells to blood vessels. Invest Ophthalmol Vis Sci. 1990 Oct;31(10):2037–40. PMID:2211000

423. Bush K, Bateman DE. Papilloedema secondary to a spinal paraganglioma. Pract Neurol. 2014 Jun;14(3):179–81. PMID:23918468

424. Bush ZM, Longtine JA, Cunningham T, et al. Temozolomide treatment for aggressive pituitary tumors: correlation of clinical outcome with O(6)-methylguanine methyltransferase (MGMT) promoter methylation and expression. J Clin Endocrinol Metab. 2010 Nov;95(11):E280–90. PMID:20668043

425. Buslei R, Hölsken A, Hofmann B, et al. Nuclear beta-catenin accumulation associates with epithelial morphogenesis in craniopharyngiomas. Acta Neuropathol. 2007 May;113(5):585–90. PMID:17221204

426. Buslei R, Nolde M, Hofmann B, et al. Common mutations of beta-catenin in adamantinomatous craniopharyngiomas but not in other tumours originating from the sellar region. Acta Neuropathol. 2005 Jun;109(6):589–97. PMID:15891929

427. Butler MG, Dasouki MJ, Zhou XP, et al. Subset of individuals with autism spectrum disorders and extreme macrocephaly associated with germline PTEN tumour suppressor gene mutations. J Med Genet. 2005 Apr;42(4):318–21. PMID:15805158

428. Byeon SJ, Cho HJ, Baek HW, et al. Rhabdoid glioblastoma is distinguishable from classical glioblastoma by cytogenetics and molecular genetics. Hum Pathol. 2014 Mar;45(3):611–20. PMID:24457079

429. Byun J, Hong SH, Yoon MJ, et al. Prognosis and treatment outcomes of central neurocytomas: clinical interrogation based on a single center experience. J Neurooncol. 2018 Dec;140(3):669–77. PMID:30225773

430. Cabanillas R, Astudillo A, Valle M, et al. Novel germline CDKN2A mutation associated with head and neck squamous cell carcinomas and melanomas. Head Neck. 2013 Mar;35(3):E80–4. PMID:22083977

431. Cabaret O, Perron E, Bressac-de Paillerets B, et al. Occurrence of BAP1 germline mutations in cutaneous melanocytic tumors with loss of BAP1-expression: a pilot study. Genes Chromosomes Cancer. 2017 Sep;56(9):691–4. PMID:28560743

432. Caccamo DV, Ho KL, Garcia JH. Cauda equina tumor with ependymal and paraganglionic differentiation. Hum Pathol. 1992 Jul;23(7):835–8. PMID:1612583

433. Cacciola F, Conti R, Taddei GL, et al. Cerebellar liponeurocytoma. Case report with considerations on prognosis and management. Acta Neurochir (Wien). 2002 Aug;144(8):829–33. PMID:12181694

434. Cady FM, O'Neill BP, Law ME, et al. Del(6)(q22) and BCL6 rearrangements in primary CNS lymphoma are indicators of an aggressive clinical course. J Clin Oncol. 2008 Oct 10;26(29):4814–9. PMID:18645192

435. Cahill DP, Levine KK, Betensky RA, et al. Loss of the mismatch repair protein MSH6 in human glioblastomas is associated with tumor progression during temozolomide treatment. Clin Cancer Res. 2007 Apr 1;13(7):2038–45. PMID:17404084

436. Cai J, Li W, Du J, et al. Supratentorial intracerebral cerebellar liponeurocytoma: a case report and literature review. Medicine (Baltimore). 2018 Jan;97(2):e9556. PMID:29480846

437. Cai M, He H, Zhang B, et al. An ectopic recurrent craniopharyngioma of the temporal lobe: case report and review of the literature. World Neurosurg. 2019 Jun;126:216–22. PMID:30877004

438. Cairncross G, Wang M, Shaw E, et al. Phase III trial of chemoradiotherapy for anaplastic oligodendroglioma: long-term results of RTOG 9402. J Clin Oncol. 2013 Jan 20;31(3):337–43. PMID:23071247

439. Cajaiba MM, Benjamin D, Halaban R, et al. Metastatic peritoneal neurocutaneous melanocytosis. Am J Surg Pathol. 2008 Jan;32(1):156–61. PMID:18162783

440. Calaminus G, Frappaz D, Kortmann RD, et al. Outcome of patients with intracranial non-germinomatous germ cell tumors-lessons from the SIOP-CNS-GCT-96 trial. Neuro Oncol. 2017 Nov 29;19(12):1661–72. PMID:29048505

441. Calaminus G, Kortmann R, Worch J, et al. SIOP CNS GCT 96: final report of outcome of a prospective, multinational nonrandomized trial for children and adults with intracranial germinoma, comparing craniospinal irradiation alone with chemotherapy followed by focal primary site irradiation for patients with localized disease. Neuro Oncol. 2013 Jun;15(6):788–96. PMID:23460321

442. Calderon-Garcidueñas AL, Mathon B, Lévy P, et al. New clinicopathological associations and histoprognostic markers in ILAE types of hippocampal sclerosis. Brain Pathol. 2018 Sep;28(5):644–55. PMID:29476662

443. Caltabiano R, Magro G, Polizzi A, et al. A mosaic pattern of INI1/SMARCB1 protein expression distinguishes Schwannomatosis and NF2-associated peripheral schwannomas from solitary peripheral schwannomas and NF2-associated vestibular schwannomas. Childs Nerv Syst. 2017 Jun;33(6):933–40. PMID:28365909

444. Cambiaso P, Amodio D, Procaccini E, et al. Pituicytoma and Cushing's disease in a 7-year-old girl: a mere coincidence? Pediatrics. 2015 Dec;136(6):e1632–6. PMID:26553184

445. Camelo-Piragua S, Jansen M, Ganguly A, et al. A sensitive and specific diagnostic panel to distinguish diffuse astrocytoma from astrocytosis: chromosome 7 gain with mutant isocitrate dehydrogenase 1 and p53. J Neuropathol Exp Neurol. 2011 Feb;70(2):110–5. PMID:21343870

446. Camidge DR, Lee EQ, Lin NU, et al. Clinical trial design for systemic agents in patients with brain metastases from solid tumours: a guideline by the Response Assessment in Neuro-Oncology Brain Metastases working group. Lancet Oncol. 2018 Jan;19(1):e20–32. PMID:29304358

447. Campbell BB, Light N, Fabrizio D, et al. Comprehensive analysis of hypermutation in human cancer. Cell. 2017 Nov 16;171(5):1042–1056.e10. PMID:29056344

448. Campian J, Gutmann DH. CNS tumors in neurofibromatosis. J Clin Oncol. 2017 Jul 20;35(21):2378–85. PMID:28640700

449. Campos AR, Clusmann H, von Lehe M, et al. Simple and complex dysembryoplastic neuroepithelial tumors (DNT) variants: clinical profile, MRI, and histopathology. Neuroradiology. 2009 Jul;51(7):433–43. PMID:19242688

450. Can A, Gross BA, Du R. The natural history of cerebral arteriovenous malformations. Handb Clin Neurol. 2017;143:15–24. PMID:28552137

451. Cancer Genome Atlas Research Network. Comprehensive genomic characterization defines human glioblastoma genes and core pathways. Nature. 2008 Oct 23;455(7216):1061–8. PMID:18772890

452. Brat DJ, Verhaak RG, Aldape KD, et al. Comprehensive, integrative genomic analysis of diffuse lower-grade gliomas. N Engl J Med. 2015 Jun 25;372(26):2481–98. PMID:26061751

453. Cannavo S, Ragonese M, Puglisi S, et al. Acromegaly is more severe in patients with ahr or aip gene variants living in highly polluted areas. J Clin Endocrinol Metab. 2016 Apr;101(4):1872–9. PMID:26963951

454. Cannavo S, Trimarchi F, Ferraù F. Acromegaly, genetic variants of the aryl hydrocarbon receptor pathway and environmental burden. Mol Cell Endocrinol. 2017 Dec 5;457:81–8. PMID:27998805
455. Cannon DM, Mohindra P, Gondi V, et al. Choroid plexus tumor epidemiology and outcomes: implications for surgical and radiotherapeutic management. J Neurooncol. 2015 Jan;121(1):151–7. PMID:25270349
456. Canturk S, Qaddoumi I, Khetan V, et al. Survival of retinoblastoma in less-developed countries impact of socioeconomic and health-related indicators. Br J Ophthalmol. 2010 Nov;94(11):1432–6. PMID:20733021
457. Cao D, Liu A, Wang F, et al. RNA-binding protein LIN28 is a marker for primary extragonadal germ cell tumors: an immunohistochemical study of 131 cases. Mod Pathol. 2011 Feb;24(2):288–96. PMID:21057460
458. Caporlingua F, Lapadula G, Antonelli M, et al. Pleomorphic rhabdomyosarcoma of the cerebellopontine angle in an adult: a review of literature. BMJ Case Rep. 2014 Jan 30;2014:bcr2013203257. PMID:24481021
459. Capper D, Berghoff AS, Magerle M, et al. Immunohistochemical testing of BRAF V600E status in 1,120 tumor tissue samples of patients with brain metastases. Acta Neuropathol. 2012 Feb;123(2):223–33. PMID:22012135
460. Capper D, Jones DTW, Sill M, et al. DNA methylation-based classification of central nervous system tumours. Nature. 2018 Mar 22;555(7697):469–74. PMID:29539639
461. Capper D, Reuss D, Schittenhelm J, et al. Mutation-specific IDH1 antibody differentiates oligodendrogliomas and oligoastrocytomas from other brain tumors with oligodendroglioma-like morphology. Acta Neuropathol. 2011 Feb;121(2):241–52. PMID:21069360
462. Capper D, Sahm F, Hartmann C, et al. Application of mutant IDH1 antibody to differentiate diffuse glioma from nonneoplastic central nervous system lesions and therapy-induced changes. Am J Surg Pathol. 2010 Aug;34(8):1199–204. PMID:20661018
463. Capper D, Stichel D, Sahm F, et al. Practical implementation of DNA methylation and copy-number-based CNS tumor diagnostics: the Heidelberg experience. Acta Neuropathol. 2018 Aug;136(2):181–210. PMID:29967940
464. Capper D, Weissert S, Balss J, et al. Characterization of R132H mutation-specific IDH1 antibody binding in brain tumors. Brain Pathol. 2010 Jan;20(1):245–54. PMID:19903171
465. Capper D, Zentgraf H, Balss J, et al. Monoclonal antibody specific for IDH1 R132H mutation. Acta Neuropathol. 2009 Nov;118(5):599–601. PMID:19798509
466. Carbone M, Arron ST, Beutler B, et al. Tumour predisposition and cancer syndromes as models to study gene-environment interactions. Nat Rev Cancer. 2020 Sep;20(9):533–49. PMID:32472073
467. Carlson GJ, Nivatvongs S, Snover DC. Colorectal polyps in Cowden's disease (multiple hamartoma syndrome). Am J Surg Pathol. 1984 Oct;8(10):763–70. PMID:6496844
468. Carlson ML, Babovic-Vuksanovic D, Messiaen L, et al. Radiation-induced rhabdomyosarcoma of the brainstem in a patient with neurofibromatosis type 2. J Neurosurg. 2010 Jan;112(1):81–7. PMID:19575577
469. Carneiro SS, Scheithauer BW, Nascimento AG, et al. Solitary fibrous tumor of the meninges: a lesion distinct from fibrous meningioma. A clinicopathologic and immunohistochemical study. Am J Clin Pathol. 1996 Aug;106(2):217–24. PMID:8712177
470. Carney JA. Psammomatous melanotic schwannoma. A distinctive, heritable tumor with special associations, including cardiac myxoma and the Cushing syndrome. Am J Surg Pathol. 1990 Mar;14(3):206–22. PMID:2305928
471. Carney JA, Gordon H, Carpenter PC, et al. The complex of myxomas, spotty pigmentation, and endocrine overactivity. Medicine (Baltimore). 1985 Jul;64(4):270–83. PMID:4010501
472. Carpten JD, Faber AL, Horn C, et al. A transforming mutation in the pleckstrin homology domain of AKT1 in cancer. Nature. 2007 Jul 26;448(7152):439–44. PMID:17611497
473. Carrillo JA, Lai A, Nghiemphu PL, et al. Relationship between tumor enhancement, edema, IDH1 mutational status, MGMT promoter methylation, and survival in glioblastoma. AJNR Am J Neuroradiol. 2012 Aug;33(7):1349–55. PMID:22322613
474. Carrió M, Gel B, Terribas E, et al. Analysis of intratumor heterogeneity in neurofibromatosis type 1 plexiform neurofibromas and neurofibromas with atypical features: correlating histological and genomic findings. Hum Mutat. 2018 Aug;39(8):1112–25. PMID:29774626
475. Carstens PH, Johnson GS, Jelsma LF. Spinal gliosarcoma: a light, immunohistochemical and ultrastructural study. Ann Clin Lab Sci. 1995 May-Jun;25(3):241–6. PMID:7605106
476. Carter JM, O'Hara C, Dundas G, et al. Epithelioid malignant peripheral nerve sheath tumor arising in a schwannoma, in a patient with "neuroblastoma-like" schwannomatosis and a novel germline SMARCB1 mutation. Am J Surg Pathol. 2012 Jan;36(1):154–60. PMID:22082606
477. Carter JM, Wu Y, Blessing MM, et al. Recurrent genomic alterations in soft tissue perineuriomas. Am J Surg Pathol. 2018 Dec;42(12):1708–14. PMID:30303818
478. Carter M, Nicholson J, Ross F, et al. Genetic abnormalities detected in ependymomas by comparative genomic hybridisation. Br J Cancer. 2002 Mar 18;86(6):929–39. PMID:11953826
479. Carvalho JADV, Barbosa CCL, Feher O, et al. Systemic dissemination of glioblastoma: literature review. Rev Assoc Med Bras (1992). 2019 Mar;65(3):460–8. PMID:30994848
480. Casadei GP, Komori T, Scheithauer BW, et al. Intracranial parenchymal schwannoma. A clinicopathological and neuroimaging study of nine cases. J Neurosurg. 1993 Aug;79(2):217–22. PMID:8331403
481. Casar-Borota O, Bollerslev J, Pontén F. Immunohistochemistry for transcription factor T-Pit as a tool in diagnostics of corticotroph pituitary tumours. Pituitary. 2018 Aug;21(4):443. PMID:29468382
482. Cassarino DS, Auerbach A, Rushing EJ. Widely invasive solitary fibrous tumor of the sphenoid sinus, cavernous sinus, and pituitary fossa. Ann Diagn Pathol. 2003 Jun;7(3):169–73. PMID:12808569
483. Castel D, Kergrohen T, Tauziède-Espariat A, et al. Histone H3 wild-type DIPG/DMG overexpressing EZHIP extend the spectrum diffuse midline gliomas with PRC2 inhibition beyond H3-K27M mutation. Acta Neuropathol. 2020 Jun;139(6):1109–13. PMID:32193787
484. Castel D, Philippe C, Calmon R, et al. Histone H3F3A and HIST1H3B K27M mutations define two subgroups of diffuse intrinsic pontine gliomas with different prognosis and phenotypes. Acta Neuropathol. 2015 Dec;130(6):815–27. PMID:26399631
485. Castel D, Philippe C, Kergrohen T, et al. Transcriptomic and epigenetic profiling of 'diffuse midline gliomas, H3 K27M-mutant' discriminate two subgroups based on the type of histone H3 mutated and not supratentorial or infratentorial location. Acta Neuropathol Commun. 2018 Nov 5;6(1):117. PMID:30396367
486. Castellanos E, Plana A, Carrato C, et al. Early genetic diagnosis of neurofibromatosis type 2 from skin plaque plexiform schwannomas in childhood. JAMA Dermatol. 2018 Mar 1;154(3):341–6. PMID:29322178
487. Castro-Vega LJ, Buffet A, De Cubas AA, et al. Germline mutations in FH confer predisposition to malignant pheochromocytomas and paragangliomas. Hum Mol Genet. 2014 May 1;23(9):2440–6. PMID:24334767
488. Castro-Vega LJ, Letouzé E, Burnichon N, et al. Multi-omics analysis defines core genomic alterations in pheochromocytomas and paragangliomas. Nat Commun. 2015 Jan 27;6:6044. PMID:25625332
489. Cataltepe O, Marshall P, Smith TW. Dysembryoplastic neuroepithelial tumor located in pericallosal and intraventricular area in a child. Case report. J Neurosurg Pediatr. 2009 Jun;3(6):456–60. PMID:19485727
490. Cavalli FMG, Hübner JM, Sharma T, et al. Heterogeneity within the PF-EPN-B ependymoma subgroup. Acta Neuropathol. 2018 Aug;136(2):227–37. PMID:30019219
491. Cavalli FMG, Remke M, Rampasek L, et al. Intertumoral heterogeneity within medulloblastoma subgroups. Cancer Cell. 2017 Jun 12;31(6):737–754.e6. PMID:28609654
492. Cavalli G, Guglielmi B, Berti A, et al. The multifaceted clinical presentations and manifestations of Erdheim-Chester disease: comprehensive review of the literature and of 10 new cases. Ann Rheum Dis. 2013 Oct;72(10):1691–5. PMID:23396641
493. Cawthon RM, Weiss R, Xu GF, et al. A major segment of the neurofibromatosis type 1 gene: cDNA sequence, genomic structure, and point mutations. Cell. 1990 Jul 13;62(1):193–201. PMID:2114220
494. Ceccon G, Werner JM, Dunkl V, et al. Dabrafenib treatment in a patient with an epithelioid glioblastoma and BRAF V600E mutation. Int J Mol Sci. 2018 Apr 5;19(4):E1090. PMID:29621181
495. Celano E, Salehani A, Malcolm JG, et al. Spinal cord ependymoma: a review of the literature and case series of ten patients. J Neurooncol. 2016 Jul;128(3):377–86. PMID:27154165
496. Cenacchi G, Giangaspero F, Cerasoli S, et al. Ultrastructural characterization of oligodendroglial-like cells in central nervous system tumors. Ultrastruct Pathol. 1996 Nov-Dec;20(6):537–47. PMID:8940761
497. Cenacchi G, Roncaroli F, Cerasoli S, et al. Chordoid glioma of the third ventricle: an ultrastructural study of three cases with a histogenetic hypothesis. Am J Surg Pathol. 2001 Mar;25(3):401–5. PMID:11224612
498. Central Brain Tumor Registry of the United States [Internet]. Chicago (IL): CBTRUS; 2020. Available from: https://cbtrus.org/.
499. Cerase A, Vallone IM, Di Pietro G, et al. Neuroradiological follow-up of the growth of papillary tumor of the pineal region: a case report. J Neurooncol. 2009 Dec;95(3):433–5. PMID:19517065
500. Cervoni L, Celli P, Caruso R, et al. [Neurinomas and ependymomas of the cauda equina. A review of the clinical characteristics]. Minerva Chir. 1997 May;52(5):629–33. Italian. PMID:9297152
501. Chacón-Quesada T, Rodriguez GJ, Maud A, et al. Trans-arterial onyx embolization of a functional thoracic paraganglioma. Neurointervention. 2015 Feb;10(1):34–8. PMID:25763296
502. Chai RC, Zhang YW, Liu YQ, et al. The molecular characteristics of spinal cord gliomas with or without H3 K27M mutation. Acta Neuropathol Commun. 2020 Mar 30;8(1):40. PMID:32228694
503. Chainey J, Chan VK, Au K, et al. Multiple recurrences of spindle cell oncocytoma: a case report and literature review. Clin Neuropathol. 2020 Jan/Feb;39(1):32–9. PMID:31496509
504. Chakraborti S, Govindan A, Alapatt JP, et al. Primary myxopapillary ependymoma of the fourth ventricle with cartilaginous metaplasia: a case report and review of the literature. Brain Tumor Pathol. 2012 Jan;29(1):25–30. PMID:21837503
505. Chalasani S, Hennick MR, Hocking WG, et al. Unusual presentation of a rare cancer: histiocytic sarcoma in the brain 16 years after treatment for acute lymphoblastic leukemia. Clin Med Res. 2013 Feb;11(1):31–5. PMID:22997353
506. Chamberlain M, Soffietti R, Raizer J, et al. Leptomeningeal metastasis: a Response Assessment in Neuro-Oncology critical review of endpoints and response criteria of published randomized clinical trials. Neuro Oncol. 2014 Sep;16(9):1176–85. PMID:24867803
507. Chan AK, Han SJ, Choy W, et al. Familial melanoma-astrocytoma syndrome: synchronous diffuse astrocytoma and pleomorphic xanthoastrocytoma in a patient with germline CDKN2A/B deletion and a significant family history. Clin Neuropathol. 2017 Sep/Oct;36(5):213–21. PMID:28699883
508. Chan AK, Pang JC, Chung NY, et al. Loss of CIC and FUBP1 expressions are potential markers of shorter time to recurrence in oligodendroglial tumors. Mod Pathol. 2014 Mar;27(3):332–42. PMID:24030748
509. Chan CC, Koch CA, Kaiser-Kupfer MI, et al. Loss of heterozygosity for the NF2 gene in retinal and optic nerve lesions of patients with neurofibromatosis 2. J Pathol. 2002 Sep;198(1):14–20. PMID:12210058
510. Chan E, Bollen AW, Sirohi D, et al. Angiocentric glioma with MYB-QKI fusion located in the brainstem, rather than cerebral cortex. Acta Neuropathol. 2017 Oct;134(4):671–3. PMID:28776091
511. Chan GL, Little JB. Cultured diploid fibroblasts from patients with the nevoid basal cell carcinoma syndrome are hypersensitive to killing by ionizing radiation. Am J Pathol. 1983 Apr;111(1):50–5. PMID:6837723
512. Chan JA, Zhang H, Roberts PS, et al. Pathogenesis of tuberous sclerosis subependymal giant cell astrocytomas: biallelic inactivation of TSC1 or TSC2 leads to mTOR activation. J Neuropathol Exp Neurol. 2004 Dec;63(12):1236–42. PMID:15624760
513. Chan JK, Lamant L, Algar E, et al. ALK+ histiocytosis: a novel type of systemic histiocytic proliferative disorder of early infancy. Blood. 2008 Oct 1;112(7):2965–8. PMID:18660380
514. Chan KM, Fang D, Gan H, et al. The histone H3.3K27M mutation in pediatric glioma reprograms H3K27 methylation and gene expression. Genes Dev. 2013 May 1;27(9):985–90. PMID:23603901
515. Chan V, Marro A, Findlay JM, et al. A systematic review of atypical teratoid rhabdoid tumor in adults. Front Oncol. 2018 Nov 28;8:567. PMID:30547013
516. Chaney M, Vajtai I. Late development of third ventricular subependymoma following surgery for craniopharyngioma. Clin Neuropathol. 2007 Jan-Feb;26(1):37–9. PMID:17290937
517. Chang AH, Fuller GN, Debnam JM, et al. MR imaging of papillary tumor of the pineal region. AJNR Am J Neuroradiol. 2008 Jan;29(1):187–9. PMID:17925365
518. Chang AL, Miska J, Wainwright DA, et al. CCL2 produced by the glioma microenvironment is essential for the recruitment of regulatory T cells and myeloid-derived suppressor cells. Cancer Res. 2016 Oct 1;76(19):5671–82. PMID:27530322
519. Chang CH, Housepian EM, Herbert C Jr. An operative staging system and a megavoltage radiotherapeutic technic for cerebellar medulloblastomas. Radiology. 1969

Dec;93(6):1351–9. PMID:4983156
520. Chang KTE, Tay AZE, Kuick CH, et al. ALK-positive histiocytosis: an expanded clinicopathologic spectrum and frequent presence of KIF5B-ALK fusion. Mod Pathol. 2019 May;32(5):598–608. PMID:30573850
521. Chang SM, Lillis-Hearne PK, Larson DA, et al. Pineoblastoma in adults. Neurosurgery. 1995 Sep;37(3):383–90. PMID:7501100
522. Chao L, Tao XB, Jun YK, et al. Recurrence and histological evolution of dysembryoplastic neuroepithelial tumor: a case report and review of the literature. Oncol Lett. 2013 Oct;6(4):907–14. PMID:24137435
523. Chappé C, Padovani L, Scavarda D, et al. Dysembryoplastic neuroepithelial tumors share with pleomorphic xanthoastrocytomas and gangliogliomas BRAF(V600E) mutation and expression. Brain Pathol. 2013 Sep;23(5):574–83. PMID:23442159
524. Charifa A, Paulson N, Levy L, et al. Intravascular large B-cell lymphoma: clinical and histopathologic findings. Yale J Biol Med. 2020 Mar 27;93(1):35–40. PMID:32226333
525. Chatterjee D, Garg C, Singla N, et al. Desmoplastic non-infantile astrocytoma/ganglioglioma: rare low-grade tumor with frequent BRAF V600E mutation. Hum Pathol. 2018 Oct;80:186–91. PMID:29902580
526. Chatzellis E, Alexandraki KI, Androulakis II, et al. Aggressive pituitary tumors. Neuroendocrinology. 2015;101(2):87–104. PMID:25571935
527. Chau C, van Doorn R, van Poppelen NM, et al. Families with BAP1-tumor predisposition syndrome in the Netherlands: path to identification and a proposal for genetic screening guidelines. Cancers (Basel). 2019 Aug 4;11(8):E1114. PMID:31382694
528. Chaudhry NS, Ahmad F, Blieden C, et al. Suprasellar and sellar paraganglioma presenting as a nonfunctioning pituitary macroadenoma. J Clin Neurosci. 2013 Nov;20(11):1615–8. PMID:23876285
529. Chawla B, Tomar A, Sen S, et al. Intraocular fine needle aspiration cytology as a diagnostic modality for retinoblastoma. Int J Ophthalmol. 2016 Aug 18;9(8):1233–5. PMID:27588281
530. Cheadle JP, Reeve MP, Sampson JR, et al. Molecular genetic advances in tuberous sclerosis. Hum Genet. 2000 Aug;107(2):97–114. PMID:11030407
531. Cheah AL, Billings SD, Goldblum JR, et al. STAT6 rabbit monoclonal antibody is a robust diagnostic tool for the distinction of solitary fibrous tumour from its mimics. Pathology. 2014 Aug;46(5):389–95. PMID:24977739
532. Chebib I, Hornicek FJ, Nielsen GP, et al. Cytomorphologic features that distinguish schwannoma from other low-grade spindle cell lesions. Cancer Cytopathol. 2015 Mar;123(3):171–9. PMID:25641870
533. Chelliah D, Mensah Sarfo-Poku C, Stea BD, et al. Medulloblastoma with extensive nodularity undergoing post-therapeutic maturation to a gangliocytoma: a case report and literature review. Pediatr Neurosurg. 2010;46(5):381–4. PMID:21389751
534. Chen CJ, Williams EA, McAneney TE, et al. Histiocytic sarcoma of the cavernous sinus: case report and literature review. Brain Tumor Pathol. 2015 Jan;32(1):66–71. PMID:24807104
535. Chen CW, Chen IH, Hu MH, et al. Primary intradural extramedullary spinal mesenchymal chondrosarcoma: case report and literature review. BMC Musculoskelet Disord. 2019 Sep 4;20(1):408. PMID:31484514
536. Chen G, Luo Z, Liu T, et al. Functioning paraganglioma of the cervical spine. Orthopedics. 2011 Oct 5;34(10):e700–2. PMID:21956072
537. Chen H, Thomas C, Munoz FA, et al. Polysomy is associated with poor outcome in 1p/19q codeleted oligodendroglial tumors. Neuro Oncol. 2019 Sep 6;21(9):1164–74. PMID:31140557
538. Chen J, Jian X, Deng S, et al. Identification of recurrent USP48 and BRAF mutations in Cushing's disease. Nat Commun. 2018 Aug 9;9(1):3171. PMID:30093687
539. Chen L, Voronovich Z, Clark K, et al. Predicting the likelihood of an isocitrate dehydrogenase 1 or 2 mutation in diagnoses of infiltrative glioma. Neuro Oncol. 2014 Nov;16(11):1478–83. PMID:24860178
540. Chen R, Nishimura MC, Kharbanda S, et al. Hominoid-specific enzyme GLUD2 promotes growth of IDH1R132H glioma. Proc Natl Acad Sci U S A. 2014 Sep 30;111(39):14217–22. PMID:25225364
541. Chen S, Deniz K, Sung YS, et al. Ewing sarcoma with ERG gene rearrangements: a molecular study focusing on the prevalence of FUS-ERG and common pitfalls in detecting EWSR1-ERG fusions by FISH. Genes Chromosomes Cancer. 2016 Apr;55(4):340–9. PMID:26690869
542. Chen S, Wang Y, Su G, et al. Primary intraspinal dumbbell-shaped mesenchymal chondrosarcoma with massive calcifications: a case report and review of the literature. World J Surg Oncol. 2016 Aug 3;14(1):203. PMID:27487949
543. Chen SC, Lin DS, Lee CC, et al. Rhabdoid glioblastoma: a recently recognized subtype of glioblastoma. Acta Neurochir (Wien). 2013 Aug;155(8):1443–8. PMID:23812963
544. Chen T, Jiang B, Zheng Y, et al. Differentiating intracranial solitary fibrous tumor/hemangiopericytoma from meningioma using diffusion-weighted imaging and susceptibility-weighted imaging. Neuroradiology. 2020 Feb;62(2):175–84. PMID:31673748
545. Chen TJ, Chen SS. Effects of non-pathological factors on brain stem auditory evoked potentials in rats. Gaoxiong Yi Xue Ke Xue Za Zhi. 1988 Oct;4(10):553–64. PMID:3230601
546. Chen W, Soon YY, Pratiseyo PD, et al. Central nervous system neuroepithelial tumors with MN1-alteration: an individual patient data meta-analysis of 73 cases. Brain Tumor Pathol. 2020 Oct;37(4):145–53. PMID:32601775
547. Chen WC, Magill ST, Wu A, et al. Histopathological features predictive of local control of atypical meningioma after surgery and adjuvant radiotherapy. J Neurosurg. 2018 Apr 6;130(2):443–50. PMID:29624151
548. Chen X, Pan C, Zhang P, et al. BRAF V600E mutation is a significant prognosticator of the tumour regrowth rate in brainstem gangliogliomas. J Clin Neurosci. 2017 Dec;46:50–7. PMID:28986151
549. Chen Y, Tian T, Guo X, et al. Polymorphous low-grade neuroepithelial tumor of the young: case report and review focus on the radiological features and genetic alterations. BMC Neurol. 2020 Apr 6;20(1):123. PMID:32252664
550. Chen Y, Wang F, Han A. Fat-forming solitary fibrous tumor of the kidney: a case report and literature review. Int J Clin Exp Pathol. 2015 Jul 1;8(7):8632–5. PMID:26339447
551. Chen YY, Yen HH, Soon MS. Solitary gastric melanotic schwannoma: sonographic findings. J Clin Ultrasound. 2007 Jan;35(1):52–4. PMID:17111368
552. Chen Z, Liu C, Patel AJ, et al. Cells of origin in the embryonic nerve roots for NF1-associated plexiform neurofibroma. Cancer Cell. 2014 Nov 10;26(5):695–706. PMID:25446898
553. Chen Z, Mo J, Brosseau JP, et al. Spatiotemporal loss of NF1 in Schwann cell lineage leads to different types of cutaneous neurofibroma susceptible to modification by the Hippo pathway. Cancer Discov. 2019 Jan;9(1):114–29. PMID:30348677
554. Cheng Z, Cheung P, Kuo AJ, et al. A molecular threading mechanism underlies Jumonji lysine demethylase KDM2A regulation of methylated H3K36. Genes Dev. 2014 Aug 15;28(16):1758–71. PMID:25128496
555. Chentli F, Belhimer F, Kessaci F, et al. Congenital craniopharyngioma: a case report and literature review. J Pediatr Endocrinol Metab. 2012;25(11-12):1181–3. PMID:23329768
556. Chetty R. Cytokeratin expression in cauda equina paragangliomas. Am J Surg Pathol. 1999 Apr;23(4):491. PMID:10199484
557. Chetty R, Vajpeyi R, Penwick JL. Psammomatous melanotic schwannoma presenting as colonic polyps. Virchows Arch. 2007 Sep;451(3):717–20. PMID:17622556
558. Cheuk W, Walford N, Lou J, et al. Primary histiocytic lymphoma of the central nervous system: a neoplasm frequently overshadowed by a prominent inflammatory component. Am J Surg Pathol. 2001 Nov;25(11):1372–9. PMID:11684953
559. Cheung M, Kadariya Y, Talarchek J, et al. Germline BAP1 mutation in a family with high incidence of multiple primary cancers and a potential gene-environment interaction. Cancer Lett. 2015 Dec 28;369(2):261–5. PMID:26409435
560. Cheung M, Testa JR. BAP1, a tumor suppressor gene driving malignant mesothelioma. Transl Lung Cancer Res. 2017 Jun;6(3):270–8. PMID:28713672
561. Chévez-Barrios P, Eagle RC Jr, Krailo M, et al. Study of unilateral retinoblastoma with and without histopathologic high-risk features and the role of adjuvant chemotherapy: a Children's Oncology Group study. J Clin Oncol. 2019 Nov 1;37(31):2883–91. PMID:31539297
562. Chhuon Y, Weon YC, Park G, et al. Pituitary blastoma in a 19-year-old woman: a case report and review of literature. World Neurosurg. 2020 Jul;139:310–3. PMID:32339720
563. Chi SN, Zimmerman MA, Yao X, et al. Intensive multimodality treatment for children with newly diagnosed CNS atypical teratoid rhabdoid tumor. J Clin Oncol. 2009 Jan 20;27(3):385–9. PMID:19064966
564. Chiang J, Dalton J, Upadhyaya SA, et al. Chromosome arm 1q gain is an adverse prognostic factor in localized and diffuse leptomeningeal glioneuronal tumors with BRAF gene fusion and 1p deletion. Acta Neuropathol. 2019 Jan;137(1):179–81. PMID:30465258
565. Chiang J, Diaz AK, Makepeace L, et al. Clinical, imaging, and molecular analysis of pediatric pontine tumors lacking characteristic imaging features of DIPG. Acta Neuropathol Commun. 2020 Apr 23;8(1):57. PMID:32326973
566. Chiang J, Harreld JH, Tinkle CL, et al. A single-center study of the clinicopathologic correlates of gliomas with a MYB or MYBL1 alteration. Acta Neuropathol. 2019 Dec;138(6):1091–2. PMID:31595312
567. Chiang J, Li X, Liu APY, et al. Tectal glioma harbors high rates of KRAS G12R and concomitant KRAS and BRAF alterations. Acta Neuropathol. 2020 Mar;139(3):601–2. PMID:31822998
568. Chiang JCH, Harreld JH, Orr BA, et al. Low-grade spinal glioneuronal tumors with BRAF gene fusion and 1p deletion but without leptomeningeal dissemination. Acta Neuropathol. 2017 Jul;134(1):159–62. PMID:28547128
569. Chiang JCH, Harreld JH, Tanaka R, et al. Septal dysembryoplastic neuroepithelial tumor: a comprehensive clinical, imaging, histopathologic, and molecular analysis. Neuro Oncol. 2019 Jun 10;21(6):800–8. PMID:30726976
570. Chiaramonte C, Rabaste S, Jacquesson T, et al. Liponeurocytoma of the cerebellopontine angle. World Neurosurg. 2018 Apr;112:18–24. PMID:29325939
571. Chiechi MV, Smirniotopoulos JG, Mena H. Pineal parenchymal tumors: CT and MR features. J Comput Assist Tomogr. 1995 Jul-Aug;19(4):509–17. PMID:7622675
572. Chikai K, Ohnishi A, Kato T, et al. Clinico-pathological features of pilomyxoid astrocytoma of the optic pathway. Acta Neuropathol. 2004 Aug;108(2):109–14. PMID:15168135
573. Chinot OL, Wick W, Mason W, et al. Bevacizumab plus radiotherapy-temozolomide for newly diagnosed glioblastoma. N Engl J Med. 2014 Feb 20;370(8):709–22. PMID:24552318
574. Chittaranjan S, Chan S, Yang C, et al. Mutations in CIC and IDH1 cooperatively regulate 2-hydroxyglutarate levels and cell clonogenicity. Oncotarget. 2014 Sep 15;5(17):7960–79. PMID:25277207
575. Chkheidze R, Cimino PJ, Hatanpaa KJ, et al. Distinct expression patterns of carbonic anhydrase ix in clear cell, microcystic, and angiomatous meningiomas. J Neuropathol Exp Neurol. 2019 Dec 1;78(12):1081–8. PMID:31589317
576. Chmara M, Wernstedt A, Wasag B, et al. Multiple pilomatricomas with somatic CTNNB1 mutations in children with constitutive mismatch repair deficiency. Genes Chromosomes Cancer. 2013 Jul;52(7):656–64. PMID:23629955
577. Chmielecki J, Crago AM, Rosenberg M, et al. Whole-exome sequencing identifies a recurrent NAB2-STAT6 fusion in solitary fibrous tumors. Nat Genet. 2013 Feb;45(2):131–2. PMID:23313954
578. Cho BK, Wang KC, Nam DH, et al. Pineal tumors: experience with 48 cases over 10 years. Childs Nerv Syst. 1998 Jan-Feb;14(1-2):53–8. PMID:9548342
579. Cho J, Pastorino S, Zeng Q, et al. Glioblastoma-derived epidermal growth factor receptor carboxyl-terminal deletion mutants are transforming and are sensitive to EGFR-directed therapies. Cancer Res. 2011 Dec 15;71(24):7587–96. PMID:22001862
580. Choi C, Ganji SK, DeBerardinis RJ, et al. 2-hydroxyglutarate detection by magnetic resonance spectroscopy in IDH-mutated patients with gliomas. Nat Med. 2012 Jan 26;18(4):624–9. PMID:22281806
581. Choi E, Kim SI, Won JK, et al. Clinicopathological and molecular analysis of multinodular and vacuolating neuronal tumors of the cerebrum. Hum Pathol. 2019 Apr;86:203–12. PMID:30550736
582. Choi EJ, Sloma EA, Miller AD. Kir7.1 immunoreactivity in canine choroid plexus tumors. J Vet Diagn Invest. 2016 Jul;28(4):464–8. PMID:27216721
583. Choi JS, Nam DH, Ko YH, et al. Primary central nervous system lymphoma in Korea: comparison of B- and T-cell lymphomas. Am J Surg Pathol. 2003 Jul;27(7):919–28. PMID:12826884
584. Choi JW, Lee JY, Phi JH, et al. Clinical course of vestibular schwannoma in pediatric neurofibromatosis Type 2. J Neurosurg Pediatr. 2014 Jun;13(6):650–7. PMID:24724714
585. Choi JY, Chung JH, Park YJ, et al. Extranodal marginal zone B-cell lymphoma of mucosa-associated tissue type involving the dura. Cancer Res Treat. 2016 Apr;48(2):859–63. PMID:26194368
586. Choi Y, Nam Y, Lee YS, et al. IDH1 mutation prediction using MR-based radiomics in glioblastoma: comparison between manual and fully automated deep learning-based approach of tumor segmentation. Eur J Radiol. 2020 Jul;128:109031. PMID:32417712
587. Chompret A, Abel A, Stoppa-Lyonnet D, et

al. Sensitivity and predictive value of criteria for p53 germline mutation screening. J Med Genet. 2001 Jan;38(1):43–7. PMID:11332399
588. Chong AS, Fahiminiya S, Strother D, et al. Revisiting pleuropulmonary blastoma and atypical choroid plexus papilloma in a young child: DICER1 syndrome or not? Pediatr Blood Cancer. 2018 Oct;65(10):e27294. PMID:29943907
589. Chow E, Jenkins JJ, Burger PC, et al. Malignant evolution of choroid plexus papilloma. Pediatr Neurosurg. 1999 Sep;31(3):127–30. PMID:10708353
590. Choy W, Ampie L, Lamano JB, et al. Predictors of recurrence in the management of chordoid meningioma. J Neurooncol. 2016 Jan;126(1):107–16. PMID:26409888
591. Christensen BC, Smith AA, Zheng S, et al. DNA methylation, isocitrate dehydrogenase mutation, and survival in glioma. J Natl Cancer Inst. 2011 Jan 19;103(2):143–53. PMID:21163902
592. Christiaans I, Kenter SB, Brink HC, et al. Germline SMARCB1 mutation and somatic NF2 mutations in familial multiple meningiomas. J Med Genet. 2011 Feb;48(2):93–7. PMID:20930055
593. Christoforidis M, Buhl R, Paulus W, et al. Intraneural perineurioma of the VIIIth cranial nerve: case report. Neurosurgery. 2007 Sep;61(3):E652. PMID:17881938
594. Chu LC, Eberhart CG, Grossman SA, et al. Epigenetic silencing of multiple genes in primary CNS lymphoma. Int J Cancer. 2006 Nov 15;119(10):2487–91. PMID:16858686
595. Chun HE, Johann PD, Milne K, et al. Identification and analyses of extra-cranial and cranial rhabdoid tumor molecular subgroups reveal tumors with cytotoxic T cell infiltration. Cell Rep. 2019 Nov 19;29(8):2338–2354.e7. PMID:31708418
596. Cimino PJ, Holland EC. Targeted copy number analysis outperforms histologic grading in predicting patient survival for WHO grades II/III IDH-mutant astrocytomas. Neuro Oncol. 2019 Jun 10;21(6):819–21. PMID:30918961
597. Cimino PJ, Zager M, McFerrin L, et al. Multidimensional scaling of diffuse gliomas: application to the 2016 World Health Organization classification system with prognostically relevant molecular subtype discovery. Acta Neuropathol Commun. 2017 May 22;5(1):39. PMID:28532485
598. Ciriello G, Miller ML, Aksoy BA, et al. Emerging landscape of oncogenic signatures across human cancers. Nat Genet. 2013 Oct;45(10):1127–33. PMID:24071851
599. Clara CA, Marie SK, de Almeida JR, et al. Angiogenesis and expression of PDGF-C, VEGF, CD105 and HIF-1α in human glioblastoma. Neuropathology. 2014 Aug;34(4):343–52. PMID:24612214
600. Clark AJ, Sughrue ME, Ivan ME, et al. Factors influencing overall survival rates for patients with pineocytoma. J Neurooncol. 2010 Nov;100(2):255–60. PMID:20461445
601. Clark VE, Erson-Omay EZ, Serin A, et al. Genomic analysis of non-NF2 meningiomas reveals mutations in TRAF7, KLF4, AKT1, and SMO. Science. 2013 Mar 1;339(6123):1077–80. PMID:23348505
602. Clark VE, Harmancı AS, Bai H, et al. Recurrent somatic mutations in POLR2A define a distinct subset of meningiomas. Nat Genet. 2016 Oct;48(10):1253–9. PMID:27548314
603. Clarke M, Mackay A, Ismer B, et al. Infant high grade gliomas comprise multiple subgroups characterized by novel targetable gene fusions and favorable outcomes. Cancer Discov. 2020 Jul;10(7):942–63. PMID:32238360
604. Clarke MJ, Foy AB, Wetjen N, et al. Imaging characteristics and growth of subependymal giant cell astrocytomas. Neurosurg Focus. 2006 Jan 15;20(1):E5. PMID:16459995
605. Claus EB, Calvocoressi L, Bondy ML, et al. Exogenous hormone use, reproductive factors, and risk of intracranial meningioma in females. J Neurosurg. 2013 Mar;118(3):649–56. PMID:23101448
606. Claus EB, Calvocoressi L, Bondy ML, et al. Family and personal medical history and risk of meningioma. J Neurosurg. 2011 Dec;115(6):1072–7. PMID:21780859
607. Claus EB, Cornish AJ, Broderick P, et al. Genome-wide association analysis identifies a meningioma risk locus at 11p15.5. Neuro Oncol. 2018 Oct 9;20(11):1485–93. PMID:29762745
608. Cleven AH, Sannaa GA, Briaire-de Bruijn I, et al. Loss of H3K27 tri-methylation is a diagnostic marker for malignant peripheral nerve sheath tumors and an indicator for an inferior survival. Mod Pathol. 2016 Jun;29(6):582–90. PMID:26990975
609. Clifford SC, Lusher ME, Lindsey JC, et al. Wnt/Wingless pathway activation and chromosome 6 loss characterize a distinct molecular sub-group of medulloblastomas associated with a favorable prognosis. Cell Cycle. 2006 Nov;5(22):2666–70. PMID:17172831
610. ClinicalTrials.gov [Internet]. Bethesda (MD): U.S. National Library of Medicine; 2021. Identifier NCT03224767, Vemurafenib and cobimetinib in treating patients with BRAF V600E mutation positive craniopharyngioma; first posted 2017 Jul 21 [updated 2021 Mar 8]. Available from: https://clinicaltrials.gov/ct2/show/NCT03224767.
611. Clynes D, Higgs DR, Gibbons RJ. The chromatin remodeller ATRX: a repeat offender in human disease. Trends Biochem Sci. 2013 Sep;38(9):461–6. PMID:23916100
612. Coakley KJ, Huston J 3rd, Scheithauer BW, et al. Pilocytic astrocytomas: well-demarcated magnetic resonance appearance despite frequent infiltration histologically. Mayo Clin Proc. 1995 Aug;70(8):747–51. PMID:7630212
613. Cobbers JM, Wolter M, Reifenberger J, et al. Frequent inactivation of CDKN2A and rare mutation of TP53 in PCNSL. Brain Pathol. 1998 Apr;8(2):263–76. PMID:9546285
614. Cobo F, Talavera P, Busquier H, et al. CNK/T-cell brain lymphoma associated with Epstein-Barr virus in a patient with AIDS. Neuropathology. 2007 Aug;27(4):396–402. PMID:17899696
615. Coca S, Vaquero J, Escandon J, et al. Immunohistochemical characterization of pineocytomas. Clin Neuropathol. 1992 Nov-Dec;11(6):298–303. PMID:1473313
616. Coccé MC, Mardin BR, Bens S, et al. Identification of ZCCHC8 as fusion partner of ROS1 in a case of congenital glioblastoma multiforme with a t(6;12)(q21;q24.3). Genes Chromosomes Cancer. 2016 Sep;55(9):677–87. PMID:27121553
617. Cogliano VJ, Baan R, Straif K, et al. Preventable exposures associated with human cancers. J Natl Cancer Inst. 2011 Dec 21;103(24):1827–39. PMID:22158127
618. Cohen M, Guger S, Hamilton J. Long term sequelae of pediatric craniopharyngioma - literature review and 20 years of experience. Front Endocrinol (Lausanne). 2011 Nov 28;2:81. PMID:22645511
619. Coiré CI, Horvath E, Smyth HS, et al. Rapidly recurring folliculostellate cell tumor of the adenohypophysis with the morphology of a spindle cell oncocytoma: case report with electron microscopic studies. Clin Neuropathol. 2009 Jul-Aug;28(4):303–8. PMID:19642510
620. Colafati GS, Voicu IP, Carducci C, et al. MRI features as a helpful tool to predict the molecular subgroups of medulloblastoma: state of the art. Ther Adv Neurol Disord. 2018 Jun 18;11:1756286418775375. PMID:29977341
621. Collins VP, Jones DT, Giannini C. Pilocytic astrocytoma: pathology, molecular mechanisms and markers. Acta Neuropathol. 2015 Jun;129(6):775–88. PMID:25792358
622. Combs SE, Schulz-Ertner D, Debus J, et al. Improved correlation of the neuropathologic classification according to adapted world health organization classification and outcome after radiotherapy in patients with atypical and anaplastic meningiomas. Int J Radiat Oncol Biol Phys. 2011 Dec 1;81(5):1415–21. PMID:20932661
623. Commins DL, Hinton DR. Cytologic features of hemangioblastoma: comparison with meningioma, anaplastic astrocytoma and renal cell carcinoma. Acta Cytol. 1998 Sep-Oct;42(5):1104–10. PMID:9755665
624. Compton JJ, Laack NN, Eckel LJ, et al. Long-term outcomes for low-grade intracranial ganglioglioma: 30-year experience from the Mayo Clinic. J Neurosurg. 2012 Nov;117(5):825–30. PMID:22957524
625. Conboy E, Dhamija R, Wang M, et al. Paraspinal neurofibromas and hypertrophic neuropathy in Noonan syndrome with multiple lentigines. J Med Genet. 2016 Feb;53(2):123–6. PMID:26337637
626. Connor JM, Pirrit LA, Yates JR, et al. Linkage of the tuberous sclerosis locus to a DNA polymorphism detected by v-abl. J Med Genet. 1987 Sep;24(9):544–6. PMID:2889832
627. Constantini S, Soffer D, Siegel T, et al. Paraganglioma of the thoracic spinal cord with cerebrospinal fluid metastasis. Spine (Phila Pa 1976). 1989 Jun;14(6):643–5. PMID:2749382
628. Conte D, Huh M, Goodall E, et al. Loss of Atrx sensitizes cells to DNA damaging agents through p53-mediated death pathways. PLoS One. 2012;7(12):e52167. PMID:23284920
629. Conti P, Mouchaty H, Spacca B, et al. Thoracic extradural paragangliomas: a case report and review of the literature. Spinal Cord. 2006 Feb;44(2):120–5. PMID:16130022
630. Conway E, Healy E, Bracken AP. PRC2 mediated H3K27 methylations in cellular identity and cancer. Curr Opin Cell Biol. 2015 Dec;37:42–8. PMID:26497635
631. Conway JE, Chou D, Clatterbuck RE, et al. Hemangioblastomas of the central nervous system in von Hippel-Lindau syndrome and sporadic disease. Neurosurgery. 2001 Jan;48(1):55–62. PMID:11152361
632. Coons SW, Johnson PC. Regional heterogeneity in the proliferative activity of human gliomas as measured by the Ki-67 labeling index. J Neuropathol Exp Neurol. 1993 Nov;52(6):609–18. PMID:8229080
633. Coons SW, Pearl DK. Mitosis identification in diffuse gliomas: implications for tumor grading. Cancer. 1998 Apr 15;82(8):1550–5. PMID:9554533
634. Coons SW, Rekate HL, Prenger EC, et al. The histopathology of hypothalamic hamartomas: study of 57 cases. J Neuropathol Exp Neurol. 2007 Feb;66(2):131–41. PMID:17278998
635. Cooper O, Ben-Shlomo A, Bonert V, et al. Silent corticogonadotroph adenomas: clinical and cellular characteristics and long-term outcomes. Horm Cancer. 2010 Apr;1(2):80–92. PMID:20717480
636. Cordero FJ, Huang Z, Grenier C, et al. Histone H3.3K27M represses p16 to accelerate gliomagenesis in a murine model of DIPG. Mol Cancer Res. 2017 Sep;15(9):1243–54. PMID:28522693
637. Cornejo KM, Hutchinson L, Cosar EF, et al. Is it a primary or metastatic melanocytic neoplasm of the central nervous system?: A molecular based approach. Pathol Int. 2013 Nov;63(11):559–64. PMID:24274719
638. Coroller TP, Bi WL, Huynh E, et al. Radiographic prediction of meningioma grade by semantic and radiomic features. PLoS One. 2017 Nov 16;12(11):e0187908. PMID:29145421
639. Corssmit EPM, Snel M, Kapiteijn E. Malignant pheochromocytoma and paraganglioma: management options. Curr Opin Oncol. 2020 Jan;32(1):20–6. PMID:31599769
640. Corti ME, Yampolsky C, Metta H, et al. Oligodendroglioma in a patient with AIDS: case report and review of the literature. Rev Inst Med Trop Sao Paulo. 2004 Jul-Aug;46(4):195–7. PMID:15361970
641. Cosar M, Iplikcioglu AC, Bek S, et al. Intracranial falcine and convexity chondromas: two case reports. Br J Neurosurg. 2005 Jun;19(3):241–3. PMID:16455525
642. Couce ME, Aker FV, Scheithauer BW. Chordoid meningioma: a clinicopathologic study of 42 cases. Am J Surg Pathol. 2000 Jul;24(7):899–905. PMID:10895812
643. Coulam CB, Annegers JF, Abboud CF, et al. Pituitary adenoma and oral contraceptives: a case-control study. Fertil Steril. 1979 Jan;31(1):25–8. PMID:369889
644. Couldwell WT, Cannon-Albright LA. A description of familial clustering of meningiomas in the Utah population. Neuro Oncol. 2017 Nov 29;19(12):1683–7. PMID:29016976
645. Courts C, Montesinos-Rongen M, Brunn A, et al. Recurrent inactivation of the PRDM1 gene in primary central nervous system lymphoma. J Neuropathol Exp Neurol. 2008 Jul;67(7):720–7. PMID:18596541
646. Covington DB, Rosenblum MK, Brathwaite CD, et al. Angiocentric glioma-like tumor of the midbrain. Pediatr Neurosurg. 2009;45(6):429–33. PMID:20110754
647. Covington MF, Chin SS, Osborn AG. Pituicytoma, spindle cell oncocytoma, and granular cell tumor: clarification and meta-analysis of the world literature since 1893. AJNR Am J Neuroradiol. 2011 Dec;32(11):2067–72. PMID:21960498
648. Cox EM, Bambakidis NC, Cohen ML. Pathology of cavernous malformations. Handb Clin Neurol. 2017;143:267–77. PMID:28552149
649. Coy S, Du Z, Sheu SH, et al. Distinct patterns of primary and motile cilia in Rathke's cleft cysts and craniopharyngioma subtypes. Mod Pathol. 2016 Dec;29(12):1446–59. PMID:27562488
650. Coy S, Dubuc AM, Dahiya S, et al. Nuclear CRX and FOXJ1 expression differentiates non-germ cell pineal region tumors and supports the ependymal differentiation of papillary tumor of the pineal region. Am J Surg Pathol. 2017 Oct;41(10):1410–21. PMID:28719464
651. Coy S, Rashid R, Lin JR, et al. Multiplexed immunofluorescence reveals potential PD-1/PD-L1 pathway vulnerabilities in craniopharyngioma. Neuro Oncol. 2018 Jul 5;20(8):1101–12. PMID:29509940
652. Coy S, Rashid R, Stemmer-Rachamimov A, et al. An update on the CNS manifestations of neurofibromatosis type 2. Acta Neuropathol. 2020 Apr;139(4):643–65. PMID:31161239
653. Crescenzo R, Abate F, Lasorsa E, et al. Convergent mutations and kinase fusions lead to oncogenic STAT3 activation in anaplastic large cell lymphoma. Cancer Cell. 2015 Apr 13;27(4):516–32. PMID:25873174
654. Crino PB, Mehta R, Vinters HV. Pathogenesis of TSC in the brain. In: Kwiatkowski DJ, Whittemore VH, Thiele EA, editors. Tuberous sclerosis complex: genes, clinical features, and therapeutics. Weinheim (Germany): Wiley-Blackwell; 2010. pp. 161–85.
655. Crino PB, Trojanowski JQ, Dichter MA, et al. Embryonic neuronal markers in tuberous sclerosis: single-cell molecular pathology. Proc Natl Acad Sci U S A. 1996 Nov

26;93(24):14152–7. PMID:8943076

656. Crocetti E, Trama A, Stiller C, et al. Epidemiology of glial and non-glial brain tumours in Europe. Eur J Cancer. 2012 Jul;48(10):1532–42. PMID:22227039

657. Crotty TB, Scheithauer BW, Young WF Jr, et al. Papillary craniopharyngioma: a clinicopathological study of 48 cases. J Neurosurg. 1995 Aug;83(2):206–14. PMID:7616262

658. Cunha MLVD, Maldaun MVC. Metastasis from glioblastoma multiforme: a meta-analysis. Rev Assoc Med Bras (1992). 2019 Mar;65(3):424–33. PMID:30994843

659. Curatolo P, Franz DN, Lawson JA, et al. Adjunctive everolimus for children and adolescents with treatment-refractory seizures associated with tuberous sclerosis complex: post-hoc analysis of the phase 3 EXIST-3 trial. Lancet Child Adolesc Health. 2018 Jul;2(7):495–504. PMID:30169322

660. Curatolo P, Moavero R. mTOR inhibitors in tuberous sclerosis complex. Curr Neuropharmacol. 2012 Dec;10(4):404–15. PMID:23730262

661. Curless RG, Toledano SR, Ragheb J, et al. Hematogenous brain metastasis in children. Pediatr Neurol. 2002 Mar;26(3):219–21. PMID:11955930

662. Dabora SL, Jozwiak S, Franz DN, et al. Mutational analysis in a cohort of 224 tuberous sclerosis patients indicates increased severity of TSC2, compared with TSC1, disease in multiple organs. Am J Hum Genet. 2001 Jan;68(1):64–80. PMID:11112665

663. Daghistani R, Miller E, Kulkarni AV, et al. Atypical characteristics and behavior of dysembryoplastic neuroepithelial tumors. Neuroradiology. 2013 Feb;55(2):217–24. PMID:23314798

664. Dagrada GP, Spagnuolo RD, Mauro V, et al. Solitary fibrous tumors: loss of chimeric protein expression and genomic instability mark dedifferentiation. Mod Pathol. 2015 Aug;28(8):1074–83. PMID:26022454

665. Dahia PL, Aguiar RC, Alberta J, et al. PTEN is inversely correlated with the cell survival factor Akt/PKB and is inactivated via multiple mechanismsin haematological malignancies. Hum Mol Genet. 1999 Feb;8(2):185–93. PMID:9931326

666. Dahiya S, Haydon DH, Alvarado D, et al. BRAF(V600E) mutation is a negative prognosticator in pediatric ganglioglioma. Acta Neuropathol. 2013 Jun;125(6):901–10. PMID:23609006

667. Dahiya S, Sarkar C, Hedley-Whyte ET, et al. Spindle cell oncocytoma of the adenohypophysis: report of two cases. Acta Neuropathol. 2005 Jul;110(1):97–9. PMID:15973544

668. Dahl NA, Luebbert T, Loi M, et al. Chordoma occurs in young children with tuberous sclerosis. J Neuropathol Exp Neurol. 2017 Jun 1;76(6):418–23. PMID:28498973

669. Dahlback HS, Gorunova L, Micci F, et al. Molecular cytogenetic analysis of a gliosarcoma with osseous metaplasia. Cytogenet Genome Res. 2011;134(2):88–95. PMID:21555877

670. Dalle Ore CL, Magill ST, Yen AJ, et al. Meningioma metastases: incidence and proposed screening paradigm. J Neurosurg. 2019 Apr 5;132(5):1447–55. PMID:30952122

671. Daly AF, Rixhon M, Adam C, et al. High prevalence of pituitary adenomas: a cross-sectional study in the province of Liege, Belgium. J Clin Endocrinol Metab. 2006 Dec;91(12):4769–75. PMID:16968795

672. Damodaran O, Robbins P, Knuckey N, et al. Primary intracranial haemangiopericytoma: comparison of survival outcomes and metastatic potential in WHO grade II and III variants. J Clin Neurosci. 2014 Aug;21(8):1310–4. PMID:24726230

673. Dandurand C, Sepehry AA, Asadi Lari MH, et al. Adult craniopharyngioma: case series, systematic review, and meta-analysis. Neurosurgery. 2018 Oct 1;83(4):631–41. PMID:29267973

674. Dang L, White DW, Gross S, et al. Cancer-associated IDH1 mutations produce 2-hydroxyglutarate. Nature. 2009 Dec 10;462(7274):739–44. PMID:19935646

675. D'Angelo F, Ceccarelli M, Tala, et al. The molecular landscape of glioma in patients with Neurofibromatosis 1. Nat Med. 2019 Jan;25(1):176–87. PMID:30531922

676. D'Arcy CE, Nobre LF, Arnaldo A, et al. Immunohistochemical and NanoString-based subgrouping of clinical medulloblastoma samples. J Neuropathol Exp Neurol. 2020 Apr 1;79(4):437–47. PMID:32053195

677. Darlix A, Zouaoui S, Rigau V, et al. Epidemiology for primary brain tumors: a nationwide population-based study. J Neurooncol. 2017 Feb;131(3):525–46. PMID:27853959

678. D'Aronco L, Rouleau C, Gayden T, et al. Brainstem angiocentric gliomas with MYB-QKI rearrangements. Acta Neuropathol. 2017 Oct;134(4):667–9. PMID:28803398

679. Das A, Roy P, Modi SK, et al. Germline DICER1-mutant intracranial sarcoma with dual chondroid and spindle cell morphology and pulmonary metastases treated with multimodal therapy. Pediatr Blood Cancer. 2019 Jul;66(7):e27744. PMID:30989777

680. Das P, Soni P, Jones J, et al. Descriptive epidemiology of chordomas in the United States. J Neurooncol. 2020 May;148(1):173–8. PMID:32342333

681. Dasgupta A, Gupta T, Pungavkar S, et al. Nomograms based on preoperative multiparametric magnetic resonance imaging for prediction of molecular subgrouping in medulloblastoma: results from a radiogenomics study of 111 patients. Neuro Oncol. 2019 Jan 1;21(1):115–24. PMID:29846693

682. Dauden MI, Jaciuk M, Weis F, et al. Molecular basis of tRNA recognition by the Elongator complex. Sci Adv. 2019 Jul 10;5(7):eaaw2326. PMID:31309145

683. Daumas-Duport C. Dysembryoplastic neuroepithelial tumours. Brain Pathol. 1993 Jul;3(3):283–95. PMID:8293188

684. Daumas-Duport C, Scheithauer B, O'Fallon J, et al. Grading of astrocytomas. A simple and reproducible method. Cancer. 1988 Nov 15;62(10):2152–65. PMID:3179928

685. Daumas-Duport C, Scheithauer BW, Chodkiewicz JP, et al. Dysembryoplastic neuroepithelial tumor: a surgically curable tumor of young patients with intractable partial seizures. Report of thirty-nine cases. Neurosurgery. 1988 Nov;23(5):545–56. PMID:3143922

686. Daumas-Duport C, Varlet P. [Dysembryoplastic neuroepithelial tumors]. Rev Neurol (Paris). 2003 Jul;159(6-7 Pt 1):622–36. French. PMID:12910070

687. Daumas-Duport C, Varlet P, Bacha S, et al. Dysembryoplastic neuroepithelial tumors: nonspecific histological forms – a study of 40 cases. J Neurooncol. 1999 Feb;41(3):267–80. PMID:10359147

688. d'Avella E, Solari D, Somma T, et al. The endoscopic endonasal approach for pediatric craniopharyngiomas: the key lessons learned. Childs Nerv Syst. 2019 Nov;35(11):2147–55. PMID:31055620

689. Davids A. Childhood psychosis. The problem of differential diagnosis. J Autism Child Schizophr. 1975 Jun;5(2):129–38. PMID:1174116

690. Davies BR, Guan N, Logie A, et al. Tumors with AKT1E17K mutations are rational targets for single agent or combination therapy with AKT inhibitors. Mol Cancer Ther. 2015 Nov;14(11):2441–51. PMID:26351323

691. Davis AA, Patel VG. The role of PD-L1 expression as a predictive biomarker: an analysis of all US Food and Drug Administration (FDA) approvals of immune checkpoint inhibitors. J Immunother Cancer. 2019 Oct 26;7(1):278. PMID:31655605

692. Davis FG, Smith TR, Gittleman HR, et al. Glioblastoma incidence rate trends in Canada and the United States compared with England, 1995-2015. Neuro Oncol. 2020 Feb 20;22(2):301–2. PMID:31786602

693. Davis RJ, D'Cruz CM, Lovell MA, et al. Fusion of PAX7 to FKHR by the variant t(1;13)(p36;q14) translocation in alveolar rhabdomyosarcoma. Cancer Res. 1994 Jun 1;54(11):2869–72. PMID:8187070

694. de Almeida Verdolin A, Lamback EB, Ventura N, et al. Collision sellar lesions: coexistence of pituitary adenoma and Rathke cleft cyst-a single-center experience. Endocrine. 2020 Apr;68(1):174–81. PMID:31802354

695. de Andrade KC, Frone MN, Wegman-Ostrosky T, et al. Response to: Concern regarding classification of germlineTP53 variants as likely pathogenic. Hum Mutat. 2019 Jun;40(6):832–3. PMID:30997946

696. de Andrade KC, Frone MN, Wegman-Ostrosky T, et al. Variable population prevalence estimates of germline TP53 variants: a gnomAD-based analysis. Hum Mutat. 2019 Jan;40(1):97–105. PMID:30352134

697. de Andrade KC, Mirabello L, Stewart DR, et al. Higher-than-expected population prevalence of potentially pathogenic germline TP53 variants in individuals unselected for cancer history. Hum Mutat. 2017 Dec;38(12):1723–30. PMID:28861920

698. De B, Khakoo Y, Souweidane MM, et al. Patterns of relapse for children with localized intracranial ependymoma. J Neurooncol. 2018 Jun;138(2):435–45. PMID:29511977

699. De B, Kinnaman MD, Wexler LH, et al. Central nervous system relapse of rhabdomyosarcoma. Pediatr Blood Cancer. 2018 Jan;65(1). PMID:28696016

700. de Chadarévian JP, Montes JL, O'Gorman AM, et al. Maturation of cerebellar neuroblastoma into ganglioneuroma with melanosis. A histologic, immunocytochemical, and ultrastructural study. Cancer. 1987 Jan 1;59(1):69–76. PMID:3539310

701. de Cubas AA, Leandro-García LJ, Schiavi F, et al. Integrative analysis of miRNA and mRNA expression profiles in pheochromocytoma and paraganglioma identifies genotype-specific markers and potentially regulated pathways. Endocr Relat Cancer. 2013 Jun 24;20(4):477–93. PMID:23660872

702. de Groot JF, Fuller G, Kumar AJ, et al. Tumor invasion after treatment of glioblastoma with bevacizumab: radiographic and pathologic correlation in humans and mice. Neuro Oncol. 2010 Mar;12(3):233–42. PMID:20167811

703. de Jong MC, Kors WA, de Graaf P, et al. Trilateral retinoblastoma: a systematic review and meta-analysis. Lancet Oncol. 2014 Sep;15(10):1157–67. PMID:25126964

704. de Kock L, Geoffrion D, Rivera B, et al. Multiple DICER1-related tumors in a child with a large interstitial 14q32 deletion. Genes Chromosomes Cancer. 2018 May;57(5):223–30. PMID:29315962

705. de Kock L, Priest JR, Foulkes WD, et al. An update on the central nervous system manifestations of DICER1 syndrome. Acta Neuropathol. 2020 Apr;139(4):689–701. PMID:30953130

706. de Kock L, Sabbaghian N, Druker H, et al. Germ-line and somatic DICER1 mutations in pineoblastoma. Acta Neuropathol. 2014 Oct;128(4):583–95. PMID:25022261

707. de Kock L, Sabbaghian N, Plourde F, et al. Pituitary blastoma: a pathognomonic feature of germ-line DICER1 mutations. Acta Neuropathol. 2014 Jul;128(1):111–22. PMID:24839956

708. de la Fouchardière A, Cabaret O, Pètre J, et al. Primary leptomeningeal melanoma is part of the BAP1-related cancer syndrome. Acta Neuropathol. 2015 Jun;129(6):921–3. PMID:25900292

709. de la Fuente MI, Haggiagi A, Moul A, et al. Marginal zone dural lymphoma: the Memorial Sloan Kettering Cancer Center and University of Miami experiences. Leuk Lymphoma. 2017 Apr;58(4):882–8. PMID:27649904

710. De Lima L, Sürme MB, Gessi M, et al. Central nervous system high-grade neuroepithelial tumor with BCOR alteration (CNS HGNET-BCOR)-case-based reviews. Childs Nerv Syst. 2020 Aug;36(8):1589–99. PMID:32542405

711. De Munnynck K, Van Gool S, Van Calenbergh F, et al. Desmoplastic infantile ganglioglioma: a potentially malignant tumor? Am J Surg Pathol. 2002 Nov;26(11):1515–22. PMID:12409729

712. De Raedt T, Beert E, Pasmant E, et al. PRC2 loss amplifies Ras-driven transcription and confers sensitivity to BRD4-based therapies. Nature. 2014 Oct 9;514(7521):247–51. PMID:25119042

713. de Ribaupierre S, Dorfmüller G, Bulteau C, et al. Subependymal giant-cell astrocytomas in pediatric tuberous sclerosis disease: when should we operate? Neurosurgery. 2007 Jan;60(1):83–9. PMID:17228255

714. de Vries NA, Hulsman D, Akhtar W, et al. Prolonged Ezh2 depletion in glioblastoma causes a robust switch in cell fate resulting in tumor progression. Cell Rep. 2015 Jan 20;10(3):383–97. PMID:25600873

715. Dearnaley DP, A'Hern RP, Whittaker S, et al. Pineal and CNS germ cell tumors: Royal Marsden Hospital experience 1962-1987. Int J Radiat Oncol Biol Phys. 1990 Apr;18(4):773–81. PMID:2323968

716. Deb P, Sharma MC, Gaikwad S, et al. Cerebellopontine angle paraganglioma - report of a case and review of literature. J Neurooncol. 2005 Aug;74(1):65–9. PMID:16078110

717. de Chadarévian JP, Vekemans M, Bernstein M. Fanconi's anemia, medulloblastoma, Wilms' tumor, horseshoe kidney, and gonadal dysgenesis. Arch Pathol Lab Med. 1985 Apr;109(4):367–9. PMID:2985019

718. Deckert M, Brunn A, Montesinos-Rongen M, et al. Primary lymphoma of the central nervous system–a diagnostic challenge. Hematol Oncol. 2014 Jun;32(2):57–67. PMID:23949943

719. Deckert M, Engert A, Brück W, et al. Modern concepts in the biology, diagnosis, differential diagnosis and treatment of primary central nervous system lymphoma. Leukemia. 2011 Dec;25(12):1797–807. PMID:21818113

720. DeDavid M, Orlow SJ, Provost N, et al. Neurocutaneous melanosis: clinical features of large congenital melanocytic nevi in patients with manifest central nervous system melanosis. J Am Acad Dermatol. 1996 Oct;35(4):529–38. PMID:8859278

721. Dedeurwaerdere F, Giannini C, Sciot R, et al. Primary peripheral PNET/Ewing's sarcoma of the dura: a clinicopathologic entity distinct from central PNET. Mod Pathol. 2002 Jun;15(6):673–8. PMID:12065782

722. Deisch JK, Patel R, Koral K, et al. Juvenile xanthogranulomas of the nervous system: a report of two cases and review of the literature. Neuropathology. 2013 Feb;33(1):39–46. PMID:22640164

723. Dekkers OM, Karavitaki N, Pereira AM. The epidemiology of aggressive pituitary tumors (and its challenges). Rev Endocr Metab Disord. 2020 Jun;21(2):209–12. PMID:32361816

724. de Kock L, Rivera B, Foulkes WD.

Pineoblastoma is uniquely tolerant of mutually exclusive loss of DICER1, DROSHA or DGCR8. Acta Neuropathol. 2020 Jun;139(6):1115–8. PMID:32124011

725. del Bufalo F, Carai A, Figà-Talamanca L, et al. Response of recurrent BRAFV600E mutated ganglioglioma to Vemurafenib as single agent. J Transl Med. 2014 Dec 19;12:356. PMID:25524464

726. Del Valle L, Enam S, Lara C, et al. Detection of JC polyomavirus DNA sequences and cellular localization of T-antigen and agnoprotein in oligodendrogliomas. Clin Cancer Res. 2002 Nov;8(11):3332–40. PMID:12429619

727. de Leeuw CN, Prayson RA. Primary intracranial rhabdomyosarcoma in an NF1 patient. Clin Neuropathol. 2019 Mar/Apr;38(2):84–6. PMID:30563612

728. Delgado-López PD, Corrales-García EM, Alonso-García E, et al. Central nervous system ependymoma: clinical implications of the new molecular classification, treatment guidelines and controversial issues. Clin Transl Oncol. 2019 Nov;21(11):1450–63. PMID:30868390

729. Delgrange E, Vasiljevic A, Wierinckx A, et al. Expression of estrogen receptor alpha is associated with prolactin pituitary tumor prognosis and supports the sex-related difference in tumor growth. Eur J Endocrinol. 2015 Jun;172(6):791–801. PMID:25792376

730. Delnatte C, Sanlaville D, Mougenot JF, et al. Contiguous gene deletion within chromosome arm 10q is associated with juvenile polyposis of infancy, reflecting cooperation between the BMPR1A and PTEN tumor-suppressor genes. Am J Hum Genet. 2006 Jun;78(6):1066–74. PMID:16685657

731. Demicco EG, Wani K, Ingram D, et al. TERT promoter mutations in solitary fibrous tumour. Histopathology. 2018 Nov;73(5):843–51. PMID:29895536

732. Demirçivi Ozer F, Aydin M, Bezircioğlu H, et al. Paraganglioma of the cauda equina: a highly vascular tumour. J Clin Neurosci. 2010 Nov;17(11):1445–7. PMID:20637630

733. Démurger F, Ichkou A, Mougou-Zerelli S, et al. New insights into genotype-phenotype correlation for GLI3 mutations. Eur J Hum Genet. 2015 Jan;23(1):92–102. PMID:24736735

734. Demuth T, Berens ME. Molecular mechanisms of glioma cell migration and invasion. J Neurooncol. 2004 Nov;70(2):217–28. PMID:15674479

735. den Dunnen JT, Dalgleish R, Maglott DR, et al. HGVS recommendations for the description of sequence variants: 2016 Update. Hum Mutat. 2016 Jun;37(6):564–9. PMID:26931183

736. Deng MY, Sill M, Chiang J, et al. Molecularly defined diffuse leptomeningeal glioneuronal tumor (DLGNT) comprises two subgroups with distinct clinical and genetic features. Acta Neuropathol. 2018 Aug;136(2):239–53. PMID:29766299

737. Deng MY, Sill M, Sturm D, et al. Diffuse glioneuronal tumour with oligodendroglioma-like features and nuclear clusters (DGONC) - a molecularly defined glioneuronal CNS tumour class displaying recurrent monosomy 14. Neuropathol Appl Neurobiol. 2020 Aug;46(5):422–30. PMID:31867747

738. Deora H, Prabhuraj AR, Saini J, et al. Cerebellar liponeurocytoma: a rare fatty tumor and its literature review. J Neurosci Rural Pract. 2019 Apr-Jun;10(2):360–3. PMID:31001037

739. Dermawan JK, Mukhopadhyay S, Shah AA. Frequency and extent of cytokeratin expression in paraganglioma: an immunohistochemical study of 60 cases from 5 anatomic sites and review of the literature. Hum Pathol. 2019 Nov;93:16–22. PMID:31442521

740. Desai KB, Mella D, Pan E. An adult patient with rare primary intracranial alveolar rhabdomyosarcoma. Anticancer Res. 2019 Jun;39(6):3067–70. PMID:31177150

741. de Saint Aubain Somerhausen N, Rubin BP, Fletcher CD. Myxoid solitary fibrous tumor: a study of seven cases with emphasis on differential diagnosis. Mod Pathol. 1999 May;12(5):463–71. PMID:10349983

742. Deshmukh H, Yu J, Shaik J, et al. Identification of transcriptional regulatory networks specific to pilocytic astrocytoma. BMC Med Genomics. 2011 Jul 11;4:57. PMID:21745356

743. Desouza RM, Bodi I, Thomas N, et al. Chordoid glioma: ten years of a low-grade tumor with high morbidity. Skull Base. 2010 Mar;20(2):125–38. PMID:20808539

744. Dewan R, Pemov A, Kim HJ, et al. Evidence of polyclonality in neurofibromatosis type 2-associated multilobulated vestibular schwannomas. Neuro Oncol. 2015 Apr;17(4):566–73. PMID:25452392

745. Dewire MD, Ellison DW, Patay Z, et al. Fanconi anemia and biallelic BRCA2 mutation diagnosed in a young child with an embryonal CNS tumor. Pediatr Blood Cancer. 2009 Dec;53(6):1140–2. PMID:19530235

746. DeWitt JC, Jordan JT, Frosch MP, et al. Cost-effectiveness of IDH testing in diffuse gliomas according to the 2016 WHO classification of tumors of the central nervous system recommendations. Neuro Oncol. 2017 Nov 29;19(12):1640–50. PMID:29016871

747. Dho YS, Jung KW, Ha J, et al. An updated nationwide epidemiology of primary brain tumors in Republic of Korea, 2013. Brain Tumor Res Treat. 2017 Apr;5(1):16–23. PMID:28516074

748. Di Cristofano A, Pesce B, Cordon-Cardo C, et al. Pten is essential for embryonic development and tumour suppression. Nat Genet. 1998 Aug;19(4):348–55. PMID:9697695

749. Di Ieva A, Davidson JM, Syro LV, et al. Crooke's cell tumors of the pituitary. Neurosurgery. 2015 May;76(5):616–22. PMID:25635886

750. Di Ieva A, Rotondo F, Syro LV, et al. Aggressive pituitary adenomas–diagnosis and emerging treatments. Nat Rev Endocrinol. 2014 Jul;10(7):423–35. PMID:24821329

751. Di Stefano AL, Fucci A, Frattini V, et al. Detection, characterization, and inhibition of FGFR-TACC fusions in IDH wild-type glioma. Clin Cancer Res. 2015 Jul 15;21(14):3307–17. PMID:25609060

752. Di Stefano AL, Picca A, Saragoussi E, et al. Clinical, molecular, and radiomic profile of gliomas with FGFR3-TACC3 fusions. Neuro Oncol. 2020 Nov 26;22(11):1614–24. PMID:32413119

753. Diamond EL, Durham BH, Haroche J, et al. Diverse and targetable kinase alterations drive histiocytic neoplasms. Cancer Discov. 2016 Feb;6(2):154–65. PMID:26566875

754. Diamond EL, Hatzoglou V, Patel S, et al. Diffuse reduction of cerebral grey matter volumes in Erdheim-Chester disease. Orphanet J Rare Dis. 2016 Aug 2;11(1):109. PMID:27484739

755. Diamond EL, Subbiah V, Lockhart AC, et al. Vemurafenib for BRAF V600-mutant Erdheim-Chester disease and Langerhans cell histiocytosis: analysis of data from the histology-independent, phase 2, open-label VE-BASKET study. JAMA Oncol. 2018 Mar 1;4(3):384–8. PMID:29188284

756. Dias-Santagata D, Lam Q, Vernovsky K, et al. BRAF V600E mutations are common in pleomorphic xanthoastrocytoma: diagnostic and therapeutic implications. PLoS One. 2011 Mar 9;6(3):e17948. PMID:21479234

757. Dimaras H, Khetan V, Halliday W, et al. Loss of RB1 induces non-proliferative retinoma: increasing genomic instability correlates with progression to retinoblastoma. Hum Mol Genet. 2008 May 15;17(10):1363–72. PMID:18211953

758. Ding H, Shannon P, Lau N, et al. Oligodendrogliomas result from the expression of an activated mutant epidermal growth factor receptor in a RAS transgenic mouse astrocytoma model. Cancer Res. 2003 Mar 1;63(5):1106–13. PMID:12615729

759. Ding X, Wang Z, Chen D, et al. The prognostic value of maximal surgical resection is attenuated in oligodendroglioma subgroups of adult diffuse glioma: a multicenter retrospective study. J Neurooncol. 2018 Dec;140(3):591–603. PMID:30206763

760. Dirks MS, Butman JA, Kim HJ, et al. Long-term natural history of neurofibromatosis type 2-associated intracranial tumors. J Neurosurg. 2012 Jul;117(1):109–17. PMID:22503123

761. Di Rocco C, Iannelli A. Bilateral thalamic tumors in children. Childs Nerv Syst. 2002 Aug;18(8):440–4. PMID:12192503

762. Djukic M, Trimmel R, Nagel I, et al. Cerebrospinal fluid abnormalities in meningeosis neoplastica: a retrospective 12-year analysis. Fluids Barriers CNS. 2017 Mar 28;14(1):7. PMID:28351400

763. do Nascimento A, Maranha LA, Corredato RA, et al. 33 year-old woman with a large sellar tumor. Brain Pathol. 2012 Nov;22(6):869–70. PMID:23050874

764. Dobbins SE, Broderick P, Melin B, et al. Common variation at 10p12.31 near MLLT10 influences meningioma risk. Nat Genet. 2011 Jul 31;43(9):825–7. PMID:21804547

765. Dobes M, Khurana VG, Shadbolt B, et al. Increasing incidence of glioblastoma multiforme and meningioma, and decreasing incidence of schwannoma (2000-2008): findings of a multicenter Australian study. Surg Neurol Int. 2011;2:176. PMID:22276231

766. Dodgshun AJ, Fukuoka K, Edwards M, et al. Germline-driven replication repair-deficient high-grade gliomas exhibit unique hypomethylation patterns. Acta Neuropathol. 2020 Nov;140(5):765–76. PMID:32895736

767. Dodgshun AJ, Maixner WJ, Hansford JR, et al. Low rates of recurrence and slow progression of pediatric pilocytic astrocytoma after gross-total resection: justification for reducing surveillance imaging. J Neurosurg Pediatr. 2016 May;17(5):569–72. PMID:26722760

768. Dodgshun AJ, SantaCruz N, Hwang J, et al. Disseminated glioneuronal tumors occurring in childhood: treatment outcomes and BRAF alterations including V600E mutation. J Neurooncol. 2016 Jun;128(2):293–302. PMID:26994902

769. Dodgshun AJ, Sexton-Oates A, Saffery R, et al. Biallelic FANCD1/BRCA2 mutations predisposing to glioblastoma multiforme with multiple oncogenic amplifications. Cancer Genet. 2016 Jan-Feb;209(1-2):53–6. PMID:26740091

770. Doğanşen SÇ, Bilgiç B, Yalin GY, et al. Clinical significance of granulation pattern in corticotroph pituitary adenomas. Turk Patoloji Derg. 2019;35(1):9–14. PMID:30035294

771. Doğansen SC, Yalin GY, Tanrikulu S, et al. Clinicopathological significance of baseline T2-weighted signal intensity in functional pituitary adenomas. Pituitary. 2018 Aug;21(4):347–54. PMID:29460202

772. Doglioni C, Dell'Orto P, Coggi G, et al. Choroid plexus tumors. An immunocytochemical study with particular reference to the coexpression of intermediate filament proteins. Am J Pathol. 1987 Jun;127(3):519–29. PMID:2438940

773. Domingues PH, Sousa P, Otero Á, et al. Proposal for a new risk stratification classification for meningioma based on patient age, WHO tumor grade, size, localization, and karyotype. Neuro Oncol. 2014 May;16(5):735–47. PMID:24536048

774. Donahue JE, Yakirevich E, Zhong S, et al. Primary Spinal Epidural CIC-DUX4 Undifferentiated Sarcoma in a Child. Pediatr Dev Pathol. 2018 Jul-Aug;21(4):411–7. PMID:28474974

775. Dong S, Nutt CL, Betensky RA, et al. Histology-based expression profiling yields novel prognostic markers in human glioblastoma. J Neuropathol Exp Neurol. 2005 Nov;64(11):948–55. PMID:16254489

776. Dong X, Li J, Huo N, et al. Primary central nervous system ALK-positive anaplastic large cell lymphoma in an adult: a rare case report. Medicine (Baltimore). 2016 Dec;95(49):e5534. PMID:27930548

777. Dono A, Wang E, Lopez-Rivera V, et al. Molecular characteristics and clinical features of multifocal glioblastoma. J Neurooncol. 2020 Jun;148(2):389–97. PMID:32440969

778. Donoho D, Zada G. Imaging of central neurocytomas. Neurosurg Clin N Am. 2015 Jan;26(1):11–9. PMID:25432179

779. Donovan MJ, Yunis EJ, DeGirolami U, et al. Chromosome aberrations in choroid plexus papillomas. Genes Chromosomes Cancer 1994 Dec;11(4):267–70. PMID:7533531

780. Donson AM, Kleinschmidt-DeMasters BK, Aisner DL, et al. Pediatric brainstem gangliogliomas show BRAF(V600E) mutation in a high percentage of cases. Brain Pathol. 2014 Mar;24(2):173–83. PMID:24238153

781. Dorfman HD, Czerniak B. Bone cancers. Cancer. 1995 Jan 1;75(1 Suppl):203–10. PMID:8000997

782. Dornbos D 3rd, Kim HJ, Butman JA, et al. Review of the neurological implications of von Hippel-Lindau disease. JAMA Neurol. 2018 May 1;75(5):620–7. PMID:29379961

783. Dougherty MJ, Santi M, Brose MS, et al. Activating mutations in BRAF characterize a spectrum of pediatric low-grade gliomas. Neuro Oncol. 2010 Jul;12(7):621–30. PMID:20156809

784. Douglas-Akinwande AC, Payner TD, Hattab EM. Medulloblastoma mimicking Lhermitte-Duclos disease on MRI and CT. Clin Neurol Neurosurg. 2009 Jul;111(6):536–9. PMID:19233547

785. Doyle LA, Fletcher CD. Peripheral hemangioblastoma: clinicopathologic characterization in a series of 22 cases. Am J Surg Pathol. 2014 Jan;38(1):119–27. PMID:24145646

786. Drilon A, Siena S, Ou SI, et al. Safety and antitumor activity of the multitargeted pan-TRK, ROS1, and ALK inhibitor entrectinib: combined results from two phase I trials (ALKA-372-001 and STARTRK-1). Cancer Discov. 2017 Apr;7(4):400–9. PMID:28183697

787. Drumm MR, Dixit KS, Grimm S, et al. Extensive brainstem infiltration, not mass effect, is a common feature of end-stage cerebral glioblastomas. Neuro Oncol. 2020 Apr 15;22(4):470–9. PMID:31711239

788. Dryja TP, Cavenee W, White R, et al. Homozygosity of chromosome 13 in retinoblastoma. N Engl J Med. 1984 Mar 1;310(9):550–3. PMID:6694706

789. Du J, Wang J, Cui Y, et al. Clinicopathologic study of endolymphatic sac tumor (ELST) and differential diagnosis of papillary tumors located at the cerebellopontine angle. Neuropathology. 2015 Oct;35(5):410–20. PMID:25944396

790. Du Z, Abedalthagafi M, Aizer AA, et al. Increased expression of the immune modulatory molecule PD-L1 (CD274) in anaplastic meningioma. Oncotarget. 2015 Mar 10;6(7):4704–16. PMID:25609200

791. Du Z, Brewster R, Merrill PH, et al. Meningioma transcription factors link cell lineage with systemic metabolic cues. Neuro Oncol. 2018 Sep 3;20(10):1331–43. PMID:29660031

792. Du Z, Santagata S. Uncovering the link between systemic hormones and oncogenic signaling in the pathogenesis of meningioma. Ann Oncol. 2018 Mar 1;29(3):537–4

PMID:29346520

793. Duan K, Asa SL, Winer D, et al. Xanthomatous hypophysitis is associated with ruptured Rathke's cleft cyst. Endocr Pathol. 2017 Mar;28(1):83–90. PMID:28120170

794. Dubbink HJ, Atmodimedjo PN, Kros JM, et al. Molecular classification of anaplastic oligodendroglioma using next-generation sequencing: a report of the prospective randomized EORTC Brain Tumor Group 26951 phase III trial. Neuro Oncol. 2016 Mar;18(3):388–400. PMID:26354927

795. Dubuc AM, Remke M, Korshunov A, et al. Aberrant patterns of H3K4 and H3K27 histone lysine methylation occur across subgroups in medulloblastoma. Acta Neuropathol. 2013 Mar;125(3):373–84. PMID:23184418

796. Ducatman BS, Scheithauer BW, Piepgras DG, et al. Malignant peripheral nerve sheath tumors. A clinicopathologic study of 120 cases. Cancer. 1986 May 15;57(10):2006–21. PMID:3082508

797. Ducray F, Crinière E, Idbaih A, et al. Alpha-internexin expression identifies 1p19q codeleted gliomas. Neurology. 2009 Jan 13;72(2):156–61. PMID:19139367

798. Ducray F, Idbaih A, de Reyniès A, et al. Anaplastic oligodendrogliomas with 1p19q codeletion have a proneural gene expression profile. Mol Cancer. 2008 May 20;7:41. PMID:18492260

799. Dudley RW, Torok MR, Gallegos DR, et al. Pediatric low-grade ganglioglioma: epidemiology, treatments, and outcome analysis on 348 children from the surveillance, epidemiology, and end results database. Neurosurgery. 2015 Mar;76(3):313–9. PMID:25603107

800. Duff J, Meyer FB, Ilstrup DM, et al. Long-term outcomes for surgically resected craniopharyngiomas. Neurosurgery. 2000 Feb;46(2):291–302. PMID:10690718

801. Duffner PK, Horowitz ME, Krischer JP, et al. The treatment of malignant brain tumors in infants and very young children: an update of the Pediatric Oncology Group experience. Neuro Oncol. 1999 Apr;1(2):152–61. PMID:11554387

802. Dulai MS, Park CY, Howell WD, et al. CNS T-cell lymphoma: an under-recognized entity? Acta Neuropathol. 2008 Mar;115(3):345–56. PMID:18196250

803. Duncan VE, Nabors LB, Warren PP, et al. Primary sellar rhabdomyosarcoma arising in association with a pituitary adenoma. Int J Surg Pathol. 2016 Dec;24(8):763–6. PMID:27422470

804. Dunham C, Hussong J, Seiff M, et al. Primary intracerebral angiomatoid fibrous histiocytoma: report of a case with a t(12;22)(q13;q12) causing type 1 fusion of the EWS and ATF-1 genes. Am J Surg Pathol. 2008 Mar;32(3):478–84. PMID:10000000

805. Dunham C, McFadden D, Dahlgren L, et al. Congenital hypothalamic "hamartoblastoma" versus "hamartoma": suggestions for neuropathologic terminology emanating from a mid-gestational autopsy case of Pallister-Hall syndrome. Pediatr Dev Pathol. 2018 May-Jun;21(3):324–31. PMID:28429635

806. Dunham C, Sugo E, Tobias V, et al. Embryonal tumor with abundant neuropil and true rosettes (ETANTR): report of a case with prominent neurocytic differentiation. J Neurooncol. 2007 Aug;84(1):91–8. PMID:17332950

806A. Dunn IF, Du Z, Touat M, el al. Mismatch repair deficiency in high-grade meningioma: a rare but recurrent event associated with dramatic immune activation and clinical response to PD-1 blockade. JCO Precis Oncol. 2018;2018:PO.18.00190. PMID:30801050

807. Dunzendorfer-Matt T, Mercado EL, Maly K, et al. The neurofibromin recruitment factor Spred1 binds to the GAP related domain without affecting Ras inactivation. Proc Natl Acad Sci U S A. 2016 Jul 5;113(27):7497–502. PMID:27313208

808. Duò D, Gasverde S, Benech F, et al. MIB-1 immunoreactivity in craniopharyngiomas: a clinico-pathological analysis. Clin Neuropathol. 2003 Sep-Oct;22(5):229–34. PMID:14531547

809. Duregon E, Bertero L, Pittaro A, et al. Ki-67 proliferation index but not mitotic thresholds integrates the molecular prognostic stratification of lower grade gliomas. Oncotarget. 2016 Apr 19;7(16):21190–8. PMID:27049832

810. Durham BH, Lopez Rodrigo E, Picarsic J, et al. Activating mutations in CSF1R and additional receptor tyrosine kinases in histiocytic neoplasms. Nat Med. 2019 Dec;25(12):1839–42. PMID:31768065

811. Durno C, Boland CR, Cohen S, et al. Recommendations on surveillance and management of biallelic mismatch repair deficiency (BMMRD) syndrome: a consensus statement by the US Multi-Society Task Force on Colorectal Cancer. Gastroenterology. 2017 May;152(6):1605–14. PMID:28363489

812. Durno CA, Aronson M, Tabori U, et al. Oncologic surveillance for subjects with biallelic mismatch repair gene mutations: 10 year follow-up of a kindred. Pediatr Blood Cancer. 2012 Oct;59(4):652–6. PMID:22180144

813. Durno CA, Sherman PM, Aronson M, et al. Phenotypic and genotypic characterisation of biallelic mismatch repair deficiency (BMMR-D) syndrome. Eur J Cancer. 2015 May;51(8):977–83. PMID:25883011

814. Dyson K, Rivera-Zengotita M, Kresak J, et al. FGFR1 N546K and H3F3A K27M mutations in a diffuse leptomeningeal tumour with glial and neuronal markers. Histopathology. 2016 Oct;69(4):704–7. PMID:27061725

815. Eagle RC Jr. High-risk features and tumor differentiation in retinoblastoma: a retrospective histopathologic study. Arch Pathol Lab Med. 2009 Aug;133(8):1203–9. PMID:19653710

816. Eaton KW, Tooke LS, Wainwright LM, et al. Spectrum of SMARCB1/INI1 mutations in familial and sporadic rhabdoid tumors. Pediatr Blood Cancer. 2011 Jan;56(1):7–15. PMID:21108436

817. Eberhart CG, Brat DJ, Cohen KJ, et al. Pediatric neuroblastic brain tumors containing abundant neuropil and true rosettes. Pediatr Dev Pathol. 2000 Jul-Aug;3(4):346–52. PMID:10890250

818. Eberhart CG, Kepner JL, Goldthwaite PT, et al. Histopathologic grading of medulloblastomas: a Pediatric Oncology Group study. Cancer. 2002 Jan 15;94(2):552–60. PMID:11900240

819. Eberhart CG, Kratz J, Wang Y, et al. Histopathological and molecular prognostic markers in medulloblastoma: c-myc, N-myc, TrkC, and anaplasia. J Neuropathol Exp Neurol. 2004 May;63(5):441–9. PMID:15198123

820. Ebert C, von Haken M, Meyer-Puttlitz B, et al. Molecular genetic analysis of ependymal tumors. NF2 mutations and chromosome 22q loss occur preferentially in intramedullary spinal ependymomas. Am J Pathol. 1999 Aug;155(2):627–32. PMID:10433955

821. Ebrahimi A, Skardelly M, Bonzheim I, et al. ATRX immunostaining predicts IDH and H3F3A status in gliomas. Acta Neuropathol Commun. 2016 Jun 16;4(1):60. PMID:27311324

822. Eccher A, Girolami I, Motter JD, et al. Donor-transmitted cancer in kidney transplant recipients: a systematic review. J Nephrol. 2020 Dec;33(6):1321–32. PMID:32535833

823. Eckel-Passow JE, Drucker KL, Kollmeyer TM, et al. Adult diffuse glioma GWAS by molecular subtype identifies variants in D2HGDH and FAM20C. Neuro Oncol. 2020 Nov 26;22(11):1602–13. PMID:32386320

824. Eckel-Passow JE, Lachance DH, Molinaro AM, et al. Glioma groups based on 1p/19q, IDH, and TERT promoter mutations in tumors. N Engl J Med. 2015 Jun 25;372(26):2499–508. PMID:26061753

824A. Economides KD, Zeltser L, Capecchi MR. Hoxb13 mutations cause overgrowth of caudal spinal cord and tail vertebrae. Dev Biol. 2003 Apr 15;256(2):317–30. PMID:12679105

825. Eder N, Roncaroli F, Domart MC, et al. YAP1/TAZ drives ependymoma-like tumour formation in mice. Nat Commun. 2020 May 13;11(1):2380. PMID:32404936

826. Eeles RA. Germline mutations in the TP53 gene. Cancer Surv. 1995;25:101–24. PMID:8718514

827. Eelloo JA, Smith MJ, Bowers NL, et al. Multiple primary malignancies associated with a germline SMARCB1 pathogenic variant. Fam Cancer. 2019 Oct;18(4):445–9. PMID:31240424

828. Egan KM, Baskin R, Nabors LB, et al. Brain tumor risk according to germ-line variation in the MLLT10 locus. Eur J Hum Genet. 2015 Jan;23(1):132–4. PMID:24755950

829. Eigenbrod S, Roeber S, Thon N, et al. α-Internexin in the diagnosis of oligodendroglial tumors and association with 1p/19q status. J Neuropathol Exp Neurol. 2011 Nov;70(11):970–8. PMID:22002423

830. Elder DE, Bastian BC, Cree IA, et al. The 2018 World Health Organization classification of cutaneous, mucosal, and uveal melanoma: detailed analysis of 9 distinct subtypes defined by their evolutionary pathway. Arch Pathol Lab Med. 2020 Apr;144(4):500–22. PMID:32057276

831. El-Habr EA, Levidou G, Trigka EA, et al. Complex interactions between the components of the PI3K/AKT/mTOR pathway, and with components of MAPK, JAK/STAT and Notch-1 pathways, indicate their involvement in meningioma development. Virchows Arch. 2014 Oct;465(4):473–85. PMID:25146167

832. El Hussein S, Vincentelli C. Pituicytoma: review of commonalities and distinguishing features among TTF-1 positive tumors of the central nervous system. Ann Diagn Pathol. 2017 Aug;29:57–61. PMID:28807344

833. Ellezam B, Theeler BJ, Luthra R, et al. Recurrent PIK3CA mutations in rosette-forming glioneuronal tumor. Acta Neuropathol. 2012 Feb;123(2):285–7. PMID:21997360

834. Ellison DW. Childhood medulloblastoma: novel approaches to the classification of a heterogeneous disease. Acta Neuropathol. 2010 Sep;120(3):305–16. PMID:20652577

835. Ellison DW. Mini-symposium in medulloblastoma genomics in the modern molecular era. Brain Pathol. 2020 May;30(3):661–3. PMID:32243002

836. Ellison DW, Aldape KD, Capper D, et al. cIMPACT-NOW update 7: advancing the molecular classification of ependymal tumors. Brain Pathol. 2020 Sep;30(5):863–6. PMID:32502305

837. Ellison DW, Dalton J, Kocak M, et al. Medulloblastoma: clinicopathological correlates of SHH, WNT, and non-SHH/WNT molecular subgroups. Acta Neuropathol. 2011 Mar;121(3):381–96. PMID:21267586

838. Ellison DW, Hawkins C, Jones DTW, et al. cIMPACT-NOW update 4: diffuse gliomas characterized by MYB, MYBL1, or FGFR1 alterations or BRAFV600E mutation. Acta Neuropathol. 2019 Apr;137(4):683–7. PMID:30848347

839. Ellison DW, Kocak M, Dalton J, et al. Definition of disease-risk stratification groups in childhood medulloblastoma using combined clinical, pathologic, and molecular variables. J Clin Oncol. 2011 Apr 10;29(11):1400–7. PMID:20921458

840. Ellison DW, Kocak M, Figarella-Branger D, et al. Histopathological grading of pediatric ependymoma: reproducibility and clinical relevance in European trial cohorts. J Negat Results Biomed. 2011 May 31;10:7. PMID:21627842

841. Ellison DW, Onilude OE, Lindsey JC, et al. beta-Catenin status predicts a favorable outcome in childhood medulloblastoma: the United Kingdom Children's Cancer Study Group Brain Tumour Committee. J Clin Oncol. 2005 Nov 1;23(31):7951–7. PMID:16258095

842. Elman JS, Ni TK, Mengwasser KE, et al. Identification of FUBP1 as a long tail cancer driver and widespread regulator of tumor suppressor and oncogene alternative splicing. Cell Rep. 2019 Sep 24;28(13):3435–3449.e5. PMID:31553912

843. Elowe-Gruau E, Beltrand J, Brauner R, et al. Childhood craniopharyngioma: hypothalamus-sparing surgery decreases the risk of obesity. J Clin Endocrinol Metab. 2013 Jun;98(6):2376–82. PMID:23633208

844. Elsamadicy AA, Koo AB, David WB, et al. Comparison of epidemiology, treatments, and outcomes in pediatric versus adult ependymoma. Neurooncol Adv. 2020 Feb 21;2(1):a019. PMID:32642681

845. Emile JF, Diamond EL, Hélias-Rodzewicz Z, et al. Recurrent RAS and PIK3CA mutations in Erdheim-Chester disease. Blood. 2014 Nov 6;124(19):3016–9. PMID:25150293

846. Emmerich D, Zemojtel T, Hecht J, et al. Somatic neurofibromatosis type 1 (NF1) inactivation events in cutaneous neurofibromas of a single NF1 patient. Eur J Hum Genet. 2015 Jun;23(6):870–3. PMID:25293717

847. Emory TS, Scheithauer BW, Hirose T, et al. Intraneural perineurioma. A clonal neoplasm associated with abnormalities of chromosome 22. Am J Clin Pathol. 1995 Jun;103(6):696–704. PMID:7785653

848. Eng C. Cowden Syndrome. J Genet Couns. 1997 Jun;6(2):181–92. PMID:26142096

849. Eng C, Murday V, Seal S, et al. Cowden syndrome and Lhermitte-Duclos disease in a family: a single genetic syndrome with pleiotropy? J Med Genet. 1994 Jun;31(6):458–61. PMID:8071972

850. Eng C, Peacocke M. PTEN and inherited hamartoma-cancer syndromes. Nat Genet. 1998 Jul;19(3):223. PMID:9662392

851. Eng DY, DeMonte F, Ginsberg L, et al. Craniospinal dissemination of central neurocytoma. Report of two cases. J Neurosurg. 1997 Mar;86(3):547–52. PMID:9046315

852. Engelhard HH, Villano JL, Porter KR, et al. Clinical presentation, histology, and treatment in 430 patients with primary tumors of the spinal cord, spinal meninges, or cauda equina. J Neurosurg Spine. 2010 Jul;13(1):67–77. PMID:20594020

853. En-Nafaa I, Latib R, Fikri M, et al. [Fronto-parietal paraganglioma: a case report]. J Radiol. 2010 Dec;91(12 Pt 1):1318–9. French. PMID:21242920

854. Erdem-Eraslan L, Gravendeel LA, de Rooi J, et al. Intrinsic molecular subtypes of glioma are prognostic and predict benefit from adjuvant procarbazine, lomustine, and vincristine chemotherapy in combination with other prognostic factors in anaplastic oligodendroglial brain tumors: a report from EORTC study 26951. J Clin Oncol. 2013 Jan 20;31(3):328–36. PMID:23269986

855. Erickson D, Scheithauer B, Atkinson J, et al. Silent subtype 3 pituitary adenoma: a clinicopathologic analysis of the Mayo Clinic experience. Clin Endocrinol (Oxf). 2009 Jul;71(1):92–9. PMID:19170710

856. Erkek S, Johann PD, Finetti MA, et al. Comprehensive analysis of chromatin states in atypical teratoid/rhabdoid tumor identifies diverging roles for SWI/SNF and polycomb in gene regulation. Cancer Cell. 2019 Jan 14;35(1):95–110.e8. PMID:30595504

857. Erlich SA, Tymianski M, Kiehl TR. Cellular schwannoma of the abducens nerve: case report and review of the literature. Clin Neurol Neurosurg. 2009 Jun;111(5):467–71. PMID:19200646

858. Erson-Omay EZ, Çağlayan AO, Schultz N, et al. Somatic POLE mutations cause an ultramutated giant cell high-grade glioma subtype with better prognosis. Neuro Oncol. 2015 Oct;17(10):1356–64. PMID:25740784

859. Espiard S, Vantyghem MC, Assié G, et al. Frequency and incidence of Carney complex manifestations: a prospective multicenter study with a three-year follow-up. J Clin Endocrinol Metab. 2020 Mar 1;105(3):dgaa002. PMID:31912137

860. Esteller M, Garcia-Foncillas J, Andion E, et al. Inactivation of the DNA-repair gene MGMT and the clinical response of gliomas to alkylating agents. N Engl J Med. 2000 Nov 9;343(19):1350–4. PMID:11070098

861. Esteller M, Hamilton SR, Burger PC, et al. Inactivation of the DNA repair gene O6-methylguanine-DNA methyltransferase by promoter hypermethylation is a common event in primary human neoplasia. Cancer Res. 1999 Feb 15;59(4):793–7. PMID:10029064

862. Evans DG. Neurofibromatosis type 2 (NF2): a clinical and molecular review. Orphanet J Rare Dis. 2009 Jun 19;4:16. PMID:19545378

863. Evans DG, Baser ME, McGaughran J, et al. Malignant peripheral nerve sheath tumours in neurofibromatosis 1. J Med Genet. 2002 May;39(5):311–4. PMID:12011145

864. Evans DG, Baser ME, O'Reilly B, et al. Management of the patient and family with neurofibromatosis 2: a consensus conference statement. Br J Neurosurg. 2005 Feb;19(1):5–12. PMID:16147576

865. Evans DG, Birch JM, Ramsden RT. Paediatric presentation of type 2 neurofibromatosis. Arch Dis Child. 1999 Dec;81(6):496–9. PMID:10569966

866. Evans DG, Bowers NL, Tobi S, et al. Schwannomatosis: a genetic and epidemiological study. J Neurol Neurosurg Psychiatry. 2018 Nov;89(11):1215–9. PMID:29909380

867. Evans DG, Farndon PA. Nevoid basal cell carcinoma syndrome. In: Adam MP, Ardinger HH, Pagon RA, et al., editors. GeneReviews. Seattle (WA): University of Washington, Seattle; 2002 Jun 20 [updated 2018 Mar 29]. PMID:20301330

868. Evans DG, Hartley CL, Smith PT, et al. Incidence of mosaicism in 1055 de novo NF2 cases: much higher than previous estimates with high utility of next-generation sequencing. Genet Med. 2020 Jan;22(1):53–9. PMID:31273341

869. Evans DG, Howard E, Giblin C, et al. Birth incidence and prevalence of tumor-prone syndromes: estimates from a UK family genetic register service. Am J Med Genet A. 2010 Feb;152A(2):327–32. PMID:20082463

870. Evans DG, Huson SM, Birch JM. Malignant peripheral nerve sheath tumours in inherited disease. Clin Sarcoma Res. 2012 Oct 4;2(1):17. PMID:23036231

871. Evans DG, Huson SM, Donnai D, et al. A clinical study of type 2 neurofibromatosis. Q J Med. 1992 Aug;84(304):603–18. PMID:1484939

872. Evans DG, King AT, Bowers NL, et al. Identifying the deficiencies of current diagnostic criteria for neurofibromatosis 2 using databases of 2777 individuals with molecular testing. Genet Med. 2019 Jul;21(7):1525–33. PMID:30523344

873. Evans DG, Ladusans EJ, Rimmer S, et al. Complications of the naevoid basal cell carcinoma syndrome: results of a population based study. J Med Genet. 1993 Jun;30(6):460–4. PMID:8326488

874. Evans DG, Moran A, King A, et al. Incidence of vestibular schwannoma and neurofibromatosis 2 in the North West of England over a 10-year period: higher incidence than previously thought. Otol Neurotol. 2005 Jan;26(1):93–7. PMID:15699726

875. Evans DG, O'Hara C, Wilding A, et al. Mortality in neurofibromatosis 1: in North West England: an assessment of actuarial survival in a region of the UK since 1989. Eur J Hum Genet. 2011 Nov;19(11):1187–91. PMID:21694737

876. Evans DG, Oudit D, Smith MJ, et al. First evidence of genotype-phenotype correlations in Gorlin syndrome. J Med Genet. 2017 Aug;54(8):530–6. PMID:28596197

877. Evans DG, Ramsden RT, Shenton A, et al. Mosaicism in neurofibromatosis type 2: an update of risk based on uni/bilaterality of vestibular schwannoma at presentation and sensitive mutation analysis including multiple ligation-dependent probe amplification. J Med Genet. 2007 Jul;44(7):424–8. PMID:17307835

878. Evans DG, Wallace AJ, Wu CL, et al. Somatic mosaicism: a common cause of classic disease in tumor-prone syndromes? Lessons from type 2 neurofibromatosis. Am J Hum Genet. 1998 Sep;63(3):727–36. PMID:9718334

879. Evans DGR, Salvador H, Chang VY, et al. Cancer and central nervous system tumor surveillance in pediatric neurofibromatosis 1. Clin Cancer Res. 2017 Jun 15;23(12):e46–53. PMID:28620004

880. Eveslage M, Calaminus G, Warmuth-Metz M, et al. The postoperative quality of life in children and adolescents with craniopharyngioma. Dtsch Arztebl Int. 2019 May 3;116(18):321–8. PMID:31219033

881. Exner ND, Valenzuela JAC, Abou-El-Ardat K, et al. Deep sequencing of a recurrent oligodendroglioma and the derived xenografts reveals new insights into the evolution of human oligodendroglioma and candidate driver genes. Oncotarget. 2019 Jun 4;10(38):3641–53. PMID:31217899

882. Ezzat S, Asa SL, Couldwell WT, et al. The prevalence of pituitary adenomas: a systematic review. Cancer. 2004 Aug 1;101(3):613–9. PMID:15274075

883. Ezzat S, Cheng S, Asa SL. Epigenetics of pituitary tumors: pathogenetic and therapeutic implications. Mol Cell Endocrinol. 2018 Jul 5;469:70–6. PMID:28711607

884. Ezzat S, Zhu X, Loeper S, et al. Tumor-derived Ikaros 6 acetylates the Bcl-XL promoter to up-regulate a survival signal in pituitary cells. Mol Endocrinol. 2006 Nov;20(11):2976–86. PMID:16873443

885. Fakhran S, Escott EJ. Pineocytoma mimicking a pineal cyst on imaging: true diagnostic dilemma or a case of incomplete imaging? AJNR Am J Neuroradiol. 2008 Jan;29(1):159–63. PMID:17925371

886. Fallon KB, Palmer CA, Roth KA, et al. Prognostic value of 1p, 19q, 9p, 10q, and EGFR-FISH analyses in recurrent oligodendrogliomas. J Neuropathol Exp Neurol. 2004 Apr;63(4):314–22. PMID:15099021

887. Fan Z, Li J, Du J, et al. A missense mutation in PTCH2 underlies dominantly inherited NBCCS in a Chinese family. J Med Genet. 2008 May;45(5):303–8. PMID:18285427

888. Fanburg-Smith JC, Auerbach A, Marwaha JS, et al. Immunoprofile of mesenchymal chondrosarcoma: aberrant desmin and EMA expression, retention of INI1, and negative estrogen receptor in 22 female-predominant central nervous system and musculoskeletal cases. Ann Diagn Pathol. 2010 Feb;14(1):8–14. PMID:20123451

889. Fanburg-Smith JC, Auerbach A, Marwaha JS, et al. Reappraisal of mesenchymal chondrosarcoma: novel morphologic observations of the hyaline cartilage and endochondral ossification and beta-catenin, Sox9, and osteocalcin immunostaining of 22 cases. Hum Pathol. 2010 May;41(5):653–62. PMID:20138330

890. Fanburg-Smith JC, Majidi M, Miettinen M. Keratin expression in schwannoma; a study of 115 retroperitoneal and 22 peripheral schwannomas. Mod Pathol. 2006 Jan;19(1):115–21. PMID:16357842

891. Fang J, Huang Y, Mao G, et al. Cancer-driving H3G34V/R/D mutations block H3K36 methylation and H3K36me3-MutSα interaction. Proc Natl Acad Sci U S A. 2018 Sep 18;115(38):9598–603. PMID:30181289

892. Fargeot G, Stefanizzi S, Depuydt S, et al. Association between ischemic stroke and Erdheim-Chester disease: a case report and review of literature. J Stroke Cerebrovasc Dis. 2017 Aug;26(8):e153–5. PMID:28623120

893. Farnia B, Allen PK, Brown PD, et al. Clinical outcomes and patterns of failure in pineoblastoma: a 30-year, single-institution retrospective review. World Neurosurg. 2014 Dec;82(6):1232–41. PMID:25045788

894. Fassnacht M, Kroiss M, Allolio B. Update in adrenocortical carcinoma. J Clin Endocrinol Metab. 2013 Dec;98(12):4551–64. PMID:24081734

895. Fauchon F, Hasselblatt M, Jouvet A, et al. Role of surgery, radiotherapy and chemotherapy in papillary tumors of the pineal region: a multicenter study. J Neurooncol. 2013 Apr;112(2):223–31. PMID:23314823

896. Fauchon F, Jouvet A, Paquis P, et al. Parenchymal pineal tumors: a clinicopathological study of 76 cases. Int J Radiat Oncol Biol Phys. 2000 Mar 1;46(4):959–68. PMID:10705018

897. Faucz FR, Tirosh A, Tatsi C, et al. Somatic USP8 gene mutations are a common cause of pediatric cushing disease. J Clin Endocrinol Metab. 2017 Aug 1;102(8):2836–43. PMID:28505279

898. Feany MB, Anthony DC, Fletcher CD. Nerve sheath tumours with hybrid features of neurofibroma and schwannoma: a conceptual challenge. Histopathology. 1998 May;32(5):405–10. PMID:9639114

899. Feiden W, Milutinovic S. [Primary CNS lymphomas. Morphology and diagnosis]. Pathologe. 2002 Jul;23(4):284–91. German. PMID:12185781

900. Feliciano DM, Quon JL, Su T, et al. Postnatal neurogenesis generates heterotopias, olfactory micronodules and cortical infiltration following single-cell Tsc1 deletion. Hum Mol Genet. 2012 Feb 15;21(4):799–810. PMID:22068588

901. Felix I, Becker LE. Intracranial germ cell tumors in children: an immunohistochemical and electron microscopic study. Pediatr Neurosurg. 1990-1991-1991;16(3):156–62. PMID:1966857

902. Felix IA, Horvath E, Kovacs K, et al. Mammosomatotroph adenoma of the pituitary associated with gigantism and hyperprolactinemia. A morphological study including immunoelectron microscopy. Acta Neuropathol. 1986;71(1-2):76–82. PMID:3776476

903. Fellah S, Caudal D, De Paula AM, et al. Multimodal MR imaging (diffusion, perfusion, and spectroscopy): is it possible to distinguish oligodendroglial tumor grade and 1p/19q codeletion in the pretherapeutic diagnosis? AJNR Am J Neuroradiol. 2013 Jul;34(7):1326–33. PMID:23221948

904. Feller C, Felix M, Weiss T, et al. Histone epiproteomic profiling distinguishes oligodendroglioma, IDH-mutant and 1p/19q co-deleted from IDH-mutant astrocytoma and reveals less tri-methylation of H3K27 in oligodendrogliomas. Acta Neuropathol. 2020 Jan;139(1):211–3. PMID:31773240

905. Felsberg J, Erkwoh A, Sabel MC, et al. Oligodendroglial tumors: refinement of candidate regions on chromosome arm 1p and correlation of 1p/19q status with survival. Brain Pathol. 2004 Apr;14(2):121–30. PMID:15193024

906. Felsberg J, Hentschel B, Kaulich K, et al. Epidermal growth factor receptor variant III (EGFRvIII) positivity in EGFR-amplified glioblastomas: prognostic role and comparison between primary and recurrent tumors. Clin Cancer Res. 2017 Nov 15;23(22):6846–55. PMID:28855349

907. Ferguson SD, Zhou S, Huse JT, et al. Targetable gene fusions associate with the IDH wild-type astrocytic lineage in adult gliomas. J Neuropathol Exp Neurol. 2018 Jun 1;77(6):437–42. PMID:29718398

908. Ferlay J, Ervik M, Lam F, et al. Global Cancer Observatory: Cancer Today [Internet]. Lyon (France): International Agency for Research on Cancer; 2018. Available from: https://gco.iarc.fr/today.

909. Fernandez A, Karavitaki N, Wass JA. Prevalence of pituitary adenomas: a community-based, cross-sectional study in Banbury (Oxfordshire, UK). Clin Endocrinol (Oxf). 2010 Mar;72(3):377–82. PMID:19650784

910. Fernandez C, Figarella-Branger D, Girard N, et al. Pilocytic astrocytomas in children: prognostic factors–a retrospective study of 80 cases. Neurosurgery. 2003 Sep;53(3):544–53. PMID:12943571

911. Fernandez C, Girard N, Paz Paredes A, et al. The usefulness of MR imaging in the diagnosis of dysembryoplastic neuroepithelial tumor in children: a study of 14 cases. AJNR Am J Neuroradiol. 2003 May;24(5):829–34. PMID:12748079

912. Ferner RE, Gutmann DH. International consensus statement on malignant peripheral nerve sheath tumors in neurofibromatosis. Cancer Res. 2002 Mar 1;62(5):1573–7. PMID:11894862

913. Ferraresi S, Garozzo D, Bianchini E, et al. Perineurioma of the sciatic nerve: a possible cause of idiopathic foot drop in children: report of 4 cases. J Neurosurg Pediatr. 2010 Nov;6(5):506–10. PMID:21039177

914. Ferreri AJ, Blay JY, Reni M, et al. Prognostic scoring system for primary CNS lymphomas: the International Extranodal Lymphoma Study Group experience. J Clin Oncol. 2003 Jan 15;21(2):266–72. PMID:12525518

915. Ferreri AJ, Dell'Oro S, Capello D, et al. Aberrant methylation in the promoter region of the reduced folate carrier gene is a potential mechanism of resistance to methotrexate in primary central nervous system lymphomas. Br J Haematol. 2004 Sep;126(5):657–64. PMID:15327516

916. Ferreri AJ, Reni M, Pasini F, et al. A multicenter study of treatment of primary CNS lymphoma. Neurology. 2002 May 28;58(10):1513–20. PMID:12034789

917. Ferris SP, Goode B, Joseph NM, et al. IDH1 mutation can be present in diffuse astrocytomas and giant cell glioblastomas of young children under 10 years of age. Acta Neuropathol. 2016 Jul;132(1):153–5. PMID:27161253

918. Ferris SP, Velazquez Vega J, Aboian M, et al. High-grade neuroepithelial tumor with BCOR exon 15 internal tandem duplication-a comprehensive clinical, radiographic, pathologic, and genomic analysis. Brain Pathol. 2020 Jan;30(1):46–62. PMID:31104347

919. Fetsch JF, Miettinen M. Sclerosing perineurioma: a clinicopathologic study of 19 cases of a distinctive soft tissue lesion with a predilection for the fingers and palms of young adults.

Am J Surg Pathol. 1997 Dec;21(12):1433–42. PMID:9414186
920. Fèvre Montange M, Vasiljevic A, Bergemer Fouquet AM, et al. Histopathologic and ultrastructural features and claudin expression in papillary tumors of the pineal region: a multicenter analysis. Am J Surg Pathol. 2012 Jun;36(6):916–28. PMID:22588068
921. Fèvre Montange M, Vasiljevic A, Champier J, et al. Papillary tumor of the pineal region: histopathological characterization and review of the literature. Neurochirurgie. 2015 Apr-Jun;61(2-3):138–42. PMID:24556386
922. Fèvre-Montange M, Champier J, Szathmari A, et al. Microarray analysis reveals differential gene expression patterns in tumors of the pineal region. J Neuropathol Exp Neurol. 2006 Jul;65(7):675–84. PMID:16825954
923. Fèvre-Montange M, Hasselblatt M, Figarella-Branger D, et al. Prognosis and histopathologic features in papillary tumors of the pineal region: a retrospective multicenter study of 31 cases. J Neuropathol Exp Neurol. 2006 Oct;65(10):1004–11. PMID:17021405
924. Fèvre-Montange M, Szathmari A, Champier J, et al. Pineocytoma and pineal parenchymal tumors of intermediate differentiation presenting cytologic pleomorphism: a multicenter study. Brain Pathol. 2008 Jul;18(3):354–9. PMID:18371183
925. Fèvre-Montange M, Vasiljevic A, Frappaz D, et al. Utility of Ki67 immunostaining in the grading of pineal parenchymal tumours: a multicentre study. Neuropathol Appl Neurobiol. 2012 Feb;38(1):87–94. PMID:21696422
926. Figarella-Branger D, Lechapt-Zalcman E, Tabouret E, et al. Supratentorial clear cell ependymomas with branching capillaries demonstrate characteristic clinicopathological features and pathological activation of nuclear factor-kappaB signaling. Neuro Oncol. 2016 Jul;18(7):919–27. PMID:26984744
927. Figarella-Branger D, Lepidi H, Poncet C, et al. Differential expression of cell adhesion molecules (CAM), neural CAM and epithelial cadherin in ependymomas and choroid plexus tumors. Acta Neuropathol. 1995;89(3):248–57. PMID:7754745
928. Figarella-Branger D, Mokhtari K, Dehais C, et al. Mitotic index, microvascular proliferation, and necrosis define 3 groups of 1p/19q codeleted anaplastic oligodendrogliomas associated with different genomic alterations. Neuro Oncol. 2014 Sep;16(9):1244–54. PMID:24723566
929. Figarella-Branger D, Mokhtari K, Dehais C, et al. Mitotic index, microvascular proliferation, and necrosis define 3 pathological subgroups of prognostic relevance among 1p/19q co-deleted anaplastic oligodendrogliomas. Neuro Oncol. 2016 Jun;18(6):888–90. PMID:27175000
930. Figarella-Branger D, Pellissier JF, Daumas-Duport C, et al. Central neurocytomas. Critical evaluation of a small-cell neuronal tumor. Am J Surg Pathol. 1992 Feb;16(2):97–109. PMID:1370756
931. Figueroa ME, Abdel-Wahab O, Lu C, et al. Leukemic IDH1 and IDH2 mutations result in a hypermethylation phenotype, disrupt TET2 function, and impair hematopoietic differentiation. Cancer Cell. 2010 Dec 14;18(6):553–67. PMID:21130701
932. Filbin MG, Tirosh I, Hovestadt V, et al. Developmental and oncogenic programs in H3K27M gliomas dissected by single-cell RNA-seq. Science. 2018 Apr 20;360(6386):331–5. PMID:29674595
933. Filipski K, Braun Y, Zinke J, et al. Lack of H3K27 trimethylation is associated with 1p/19q codeletion in diffuse gliomas. Acta Neuropathol. 2019 Aug;138(2):331–4. PMID:31065834
934. Fina F, Barets D, Colin C, et al. Droplet digital PCR is a powerful technique to demonstrate frequent FGFR1 duplication in dysembryoplastic neuroepithelial tumors. Oncotarget. 2017 Jan 10;8(2):2104–13. PMID:27791984
935. Finzi G, Cerati M, Marando A, et al. Mixed pituitary adenoma/craniopharyngioma: clinical, morphological, immunohistochemical and ultrastructural study of a case, review of the literature, and pathogenetic and nosological considerations. Pituitary. 2014 Feb;17(1):53–9. PMID:23344977
936. Fioravanzo A, Caffo M, Di Bonaventura R, et al. A risk score based on 5 clinico-pathological variables predicts recurrence of atypical meningiomas. J Neuropathol Exp Neurol. 2020 May 1;79(5):500–7. PMID:32232472
937. Fischer SB, Attenhofer M, Gultekin SH, et al. TRPS1 gene alterations in human subependymoma. J Neurooncol. 2017 Aug;134(1):133–8. PMID:28528424
938. Fish C, Sy J, Wong J. High mitotic activity in a capillary hemangioma of the cauda equina: case report and review of the literature. Clin Neuropathol. 2020 May/Jun;39(3):135–8. PMID:32049625
939. Fishbein L, Leshchiner I, Walter V, et al. Comprehensive molecular characterization of pheochromocytoma and paraganglioma. Cancer Cell. 2017 Feb 13;31(2):181–93. PMID:28162975
940. Fishbein L, Nathanson KL. Pheochromocytoma and paraganglioma susceptibility genes: estimating the associated risk of disease. JAMA Oncol. 2017 Sep 1;3(9):1212–3. PMID:28384677
941. Fite JJ, Maleki Z. Paraganglioma: cytomorphologic features, radiologic and clinical findings in 12 cases. Diagn Cytopathol. 2018 Jun;46(6):473–81. PMID:29575826
942. Fjalldal S, Holmer H, Rylander L, et al. Hypothalamic involvement predicts cognitive performance and psychosocial health in long-term survivors of childhood craniopharyngioma. J Clin Endocrinol Metab. 2013 Aug;98(8):3253–62. PMID:23771923
943. Flamme I, Krieg M, Plate KH. Up-regulation of vascular endothelial growth factor in stromal cells of hemangioblastomas is correlated with up-regulation of the transcription factor HRF/HIF-2alpha. Am J Pathol. 1998 Jul;153(1):25–9. PMID:9665461
944. Flannery T, Cawley D, Zulfiger A, et al. Familial occurrence of oligodendroglial tumours. Br J Neurosurg. 2008 Jun;22(3):436–8. PMID:18568735
945. Flavahan WA, Drier Y, Liau BB, et al. Insulator dysfunction and oncogene activation in IDH mutant gliomas. Nature. 2016 Jan 7;529(7584):110–4. PMID:26700815
946. Flemming KD, Lanzino G. Cerebral cavernous malformation: what a practicing clinician should know. Mayo Clin Proc. 2020 Sep;95(9):2005–20. PMID:32605781
947. Fletcher CD, Davies SE. Benign plexiform (multinodular) schwannoma: a rare tumour unassociated with neurofibromatosis. Histopathology. 1986 Sep;10(9):971–80. PMID:3096870
948. Fletcher JS, Wu J, Jessen WJ, et al. Cxcr3-expressing leukocytes are necessary for neurofibroma formation in mice. JCI Insight. 2019 Feb 7;4(3):98601. PMID:30728335
949. Flint-Richter P, Sadetzki S. Genetic predisposition for the development of radiation-associated meningioma: an epidemiological study. Lancet Oncol. 2007 May;8(5):403–10. PMID:17466897
950. Foley KM, Woodruff JM, Ellis FT, et al. Radiation-induced malignant and atypical peripheral nerve sheath tumors. Ann Neurol. 1980 Apr;7(4):311–8. PMID:7377756
951. Folpe AL, Billings SD, McKenney JK, et al. Expression of claudin-1, a recently described tight junction-associated protein, distinguishes soft tissue perineurioma from potential mimics. Am J Surg Pathol. 2002 Dec;26(12):1620–6. PMID:12459629
952. Folpe AL, Devaney K, Weiss SW. Lipomatous hemangiopericytoma: a rare variant of hemangiopericytoma that may be confused with liposarcoma. Am J Surg Pathol. 1999 Oct;23(10):1201–7. PMID:10524520
953. Folpe AL, Graham RP, Martinez A, et al. Mesenchymal chondrosarcomas showing immunohistochemical evidence of rhabdomyoblastic differentiation: a potential diagnostic pitfall. Hum Pathol. 2018 Jul;77:28–34. PMID:29559236
954. Fonkem E, Lok E, Robison D, et al. The natural history of intravascular lymphomatosis. Cancer Med. 2014 Aug;3(4):1010–24. PMID:24931821
955. Fontana E, Gaillard R. [Epidemiology of pituitary adenoma: results of the first Swiss study]. Rev Med Suisse. 2009 Oct 28;5(223):2172–4. French. PMID:19968031
956. Fontana M, Stanton C, Pompili A, et al. Late multifocal gliomas in adolescents previously treated for acute lymphoblastic leukemia. Cancer. 1987 Oct 1;60(7):1510–8. PMID:3476182
957. Fontebasso AM, Papillon-Cavanagh S, Schwartzentruber J, et al. Recurrent somatic mutations in ACVR1 in pediatric midline high-grade astrocytoma. Nat Genet. 2014 May;46(5):462–6. PMID:24705250
958. Fontebasso AM, Schwartzentruber J, Khuong-Quang DA, et al. Mutations in SETD2 and genes affecting histone H3K36 methylation target hemispheric high-grade gliomas. Acta Neuropathol. 2013 May;125(5):659–69. PMID:23417712
959. Forbes JA, Ordóñez-Rubiano EG, Tomasiewicz HC, et al. Endonasal endoscopic transsphenoidal resection of intrinsic third ventricular craniopharyngioma: surgical results. J Neurosurg. 2018 Nov 1:1–11. PMID:30497140
960. Forés M, Simón-Carrasco L, Ajuria L, et al. A new mode of DNA binding distinguishes Capicua from other HMG-box factors and explains its mutation patterns in cancer. PLoS Genet. 2017 Mar 9;13(3):e1006622. PMID:28278156
961. Forest F, David A, Arrufat S, et al. Conventional chondrosarcoma in a survivor of rhabdoid tumor: enlarging the spectrum of tumors associated with SMARCB1 germline mutations. Am J Surg Pathol. 2012 Dec;36(12):1892–6. PMID:23154773
962. Forshew T, Tatevossian RG, Lawson AR, et al. Activation of the ERK/MAPK pathway: a signature genetic defect in posterior fossa pilocytic astrocytomas. J Pathol. 2009 Jun;218(2):172–81. PMID:19373855
963. Fortunati N, Guaraldi F, Zunino V, et al. Effects of environmental pollutants on signaling pathways in rat pituitary GH3 adenoma cells. Environ Res. 2017 Oct;158:660–8. PMID:28732322
964. Fossey M, Li H, Afzal S, et al. Atypical teratoid rhabdoid tumor in the first year of life: the Canadian ATRT registry experience and review of the literature. J Neurooncol. 2017 Mar;132(1):155–62. PMID:28102486
965. Foster RD, Williams ML, Barkovich AJ, et al. Giant congenital melanocytic nevi: the significance of neurocutaneous melanosis in neurologically asymptomatic children. Plast Reconstr Surg. 2001 Apr 1;107(4):933–41. PMID:11252085
966. Foulkes WD, Bahubeshi A, Hamel N, et al. Extending the phenotypes associated with DICER1 mutations. Hum Mutat. 2011 Dec;32(12):1381–4. PMID:21882293
967. Foulkes WD, Clarke BA, Hasselblatt M, et al. No small surprise - small cell carcinoma of the ovary, hypercalcaemic type, is a malignant rhabdoid tumour. J Pathol. 2014 Jul;233(3):209–14. PMID:24752781
968. Foulkes WD, Kamihara J, Evans DGR, et al. Cancer surveillance in Gorlin syndrome and rhabdoid tumor predisposition syndrome. Clin Cancer Res. 2017 Jun 15;23(12):e62–7. PMID:28620006
969. Foulkes WD, Priest JR, Duchaine TF. DICER1: mutations, microRNAs and mechanisms. Nat Rev Cancer. 2014 Oct;14(10):662–72. PMID:25176334
970. Fountas KN, Karampelas I, Nikolakakos LG, et al. Primary spinal cord oligodendroglioma: case report and review of the literature. Childs Nerv Syst. 2005 Feb;21(2):171–5. PMID:15138790
971. Fowler M, Simpson DA. A malignant melanin-forming tumour of the cerebellum. J Pathol Bacteriol. 1962 Oct;84:307–11. PMID:13958991
972. Fox BD, Cheung VJ, Patel AJ, et al. Epidemiology of metastatic brain tumors. Neurosurg Clin N Am. 2011 Jan;22(1):1–6. PMID:21109143
973. Franceschi E, Hofer S, Brandes AA, et al. EANO-EURACAN clinical practice guideline for diagnosis, treatment, and follow-up of post-pubertal and adult patients with medulloblastoma. Lancet Oncol. 2019 Dec;20(12):e715–28. PMID:31797797
974. Franceschi E, Tosoni A, Bartolini S, et al. Histopathological grading affects survival in patients with IDH-mutant grade II and grade III diffuse gliomas. Eur J Cancer. 2020 Sep;137:10–7. PMID:32721633
975. Frandsen S, Broholm H, Larsen VA, et al. Clinical characteristics of gliosarcoma and outcomes from standardized treatment relative to conventional glioblastoma. Front Oncol. 2019 Dec 17;9:1425. PMID:31921679
976. Franz DN, Belousova E, Sparagana S, et al. Efficacy and safety of everolimus for subependymal giant cell astrocytomas associated with tuberous sclerosis complex (EXIST-1): a multicentre, randomised, placebo-controlled phase 3 trial. Lancet. 2013 Jan 12;381(9861):125–32. PMID:23158522
977. Franz DN, Belousova E, Sparagana S, et al. Everolimus for subependymal giant cell astrocytoma in patients with tuberous sclerosis complex: 2-year open-label extension of the randomised EXIST-1 study. Lancet Oncol. 2014 Dec;15(13):1513–20. PMID:25456370
978. Franz DN, Belousova E, Sparagana S, et al. Long-term use of everolimus in patients with tuberous sclerosis complex: final results from the EXIST-1 study. PLoS One. 2016 Jun 28;11(6):e0158476. PMID:27351628
979. Frappart PO, Lee Y, Lamont J, et al. BRCA2 is required for neurogenesis and suppression of medulloblastoma. EMBO J. 2007 Jun 6;26(11):2732–42. PMID:17476307
980. Frappaz D, Ricci AC, Kohler R, et al. Diffuse brain stem tumor in an adolescent with multiple enchondromatosis (Ollier's disease). Childs Nerv Syst. 1999 May;15(5):222–5. PMID:10392492
981. Frattini V, Trifonov V, Chan JM, et al. The integrated landscape of driver genomic alterations in glioblastoma. Nat Genet. 2013 Oct;45(10):1141–9. PMID:23917401
982. Freilich RJ, Thompson SJ, Walker RW, et al. Adenocarcinomatous transformation of intracranial germ cell tumors. Am J Surg Pathol. 1995 May;19(5):537–44. PMID:7726363
983. Freudenstein D, Wagner A, Bornemann A, et al. Primary melanocytic lesions of the CNS: report of five cases. Zentralbl Neurochir. 2004;65(3):146–53. PMID:15306980
984. Friedmann-Morvinski D, Bushong EA, Ke E, et al. Dedifferentiation of neurons and

astrocytes by oncogenes can induce gliomas in mice. Science. 2012 Nov 23;338(6110):1080–4. PMID:23087000

985. Friend KE, Chiou YK, Laws ER Jr, et al. Pit-1 messenger ribonucleic acid is differentially expressed in human pituitary adenomas. J Clin Endocrinol Metab. 1993 Nov;77(5):1281–6. PMID:8077322

986. Friend KE, Chiou YK, Lopes MB, et al. Estrogen receptor expression in human pituitary: correlation with immunohistochemistry in normal tissue, and immunohistochemistry and morphology in macroadenomas. J Clin Endocrinol Metab. 1994 Jun;78(6):1497–504. PMID:7515390

987. Frigerio S, Disciglio V, Manoukian S, et al. A large de novo 9p21.3 deletion in a girl affected by astrocytoma and multiple melanoma. BMC Med Genet. 2014 May 17;15:59. PMID:24884915

988. Fritchie K, Jensch K, Moskalev EA, et al. The impact of histopathology and NAB2-STAT6 fusion subtype in classification and grading of meningeal solitary fibrous tumor/hemangiopericytoma. Acta Neuropathol. 2019 Feb;137(2):307–19. PMID:30584643

989. Fritchie KJ, Jin L, Rubin BP, et al. NAB2-STAT6 Gene fusion in meningeal hemangiopericytoma and solitary fibrous tumor. J Neuropathol Exp Neurol. 2016 Mar;75(3):263–71. PMID:26883114

990. Fritz A, Percy C, Jack A, et al., editors. International classification of diseases for oncology (ICD-O). 3rd ed. 1st rev. Geneva (Switzerland): World Health Organization; 2013.

991. Fruehwald-Pallamar J, Puchner SB, Rossi A, et al. Magnetic resonance imaging spectrum of medulloblastoma. Neuroradiology. 2011 Jun;53(6):387–96. PMID:21279509

992. Frühwald MC, Hasselblatt M, Nemes K, et al. Age and DNA methylation subgroup as potential independent risk factors for treatment stratification in children with atypical teratoid/rhabdoid tumors. Neuro Oncol. 2020 Jul 7;22(7):1006–17. PMID:31883020

993. Fujii K, Miyashita T. Gorlin syndrome (nevoid basal cell carcinoma syndrome): update and literature review. Pediatr Int. 2014 Oct;56(5):667–74. PMID:25131638

994. Fujii K, Ohashi H, Suzuki M, et al. Frameshift mutation in the PTCH2 gene can cause nevoid basal cell carcinoma syndrome. Fam Cancer. 2013 Dec;12(4):611–4. PMID:23479190

995. Fujimaki T, Matsutani M, Funada N, et al. CT and MRI features of intracranial germ cell tumors. J Neurooncol. 1994;19(3):217–26. PMID:7807172

996. Fujio S, Juratli TA, Arita K, et al. A clinical rule for preoperative prediction of BRAF mutation status in craniopharyngiomas. Neurosurgery. 2019 Aug 1;85(2):204–10. PMID:30481321

997. Fujisawa H, Kurrer M, Reis RM, et al. Acquisition of the glioblastoma phenotype during astrocytoma progression is associated with loss of heterozygosity on 10q25-qter. Am J Pathol. 1999 Aug;155(2):387–94. PMID:10433932

998. Fujisawa H, Tohma Y, Muramatsu N, et al. Spindle cell oncocytoma of the adenohypophysis with marked hypervascularity. Case report. Neurol Med Chir (Tokyo). 2012;52(8):594–8. PMID:22976144

999. Fukuda T, Akiyama N, Ikegami M, et al. Expression of hydroxyindole-O-methyltransferase enzyme in the human central nervous system and in pineal parenchymal cell tumors. J Neuropathol Exp Neurol. 2010 May;69(5):498–510. PMID:20418777

1000. Fukuda T, Igarashi T, Hiraki H, et al. Abnormal pigmentation of schwannoma attributed to excess production of neuromelanin-like pigment. Pathol Int. 2000 Mar;50(3):230–7. PMID:10792787

1001. Fukuda T, Yasumichi K, Suzuki T. Immunohistochemistry of gliosarcoma with liposarcomatous differentiation. Pathol Int. 2008 Jun;58(6):396–401. PMID:18477220

1002. Fukuoka K, Kanemura Y, Shofuda T, et al. Significance of molecular classification of ependymomas: C11orf95-RELA fusion-negative supratentorial ependymomas are a heterogeneous group of tumors. Acta Neuropathol Commun. 2018 Dec 4;6(1):134. PMID:30514397

1003. Fukuoka K, Mamatjan Y, Ryall S, et al. BRAF V600E mutant oligodendroglioma-like tumors with chromosomal instability in adolescents and young adults. Brain Pathol. 2020 May;30(3):515–23. PMID:31630459

1004. Fukuoka K, Mamatjan Y, Tatevossian R, et al. Clinical impact of combined epigenetic and molecular analysis of pediatric low-grade gliomas. Neuro Oncol. 2020 Oct 14;22(10):1474–83. PMID:32242226

1005. Fukushima S, Otsuka A, Suzuki T, et al. Mutually exclusive mutations of KIT and RAS are associated with KIT mRNA expression and chromosomal instability in primary intracranial pure germinomas. Acta Neuropathol. 2014;127(6):911–25. PMID:24452629

1006. Fukushima S, Yamashita S, Kobayashi H, et al. Genome-wide methylation profiles in primary intracranial germ cell tumors indicate a primordial germ cell origin for germinomas. Acta Neuropathol. 2017 Mar;133(3):445–62. PMID:28078450

1007. Fuld AD, Speck ME, Harris BT, et al. Primary melanoma of the spinal cord: a case report, molecular footprint, and review of the literature. J Clin Oncol. 2011 Jun 10;29(17):e499–502. PMID:21444862

1008. Fuller GN, Bigner SH. Amplified cellular oncogenes in neoplasms of the human central nervous system. Mutat Res. 1992 May;276(3):299–306. PMID:1374522

1009. Fuller GN, Hess KR, Rhee CH, et al. Molecular classification of human diffuse gliomas by multidimensional scaling analysis of gene expression profiles parallels morphology-based classification, correlates with survival, and reveals clinically-relevant novel glioma subsets. Brain Pathol. 2002 Jan;12(1):108–16. PMID:11771519

1010. Funato K, Major T, Lewis PW, et al. Use of human embryonic stem cells to model pediatric gliomas with H3.3K27M histone mutation. Science. 2014 Dec 19;346(6216):1529–33. PMID:25525250

1011. Fung KM, Fang W, Norton RE, et al. Cerebellar central liponeurocytoma. Ultrastruct Pathol. 2003 Mar-Apr;27(2):109–14. PMID:12746202

1012. Furey C, Antwi P, Duran D, et al. 9p24 triplication in syndromic hydrocephalus with diffuse villous hyperplasia of the choroid plexus. Cold Spring Harb Mol Case Stud. 2018 Oct 1;4(5):a003145. PMID:29895553

1013. Furnari FB, Huang HJ, Cavenee WK. The phosphoinositol phosphatase activity of PTEN mediates a serum-sensitive G1 growth arrest in glioma cells. Cancer Res. 1998 Nov 15;58(22):5002–8. PMID:9823298

1014. Furnari FB, Lin H, Huang HS, et al. Growth suppression of glioma cells by PTEN requires a functional phosphatase catalytic domain. Proc Natl Acad Sci U S A. 1997 Nov 11;94(23):12479–84. PMID:9356475

1015. Furtado A, Arantes M, Silva R, et al. Comprehensive review of extraventricular neurocytoma with report of two cases, and comparison with central neurocytoma. Clin Neuropathol. 2010 May-Jun;29(3):134–40. PMID:20423686

1016. Furuta T, Moritsubo M, Muta H, et al. Central nervous system neuroblastic tumor with FOXR2 activation presenting both neuronal and glial differentiation: a case report. Brain Tumor Pathol. 2020 Jul;37(3):100–4. PMID:32535663

1017. Furuya K, Takanashi S, Ogawa A, et al. High-dose methotrexate monotherapy followed by radiation for CD30-positive, anaplastic lymphoma kinase-1-positive anaplastic large-cell lymphoma in the brain of a child. J Neurosurg Pediatr. 2014 Sep;14(3):311–5. PMID:25014324

1018. Gabeau-Lacet D, Aghi M, Betensky RA, et al. Bone involvement predicts poor outcome in atypical meningioma. J Neurosurg. 2009 Sep;111(3):464–71. PMID:19267533

1019. Gabel BC, Cleary DR, Martin JR, et al. Unusual and rare locations for craniopharyngiomas: clinical significance and review of the literature. World Neurosurg. 2017 Feb;98:381–7. PMID:27908738

1020. Gadish T, Tulchinsky H, Deutsch AA, et al. Pinealoblastoma in a patient with familial adenomatous polyposis: variant of Turcot syndrome type 2? Report of a case and review of the literature. Dis Colon Rectum. 2005 Dec;48(12):2343–6. PMID:16400511

1021. Gaffney EF, Doorly T, Dinn JJ. Aggressive oncocytic neuroendocrine tumour ('oncocytic paraganglioma') of the cauda equina. Histopathology. 1986 Mar;10(3):311–9. PMID:2422107

1022. Gajjar A, Pfister SM, Taylor MD, et al. Molecular insights into pediatric brain tumors have the potential to transform therapy. Clin Cancer Res. 2014 Nov 15;20(22):5630–40. PMID:25398846

1023. Galanis E, Buckner JC, Dinapoli RP, et al. Clinical outcome of gliosarcoma compared with glioblastoma multiforme: North Central Cancer Treatment Group results. J Neurosurg. 1998 Sep;89(3):425–30. PMID:9724117

1024. Galili N, Davis RJ, Fredericks WJ, et al. Fusion of a fork head domain gene to PAX3 in the solid tumour alveolar rhabdomyosarcoma. Nat Genet. 1993 Nov;5(3):230–5. PMID:8275086

1025. Gallina P, Buccoliero AM, Mariotti F, et al. Oncocytic meningiomas: cases with benign histopathological features and a favorable clinical course. J Neurosurg. 2006 Nov;105(5):736–8. PMID:17121136

1026. Gallon R, Mühlegger B, Wenzel SS, et al. A sensitive and scalable microsatellite instability assay to diagnose constitutional mismatch repair deficiency by sequencing of peripheral blood leukocytes. Hum Mutat. 2019 May;40(5):649–55. PMID:30740824

1027. Gambella A, Senetta R, Collemi G, et al. NTRK fusions in central nervous system tumors: a rare, but worthy target. Int J Mol Sci. 2020 Jan 23;21(3):E753. PMID:31979374

1028. Gamboa NT, Karsy M, Gamboa JT, et al. Preoperative and intraoperative perfusion magnetic resonance imaging in a RELA fusion-positive anaplastic ependymoma: a case report. Surg Neurol Int. 2018 Jul 24;9:144. PMID:30105138

1029. Ganapathi KA, Jobanputra V, Iwamoto F, et al. The genetic landscape of dural marginal zone lymphomas. Oncotarget. 2016 Jul 12;7(28):43052–61. PMID:27248180

1030. Gao L, Han F, Jin Y, et al. Imaging features of rosette-forming glioneuronal tumours. Clin Radiol. 2018 Mar;73(3):275–82. PMID:29146003

1031. Gao Q, Liang WW, Foltz SM, et al. Driver fusions and their implications in the development and treatment of human cancers. Cell Rep. 2018 Apr 3;23(1):227–238.e3. PMID:29617662

1032. Gao S, Shi X, Wang Y, et al. Malignant transformation of craniopharyngioma: case report and review of the literature. J Neuroon col. 2011 Jul;103(3):719–25. PMID:20872276

1033. Gao X, Zhang Y, Arrazola P, et al. Ts tumour suppressor proteins antagonize ami no-acid-TOR signalling. Nat Cell Biol. 200 Sep;4(9):699–704. PMID:12172555

1034. Gao Y, Jiang J, Liu Q. Clinicopathologica and immunohistochemical features of primar central nervous system germ cell tumors: 24-years experience. Int J Clin Exp Patho 2014 Sep 15;7(10):6965–72. PMID:25400782

1035. Garcia C, Gutmann DH. Nf2/Merlin con trols spinal cord neural progenitor function i a Rac1/ErbB2-dependent manner. PLoS One 2014 May 9;9(5):e97320. PMID:24817309

1036. Garcia Pulido P, Neal J, Halpin S, et a Multicentric oligodendroglioma: case repor and review of the literature. Seizure. 201 Jul;22(6):480–2. PMID:23528979

1037. Garcia-Lavandeira M, Saez C, Diaz-Ro driguez E, et al. Craniopharyngiomas expres embryonic stem cell markers (SOX2, OCT4 KLF4, and SOX9) as pituitary stem cells bu do not coexpress RET/GFRA3 receptors. Clin Endocrinol Metab. 2012 Jan;97(1):E80–7 PMID:22031517

1038. Gardiman MP, Fassan M, Orvieto E, et a Diffuse leptomeningeal glioneuronal tumors: new entity? Brain Pathol. 2010 Mar;20(2):361-6. PMID:19486008

1039. Gareton A, Pierron G, Mokhtari K, et a ESWR1-CREM fusion in an intracranial myxoi angiomatoid fibrous histiocytoma-like tumor a case report and literature review. J Neuro pathol Exp Neurol. 2018 Jul 1;77(7):537–41 PMID:29788195

1040. Gareton A, Tauziède-Espariat A, Dan gouloff-Ros V, et al. The histomolecular criteri established for adult anaplastic pilocytic astro cytoma are not applicable to the pediatric popu lation. Acta Neuropathol. 2020 Feb;139(2):287-303. PMID:31677015

1041. Garnier L, Ducray F, Verlut C, et al. Pro longed response induced by single agent vemu rafenib in a BRAF V600E spinal ganglioglioma a case report and review of the literature. Fror Oncol. 2019 Mar 26;9:177. PMID:30984614

1042. Garrè ML, Cama A, Bagnasco F, et a Medulloblastoma variants: age-dependen occurrence and relation to Gorlin syndrome– new clinical perspective. Clin Cancer Res. 200 Apr 1;15(7):2463–71. PMID:19276247

1043. Garvin JH Jr, Selch MT, Holmes E, et a Phase II study of pre-irradiation chemotherap for childhood intracranial ependymoma. Chil dren's Cancer Group protocol 9942: a repo from the Children's Oncology Group. Pedia Blood Cancer. 2012 Dec 15;59(7):1183–9 PMID:22949057

1044. Garzia L, Kijima N, Morrissy AS, et a A hematogenous route for medulloblastom leptomeningeal metastases. Cell. 2018 Fe 22;172(5):1050–1062.e14. PMID:29474906

1045. Garzon-Muvdi T, Yang W, Lim M, et a Atypical and anaplastic meningioma: outcome in a population based study. J Neuroonco 2017 Jun;133(2):321–30. PMID:28429237

1046. Gasco J, Franklin B, Fuller GN, et a Multifocal epithelioid glioblastoma mimick ing cerebral metastasis: case report. Neu rocirugia (Astur). 2009 Dec;20(6):550–4 PMID:19967320

1047. Gaston-Massuet C, Andoniadou CL Signore M, et al. Increased Wingless (Wnt signaling in pituitary progenitor/stem cell gives rise to pituitary tumors in mice an humans. Proc Natl Acad Sci U S A. 2011 Ju 12;108(28):11482–7. PMID:21636786

1048. Gauchotte G, Peyre M, Pouget C, et a Prognostic value of histopathological feature and loss of H3K27me3 immunolabeling in ana plastic meningioma: a multicenter retrospective study. J Neuropathol Exp Neurol. 2020 Jul 1;79(7):754–62. PMID:32447376

1049. Gavrilovic IT, Posner JB. Brain metastases: epidemiology and pathophysiology. J Neurooncol. 2005 Oct;75(1):5–14. PMID:16215811

1050. Gazzola DM, Arbini AA, Haglof K, et al. Primary marginal zone lymphoma of the cns presenting as a diffuse leptomeningeal process. Neurology. 2010 Dec 13;07(11):1180 J. PMID:27521434

1051. Geddes JF, Thom M, Robinson SF, et al. Granular cell change in astrocytic tumors. Am J Surg Pathol. 1996 Jan;20(1):55–63. PMID:8540609

1052. Gelabert-González M. Paragangliomas of the lumbar region. Report of two cases and review of the literature. J Neurosurg Spine. 2005 Mar;2(3):354–65. PMID:15796363

1053. Geller JI, Roth JJ, Biegel JA. Biology and treatment of rhabdoid tumor. Crit Rev Oncog. 2015;20(3-4):199–216. PMID:26349416

1054. Gembruch O, Junker A, Mönninghoff C, et al. Liponeurocytoma: systematic review of a rare entity. World Neurosurg. 2018 Dec;120:214–33. PMID:30205225

1055. Gempt J, Baldawa SS, Weirich G, et al. Recurrent multiple spinal paragangliomas as a manifestation of a metastatic composite paraganglioma-ganglioneuroblastoma. Acta Neurochir (Wien). 2013 Jul;155(7):1241–2. PMID:23532344

1056. Gempt J, Ringel F, Oexle K, et al. Familial pineocytoma. Acta Neurochir (Wien). 2012 Aug;154(8):1413–6. PMID:22699425

1057. George DH, Scheithauer BW, Aker FV, et al. Primary anaplastic large cell lymphoma of the central nervous system: prognostic effect of ALK-1 expression. Am J Surg Pathol. 2003 Apr;27(4):487–93. PMID:12657933

1058. George DH, Scheithauer BW, Kovacs K, et al. Crooke's cell adenoma of the pituitary: an aggressive variant of corticotroph adenoma. Am J Surg Pathol. 2003 Oct;27(10):1330–6. PMID:14508394

1059. Georgescu MM, Olar A, Mobley BC, et al. Epithelial differentiation with microlumen formation in meningioma: diagnostic utility of NHERF1/EBP50 immunohistochemistry. Oncotarget. 2018 Jun 19;9(47):28652–65. PMID:29983887

1060. Gerber NU, von Hoff K, von Bueren AO, et al. Outcome of 11 children with ependymoblastoma treated within the prospective HIT-trials between 1991 and 2006. J Neurooncol. 2011 May;102(3):459–69. PMID:21308398

1061. Gerkes EH, Fock JM, den Dunnen WF, et al. A heritable form of SMARCE1-related meningiomas with important implications for follow-up and family screening. Neurogenetics. 2016 Apr;17(2):83–9. PMID:26803492

1062. Gerson SL. MGMT: its role in cancer aetiology and cancer therapeutics. Nat Rev Cancer. 2004 Apr;4(4):296–307. PMID:15057289

1063. Gerstner E, Batchelor T. Primary CNS lymphoma. Expert Rev Anticancer Ther. 2007 May;7(5):689–700. PMID:17492932

1064. Gerstner ER, Abrey LE, Schiff D, et al. CNS Hodgkin lymphoma. Blood. 2008 Sep 1;112(5):1658–61. PMID:18591379

1065. Gessi M, Capper D, Sahm F, et al. Evidence of H3 K27M mutations in posterior fossa ependymomas. Acta Neuropathol. 2016 Oct;132(4):635–7. PMID:27539613

1066. Gessi M, Dörner E, Dreschmann V, et al. Intramedullary gangliogliomas: histopathologic and molecular features of 25 cases. Hum Pathol. 2016 Mar;49:107–13. PMID:26826417

1067. Gessi M, Giagnacovo M, Modena P, et al. Role of immunohistochemistry in the identification of supratentorial c11orf95-rela fused ependymoma in routine neuropathology. Am J Surg Pathol. 2019 Jan;43(1):56–63. PMID:29266023

1068. Gessi M, Giangaspero F, Lauriola L, et al. Embryonal tumors with abundant neuropil and true rosettes: a distinctive CNS primitive neuroectodermal tumor. Am J Surg Pathol. 2009 Feb;33(2):211–7. PMID:18987548

1069. Gessi M, Giangaspero F, Pietsch T. Atypical teratoid/rhabdoid tumors and choroid plexus tumors; when genetics "surprise" pathology. Brain Pathol. 2003 Jul;13(3):409–14. PMID:12946029

1070. Gessi M, Gielen GH, Dreschmann V, et al. High frequency of H3F3A (K27M) mutations characterizes pediatric and adult high-grade gliomas of the spinal cord. Acta Neuropathol. 2015 Sep;130(3):435–7. PMID:26231952

1071. Gessi M, Hammes J, Lauriola L, et al. GNA11 and N-RAS mutations: alternatives for MAPK pathway activating GNAQ mutations in primary melanocytic tumours of the central nervous system. Neuropathol Appl Neurobiol. 2013 Jun;39(4):417–25. PMID:22758774

1072. Gessi M, Hattingen E, Dörner E, et al. Dysembryoplastic neuroepithelial tumor of the septum pellucidum and the supratentorial midline: histopathologic, neuroradiologic, and molecular features of 7 cases. Am J Surg Pathol. 2016 Jun;40(6):806–11. PMID:26796505

1073. Gessi M, Japp AS, Dreschmann V, et al. High-resolution genomic analysis of cribriform neuroepithelial tumors of the central nervous system. J Neuropathol Exp Neurol. 2015 Oct;74(10):970–4. PMID:26352987

1074. Gessi M, Moneim YA, Hammes J, et al. FGFR1 mutations in Rosette-forming glioneuronal tumors of the fourth ventricle. J Neuropathol Exp Neurol. 2014 Jun;73(6):580–4. PMID:24806303

1075. Gessi M, van de Nes J, Griewank K, et al. Absence of TERT promoter mutations in primary melanocytic tumours of the central nervous system. Neuropathol Appl Neurobiol. 2014 Oct;40(6):794–7. PMID:24645797

1076. Gessi M, von Bueren A, Treszl A, et al. MYCN amplification predicts poor outcome for patients with supratentorial primitive neuroectodermal tumors of the central nervous system. Neuro Oncol. 2014 Jul;16(7):924–32. PMID:24470553

1077. Gessi M, Zur Mühlen A, Hammes J, et al. Genome-wide DNA copy number analysis of desmoplastic infantile astrocytomas and desmoplastic infantile gangliogliomas. J Neuropathol Exp Neurol. 2013 Sep;72(9):807–15. PMID:23965740

1078. Ghanbari N, Lam A, Wycoco V, et al. Intracranial myxoid variant of angiomatoid fibrous histiocytoma: a case report and literature review. Cureus. 2019 Mar 18;11(3):e4261. PMID:31139520

1079. Ghasemi DR, Sill M, Okonechnikov K, et al. MYCN amplification drives an aggressive form of spinal ependymoma. Acta Neuropathol. 2019 Dec;138(6):1075–89. PMID:31414211

1080. Gherardi R, Baudrimont M, Nguyen JP, et al. Monstrocellular heavily lipidized malignant glioma. Acta Neuropathol. 1986;69(1-2):28–32. PMID:3515829

1081. Gheyi V, Hui FK, Doppenberg EM, et al. Glioblastoma multiforme causing calvarial destruction: an unusual manifestation revisited. AJNR Am J Neuroradiol. 2004 Oct;25(9):1533–7. PMID:15502132

1082. Giacomelli AO, Yang X, Lintner RE, et al. Mutational processes shape the landscape of TP53 mutations in human cancer. Nat Genet. 2018 Oct;50(10):1381–7. PMID:30224644

1083. Giagnacovo M, Antonelli M, Biassoni V, et al. Retrospective analysis on the consistency of MRI features with histological and molecular markers in diffuse intrinsic pontine glioma (DIPG). Childs Nerv Syst. 2020 Apr;36(4):697–704. PMID:31848724

1084. Giangaspero F, Cenacchi G, Losi L, et al. Extraventricular neoplasms with neurocytoma features. A clinicopathological study of 11 cases. Am J Surg Pathol. 1997 Feb;21(2):206–12. PMID:9042288

1085. Giangaspero F, Cenacchi G, Roncaroli F, et al. Medulloblastoma (lipidized medulloblastoma). A cerebellar neoplasm of adults with favorable prognosis. Am J Surg Pathol. 1996 Jun;20(6):656–64. PMID:8651344

1086. Giangaspero F, Chieco P, Ceccarelli C, et al. "Desmoplastic" versus "classic" medulloblastoma: comparison of DNA content, histopathology and differentiation. Virchows Arch A Pathol Anat Histopathol. 1991;418(3):207–14. PMID:1900966

1087. Giangaspero F, Guiducci A, Lenz FA, et al. Meningioma with meningioangiomatosis: a condition mimicking invasive meningiomas in children and young adults: report of two cases and review of the literature. Am J Surg Pathol. 1999 Aug;23(8):872–5. PMID:10435554

1088. Giangaspero F, Perilongo G, Fondelli MP, et al. Medulloblastoma with extensive nodularity: a variant with favorable prognosis. J Neurosurg. 1999 Dec;91(6):971–7. PMID:10584843

1089. Giangaspero F, Rigobello L, Badiali M, et al. Large-cell medulloblastoma. A distinct variant with highly aggressive behavior. Am J Surg Pathol. 1992 Jul;16(7):687–93. PMID:1530108

1090. Giannini C, Hebrink D, Scheithauer BW, et al. Analysis of p53 mutation and expression in pleomorphic xanthoastrocytoma. Neurogenetics. 2001 Jul;3(3):159–62. PMID:11523567

1091. Giannini C, Scheithauer BW, Burger PC, et al. Cellular proliferation in pilocytic and diffuse astrocytomas. J Neuropathol Exp Neurol. 1999 Jan;58(1):46–53. PMID:10068313

1092. Giannini C, Scheithauer BW, Burger PC, et al. Pleomorphic xanthoastrocytoma: what do we really know about it? Cancer. 1999 May 1;85(9):2033–45. PMID:10223246

1093. Giannini C, Scheithauer BW, Jenkins RB, et al. Soft-tissue perineurioma. Evidence for an abnormality of chromosome 22, criteria for diagnosis, and review of the literature. Am J Surg Pathol. 1997 Feb;21(2):164–73. PMID:9042282

1094. Giannini C, Scheithauer BW, Lopes MB, et al. Immunophenotype of pleomorphic xanthoastrocytoma. Am J Surg Pathol. 2002 Apr;26(4):479–85. PMID:11914626

1095. Giannini C, Scheithauer BW, Steinberg J, et al. Intraventricular perineurioma: case report. Neurosurgery. 1998 Dec;43(6):1478–81. PMID:9848865

1096. Giannini C, Scheithauer BW, Weaver AL, et al. Oligodendrogliomas: reproducibility and prognostic value of histologic diagnosis and grading. J Neuropathol Exp Neurol. 2001 Mar;60(3):248–62. PMID:11245209

1097. Gianno F, Antonelli M, Ferretti E, et al. Pediatric high-grade glioma: a heterogeneous group of neoplasms with different molecular drivers. Glioma. 2018 1;117–24. doi:10.4103/glioma.glioma_27_18.

1098. Giannini Larsen AM, Cote DJ, Zaidi HA, et al. Spindle cell oncocytoma of the pituitary gland. J Neurosurg. 2018 Oct 19;131(2):517–25. PMID:30485213

1099. Gibson P, Tong Y, Robinson G, et al. Subtypes of medulloblastoma have distinct developmental origins. Nature. 2010 Dec 23;468(7327):1095–9. PMID:21150909

1100. Gielen PR, Schulte BM, Kers-Rebel ED, et al. Increase in both CD14-positive and CD15-positive myeloid-derived suppressor cell subpopulations in the blood of patients with glioma but predominance of CD15-positive myeloid-derived suppressor cells in glioma tissue. J Neuropathol Exp Neurol. 2015 May;74(5):390–400. PMID:25853692

1101. Giese A, Bjerkvig R, Berens ME, et al. Cost of migration: invasion of malignant gliomas and implications for treatment. J Clin Oncol. 2003 Apr 15;21(8):1624–36. PMID:12697889

1102. Giese A, Loo MA, Tran N, et al. Dichotomy of astrocytoma migration and proliferation. Int J Cancer. 1996 Jul 17;67(2):275–82. PMID:8760599

1103. Gilbert AR, Zaky W, Gokden M, et al. Extending the neuroanatomic territory of diffuse midline glioma, K27M mutant: pineal region origin. Pediatr Neurosurg. 2018;53(1):59–63. PMID:29131126

1104. Gilbert MR, Dignam JJ, Armstrong TS, et al. A randomized trial of bevacizumab for newly diagnosed glioblastoma. N Engl J Med. 2014 Feb 20;370(8):699–708. PMID:24552317

1105. Gilbert MR, Wang M, Aldape KD, et al. Dose-dense temozolomide for newly diagnosed glioblastoma: a randomized phase III clinical trial. J Clin Oncol. 2013 Nov 10;31(32):4085–91. PMID:24101040

1106. Gil-Gouveia R, Cristino N, Farias JP, et al. Pleomorphic xanthoastrocytoma of the cerebellum: illustrated review. Acta Neurochir (Wien). 2004 Nov;146(11):1241–4. PMID:15455217

1107. Gill AJ, Benn DE, Chou A, et al. Immunohistochemistry for SDHB triages genetic testing of SDHB, SDHC, and SDHD in paraganglioma-pheochromocytoma syndromes. Hum Pathol. 2010 Jun;41(6):805–14. PMID:20236688

1108. Gillet E, Alentorn A, Doukouré B, et al. TP53 and p53 statuses and their clinical impact in diffuse low grade gliomas. J Neurooncol. 2014 May;118(1):131–9. PMID:24590827

1109. Gimenez-Roqueplo AP, Dahia PL, Robledo M. An update on the genetics of paraganglioma, pheochromocytoma, and associated hereditary syndromes. Horm Metab Res. 2012 May;44(5):328–33. PMID:22328163

1110. Gimm O, Attié-Bitach T, Lees JA, et al. Expression of the PTEN tumour suppressor protein during human development. Hum Mol Genet. 2000 Jul 1;9(11):1633–9. PMID:10861290

1111. Gimple RC, Bhargava S, Dixit D, et al. Glioblastoma stem cells: lessons from the tumor hierarchy in a lethal cancer. Genes Dev. 2019 Jun 1;33(11-12):591–609. PMID:31160393

1112. Giorgianni A, Pellegrino C, De Benedictis A, et al. Lhermitte-Duclos disease. A case report. Neuroradiol J. 2013 Dec;26(6):655–60. PMID:24355184

1113. Gire J, Deveze A, Garcia S, et al. [Paraganglioma of the cerebellopontine angle: report of two cases]. Rev Laryngol Otol Rhinol (Bord). 2008;129(3):213–6. French. PMID:19694167

1114. Giussani C, Isimbaldi G, Massimino M, et al. Ganglioglioma of the spinal cord in neurofibromatosis type 1. Pediatr Neurosurg. 2013;49(1):50–4. PMID:24192615

1114A. Gläsker S, Bender BU, Apel TW, et al. Reconsideration of biallelic inactivation of the VHL tumour suppressor gene in hemangioblastomas of the central nervous system. J Neurol Neurosurg Psychiatry. 2001 May;70(5):644–8. PMID:11309459

1115. Gläsker S, Bender BU, Apel TW, et al. The impact of molecular genetic analysis of the VHL gene in patients with haemangioblastomas of the central nervous system. J Neurol Neurosurg Psychiatry. 1999 Dec;67(6):758–62. PMID:10567493

1116. Gläsker S, Berlis A, Pagenstecher A, et al. Characterization of hemangioblastomas of spinal nerves. Neurosurgery. 2005 Mar;56(3):503–9. PMID:15730575

1117. Gläsker S, Krüger MT, Klingler JH, et al. Hemangioblastomas and neurogenic polyglobulia. Neurosurgery. 2013 Jun;72(6):930–5.

PMID:23407287
1118. Gläsker S, Lonser RR, Tran MG, et al. Effects of VHL deficiency on endolymphatic duct and sac. Cancer Res. 2005 Dec 1;65(23):10847–53. PMID:16322231
1119. Gleissner B, Chamberlain MC. Neoplastic meningitis. Lancet Neurol. 2006 May;5(5):443–52. PMID:16632315
1120. Gleize V, Alentorn A, Connen de Kérillis L, et al. CIC inactivating mutations identify aggressive subset of 1p19q codeleted gliomas. Ann Neurol. 2015 Sep;78(3):355–74. PMID:26017892
1121. Glick R, Baker C, Husain S, et al. Primary melanocytomas of the spinal cord: a report of seven cases. Clin Neuropathol. 1997 May-Jun;16(3):127–32. PMID:9197936
1122. Gnekow AK, Walker DA, Kandels D, et al. A European randomised controlled trial of the addition of etoposide to standard vincristine and carboplatin induction as part of an 18-month treatment programme for childhood (≤16 years) low grade glioma - A final report. Eur J Cancer. 2017 Aug;81:206–25. PMID:28649001
1123. Godfraind C, Kaczmarska JM, Kocak M, et al. Distinct disease-risk groups in pediatric supratentorial and posterior fossa ependymomas. Acta Neuropathol. 2012 Aug;124(2):247–57. PMID:22526017
1124. Goebel HH, Cravioto H. Ultrastructure of human and experimental ependymomas. A comparative study. J Neuropathol Exp Neurol. 1972 Jan;31(1):54–71. PMID:5060130
1125. Goellner JR, Laws ER Jr, Soule EH, et al. Hemangiopericytoma of the meninges. Mayo Clinic experience. Am J Clin Pathol. 1978 Sep;70(3):375–80. PMID:707404
1126. Goffena J, Lefcort F, Zhang Y, et al. Elongator and codon bias regulate protein levels in mammalian peripheral neurons. Nat Commun. 2018 Mar 1;9(1):889. PMID:29497044
1127. Goh S, Butler W, Thiele EA. Subependymal giant cell tumors in tuberous sclerosis complex. Neurology. 2004 Oct 26;63(8):1457–61. PMID:15505165
1128. Gokden M, Mrak RE. Pituitary adenoma with craniopharyngioma component. Hum Pathol. 2009 Aug;40(8):1189–93. PMID:19427020
1129. Goldman-Lévy G, Rigau V, Bléchet C, et al. Primary melanoma of the leptomeninges with BAP1 expression-loss in the setting of a nevus of Ota: a clinical, morphological and genetic study of 2 cases. Brain Pathol. 2016 Jul;26(4):547–50. PMID:26834043
1130. Goldstein HE, Solomon RA. Epidemiology of cavernous malformations. Handb Clin Neurol. 2017;143:241–7. PMID:28552146
1131. Gomez DR, Missett BT, Wara WM, et al. High failure rate in spinal ependymomas with long-term follow-up. Neuro Oncol. 2005 Jul;7(3):254–9. PMID:16053700
1132. Gomez MR. Phenotypes of the tuberous sclerosis complex with a revision of diagnostic criteria. Ann N Y Acad Sci. 1991;615:1–7. PMID:2039135
1133. Gomez-Hernandez K, Ezzat S, Asa SL, et al. Clinical implications of accurate subtyping of pituitary adenomas: perspectives from the treating physician. Turk Patoloji Derg. 2015;31 Suppl 1:4–17. PMID:26177314
1134. Gonzalez KD, Noltner KA, Buzin CH, et al. Beyond Li Fraumeni syndrome: clinical characteristics of families with p53 germline mutations. J Clin Oncol. 2009 Mar 10;27(8):1250–6. PMID:19204208
1135. González-Acosta M, Marín F, Puliafito B, et al. High-sensitivity microsatellite instability assessment for the detection of mismatch repair defects in normal tissue of biallelic germline mismatch repair mutation carriers. J Med Genet. 2020 Apr;57(4):269–73. PMID:31494577
1136. Gonzalez-Aguilar A, Idbaih A, Boisselier B, et al. Recurrent mutations of MYD88 and TBL1XR1 in primary central nervous system lymphomas. Clin Cancer Res. 2012 Oct 1;18(19):5203–11. PMID:22837180
1137. González-Cámpora R, Weller RO. Lipidized mature neuroectodermal tumour of the cerebellum with myoid differentiation. Neuropathol Appl Neurobiol. 1998 Oct;24(5):397–402. PMID:9821171
1138. Gonzalez-Meljem JM, Haston S, Carreno G, et al. Stem cell senescence drives age-attenuated induction of pituitary tumours in mouse models of paediatric craniopharyngioma. Nat Commun. 2017 Nov 28;8(1):1819. PMID:29180744
1139. Goode B, Mondal G, Hyun M, et al. A recurrent kinase domain mutation in PRKCA defines chordoid glioma of the third ventricle. Nat Commun. 2018 Feb 23;9(1):810. PMID:29476136
1140. Goodrich LV, Scott MP. Hedgehog and patched in neural development and disease. Neuron. 1998 Dec;21(6):1243–57. PMID:9883719
1141. Gore AC. Neuroendocrine targets of endocrine disruptors. Hormones (Athens). 2010 Jan-Mar;9(1):16–27. PMID:20363718
1142. Gorelyshev A, Mazerkina N, Medvedeva O, et al. Second-hit APC mutation in a familial adamantinomatous craniopharyngioma. Neuro Oncol. 2020 Jun 9;22(6):889–91. PMID:32170310
1143. Gorlia T, Delattre JY, Brandes AA, et al. New clinical, pathological and molecular prognostic models and calculators in patients with locally diagnosed anaplastic oligodendroglioma or oligoastrocytoma. A prognostic factor analysis of European Organisation for Research and Treatment of Cancer Brain Tumour Group Study 26951. Eur J Cancer. 2013 Nov;49(16):3477–85. PMID:23896377
1144. Gorlin RJ. Nevoid basal-cell carcinoma syndrome. Medicine (Baltimore). 1987 Mar;66(2):98–113. PMID:3547011
1145. Gorovets D, Kannan K, Shen R, et al. IDH mutation and neuroglial developmental features define clinically distinct subclasses of lower grade diffuse astrocytic glioma. Clin Cancer Res. 2012 May 1;18(9):2490–501. PMID:22415316
1146. Goschzik T, Gessi M, Denkhaus D, et al. PTEN mutations and activation of the PI3K/Akt/mTOR signaling pathway in papillary tumors of the pineal region. J Neuropathol Exp Neurol. 2014 Aug;73(8):747–51. PMID:25003235
1147. Goschzik T, Gessi M, Dreschmann V, et al. Genomic alterations of adamantinomatous and papillary craniopharyngioma. J Neuropathol Exp Neurol. 2017 Feb 1;76(2):126–34. PMID:28069929
1148. Goschzik T, Schwalbe EC, Hicks D, et al. Prognostic effect of whole chromosomal aberration signatures in standard-risk, non-WNT/non-SHH medulloblastoma: a retrospective, molecular analysis of the HIT-SIOP PNET 4 trial. Lancet Oncol. 2018 Dec;19(12):1602–16. PMID:30392813
1149. Goss JA, Huang AY, Smith E, et al. Somatic mutations in intracranial arteriovenous malformations. PLoS One. 2019 Dec 31;14(12):e0226852. PMID:31891627
1150. Gossage L, Eisen T, Maher ER. VHL, the story of a tumour suppressor gene. Nat Rev Cancer. 2015 Jan;15(1):55–64. PMID:25533676
1151. Götze S, Wolter M, Reifenberger G, et al. Frequent promoter hypermethylation of Wnt pathway inhibitor genes in malignant astrocytic gliomas. Int J Cancer. 2010 Jun 1;126(11):2584–93. PMID:19847810
1152. Goutagny S, Nault JC, Mallet M, et al. High incidence of activating TERT promoter mutations in meningiomas undergoing malignant progression. Brain Pathol. 2014 Mar;24(2):184–9. PMID:24261697
1153. Goutagny S, Yang HW, Zucman-Rossi J, et al. Genomic profiling reveals alternative genetic pathways of meningioma malignant progression dependent on the underlying NF2 status. Clin Cancer Res. 2010 Aug 15;16(16):4155–64. PMID:20682713
1154. Governale LS, Vortmeyer AO, Zhuang Z, et al. Fibrous meningioma in a patient with von Hippel-Lindau disease: a genetic analysis. J Neurosurg. 2001 Dec;95(6):1045–9. PMID:11765821
1155. Goyal G, Heaney ML, Collin M, et al. Erdheim-Chester disease: consensus recommendations for evaluation, diagnosis, and treatment in the molecular era. Blood. 2020 May 28;135(22):1929–45. PMID:32187362
1156. Goyal G, Young JR, Koster MJ, et al. The Mayo Clinic Histiocytosis Working Group consensus statement for the diagnosis and evaluation of adult patients with histiocytic neoplasms: Erdheim-Chester disease, Langerhans cell histiocytosis, and Rosai-Dorfman disease. Mayo Clin Proc. 2019 Oct;94(10):2054–71. PMID:31472931
1157. Gozali AE, Britt B, Shane L, et al. Choroid plexus tumors; management, outcome, and association with the Li-Fraumeni syndrome: the Children's Hospital Los Angeles (CHLA) experience, 1991-2010. Pediatr Blood Cancer. 2012 Jun;58(6):905–9. PMID:21990040
1158. Graadt van Roggen JF, McMenamin ME, Belchis DA, et al. Reticular perineurioma: a distinctive variant of soft tissue perineurioma. Am J Surg Pathol. 2001 Apr;25(4):485–93. PMID:11257623
1159. Grabb PA, Albright AL, Pang D. Dissemination of supratentorial malignant gliomas via the cerebrospinal fluid in children. Neurosurgery. 1992 Jan;30(1):64–71. PMID:1738457
1160. Grahovac G, Alden T, Nitin W. Mixed pineal mature teratoma and germinoma in two brothers of the fraternal triplets. Childs Nerv Syst. 2017 May;33(5):859–63. PMID:28236067
1161. Grajkowska W, Kotulska K, Jurkiewicz E, et al. Subependymal giant cell astrocytomas with atypical histological features mimicking malignant gliomas. Folia Neuropathol. 2011;49(1):39–46. PMID:21455842
1162. Gravendeel LA, Kouwenhoven MC, Gevaert O, et al. Intrinsic gene expression profiles of gliomas are a better predictor of survival than histology. Cancer Res. 2009 Dec 1;69(23):9065–72. PMID:19920198
1163. Greer A, Foreman NK, Donson A, et al. Desmoplastic infantile astrocytoma/ganglioglioma with rare BRAF V600D mutation. Pediatr Blood Cancer. 2017 Jun;64(6). PMID:27860162
1164. Griewank KG, Koelsche C, van de Nes JAP, et al. Integrated genomic classification of melanocytic tumors of the central nervous system using mutation analysis, copy number alterations, and dna methylation Profiling. Clin Cancer Res. 2018 Sep 15;24(18):4494–504. PMID:29891723
1165. Griffin CA, Burger P, Morsberger L, et al. Identification of der(1;19)(q10;p10) in five oligodendrogliomas suggests mechanism of concurrent 1p and 19q loss. J Neuropathol Exp Neurol. 2006 Oct;65(10):988–94. PMID:17021403
1166. Griffith JL, Morris SM, Mahdi J, et al. Increased prevalence of brain tumors classified as T2 hyperintensities in neurofibromatosis 1. Neurol Clin Pract. 2018 Aug;8(4):283–91. PMID:30140579
1167. Grimm F, Maurus R, Beschorner R, et al. Ki-67 labeling index and expression of p53 are non-predictive for invasiveness and tumor size in functional and nonfunctional pituitary adenomas. Acta Neurochir (Wien). 2019 Jun;161(6):1149–56. PMID:31037500
1168. Grois N, Fahrner B, Arceci RJ, et al. Central nervous system disease in Langerhans cell histiocytosis. J Pediatr. 2010 Jun;156(6):873–881.e1. PMID:20434166
1169. Grommes C, Pastore A, Palaskas N, et al. Ibrutinib unmasks critical role of Bruton tyrosine kinase in primary CNS lymphoma. Cancer Discov. 2017 Sep;7(9):1018–29. PMID:28619981
1170. Gross AM, Wolters PL, Dombi E, et al. Selumetinib in children with inoperable plexiform neurofibromas. N Engl J Med. 2020 Apr 9;382(15):1430–42. PMID:32187457
1171. Groussin L, Kirschner LS, Vincent-Dejean C, et al. Molecular analysis of the cyclic AMP-dependent protein kinase A (PKA) regulatory subunit 1A (PRKAR1A) gene in patients with Carney complex and primary pigmented nodular adrenocortical disease (PPNAD) reveals novel mutations and clues for pathophysiology: augmented PKA signaling is associated with adrenal tumorigenesis in PPNAD. Am J Hum Genet. 2002 Dec;71(6):1433–42. PMID:12424709
1172. Grünewald TGP, Cidre-Aranaz F, Surdez D, et al. Ewing sarcoma. Nat Rev Dis Primers. 2018 Jul 5;4(1):5. PMID:29977059
1173. Gu J, Tamura M, Yamada KM. Tumor suppressor PTEN inhibits integrin- and growth factor-mediated mitogen-activated protein (MAP) kinase signaling pathways. J Cell Biol. 1998 Nov 30;143(5):1375–83. PMID:9832564
1174. Guadagno E, Cervasio M, Di Somma A, et al. Essential role of ultrastructural examination for spindle cell oncocytoma: case report of a rare neoplasm and review of the literature. Ultrastruct Pathol. 2016;40(2):121–4. PMID:27031178
1175. Guan H, Huang Y, Wen W, et al. Primary central nervous system extranodal NK/T-cell lymphoma, nasal type: case report and review of the literature. J Neurooncol. 2011 Jun;103(2):387–91. PMID:20845062
1176. Gucer H, Mete O. Endobronchial gangliocytic paraganglioma: not all keratin-positive endobronchial neuroendocrine neoplasms are pulmonary carcinoids. Endocr Pathol. 2014 Sep;25(3):356–8. PMID:23912549
1177. Gudowius S, Engelbrecht V, Messing-Jünger M, et al. Diagnostic difficulties in childhood bilateral thalamic astrocytomas. Neuropediatrics. 2002 Dec;33(6):331–5. PMID:12571791
1178. Guermazi A, De Kerviler E, Zagdanski AM, et al. Diagnostic imaging of choroid plexus disease. Clin Radiol. 2000 Jul;55(7):503–16. PMID:10924373
1179. Guerreiro Stucklin AS, Ryall S, Fukuoka K, et al. Alterations in ALK/ROS1/NTRK/MET drive a group of infantile hemispheric gliomas. Nat Commun. 2019 Sep 25;10(1):4343. PMID:31554817
1180. Guerrero-Pérez F, Marengo AP, Vidal N, et al. Primary tumors of the posterior pituitary: a systematic review. Rev Endocr Metab Disord. 2019 Jun;20(2):219–38. PMID:30864049
1181. Guerrero-Pérez F, Vidal N, Marengo AP, et al. Posterior pituitary tumours: the spectrum of a unique entity. A clinical and histological study of a large case series. Endocrine. 2019 Jan;63(1):36–43. PMID:30276594
1182. Guerrini-Rousseau L, Dufour C, Varlet P, et al. Germline SUFU mutation carriers and medulloblastoma: clinical characteristics, cancer risk, and prognosis. Neuro Oncol. 2018 Jul 5;20(8):1122–32. PMID:29186568
1183. Guerrini-Rousseau L, Varlet P, Colas C, et al. Constitutional mismatch repair deficiency-associated brain tumors: report from the European C4CMMRD consortium. Neurooncol

Adv. 2019 Dec 2;1(1):vdz033. PMID:32642664
1184. Guesmi H, Houtteville JP, Courthéoux P, et al. [Dysembryoplastic neuroepithelial tumors. Report of 8 cases including two with unusual localization]. Neurochirurgie. 1999 Sep;45(3):190–200. French. PMID:10567958
1185. Gugel I, Grimm F, Teuber C, et al. Presenting symptoms in children with neurofibromatosis type 2. Childs Nerv Syst. 2020 Oct;36(10):2463–70. PMID:32537663
1186. Guillou L, Gebhard S, Coindre JM. Lipomatous hemangiopericytoma: a fat-containing variant of solitary fibrous tumor? Clinicopathologic, immunohistochemical, and ultrastructural analysis of a series in favor of a unifying concept. Hum Pathol. 2000 Sep;31(9):1108–15. PMID:11014579
1187. Guo J, He H, Liu Q, et al. Identification and epigenetic analysis of a maternally imprinted gene Qpct. Mol Cells. 2015 Oct;38(10):859–65. PMID:26447138
1188. Guo R, Zhang X, Niu C, et al. Primary central nervous system small lymphocytic lymphoma in the bilateral ventricles: two case reports. BMC Neurol. 2019 Aug 19;19(1):200. PMID:31426757
1189. Gupta K, Harreld JH, Sabin ND, et al. Massively calcified low-grade glioma - a rare and distinctive entity. Neuropathol Appl Neurobiol. 2014 Feb;40(2):221–4. PMID:23927783
1190. Gupta K, Orisme W, Harreld JH, et al. Posterior fossa and spinal gangliogliomas form two distinct clinicopathologic and molecular subgroups. Acta Neuropathol Commun. 2014 Feb 14;2:18. PMID:24529209
1191. Gupta MP, Lane AM, DeAngelis MM, et al. Clinical characteristics of uveal melanoma in patients with germline BAP1 mutations. JAMA Ophthalmol. 2015 Aug;133(8):881–7. PMID:25974357
1192. Gupta N, Nasim M, Spitzer SG, et al. Primary central nervous system T-cell lymphoma with aberrant expression of CD20 and CD79a: a diagnostic pitfall. Int J Surg Pathol. 2017 Oct;25(7):599–603. PMID:28612004
1193. Gupta VR, Giller C, Kolhe R, et al. Polymorphous low-grade neuroepithelial tumor of the young: a case report with genomic findings. World Neurosurg. 2019 Dec;132:347–55. PMID:31520766
1194. Gusella JF, Ramesh V, MacCollin M, et al. Merlin: the neurofibromatosis 2 tumor suppressor. Biochim Biophys Acta. 1999 Mar 25;1423(2):M29–36. PMID:10214350
1195. Gusella JF, Ramesh V, MacCollin M, et al. Neurofibromatosis 2: loss of merlin's protective spell. Curr Opin Genet Dev. 1996 Feb;6(1):87–92. PMID:8791482
1196. Gutenberg A, Brandis A, Hong B, et al. Common molecular cytogenetic pathway in papillary tumors of the pineal region (PTPR). Brain Pathol. 2011 Nov;21(6):672–7. PMID:21470326
1197. Gutmann DH, Aylsworth A, Carey JC, et al. The diagnostic evaluation and multidisciplinary management of neurofibromatosis 1 and neurofibromatosis 2. JAMA. 1997 Jul 2;278(1):51–7. PMID:9207339
1198. Gutmann DH, Donahoe J, Brown T, et al. Loss of neurofibromatosis 1 (NF1) gene expression in NF1-associated pilocytic astrocytomas. Neuropathol Appl Neurobiol. 2000 Aug;26(4):361–7. PMID:10931370
1199. Gutmann DH, Ferner RE, Listernick RH, et al. Neurofibromatosis type 1. Nat Rev Dis Primers. 2017 Feb 23;3:17004. PMID:28230061
1200. Gutmann DH, Kettenmann H. Microglia/brain macrophages as central drivers of brain tumor pathobiology. Neuron. 2019 Nov 6;104(3):442–9. PMID:31697921
1201. Gutmann DH, McLellan MD, Hussain I, et al. Somatic neurofibromatosis type 1 (NF1) inactivation characterizes NF1-associated pilocytic astrocytoma. Genome Res. 2013 Mar;23(3):431–9. PMID:23222849
1202. Guyot A, Duchesne M, Robert S, et al. Analysis of CDKN2A gene alterations in recurrent and non-recurrent meningioma. J Neurooncol. 2019 Dec;145(3):449–59. PMID:31729637
1203. Guyot-Goubin A, Donadieu J, Barkaoui M, et al. Descriptive epidemiology of childhood Langerhans cell histiocytosis in France, 2000-2004. Pediatr Blood Cancer. 2008 Jul;51(1):71–5. PMID:18260117
1204. Gyure KA, Morrison AL. Cytokeratin 7 and 20 expression in choroid plexus tumors: utility in differentiating these neoplasms from metastatic carcinomas. Mod Pathol. 2000 Jun;13(6):638–43. PMID:10874668
1205. Gyure KA, Prayson RA. Subependymal giant cell astrocytoma: a clinicopathologic study with HMB45 and MIB-1 immunohistochemical analysis. Mod Pathol. 1997 Apr;10(4):313–7. PMID:9110292
1206. Habek M, Brinar VV, Mubrin Z, et al. Bilateral thalamic astrocytoma. J Neurooncol. 2007 Sep;84(2):175–7. PMID:17522784
1207. Haberler C, Jarius C, Lang S, et al. Fibrous meningeal tumours with extensive non-calcifying collagenous whorls and glial fibrillary acidic protein expression: the whorling-sclerosing variant of meningioma. Neuropathol Appl Neurobiol. 2002 Feb;28(1):42–7. PMID:11849562
1208. Haberler C, Laggner U, Slavc I, et al. Immunohistochemical analysis of INI1 protein in malignant pediatric CNS tumors: lack of INI1 in atypical teratoid/rhabdoid tumors and in a fraction of primitive neuroectodermal tumors without rhabdoid phenotype. Am J Surg Pathol. 2006 Nov;30(11):1462–8. PMID:17063089
1209. Haberler C, Reiniger L, Rajnai H, et al. Case of the month 1-2019: CNS high-grade neuroepithelial tumor with BCOR alteration. Clin Neuropathol. 2019 Jan/Feb;38(1):4–7. PMID:30526817
1210. Haddad AF, Young JS, Oh T, et al. Clinical characteristics and outcomes of null-cell versus silent gonadotroph adenomas in a series of 1166 pituitary adenomas from a single institution. Neurosurg Focus. 2020 Jun;48(6):E13. PMID:32480370
1211. Haddad SF, Moore SA, Schelper RL, et al. Vascular smooth muscle hyperplasia underlies the formation of glomeruloid vascular structures of glioblastoma multiforme. J Neuropathol Exp Neurol. 1992 Sep;51(5):488–92. PMID:1381413
1212. Hadfield KD, Newman WG, Bowers NL, et al. Molecular characterisation of SMARCB1 and NF2 in familial and sporadic schwannomatosis. J Med Genet. 2008 Jun;45(6):332–9. PMID:18285426
1213. Hadfield KD, Smith MJ, Urquhart JE, et al. Rates of loss of heterozygosity and mitotic recombination in NF2 schwannomas, sporadic vestibular schwannomas and schwannomatosis schwannomas. Oncogene. 2010 Nov 25;29(47):6216–21. PMID:20729918
1214. Hafezi F, Perez Bercoff D. The Solo play of TERT promoter mutations. Cells. 2020 Mar 19;9(3):E749. PMID:32204305
1215. Hagel C, Buslei R, Buchfelder M, et al. Immunoprofiling of glial tumours of the neurohypophysis suggests a common pituicytic origin of neoplastic cells. Pituitary. 2017 Apr;20(2):211–7. PMID:27744503
1216. Hagel C, Stemmer-Rachamimov AO, Bornemann A, et al. Clinical presentation, immunohistochemistry and electron microscopy indicate neurofibromatosis type 2-associated gliomas to be spinal ependymomas. Neuropathology. 2012 Dec;32(6):611–6. PMID:22394059
1217. Hahn H, Wicking C, Zaphiropoulous PG, et al. Mutations of the human homolog of Drosophila patched in the nevoid basal cell carcinoma syndrome. Cell. 1996 Jun 14;85(6):841–51. PMID:8681379
1218. Hair LS, Symmans F, Powers JM, et al. Immunohistochemistry and proliferative activity in Lhermitte-Duclos disease. Acta Neuropathol. 1992;84(5):570–3. PMID:1462769
1219. Hajnsek S, Paladino J, Gadze ZP, et al. Clinical and neurophysiological changes in patients with pineal region expansions. Coll Antropol. 2013 Mar;37(1):35–40. PMID:23697248
1220. Hakimi AA, Ostrovnaya I, Reva B, et al. Adverse outcomes in clear cell renal cell carcinoma with mutations of 3p21 epigenetic regulators BAP1 and SETD2: a report by MSKCC and the KIRC TCGA research network. Clin Cancer Res. 2013 Jun 15;19(12):3259–67. PMID:23620406
1221. Halani SH, Yousefi S, Velazquez Vega J, et al. Multi-faceted computational assessment of risk and progression in oligodendroglioma implicates NOTCH and PI3K pathways. NPJ Precis Oncol. 2018 Nov 6;2:24. PMID:30417117
1222. Haller F, Moskalev EA, Faucz FR, et al. Aberrant DNA hypermethylation of SDHC: a novel mechanism of tumor development in Carney triad. Endocr Relat Cancer. 2014 Aug;21(4):567–77. PMID:24859990
1223. Hamidi O, Young WF Jr, Gruber L, et al. Outcomes of patients with metastatic phaeochromocytoma and paraganglioma: a systematic review and meta-analysis. Clin Endocrinol (Oxf). 2017 Nov;87(5):440–50. PMID:28746746
1224. Hamilton JD, Rapp M, Schneiderhan T, et al. Glioblastoma multiforme metastasis outside the CNS: three case reports and possible mechanisms of escape. J Clin Oncol. 2014 Aug 1;32(22):e80–4. PMID:24567434
1225. Hamilton SR, Liu B, Parsons RE, et al. The molecular basis of Turcot's syndrome. N Engl J Med. 1995 Mar 30;332(13):839–47. PMID:7661930
1226. Han SJ, Yang I, Otero JJ, et al. Secondary gliosarcoma after diagnosis of glioblastoma: clinical experience with 30 consecutive patients. J Neurosurg. 2010 May;112(5):990–6. PMID:19817543
1227. Han SJ, Yang I, Tihan T, et al. Primary gliosarcoma: key clinical and pathologic distinctions from glioblastoma with implications as a unique oncologic entity. J Neurooncol. 2010 Feb;96(3):313–20. PMID:19618114
1228. Han Z, Kang P, Zhang H, et al. Prognostic value of H3K27me3 in children with ependymoma. Pediatr Blood Cancer. 2020 Mar;67(3):e28121. PMID:31850684
1229. Hang JF, Hsu CY, Lin SC, et al. Thyroid transcription factor-1 distinguishes subependymal giant cell astrocytoma from its mimics and supports its cell origin from the progenitor cells in the medial ganglionic eminence. Mod Pathol. 2017 Mar;30(3):318–28. PMID:27910945
1230. Hansen JM, Larsen VA, Scheie D, et al. Primary intracranial angiomatoid fibrous histiocytoma presenting with anaemia and migraine-like headaches and aura as early clinical features. Cephalalgia. 2015 Dec;35(14):1334–6. PMID:25900984
1231. Hansen TH, Myers NB, Lee DR. Studies of two antigenic forms of Ld with disparate beta 2-microglobulin (beta 2m) associations suggest that beta 2m facilitate the folding of the alpha 1 and alpha 2 domains during de novo synthesis. J Immunol. 1988 May 15;140(10):3522–7. PMID:2452190
1232. Hanssen AM, Fryns JP. Cowden syndrome. J Med Genet. 1995 Feb;32(2):117–9. PMID:7760320
1233. Hao S, Huang G, Feng J, et al. Non-NF2 mutations have a key effect on inhibitory immune checkpoints and tumor pathogenesis in skull base meningiomas. J Neurooncol. 2019 Aug;144(1):11–20. PMID:31177425
1234. Hara T, Akutsu H, Takano S, et al. Clinical and biological significance of adamantinomatous craniopharyngioma with CTNNB1 mutation. J Neurosurg. 2018 Aug 3;131(1):217–26. PMID:30074466
1235. Harbour JW, Onken MD, Roberson ED, et al. Frequent mutation of BAP1 in metastasizing uveal melanomas. Science. 2010 Dec 3;330(6009):1410–3. PMID:21051595
1236. Hardell L, Carlberg M. Mobile phone and cordless phone use and the risk for glioma - Analysis of pooled case-control studies in Sweden, 1997-2003 and 2007-2009. Pathophysiology. 2015 Mar;22(1):1–13. PMID:25466607
1237. Harder A, Wesemann M, Hagel C, et al. Hybrid neurofibroma/schwannoma is overrepresented among schwannomatosis and neurofibromatosis patients. Am J Surg Pathol. 2012 May;36(5):702–9. PMID:22446939
1238. Haresh KP, Prabhakar R, Anand Rajan KD, et al. A rare case of paraganglioma of the sella with bone metastases. Pituitary. 2009;12(3):276–9. PMID:18320326
1239. Hargrave DR, Bouffet E, Tabori U, et al. Efficacy and safety of dabrafenib in pediatric patients with BRAF V600 mutation-positive relapsed or refractory low-grade glioma: results from a phase I/IIa study. Clin Cancer Res. 2019 Dec 15;25(24):7303–11. PMID:31811016
1240. Hariri OR, Khachekian A, Muilli D, et al. Acute-onset cerebellar symptoms in Lhermitte-Duclos disease: case report. Cerebellum. 2013 Feb;12(1):127–30. PMID:22692559
1241. Haroche J, Charlotte F, Arnaud L, et al. High prevalence of BRAF V600E mutations in Erdheim-Chester disease but not in other non-Langerhans cell histiocytoses. Blood. 2012 Sep 27;120(13):2700–3. PMID:22879539
1242. Hart J, Gardner JM, Edgar M, et al. Epithelioid schwannomas: an analysis of 58 cases including atypical variants. Am J Surg Pathol. 2016 May;40(5):704–13. PMID:26752543
1243. Harter DH, Omeis I, Forman S, et al. Endoscopic resection of an intraventricular dysembryoplastic neuroepithelial tumor of the septum pellucidum. Pediatr Neurosurg. 2006;42(2):105–7. PMID:16465080
1244. Hartmann C, Hentschel B, Simon M, et al. Long-term survival in primary glioblastoma with versus without isocitrate dehydrogenase mutations. Clin Cancer Res. 2013 Sep 15;19(18):5146–57. PMID:23918605
1245. Hartmann C, Hentschel B, Wick W, et al. Patients with IDH1 wild type anaplastic astrocytomas exhibit worse prognosis than IDH1-mutated glioblastomas, and IDH1 mutation status accounts for the unfavorable prognostic effect of higher age: implications for classification of gliomas. Acta Neuropathol. 2010 Dec;120(6):707–18. PMID:21088844
1246. Hartmann C, Meyer J, Balss J, et al. Type and frequency of IDH1 and IDH2 mutations are related to astrocytic and oligodendroglial differentiation and age: a study of 1,010 diffuse gliomas. Acta Neuropathol. 2009 Oct;118(4):469–74. PMID:19554337
1247. Harutyunyan AS, Krug B, Chen H, et al. H3K27M induces defective chromatin spread of PRC2-mediated repressive H3K27me2/me3 and is essential for glioma tumorigenesis. Nat Commun. 2019 Mar 19;10(1):1262. PMID:30890717
1248. Hashimoto N, Handa H, Nishi S. Intracranial and intraspinal dissemination from a growth hormone-secreting pituitary tumor. Case report. J Neurosurg. 1986 Jan;64(1):140–4. PMID:3941337

1249. Hasselblatt M, Blümcke I, Jeibmann A, et al. Immunohistochemical profile and chromosomal imbalances in papillary tumours of the pineal region. Neuropathol Appl Neurobiol. 2006 Jun;32(3):278–83. PMID:16640646
1250. Hasselblatt M, Böhm C, Tatenhorst L, et al. Identification of novel diagnostic markers for choroid plexus tumors: a microarray-based approach. Am J Surg Pathol. 2006 Jan;30(1):66–74. PMID:16330944
1251. Hasselblatt M, Gesk S, Oyen F, et al. Nonsense mutation and inactivation of SMARCA4 (BRG1) in an atypical teratoid/rhabdoid tumor showing retained SMARCB1 (INI1) expression. Am J Surg Pathol. 2011 Jun;35(6):933–5. PMID:21566516
1252. Hasselblatt M, Isken S, Linge A, et al. High-resolution genomic analysis suggests the absence of recurrent genomic alterations other than SMARCB1 aberrations in atypical teratoid/rhabdoid tumors. Genes Chromosomes Cancer. 2013 Feb;52(2):185–90. PMID:23074045
1253. Hasselblatt M, Jeibmann A, Guerry M, et al. Choroid plexus papilloma with neuropil-like islands. Am J Surg Pathol. 2008 Jan;32(1):162–6. PMID:18162784
1254. Hasselblatt M, Nagel I, Oyen F, et al. SMARCA4-mutated atypical teratoid/rhabdoid tumors are associated with inherited germline alterations and poor prognosis. Acta Neuropathol. 2014 Sep;128(3):453–6. PMID:25060813
1255. Hasselblatt M, Oyen F, Gesk S, et al. Cribriform neuroepithelial tumor (CRINET): a nonrhabdoid ventricular tumor with INI1 loss and relatively favorable prognosis. J Neuropathol Exp Neurol. 2009 Dec;68(12):1249–55. PMID:19915490
1256. Hasselblatt M, Paulus W. Sensitivity and specificity of epithelial membrane antigen staining patterns in ependymomas. Acta Neuropathol. 2003 Oct;106(4):385–8. PMID:12898159
1257. Hasselblatt M, Sepehrnia A, von Falkenhausen M, et al. Intracranial follicular dendritic cell sarcoma. Case report. J Neurosurg. 2003 Dec;99(6):1089–90. PMID:14705740
1258. Hasselblatt M, Thomas C, Hovestadt V, et al. Poorly differentiated chordoma with SMARCB1/INI1 loss: a distinct molecular entity with dismal prognosis. Acta Neuropathol. 2016 Jul;132(1):149–51. PMID:27067307
1259. Hasselblatt M, Thomas C, Nemes K, et al. Tyrosinase immunohistochemistry can be employed for the diagnosis of atypical teratoid/rhabdoid tumours of the tyrosinase subgroup (ATRT-TYR). Neuropathol Appl Neurobiol. 2020 Feb;46(2):186–9. PMID:31077608
1260. Hassn Mesrati M, Behrooz AB, Y Abuhamad A, et al. Understanding glioblastoma biomarkers: knocking a mountain with a hammer. Cells. 2020 May 16;9(5):E1236. PMID:32429463
1261. Hassoun J, Gambarelli D, Peragut JC, et al. Specific ultrastructural markers of human pinealomas. A study of four cases. Acta Neuropathol. 1983;62(1-2):31–40. PMID:6318505
1262. Hassoun J, Söylemezoglu F, Gambarelli D, et al. Central neurocytoma: a synopsis of clinical and histological features. Brain Pathol. 1993 Jul;3(3):297–306. PMID:8293189
1263. Haston S, Pozzi S, Carreno G, et al. MAPK pathway control of stem cell proliferation and differentiation in the embryonic pituitary provides insights into the pathogenesis of papillary craniopharyngioma. Development. 2017 Jun 15;144(12):2141–52. PMID:28506993
1264. Hasturk AE, Gokce EC, Elbir C, et al. A very rare spinal cord tumor primary spinal oligodendroglioma: a review of sixty cases in the literature. J Craniovertebr Junction Spine. 2017 Jul-Sep;8(3):253–62. PMID:29021677
1265. Hattori K, Sakata-Yanagimoto M, Suehara Y, et al. Clinical significance of disease-specific MYD88 mutations in circulating DNA in primary central nervous system lymphoma. Cancer Sci. 2018 Jan;109(1):225–30. PMID:29151258
1266. Haugh AM, Njauw CN, Bubley JA, et al. Genotypic and phenotypic features of BAP1 cancer syndrome: a report of 8 new families and review of cases in the literature. JAMA Dermatol. 2017 Oct 1;153(10):999–1006. PMID:28793149
1267. Hauser BM, Lau A, Gupta S, et al. The epigenomics of pituitary adenoma. Front Endocrinol (Lausanne). 2019 May 14;10:290. PMID:31139150
1268. Håvik AL, Bruland O, Myrseth E, et al. Genetic landscape of sporadic vestibular schwannoma. J Neurosurg. 2018 Mar;128(3):911–22. PMID:28409725
1269. Hawkins C, Muller P, Bilbao JM. April 1999–44 year old man with a bleeding intracerebral tumor. Brain Pathol. 1999 Oct;9(4):741–2. PMID:10517512
1270. Hayashi K, Inoshita N, Kawaguchi K, et al. The USP8 mutational status may predict drug susceptibility in corticotroph adenomas of Cushing's disease. Eur J Endocrinol. 2016 Feb;174(2):213–26. PMID:26578638
1271. Hayashi K, Ohara N, Jeon HJ, et al. Gliosarcoma with features of chondroblastic osteosarcoma. Cancer. 1993 Aug 1;72(3):850–5. PMID:8334639
1272. He C, Wang Y, Zhang L, et al. Isolated lymphomatoid granulomatosis of the central nervous system: a case report and literature review. Neuropathology. 2019 Dec;39(6):479–88. PMID:31746046
1273. He J, Mokhtari K, Sanson M, et al. Glioblastomas with an oligodendroglial component: a pathological and molecular study. J Neuropathol Exp Neurol. 2001 Sep;60(9):863–71. PMID:11556543
1274. Heald B, Mester J, Rybicki L, et al. Frequent gastrointestinal polyps and colorectal adenocarcinomas in a prospective series of PTEN mutation carriers. Gastroenterology. 2010 Dec;139(6):1927–33. PMID:20600018
1275. Heaney AP. Clinical review: pituitary carcinoma: difficult diagnosis and treatment. J Clin Endocrinol Metab. 2011 Dec;96(12):3649–60. PMID:21956419
1276. Heaphy CM, de Wilde RF, Jiao Y, et al. Altered telomeres in tumors with ATRX and DAXX mutations. Science. 2011 Jul 22;333(6041):425. PMID:21719641
1277. Heath JA, Ng J, Beshay V, et al. Anaplastic oligodendroglioma in an adolescent with Lynch syndrome. Pediatr Blood Cancer. 2013 Jun;60(6):E13–5. PMID:23255519
1278. Heck A, Emblem KE, Casar-Borota O, et al. Quantitative analyses of T2-weighted MRI as a potential marker for response to somatostatin analogs in newly diagnosed acromegaly. Endocrine. 2016 May;52(2):333–43. PMID:26475495
1279. Hegi ME, Diserens AC, Gorlia T, et al. MGMT gene silencing and benefit from temozolomide in glioblastoma. N Engl J Med. 2005 Mar 10;352(10):997–1003. PMID:15758010
1280. Heiland DH, Staszewski O, Hirsch M, et al. Malignant transformation of a dysembryoplastic neuroepithelial tumor (DNET) characterized by genome-wide methylation analysis. J Neuropathol Exp Neurol. 2016 Apr;75(4):358–65. PMID:26921879
1281. Heim S, Beschorner R, Mittelbronn M, et al. Increased mitotic and proliferative activity are associated with worse prognosis in papillary tumors of the pineal region. Am J Surg Pathol. 2014 Jan;38(1):106–10. PMID:24121176
1282. Heim S, Coras R, Ganslandt O, et al. Papillary tumor of the pineal region with anaplastic small cell component. J Neurooncol. 2013 Oct;115(1):127–30. PMID:23817812
1283. Heim S, Sill M, Jones DT, et al. Papillary tumor of the pineal region: a distinct molecular entity. Brain Pathol. 2016 Mar;26(2):199–205. PMID:26113311
1284. Heimberger AB, Abou-Ghazal M, Reina-Ortiz C, et al. Incidence and prognostic impact of FoxP3+ regulatory T cells in human gliomas. Clin Cancer Res. 2008 Aug 15;14(16):5166–72. PMID:18698034
1285. Heimdal K, Evensen SA, Fosså SD, et al. Karyotyping of a hematologic neoplasia developing shortly after treatment for cerebral extragonadal germ cell tumor. Cancer Genet Cytogenet. 1991 Nov;57(1):41–6. PMID:1756483
1286. Helal A, Graffeo CS, Perry A, et al. Capicua transcriptional repressor-rearranged undifferentiated round cell sarcoma metastatic to the brain treated with surgery and stereotactic radiosurgery. World Neurosurg. 2020 Jul;139:12–9. PMID:32251827
1287. Helgager J, Lidov HG, Mahadevan NR, et al. A novel GIT2-BRAF fusion in pilocytic astrocytoma. Diagn Pathol. 2017 Nov 15;12(1):82. PMID:29141672
1288. Hemminki K, Liu X, Försti A, et al. Subsequent brain tumors in patients with autoimmune disease. Neuro Oncol. 2013 Sep;15(9):1142–50. PMID:23757294
1289. Hennessy MJ, Elwes RD, Rabe-Hesketh S, et al. Prognostic factors in the surgical treatment of medically intractable epilepsy associated with mesial temporal sclerosis. Acta Neurol Scand. 2001 Jun;103(6):344–50. PMID:11421846
1290. Henske EP, Wessner LL, Golden J, et al. Loss of tuberin in both subependymal giant cell astrocytomas and angiomyolipomas supports a two-hit model for the pathogenesis of tuberous sclerosis tumors. Am J Pathol. 1997 Dec;151(6):1639–47. PMID:9403714
1291. Héritier S, Barkaoui MA, Miron J, et al. Incidence and risk factors for clinical neurodegenerative Langerhans cell histiocytosis: a longitudinal cohort study. Br J Haematol. 2018 Nov;183(4):608–17. PMID:30421536
1292. Héritier S, Saffroy R, Radosevic-Robin N, et al. Common cancer-associated PIK3CA activating mutations rarely occur in Langerhans cell histiocytosis. Blood. 2015 Apr 9;125(15):2448–9. PMID:25858893
1293. Herman V, Fagin J, Gonsky R, et al. Clonal origin of pituitary adenomas. J Clin Endocrinol Metab. 1990 Dec;71(6):1427–33. PMID:1977759
1294. Hernández-Ramírez LC, Gam R, Valdés N, et al. Loss-of-function mutations in the CABLES1 gene are a novel cause of Cushing's disease. Endocr Relat Cancer. 2017 Aug;24(8):379–92. PMID:28533356
1295. Herpers MJ, Budka H. Glial fibrillary acidic protein (GFAP) in oligodendroglial tumors: gliofibrillary oligodendroglioma and transitional oligoastrocytoma as subtypes of oligodendroglioma. Acta Neuropathol. 1984;64(4):265–72. PMID:6391068
1296. Herpers MJ, Ramaekers FC, Aldeweireldt J, et al. Co-expression of glial fibrillary acidic protein- and vimentin-type intermediate filaments in human astrocytomas. Acta Neuropathol. 1986;70(3-4):333–9. PMID:3020864
1297. Herrick MK, Rubinstein LJ. The cytological differentiating potential of pineal parenchymal neoplasms (true pinealomas). A clinicopathological study of 28 tumours. Brain. 1979 Jun;102(2):289–320. PMID:88244
1298. Herrlinger U, Jones DTW, Glas M, et al. Gliomatosis cerebri: no evidence for a separate brain tumor entity. Acta Neuropathol. 2016 Feb;131(2):309–19. PMID:26493382
1299. Herrlinger U, Tzaridis T, Mack F, et al. Lomustine-temozolomide combination therapy versus standard temozolomide therapy in patients with newly diagnosed glioblastoma with methylated MGMT promoter (CeTeG/NOA-09): a randomised, open-label, phase 3 trial. Lancet. 2019 Feb 16;393(10172):678–88. PMID:30782343
1300. Hervier B, Haroche J, Arnaud L, et al. Association of both Langerhans cell histiocytosis and Erdheim-Chester disease linked to the BRAFV600E mutation. Blood. 2014 Aug 14;124(7):1119–26. PMID:24894769
1301. Hewer E, Beck J, Murek M, et al. Polymorphous oligodendroglioma of Zülch revisited: a genetically heterogeneous group of anaplastic gliomas including tumors of bona fide oligodendroglial differentiation. Neuropathology. 2014 Aug;34(4):323–32. PMID:24444336
1302. Hewer E, Knecht U, Ulrich CT. Two adult cases of massively calcified low-grade glioma: expanding clinical spectrum of an emerging entity. Neuropathology. 2016 Oct;36(5):508–9. PMID:26991895
1303. Hewer E, Vajtai I. Consistent nuclear expression of thyroid transcription factor 1 in subependymal giant cell astrocytomas suggests lineage-restricted histogenesis. Clin Neuropathol. 2015 May-Jun;34(3):128–31. PMID:25669749
1303A. Hicks D, Rafiee G, Schwalbe EC, et al. The molecular landscape and associated clinical experience in infant medulloblastoma: prognostic significance of second-generation subtypes. Neuropathol Appl Neurobiol. 2021 Feb;47(2):236–50. PMID:32779246
1304. Hidalgo ET, Orillac C, Kvint S, et al. Quality of life, hypothalamic obesity, and sexual function in adulthood two decades after primary gross-total resection for childhood craniopharyngioma. Childs Nerv Syst. 2020 Feb;36(2):281–9. PMID:31222446
1305. Hiemcke-Jiwa LS, Leguit RJ, Snijders TJ, et al. MYD88 p.(L265P) detection on cell-free DNA in liquid biopsies of patients with primary central nervous system lymphoma. Br J Haematol. 2019 Jun;185(5):974–7. PMID:30408153
1306. Hiemcke-Jiwa LS, Minnema MC, Radersma-van Loon JH, et al. The use of droplet digital PCR in liquid biopsies: a highly sensitive technique for MYD88 p.(L265P) detection in cerebrospinal fluid. Hematol Oncol. 2018 Apr;36(2):429–35. PMID:29210102
1307. Higham CS, Dombi E, Rogiers A, et al. The characteristics of 76 atypical neurofibromas as precursors to neurofibromatosis 1 associated malignant peripheral nerve sheath tumors. Neuro Oncol. 2018 May 18;20(6):818–25. PMID:29409029
1308. Hildebrand MS, Griffin NG, Damiano JA, et al. Mutations of the sonic hedgehog pathway underlie hypothalamic hamartoma with gelastic epilepsy. Am J Hum Genet. 2016 Aug 4;99(2):423–9. PMID:27453577
1309. Hill DA, Ivanovich J, Priest JR, et al. DICER1 mutations in familial pleuropulmonary blastoma. Science. 2009 Aug 21;325(5943):965. PMID:19556464
1309A. Hill RM, Richardson S, Schwalbe EC, et al. Time, pattern, and outcome of medulloblastoma relapse and their association with tumour biology at diagnosis and therapy: a multicentre cohort study. Lancet Child Adolesc Health. 2020 Dec;4(12):865–74. PMID:33222802
1310. Hiniker A, Hagenkord JM, Powers MP, et al. Gliosarcoma arising from an oligodendroglioma (oligosarcoma). Clin Neuropathol. 2013 May-Jun;32(3):165–70. PMID:23254140
1311. Hinkes BG, von Hoff K, Deinlein F, et al.

Childhood pineoblastoma: experiences from the prospective multicenter trials HIT-SKK87, HIT-SKK92 and HIT91. J Neurooncol. 2007 Jan;81(2):217–23. PMID:16941074

1312. Hinrichs BH, Newman S, Appin CL, et al. Farewell to GBM-O: genomic and transcriptomic profiling of glioblastoma with oligodendroglioma component reveals distinct molecular subgroups. Acta Neuropathol Commun. 2016 Jan 13;4:4. PMID:26757882

1313. Hirata Y, Brems H, Suzuki M, et al. Interaction between a domain of the negative regulator of the Ras-ERK Pathway, SPRED1 Protein, and the GTPase-activating protein-related domain of neurofibromin is implicated in legius syndrome and neurofibromatosis type 1. J Biol Chem. 2016 Feb 12;291(7):3124–34. PMID:26635368

1314. Hirose T, Giannini C, Scheithauer BW. Ultrastructural features of pleomorphic xanthoastrocytoma: a comparative study with glioblastoma multiforme. Ultrastruct Pathol. 2001 Nov-Dec;25(6):469–78. PMID:11783911

1315. Hirose T, Nobusawa S, Sugiyama K, et al. Astroblastoma: a distinct tumor entity characterized by alterations of the X chromosome and MN1 rearrangement. Brain Pathol. 2018 Sep;28(5):684–94. PMID:28990708

1316. Hirose T, Scheithauer BW, Lopes MB, et al. Ganglioglioma: an ultrastructural and immunohistochemical study. Cancer. 1997 Mar 1;79(5):989–1003. PMID:9041162

1317. Hirose T, Scheithauer BW, Lopes MB, et al. Tuber and subependymal giant cell astrocytoma associated with tuberous sclerosis: an immunohistochemical, ultrastructural, and immunoelectron and microscopic study. Acta Neuropathol. 1995;90(4):387–99. PMID:8546029

1318. Hirose T, Scheithauer BW, Sano T. Perineurial malignant peripheral nerve sheath tumor (MPNST): a clinicopathologic, immunohistochemical, and ultrastructural study of seven cases. Am J Surg Pathol. 1998 Nov;22(11):1368–78. PMID:9808129

1319. Hirsch B, Shimamura A, Moreau L, et al. Association of biallelic BRCA2/FANCD1 mutations with spontaneous chromosomal instability and solid tumors of childhood. Blood. 2004 Apr 1;103(7):2554–9. PMID:14670928

1320. Ho B, Johann PD, Grabovska Y, et al. Molecular subgrouping of atypical teratoid/rhabdoid tumors-a reinvestigation and current consensus. Neuro Oncol. 2020 May 15;22(5):613–24. PMID:31889194

1321. Ho DM, Liu HC. Primary intracranial germ cell tumor. Pathologic study of 51 patients. Cancer. 1992 Sep 15;70(6):1577–84. PMID:1325276

1321A. Hoang MP, Amirkhan RH. Inhibin alpha distinguishes hemangioblastoma from clear cell renal cell carcinoma. Am J Surg Pathol. 2003 Aug;27(8):1152–6. PMID:12883249

1322. Hoang-Xuan K, Capelle L, Kujas M, et al. Temozolomide as initial treatment for adults with low-grade oligodendrogliomas or oligoastrocytomas and correlation with chromosome 1p deletions. J Clin Oncol. 2004 Aug 1;22(15):3133–8. PMID:15284265

1323. Hodges TR, Ott M, Xiu J, et al. Mutational burden, immune checkpoint expression, and mismatch repair in glioma: implications for immune checkpoint immunotherapy. Neuro Oncol. 2017 Aug 1;19(8):1047–57. PMID:28371827

1324. Hoei-Hansen CE, Sehested A, Juhler M, et al. New evidence for the origin of intracranial germ cell tumours from primordial germ cells: expression of pluripotency and cell differentiation markers. J Pathol. 2006 May;209(1):25–33. PMID:16456896

1325. Hoffman DI, Abdullah KG, McCoskey M, et al. Negative prognostic impact of epidermal growth factor receptor copy number gain in young adults with isocitrate dehydrogenase wild-type glioblastoma. J Neurooncol. 2019 Nov;145(2):321–8. PMID:31542863

1326. Hoffman HJ, Otsubo H, Hendrick EB, et al. Intracranial germ-cell tumors in children. J Neurosurg. 1991 Apr;74(4):545–51. PMID:1848284

1327. Hoffman LM, DeWire M, Ryall S, et al. Spatial genomic heterogeneity in diffuse intrinsic pontine and midline high-grade glioma: implications for diagnostic biopsy and targeted therapeutics. Acta Neuropathol Commun. 2016 Jan 4;4:1. PMID:26727948

1328. Hoffman LM, Richardson EA, Ho B, et al. Advancing biology-based therapeutic approaches for atypical teratoid rhabdoid tumors. Neuro Oncol. 2020 Jul 7;22(7):944–54. PMID:32129445

1329. Hoffman LM, Veldhuijzen van Zanten SEM, Colditz N, et al. Clinical, radiologic, pathologic, and molecular characteristics of long-term survivors of diffuse intrinsic pontine glioma (DIPG): a collaborative report from the international and european society for pediatric oncology DIPG registries. J Clin Oncol. 2018 Jul 1;36(19):1963–72. PMID:29746225

1330. Hoffmann A, Boekhoff S, Gebhardt U, et al. History before diagnosis in childhood craniopharyngioma: associations with initial presentation and long-term prognosis. Eur J Endocrinol. 2015 Dec;173(6):853–62. PMID:26392473

1331. Hoffmann A, Brentrup A, Müller HL. First report on spinal metastasis in childhood-onset craniopharyngioma. J Neurooncol. 2016 Aug;129(1):193–4. PMID:27278607

1332. Hofman S, Heeg M, Klein JP, et al. Simultaneous occurrence of a supra- and an infratentorial glioma in a patient with Ollier's disease: more evidence for non-mesodermal tumor predisposition in multiple enchondromatosis. Skeletal Radiol. 1998 Dec;27(12):688–91. PMID:9921931

1333. Holland EC, Hively WP, DePinho RA, et al. A constitutively active epidermal growth factor receptor cooperates with disruption of G1 cell-cycle arrest pathways to induce glioma-like lesions in mice. Genes Dev. 1998 Dec 1;12(23):3675–85. PMID:9851974

1334. Hölsken A, Kreutzer J, Hofmann BM, et al. Target gene activation of the Wnt signaling pathway in nuclear beta-catenin accumulating cells of adamantinomatous craniopharyngiomas. Brain Pathol. 2009 Jul;19(3):357–64. PMID:18540944

1335. Hölsken A, Sill M, Merkle J, et al. Adamantinomatous and papillary craniopharyngiomas are characterized by distinct epigenomic as well as mutational and transcriptomic profiles. Acta Neuropathol Commun. 2016 Feb 29;4:20. PMID:26927026

1336. Holsten T, Lubieniecki F, Spohn M, et al. Detailed clinical and histopathological description of 8 cases of molecularly defined CNS neuroblastomas. J Neuropathol Exp Neurol. 2021 Jan 1;80(1):52–9. PMID:33270865

1337. Homma T, Fukushima T, Vaccarella S, et al. Correlation among pathology, genotype, and patient outcomes in glioblastoma. J Neuropathol Exp Neurol. 2006 Sep;65(9):846–54. PMID:16957578

1338. Honavar M, Janota I, Polkey CE. Histological heterogeneity of dysembryoplastic neuroepithelial tumour: identification and differential diagnosis in a series of 74 cases. Histopathology. 1999 Apr;34(4):342–56. PMID:10231402

1339. Honeyman SI, Warr W, Curran OE, et al. Paraganglioma of the lumbar spine: a case report and literature review. Neurochirurgie. 2019 Dec;65(6):387–92. PMID:31247160

1340. Horbinski C, Kofler J, Yeaney G, et al. Isocitrate dehydrogenase 1 analysis differentiates gangliogliomas from infiltrative gliomas. Brain Pathol. 2011 Sep;21(5):564–74. PMID:21314850

1341. Horbinski C, Miller CR, Perry A. Gone FISHing: clinical lessons learned in brain tumor molecular diagnostics over the last decade. Brain Pathol. 2011 Jan;21(1):57–73. PMID:21129060

1342. Horiguchi H, Hirose T, Sano T, et al. Meningioma with granulofilamentous inclusions. Ultrastruct Pathol. 2000 Jul-Aug;24(4):267–71. PMID:11013967

1343. Horn S, Figl A, Rachakonda PS, et al. TERT promoter mutations in familial and sporadic melanoma. Science. 2013 Feb 22;339(6122):959–61. PMID:23348503

1344. Hornick JL, Bundock EA, Fletcher CD. Hybrid schwannoma/perineurioma: clinicopathologic analysis of 42 distinctive benign nerve sheath tumors. Am J Surg Pathol. 2009 Oct;33(10):1554–61. PMID:19623031

1345. Hornick JL, Fletcher CD. Soft tissue perineurioma: clinicopathologic analysis of 81 cases including those with atypical histologic features. Am J Surg Pathol. 2005 Jul;29(7):845–58. PMID:15958848

1346. Horstmann S, Perry A, Reifenberger G, et al. Genetic and expression profiles of cerebellar liponeurocytomas. Brain Pathol. 2004 Jul;14(3):281–9. PMID:15446583

1347. Horten BC, Rubinstein LJ. Primary cerebral neuroblastoma. A clinicopathological study of 35 cases. Brain. 1976 Dec;99(4):735–56. PMID:1030655

1348. Horvath E, Kovacs K, Killinger DW, et al. Mammosomatotroph cell adenoma of the human pituitary: a morphologic entity. Virchows Arch A Pathol Anat Histopathol. 1983;398(3):277–89. PMID:6402839

1349. Horvath E, Kovacs K, Singer W, et al. Acidophil stem cell adenoma of the human pituitary. Arch Pathol Lab Med. 1977 Nov;101(11):594–9. PMID:199135

1350. Horvath E, Kovacs K, Singer W, et al. Acidophil stem cell adenoma of the human pituitary: clinicopathologic analysis of 15 cases. Cancer. 1981 Feb 15;47(4):761–71. PMID:6261917

1351. Horvath E, Kovacs K, Smyth HS, et al. Silent adenoma subtype 3 of the pituitary–immunohistochemical and ultrastructural classification: a review of 29 cases. Ultrastruct Pathol. 2005 Nov-Dec;29(6):511–24. PMID:16316952

1352. Horwitz M, Dufour C, Leblond P, et al. Embryonal tumors with multilayered rosettes in children: the SFCE experience. Childs Nerv Syst. 2016 Feb;32(2):299–305. PMID:26438544

1353. Hosono J, Nitta M, Masui K, et al. Role of a promoter mutation in TERT in malignant transformation of pleomorphic xanthoastrocytoma. World Neurosurg. 2019 Jun;126:624–30. PMID:30599247

1354. Hou Y, Pinheiro J, Sahm F, et al. Papillary glioneuronal tumor (PGNT) exhibits a characteristic methylation profile and fusions involving PRKCA. Acta Neuropathol. 2019 May;137(5):837–46. PMID:30759284

1355. Hovestadt V, Ayrault O, Swartling FJ, et al. Medulloblastomics revisited: biological and clinical insights from thousands of patients. Nat Rev Cancer. 2020 Jan;20(1):42–56. PMID:31819232

1356. Hovestadt V, Remke M, Kool M, et al. Robust molecular subgrouping and copy-number profiling of medulloblastoma from small amounts of archival tumour material using high-density DNA methylation arrays. Acta Neuropathol. 2013 Jun;125(6):913–6. PMID:23670100

1357. Hovestadt V, Smith KS, Bihannic L, et al. Resolving medulloblastoma cellular architecture by single-cell genomics. Nature. 2019 Aug;572(7767):74–9. PMID:31341285

1358. Howe JR, Ringold JC, Summers RW, et al. A gene for familial juvenile polyposis maps to chromosome 18q21.1. Am J Hum Genet. 1998 May;62(5):1129–36. PMID:9545410

1359. Howe JR, Roth S, Ringold JC, et al. Mutations in the SMAD4/DPC4 gene in juvenile polyposis. Science. 1998 May 15;280(5366):1086–8. PMID:9582123

1360. Hoyt WF, Baghdassarian SA. Optic glioma of childhood. Natural history and rationale for conservative management. Br J Ophthalmol. 1969 Dec;53(12):793–8. PMID:5386369

1361. Hsiao SJ, Karajannis MA, Diolaiti D, et al. A novel, potentially targetable TMEM106B-BRAF fusion in pleomorphic xanthoastrocytoma. Cold Spring Harb Mol Case Stud. 2017 Mar;3(2):a001396. PMID:28299358

1362. Hu H, Mu Q, Bao Z, et al. Mutational landscape of secondary glioblastoma guides MET-targeted trial in brain tumor. Cell. 2018 Nov 29;175(6):1665–1678.e18. PMID:30343896

1363. Huang B, Johansson MJ, Byström AS. An early step in wobble uridine tRNA modification requires the Elongator complex. RNA. 2005 Apr;11(4):424–36. PMID:15769872

1364. Huang H, Reis R, Yonekawa Y, et al. Identification in human brain tumors of DNA sequences specific for SV40 large T antigen. Brain Pathol. 1999 Jan;9(1):33–42. PMID:9989448

1365. Huang HY, Park N, Erlandson RA, et al. Immunohistochemical and ultrastructural comparative study of external lamina structure in 31 cases of cellular, classical, and melanotic schwannomas. Appl Immunohistochem Mol Morphol. 2004 Mar;12(1):50–8. PMID:15163020

1366. Huang J, Grotzer MA, Watanabe T, et al. Mutations in the Nijmegen breakage syndrome gene in medulloblastomas. Clin Cancer Res. 2008 Jul 1;14(13):4053–8. PMID:18593981

1367. Huang JF, Chen D, Zheng XQ, et al. Conditional survival and changing risk profile in patients with chordoma: a population-based longitudinal cohort study. J Orthop Surg Res. 2019 Jun 17;14(1):181. PMID:31208441

1368. Huang MC, Kubo O, Tajika Y, et al. A clinico-immunohistochemical study of giant cell glioblastoma. Noshuyo Byori. 1996 Apr;13(1):11–6. PMID:8916121

1369. Huang Q, Li F, Chen Y, et al. Prognostic factors and clinical outcomes in adult primary gliosarcoma patients: a Surveillance, Epidemiology, and End Results (SEER) analysis from 2004 to 2015. Br J Neurosurg. 2020 Apr;34(2):161–7. PMID:31829033

1370. Huang QL, Cao X, Chai X, et al. The radiological imaging features of easily misdiagnosed epithelioid glioblastoma in seven patients. World Neurosurg. 2019 Jan 4:S1878-8750(18)32951-6. PMID:30611946

1371. Huang SC, Zhang L, Sung YS, et al. Recurrent CIC gene abnormalities in angiosarcomas: a molecular study of 120 cases with concurrent investigation of PLCG1, KDR, MYC, and FLT4 gene alterations. Am J Surg Pathol. 2016 May;40(5):645–55. PMID:26735859

1372. Huang T, Garcia R, Qi J, et al. Detection of histone H3 K27M mutation and post-translational modifications in pediatric diffuse midline glioma via tissue immunohistochemistry informs diagnosis and clinical outcomes. Oncotarget. 2018 Dec 14;9(98):37112–24. PMID:30647848

1373. Huang Y, Chan L, Bai HX, et al. Assessment of care pattern and outcome in hemangioblastoma. Sci Rep. 2018 Jul 24;8(1):11144. PMID:30042517

1374. Hübner JM, Müller T, Papageorgiou DN, et al. EZHIP/CXorf67 mimics K27M mutated oncohistones and functions as an intrinsic inhibitor of PRC2 function in aggressive posterior fossa ependymoma. Neuro Oncol. 2019 Jul 11;21(7):878–89. PMID:30923826

1375. Huizenga NA, de Lange P, Koper JW, et al. Human adrenocorticotropin-secreting pituitary adenomas show frequent loss of heterozygosity at the glucocorticoid receptor gene locus. J Clin Endocrinol Metab. 1998 Mar;83(3):917–21. PMID:9506748

1376. Hulsebos TJ, Kenter S, Baas F, et al. Type 1 papillary renal cell carcinoma in a patient with schwannomatosis: mosaic versus loss of SMARCB1 expression in respectively schwannoma and renal tumor cells. Genes Chromosomes Cancer. 2016 Apr;55(4):350–4. PMID:26799435

1377. Hulsebos TJ, Kenter S, Siebers-Renelt U, et al. SMARCB1 involvement in the development of leiomyoma in a patient with schwannomatosis. Am J Surg Pathol. 2014 Mar;38(3):421–5. PMID:24525513

1378. Hulsebos TJ, Plomp AS, Wolterman RA, et al. Germline mutation of INI1/SMARCB1 in familial schwannomatosis. Am J Hum Genet. 2007 Apr;80(4):805–10. PMID:17357086

1379. Hung YP, Diaz-Perez JA, Cote GM, et al. Dedifferentiated chordoma: clinicopathologic and molecular characteristics with integrative analysis. Am J Surg Pathol. 2020 Sep;44(9):1213–23. PMID:32427623

1380. Hunter C, Smith R, Cahill DP, et al. A hypermutation phenotype and somatic MSH6 mutations in recurrent human malignant gliomas after alkylator chemotherapy. Cancer Res. 2006 Apr 15;66(8):3987–91. PMID:16618716

1381. Huq AJ, Walsh M, Rajagopalan B, et al. Mutations in SUFU and PTCH1 genes may cause different cutaneous cancer predisposition syndromes: similar, but not the same. Fam Cancer. 2018 Oct;17(4):601–6. PMID:29356994

1382. Huse JT, Diamond EL, Wang L, et al. Mixed glioma with molecular features of composite oligodendroglioma and astrocytoma: a true "oligoastrocytoma"? Acta Neuropathol. 2015 Jan;129(1):151–3. PMID:25359109

1383. Huse JT, Edgar M, Halliday J, et al. Multinodular and vacuolating neuronal tumors of the cerebrum: 10 cases of a distinctive seizure-associated lesion. Brain Pathol. 2013 Sep;23(5):515–24. PMID:23324039

1384. Huse JT, Snuderl M, Jones DT, et al. Polymorphous low-grade neuroepithelial tumor of the young (PLNTY): an epileptogenic neoplasm with oligodendroglioma-like components, aberrant CD34 expression, and genetic alterations involving the MAP kinase pathway. Acta Neuropathol. 2017 Mar;133(3):417–29. PMID:27812792

1385. Hussain N, Curran A, Pilling D, et al. Congenital subependymal giant cell astrocytoma diagnosed on fetal MRI. Arch Dis Child. 2006 Jun;91(6):520. PMID:16714726

1386. Husseini L, Saleh A, Reifenberger G, et al. Inflammatory demyelinating brain lesions heralding primary CNS lymphoma. Can J Neurol Sci. 2012 Jan;39(1):6–10. PMID:22384490

1387. Huttenlocher PR, Heydemann PT. Fine structure of cortical tubers in tuberous sclerosis: a Golgi study. Ann Neurol. 1984 Nov;16(5):595–602. PMID:6508241

1388. Hutter S, Piro RM, Reuss DE, et al. Whole exome sequencing reveals that the majority of schwannomatosis cases remain unexplained after excluding SMARCB1 and LZTR1 germline variants. Acta Neuropathol. 2014 Sep;128(3):449–52. PMID:25008767

1389. Hwang EI, Kool M, Burger PC, et al. Extensive molecular and clinical heterogeneity in patients with histologically diagnosed CNS-PNET treated as a single entity: a report from the Children's Oncology Group randomized ACNS0332 trial. J Clin Oncol. 2018 Oct 17;JCO2017764720. PMID:30332335

1390. Hwang I, Cao D, Na Y, et al. Far upstream element-binding protein 1 regulates LSD1 alternative splicing to promote terminal differentiation of neural progenitors. Stem Cell Reports. 2018 Apr 10;10(4):1208–21. PMID:29606613

1391. Hyer W, Cohen S, Attard T, et al. Management of familial adenomatous polyposis in children and adolescents: position paper from the ESPGHAN Polyposis Working Group. J Pediatr Gastroenterol Nutr. 2019 Mar;68(3):428–41. PMID:30585891

1392. Hyrcza MD, Ezzat S, Mete O, et al. Pituitary adenomas presenting as sinonasal or nasopharyngeal masses: a case series illustrating potential diagnostic pitfalls. Am J Surg Pathol. 2017 Apr;41(4):525–34. PMID:28009611

1393. Iacovazzo D, Carlsen E, Lugli F, et al. Factors predicting pasireotide responsiveness in somatotroph pituitary adenomas resistant to first-generation somatostatin analogues: an immunohistochemical study. Eur J Endocrinol. 2016 Feb;174(2):241–50. PMID:26586796

1394. IARC TP53 Database [Internet]. Lyon (France): International Agency for Research on Cancer; 2019. Version R20, July 2019. Available from: https://p53.iarc.fr/.

1395. Ibrahim GM, Huang A, Halliday W, et al. Cribriform neuroepithelial tumour: novel clinicopathological, ultrastructural and cytogenetic findings. Acta Neuropathol. 2011 Oct;122(4):511–4. PMID:21918902

1396. Ichikawa T, Otani Y, Kurozumi K, et al. Phenotypic Transition as a Survival Strategy of Glioma. Neurol Med Chir (Tokyo). 2016 Jul 15;56(7):387–95. PMID:27169497

1397. Ichimura K, Fukushima S, Totoki Y, et al. Recurrent neomorphic mutations of MTOR in central nervous system and testicular germ cell tumors may be targeted for therapy. Acta Neuropathol. 2016 Jun;131(6):889–901. PMID:26956871

1398. Ichimura K, Narita Y, Hawkins CE. Diffusely infiltrating astrocytomas: pathology, molecular mechanisms and markers. Acta Neuropathol. 2015 Jun;129(6):789–808. PMID:25975377

1399. Iczkowski KA, Butler SL, Shanks JH, et al. Trials of new germ cell immunohistochemical stains in 93 extragonadal and metastatic germ cell tumors. Hum Pathol. 2008 Feb;39(2):275–81. PMID:18045648

1400. Ida CM, Rodriguez FJ, Burger PC, et al. Pleomorphic xanthoastrocytoma: natural history and long-term follow-up. Brain Pathol. 2015 Sep;25(5):575–86. PMID:25318587

1401. Ida CM, Vrana JA, Rodriguez FJ, et al. Immunohistochemistry is highly sensitive and specific for detection of BRAF V600E mutation in pleomorphic xanthoastrocytoma. Acta Neuropathol Commun. 2013 May 30;1:20. PMID:24252190

1402. Iglesias P, Guerrero-Pérez F, Villabona C, et al. Adenohypophyseal hyperfunction syndromes and posterior pituitary tumors: prevalence, clinical characteristics, and pathophysiological mechanisms. Endocrine. 2020 Oct;70(1):15–23. PMID:32613546

1403. Iida M, Harari PM, Wheeler DL, et al. Targeting AKT/PKB to improve treatment outcomes for solid tumors. Mutat Res. 2020 Jan-Apr;819-820:111690. PMID:32120136

1404. Ikeda J, Sawamura Y, van Meir EG. Pineoblastoma presenting in familial adenomatous polyposis (FAP): random association, FAP variant or Turcot syndrome? Br J Neurosurg. 1998 Dec;12(6):576–8. PMID:10070471

1405. Ikemura M, Shibahara J, Mukasa A, et al. Utility of ATRX immunohistochemistry in diagnosis of adult diffuse gliomas. Histopathology. 2016 Aug;69(2):260–7. PMID:26741321

1406. Illerhaus G, Schorb E, Kasenda B. Novel agents for primary central nervous system lymphoma: evidence and perspectives. Blood. 2018 Aug 16;132(7):681–8. PMID:29986908

1407. Imashuku S, Okazaki N, Nakayama M, et al. Treatment of neurodegenerative CNS disease in Langerhans cell histiocytosis with a combination of intravenous immunoglobulin and chemotherapy. Pediatr Blood Cancer. 2008 Feb;50(2):308–11. PMID:17458874

1408. Imber BS, Braunstein SE, Wu FY, et al. Clinical outcome and prognostic factors for central neurocytoma: twenty year institutional experience. J Neurooncol. 2016 Jan;126(1):193–200. PMID:26493740

1409. Imperiale A, Moussallieh FM, Roche P, et al. Metabolome profiling by HRMAS NMR spectroscopy of pheochromocytomas and paragangliomas detects SDH deficiency: clinical and pathophysiological implications. Neoplasia. 2015 Jan;17(1):55–65. PMID:25622899

1410. Inatomi Y, Ito T, Nagae K, et al. Hybrid perineurioma-neurofibroma in a patient with neurofibromatosis type 1, clinically mimicking malignant peripheral nerve sheath tumor. Eur J Dermatol. 2014 May-Jun;24(3):412–3. PMID:24751814

1411. Indraccolo S, Lombardi G, Fassan M, et al. Genetic, epigenetic, and immunologic profiling of MMR-deficient relapsed glioblastoma. Clin Cancer Res. 2019 Mar 15;25(6):1828–37. PMID:30514778

1412. Ingham PW. The patched gene in development and cancer. Curr Opin Genet Dev. 1998 Feb;8(1):88–94. PMID:9529611

1413. Inoue Y, Nemoto Y, Murata R, et al. CT and MR imaging of cerebral tuberous sclerosis. Brain Dev. 1998 Jun;20(4):209–21. PMID:9661965

1414. International Association of Cancer Registries (IACR) [Internet]. Lyon (France): International Agency for Research on Cancer; 2021. International Classification of Diseases for Oncology (ICD-O) – ICD-O-3.2; updated 2021 Jan 25. Available from: http://www.iacr.com.fr/index.php?option=com_content&view=category&layout=blog&id=100&Itemid=577.

1415. International Cancer Genome Consortium PedBrain Tumor Project. Recurrent MET fusion genes represent a drug target in pediatric glioblastoma. Nat Med. 2016 Nov;22(11):1314–20. PMID:27748748

1416. Ironside JW, Jefferson AA, Royds JA, et al. Carcinoid tumour arising in a recurrent intradural spinal teratoma. Neuropathol Appl Neurobiol. 1984 Nov-Dec;10(6):479–89. PMID:6084821

1417. Isaacs H Jr. Fetal intracranial teratoma. A review. Fetal Pediatr Pathol. 2014 Oct-Dec;33(5-6):289–92. PMID:25353702

1418. Ishi Y, Yamaguchi S, Iguchi A, et al. Primary pineal rhabdomyosarcoma successfully treated by high-dose chemotherapy followed by autologous peripheral blood stem cell transplantation: case report. J Neurosurg Pediatr. 2016 Jul;18(1):41–5. PMID:26942266

1419. Ishiuchi S, Nakazato Y, Iino M, et al. In vitro neuronal and glial production and differentiation of human central neurocytoma cells. J Neurosci Res. 1998 Feb 15;51(4):526–35. PMID:9514206

1420. Ishizawa K, Komori T, Hirose T. Stromal cells in hemangioblastoma: neuroectodermal differentiation and morphological similarities to ependymoma. Pathol Int. 2005 Jul;55(7):377–85. PMID:15982211

1421. Ishizawa K, Komori T, Shimada S, et al. Olig2 and CD99 are useful negative markers for the diagnosis of brain tumors. Clin Neuropathol. 2008 May-Jun;27(3):118–28. PMID:18552083

1422. Ishizawa K, Tsukamoto Y, Ikeda S, et al. 'Papillary' solitary fibrous tumor/hemangiopericytoma with nuclear STAT6 expression and NAB2-STAT6 fusion. Brain Tumor Pathol. 2016 Apr;33(2):151–6. PMID:26746203

1423. Isler C, Erturk Cetin O, Ugurlar D, et al. Dysembryoplastic neuroepithelial tumours: clinical, radiological, pathological features and outcome. Br J Neurosurg. 2018 Aug;32(4):436–41. PMID:29792345

1424. Italiano A, Sung YS, Zhang L, et al. High prevalence of CIC fusion with double-homeobox (DUX4) transcription factors in EWSR1-negative undifferentiated small blue round cell sarcomas. Genes Chromosomes Cancer. 2012 Mar;51(3):207–18. PMID:22072439

1425. Ito J, Nakano Y, Shima H, et al. Central nervous system ganglioneuroblastoma harboring MYO5A-NTRK3 fusion. Brain Tumor Pathol. 2020 Jul;37(3):105–10. PMID:32556925

1426. Ito M, Ishikawa M, Kitajima M, et al. A case report of CIC-rearranged undifferentiated small round cell sarcoma in the cerebrum. Diagn Cytopathol. 2016 Oct;44(10):828–32. PMID:27324529

1427. Ito T, Kanno H, Sato K, et al. Clinicopathologic study of pineal parenchymal tumors of intermediate differentiation. World Neurosurg. 2014 May-Jun;81(5-6):783–9. PMID:23396072

1428. Iwamoto FM, DeAngelis LM, Abrey LE. Primary dural lymphomas: a clinicopathologic study of treatment and outcome in eight patients. Neurology. 2006 Jun 13;66(11):1763–5. PMID:16769960

1429. Jääskeläinen J. Seemingly complete removal of histologically benign intracranial meningioma: late recurrence rate and factors predicting recurrence in 657 patients. A multivariate analysis. Surg Neurol. 1986 Nov;26(5):461–9. PMID:3764651

1430. Jääskeläinen J, Haltia M, Servo A. Atypical and anaplastic meningiomas: radiology, surgery, radiotherapy, and outcome. Surg Neurol. 1986 Mar;25(3):233–42. PMID:3945904

1431. Jääskeläinen J, Paetau A, Pyykkö I, et al. Interface between the facial nerve and large acoustic neurinomas. Immunohistochemical study of the cleavage plane in NF2 and non-NF2 cases. J Neurosurg. 1994 Mar;80(3):541–7. PMID:8113868

1432. Jackson CG. Glomus tympanicum and glomus jugulare tumors. Otolaryngol Clin North Am. 2001 Oct;34(5):941–70. PMID:11557448

1433. Jackson TR, Regine WF, Wilson D, et al. Cerebellar liponeurocytoma. Case report and review of the literature. J Neurosurg. 2001 Oct;95(4):700–3. PMID:11596966

1434. Jacobs DI, Fukumura K, Bainbridge MN, et al. Elucidating the molecular pathogenesis of glioma: integrated germline and somatic profiling of a familial glioma case series. Neuro Oncol. 2018 Nov 12;20(12):1625–33. PMID:30165405

1435. Jacobs JJ, Rosenberg AE. Extracranial skeletal metastasis from a pinealoblastoma. A case report and review of the literature. Clin Orthop Relat Res. 1989 Oct; (247):256–60. PMID:2676297

1436. Jacoby LB, Jones D, Davis K, et al. Molecular analysis of the NF2 tumor-suppressor gene in schwannomatosis. Am J Hum Genet. 1997 Dec;61(6):1293–302. PMID:9399891

1437. Jacoby LB, MacCollin M, Barone R, et al. Frequency and distribution of NF2 mutations in schwannomas. Genes Chromosomes Cancer. 1996 Sep;17(1):45–55. PMID:8889506

1438. Jacques TS, Eldridge C, Patel A, et al. Mixed glioneuronal tumour of the fourth ventricle with prominent rosette formation. Neuropathol Appl Neurobiol. 2006 Apr;32(2):217–20. PMID:16599951

1439. Jacques TS, Valentine A, Bradford R, et al. December 2003: a 70-year-old woman with a recurrent meningeal mass. Recurrent meningioma with rhabdomyosarcomatous differentiation. Brain Pathol. 2004 Apr;14(2):229–30. PMID:15193039

1440. Jaeckle KA, Decker PA, Ballman KV, et al. Transformation of low grade glioma and correlation with outcome: an NCCTG database analysis. J Neurooncol. 2011 Aug;104(1):253–9. PMID:21153680

1441. Jager B, Schuhmann MU, Schober R, et al. Induction of gliosarcoma and atypical meningioma 13 years after radiotherapy of residual pilocytic astrocytoma in childhood. Pediatr Neurosurg. 2008;44(2):153–8. PMID:18230932

1442. Jager MJ, Shields CL, Cebulla CM, et al. Uveal melanoma. Nat Rev Dis Primers. 2020 Apr 9;6(1):24. PMID:32273508

1443. Jahanseir K, Folpe AL, Graham RP, et al. Ewing sarcoma in older adults: a clinicopathologic study of 50 cases occurring in patients aged ≥40 years, with emphasis on histologic mimics. Int J Surg Pathol. 2020 Jun;28(4):352–60. PMID:31847636

1444. Jahnke K, Korfel A, Komm J, et al. Intraocular lymphoma 2000-2005: results of a retrospective multicentre trial. Graefes Arch Clin Exp Ophthalmol. 2006 Jun;244(6):663–9. PMID:16228920

1445. Jahnke K, Thiel E, Martus P, et al. Relapse of primary central nervous system lymphoma: clinical features, outcome and prognostic factors. J Neurooncol. 2006 Nov;80(2):159–65. PMID:16699873

1446. Jahnke K, Thiel E, Schilling A, et al. Low-grade primary central nervous system lymphoma in immunocompetent patients. Br J Haematol. 2005 Mar;128(5):616–24. PMID:15725082

1447. Jain P, Mohamed A, Sigamani E, et al. Bilateral thalamic lesions in a child. Eur Neurol. 2013;70(1-2):33–4. PMID:23689275

1448. Jain SU, Do TJ, Lund PJ, et al. PFA ependymoma-associated protein EZHIP inhibits PRC2 activity through a H3 K27M-like mechanism. Nat Commun. 2019 May 13;10(1):2146. PMID:31086175

1449. Jaiswal S, Vij M, Jaiswal AK, et al. Squash cytology of subependymal giant cell astrocytoma: report of four cases with brief review of literature. Diagn Cytopathol. 2012 Apr;40(4):333–6. PMID:22431322

1450. Jaju A, Hwang EI, Kool M, et al. MRI features of histologically diagnosed supratentorial primitive neuroectodermal tumors and pineoblastomas in correlation with molecular diagnoses and outcomes: a report from the Children's Oncology Group ACNS0332 trial. AJNR Am J Neuroradiol. 2019 Nov;40(11):1796–803. PMID:31601576

1451. Jakacki RI, Burger PC, Koçak M, et al. Outcome and prognostic factors for children with supratentorial primitive neuroectodermal tumors treated with carboplatin during radiotherapy: a report from the Children's Oncology Group. Pediatr Blood Cancer. 2015 May;62(5):776–83. PMID:25704363

1452. Jänisch W, Staneczek W. [Primary tumors of the choroid plexus. Frequency, localization and age]. Zentralbl Allg Pathol. 1989;135(3):235–40. German. PMID:2773602

1453. Janson K, Nedzi LA, David O, et al. Predisposition to atypical teratoid/rhabdoid tumor due to an inherited INI1 mutation. Pediatr Blood Cancer. 2006 Sep;47(3):279–84. PMID:16261613

1454. Janzarik WG, Kratz CP, Loges NT, et al. Further evidence for a somatic KRAS mutation in a pilocytic astrocytoma. Neuropediatrics. 2007 Apr;38(2):61–3. PMID:17712732

1455. Japp AS, Gessi M, Messing-Jünger M, et al. High-resolution genomic analysis does not qualify atypical plexus papilloma as a separate entity among choroid plexus tumors. J Neuropathol Exp Neurol. 2015 Feb;74(2):110–20. PMID:25575132

1456. Jaramillo S, Grosshans DR, Philip N, et al. Radiation for ETMR: literature review and case series of patients treated with proton therapy. Clin Transl Radiat Oncol. 2018 Nov 7;15:31–7. PMID:30582019

1457. Jaros E, Perry RH, Adam L, et al. Prognostic implications of p53 protein, epidermal growth factor receptor, and Ki-67 labelling in brain tumours. Br J Cancer. 1992 Aug;66(2):373–85. PMID:1503912

1458. Jaunmuktane Z, Capper D, Jones DTW, et al. Methylation array profiling of adult brain tumours: diagnostic outcomes in a large, single centre. Acta Neuropathol Commun. 2019 Feb 20;7(1):24. PMID:30786920

1459. Javahery RJ, Davidson L, Fangusaro J, et al. Aggressive variant of a papillary glioneuronal tumor. Report of 2 cases. J Neurosurg Pediatr. 2009 Jan;3(1):46–52. PMID:19119904

1460. Jay V, Squire J, Becker LE, et al. Malignant transformation in a ganglioglioma with anaplastic neuronal and astrocytic components. Report of a case with flow cytometric and cytogenetic analysis. Cancer. 1994 Jun 1;73(11):2862–8. PMID:8194028

1461. Jeffs GJ, Lee GY, Wong GT. Functioning paraganglioma of the thoracic spine: case report. Neurosurgery. 2003 Oct;53(4):992–4. PMID:14519233

1462. Jeibmann A, Eikmeier K, Linge A, et al. Identification of genes involved in the biology of atypical teratoid/rhabdoid tumours using Drosophila melanogaster. Nat Commun. 2014 Jun 3;5:4005. PMID:24892285

1463. Jeibmann A, Hasselblatt M, Gerss J, et al. Prognostic implications of atypical histologic features in choroid plexus papilloma. J Neuropathol Exp Neurol. 2006 Nov;65(11):1069–73. PMID:17086103

1464. Jeibmann A, Wrede B, Peters O, et al. Malignant progression in choroid plexus papillomas. J Neurosurg. 2007 Sep;107(3 Suppl):199–202. PMID:17918524

1465. Jenkins RB, Blair H, Ballman KV, et al. A t(1;19)(q10;p10) mediates the combined deletions of 1p and 19q and predicts a better prognosis of patients with oligodendroglioma. Cancer Res. 2006 Oct 15;66(20):9852–61. PMID:17047046

1466. Jenkins RB, Xiao Y, Sicotte H, et al. A low-frequency variant at 8q24.21 is strongly associated with risk of oligodendroglial tumors and astrocytomas with IDH1 or IDH2 mutation. Nat Genet. 2012 Oct;44(10):1122–5. PMID:22922872

1467. Jenkinson MD, Bosma JJ, Du Plessis D, et al. Cerebellar liponeurocytoma with an unusually aggressive clinical course: case report. Neurosurgery. 2003 Dec;53(6):1425–7. PMID:14633310

1468. Jensen DE, Proctor M, Marquis ST, et al. BAP1: a novel ubiquitin hydrolase which binds to the BRCA1 RING finger and enhances BRCA1-mediated cell growth suppression. Oncogene. 1998 Mar 5;16(9):1097–112. PMID:9528852

1469. Jensen RL, Caamano E, Jensen EM, et al. Development of contrast enhancement after long-term observation of a dysembryoplastic neuroepithelial tumor. J Neurooncol. 2006 May;78(1):59–62. PMID:16314940

1470. Jentoft M, Giannini C, Rossi S, et al. Oligodendroglial tumors with marked desmoplasia: clinicopathologic and molecular features of 7 cases. Am J Surg Pathol. 2011 Jun;35(6):845–52. PMID:21552114

1471. Jeon YK, Cheon JE, Kim SK, et al. Clinicopathological features and global genomic copy number alterations of pilomyxoid astrocytoma in the hypothalamus/optic pathway: comparative analysis with pilocytic astrocytoma using array-based comparative genomic hybridization. Mod Pathol. 2008 Nov;21(11):1345–56. PMID:18622384

1472. Jessa S, Blanchet-Cohen A, Krug B, et al. Stalled developmental programs at the root of pediatric brain tumors. Nat Genet. 2019 Dec;51(12):1702–13. PMID:31768071

1473. Jiang M, Long L, Zeng J, et al. Imaging characteristics of cerebral extraventricular neurocytoma with pathological correlation. J Neurooncol. 2018 Nov;140(2):289–96. PMID:30062611

1474. Jiao Y, Killela PJ, Reitman ZJ, et al. Frequent ATRX, CIC, FUBP1 and IDH1 mutations refine the classification of malignant gliomas. Oncotarget. 2012 Jul;3(7):709–22. PMID:22869205

1475. Jiménez-Heffernan JA, Freih Fraih A, Álvarez F, et al. Cytologic features of pleomorphic xanthoastrocytoma, WHO grade II. A comparative study with glioblastoma. Diagn Cytopathol. 2017 Apr;45(4):339–44. PMID:28084690

1476. Jimsheleishvili S, Alshareef AT, Papadimitriou K, et al. Extracranial glioblastoma in transplant recipients. J Cancer Res Clin Oncol. 2014 May;140(5):801–7. PMID:24595597

1477. Jinkala SR, Muthalagan E, Badhe BA. Granulomatous response in intracranial germinomas: diagnostic problems. Int J Appl Basic Med Res. 2018 Jan-Mar;8(1):51–3. PMID:29552538

1478. Jo VY, Fletcher CD. Epithelioid malignant peripheral nerve sheath tumor: clinicopathologic analysis of 63 cases. Am J Surg Pathol. 2015 May;39(5):673–82. PMID:25602794

1479. Jo VY, Fletcher CDM. SMARCB1/INI1 loss in epithelioid schwannoma: a clinicopathologic and immunohistochemical study of 65 cases. Am J Surg Pathol. 2017 Aug;41(8):1013–22. PMID:28368924

1480. Johann PD, Bens S, Oyen F, et al. Sellar region atypical teratoid/rhabdoid tumors (ATRT) in adults display DNA methylation profiles of the ATRT-MYC subgroup. Am J Surg Pathol. 2018 Apr;42(4):506–11. PMID:29324471

1481. Johann PD, Erkek S, Zapatka M, et al. Atypical teratoid/rhabdoid tumors are comprised of three epigenetic subgroups with distinct enhancer landscapes. Cancer Cell. 2016 Mar 14;29(3):379–93. PMID:26923874

1482. Johann PD, Hovestadt V, Thomas C, et al. Cribriform neuroepithelial tumor: molecular characterization of a SMARCB1-deficient non-rhabdoid tumor with favorable long-term outcome. Brain Pathol. 2017 Jul;27(4):411–8. PMID:27380723

1483. Johanns TM, Miller CA, Dorward IG, et al. Immunogenomics of hypermutated glioblastoma: a patient with germline POLE deficiency treated with checkpoint blockade immunotherapy. Cancer Discov. 2016 Nov;6(11):1230–6. PMID:27683556

1484. Johannsson O, Ostermeyer EA, Håkansson S, et al. Founding BRCA1 mutations in hereditary breast and ovarian cancer in southern Sweden. Am J Hum Genet. 1996 Mar;58(3):441–50. PMID:8644702

1485. Johnson DR, Giannini C, Jenkins RB, et al. Plenty of calcification: imaging characterization of polymorphous low-grade neuroepithelial tumor of the young. Neuroradiology. 2019 Nov;61(11):1327–32. PMID:31396664

1486. Johnson LN, Hepler RS, Yee RD, et al. Magnetic resonance imaging of craniopharyngioma. Am J Ophthalmol. 1986 Aug 15;102(2):242–4. PMID:3740186

1487. Johnson MW, Eberhart CG, Perry A, et al. Spectrum of pilomyxoid astrocytomas: intermediate pilomyxoid tumors. Am J Surg Pathol. 2010 Dec;34(12):1783–91. PMID:21107083

1488. Johnson MW, Emelin JK, Park SH, et al. Co-localization of TSC1 and TSC2 gene products in tubers of patients with tuberous sclerosis. Brain Pathol. 1999 Jan;9(1):45–54. PMID:9989450

1489. Johnson MW, Kerfoot C, Bushnell T, et al. Hamartin and tuberin expression in human tissues. Mod Pathol. 2001 Mar;14(3):202–10. PMID:11266527

1490. Johnson RA, Wright KD, Poppleton H, et al. Cross-species genomics matches driver mutations and cell compartments to model ependymoma. Nature. 2010 Jul 29;466(7306):632–6. PMID:20639864

1491. Johnson RL, Rothman AL, Xie J, et al. Human homolog of patched, a candidate gene for the basal cell nevus syndrome. Science. 1996 Jun 14;272(5268):1668–71. PMID:8658145

1492. Jones AC, Shyamsundar MM, Thomas MW, et al. Comprehensive mutation analysis of TSC1 and TSC2-and phenotypic correlations in 150 families with tuberous sclerosis. Am J Hum Genet. 1999 May;64(5):1305–15. PMID:10205261

1493. Jones DT, Hutter B, Jäger N, et al. Recurrent somatic alterations of FGFR1 and NTRK2 in pilocytic astrocytoma. Nat Genet. 2013 Aug;45(8):927–32. PMID:23817572

1494. Jones DT, Ichimura K, Liu L, et al. Genomic analysis of pilocytic astrocytomas at 0.97 Mb resolution shows an increasing tendency toward chromosomal copy number change with age. J Neuropathol Exp Neurol. 2006 Nov;65(11):1049–58. PMID:17086101

1495. Jones DT, Kocialkowski S, Liu L, et al. Oncogenic RAF1 rearrangement and a novel BRAF mutation as alternatives to KIAA1549:BRAF fusion in activating the MAPK pathway in pilocytic astrocytoma. Oncogene. 2009 May 21;28(20):2119–23. PMID:19363522

1496. Jones DT, Kocialkowski S, Liu L, et al. Tandem duplication producing a novel oncogenic BRAF fusion gene defines the majority of pilocytic astrocytomas. Cancer Res. 2008 Nov 1;68(21):8673–7. PMID:18974108

1497. Jones DT, Northcott PA, Kool M, et al. The role of chromatin remodeling in medulloblastoma. Brain Pathol. 2013 Mar;23(2):193–9. PMID:23432644

1498. Jones RT, Abedalthagafi MS, Brahmandam M, et al. Cross-reactivity of the BRAF VE1 antibody with epitopes in axonemal dyneins leads to staining of cilia. Mod Pathol. 2015 Apr;28(4):596–606. PMID:25412847

1499. Jordanova ES, Riemersma SA, Philippo K, et al. Hemizygous deletions in the HLA region account for loss of heterozygosity in the majority of diffuse large B-cell lymphomas of the testis and the central nervous system. Genes Chromosomes Cancer. 2002 Sep;35(1):38–48. PMID:12203788

1500. Joseph NM, Phillips J, Dahiya S, et al. Diagnostic implications of IDH1-R132H and OLIG2 expression patterns in rare and challenging glioblastoma variants. Mod Pathol. 2013 Mar;26(3):315–26. PMID:23041832

1501. Jour G, Serrano J, Koelsche C, et al. Primary CNS alveolar rhabdomyosarcoma: importance of epigenetic and transcriptomic assays for accurate diagnosis. J Neuropathol Exp Neurol. 2019 Nov 1;78(11):1073–5. PMID:31553442

1502. Jouvet A, Fauchon F, Liberski P, et al. Papillary tumor of the pineal region. Am J Surg Pathol. 2003 Apr;27(4):505–12. PMID:12657936

1503. Jouvet A, Fèvre-Montange M, Besançon R, et al. Structural and ultrastructural

characteristics of human pineal gland, and pineal parenchymal tumors. Acta Neuropathol. 1994;88(4):334–48. PMID:7839826
1504. Jouvet A, Lellouch-Tubiana A, Boddaert N, et al. Fourth ventricle neurocytoma with lipomatous and ependymal differentiation. Acta Neuropathol. 2005 Mar;109(3):346–51. PMID:15627205
1505. Jouvet A, Saint-Pierre G, Fauchon F, et al. Pineal parenchymal tumors: a correlation of histological features with prognosis in 66 cases. Brain Pathol. 2000 Jan;10(1):49–60. PMID:10668895
1506. Jozwiak J, Jozwiak S, Skopinski P. Immunohistochemical and microscopic studies on giant cells in tuberous sclerosis. Histol Histopathol. 2005 Oct;20(4):1321–6. PMID:16136513
1507. Jóźwiak S, Kwiatkowski D, Kotulska K, et al. Tuberin and hamartin expression is reduced in the majority of subependymal giant cell astrocytomas in tuberous sclerosis complex consistent with a two-hit model of pathogenesis. J Child Neurol. 2004 Feb;19(2):102–6. PMID:15072102
1508. Juco J, Horvath E, Smyth H, et al. Hemangiopericytoma of the sella mimicking pituitary adenoma: case report and review of the literature. Clin Neuropathol. 2007 Nov-Dec;26(6):288–93. PMID:18232595
1509. Judkins AR, Burger PC, Hamilton RL, et al. INI1 protein expression distinguishes atypical teratoid/rhabdoid tumor from choroid plexus carcinoma. J Neuropathol Exp Neurol. 2005 May;64(5):391–7. PMID:15892296
1510. Judkins AR, Ellison DW. Ependymoblastoma: dear, damned, distracting diagnosis, farewell!*. Brain Pathol. 2010 Jan;20(1):133–9. PMID:19120373
1511. Judkins AR, Mauger J, Ht A, et al. Immunohistochemical analysis of hSNF5/INI1 in pediatric CNS neoplasms. Am J Surg Pathol. 2004 May;28(5):644–50. PMID:15105654
1512. Jünger ST, Andreiuolo F, Mynarek M, et al. CDKN2A deletion in supratentorial ependymoma with RELA alteration indicates a dismal prognosis: a retrospective analysis of the HIT ependymoma trial cohort. Acta Neuropathol. 2020 Sep;140(3):405–7. PMID:32514758
1513. Jünger ST, Mynarek M, Wohlers I, et al. Improved risk-stratification for posterior fossa ependymoma of childhood considering clinical, histological and genetic features - a retrospective analysis of the HIT ependymoma trial cohort. Acta Neuropathol Commun. 2019 Nov 14;7(1):181. PMID:31727173
1514. Jungk C, Scherer M, Mock A, et al. Prognostic value of the extent of resection in supratentorial WHO grade II astrocytomas stratified for IDH1 mutation status: a single-center volumetric analysis. J Neurooncol. 2016 Sep;129(2):319–28. PMID:27344556
1515. Juratli TA, Jones PS, Wang N, et al. Targeted treatment of papillary craniopharyngiomas harboring BRAF V600E mutations. Cancer. 2019 Sep 1;125(17):2910–4. PMID:31314136
1516. Juratli TA, McCabe D, Nayyar N, et al. DMD genomic deletions characterize a subset of progressive/higher-grade meningiomas with poor outcome. Acta Neuropathol. 2018 Nov;136(5):779–92. PMID:30123936
1517. Juratli TA, Thiede C, Koerner MVA, et al. Intratumoral heterogeneity and TERT promoter mutations in progressive/higher-grade meningiomas. Oncotarget. 2017 Nov 24;8(65):109228–37. PMID:29312603
1518. Juratli TA, Tummala SS, Riedl A, et al. Radiographic assessment of contrast enhancement and T2/FLAIR mismatch sign in lower grade gliomas: correlation with molecular groups. J Neurooncol. 2019 Jan;141(2):327–35. PMID:30536195
1519. Justin N, Zhang Y, Tarricone C, et al. Structural basis of oncogenic histone H3K27M inhibition of human polycomb repressive complex 2. Nat Commun. 2016 Apr 28;7:11316. PMID:27121947
1520. Kaatsch P, Rickert CH, Kühl J, et al. Population-based epidemiologic data on brain tumors in German children. Cancer. 2001 Dec 15;92(12):3155–64. PMID:11753995
1521. Kacerovska D, Michal M, Kuroda N, et al. Hybrid peripheral nerve sheath tumors, including a malignant variant in type 1 neurofibromatosis. Am J Dermatopathol. 2013 Aug;35(6):641–9. PMID:23676318
1522. Kadoch C, Williams RT, Calarco JP, et al. Dynamics of BAF-Polycomb complex opposition on heterochromatin in normal and oncogenic states. Nat Genet. 2017 Feb;49(2):213–22. PMID:27941796
1523. Kadonaga JN, Frieden IJ. Neurocutaneous melanosis: definition and review of the literature. J Am Acad Dermatol. 1991 May;24(5 Pt 1):747–55. PMID:1869648
1524. Kaelin WG Jr. The VHL tumor suppressor gene: insights into oxygen sensing and cancer. Trans Am Clin Climatol Assoc. 2017;128:298–307. PMID:28790514
1525. Kageji T, Miyamoto T, Kotani Y, et al. Congenital craniopharyngioma treated by radical surgery: case report and review of the literature. Childs Nerv Syst. 2017 Feb;33(2):357–62. PMID:27669698
1526. Kaido T, Sasaoka Y, Hashimoto H, et al. De novo germinoma in the brain in association with Klinefelter's syndrome: case report and review of the literature. Surg Neurol. 2003 Dec;60(6):553–8. PMID:14670679
1527. Kakkar A, Biswas A, Kalyani N, et al. Intracranial germ cell tumors: a multi-institutional experience from three tertiary care centers in India. Childs Nerv Syst. 2016 Nov;32(11):2173–80. PMID:27476038
1528. Kakkar A, Majumdar A, Kumar A, et al. Alterations in BRAF gene, and enhanced mTOR and MAPK signaling in dysembryoplastic neuroepithelial tumors (DNTs). Epilepsy Res. 2016 Nov;127:141–51. PMID:27599148
1529. Kakkar A, Sable M, Suri V, et al. Cerebellar liponeurocytoma, an unusual tumor of the central nervous system–ultrastructural examination. Ultrastruct Pathol. 2015;39(6):419–23. PMID:26107691
1530. Kalamarides M, Niwa-Kawakita M, Leblois H, et al. Nf2 gene inactivation in arachnoidal cells is rate-limiting for meningioma development in the mouse. Genes Dev. 2002 May 1;16(9):1060–5. PMID:12000789
1531. Kaleta M, Wakulińska A, Karkucińska-Więckowska A, et al. OLIG2 is a novel immunohistochemical marker associated with the presence of PAX3/7-FOXO1 translocation in rhabdomyosarcomas. Diagn Pathol. 2019 Sep 7;14(1):103. PMID:31493794
1532. Kamb A, Shattuck-Eidens D, Eeles R, et al. Analysis of the p16 gene (CDKN2) as a candidate for the chromosome 9p melanoma susceptibility locus. Nat Genet. 1994 Sep;8(1):23–6. PMID:7987388
1533. Kambe A, Nakada S, Nagao Y, et al. A dedifferentiated intracranial solitary fibrous tumor with osteosarcoma components: rapid tumor progression and lethal clinical course. Brain Tumor Pathol. 2020 Oct;37(4):165–70. PMID:32740753
1534. Kambham N, Chang Y, Matsushima AY. Primary low-grade B-cell lymphoma of mucosa-associated lymphoid tissue (MALT) arising in dura. Clin Neuropathol. 1998 Nov-Dec;17(6):311–7. PMID:9832258
1535. Kamihara J, Paulson V, Breen MA, et al. DICER1-associated central nervous system sarcoma in children: comprehensive clinicopathologic and genetic analysis of a newly described rare tumor. Mod Pathol. 2020 Oct;33(10):1910–21. PMID:32291395
1536. Kamoshima Y, Sawamura Y, Sugiyama T, et al. Primary central nervous system mucosa-associated lymphoid tissue lymphoma–case report. Neurol Med Chir (Tokyo). 2011;51(7):527–30. PMID:21785250
1537. Kamoun A, Idbaih A, Dehais C, et al. Integrated multi-omics analysis of oligodendroglial tumours identifies three subgroups of 1p/19q co-deleted gliomas. Nat Commun. 2016 Apr 19;7:11263. PMID:27090007
1538. Kandt RS, Haines JL, Smith M, et al. Linkage of an important gene locus for tuberous sclerosis to a chromosome 16 marker for polycystic kidney disease. Nat Genet. 1992 Sep;2(1):37–41. PMID:1303246
1539. Kane AJ, Sughrue ME, Rutkowski MJ, et al. Anatomic location is a risk factor for atypical and malignant meningiomas. Cancer. 2011 Mar 15;117(6):1272–8. PMID:21381014
1540. Kane AJ, Sughrue ME, Rutkowski MJ, et al. Atypia predicting prognosis for intracranial extraventricular neurocytomas. J Neurosurg. 2012 Feb;116(2):349–54. PMID:22054208
1541. Kane LA, Leinung MC, Scheithauer BW, et al. Pituitary adenomas in childhood and adolescence. J Clin Endocrinol Metab. 1994 Oct;79(4):1135–40. PMID:7525627
1542. Kane PJ, Phipps KP, Harkness WF, et al. Intracranial neoplasms in the first year of life: results of a second cohort of patients from a single institution. Br J Neurosurg. 1999 Jun;13(3):294–8. PMID:10562841
1543. Kaneko M, Fukaya M, Nakayama K, et al. Holoprosencephaly: report of a case. Aichi Gakuin Dent Sci. 1989;2:29–37. PMID:2641432
1544. Kanemaru Y, Natsumeda M, Okada M, et al. Dramatic response of BRAF V600E-mutant epithelioid glioblastoma to combination therapy with BRAF and MEK inhibitor: establishment and xenograft of a cell line to predict clinical efficacy. Acta Neuropathol Commun. 2019 Jul 25;7(1):119. PMID:31345255
1545. Kang JH, Buckley AF, Nagpal S, et al. A diffuse leptomeningeal glioneuronal tumor without diffuse leptomeningeal involvement: detailed molecular and clinical characterization. J Neuropathol Exp Neurol. 2018 Sep 1;77(9):751–6. PMID:29931222
1546. Kang JM, Ha J, Hong EK, et al. A nationwide, population-based epidemiologic study of childhood brain tumors in Korea, 2005-2014: a comparison with United States data. Cancer Epidemiol Biomarkers Prev. 2019 Feb;28(2):409–16. PMID:30348678
1547. Kannan K, Inagaki A, Silber J, et al. Whole-exome sequencing identifies ATRX mutation as a key molecular determinant in lower-grade glioma. Oncotarget. 2012 Oct;3(10):1194–203. PMID:23104868
1548. Kanno H, Nishihara H, Oikawa M, et al. Expression of O6-methylguanine DNA methyltransferase (MGMT) and immunohistochemical analysis of 12 pineal parenchymal tumors. Neuropathology. 2012 Dec;32(6):647–53. PMID:22458700
1549. Kanno H, Yamamoto I, Yoshida M, et al. Meningioma showing VHL gene inactivation in a patient with von Hippel-Lindau disease. Neurology. 2003 Apr 8;60(7):1197–9. PMID:12682336
1550. Kansal R, Quintanilla-Martinez L, Datta V, et al. Identification of the V600D mutation in Exon 15 of the BRAF oncogene in congenital, benign langerhans cell histiocytosis. Genes Chromosomes Cancer. 2013 Jan;52(1):99–106. PMID:22996177
1551. Kao YC, Sung YS, Chen CL, et al. ETV transcriptional upregulation is more reliable than RNA sequencing algorithms and FISH in diagnosing round cell sarcomas with CIC gene rearrangements. Genes Chromosomes Cancer. 2017 Jun;56(6):501–10. PMID:28233365
1552. Kao YC, Sung YS, Zhang L, et al. EWSR1 Fusions With CREB Family Transcription Factors Define a Novel Myxoid Mesenchymal Tumor With Predilection for Intracranial Location. Am J Surg Pathol. 2017 Apr;41(4):482–90. PMID:28009602
1553. Kao YC, Sung YS, Zhang L, et al. Recurrent BCOR internal tandem duplication and YWHAE-NUTM2B fusions in soft tissue undifferentiated round cell sarcoma of infancy: overlapping genetic features with clear cell sarcoma of kidney. Am J Surg Pathol. 2016 Aug;40(8):1009–20. PMID:26945340
1554. Kaplan KJ, Perry A. Gliosarcoma with primitive neuroectodermal differentiation: case report and review of the literature. J Neurooncol. 2007 Jul;83(3):313–8. PMID:17406789
1555. Karafin M, Jallo GI, Ayars M, et al. Rosette forming glioneuronal tumor in association with Noonan syndrome: pathobiological implications. Clin Neuropathol. 2011 Nov-Dec;30(6):297–300. PMID:22011734
1556. Karamchandani JR, Nielsen TO, van de Rijn M, et al. Sox10 and S100 in the diagnosis of soft-tissue neoplasms. Appl Immunohistochem Mol Morphol. 2012 Oct;20(5):445–50. PMID:22495377
1557. Karamitopoulou E, Perentes E, Diamantis I, et al. Ki-67 immunoreactivity in human central nervous system tumors: a study with MIB 1 monoclonal antibody on archival material. Acta Neuropathol. 1994;87(1):47–54. PMID:7511316
1558. Karavitaki N, Brufani C, Warner JT, et al. Craniopharyngiomas in children and adults: systematic analysis of 121 cases with long-term follow-up. Clin Endocrinol (Oxf). 2005 Apr;62(4):397–409. PMID:15807869
1559. Karimi S, Zuccato JA, Mamatjan Y, et al. The central nervous system tumor methylation classifier changes neuro-oncology practice for challenging brain tumor diagnoses and directly impacts patient care. Clin Epigenetics. 2019 Dec 5;11(1):185. PMID:31806041
1560. Karmakar S, Reilly KM. The role of the immune system in neurofibromatosis type 1-associated nervous system tumors. CNS Oncol. 2017 Jan;6(1):45–60. PMID:28001089
1561. Karremann M, Butenhoff S, Rausche U, et al. Pediatric giant cell glioblastoma: new insights into a rare tumor entity. Neuro Oncol. 2009 Jun;11(3):323–9. PMID:19050301
1562. Karremann M, Pietsch T, Janssen G, et al. Anaplastic ganglioglioma in children. J Neurooncol. 2009 Apr;92(2):157–63. PMID:19043777
1563. Karremann M, Rausche U, Fleischhack G, et al. Clinical and epidemiological characteristics of pediatric gliosarcomas. J Neurooncol. 2010 Apr;97(2):257–65. PMID:19806321
1564. Karschnia P, Batchelor TT, Jordan JT, et al. Primary dural lymphomas: clinical presentation, management, and outcome. Cancer. 2020 Jun 15;126(12):2811–20. PMID:32176324
1565. Kasper LH, Baker SJ. Invited Review: Emerging functions of histone H3 mutations in paediatric diffuse high-grade gliomas. Neuropathol Appl Neurobiol. 2020 Feb;46(1):73–85. PMID:31859390
1566. Kastenhuber ER, Lowe SW. Putting p53 in Context. Cell. 2017 Sep 7;170(6):1062–78. PMID:28886379
1567. Kato K, Nakatani Y, Kanno H, et al. Possible linkage between specific histological structures and aberrant reactivation of the Wnt pathway in adamantinomatous craniopharyngioma. J Pathol. 2004 Jul;203(3):814–21. PMID:15221941
1568. Kato S, Han SY, Liu W, et al.

Understanding the function-structure and function-mutation relationships of p53 tumor suppressor protein by high-resolution missense mutation analysis. Proc Natl Acad Sci U S A. 2003 Jul 8;100(14):8424–9. PMID:12826609

1569. Katz LM, Hielscher T, Liechty B, et al. Loss of histone H3K27me3 identifies a subset of meningiomas with increased risk of recurrence. Acta Neuropathol. 2018 Jun;135(6):955–63. PMID:29627952

1570. Katzenstein AL, Carrington CB, Liebow AA. Lymphomatoid granulomatosis: a clinicopathologic study of 152 cases. Cancer. 1979 Jan;43(1):360–73. PMID:761171

1571. Kaufman DK, Kimmel DW, Parisi JE, et al. A familial syndrome with cutaneous malignant melanoma and cerebral astrocytoma. Neurology. 1993 Sep;43(9):1728–31. PMID:8414022

1572. Kaufman DL, Heinrich BS, Willett C, et al. Somatic instability of the NF2 gene in schwannomatosis. Arch Neurol. 2003 Sep;60(9):1317–20. PMID:12975302

1573. Kaulich K, Blaschke B, Nümann A, et al. Genetic alterations commonly found in diffusely infiltrating cerebral gliomas are rare or absent in pleomorphic xanthoastrocytomas. J Neuropathol Exp Neurol. 2002 Dec;61(12):1092–9. PMID:12484572

1574. Kaur B, Khwaja FW, Severson EA, et al. Hypoxia and the hypoxia-inducible-factor pathway in glioma growth and angiogenesis. Neuro Oncol. 2005 Apr;7(2):134–53. PMID:15831232

1575. Kaur K, Jha P, Pathak P, et al. Approach to molecular subgrouping of medulloblastomas: comparison of NanoString nCounter assay versus combination of immunohistochemistry and fluorescence in-situ hybridization in resource constrained centres. J Neurooncol. 2019 Jul;143(3):393–403. PMID:31104222

1576. Kaur K, Kakkar A, Kumar A, et al. Integrating molecular subclassification of medulloblastomas into routine clinical practice: a simplified approach. Brain Pathol. 2016 May;26(3):334–43. PMID:26222673

1577. Kawaguchi T, Kumabe T, Kanamori M, et al. Logarithmic decrease of serum alpha-fetoprotein or human chorionic gonadotropin in response to chemotherapy can distinguish a subgroup with better prognosis among highly malignant intracranial non-germinomatous germ cell tumors. J Neurooncol. 2011 Sep;104(3):779–87. PMID:21359564

1578. Kawamura-Saito M, Yamazaki Y, Kaneko K, et al. Fusion between CIC and DUX4 up-regulates PEA3 family genes in Ewing-like sarcomas with t(4;19)(q35;q13) translocation. Hum Mol Genet. 2006 Jul 1;15(13):2125–37. PMID:16717057

1579. Kawano N, Yasui Y, Utsuki S, et al. Light microscopic demonstration of the microlumen of ependymoma: a study of the usefulness of antigen retrieval for epithelial membrane antigen (EMA) immunostaining. Brain Tumor Pathol. 2004;21(1):17–21. PMID:15696964

1580. Kawauchi D, Ogg RJ, Liu L, et al. Novel MYC-driven medulloblastoma models from multiple embryonic cerebellar cells. Oncogene. 2017 Sep 14;36(37):5231–42. PMID:28504719

1581. Kayani B, Sewell MD, Hanna SA, et al. Prognostic factors in the operative management of dedifferentiated sacral chordomas. Neurosurgery. 2014 Sep;75(3):269–75. PMID:24867206

1582. Kebir S, Kuchelmeister K, Niehusmann P, et al. Intravascular CNS lymphoma: successful therapy using high-dose methotrexate-based polychemotherapy. Exp Hematol Oncol. 2012 Dec 5;1(1):37. PMID:23217063

1583. Kehrer-Sawatzki H, Farschtschi S, Mautner VF, et al. The molecular pathogenesis of schwannomatosis, a paradigm for the co-involvement of multiple tumour suppressor genes in tumorigenesis. Hum Genet. 2017 Feb;136(2):129–48. PMID:27921248

1584. Kehrer-Sawatzki H, Kordes U, Seiffert S, et al. Co-occurrence of schwannomatosis and rhabdoid tumor predisposition syndrome 1. Mol Genet Genomic Med. 2018 May 20;6(4):627–37. PMID:29770240

1585. Kelley MJ, Shi J, Ballew B, et al. Characterization of T gene sequence variants and germline duplications in familial and sporadic chordoma. Hum Genet. 2014 Oct;133(10):1289–97. PMID:24990759

1586. Kelley TW, Prayson RA, Barnett GH, et al. Extranodal marginal zone B-cell lymphoma of mucosa-associated lymphoid tissue arising in the lateral ventricle. Leuk Lymphoma. 2005 Oct;46(10):1423–7. PMID:16194887

1587. Kelsey KT, Wrensch M, Zuo ZF, et al. A population-based case-control study of the CYP2D6 and GSTT1 polymorphisms and malignant brain tumors. Pharmacogenetics. 1997 Dec;7(6):463–8. PMID:9429231

1588. Kemp S, Achan A, Ng T, et al. Rosette-forming glioneuronal tumour of the lateral ventricle in a patient with neurofibromatosis 1. J Clin Neurosci. 2012 Aug;19(8):1180–1. PMID:22613490

1589. Kepes JJ. Astrocytomas: old and newly recognized variants, their spectrum of morphology and antigen expression. Can J Neurol Sci. 1987 May;14(2):109–21. PMID:3607613

1590. Kepes JJ, Chen WY, Connors MH, et al. "Chordoid" meningeal tumors in young individuals with peritumoral lymphoplasmacellular infiltrates causing systemic manifestations of the Castleman syndrome. A report of seven cases. Cancer. 1988 Jul 15;62(2):391–406. PMID:3383139

1591. Kepes JJ, Fulling KH, Garcia JH. The clinical significance of "adenoid" formations of neoplastic astrocytes, imitating metastatic carcinoma, in gliosarcomas. A review of five cases. Clin Neuropathol. 1982;1(4):139–50. PMID:6188569

1592. Kepes JJ, Moral LA, Wilkinson SB, et al. Rhabdoid transformation of tumor cells in meningiomas: a histologic indication of increased proliferative activity: report of four cases. Am J Surg Pathol. 1998 Feb;22(2):231–8. PMID:9500225

1593. Kepes JJ, Rengachary SS, Lee SH. Astrocytes in hemangioblastomas of the central nervous system and their relationship to stromal cells. Acta Neuropathol. 1979 Jul 13;47(2):99–104. PMID:573044

1594. Kepes JJ, Rubinstein LJ. Malignant gliomas with heavily lipidized (foamy) tumor cells: a report of three cases with immunoperoxidase study. Cancer. 1981 May 15;47(10):2451–9. PMID:7023643

1595. Kepes JJ, Rubinstein LJ, Eng LF. Pleomorphic xanthoastrocytoma: a distinctive meningocerebral glioma of young subjects with relatively favorable prognosis. A study of 12 cases. Cancer. 1979 Nov;44(5):1839–52. PMID:498051

1596. Kerfoot C, Wienecke R, Menchine M, et al. Localization of tuberous sclerosis 2 mRNA and its protein product tuberin in normal human brain and in cerebral lesions of patients with tuberous sclerosis. Brain Pathol. 1996 Oct;6(4):367–75. PMID:8944308

1597. Kerr K, Qualmann K, Esquenazi Y, et al. Familial syndromes involving meningiomas provide mechanistic insight into sporadic disease. Neurosurgery. 2018 Dec 1;83(6):1107–18. PMID:29660026

1598. Kesari S, Schiff D, Drappatz J, et al. Phase II study of protracted daily temozolomide for low-grade gliomas in adults. Clin Cancer Res. 2009 Jan 1;15(1):330–7. PMID:19118062

1599. Ketter R, Kim YJ, Storck S, et al. Hyperdiploidy defines a distinct cytogenetic entity of meningiomas. J Neurooncol. 2007 Jun;83(2):213–21. PMID:17225936

1600. Khalid L, Carone M, Dumrongpisutikul N, et al. Imaging characteristics of oligodendrogliomas that predict grade. AJNR Am J Neuroradiol. 2012 May;33(5):852–7. PMID:22268087

1601. Khan NE, Bauer AJ, Schultz KAP, et al. Quantification of thyroid cancer and multinodular goiter risk in the DICER1 syndrome: a family-based cohort study. J Clin Endocrinol Metab. 2017 May 1;102(5):1614–22. PMID:28323992

1602. Khandpur U, Huntoon K, Smith-Cohn M, et al. Bilateral recurrent dysplastic cerebellar gangliocytoma (Lhermitte-Duclos disease) in Cowden syndrome: a case report and literature review. World Neurosurg. 2019 Jul;127:319–25. PMID:30905649

1603. Khanna M, Siraj F, Chopra P, et al. Gliosarcoma with prominent smooth muscle component (gliomyosarcoma): a report of 10 cases. Indian J Pathol Microbiol. 2011 Jan-Mar;54(1):51–4. PMID:21393877

1604. Khanna V, Achey RL, Ostrom QT, et al. Incidence and survival trends for medulloblastomas in the United States from 2001 to 2013. J Neurooncol. 2017 Dec;135(3):433–41. PMID:28828582

1605. Khater F, Langlois S, Cassart P, et al. Recurrent somatic BRAF insertion (p.V504_R506dup): a tumor marker and a potential therapeutic target in pilocytic astrocytoma. Oncogene. 2019 Apr;38(16):2994–3002. PMID:30575814

1606. Khatri D, Bhaisora KS, Das KK, et al. Cerebellar liponeurocytoma: the dilemma of multifocality. World Neurosurg. 2018 Dec;120:131–7. PMID:30172975

1607. Khoo M, Pressney I, Hargunani R, et al. Melanotic schwannoma: an 11-year case series. Skeletal Radiol. 2016 Jan;45(1):29–34. PMID:26386847

1608. Kickingereder P, Neuberger U, Bonekamp D, et al. Radiomic subtyping improves disease stratification beyond key molecular, clinical, and standard imaging characteristics in patients with glioblastoma. Neuro Oncol. 2018 May 18;20(6):848–57. PMID:29036412

1609. Kienast Y, von Baumgarten L, Fuhrmann M, et al. Real-time imaging reveals the single steps of brain metastasis formation. Nat Med. 2010 Jan;16(1):116–22. PMID:20023634

1610. Kijima C, Miyashita T, Suzuki M, et al. Two cases of nevoid basal cell carcinoma syndrome associated with meningioma caused by a PTCH1 or SUFU germline mutation. Fam Cancer. 2012 Dec;11(4):565–70. PMID:22829011

1611. Kilday JP, Mitra B, Domerg C, et al. Copy number gain of 1q25 predicts poor progression-free survival for pediatric intracranial ependymomas and enables patient risk stratification: a prospective European clinical trial cohort analysis on behalf of the Children's Cancer Leukaemia Group (CCLG), Societe Francaise d'Oncologie Pediatrique (SFOP), and International Society for Pediatric Oncology (SIOP). Clin Cancer Res. 2012 Apr 1;18(7):2001–11. PMID:22338015

1612. Kilicksmez O, Sanal HT, Haholu A, et al. Coexistence of pleomorphic xanthoastrocytoma with Sturge-Weber syndrome: MRI features. Pediatr Radiol. 2005 Sep;35(9):910–3. PMID:15883827

1613. Killela PJ, Pirozzi CJ, Healy P, et al. Mutations in IDH1, IDH2, and in the TERT promoter define clinically distinct subgroups of adult malignant gliomas. Oncotarget. 2014 Mar 30;5(6):1515–25. PMID:24722048

1614. Killela PJ, Reitman ZJ, Jiao Y, et al. TERT promoter mutations occur frequently in gliomas and a subset of tumors derived from cells with low rates of self-renewal. Proc Natl Acad Sci U S A. 2013 Apr 9;110(15):6021–6. PMID:23530248

1615. Kilpatrick SE, Reith JD, Rubin B. Ewing sarcoma and the history of similar and possibly related small round cell tumors: from whence have we come and where are we going? Adv Anat Pathol. 2018 Sep;25(5):314–26. PMID:29911999

1616. Kim B, Tabori U, Hawkins C. An update on the CNS manifestations of brain tumor polyposis syndromes. Acta Neuropathol. 2020 Apr;139(4):703–15. PMID:31970492

1617. Kim CY, Choi JW, Lee JY, et al. Intracranial growing teratoma syndrome: clinical characteristics and treatment strategy. J Neurooncol. 2011 Jan;101(1):109–15. PMID:20532955

1618. Kim DG, Lee DY, Paek SH, et al. Supratentorial primitive neuroectodermal tumors in adults. J Neurooncol. 2002 Oct;60(1):43–52. PMID:12416545

1619. Kim ES, Kwon MJ, Song JH, et al. Adenocarcinoma arising from intracranial recurrent mature teratoma and featuring mutated KRAS and wild-type BRAF genes. Neuropathology. 2015 Feb;35(1):44–9. PMID:25039399

1620. Kim I. Lymphomatoid granulomatosis with spinal involvement after childhood acute lymphoblastic leukemia. Korean J Spine. 2012 Mar;9(1):32–6. PMID:25983786

1621. Kim J, Field A, Schultz KAP, et al. The prevalence of DICER1 pathogenic variation in population databases. Int J Cancer. 2017 Nov 15;141(10):2030–6. PMID:28748527

1622. Kim JH, Paulus W, Heim S. BRAF V600E mutation is a useful marker for differentiating Rathke's cleft cyst with squamous metaplasia from papillary craniopharyngioma. J Neurooncol. 2015 May;123(1):189–91. PMID:25820214

1623. Kim JY, Jung KC, Park SH, et al. Primary lymphomatoid granulomatosis in the central nervous system: a report of three cases. Neuropathology. 2018 Apr 10. PMID:29635846

1624. Kim KH, Roberts CW. Mechanisms by which SMARCB1 loss drives rhabdoid tumor growth. Cancer Genet. 2014 Sep;207(9):365–72. PMID:24853101

1625. Kim SI, Lee Y, Kim SK, et al. Aggressive supratentorial ependymoma, RELA fusion-positive with extracranial metastasis: a case report. J Pathol Transl Med. 2017 Nov;51(6):588–93. PMID:29161788

1626. Kim Y, Lee SY, Yi KS, et al. Infratentorial and intraparenchymal subependymoma in the cerebellum: case report. Korean J Radiol. 2014 Jan-Feb;15(1):151–5. PMID:24497806

1627. Kim YH, Kim JW, Park CK, et al. Papillary tumor of pineal region presenting with leptomeningeal seeding. Neuropathology. 2010 Dec;30(6):654–60. PMID:20374498

1628. Kim YH, Nonoguchi N, Paulus W, et al. Frequent BRAF gain in low-grade diffuse gliomas with 1p/19q loss. Brain Pathol. 2012 Nov;22(6):834–40. PMID:22568401

1629. Kim YH, Ohta T, Oh JE, et al. TP53, MSH4, and LATS1 germline mutations in a family with clustering of nervous system tumors. Am J Pathol. 2014 Sep;184(9):2374–81. PMID:25041856

1630. Kim YH, Yie GT, Kim NR, et al. Pediatric intracerebral histiocytic sarcoma with rhabdoid features: case report and literature review. Neuropathology. 2017 Dec;37(6):560–8. PMID:28748542

1631. Kimonis VE, Goldstein AM, Pastakia B, et al. Clinical manifestations in 105 persons with nevoid basal cell carcinoma syndrome. Am J Med Genet. 1997 Mar 31;69(3):299–308. PMID:9096761

1632. Kimura N, Takekoshi K, Horii A, et al. Clinicopathological study of SDHB mutation-related pheochromocytoma and sympathetic paraganglioma. Endocr Relat Cancer. 2014 May 6;21(3):L13–6. PMID:24659481

1633. Kimura T, Budka H, Soler-Federsppiel S. An immunocytochemical comparison of the glia-associated proteins glial fibrillary acidic protein (GFAP) and S-100 protein (S100P) in human brain tumors. Clin Neuropathol. 1986 Jan-Feb;5(1):21–7. PMID:3512139

1634. Kinnersley B, Houlston RS, Bondy ML. Genome-Wide Association Studies in Glioma. Cancer Epidemiol Biomarkers Prev. 2018 Apr;27(4):418–28. PMID:29382702

1635. Kinsler VA, O'Hare P, Jacques T, et al. MEK inhibition appears to improve symptom control in primary NRAS-driven CNS melanoma in children. Br J Cancer. 2017 Apr 11;116(8):990–3. PMID:28253523

1636. Kinsler VA, Polubothu S, Calonje JE, et al. Copy number abnormalities in new or progressive 'neurocutaneous melanosis' confirm it to be primary CNS melanoma. Acta Neuropathol. 2017 Feb;133(2):329–31. PMID:27933403

1637. Kinsler VA, Thomas AC, Ishida M, et al. Multiple congenital melanocytic nevi and neurocutaneous melanosis are caused by postzygotic mutations in codon 61 of NRAS. J Invest Dermatol. 2013 Sep;133(9):2229–36. PMID:23392294

1638. Kirkman MA, Pickles JC, Fairchild AR, et al. Early wound site seeding in a patient with central nervous system high-grade neuroepithelial tumor with BCOR alteration. World Neurosurg. 2018 Aug;116:279–84. PMID:29859355

1639. Kirschner LS, Carney JA, Pack SD, et al. Mutations of the gene encoding the protein kinase A type I-alpha regulatory subunit in patients with the Carney complex. Nat Genet. 2000 Sep;26(1):89–92. PMID:10973256

1640. Kiseljak-Vassiliades K, Xu M, Mills TS, et al. Differential somatostatin receptor (SSTR) 1-5 expression and downstream effectors in histologic subtypes of growth hormone pituitary tumors. Mol Cell Endocrinol. 2015 Dec 5;417:73–83. PMID:26391562

1641. Kishore M, Gupta P, Bhardwaj M. Cerebrospinal fluid cytology of choroid plexus tumor: a report of two cases. Cytojournal. 2019 Apr 22;16:9. PMID:31080487

1642. Kissil JL, Wilker EW, Johnson KC, et al. Merlin, the product of the Nf2 tumor suppressor gene, is an inhibitor of the p21-activated kinase, Pak1. Mol Cell. 2003 Oct;12(4):841–9. PMID:14580336

1643. Kitamura Y, Komori T, Shibuya M, et al. Comprehensive genetic characterization of rosette-forming glioneuronal tumors: independent component analysis by tissue microdissection. Brain Pathol. 2018 Jan;28(1):87–93. PMID:27893178

1644. Kitamura Y, Sasaki H, Yoshida K. Genetic aberrations and molecular biology of skull base chordoma and chondrosarcoma. Brain Tumor Pathol. 2017 Apr;34(2):78–90. PMID:28432450

1645. Kivelä T. The epidemiological challenge of the most frequent eye cancer: retinoblastoma, an issue of birth and death. Br J Ophthalmol. 2009 Sep;93(9):1129–31. PMID:19704035

1646. Kivelä T. Trilateral retinoblastoma: a meta-analysis of hereditary retinoblastoma associated with primary ectopic intracranial retinoblastoma. J Clin Oncol. 1999 Jun;17(6):1829–37. PMID:10561222

1647. Kleihues P, Kiessling M, Janzer RC. Morphological markers in neuro-oncology. Curr Top Pathol. 1987;77:307–38. PMID:2827963

1648. Kleihues P, Schäuble B, zur Hausen A, et al. Tumors associated with p53 germline mutations: a synopsis of 91 families. Am J Pathol. 1997 Jan;150(1):1–13. PMID:9006316

1649. Klein CJ, Wu Y, Jentoft ME, et al. Genomic analysis reveals frequent TRAF7 mutations in intraneural perineuriomas. Ann Neurol. 2017

Feb;81(2):316–21. PMID:28019650

1650. Kleinman CL, Gerges N, Papillon-Cavanagh S, et al. Fusion of TTYH1 with the C19MC microRNA cluster drives expression of a brain-specific DNMT3B isoform in the embryonal brain tumor ETMR. Nat Genet. 2014 Jan;46(1):39–44. PMID:24316981

1651. Kleinschmidt-DeMasters BK, Aisner DL, Birks DK, et al. Epithelioid GBMs show a high percentage of BRAF V600E mutation. Am J Surg Pathol. 2013 May;37(5):685–98. PMID:23552385

1652. Kleinschmidt-DeMasters BK, Aisner DL. Foreman NK. BRAF VE1 immunoreactivity patterns in epithelioid glioblastomas positive for BRAF V600E mutation. Am J Surg Pathol. 2015 Apr;39(4):528–40. PMID:25581727

1653. Kleinschmidt-DeMasters BK, Alassiri AH, Birks DK, et al. Epithelioid versus rhabdoid glioblastomas are distinguished by monosomy 22 and immunohistochemical expression of INI-1 but not claudin 6. Am J Surg Pathol. 2010 Mar;34(3):341–54. PMID:20118769

1654. Kleinschmidt-DeMasters BK, Donson A. Foreman NK, et al. H3 K27M mutation in gangliogliomas can be associated with poor prognosis. Brain Pathol. 2017 Nov;27(6):846–50. PMID:28378357

1655. Kleinschmidt-DeMasters BK, Donson AM, Richmond AM, et al. SOX10 distinguishes pilocytic and pilomyxoid astrocytomas from ependymomas but shows no differences in expression level in ependymomas from infants versus older children or among molecular subgroups. J Neuropathol Exp Neurol. 2016 Apr;75(4):295–8. PMID:26945037

1656. Kleinschmidt-DeMasters BK, Donson AM, Vogel H, et al. Pilomyxoid Astrocytoma (PMA) shows significant differences in gene expression vs. Pilocytic Astrocytoma (PA) and variable tendency toward maturation to PA. Brain Pathol. 2015 Jul;25(4):429–40. PMID:25521223

1657. Kleinschmidt-DeMasters BK, Lillehei KO, Hankinson TC. Review of xanthomatous lesions of the sella. Brain Pathol. 2017 May;27(3):377–95. PMID:28236350

1658. Kleinschmidt-DeMasters BK, Lopes MB. Update on hypophysitis and TTF-1 expressing sellar region masses. Brain Pathol. 2013 Sep;23(5):495–514. PMID:23701182

1659. Klemm F, Maas RR, Bowman RL, et al. Interrogation of the microenvironmental landscape in brain tumors reveals disease-specific alterations of immune cells. Cell. 2020 Jun 25;181(7):1643–1660.e17. PMID:32470396

1660. Klesse LJ, Jordan JT, Radtke HB, et al. The use of MEK inhibitors in neurofibromatosis type 1-associated tumors and management of toxicities. Oncologist. 2020 Jul;25(7):e1109–16. PMID:32272491

1661. Kliewer KE, Cochran AJ. A review of the histology, ultrastructure, immunohistology, and molecular biology of extra-adrenal paragangliomas. Arch Pathol Lab Med. 1989 Nov;113(11):1209–18. PMID:2684087

1662. Kline CN, Joseph NM, Grenert JP, et al. Targeted next-generation sequencing of pediatric neuro-oncology patients improves diagnosis, identifies pathogenic germline mutations, and directs targeted therapy. Neuro Oncol. 2017 May 1;19(5):699–709. PMID:28453743

1663. Kloub O, Perry A, Tu PH, et al. Spindle cell oncocytoma of the adenohypophysis: report of two recurrent cases. Am J Surg Pathol. 2005 Feb;29(2):247–53. PMID:15644783

1664. Kluwe L, MacCollin M, Tatagiba M, et al. Phenotypic variability associated with 14 splice-site mutations in the NF2 gene. Am J Med Genet. 1998 May 18;77(3):228–33. PMID:9605590

1665. Kluwe L, Mautner V, Heinrich B, et al.

Molecular study of frequency of mosaicism in neurofibromatosis 2 patients with bilateral vestibular schwannomas. J Med Genet. 2003 Feb;40(2):109–14. PMID:12566519

1666. Kluwe L, Mautner VF. Mosaicism in sporadic neurofibromatosis 2 patients. Hum Mol Genet. 1998 Dec;7(13):2051–5. PMID:9817921

1667. Knappe UJ, Tischoff I, Tannapfel A, et al. Intraventricular melanocytoma diagnosis confirmed by gene mutation profile. Neuropathology. 2018 Jun;38(3):288–92. PMID:29226425

1668. Knosp E, Steiner E, Kitz K, et al. Pituitary adenomas with invasion of the cavernous sinus space: a magnetic resonance imaging classification compared with surgical findings. Neurosurgery. 1993 Oct;33(4):610–7. PMID:8232800

1669. Knowles DM. Immunodeficiency-associated lymphoproliferative disorders. Mod Pathol. 1999 Feb;12(2):200–17. PMID:10071343

1670. Kobayashi C, Oda Y, Takahira T, et al. Chromosomal aberrations and microsatellite instability of malignant peripheral nerve sheath tumors: a study of 10 tumors from nine patients. Cancer Genet Cytogenet. 2006 Mar;165(2):98–105. PMID:16527603

1671. Koch CA, Mauro D, Walther MM, et al. Pheochromocytoma in von hippel-lindau disease: distinct histopathologic phenotype compared to pheochromocytoma in multiple endocrine neoplasia type 2. Endocr Pathol. 2002 Spring;13(1):17–27. PMID:12114747

1672. Koczkowska M, Callens T, Gomes A, et al. Expanding the clinical phenotype of individuals with a 3-bp in-frame deletion of the NF1 gene (c.2970_2972del): an update of genotype-phenotype correlation. Genet Med. 2019 Apr;21(4):867–76. PMID:30190611

1673. Koczkowska M, Chen Y, Callens T, et al. Genotype-phenotype correlation in NF1: evidence for a more severe phenotype associated with missense mutations affecting NF1 codons 844-848. Am J Hum Genet. 2018 Jan 4;102(1):69–87. PMID:29290338

1674. Koeller KK, Rosenblum RS, Morrison AL. Neoplasms of the spinal cord and filum terminale: radiologic-pathologic correlation. Radiographics. 2000 Nov-Dec;20(6):1721–49. PMID:11112826

1675. Koelsche C, Hartmann W, Schrimpf D, et al. Array-based DNA-methylation profiling in sarcomas with small blue round cell histology provides valuable diagnostic information. Mod Pathol. 2018 Aug;31(8):1246–56. PMID:29572501

1676. Koelsche C, Hovestadt V, Jones DT, et al. Melanotic tumors of the nervous system are characterized by distinct mutational, chromosomal and epigenomic profiles. Brain Pathol. 2015 Mar;25(2):202–8. PMID:25399693

1677. Koelsche C, Mynarek M, Schrimpf D, et al. Primary intracranial spindle cell sarcoma with rhabdomyosarcoma-like features share a highly distinct methylation profile and DICER1 mutations. Acta Neuropathol. 2018 Aug;136(2):327–37. PMID:29881993

1678. Koelsche C, Sahm F, Capper D, et al. Distribution of TERT promoter mutations in pediatric and adult tumors of the nervous system. Acta Neuropathol. 2013 Dec;126(6):907–15. PMID:24154961

1679. Koelsche C, Sahm F, Paulus W, et al. BRAF V600E expression and distribution in desmoplastic infantile astrocytoma/ganglioglioma. Neuropathol Appl Neurobiol. 2014 Apr;40(3):337–44. PMID:23822828

1680. Koelsche C, Sahm F, Wöhrer A, et al. BRAF-mutated pleomorphic xanthoastrocytoma is associated with temporal location, reticulin fiber deposition and CD34 expression. Brain Pathol. 2014 Apr;24(3):221–9. PMID:24345274

1681. Koelsche C, Schweizer L, Renner M, et

al. Nuclear relocation of STAT6 reliably predicts NAB2-STAT6 fusion for the diagnosis of solitary fibrous tumour. Histopathology. 2014 Nov;65(5):613–22. PMID:24702701

1682. Koelsche C, Wöhrer A, Jeibmann A, et al. Mutant BRAF V600E protein in ganglioglioma is predominantly expressed by neuronal tumor cells. Acta Neuropathol. 2013 Jun;125(6):891–900. PMID:23435618

1683. Koen JL, McLendon RE, George TM. Intradural spinal teratoma: evidence for a dysembryogenic origin. Report of four cases. J Neurosurg. 1998 Nov;89(5):844–51. PMID:9817426

1684. Koenigsmann M, Jautzke G, Unger M, et al. June 2002: 57-year-old male with leptomeningeal and liver tumors. Brain Pathol. 2002 Oct;12(4):519–21. PMID:12408241

1685. Koga T, Chaim IA, Benitez JA, et al. Longitudinal assessment of tumor development using cancer avatars derived from genetically engineered pluripotent stem cells. Nat Commun. 2020 Jan 28;11(1):550. PMID:31992716

1686. Koga Y, Hamada S, Saito H, et al. Intracranial, intra-parenchymal capillary hemangioma - Case report. NMC Case Rep J. 2020 Mar 24;7(2):43–6. PMID:32322449

1687. Koh HY, Kim SH, Jang J, et al. BRAF somatic mutation contributes to intrinsic epileptogenicity in pediatric brain tumors. Nat Med. 2018 Nov;24(11):1662–8. PMID:30224756

1688. Kohno D, Inoue A, Fukushima M, et al. Epithelioid glioblastoma presenting as multicentric glioma: a case report and review of the literature. Surg Neurol Int. 2020 Jan 17;11:8. PMID:31966927

1689. Kolin DL, Geddie WR, Ko HM. CSF cytology diagnosis of NRAS-mutated primary leptomeningeal melanomatosis with neurocutaneous melanosis. Cytopathology. 2017 Jun;28(3):235–8. PMID:27696542

1690. Komakula S, Warmuth-Metz M, Hildenbrand P, et al. Pineal parenchymal tumor of intermediate differentiation: imaging spectrum of an unusual tumor in 11 cases. Neuroradiology. 2011 Aug;53(8):577–84. PMID:21080159

1691. Komatsu M, Yoshida A, Tanaka K, et al. Intracranial myxoid mesenchymal tumor with EWSR1-CREB1 gene fusion: a case report and literature review. Brain Tumor Pathol. 2020 Apr;37(2):76–80. PMID:32215804

1692. Komori T, Scheithauer BW, Anthony DC, et al. Papillary glioneuronal tumor: a new variant of mixed neuronal-glial neoplasm. Am J Surg Pathol. 1998 Oct;22(10):1171–83. PMID:9777979

1693. Komori T, Scheithauer BW, Hirose T. A rosette-forming glioneuronal tumor of the fourth ventricle: infratentorial form of dysembryoplastic neuroepithelial tumor? Am J Surg Pathol. 2002 May;26(5):582–91. PMID:11979088

1694. Komotar RJ, Burger PC, Carson BS, et al. Pilocytic and pilomyxoid hypothalamic/chiasmatic astrocytomas. Neurosurgery. 2004 Jan;54(1):72–9. PMID:14683543

1695. Komura S, Akiyama Y, Suzuki H, et al. Far-anterior interhemispheric transcallosal approach for a central neurocytoma in the lateral ventricle. Neurol Med Chir (Tokyo). 2019 Dec 15;59(12):511–6. PMID:31656237

1696. Kondziolka D, Parry PV, Lunsford LD, et al. The accuracy of predicting survival in individual patients with cancer. J Neurosurg. 2014 Jan;120(1):24–30. PMID:24160479

1697. Kong LY, Wei J, Haider AS, et al. Therapeutic targets in subependymoma. J Neuroimmunol. 2014 Dec 15;277(1-2):168–75. PMID:25465288

1698. Konno S, Oka H, Utsuki S, et al. Germinoma with a granulomatous reaction. Problems of differential diagnosis. Clin Neuropathol. 2002 Nov-Dec;21(6):248–51. PMID:12489672

1699. Konovalov AN, Konovalov NA, Pronin IN, et al. Multiple primary liponeurocytoma of the central nervous system. Zh Vopr Neirokhir Im N N Burdenko. 2015;79(2):87–96. English, Russian. PMID:26146048

1700. Konovalov AN, Pitskhelauri DI. Principles of treatment of the pineal region tumors. Surg Neurol. 2003 Apr;60(4):250–68. PMID:12748006

1701. Konstantinidis A, Cheesman E, O'Sullivan J, et al. Intracranial angiomatoid fibrous histiocytoma with EWSR1-CREB family fusions: a report of 2 pediatric cases. World Neurosurg. 2019 Jun;126:113–9. PMID:30831299

1702. Kool M, Jones DT, Jäger N, et al. Genome sequencing of SHH medulloblastoma predicts genotype-related response to smoothened inhibition. Cancer Cell. 2014 Mar 17;25(3):393–405. PMID:24651015

1703. Kool M, Korshunov A, Remke M, et al. Molecular subgroups of medulloblastoma: an international meta-analysis of transcriptome, genetic aberrations, and clinical data of WNT, SHH, Group 3, and Group 4 medulloblastomas. Acta Neuropathol. 2012 Apr;123(4):473–84. PMID:22358457

1704. Koopmans AE, Verdijk RM, Brouwer RW, et al. Clinical significance of immunohistochemistry for detection of BAP1 mutations in uveal melanoma. Mod Pathol. 2014 Oct;27(10):1321–30. PMID:24633195

1705. Koral K, Koral KM, Sklar F. Angiocentric glioma in a 4-year-old boy: imaging characteristics and review of the literature. Clin Imaging. 2012 Jan-Feb;36(1):61–4. PMID:22226445

1706. Kordek R, Biernat W, Sapieja W, et al. Pleomorphic xanthoastrocytoma with a gangliomatous component: an immunohistochemical and ultrastructural study. Acta Neuropathol. 1995;89(2):194–7. PMID:7732793

1707. Kordes M, Röring M, Heining C, et al. Cooperation of BRAF(F595L) and mutant HRAS in histiocytic sarcoma provides new insights into oncogenic BRAF signaling. Leukemia. 2016 Apr;30(4):937–46. PMID:26582644

1708. Kordes U, Flitsch J, Hagel C, et al. Ectopic craniopharyngioma. Klin Padiatr. 2011 May;223(3):176–7. PMID:21462099

1709. Korfel A, Schlegel U. Diagnosis and treatment of primary CNS lymphoma. Nat Rev Neurol. 2013 Jun;9(6):317–27. PMID:23670107

1710. Korfel A, Weller M, Martus P, et al. Prognostic impact of meningeal dissemination in primary CNS lymphoma (PCNSL): experience from the G-PCNSL-SG1 trial. Ann Oncol. 2012 Sep;23(9):2374–80. PMID:22396446

1711. Kornreich L, Blaser S, Schwarz M, et al. Optic pathway glioma: correlation of imaging findings with the presence of neurofibromatosis. AJNR Am J Neuroradiol. 2001 Nov-Dec;22(10):1963–9. PMID:11733333

1712. Korpershoek E, Favier J, Gaal J, et al. SDHA immunohistochemistry detects germline SDHA gene mutations in apparently sporadic paragangliomas and pheochromocytomas. J Clin Endocrinol Metab. 2011 Sep;96(9):E1472–6. PMID:21752896

1713. Korshunov A, Capper D, Reuss D, et al. Histologically distinct neuroepithelial tumors with histone 3 G34 mutation are molecularly similar and comprise a single nosologic entity. Acta Neuropathol. 2016 Jan;131(1):137–46. PMID:26482474

1714. Korshunov A, Casalini B, Chavez L, et al. Integrated molecular characterization of IDH-mutant glioblastomas. Neuropathol Appl Neurobiol. 2019 Feb;45(2):108–18. PMID:30326163

1715. Korshunov A, Chavez L, Northcott PA, et al. DNA-methylation profiling discloses significant advantages over NanoString method for molecular classification of medulloblastoma.

1716. Korshunov A, Chavez L, Sharma T, et al. Epithelioid glioblastomas stratify into established diagnostic subsets upon integrated molecular analysis. Brain Pathol. 2018 Sep;28(5):656–62. PMID:28990704

1717. Korshunov A, Golanov A. The prognostic significance of DNA topoisomerase II-alpha (Ki-S1), p21/Cip-1, and p27/Kip-1 protein immunoexpression in oligodendrogliomas. Arch Pathol Lab Med. 2001 Jul;125(7):892–8. PMID:11419973

1718. Korshunov A, Okonechnikov K, Sahm F, et al. Molecular progression of SHH-activated medulloblastomas. Acta Neuropathol. 2019 Aug;138(2):327–30. PMID:31030238

1719. Korshunov A, Okonechnikov K. Sahm F, et al. Transcriptional profiling of medulloblastoma with extensive nodularity (MBEN) reveals two clinically relevant tumor subsets with VSNL1 as potent prognostic marker. Acta Neuropathol. 2020 Mar;139(3):583–96. PMID:31781912

1720. Korshunov A, Remke M, Werft W, et al. Adult and pediatric medulloblastomas are genetically distinct and require different algorithms for molecular risk stratification. J Clin Oncol. 2010 Jun 20;28(18):3054–60. PMID:20479417

1721. Korshunov A, Ryzhova M, Hovestadt V, et al. Integrated analysis of pediatric glioblastoma reveals a subset of biologically favorable tumors with associated molecular prognostic markers. Acta Neuropathol. 2015 May;129(5):669–78. PMID:25752754

1722. Korshunov A, Sahm F, Okonechnikov K, et al. Desmoplastic/nodular medulloblastoma (DNMB) and medulloblastoma with extensive nodularity (MBEN) disclose similar epigenetic signatures but different transcriptional profiles. Acta Neuropathol. 2019 Jun;137(6):1003–15. PMID:30826918

1723. Korshunov A, Schrimpf D, Ryzhova M, et al. H3-/IDH-wild type pediatric glioblastoma is comprised of molecularly and prognostically distinct subtypes with associated oncogenic drivers. Acta Neuropathol. 2017 Sep;134(3):507–16. PMID:28401334

1724. Korshunov A, Shishkina L, Golanov A. Immunohistochemical analysis of p16INK4a, p14ARF, p18INK4c, p21CIP1, p27KIP1 and p73 expression in 271 meningiomas correlation with tumor grade and clinical outcome. Int J Cancer. 2003 May 10;104(6):728–34. PMID:12640680

1725. Korshunov A, Sturm D, Ryzhova M, et al. Embryonal tumor with abundant neuropil and true rosettes (ETANTR), ependymoblastoma, and medulloepithelioma share molecular similarity and comprise a single clinicopathological entity. Acta Neuropathol. 2014 Aug;128(2):279–89. PMID:24337497

1726. Korshunov A, Sycheva R, Golanov A. Recurrent cytogenetic aberrations in central neurocytomas and their biological relevance. Acta Neuropathol. 2007 Mar;113(3):303–12. PMID:17123091

1727. Kotler E, Segal E, Oren M. Functional characterization of the p53 "mutome". Mol Cell Oncol. 2018 Sep 25;5(6):e1511207. PMID:30525089

1728. Koubaa Mahjoub W, Jouini R, Khanchel F, et al. Neuroblastoma-like schwannoma with giant rosette: a potential diagnostic pitfall for hyalinizing spindle cell tumor. J Cutan Pathol. 2019 Mar;46(3):234–7. PMID:30582192

1729. Koutourousiou M, Georgakoulias N, Kontogeorgos G, et al. Subependymomas of the lateral ventricle: tumor recurrence correlated with increased Ki-67 labeling index. Neurol India. 2009 Mar-Apr;57(2):191–3. PMID:19439853

1730. Kozak KR, Mahadevan A, Moody JS. Adult gliosarcoma: epidemiology, natural history, and factors associated with outcome. Neuro Oncol. 2009 Apr;11(2):183–91. PMID:18780813

1731. Kozak KR, Moody JS. Giant cell glioblastoma: a glioblastoma subtype with distinct epidemiology and superior prognosis. Neuro Oncol. 2009 Dec;11(6):833–41. PMID:19332771

1732. Kraan W, Horlings HM, van Keimpema M, et al. High prevalence of oncogenic MYD88 and CD79B mutations in diffuse large B-cell lymphomas presenting at immune-privileged sites. Blood Cancer J. 2013 Sep 6;3:e139. PMID:24013661

1733. Kratz CP, Achatz MI, Brugières L, et al. Cancer screening recommendations for individuals with Li-Fraumeni syndrome. Clin Cancer Res. 2017 Jun 1;23(11):e38–45. PMID:28572266

1734. Kraus JA, Lamszus K, Glesmann N, et al. Molecular genetic alterations in glioblastomas with oligodendroglial component. Acta Neuropathol. 2001 Apr;101(4):311–20. PMID:11355302

1735. Krauss T, Ferrara AM, Links TP, et al. Preventive medicine of von Hippel-Lindau disease-associated pancreatic neuroendocrine tumors. Endocr Relat Cancer. 2018 Sep;25(9):783–93. PMID:29748190

1736. Kreutzer J, Vance ML, Lopes MB, et al. Surgical management of GH-secreting pituitary adenomas: an outcome study using modern remission criteria. J Clin Endocrinol Metab. 2001 Sep;86(9):4072–7. PMID:11549628

1737. Krieg M, Marti HH, Plate KH. Coexpression of erythropoietin and vascular endothelial growth factor in nervous system tumors associated with von Hippel-Lindau tumor suppressor gene loss of function. Blood. 1998 Nov 1;92(9):3388–93. PMID:9787178

1738. Krishnan S, Brown PD, Scheithauer BW, et al. Choroid plexus papillomas: a single institutional experience. J Neurooncol. 2004 May;68(1):49–55. PMID:15174521

1739. Krishnatry R, Zhukova N, Guerreiro Stucklin AS, et al. Clinical and treatment factors determining long-term outcomes for adult survivors of childhood low-grade glioma: a population-based study. Cancer. 2016 Apr 15;122(8):1261–9. PMID:26970559

1740. Kristensen MH, Nielsen S, Vyberg M. Thyroid transcription factor-1 in primary CNS tumors. Appl Immunohistochem Mol Morphol. 2011 Oct;19(5):437–43. PMID:21325940

1741. Krokker L, Nyírő G, Reiniger L, et al. Differentially expressed miRNAs influence metabolic processes in pituitary oncocytoma. Neurochem Res. 2019 Oct;44(10):2360–71. PMID:30945144

1742. Kros JM, Delwel EJ, de Jong TH, et al. Desmoplastic infantile astrocytoma and ganglioglioma: a search for genomic characteristics. Acta Neuropathol. 2002 Aug;104(2):144–8. PMID:12111357

1743. Kros JM, van den Brink WA, van Loon-van Luyt JJ, et al. Signet-ring cell oligodendroglioma—report of two cases and discussion of the differential diagnosis. Acta Neuropathol. 1997 Jun;93(6):638–43. PMID:9194905

1744. Krouwer HG, Davis RL, Silver P, et al. Gemistocytic astrocytomas: a reappraisal. J Neurosurg. 1991 Mar;74(3):399–406. PMID:1993905

1745. Krueger DA, Northrup H, International Tuberous Sclerosis Complex Consensus Group. Tuberous sclerosis complex surveillance and management: recommendations of the 2012 International Tuberous Sclerosis Complex Consensus Conference. Pediatr Neurol. 2013 Oct;49(4):255–65. PMID:24053983

1746. Krutilkova V, Trkova M, Fleitz J, et al. Identification of five new families strengthens the link between childhood choroid plexus carcinoma and germline TP53 mutations. Eur J Cancer. 2005 Jul;41(11):1597–603. PMID:15925506

1747. Kubo O, Oasahara A, Tajika Y, et al. Pleomorphic xanthoastrocytoma with neurofibromatosis type 1: case report. Noshuyo Byori. 1996 Apr;13(1):79–83. PMID:8916131

1748. Kubota T, Hayashi M, Yamamoto S. Primary intracranial mesenchymal chondrosarcoma: case report with review of the literature. Neurosurgery. 1982 Jan;10(1):105–10. PMID:7057966

1749. Kubota T, Sato K, Arishima H, et al. Astroblastoma: immunohistochemical and ultrastructural study of distinctive epithelial and probable tanycytic differentiation. Neuropathology. 2006 Feb;26(1):72–81. PMID:16521483

1750. Kuchelmeister K, Hügens-Penzel M, Jödicke A, et al. Papillary tumour of the pineal region: histodiagnostic considerations. Neuropathol Appl Neurobiol. 2006 Apr;32(2):203–8. PMID:16599948

1751. Kuchelmeister K, von Borcke IM, Klein H, et al. Pleomorphic pineocytoma with extensive neuronal differentiation: report of two cases. Acta Neuropathol. 1994;88(5):448–53. PMID:7847074

1752. Kuentz P, St-Onge J, Duffourd Y, et al. Molecular diagnosis of PIK3CA-related overgrowth spectrum (PROS) in 162 patients and recommendations for genetic testing. Genet Med. 2017 Sep;19(9):989–97. PMID:28151489

1753. Kuhlmann T, Lassmann H, Brück W. Diagnosis of inflammatory demyelination in biopsy specimens: a practical approach. Acta Neuropathol. 2008 Mar;115(3):275–87. PMID:18175128

1754. Kujas M, Faillot T, Lalam T, et al. Astroblastomas revisited. Report of two cases with immunocytochemical and electron microscopic study. Histogenetic considerations. Neuropathol Appl Neurobiol. 2000 Jun;26(3):295–8. PMID:10866687

1755. Küker W, Nägele T, Korfel A, et al. Primary central nervous system lymphomas (PCNSL): MRI features at presentation in 100 patients. J Neurooncol. 2005 Apr;72(2):169–77. PMID:15925998

1756. Kulac I, Tihan T. Pilomyxoid astrocytomas: a short review. Brain Tumor Pathol. 2019 Apr;36(2):52–5. PMID:30945015

1757. Kumar R, Liu APY, Northcott PA. Medulloblastoma genomics in the modern molecular era. Brain Pathol. 2020 May;30(3):679–90. PMID:31799776

1758. Kumar RM, Finn M. Primary multifocal gliosarcoma of the spinal cord. Rare Tumors. 2016 Mar 21;8(1):6102. PMID:27134708

1759. Kumar S, Kumar D, Kaldjian EP, et al. Primary low-grade B-cell lymphoma of the dura: a mucosa associated lymphoid tissue-type lymphoma. Am J Surg Pathol. 1997 Jan;21(1):81–7. PMID:8990144

1760. Kuntegowdenahalli LC, Jacob LA, Komaranchath AS, et al. A rare case of primary anaplastic large cell lymphoma of the central nervous system. J Cancer Res Ther. 2015 Oct-Dec;11(4):943–5. PMID:26881551

1761. Kuo KL, Lin CL, Wu CH, et al. Meningeal melanocytoma associated with nevus of ota: analysis of twelve reported cases. World Neurosurg. 2019 Jul;127:e311–20. PMID:30904806

1762. Kuroki S, Akiyoshi M, Tokura M, et al. JMJD1C, a JmjC domain-containing protein, is required for long-term maintenance of male germ cells in mice. Biol Reprod. 2013 Oct 17;89(4):93. PMID:24006281

1763. Kurosaki M, Saeger W, Lüdecke DK. Immunohistochemical localisation of

cytokeratins in craniopharyngioma. Acta Neurochir (Wien). 2001;143(2):147–51. PMID:11459086
1764. Kurose K, Araki T, Matsunaka T, et al. Variant manifestation of Cowden disease in Japan: hamartomatous polyposis of the digestive tract with mutation of the PTEN gene. Am J Hum Genet. 1999 Jan;64(1):308–10. PMID:9915974
1765. Kurt E, Zheng PP, Hop WC, et al. Identification of relevant prognostic histopathologic features in 69 intracranial ependymomas, excluding myxopapillary ependymomas and subependymomas. Cancer. 2006 Jan 15;106(2):388–95. PMID:16342252
1766. Kurtkaya-Yapicier O, Scheithauer BW, Woodruff JM, et al. Schwannoma with rhabdomyoblastic differentiation: a unique variant of malignant triton tumor. Am J Surg Pathol. 2003 Jun;27(6):848–53. PMID:12766593
1767. Kurtulmus N, Mert M, Tanakol R, et al. The pituitary gland in patients with Langerhans cell histiocytosis: a clinical and radiological evaluation. Endocrine. 2015 Apr;48(3):949–56. PMID:25209890
1768. Kurzwelly D, Glas M, Roth P, et al. Primary CNS lymphoma in the elderly: temozolomide therapy and MGMT status. J Neurooncol. 2010 May;97(3):389–92. PMID:19841864
1769. Küsters-Vandevelde HV, Creytens D, van Engen-van Grunsven AC, et al. SF3B1 and EIF1AX mutations occur in primary leptomeningeal melanocytic neoplasms; yet another similarity to uveal melanomas. Acta Neuropathol Commun. 2016 Jan 15;4:5. PMID:26769193
1770. Küsters-Vandevelde HV, Klaasen A, Küsters B, et al. Activating mutations of the GNAQ gene: a frequent event in primary melanocytic neoplasms of the central nervous system. Acta Neuropathol. 2010 Mar;119(3):317–23. PMID:19936769
1771. Küsters-Vandevelde HV, Kruse V, Van Maerken T, et al. Copy number variation analysis and methylome profiling of a GNAQ-mutant primary meningeal melanocytic tumor and its liver metastasis. Exp Mol Pathol. 2017 Feb;102(1):25–31. PMID:27974237
1772. Küsters-Vandevelde HV, Küsters B, van Engen-van Grunsven AC, et al. Primary melanocytic tumors of the central nervous system: a review with focus on molecular aspects. Brain Pathol. 2015 Mar;25(2):209–26. PMID:25534128
1773. Küsters-Vandevelde HV, van Engen-van Grunsven IA, Coupland SE, et al. Mutations in g protein encoding genes and chromosomal alterations in primary leptomeningeal melanocytic neoplasms. Pathol Oncol Res. 2015 Apr;21(2):439–47. PMID:25315378
1774. Küsters-Vandevelde HV, van Engen-van Grunsven IA, Küsters B, et al. Improved discrimination of melanotic schwannoma from melanocytic lesions by combined morphological and GNAQ mutational analysis. Acta Neuropathol. 2010 Dec;120(6):755–64. PMID:20865267
1775. Kuznetsov JN, Aguero TH, Owens DA, et al. BAP1 regulates epigenetic switch from pluripotency to differentiation in developmental lineages giving rise to BAP1-mutant cancers. Sci Adv. 2019 Sep 18;5(9):eaax1738. PMID:31555735
1776. Kwon CH, Zhu X, Zhang J, et al. Pten regulates neuronal soma size: a mouse model of Lhermitte-Duclos disease. Nat Genet. 2001 Dec;29(4):404–11. PMID:11726927
1777. La Corte E, Younus I, Pivari F, et al. BRAF V600E mutant papillary craniopharyngiomas: a single-institutional case series. Pituitary. 2018 Dec;21(6):571–83. PMID:30187175
1778. Labreche K, Simeonova I, Kamoun A, et al. TCF12 is mutated in anaplastic oligodendroglioma. Nat Commun. 2015 Jun 12;6:7207. PMID:26068201
1779. Labussière M, Boisselier B, Mokhtari K, et al. Combined analysis of TERT, EGFR, and IDH status defines distinct prognostic glioblastoma classes. Neurology. 2014 Sep 23;83(13):1200–6. PMID:25150284
1780. Labussière M, Di Stefano AL, Gleize V, et al. TERT promoter mutations in gliomas, genetic associations and clinico-pathological correlations. Br J Cancer. 2014 Nov 11;111(10):2024–32. PMID:25314060
1781. Lachenal F, Cotton F, Desmurs-Clavel H, et al. Neurological manifestations and neuroradiological presentation of Erdheim-Chester disease: report of 6 cases and systematic review of the literature. J Neurol. 2006 Oct;253(10):1267–77. PMID:17063320
1782. Lack EE. Paragangliomas. In: Sternberg SS, editor. Diagnostic surgical pathology. 2nd ed. New York (NY): Raven Press; 1994. pp. 559–621.
1783. Lafay-Cousin L, Bouffet E, Strother D, et al. Phase II study of nonmetastatic desmoplastic medulloblastoma in children younger than 4 years of age: a report of the Children's Oncology Group (ACNS1221). J Clin Oncol. 2020 Jan 20;38(3):223–31. PMID:31774708
1784. Lafay-Cousin L, Hader W, Wei XC, et al. Post-chemotherapy maturation in supratentorial primitive neuroectodermal tumors. Brain Pathol. 2014 Mar;24(2):166–72. PMID:24033491
1785. Lafay-Cousin L, Hawkins C, Carret AS, et al. Central nervous system atypical teratoid rhabdoid tumours: the Canadian Paediatric Brain Tumour Consortium experience. Eur J Cancer. 2012 Feb;48(3):353–9. PMID:22023887
1786. Lafay-Cousin L, Keene D, Carret AS, et al. Choroid plexus tumors in children less than 36 months: the Canadian Pediatric Brain Tumor Consortium (CPBTC) experience. Childs Nerv Syst. 2011 Feb;27(2):259–64. PMID:20809071
1787. Laghari AA, Javed G, Khan MF, et al. Spontaneous intraventricular hemorrhage: a rare presentation of a skull base mesenchymal chondrosarcoma. World Neurosurg. 2017 Mar;99:811.e1–5. PMID:28042016
1788. Laguesse S, Creppe C, Nedialkova DD, et al. A dynamic unfolded protein response contributes to the control of cortical neurogenesis. Dev Cell. 2015 Dec 7;35(5):553–67. PMID:26651292
1789. Lai A, Kharbanda S, Pope WB, et al. Evidence for sequenced molecular evolution of IDH1 mutant glioblastoma from a distinct cell of origin. J Clin Oncol. 2011 Dec 1;29(34):4482–90. PMID:22025148
1790. Laigle-Donadey F, Martin-Duverneuil N, Lejeune J, et al. Correlations between molecular profile and radiologic pattern in oligodendroglial tumors. Neurology. 2004 Dec 28;63(12):2360–2. PMID:15623700
1791. Laigle-Donadey F, Taillibert S, Mokhtari K, et al. Dural metastases. J Neurooncol. 2005 Oct;75(1):57–61. PMID:16215816
1792. Lake JA, Donson AM, Prince E, et al. Targeted fusion analysis can aid in the classification and treatment of pediatric glioma, ependymoma, and glioneuronal tumors. Pediatr Blood Cancer. 2020 Jan;67(1):e28028. PMID:31595628
1793. Lal A, Dahiya S, Gonzales M, et al. IgG4 overexpression is rare in meningiomas with a prominent inflammatory component: a review of 16 cases. Brain Pathol. 2014 Jul;24(4):352–9. PMID:24467316
1794. Lam SW, Cleton-Jansen AM, Cleven AHG, et al. Molecular analysis of gene fusions in bone and soft tissue tumors by anchored multiplex PCR-based targeted next-generation sequencing. J Mol Diagn. 2018 Sep;20(5):653–63. PMID:30139549
1795. Lambert SR, Witt H, Hovestadt V, et al. Differential expression and methylation of brain developmental genes define location-specific subsets of pilocytic astrocytoma. Acta Neuropathol. 2013 Aug;126(2):291–301. PMID:23660940
1796. Lambiv WL, Vassallo I, Delorenzi M, et al. The Wnt inhibitory factor 1 (WIF1) is targeted in glioblastoma and has a tumor suppressing function potentially by induction of senescence. Neuro Oncol. 2011 Jul;13(7):736–47. PMID:21642372
1797. Lambo S, Gröbner SN, Rausch T, et al. The molecular landscape of ETMR at diagnosis and relapse. Nature. 2019 Dec;576(7786):274–80. PMID:31802000
1798. Lambo S, von Hoff K, Korshunov A, et al. ETMR: a tumor entity in its infancy. Acta Neuropathol. 2020 Sep;140(3):249–66. PMID:32601913
1799. Lamzabi I, Arvanitis LD, Reddy VB, et al. Immunophenotype of myxopapillary ependymomas. Appl Immunohistochem Mol Morphol. 2013 Dec;21(6):485–9. PMID:23455181
1800. Landis CA, Masters SB, Spada A, et al. GTPase inhibiting mutations activate the alpha chain of Gs and stimulate adenylyl cyclase in human pituitary tumours. Nature. 1989 Aug 31;340(6236):692–6. PMID:2549426
1801. Lang FF, Epstein FJ, Ransohoff J, et al. Central nervous system gangliogliomas. Part 2: clinical outcome. J Neurosurg. 1993 Dec;79(6):867–73. PMID:8246055
1802. Lang SS, Beslow LA, Gabel B, et al. Surgical treatment of brain tumors in infants younger than six months of age and review of the literature. World Neurosurg. 2012 Jul;78(1-2):137–44. PMID:22120270
1803. Larkin SJ, Preda V, Karavitaki N, et al. BRAF V600E mutations are characteristic for papillary craniopharyngioma and may coexist with CTNNB1-mutated adamantinomatous craniopharyngioma. Acta Neuropathol. 2014;127(6):927–9. PMID:24715106
1804. Larson JD, Kasper LH, Paugh BS, et al. Histone H3.3 K27M accelerates spontaneous brainstem glioma and drives restricted changes in bivalent gene expression. Cancer Cell. 2019 Jan 14;35(1):140–155.e7. PMID:30595505
1805. Lashner BA, Riddell RH, Winans CS. Ganglioneuromatosis of the colon and extensive glycogenic acanthosis in Cowden's disease. Dig Dis Sci. 1986 Feb;31(2):213–6. PMID:3943449
1806. Lassaletta A, Zapotocky M, Mistry M, et al. Therapeutic and prognostic implications of BRAF V600E in pediatric low-grade gliomas. J Clin Oncol. 2017 Sep 1;35(25):2934–41. PMID:28727518
1807. Lassaletta L, Torres-Martín M, Peña-Granero C, et al. NF2 genetic alterations in sporadic vestibular schwannomas: clinical implications. Otol Neurotol. 2013 Sep;34(7):1355–61. PMID:23921927
1808. Łastowska M, Trubicka J, Sobocińska A, et al. Molecular identification of CNS NB-FOXR2, CNS EFT-CIC, CNS HGNET-MN1 and CNS HGNET-BCOR pediatric brain tumors using tumor-specific signature genes. Acta Neuropathol Commun. 2020 Jul 10;8(1):105. PMID:32650833
1809. Latta S, Myint ZW, Jallad B, et al. Primary central nervous system T-cell lymphoma in aids patients: case report and literature review. Curr Oncol. 2010 Oct;17(5):63–6. PMID:20975881
1810. Latysheva A, Emblem KE, Brandal P, et al. Dynamic susceptibility contrast and diffusion MR imaging identify oligodendroglioma as defined by the 2016 WHO classification for brain tumors: histogram analysis approach. Neuroradiology. 2019 May;61(5):545–55. PMID:30712139
1811. Lau D, La Marca F, Camelo-Piragua S, et al. Metastatic paraganglioma of the spine: case report and review of the literature. Clin Neurol Neurosurg. 2013 Sep;115(9):1571–4. PMID:23398849
1812. Lau SK, Cykowski MD, Desai S, et al. Primary rhabdomyosarcoma of the pineal gland. Am J Clin Pathol. 2015 May;143(5):728–33. PMID:25873508
1813. Launbjerg K, Bache I, Galanakis M, et al. von Hippel-Lindau development in children and adolescents. Am J Med Genet A. 2017 Sep;173(9):2381–94. PMID:28650583
1814. Lauretta R, Sansone A, Sansone M, et al. Endocrine disrupting chemicals: effects on endocrine glands. Front Endocrinol (Lausanne). 2019 Mar 21;10:178. PMID:30984107
1815. Le BH, Towfighi J, Kapadia SB, et al. Comparative immunohistochemical assessment of craniopharyngioma and related lesions. Endocr Pathol. 2007 Spring;18(1):23–30. PMID:17652797
1816. Le DT, Uram JN, Wang H, et al. PD-1 Blockade in tumors with mismatch-repair deficiency. N Engl J Med. 2015 Jun 25;372(26):2509–20. PMID:26028255
1817. Le Guellec S, Decouvelaere AV, Filleron T, et al. Malignant peripheral nerve sheath tumor is a challenging diagnosis: a systematic pathology review, immunohistochemistry, and molecular analysis in 160 patients from the French Sarcoma Group database. Am J Surg Pathol. 2016 Jul;40(7):896–908. PMID:27158754
1818. Le Loarer F, Pissaloux D, Watson S, et al. Clinicopathologic features of CIC-NUTM1 sarcomas, a new molecular variant of the family of CIC-fused sarcomas. Am J Surg Pathol. 2019 Feb;43(2):268–76. PMID:30407212
1819. Le LQ, Shipman T, Burns DK, et al. Cell of origin and microenvironment contribution for NF1-associated dermal neurofibromas. Cell Stem Cell. 2009 May 8;4(5):453–63. PMID:19427294
1820. Le Rhun E, Devos P, Boulanger T, et al. The RANO Leptomeningeal Metastasis Group proposal to assess response to treatment: lack of feasibility and clinical utility and a revised proposal. Neuro Oncol. 2019 May 6;21(5):648–58. PMID:30715514
1821. Le Rhun E, Preusser M, Roth P, et al. Molecular targeted therapy of glioblastoma. Cancer Treat Rev. 2019 Nov;80:101896. PMID:31541850
1822. Le Rhun E, Weller M, Brandsma D, et al. EANO-ESMO Clinical Practice Guidelines for diagnosis, treatment and follow-up of patients with leptomeningeal metastasis from solid tumours. Ann Oncol. 2017 Jul 1;28 (suppl_4):iv84–99. PMID:28881917
1823. LeBlanc VG, Firme M, Song J, et al. Comparative transcriptome analysis of isogenic cell line models and primary cancers links capicua (CIC) loss to activation of the MAPK signalling cascade. J Pathol. 2017 Jun;242(2):206–20. PMID:28295365
1824. Lebrun C, Fontaine D, Ramaioli A, et al. Long-term outcome of oligodendrogliomas. Neurology. 2004 May 25;62(10):1783–7. PMID:15159478
1825. Lechapt-Zalcman E, Chapon F, Guillamo JS, et al. Long-term clinicopathological observations on a papillary tumour of the pineal region. Neuropathol Appl Neurobiol. 2011 Jun;37(4):431–5. PMID:20942871
1826. Lee CH, Jung KW, Yoo H, et al. Epidemiology of primary brain and central nervous system tumors in Korea. J Korean Neurosurg Soc. 2010 Aug;48(2):145–52. PMID:20856664
1827. Lee CH, Yu JR, Granat J, et al. Automethylation of PRC2 promotes H3K27 methylation

and is impaired in H3K27M pediatric glioma. Genes Dev. 2019 Oct 1;33(19-20):1428–40. PMID:31488577

1828. Lee D, Cho YH, Kang SY, et al. BRAF V600E mutations are frequent in dysembryoplastic neuroepithelial tumors and subependymal giant cell astrocytomas. J Surg Oncol. 2015 Mar;111(3):359–64. PMID:25346165

1829. Lee EB, Tihan T, Scheithauer BW, et al. Thyroid transcription factor 1 expression in sellar tumors: a histogenetic marker? J Neuropathol Exp Neurol. 2009 May;68(5):482–8. PMID:19525896

1830. Lee EQ. Nervous system metastases from systemic cancer. Continuum (Minneap Minn). 2015 Apr;21(2 Neuro-oncology):415–28. PMID:25837904

1831. Lee HJ, Wu CC, Wu HM, et al. Pretreatment diagnosis of suprasellar papillary craniopharyngioma and germ cell tumors of adult patients. AJNR Am J Neuroradiol. 2015 Mar;36(3):508–17. PMID:25339645

1832. Lee HY, Yoon CS, Sevenet N, et al. Rhabdoid tumor of the kidney is a component of the rhabdoid predisposition syndrome. Pediatr Dev Pathol. 2002 Jul-Aug;5(4):395–9. PMID:12016529

1833. Lee J, Putnam AR, Chesier SH, et al. Oligodendrogliomas, IDH-mutant and 1p/19q-codeleted, arising during teenage years often lack TERT promoter mutation that is typical of their adult counterparts. Acta Neuropathol Commun. 2018 Sep 19;6(1):95. PMID:30231927

1834. Lee JC, Mazor T, Lao R, et al. Recurrent KBTBD4 small in-frame insertions and absence of DROSHA deletion or DICER1 mutation differentiate pineal parenchymal tumor of intermediate differentiation (PPTID) from pineoblastoma. Acta Neuropathol. 2019 May;137(5):851–4. PMID:30877433

1835. Lee JC, Sharifai N, Dahiya S, et al. Clinicopathologic features of anaplastic myxopapillary ependymomas. Brain Pathol. 2019 Jan;29(1):75–84. PMID:30417460

1836. Lee JC, Villanueva-Meyer JE, Ferris SP, et al. Primary intracranial sarcomas with DICER1 mutation often contain prominent eosinophilic cytoplasmic globules and can occur in the setting of neurofibromatosis type 1. Acta Neuropathol. 2019 Mar;137(3):521–5. PMID:30649606

1837. Lee JH, Lee JE, Kahng JY, et al. Human glioblastoma arises from subventricular zone cells with low-level driver mutations. Nature. 2018 Aug;560(7717):243–7. PMID:30069053

1837A. Lee JY, Dong SM, Park WS, et al. Loss of heterozygosity and somatic mutations of the VHL tumor suppressor gene in sporadic cerebellar hemangioblastomas. Cancer Res. 1998 Feb 1;58(3):504–8. PMID:9458097

1838. Lee JY, Wakabayashi T, Yoshida J. Management and survival of pineoblastoma: an analysis of 34 adults from the brain tumor registry of Japan. Neurol Med Chir (Tokyo). 2005 Mar;45(3):132–41. PMID:15782004

1839. Lee LH, Bos GD, Marsh WL Jr, et al. Fine-needle aspiration cytology of sclerosing perineurioma. Ann Diagn Pathol. 2004 Apr;8(2):80–6. PMID:15060885

1840. Lee RS, Stewart C, Carter SL, et al. A remarkably simple genome underlies highly malignant pediatric rhabdoid cancers. J Clin Invest. 2012 Aug;122(8):2983–8. PMID:22797305

1841. Lee S, Kim NR, Chung DH, et al. Squash cytology of a dural-based high-grade chondrosarcoma may mimic that of glioblastoma in the central nervous system. Acta Cytol. 2015;59(2):219–24. PMID:25997403

1842. Lee W, Teckie S, Wiesner T, et al. PRC2 is recurrently inactivated through EED or SUZ12 loss in malignant peripheral nerve sheath tumors. Nat Genet. 2014 Nov;46(11):1227–32. PMID:25240281

1843. Lee YR, Yehia L, Kishikawa T, et al. WWP1 gain-of-function inactivation of PTEN in cancer predisposition. N Engl J Med. 2020 May 28;382(22):2103–16. PMID:32459922

1844. Leeds NE, Lang FF, Ribalta T, et al. Origin of chordoid glioma of the third ventricle. Arch Pathol Lab Med. 2006 Apr;130(4):460–4. PMID:16594739

1845. Leenstra JL, Rodriguez FJ, Frechette CM, et al. Central neurocytoma: management recommendations based on a 35-year experience. Int J Radiat Oncol Biol Phys. 2007 Mar 15;67(4):1145–54. PMID:17187939

1846. Legius E, Marchuk DA, Collins FS, et al. Somatic deletion of the neurofibromatosis type 1 gene in a neurofibrosarcoma supports a tumour suppressor gene hypothesis. Nat Genet. 1993 Feb;3(2):122–6. PMID:8499945

1847. Lehman NL, Horoupian DS, Warnke RA, et al. Dural marginal zone lymphoma with massive amyloid deposition: rare low-grade primary central nervous system B-cell lymphoma. Case report. J Neurosurg. 2002 Feb;96(2):368–72. PMID:11838814

1848. Lehman NL, Usubalieva A, Lin T, et al. Genomic analysis demonstrates that histologically-defined astroblastomas are molecularly heterogeneous and that tumors with MN1 rearrangement exhibit the most favorable prognosis. Acta Neuropathol Commun. 2019 Mar 15;7(1):42. PMID:30876455

1849. Leiden University Medical Center. LOVD v.3.0 - Leiden Open Variation Database [Internet]. Leiden (Netherlands): Leiden University Medical Center; 2021. The TSC1 gene homepage; updated 2021 Mar 9. Available from: https://databases.lovd.nl/shared/genes/TSC1.

1850. Leiden University Medical Center. LOVD v.3.0 - Leiden Open Variation Database [Internet]. Leiden (Netherlands): Leiden University Medical Center; 2021. The TSC2 gene homepage; updated 2021 Mar 9. Available from: https://databases.lovd.nl/shared/genes/TSC2.

1851. Lekanne Deprez RH, Riegman PH, van Drunen E, et al. Cytogenetic, molecular genetic and pathological analyses in 126 meningiomas. J Neuropathol Exp Neurol. 1995 Mar;54(2):224–35. PMID:7876890

1852. Lellouch-Tubiana A, Boddaert N, Bourgeois M, et al. Angiocentric neuroepithelial tumor (ANET): a new epilepsy-related clinicopathological entity with distinctive MRI. Brain Pathol. 2005 Oct;15(4):281–6. PMID:16389940

1853. Lellouch-Tubiana A, Bourgeois M, Vekemans M, et al. Dysembryoplastic neuroepithelial tumors in two children with neurofibromatosis type 1. Acta Neuropathol. 1995;90(3):319–22. PMID:8525807

1854. Lelotte J, Mourin A, Fomekong E, et al. Both invasiveness and proliferation criteria predict recurrence of non-functioning pituitary macroadenomas after surgery: a retrospective analysis of a monocentric cohort of 120 patients. Eur J Endocrinol. 2018 Mar;178(3):237–46. PMID:29259039

1855. Leoz ML, Carballal S, Moreira L, et al. The genetic basis of familial adenomatous polyposis and its implications for clinical practice and risk management. Appl Clin Genet. 2015 Apr 16;8:95–107. PMID:25931827

1856. Leruste A, Tosello J, Ramos RN, et al. Clonally expanded T cells reveal immunogenicity of rhabdoid tumors. Cancer Cell. 2019 Dec 9;36(6):597–612.e8. PMID:31708437

1856A. Leske H, Dalgleish R, Lazar AJ, et al. A common classification framework for histone sequence alterations in tumours: an expert consensus proposal. J Pathol. 2021 Jun;254(2):109–20. PMID:33779999

1857. Leske H, Rushing E, Budka H, et al. K27/G34 versus K28/G35 in histone H3-mutant gliomas: a note of caution. Acta Neuropathol. 2018 Jul;136(1):175–6. PMID:29766298

1858. Letouzé E, Martinelli C, Loriot C, et al. SDH mutations establish a hypermethylator phenotype in paraganglioma. Cancer Cell. 2013 Jun 10;23(6):739–52. PMID:23707781

1859. Levin N, Lavon I, Zelikovitsh B, et al. Progressive low-grade oligodendrogliomas: response to temozolomide and correlation between genetic profile and O6-methylguanine DNA methyltransferase protein expression. Cancer. 2006 Apr 15;106(8):1759–65. PMID:16541434

1860. Levine AJ. p53: 800 million years of evolution and 40 years of discovery. Nat Rev Cancer. 2020 Aug;20(8):471–80. PMID:32404993

1861. Levy RA. Paraganglioma of the filum terminale: MR findings. AJR Am J Roentgenol. 1993 Apr;160(4):851–2. PMID:8456679

1862. Lewis PW, Müller MM, Koletsky MS, et al. Inhibition of PRC2 activity by a gain-of-function H3 mutation found in pediatric glioblastoma. Science. 2013 May 17;340(6134):857–61. PMID:23539183

1863. Lhermitte J, Duclos P. Sur un ganglioneurome diffus du cortex du cervelet. Bull Assoc Fr Etud Cancer. 1920;9:99–107. French.

1864. Li B, Tao B, Bai H, et al. Papillary meningioma: an aggressive variant meningioma with clinical features and treatment: a retrospective study of 10 cases. Int J Neurosci. 2016 Oct;126(10):878–87. PMID:26299848

1865. Li BK, Vasiljevic A, Dufour C, et al. Pineoblastoma segregates into molecular subgroups with distinct clinico-pathologic features: a Rare Brain Tumor Consortium registry study. Acta Neuropathol. 2020 Feb;139(2):223–41. PMID:31820118

1866. Li D, Fu F, Lian L. Primary central nervous system extranodal nasal-type natural killer/T-cell lymphoma with CD20 expression. Neuropathology. 2018 Apr;38(2):198–204. PMID:29063643

1867. Li D, Wang JM, Li GL, et al. Clinical, radiological, and pathological features of 16 papillary glioneuronal tumors. Acta Neurochir (Wien). 2014 Apr;156(4):627–39. PMID:24553727

1868. Li DM, Sun H. TEP1, encoded by a candidate tumor suppressor locus, is a novel protein tyrosine phosphatase regulated by transforming growth factor beta. Cancer Res. 1997 Jun 1;57(11):2124–9. PMID:9187108

1869. Li FP, Fraumeni JF Jr, Mulvihill JJ, et al. A cancer family syndrome in twenty-four kindreds. Cancer Res. 1988 Sep 15;48(18):5358–62. PMID:3409256

1870. Li J, Liang R, Song C, et al. Prognostic significance of epidermal growth factor receptor expression in glioma patients. Onco Targets Ther. 2018 Feb 7;11:701–12. PMID:29445288

1871. Li J, Simpson L, Takahashi M, et al. The PTEN/MMAC1 tumor suppressor induces cell death that is rescued by the AKT/protein kinase B oncogene. Cancer Res. 1998 Dec 15;58(24):5667–72. PMID:9865719

1872. Li J, Yen C, Liaw D, et al. PTEN, a putative protein tyrosine phosphatase gene mutated in human brain, breast, and prostate cancer. Science. 1997 Mar 28;275(5308):1943–7. PMID:9072974

1873. Li JY, Langford LA, Adesina A, et al. The high mitotic count detected by phospho-histone H3 immunostain does not alter the benign behavior of angiocentric glioma. Brain Tumor Pathol. 2012 Jan;29(1):68–72. PMID:21892765

1874. Li JY, Lopez JI, Powell SZ, et al. Giant cell ependymoma-report of three cases and review of the literature. Int J Clin Exp Pathol. 2012;5(5):458–62. PMID:22808300

1875. Li KK, Shi ZF, Malta TM, et al. Identification of subsets of IDH-mutant glioblastomas with distinct epigenetic and copy number alterations and stratified clinical risks. Neurooncol Adv. 2019 May-Dec;1(1):vdz015. PMID:31667475

1876. Li L, Grausam KB, Wang J, et al. Sonic hedgehog promotes proliferation of Notch-dependent monociliated choroid plexus tumour cells. Nat Cell Biol. 2016 Apr;18(4):418–30. PMID:26999738

1877. Li MM, Datto M, Duncavage EJ, et al. Standards and guidelines for the interpretation and reporting of sequence variants in cancer: a joint consensus recommendation of the Association for Molecular Pathology, American Society of Clinical Oncology, and College of American Pathologists. J Mol Diagn. 2017 Jan;19(1):4–23. PMID:27993330

1878. Li P, James SL, Evans N, et al. Paraganglioma of the cauda equina with subarachnoid haemorrhage. Clin Radiol. 2007 Mar;62(3):277–80. PMID:17293223

1879. Li W, Cooper J, Zhou L, et al. Merlin/NF2 loss-driven tumorigenesis linked to CRL4(DCAF1)-mediated inhibition of the hippo pathway kinases Lats1 and 2 in the nucleus. Cancer Cell. 2014 Jul 14;26(1):48–60. PMID:25026211

1880. Li X, Fisher OS, Boggon TJ. The cerebral cavernous malformations proteins. Oncotarget. 2015 Oct 20;6(32):32279–80. PMID:26356566

1881. Li Y, Chen SH, Sheinberg D, et al. Imaging characteristics of a hypervascular pituitary spindle cell oncocytoma on magnetic resonance imaging and digital subtraction angiography. World Neurosurg. 2020 Jan;133:56–9. PMID:31568904

1882. Li ZJ, Lan XL, Hao FY, et al. Primary cerebellar paraganglioma: a pediatric case report and review of the literature. Pediatr Neurol. 2014 Apr;50(4):303–6. PMID:24485927

1883. Lian F, Wang LM, Qi XL, et al. MYB-QKI rearrangement in angiocentric glioma. Clin Neuropathol. 2020 Nov/Dec;39(6):263–70. PMID:32589128

1884. Liang L, Korogi Y, Sugahara T, et al. MRI of intracranial germ-cell tumours. Neuroradiology. 2002 May;44(5):382–8. PMID:12012121

1885. Liang X, Shen D, Huang Y, et al. Molecular pathology and CXCR4 expression in surgically excised retinal hemangioblastomas associated with von Hippel-Lindau disease. Ophthalmology. 2007 Jan;114(1):147–56. PMID:17070589

1886. Liang Y, Heller RS, Wu JK, et al. High p16 expression is associated with malignancy and shorter disease-free survival time in solitary fibrous tumor/hemangiopericytoma. J Neurol Surg B Skull Base. 2019 Jun;80(3):232–8. PMID:31143564

1887. Liao CP, Booker RC, Brosseau JP, et al. Contributions of inflammation and tumor microenvironment to neurofibroma tumorigenesis. J Clin Invest. 2018 Jul 2;128(7):2848–61. PMID:29596064

1888. Liao CP, Pradhan S, Chen Z, et al. The role of nerve microenvironment for neurofibroma development. Oncotarget. 2016 Sep 20;7(38):61500–8. PMID:27517146

1889. Liaw D, Marsh DJ, Li J, et al. Germline mutations of the PTEN gene in Cowden disease, an inherited breast and thyroid cancer syndrome. Nat Genet. 1997 May;16(1):64–7. PMID:9140396

1890. Licis AK, Vallorani A, Gao F, et al. Prevalence of sleep disturbances in children with neurofibromatosis type 1. J Child Neurol. 2013 Nov;28(11):1400–5. PMID:24065580

1891. Liegl B, Bennett MW, Fletcher CD. Microcystic/reticular schwannoma: a distinct variant with predilection for visceral locations. Am J Surg Pathol. 2008 Jul;32(7):1080–7. PMID:18520439

1892. Ligon KL, Alberta JA, Kho AT, et al. The oligodendroglial lineage marker OLIG2 is universally expressed in diffuse gliomas. J Neuropathol Exp Neurol. 2004 May;63(5):499–509. PMID:15198128
1893. Lillard JC, Venable GT, Khan NR, et al. Pediatric supratentorial ependymoma: surgical, clinical, and molecular analysis. Neurosurgery. 2019 Jul 1;85(1):41–9. PMID:29917116
1894. Lim JS, Gopalappa R, Kim SH, et al. Somatic mutations in TSC1 and TSC2 cause focal cortical dysplasia. Am J Hum Genet. 2017 Mar 2;100(3):454–72. PMID:28215400
1895. Limaiem F, Bellil S, Chelly I, et al. Recurrent cerebellar liponeurocytoma with supratentorial extension. Can J Neurol Sci. 2009 Sep;36(5):662–5. PMID:19831141
1896. Lin FY, Bergstrom K, Person R, et al. Integrated tumor and germline whole-exome sequencing identifies mutations in MAPK and PI3K pathway genes in an adolescent with rosette-forming glioneuronal tumor of the fourth ventricle. Cold Spring Harb Mol Case Stud. 2016 Sep;2(5):a001057. PMID:27626068
1897. Lin KM, Lin SJ, Lin JH, et al. Dysregulation of dual-specificity phosphatases by Epstein-Barr virus LMP1 and its impact on lymphoblastoid cell line survival. J Virol. 2020 Jan 31;94(4):e01837-19. PMID:31776277
1898. Lin L, Varikatt W, Dexter M, et al. Diagnostic pitfall in the diagnosis of mesenchymal chondrosarcoma arising in the central nervous system. Neuropathology. 2012 Feb;32(1):82–90. PMID:21615516
1899. Lin LL, El Naqa I, Leonard JR, et al. Long-term outcome in children treated for craniopharyngioma with and without radiotherapy. J Neurosurg Pediatr. 2008 Feb;1(2):126–30. PMID:18352781
1900. Lin YJ, Yang QX, Tian XY, et al. Unusual primary intracranial dural-based poorly differentiated synovial sarcoma with t(X; 18)(p11; q11). Neuropathology. 2013 Feb;33(1):75–82. PMID:22537253
1901. Lindberg N, Jiang Y, Xie Y, et al. Oncogenic signaling is dominant to cell of origin and dictates astrocytic or oligodendroglial tumor development from oligodendrocyte precursor cells. J Neurosci. 2014 Oct 29;34(44):14644–51. PMID:25355217
1902. Lindeman NI, Cagle PT, Aisner DL, et al. Updated molecular testing guideline for the selection of lung cancer patients for treatment with targeted tyrosine kinase inhibitors: guideline from the College of American Pathologists, the International Association for the Study of Lung Cancer, and the Association for Molecular Pathology. J Thorac Oncol. 2018 Mar;13(3):323–58. PMID:29396253
1903. Lindsey JC, Schwalbe EC, Potluri S, et al. TERT promoter mutation and aberrant hypermethylation are associated with elevated expression in medulloblastoma and characterise the majority of non-infant SHH subgroup tumours. Acta Neuropathol. 2014 Feb;127(2):307–9. PMID:24337442
1904. Lindström E, Shimokawa T, Toftgård R, et al. PTCH mutations: distribution and analyses. Hum Mutat. 2006 Mar;27(3):215–9. PMID:16419085
1905. Linglart A, Menguy C, Couvineau A, et al. Recurrent PRKAR1A mutation in acrodysostosis with hormone resistance. N Engl J Med. 2011 Jun 9;364(23):2218–26. PMID:21651393
1906. Linnebank M, Moskau S, Kowoll A, et al. Association of transcobalamin c. 776C>G with overall survival in patients with primary central nervous system lymphoma. Br J Cancer. 2012 Nov 20;107(11):1840–3. PMID:23099805
1907. Linnebank M, Schmidt S, Kölsch H, et al. The methionine synthase polymorphism D919G alters susceptibility to primary central nervous system lymphoma. Br J Cancer. 2004 May 17;90(10):1969–71. PMID:15138479
1908. Lionakis MS, Dunleavy K, Roschewski M, et al. Inhibition of B cell receptor signaling by ibrutinib in primary CNS lymphoma. Cancer Cell. 2017 Jun 12;31(6):833–843.e5. PMID:28552327
1909. Lipper S, Decker RE. Paraganglioma of the cauda equina. A histologic, immunohistochemical, and ultrastructural study and review of the literature. Surg Neurol. 1984 Oct;22(4):415–20. PMID:6474349
1910. Lirng JF, Enterline DS, Tien RD, et al. MRI of papillary meningiomas in children. Pediatr Radiol. 1995 Nov;25 Suppl 1:S9–13. PMID:8577564
1911. Listernick R, Charrow J, Greenwald M, et al. Natural history of optic pathway tumors in children with neurofibromatosis type 1: a longitudinal study. J Pediatr. 1994 Jul;125(1):63–6. PMID:8021787
1912. Listernick R, Ferner RE, Liu GT, et al. Optic pathway gliomas in neurofibromatosis-1: controversies and recommendations. Ann Neurol. 2007 Mar;61(3):189–98. PMID:17387725
1913. Liu APY, Gudenas B, Lin T, et al. Risk-adapted therapy and biological heterogeneity in pineoblastoma: integrated clinico-pathological analysis from the prospective, multi-center SJMB03 and SJYC07 trials. Acta Neuropathol. 2020 Feb;139(2):259–71. PMID:31802236
1913A. Liu APY, Li BK, Pfaff E, et al. Clinical and molecular heterogeneity of pineal parenchymal tumors: a consensus study. Acta Neuropathol. 2021 May;141(5):771–85. PMID:33619588
1914. Liu APY, Priesterbach-Ackley LP, Orr BA, et al. WNT-activated embryonal tumors of the pineal region: ectopic medulloblastomas or a novel pineoblastoma subgroup? Acta Neuropathol. 2020 Oct;140(4):595–7. PMID:32772175
1915. Liu C, Sage JC, Miller MR, et al. Mosaic analysis with double markers reveals tumor cell of origin in glioma. Cell. 2011 Jul 22;146(2):209–21. PMID:21737130
1916. Liu XY, Gerges N, Korshunov A, et al. Frequent ATRX mutations and loss of expression in adult diffuse astrocytic tumors carrying IDH1/IDH2 and TP53 mutations. Acta Neuropathol. 2012 Nov;124(5):615–25. PMID:22886134
1917. Liubinas SV, Maartens N, Drummond KJ. Primary melanocytic neoplasms of the central nervous system. J Clin Neurosci. 2010 Oct;17(10):1227–32. PMID:20558070
1918. Lloyd KM 2nd, Dennis M. Cowden's disease. A possible new symptom complex with multiple system involvement. Ann Intern Med. 1963 Jan;58:136–42. PMID:13931122
1919. Lloyd RV, Osamura RY, Klöppel G, et al., editors. WHO classification of tumours of endocrine organs. Lyon (France): International Agency for Research on Cancer; 2017. (WHO classification of tumours series, 4th ed.; vol. 10). https://publications.iarc.fr/554.
1920. Loh JK, Lieu AS, Chai CY, et al. Malignant transformation of a desmoplastic infantile ganglioglioma. Pediatr Neurol. 2011 Aug;45(2):135–7. PMID:21763958
1921. Loke BN, Lee VKM, Sudhanshi J, et al. Novel exon-exon breakpoint in CIC-DUX4 fusion sarcoma identified by anchored multiplex PCR (Archer FusionPlex Sarcoma Panel). J Clin Pathol. 2017 Aug;70(8):697–701. PMID:28137728
1922. Longatti P, Basaldella L, Orvieto E, et al. Aquaporin 1 expression in cystic hemangioblastomas. Neurosci Lett. 2006 Jan 16;392(3):178–80. PMID:16300893
1923. Longo JF, Weber SM, Turner-Ivey BP, et al. Recent advances in the diagnosis and pathogenesis of neurofibromatosis type 1 (NF1)-associated peripheral nervous system neoplasms. Adv Anat Pathol. 2018 Sep;25(5):353–68. PMID:29762158
1924. Longy M, Lacombe D. Cowden disease. Report of a family and review. Ann Genet. 1996;39(1):35–42. PMID:9297442
1925. Lopes MB, Altermatt HJ, Scheithauer BW, et al. Immunohistochemical characterization of subependymal giant cell astrocytomas. Acta Neuropathol. 1996;91(4):368–75. PMID:8928613
1926. Lopes MB, Sloan E, Polder J. Mixed gangliocytoma-pituitary adenoma: insights on the pathogenesis of a rare sellar tumor. Am J Surg Pathol. 2017 May;41(5):586–95. PMID:28079576
1927. López G, Oberheim Bush NA, Berger MS, et al. Diffuse non-midline glioma with H3F3A K27M mutation: a prognostic and treatment dilemma. Acta Neuropathol Commun. 2017 May 15;5(1):38. PMID:28506301
1928. López GY, Van Ziffle J, Onodera C, et al. The genetic landscape of gliomas arising after therapeutic radiation. Acta Neuropathol. 2019 Jan;137(1):139–50. PMID:30196423
1929. Losa M, Vimercati A, Acerno S, et al. Correlation between clinical characteristics and proliferative activity in patients with craniopharyngioma. J Neurol Neurosurg Psychiatry. 2004 Jun;75(6):889–92. PMID:15146007
1930. Lossos C, Bayraktar S, Weinzierl E, et al. LMO2 and BCL6 are associated with improved survival in primary central nervous system lymphoma. Br J Haematol. 2014 Jun;165(5):640–8. PMID:24571259
1931. Lotan I, Khlebtovsky A, Inbar E, et al. Primary brain T-cell lymphoma in an HTLV-1 serologically positive male. J Neurol Sci. 2012 Mar 15;314(1-2):163–5. PMID:22118868
1932. Louis DN, Aldape K, Brat DJ, et al. Announcing cIMPACT-NOW: the consortium to inform molecular and practical approaches to CNS tumor taxonomy. Acta Neuropathol. 2017 Jan;133(1):1–3. PMID:27909809
1933. Louis DN, Aldape K, Brat DJ, et al. cIMPACT-NOW (the consortium to inform molecular and practical approaches to CNS tumor taxonomy): a new initiative in advancing nervous system tumor classification. Brain Pathol. 2017 Nov;27(6):851–2. PMID:27997995
1934. Louis DN, Ellison DW, Brat DJ, et al. cIMPACT-NOW: a practical summary of diagnostic points from Round 1 updates. Brain Pathol. 2019 Jul;29(4):469–72. PMID:31038238
1935. Louis DN, Giannini C, Capper D, et al. cIMPACT-NOW update 2: diagnostic clarifications for diffuse midline glioma, H3 K27M-mutant and diffuse astrocytoma/anaplastic astrocytoma, IDH-mutant. Acta Neuropathol. 2018 Apr;135(4):639–42. PMID:29497819
1936. Louis DN, Hamilton AJ, Sobel RA, et al. Pseudopsammomatous meningioma with elevated serum carcinoembryonic antigen: a true secretory meningioma. Case report. J Neurosurg. 1991 Jan;74(1):129–32. PMID:1984492
1937. Louis DN, Ohgaki H, Wiestler OD, et al., editors. WHO classification of tumours of the central nervous system. Lyon (France): International Agency for Research on Cancer; 2007. (WHO classification of tumours series, 4th ed.; vol. 1). https://publications.iarc.fr/11.
1938. Louis DN, Ohgaki H, Wiestler OD, et al., editors. WHO classification of tumours of the central nervous system. Lyon (France): International Agency for Research on Cancer; 2016. (WHO classification of tumours series, 4th rev. ed.; vol. 1). https://publications.iarc.fr/543.
1939. Louis DN, Perry A, Burger P, et al. International Society of Neuropathology–Haarlem consensus guidelines for nervous system tumor classification and grading. Brain Pathol. 2014 Sep;24(5):429–35. PMID:24990071
1940. Louis DN, Perry A, Reifenberger G, et al. The 2016 World Health Organization classification of tumors of the central nervous system: a summary. Acta Neuropathol. 2016 Jun;131(6):803–20. PMID:27157931
1941. Louis DN, Ramesh V, Gusella JF. Neuropathology and molecular genetics of neurofibromatosis 2 and related tumors. Brain Pathol. 1995 Apr;5(2):163–72. PMID:7670657
1942. Louis DN, von Deimling A, Dickersin GR, et al. Desmoplastic cerebral astrocytomas of infancy: a histopathologic, immunohistochemical, ultrastructural, and molecular genetic study. Hum Pathol. 1992 Dec;23(12):1402–9. PMID:1468778
1943. Louis DN, von Deimling A. Grading of diffuse astrocytic gliomas: Broders, Kernohan, Zülch, the WHO... and Shakespeare. Acta Neuropathol. 2017 Oct;134(4):517–20. PMID:28801693
1944. Louis DN, Wesseling P, Aldape K, et al. cIMPACT-NOW update 6: new entity and diagnostic principle recommendations of the cIMPACT-Utrecht meeting on future CNS tumor classification and grading. Brain Pathol. 2020 Jul;30(4):844–56. PMID:32307792
1945. Louis DN, Wesseling P, Brandner S, et al. Data sets for the reporting of tumors of the central nervous system: recommendations from the International Collaboration on Cancer Reporting. Arch Pathol Lab Med. 2020 Feb;144(2):196–206. PMID:31219344
1946. Louis DN, Wesseling P, Paulus W, et al. cIMPACT-NOW update 1: not otherwise specified (NOS) and not elsewhere classified (NEC). Acta Neuropathol. 2018 Mar;135(3):481–4. PMID:29372318
1947. Lowder L, Hauenstein J, Woods A, et al. Gliosarcoma: distinct molecular pathways and genomic alterations identified by DNA copy number/SNP microarray analysis. J Neurooncol. 2019 Jul;143(3):381–92. PMID:31073965
1948. Lu C, Ward PS, Kapoor GS, et al. IDH mutation impairs histone demethylation and results in a block to cell differentiation. Nature. 2012 Feb 15;483(7390):474–8. PMID:22343901
1949. Lu HC, Eulo V, Apicelli AJ, et al. Aberrant ATRX protein expression is associated with poor overall survival in NF1-MPNST. Oncotarget. 2018 May 1;9(33):23018–28. PMID:29796169
1950. Lu L, Dai Z, Zhong Y, et al. Cervical intradural paraganglioma presenting as progressive cervicodynia: case report and literature review. Clin Neurol Neurosurg. 2013 Mar;115(3):359–61. PMID:22721774
1951. Lu S, Stein JE, Rimm DL, et al. Comparison of biomarker modalities for predicting response to PD-1/PD-L1 checkpoint blockade: a systematic review and meta-analysis. JAMA Oncol. 2019 Aug 1;5(8):1195–204. PMID:31318407
1952. Lucas CG, Gilani A, Solomon DA, et al. ALK-positive histiocytosis with KIF5B-ALK fusion in the central nervous system. Acta Neuropathol. 2019 Aug;138(2):335–7. PMID:31119374
1953. Lucas CG, Gupta R, Doo P, et al. Comprehensive analysis of diverse low-grade neuroepithelial tumors with FGFR1 alterations reveals a distinct molecular signature of rosette-forming glioneuronal tumor. Acta Neuropathol Commun. 2020 Aug 28;8(1):151. PMID:32859279
1954. Lucas CG, Villanueva-Meyer JE, Whipple N, et al. Myxoid glioneuronal tumor, PDGFRA p.K385-mutant: clinical, radiologic, and histopathologic features. Brain Pathol. 2020 May;30(3):479–94. PMID:31609499
1955. Lucas JT Jr, Huang AJ, Mott RT, et al. Anaplastic ganglioglioma: a report of three cases and review of the literature. J Neurooncol. 2015 May;123(1):171–7. PMID:25862009

1956. Lucchesi KM, Grant R, Kahle KT, et al. Primary spinal myxopapillary ependymoma in the pediatric population: a study from the Surveillance, Epidemiology, and End Results (SEER) database. J Neurooncol. 2016 Oct;130(1):133–40. PMID:27423644
1957. Ludwin SK, Rubinstein LJ, Russell DS. Papillary meningioma: a malignant variant of meningioma. Cancer. 1975 Oct;36(4):1363–73. PMID:1175134
1958. Lun M, Lok E, Gautam S, et al. The natural history of extracranial metastasis from glioblastoma multiforme. J Neurooncol. 2011 Nov;105(2):261–73. PMID:21512826
1959. Luyken C, Blümcke I, Fimmers R, et al. Supratentorial gangliogliomas: histopathologic grading and tumor recurrence in 184 patients with a median follow-up of 8 years. Cancer. 2004 Jul 1;101(1):146–55. PMID:15222000
1960. Luzzi S, Elia A, Del Maestro M, et al. Dysembryoplastic neuroepithelial tumors: what you need to know. World Neurosurg. 2019 Jul;127:255–65. PMID:30981794
1961. Lynch ED, Ostermeyer EA, Lee MK, et al. Inherited mutations in PTEN that are associated with breast cancer, cowden disease, and juvenile polyposis. Am J Hum Genet. 1997 Dec;61(6):1254–60. PMID:9399897
1962. Ma C, Feng R, Chen H, et al. BRAF V600E, TERT, and IDH2 mutations in pleomorphic xanthoastrocytoma: observations from a large case-series study. World Neurosurg. 2018 Dec;120:e1225–33. PMID:30240866
1963. Ma J, Benitez JA, Li J, et al. Inhibition of nuclear PTEN tyrosine phosphorylation enhances glioma radiation sensitivity through attenuated DNA repair. Cancer Cell. 2019 Mar 18;35(3):504–518.e7. PMID:30827889
1964. Ma ZY, Song ZJ, Chen JH, et al. Recurrent gain-of-function USP8 mutations in Cushing's disease. Cell Res. 2015 Mar;25(3):306–17. PMID:25675982
1965. Macagno N, Figarella-Branger D, Mokthari K, et al. Differential diagnosis of meningeal SFT-HPC and meningioma: which immunohistochemical markers should be used? Am J Surg Pathol. 2016 Feb;40(2):270–8. PMID:26448189
1966. Macagno N, Vogels R, Appay R, et al. Grading of meningeal solitary fibrous tumors/hemangiopericytomas: analysis of the prognostic value of the Marseille Grading System in a cohort of 132 patients. Brain Pathol. 2019 Jan;29(1):18–27. PMID:29600523
1967. MacCollin M, Chiocca EA, Evans DG, et al. Diagnostic criteria for schwannomatosis. Neurology. 2005 Jun 14;64(11):1838–45. PMID:15955931
1968. MacCollin M, Ramesh V, Jacoby LB, et al. Mutational analysis of patients with neurofibromatosis 2. Am J Hum Genet. 1994 Aug;55(2):314–20. PMID:7913580
1969. MacCollin M, Willett C, Heinrich B, et al. Familial schwannomatosis: exclusion of the NF2 locus as the germline event. Neurology. 2003 Jun 24;60(12):1968–74. PMID:12821741
1970. MacCollin M, Woodfin W, Kronn D, et al. Schwannomatosis: a clinical and pathologic study. Neurology. 1996 Apr;46(4):1072–9. PMID:8780094
1971. Machado I, Yoshida A, López-Guerrero JA, et al. Immunohistochemical analysis of NKX2.2, ETV4, and BCOR in a large series of genetically confirmed Ewing sarcoma family of tumors. Pathol Res Pract. 2017 Sep;213(9):1048–53. PMID:28864350
1972. Machein MR, Plate KH. VEGF in brain tumors. J Neurooncol. 2000 Oct-Nov;50(1-2):109–20. PMID:11245271
1973. Mack SC, Agnihotri S, Bertrand KC, et al. Spinal myxopapillary ependymomas demonstrate a Warburg phenotype. Clin Cancer Res. 2015 Aug 15;21(16):3750–8. PMID:25957288
1974. Mack SC, Pajtler KW, Chavez L, et al. Therapeutic targeting of ependymoma as informed by oncogenic enhancer profiling. Nature. 2018 Jan 4;553(7686):101–5. PMID:29258295
1975. Mack SC, Witt H, Piro RM, et al. Epigenomic alterations define lethal CIMP-positive ependymomas of infancy. Nature. 2014 Feb 27;506(7489):445–50. PMID:24553142
1976. Mackay A, Burford A, Carvalho D, et al. Integrated molecular meta-analysis of 1,000 pediatric high-grade and diffuse intrinsic pontine glioma. Cancer Cell. 2017 Oct 9;32(4):520–537.e5. PMID:28966033
1977. Mackay A, Burford A, Molinari V, et al. Molecular, pathological, radiological, and immune profiling of non-brainstem pediatric high-grade glioma from the HERBY phase II randomized trial. Cancer Cell. 2018 May 14;33(5):829–842.e5. PMID:29763623
1978. Macyszyn L, Akbari H, Pisapia JM, et al. Imaging patterns predict patient survival and molecular subtype in glioblastoma via machine learning techniques. Neuro Oncol. 2016 Mar;18(3):417–25. PMID:26188015
1979. Madsen PJ, Buch VP, Douglas JE, et al. Endoscopic endonasal resection versus open surgery for pediatric craniopharyngioma: comparison of outcomes and complications. J Neurosurg Pediatr. 2019 Jun 7:1–10. PMID:31174192
1980. Maehama T, Dixon JE. The tumor suppressor, PTEN/MMAC1, dephosphorylates the lipid second messenger, phosphatidylinositol 3,4,5-trisphosphate. J Biol Chem. 1998 May 29;273(22):13375–8. PMID:9593664
1981. Maekawa A, Kohashi K, Yamada Y, et al. A case of intracranial solitary fibrous tumor/hemangiopericytoma with dedifferentiated component. Neuropathology. 2015 Jun;35(3):260–5. PMID:25516114
1982. Maekawa M, Fujisawa H, Iwayama Y, et al. Giant subependymoma developed in a patient with aniridia: analyses of PAX6 and tumor-relevant genes. Brain Pathol. 2010 Nov;20(6):1033–41. PMID:20500513
1983. Magaki SD, Vinters HV. Tuberous sclerosis complex. In: Adle-Biassette H, Harding BN, Golden JA, editors. Developmental neuropathology. 2nd ed. Oxford (UK): John Wiley & Sons Ltd; 2018. pp. 117–31.
1984. Magri L, Cambiaghi M, Cominelli M, et al. Sustained activation of mTOR pathway in embryonic neural stem cells leads to development of tuberous sclerosis complex-associated lesions. Cell Stem Cell. 2011 Nov 4;9(5):447–62. PMID:22056141
1985. Mahdi J, Goyal MS, Griffith J, et al. Nonoptic pathway tumors in children with neurofibromatosis type 1. Neurology. 2020 Aug 25;95(8):e1052–9. PMID:32300062
1986. Mahdi J, Shah AC, Sato A, et al. A multi-institutional study of brainstem gliomas in children with neurofibromatosis type 1. Neurology. 2017 Apr 18;88(16):1584–9. PMID:28330960
1987. Mahler C, Verhelst J, Klaes R, et al. Cushing's disease and hyperprolactinemia due to a mixed ACTH- and prolactin-secreting pituitary macroadenoma. Pathol Res Pract. 1991 Jun;187(5):598–602. PMID:1656408
1988. Majós C, Aguilera C, Cos M, et al. In vivo proton magnetic resonance spectroscopy of intraventricular tumours of the brain. Eur Radiol. 2009 Aug;19(8):2049–59. PMID:19277673
1989. Makino K, Nakamura H, Yano S, et al. Incidence of primary central nervous system germ cell tumors in childhood: a regional survey in Kumamoto prefecture in southern Japan. Pediatr Neurosurg. 2013;49(3):155–8. PMID:24751890
1990. Makise N, Sekimizu M, Konishi E, et al. H3K27me3 deficiency defines a subset of dedifferentiated chondrosarcomas with characteristic clinicopathological features. Mod Pathol. 2019 Mar;32(3):435–45. PMID:30291346
1991. Malanga D, Belmonte S, Colelli F, et al. AKT1E17K is oncogenic in mouse lung and cooperates with chemical carcinogens in inducing lung cancer. PLoS One. 2016 Feb 9;11(2):e0147334. PMID:26859676
1992. Malgulwar PB, Nambirajan A, Pathak P, et al. C11orf95-RELA fusions and upregulated NF-KB signalling characterise a subset of aggressive supratentorial ependymomas that express L1CAM and nestin. J Neurooncol. 2018 May;138(1):29–39. PMID:29354850
1993. Malgulwar PB, Nambirajan A, Pathak P, et al. Study of β-catenin and BRAF alterations in adamantinomatous and papillary craniopharyngiomas: mutation analysis with immunohistochemical correlation in 54 cases. J Neurooncol. 2017 Jul;133(3):487–95. PMID:28500561
1994. Malik SN, Farmer PM, Hajdu SI, et al. Mesenchymal chondrosarcoma of the cerebellum. Ann Clin Lab Sci. 1996 Nov-Dec;26(6):496–500. PMID:8908319
1995. Mallereau CH, Ganau M, Todeschi J, et al. Primary brain rhabdomyosarcoma causing extracranial metastases: case report with narrative review of atypical presentations and their diagnostic challenges. World Neurosurg. 2020 Jun;138:363–8. PMID:32229305
1996. Mallick S, Benson R, Rath GK. Patterns of care and survival outcomes in patients with pineal parenchymal tumor of intermediate differentiation: an individual patient data analysis. Radiother Oncol. 2016 Nov;121(2):204–8. PMID:27865543
1997. Mallory SB. Cowden syndrome (multiple hamartoma syndrome). Dermatol Clin. 1995 Jan;13(1):27–31. PMID:7712647
1998. Malmström A, Grønberg BH, Marosi C, et al. Temozolomide versus standard 6-week radiotherapy versus hypofractionated radiotherapy in patients older than 60 years with glioblastoma: the Nordic randomised, phase 3 trial. Lancet Oncol. 2012 Sep;13(9):916–26. PMID:22877848
1999. Malzkorn B, Reifenberger G. Integrated diagnostics of diffuse astrocytic and oligodendroglial tumors. Pathologe. 2019 Jun;40(Suppl 1):9–17. PMID:31025086
2000. Man W, Wang G. Incidence, outcomes and predictors of primary central nervous system melanoma: a SEER-based study. World Neurosurg. 2019 Sep;129:e782–90. PMID:31203063
2001. Manjila S, Asmar NE, Vidalis BM, et al. Intratumoral Rathke's cleft cyst remnants within craniopharyngioma, pituitary adenoma, suprasellar dermoid, and epidermoid cysts: a ubiquitous signature of ectodermal lineage or a transitional entity? Neurosurgery. 2019 Aug 1;85(2):180–8. PMID:30010935
2002. Manjila S, Miller E, Awadallah A, et al. Ossified choroid plexus papilloma of the fourth ventricle: elucidation of the mechanism of osteogenesis in benign brain tumors. J Neurosurg Pediatr. 2013 Jul;12(1):13–20. PMID:23641963
2003. Manoharan N, Julka PK, Rath GK. Descriptive epidemiology of primary brain and CNS tumors in Delhi, 2003-2007. Asian Pac J Cancer Prev. 2012;13(2):637–40. PMID:22524838
2004. Manoranjan B, Koziarz A, Kameda-Smith MM, et al. Multiple recurrences require long-term follow-up in patients diagnosed with spindle cell oncocytoma of the sella turcica. J Clin Neurosci. 2017 Sep;43:134–46. PMID:28668473
2005. Mantilla JG, Ricciotti RW, Chen E, et al. Detecting disease-defining gene fusions in unclassified round cell sarcomas using anchored multiplex PCR/targeted RNA next-generation sequencing-Molecular and clinicopathological characterization of 16 cases. Genes Chromosomes Cancer. 2019 Oct;58(10):713–22. PMID:31033080
2006. Marano SR, Johnson PC, Spetzler RF. Recurrent Lhermitte-Duclos disease in a child. Case report. J Neurosurg. 1988 Oct;69(4):599–603. PMID:3418394
2007. Marcel V, Dichtel-Danjoy ML, Sagne C, et al. Biological functions of p53 isoforms through evolution: lessons from animal and cellular models. Cell Death Differ. 2011 Dec;18(12):1815–24. PMID:21941372
2008. Marcelis L, Antoranz A, Delsupehe AM, et al. In-depth characterization of the tumor microenvironment in central nervous system lymphoma reveals implications for immune-checkpoint therapy. Cancer Immunol Immunother. 2020 Sep;69(9):1751–66. PMID:32335702
2009. Marciscano AE, Stemmer-Rachamimov AO, Niemierko A, et al. Benign meningiomas (WHO Grade I) with atypical histological features: correlation of histopathological features with clinical outcomes. J Neurosurg. 2016 Jan;124(1):106–14. PMID:26274991
2010. Marcotte L, Aronica E, Baybis M, et al. Cytoarchitectural alterations are widespread in cerebral cortex in tuberous sclerosis complex. Acta Neuropathol. 2012 May;123(5):685–93. PMID:22327361
2011. Marees T, Moll AC, Imhof SM, et al. Risk of second malignancies in survivors of retinoblastoma: more than 40 years of follow-up. J Natl Cancer Inst. 2008 Dec 17;100(24):1771–9. PMID:19066271
2012. Margetts JC, Kalyan-Raman UP. Giant-celled glioblastoma of brain. A clinico-pathological and radiological study of ten cases (including immunohistochemistry and ultrastructure). Cancer. 1989 Feb 1;63(3):524–31. PMID:2912529
2013. Margueron R, Reinberg D. The Polycomb complex PRC2 and its mark in life. Nature. 2011 Jan 20;469(7330):343–9. PMID:21248841
2014. Marigo V, Davey RA, Zuo Y, et al. Biochemical evidence that patched is the Hedgehog receptor. Nature. 1996 Nov 14;384(6605):176–9. PMID:8906794
2015. Marks AM, Bindra RS, DiLuna ML, et al. Response to the BRAF/MEK inhibitors dabrafenib/trametinib in an adolescent with a BRAF V600E mutated anaplastic ganglioglioma intolerant to vemurafenib. Pediatr Blood Cancer. 2018 May;65(5):e26969. PMID:29380516
2016. Marsan E, Baulac S. Review: Mechanistic target of rapamycin (mTOR) pathway, focal cortical dysplasia and epilepsy. Neuropathol Appl Neurobiol. 2018 Feb;44(1):6–17. PMID:29359340
2017. Marsh A, Wicking C, Wainwright B, et al. DHPLC analysis of patients with nevoid basal cell carcinoma syndrome reveals novel PTCH missense mutations in the sterol-sensing domain. Hum Mutat. 2005 Sep;26(3):283. PMID:16088933
2018. Marsh DJ, Coulon V, Lunetta KL, et al. Mutation spectrum and genotype-phenotype analyses in Cowden disease and Bannayan-Zonana syndrome, two hamartoma syndromes with germline PTEN mutation. Hum Mol Genet. 1998 Mar;7(3):507–15. PMID:9467011
2019. Marsh DJ, Dahia PL, Caron S, et al. Germline PTEN mutations in Cowden syndrome-like families. J Med Genet. 1998 Nov;35(11):881–5. PMID:9832031
2020. Marsh DJ, Dahia PL, Zheng Z, et al. Germline mutations in PTEN are present in Bannayan-Zonana syndrome. Nat Genet. 1997 Aug;16(4):333–4. PMID:9241266
2021. Marsh DJ, Kum JB, Lunetta KL, et al. PTEN mutation spectrum and genotype-phenotype

correlations in Bannayan-Riley-Ruvalcaba syndrome suggest a single entity with Cowden syndrome. Hum Mol Genet. 1999 Aug;8(8):1461–72. PMID:10400993
2022. Marsh DJ, Roth S, Lunetta KL, et al. Exclusion of PTEN and 10q22-24 as the susceptibility locus for juvenile polyposis syndrome. Cancer Res. 1997 Nov 15;57(22):5017–21. PMID:9371495
2023. Martinez-Diaz H, Kleinschmidt-DeMasters BK, Powell SZ, et al. Giant cell glioblastoma and pleomorphic xanthoastrocytoma show different immunohistochemical profiles for neuronal antigens and p53 but share reactivity for class III beta-tubulin. Arch Pathol Lab Med. 2003 Sep;127(9):1187–91. PMID:12946225
2024. Martins R, Bugalho MJ. Paragangliomas/Pheochromocytomas: clinically oriented genetic testing. Int J Endocrinol. 2014;2014:794187. PMID:24899893
2025. Martuza RL, Eldridge R. Neurofibromatosis 2 (bilateral acoustic neurofibromatosis). N Engl J Med. 1988 Mar 17;318(11):684–8. PMID:3125435
2026. Marucci G, Di Oto E, Farnedi A, et al. Nogo-A: a useful marker for the diagnosis of oligodendroglioma and for identifying 1p19q codeletion. Hum Pathol. 2012 Mar;43(3):374–80. PMID:21835431
2027. Maruya J, Seki Y, Morita K, et al. Meningeal hemangiopericytoma manifesting as massive intracranial hemorrhage–two case reports. Neurol Med Chir (Tokyo). 2006 Feb;46(2):92–7. PMID:16498220
2028. Masciari S, Dillon DA, Rath M, et al. Breast cancer phenotype in women with TP53 germline mutations: a Li-Fraumeni syndrome consortium effort. Breast Cancer Res Treat. 2012 Jun;133(3):1125–30. PMID:22392042
2029. Masliah-Planchon J, Machet MC, Fréneaux P, et al. SMARCA4-Mutated Atypical Teratoid/Rhabdoid Tumor with Retained BRG1 Expression. Pediatr Blood Cancer. 2016 Mar;63(3):568–9. PMID:26469284
2030. Massengill JB, Sample KM, Pilarski R, et al. Analysis of the exome aggregation consortium (ExAC) database suggests that the BAP1-tumor predisposition syndrome is underreported in cancer patients. Genes Chromosomes Cancer. 2018 Sep;57(9):478–81. PMID:29761599
2031. Massimino M, Antonelli M, Gandola L, et al. Histological variants of medulloblastoma are the most powerful clinical prognostic indicators. Pediatr Blood Cancer. 2013 Feb;60(2):210–6. PMID:22693015
2032. Massimino M, Miceli R, Giangaspero F, et al. Final results of the second prospective AIEOP protocol for pediatric intracranial ependymoma. Neuro Oncol. 2016 Oct;18(10):1451–60. PMID:27194148
2033. Masuoka J, Brandner S, Paulus W, et al. Germline SDHD mutation in paraganglioma of the spinal cord. Oncogene. 2001 Aug 16;20(36):5084–6. PMID:11526495
2034. Mateus C, Palangié A, Franck N, et al. Heterogeneity of skin manifestations in patients with Carney complex. J Am Acad Dermatol. 2008 Nov;59(5):801–10. PMID:18804312
2035. Mathews JD, Forsythe AV, Brady Z, et al. Cancer risk in 680,000 people exposed to computed tomography scans in childhood or adolescence: data linkage study of 11 million Australians. BMJ. 2013 May 21;346:f2360. PMID:23694687
2036. Mathews T, Moossy J. Gliomas containing bone and cartilage. J Neuropathol Exp Neurol. 1974 Jul;33(3):456–71. PMID:4365915
2037. Mathon B, Carpentier A, Clemenceau S, et al. [Paraganglioma of the cauda equina region: report of six cases and review of the literature]. Neurochirurgie. 2012 Dec;58(6):341–5. French. PMID:22770767
2038. Matjašič A, Zupan A, Boštjančič E, et al. A novel PTPRZ1-ETV1 fusion in gliomas. Brain Pathol. 2020 Mar;30(2):226–34. PMID:31381204
2039. Matsumura N, Natsume A, Maeda S, et al. Malignant transformation of a dysembryoplastic neuroepithelial tumor verified by a shared copy number gain of the tyrosine kinase domain of FGFR1. Brain Tumor Pathol. 2020 Apr;37(2):69–75. PMID:32297014
2040. Matsumura N, Nobusawa S, Ito J, et al. Multiplex ligation-dependent probe amplification analysis is useful for detecting a copy number gain of the FGFR1 tyrosine kinase domain in dysembryoplastic neuroepithelial tumors. J Neurooncol. 2019 May;143(1):27–33. PMID:30825062
2041. Matsutani M, Japanese Pediatric Brain Tumor Study Group. Combined chemotherapy and radiation therapy for CNS germ cell tumors–the Japanese experience. J Neurooncol. 2001 Sep;54(3):311–6. PMID:11767296
2042. Matsutani M, Sano K, Takakura K, et al. Primary intracranial germ cell tumors: a clinical analysis of 153 histologically verified cases. J Neurosurg. 1997 Mar;86(3):446–55. PMID:9046301
2043. Matyakhina L, Pack S, Kirschner LS, et al. Chromosome 2 (2p16) abnormalities in Carney complex tumours. J Med Genet. 2003 Apr;40(4):268–77. PMID:12676898
2044. Mautner VF, Tatagiba M, Lindenau M, et al. Spinal tumors in patients with neurofibromatosis type 2: MR imaging study of frequency, multiplicity, and variety. AJR Am J Roentgenol. 1995 Oct;165(4):951–5. PMID:7676998
2045. May JM, Waddle MR, Miller DH, et al. Primary histiocytic sarcoma of the central nervous system: a case report with platelet derived growth factor receptor mutation and PD-L1/PD-L2 expression and literature review. Radiat Oncol. 2018 Sep 5;13(1):167. PMID:30185195
2046. Mayer R. [History of the medical campus of the Free University of Brussels]. Rev Med Brux. 1990 Nov;11(9):450–60. French. PMID:2287848
2047. McClain KL, Picarsic J, Chakraborty R, et al. CNS Langerhans cell histiocytosis: common hematopoietic origin for LCH-associated neurodegeneration and mass lesions. Cancer. 2018 Jun 15;124(12):2607–20. PMID:29624648
2048. McClatchey AI, Giovannini M. Membrane organization and tumorigenesis–the NF2 tumor suppressor, Merlin. Genes Dev. 2005 Oct 1;19(19):2265–77. PMID:16204178
2049. McCluggage WG, Foulkes WD. DICER1-associated sarcomas: towards a unified nomenclature. Mod Pathol. 2021 Jun;34(6):1226–8. PMID:32572152
2050. McCormack A, Dekkers OM, Petersenn S, et al. Treatment of aggressive pituitary tumours and carcinomas: results of a European Society of Endocrinology (ESE) survey 2016. Eur J Endocrinol. 2018 Mar;178(3):265–76. PMID:29330228
2051. McCracken JA, Gonzales MF, Phal PM, et al. Angiocentric glioma transformed into anaplastic ependymoma: review of the evidence for malignant potential. J Clin Neurosci. 2016 Dec;34:47–52. PMID:27742374
2052. McGaughran JM, Harris DI, Donnai D, et al. A clinical study of type 1 neurofibromatosis in north west England. J Med Genet. 1999 Mar;36(3):197–203. PMID:10204844
2053. McGowan-Jordan J, Hastings RJ, Moore S, editors. ISCN 2020: an international system for human cytogenomic nomenclature (2020). Basel (Switzerland): Karger Publishers; 2020.
2054. McGuire CS, Sainani KL, Fisher PG. Incidence patterns for ependymoma: a surveillance, epidemiology, and end results study. J Neurosurg. 2009 Apr;110(4):725–9. PMID:19061350
2055. McHugh BJ, Baranoski JF, Malhotra A, et al. Intracranial infantile hemangiopericytoma. J Neurosurg Pediatr. 2014 Aug;14(2):149–54. PMID:24905842
2056. McManamy CS, Lamont JM, Taylor RE, et al. Morphophenotypic variation predicts clinical behavior in childhood non-desmoplastic medulloblastomas. J Neuropathol Exp Neurol. 2003 Jun;62(6):627–32. PMID:12834107
2057. McManamy CS, Pears J, Weston CL, et al. Nodule formation and desmoplasia in medulloblastomas-defining the nodular/desmoplastic variant and its biological behavior. Brain Pathol. 2007 Apr;17(2):151–64. PMID:17388946
2058. McMenamin ME, Fletcher CD. Expanding the spectrum of malignant change in schwannomas: epithelioid malignant change, epithelioid malignant peripheral nerve sheath tumor, and epithelioid angiosarcoma: a study of 17 cases. Am J Surg Pathol. 2001 Jan;25(1):13–25. PMID:11145248
2059. McWilliams GD, SantaCruz K, Hart B, et al. Occurrence of DNET and other brain tumors in Noonan syndrome warrants caution with growth hormone therapy. Am J Med Genet A. 2016 Jan;170A(1):195–201. PMID:26377682
2060. Medhi G, Prasad C, Saini J, et al. Imaging features of rosette-forming glioneuronal tumours (RGNTs): a series of seven cases. Eur Radiol. 2016 Jan;26(1):262–70. PMID:26017735
2061. Medhkour A, Traul D, Husain M. Neonatal subependymal giant cell astrocytoma. Pediatr Neurosurg. 2002 May;36(5):271–4. PMID:12053047
2062. Mei K, Liu A, Allan RW, et al. Diagnostic utility of SALL4 in primary germ cell tumors of the central nervous system: a study of 77 cases. Mod Pathol. 2009 Dec;22(12):1628–36. PMID:19820689
2063. Meij BP, Lopes MB, Ellegala DB, et al. The long-term significance of microscopic dural invasion in 354 patients with pituitary adenomas treated with transsphenoidal surgery. J Neurosurg. 2002 Feb;96(2):195–208. PMID:11838791
2064. Melani C, Jaffe ES, Wilson WH. Pathobiology and treatment of lymphomatoid granulomatosis, a rare EBV-driven disorder. Blood. 2020 Apr 16;135(16):1344–52. PMID:32107539
2065. Melin BS, Barnholtz-Sloan JS, Wrensch MR, et al. Genome-wide association study of glioma subtypes identifies specific differences in genetic susceptibility to glioblastoma and non-glioblastoma tumors. Nat Genet. 2017 May;49(5):789–94. PMID:28346443
2066. Mena H, Ribas JL, Pezeshkpour GH, et al. Hemangiopericytoma of the central nervous system: a review of 94 cases. Hum Pathol. 1991 Jan;22(1):84–91. PMID:1985083
2067. Mena H, Rushing EJ, Ribas JL, et al. Tumors of pineal parenchymal cells: a correlation of histological features, including nucleolar organizer regions, with survival in 35 cases. Hum Pathol. 1995 Jan;26(1):20–30. PMID:7821912
2068. Méndez JC, Carrasco R, Prieto MA, et al. Paraganglioma of the cauda equina: MR and angiographic findings. Radiol Case Rep. 2019 Jul 25;14(10):1185–7. PMID:31379984
2069. Mendoza PR, Specht CS, Hubbard GB, et al. Histopathologic grading of anaplasia in retinoblastoma. Am J Ophthalmol. 2015 Apr;159(4):764–76. PMID:25528954
2070. Menke JR, Raleigh DR, Gown AM, et al. Somatostatin receptor 2a is a more sensitive diagnostic marker of meningioma than epithelial membrane antigen. Acta Neuropathol. 2015 Sep;130(3):441–3. PMID:26195322
2071. Menko FH, Kaspers GL, Meijer GA, et al. A homozygous MSH6 mutation in a child with café-au-lait spots, oligodendroglioma and rectal cancer. Fam Cancer. 2004;3(2):123–7. PMID:15340263
2072. Menon MP, Nicolae A, Meeker H, et al. Primary CNS T-cell lymphomas: a clinical, morphologic, immunophenotypic, and molecular analysis. Am J Surg Pathol. 2015 Dec;39(12):1719–29. PMID:26379152
2073. Merchant TE, Bendel AE, Sabin ND, et al. Conformal radiation therapy for pediatric ependymoma, chemotherapy for incompletely resected ependymoma, and observation for completely resected, supratentorial ependymoma. J Clin Oncol. 2019 Apr 20;37(12):974–83. PMID:30811284
2074. Merchant TE, Li C, Xiong X, et al. Conformal radiotherapy after surgery for paediatric ependymoma: a prospective study. Lancet Oncol. 2009 Mar;10(3):258–66. PMID:19274783
2075. Merchant TE, Pollack IF, Loeffler JS. Brain tumors across the age spectrum: biology, therapy, and late effects. Semin Radiat Oncol. 2010 Jan;20(1):58–66. PMID:19959032
2076. Mercuri S, Gazzeri R, Galarza M, et al. Primary meningeal pheochromocytoma: case report. J Neurooncol. 2005 Jun;73(2):169–72. PMID:15981108
2077. Mérel P, Hoang-Xuan K, Sanson M, et al. Screening for germ-line mutations in the NF2 gene. Genes Chromosomes Cancer. 1995 Feb;12(2):117–27. PMID:7535084
2078. Merfeld EC, Dahiya S, Perkins SM. Patterns of care and treatment outcomes of patients with astroblastoma: a National Cancer Database analysis. CNS Oncol. 2018 Apr;7(2):CNS13. PMID:29708401
2079. Merino DM, Shlien A, Villani A, et al. Molecular characterization of choroid plexus tumors reveals novel clinically relevant subgroups. Clin Cancer Res. 2015 Jan 1;21(1):184–92. PMID:25336695
2080. Merker VL, Esparza S, Smith MJ, et al. Clinical features of schwannomatosis: a retrospective analysis of 87 patients. Oncologist. 2012;17(10):1317–22. PMID:22927469
2081. Merlin E, Chabrier S, Verkarre V, et al. Primary leptomeningeal ALK+ lymphoma in a 13-year-old child. J Pediatr Hematol Oncol. 2008 Dec;30(12):963–7. PMID:19131793
2082. Merrell R, Nabors LB, Perry A, et al. 1p/19q chromosome deletions in metastatic oligodendroglioma. J Neurooncol. 2006 Nov;80(2):203–7. PMID:16710746
2083. Messiaen L, Yao S, Brems H, et al. Clinical and mutational spectrum of neurofibromatosis type 1-like syndrome. JAMA. 2009 Nov 18;302(19):2111–8. PMID:19920235
2084. Messiaen LM, Callens T, Mortier G, et al. Exhaustive mutation analysis of the NF1 gene allows identification of 95% of mutations and reveals a high frequency of unusual splicing defects. Hum Mutat. 2000;15(6):541–55. PMID:10862084
2085. Messinger YH, Stewart DR, Priest JR, et al. Pleuropulmonary blastoma: a report on 350 central pathology-confirmed pleuropulmonary blastoma cases by the International Pleuropulmonary Blastoma Registry. Cancer. 2015 Jan 15;121(2):276–85. PMID:25209242
2086. Messing-Jünger AM, Floeth FW, Pauleit D, et al. Multimodal target point assessment for stereotactic biopsy in children with diffuse bithalamic astrocytomas. Childs Nerv Syst. 2002 Aug;18(8):445–9. PMID:12192504
2087. Mester J, Eng C. Estimate of de novo mutation frequency in probands with PTEN hamartoma tumor syndrome. Genet Med. 2012 Sep;14(9):819–22. PMID:22595938
2088. Mete O, Alshaikh OM, Cintosun A, et al. Synchronous multiple pituitary neuroendocrine

tumors of different cell lineages. Endocr Pathol. 2018 Dec;29(4):332–8. PMID:30215160
2089. Mete O, Asa SL. Clinicopathological correlations in pituitary adenomas. Brain Pathol. 2012 Jul;22(4):443–53. PMID:22697380
2090. Mete O, Cintosun A, Pressman I, et al. Epidemiology and biomarker profile of pituitary adenohypophysial tumors. Mod Pathol. 2018 Jun;31(6):900–9. PMID:29434339
2091. Mete O, Gomez-Hernandez K, Kucharczyk W, et al. Silent subtype 3 pituitary adenomas are not always silent and represent poorly differentiated monomorphous plurihormonal Pit-1 lineage adenomas. Mod Pathol. 2016 Feb;29(2):131–42. PMID:26743473
2092. Mete O, Kefeli M, Çalışkan S, et al. GATA3 immunoreactivity expands the transcription factor profile of pituitary neuroendocrine tumors. Mod Pathol. 2019 Apr;32(4):484–9. PMID:30390035
2093. Mete O, Lopes MB. Overview of the 2017 WHO classification of pituitary tumors. Endocr Pathol. 2017 Sep;28(3):228–43. PMID:28766057
2094. Mete O, Lopes MB, Asa SL. Spindle cell oncocytomas and granular cell tumors of the pituitary are variants of pituicytoma. Am J Surg Pathol. 2013 Nov;37(11):1694–9. PMID:23887161
2095. Mete O, Tischler AS, de Krijger R, et al. Protocol for the examination of specimens from patients with pheochromocytomas and extra-adrenal paragangliomas. Arch Pathol Lab Med. 2014 Feb;138(2):182–8. PMID:24476517
2096. Metellus P, Bouvier C, Guyotat J, et al. Solitary fibrous tumors of the central nervous system: clinicopathological and therapeutic considerations of 18 cases. Neurosurgery. 2007 Apr;60(4):715–22. PMID:17415209
2097. Meyenberger C, Biener K. [Health problems of the population in an alpine valley]. Schweiz Rundsch Med Prax. 1979 Feb 20;68(8):255–9. German. PMID:419079
2098. Meyer-Puttlitz B, Hayashi Y, Waha A, et al. Molecular genetic analysis of giant cell glioblastomas. Am J Pathol. 1997 Sep;151(3):853–7. PMID:9284834
2099. Meyers SP, Khademian ZP, Biegel JA, et al. Primary intracranial atypical teratoid/rhabdoid tumors of infancy and childhood: MRI features and patient outcomes. AJNR Am J Neuroradiol. 2006 May;27(5):962–71. PMID:16687525
2100. Meyers SP, Khademian ZP, Chuang SH, et al. Choroid plexus carcinomas in children: MRI features and patient outcomes. Neuroradiology. 2004 Sep;46(9):770–80. PMID:15309348
2101. Meyronet D, Esteban-Mader M, Bonnet C, et al. Characteristics of H3 K27M-mutant gliomas in adults. Neuro Oncol. 2017 Aug 1;19(8):1127–34. PMID:28201752
2102. Mezmezian MB, Fernandez Ugazio G, Paparella ML. Histopathological features of malignant craniopharyngioma: case report and literature review. Clin Neuropathol. 2020 Jan/Feb;39(1):26–31. PMID:31661068
2103. Mhatre R, Sugur HS, Nandeesh BN, et al. MN1 rearrangement in astroblastoma: study of eight cases and review of literature. Brain Tumor Pathol. 2019 Jul;36(3):112–20. PMID:31111274
2104. Miao R, Wang H, Jacobson A, et al. Radiation-induced and neurofibromatosis-associated malignant peripheral nerve sheath tumors (MPNST) have worse outcomes than sporadic MPNST. Radiother Oncol. 2019 Aug;137:61–70. PMID:31078939
2105. Michal M, Kazakov DV, Belousova I, et al. A benign neoplasm with histopathological features of both schwannoma and retiform perineurioma (benign schwannoma-perineurioma): a report of six cases of a distinctive soft tissue tumor with a predilection for the fingers. Virchows Arch. 2004 Oct;445(4):347–53. PMID:15322875
2106. Michaud K, de Tayrac M, D'Astous M, et al. Contribution of 1p, 19q, 9p and 10q automated analysis by FISH to the diagnosis and prognosis of oligodendroglial tumors according to WHO 2016 guidelines. PLoS One. 2016 Dec 28;11(12):e0168728. PMID:28030632
2107. Micko AS, Wöhrer A, Wolfsberger S, et al. Invasion of the cavernous sinus space in pituitary adenomas: endoscopic verification and its correlation with an MRI-based classification. J Neurosurg. 2015 Apr;122(4):803–11. PMID:25658782
2108. Miele E, Mastronuzzi A, Po A, et al. Characterization of medulloblastoma in Fanconi Anemia: a novel mutation in the BRCA2 gene and SHH molecular subgroup. Biomark Res. 2015 Jun 6;3:13. PMID:26064523
2109. Miettinen MM, Antonescu CR, Fletcher CDM, et al. Histopathologic evaluation of atypical neurofibromatous tumors and their transformation into malignant peripheral nerve sheath tumor in patients with neurofibromatosis 1-a consensus overview. Hum Pathol. 2017 Sep;67:1–10. PMID:28551330
2110. Migheli A, Cavalla P, Marino S, et al. A study of apoptosis in normal and pathologic nervous tissue after in situ end-labeling of DNA strand breaks. J Neuropathol Exp Neurol. 1994 Nov;53(6):606–16. PMID:7525880
2111. Milbouw G, Born JD, Martin D, et al. Clinical and radiological aspects of dysplastic gangliocytoma (Lhermitte-Duclos disease): a report of two cases with review of the literature. Neurosurgery. 1988 Jan;22(1 Pt 1):124–8. PMID:3278250
2112. Miller CA, Torack RM. Secretory ependymoma of the filum terminale. Acta Neuropathol. 1970;15(3):240–50. PMID:4193811
2113. Miller CR, Dunham CP, Scheithauer BW, et al. Significance of necrosis in grading of oligodendroglial neoplasms: a clinicopathologic and genetic study of newly diagnosed high-grade gliomas. J Clin Oncol. 2006 Dec 1;24(34):5419–26. PMID:17135643
2114. Miller MB, Bi WL, Ramkissoon LA, et al. MAPK activation and HRAS mutation identified in pituitary spindle cell oncocytoma. Oncotarget. 2016 Jun 14;7(24):37054–63. PMID:27175596
2115. Miller S, Rogers HA, Lyon P, et al. Genome-wide molecular characterization of central nervous system primitive neuroectodermal tumor and pineoblastoma. Neuro Oncol. 2011 Aug;13(8):866–79. PMID:21798848
2116. Miller S, Ward JH, Rogers HA, et al. Loss of INI1 protein expression defines a subgroup of aggressive central nervous system primitive neuroectodermal tumors. Brain Pathol. 2013 Jan;23(1):19–27. PMID:22672440
2117. Min HS, Lee JY, Kim SK, et al. Genetic grouping of medulloblastomas by representative markers in pathologic diagnosis. Transl Oncol. 2013 Jun 1;6(3):265–72. PMID:23730405
2118. Min KW, Scheithauer BW. Pineal germinomas and testicular seminoma: a comparative ultrastructural study with special references to early carcinomatous transformation. Ultrastruct Pathol. 1990 Nov-Dec;14(6):483–96. PMID:2281547
2119. Min KW, Scheithauer BW, Bauserman SC. Pineal parenchymal tumors: an ultrastructural study with prognostic implications. Ultrastruct Pathol. 1994 Jan-Apr;18(1-2):69–85. PMID:8191649
2120. Minaguchi T, Waite KA, Eng C. Nuclear localization of PTEN is regulated by Ca(2+) through a tyrosil phosphorylation-independent conformational modification in major vault protein. Cancer Res. 2006 Dec 15;66(24):11677–82. PMID:17178862
2121. Minehan KJ, Shaw EG, Scheithauer BW, et al. Spinal cord astrocytoma: pathological and treatment considerations. J Neurosurg. 1995 Oct;83(4):590–5. PMID:7674006
2122. Mirchia K, Sathe AA, Walker JM, et al. Total copy number variation as a prognostic factor in adult astrocytoma subtypes. Acta Neuropathol Commun. 2019 Jun 10;7(1):92. PMID:31177992
2123. Mirchia K, Snuderl M, Galbraith K, et al. Establishing a prognostic threshold for total copy number variation within adult IDH-mutant grade II/III astrocytomas. Acta Neuropathol Commun. 2019 Jul 26;7(1):121. PMID:31349875
2124. Mirian C, Duun-Henriksen AK, Juratli T, et al. Poor prognosis associated with TERT gene alterations in meningioma is independent of the WHO classification: an individual patient data meta-analysis. J Neurol Neurosurg Psychiatry. 2020 Apr;91(4):378–87. PMID:32041819
2125. Mirow C, Pietsch T, Berkefeld S, et al. Children <1 year show an inferior outcome when treated according to the traditional LGG treatment strategy: a report from the German multicenter trial HIT-LGG 1996 for children with low grade glioma (LGG). Pediatr Blood Cancer. 2014 Mar;61(3):457–63. PMID:24039013
2126. Mishra T, Goel NA, Goel AH. Primary paraganglioma of the spine: a clinicopathological study of eight cases. J Craniovertebr Junction Spine. 2014 Jan;5(1):20–4. PMID:25013343
2127. Mistry M, Zhukova N, Merico D, et al. BRAF mutation and CDKN2A deletion define a clinically distinct subgroup of childhood secondary high-grade glioma. J Clin Oncol. 2015 Mar 20;33(9):1015–22. PMID:25667294
2128. Mitchell A, Scheithauer BW, Doyon J, et al. Malignant perineurioma (malignant peripheral nerve sheath tumor with perineural differentiation). Clin Neuropathol. 2012 Nov-Dec;31(6):424–9. PMID:22762889
2129. Mittal P, Gupta K, Saggar K, et al. Adult medulloblastoma mimicking Lhermitte-Duclos disease: can diffusion weighted imaging help? Neurol India. 2009 Mar-Apr;57(2):203–5. PMID:19439857
2130. Mittal P, Roberts CWM. The SWI/SNF complex in cancer - biology, biomarkers and therapy. Nat Rev Clin Oncol. 2020 Jul;17(7):435–48. PMID:32303701
2131. Miyagami M, Katayama Y, Nakamura S. Clinicopathological study of vascular endothelial growth factor (VEGF), p53, and proliferative potential in familial von Hippel-Lindau disease and sporadic hemangioblastomas. Brain Tumor Pathol. 2000;17(3):111–20. PMID:11310918
2132. Miyahara H, Toyoshima Y, Natsumeda M, et al. Anaplastic astrocytoma with angiocentric ependymal differentiation. Neuropathology. 2011 Jun;31(3):292–8. PMID:21062363
2133. Miyake Y, Adachi JI, Suzuki T, et al. Craniospinal germinomas in patient with Down syndrome successfully treated with standard-dose chemotherapy and craniospinal irradiation: case report and literature review. World Neurosurg. 2017 Dec;108:995.e9–15. PMID:28919233
2134. Miyata H, Ryufuku M, Kubota Y, et al. Adult-onset angiocentric glioma of epithelioid cell-predominant type of the mesial temporal lobe suggestive of a rare but distinct clinicopathological subset within a spectrum of angiocentric cortical ependymal tumors. Neuropathology. 2012 Oct;32(5):479–91. PMID:22151480
2135. Miyata-Takata T, Takata K, Kato S, et al. Clinicopathological analysis of primary central nervous system NK/T cell lymphoma: rare and localized aggressive tumour among extranasal NK/T cell tumours. Histopathology. 2017 Aug;71(2):287–95. PMID:28342197
2136. Mizuguchi M, Ikeda K, Takashima S. Simultaneous loss of hamartin and tuberin from the cerebrum, kidney and heart with tuberous sclerosis. Acta Neuropathol. 2000 May;99(5):503–10. PMID:10805093
2137. Mizuguchi M, Kato M, Yamanouchi H, et al. Loss of tuberin from cerebral tissues with tuberous sclerosis and astrocytoma. Ann Neurol. 1996 Dec;40(6):941–4. PMID:9007104
2138. Mizuguchi M, Takashima S. Neuropathology of tuberous sclerosis. Brain Dev. 2001 Nov;23(7):508–15. PMID:11701246
2139. Modena P, Lualdi E, Facchinetti F, et al. SMARCB1/INI1 tumor suppressor gene is frequently inactivated in epithelioid sarcomas. Cancer Res. 2005 May 15;65(10):4012–9. PMID:15899790
2140. Molitch ME. Diagnosis and treatment of pituitary adenomas: a review. JAMA. 2017 Feb 7;317(5):516–24. PMID:28170483
2141. Möllemann M, Wolter M, Felsberg J, et al. Frequent promoter hypermethylation and low expression of the MGMT gene in oligodendroglial tumors. Int J Cancer. 2005 Jan 20;113(3):379–85. PMID:15455350
2142. Momota H, Ichimiya S, Ikeda T, et al. Immunohistochemical analysis of the p53 family members in human craniopharyngiomas. Brain Tumor Pathol. 2003;20(2):73–7. PMID:14756444
2143. Momota H, Iwami K, Fujii M, et al. Rhabdoid glioblastoma in a child: case report and literature review. Brain Tumor Pathol. 2011 Feb;28(1):65–70. PMID:21213124
2144. Momota H, Narita Y, Maeshima AM, et al. Prognostic value of immunohistochemical profile and response to high-dose methotrexate therapy in primary CNS lymphoma. J Neurooncol. 2010 Jul;98(3):341–8. PMID:20012911
2145. Mondal G, Lee JC, Ravindranathan A, et al. Pediatric bithalamic gliomas have a distinct epigenetic signature and frequent EGFR exon 20 insertions resulting in potential sensitivity to targeted kinase inhibition. Acta Neuropathol. 2020 Jun;139(6):1071–88. PMID:32303840
2146. Mondello P, Mian M, Bertoni F. Primary central nervous system lymphoma: novel precision therapies. Crit Rev Oncol Hematol. 2019 Sep;141:139–45. PMID:31295667
2147. Monté AMC, D'Arco F, De Cocker LJL. Multinodular and vacuolating neuronal tumor in an adolescent with Klinefelter syndrome. Neuroradiology. 2017 Dec;59(12):1187–8. PMID:29038865
2148. Montesinos-Rongen M, Besleaga R, Heinsohn S, et al. Absence of simian virus 40 DNA sequences in primary central nervous system lymphoma in HIV-negative patients. Virchows Arch. 2004 May;444(5):436–8. PMID:15042369
2149. Montesinos-Rongen M, Brunn A, Tuchscherer A, et al. Analysis of driver mutational hot spots in blood-derived cell-free DNA of patients with primary central nervous system lymphoma obtained before intracerebral biopsy. J Mol Diagn. 2020 Oct;22(10):1300–7. PMID:32745612
2150. Montesinos-Rongen M, Godlewska E, Brunn A, et al. Activating L265P mutations of the MYD88 gene are common in primary central nervous system lymphoma. Acta Neuropathol. 2011 Dec;122(6):791–2. PMID:22020631
2151. Montesinos-Rongen M, Hans VH, Eis-Hübinger AM, et al. Human herpes virus-8 is not associated with primary central nervous system lymphoma in HIV-negative patients. Acta Neuropathol. 2001 Nov;102(5):489–95. PMID:11699563
2152. Montesinos-Rongen M, Küppers R,

Schlüter D, et al. Primary central nervous system lymphomas are derived from germinal-center B cells and show a preferential usage of the V4-34 gene segment. Am J Pathol. 1999 Dec;155(6):2077–86. PMID:10595937
2153. Montesinos-Rongen M, Schäfer E, Siebert R, et al. Genes regulating the B cell receptor pathway are recurrently mutated in primary central nervous system lymphoma. Acta Neuropathol. 2012 Dec;124(6):905–6. PMID:23138649
2154. Montesinos-Rongen M, Schmitz R, Brunn A, et al. Mutations of CARD11 but not TNFAIP3 may activate the NF-kappaB pathway in primary CNS lymphoma. Acta Neuropathol. 2010 Oct;120(4):529–35. PMID:20544211
2155. Montesinos-Rongen M, Schmitz R, Courts C, et al. Absence of immunoglobulin class switch in primary lymphomas of the central nervous system. Am J Pathol. 2005 Jun;166(6):1773–9. PMID:15920162
2156. Montesinos-Rongen M, Terrao M, May C, et al. The process of somatic hypermutation increases polyreactivity for central nervous system antigens in primary central nervous system lymphoma. Haematologica. 2021 Mar 1;106(3):708–17. PMID:32193251
2157. Montesinos-Rongen M, Van Roost D, Schaller C, et al. Primary diffuse large B-cell lymphomas of the central nervous system are targeted by aberrant somatic hypermutation. Blood. 2004 Mar 1;103(5):1869–75. PMID:14592832
2158. Montesinos-Rongen M, Zühlke-Jenisch R, Gesk S, et al. Interphase cytogenetic analysis of lymphoma-associated chromosomal breakpoints in primary diffuse large B-cell lymphomas of the central nervous system. J Neuropathol Exp Neurol. 2002 Oct;61(10):926–33. PMID:12387458
2159. Montgomery BK, Alimchandani M, Mehta GU, et al. Tumors displaying hybrid schwannoma and neurofibroma features in patients with neurofibromatosis type 2. Clin Neuropathol. 2016 Mar-Apr;35(2):78–83. PMID:26709712
2160. Mooney KL, Choy W, Woodard J, et al. Primary central nervous system gamma delta cytotoxic T-cell lymphoma. J Clin Neurosci. 2016 Apr;26:138–40. PMID:26804925
2161. Moore BD 3rd, Slopis JM, Jackson EF, et al. Brain volume in children with neurofibromatosis type 1: relation to neuropsychological status. Neurology. 2000 Feb 22;54(4):914–20. PMID:10690986
2162. Moran CA, Rush W, Mena H. Primary spinal paragangliomas: a clinicopathological and immunohistochemical study of 30 cases. Histopathology. 1997 Aug;31(2):167–73. PMID:9279569
2163. Morin O, Chen WC, Nassiri F, et al. Integrated models incorporating radiologic and radiomic features predict meningioma grade, local failure, and overall survival. Neurooncol Adv. 2019 May-Dec;1(1):vdz011. PMID:31608329
2164. Mørk SJ, Rubinstein LJ, Kepes JJ, et al. Patterns of epithelial metaplasia in malignant gliomas. II. Squamous differentiation of epithelial-like formations in gliosarcomas and glioblastomas. J Neuropathol Exp Neurol. 1988 Mar;47(2):101–18. PMID:3339369
2165. Morris SM, Acosta MT, Garg S, et al. Disease burden and symptom structure of autism in neurofibromatosis type 1: a study of the International NF1-ASD Consortium Team (INFACT). JAMA Psychiatry. 2016 Dec 1;73(12):1276–84. PMID:27760236
2165A. Morton WE. Leukemias and occupation in Sweden. Am J Ind Med. 1989;15(5):607–8. PMID:2741965
2166. Motta M, Fidan M, Bellacchio E, et al. Dominant Noonan syndrome-causing LZTR1 mutations specifically affect the Kelch domain substrate-recognition surface and enhance RAS-MAPK signaling. Hum Mol Genet. 2019 Mar 15;28(6):1007–22. PMID:30481304
2167. Mu Q, Yu J, Qu L, et al. Spindle cell oncocytoma of the adenohypophysis: two case reports and a review of the literature. Mol Med Rep. 2015 Jul;12(1):871–6. PMID:25777996
2168. Mukai K, Seljeskog EL, Dehner LP. Pituitary adenomas in patients under 20 years old. A clinicopathological study of 12 cases. J Neurooncol. 1986;4(1):79–89. PMID:3018185
2169. Müller HL. Consequences of craniopharyngioma surgery in children. J Clin Endocrinol Metab. 2011 Jul;96(7):1981–91. PMID:21508127
2170. Müller HL, Bueb K, Bartels U, et al. Obesity after childhood craniopharyngioma–German multicenter study on pre-operative risk factors and quality of life. Klin Padiatr. 2001 Jul-Aug;213(4):244–9. PMID:11528558
2171. Müller HL, Emser A, Faldum A, et al. Longitudinal study on growth and body mass index before and after diagnosis of childhood craniopharyngioma. J Clin Endocrinol Metab. 2004 Jul;89(7):3298–305. PMID:15240606
2172. Müller HL, Gebhardt U, Teske C, et al. Post-operative hypothalamic lesions and obesity in childhood craniopharyngioma: results of the multinational prospective trial KRANIOPHARYNGEOM 2000 after 3-year follow-up. Eur J Endocrinol. 2011 Jul;165(1):17–24. PMID:21490122
2173. Müller HL, Merchant TE, Warmuth-Metz M, et al. Craniopharyngioma. Nat Rev Dis Primers. 2019 Nov 7;5(1):75. PMID:31699993
2174. Müller-Scholden J, Lehrnbecher T, Müller HL, et al. Radical surgery in a neonate with craniopharyngioma. report of a case. Pediatr Neurosurg. 2000 Nov;33(5):265–9. PMID:11155065
2175. Muñoz-Hidalgo L, San-Miguel T, Megías J, et al. Somatic copy number alterations are associated with EGFR amplification and shortened survival in patients with primary glioblastoma. Neoplasia. 2020 Jan;22(1):10–21. PMID:31751860
2176. Murali R, Wiesner T, Rosenblum MK, et al. GNAQ and GNA11 mutations in melanocytomas of the central nervous system. Acta Neuropathol. 2012 Mar;123(3):457–9. PMID:22307269
2177. Murray JC, Donahue DJ, Malik SI, et al. Temporal lobe pleomorphic xanthoastrocytoma and acquired BRAF mutation in an adolescent with the constitutional 22q11.2 deletion syndrome. J Neurooncol. 2011 May;102(3):509–14. PMID:20730472
2178. Murray JM, Morgello S. Polyomaviruses and primary central nervous system lymphomas. Neurology. 2004 Oct 12;63(7):1299–301. PMID:15477558
2179. Murray MJ, Bartels U, Nishikawa R, et al. Consensus on the management of intracranial germ-cell tumours. Lancet Oncol. 2015 Sep;16(9):e470–7. PMID:26370356
2180. Murthy A, Gonzalez-Agosti C, Cordero E, et al. NHE-RF, a regulatory cofactor for Na(+)-H+ exchange, is a common interactor for merlin and ERM (MERM) proteins. J Biol Chem. 1998 Jan 16;273(3):1273–6. PMID:9430655
2181. Muscarella LA, Bisceglia M, Galliani CA, et al. Extraneuraxial hemangioblastoma: a clinicopathologic study of 10 cases with molecular analysis of the VHL gene. Pathol Res Pract. 2018 Aug;214(8):1156–65. PMID:29941223
2182. Mut M, Schiff D, Shaffrey ME. Metastasis to nervous system: spinal epidural and intramedullary metastases. J Neurooncol. 2005 Oct;75(1):43–56. PMID:16215815
2183. Muthappan M, Muthu T, Hussain Z, et al. Cervical intramedullary melanocytoma: a case report and review of literature. J Clin Neurosci. 2012 Oct;19(10):1450–3. PMID:22796275
2184. Myers KA, Mandelstam SA, Ramantani G, et al. The epileptology of Koolen-de Vries syndrome: electro-clinico-radiologic findings in 31 patients. Epilepsia. 2017 Jun;58(6):1085–94. PMID:28440867
2185. Myers MP, Stolarov JP, Eng C, et al. P-TEN, the tumor suppressor from human chromosome 10q23, is a dual-specificity phosphatase. Proc Natl Acad Sci U S A. 1997 Aug 19;94(17):9052–7. PMID:9256433
2186. Mynarek M, von Hoff K, Pietsch T, et al. Nonmetastatic medulloblastoma of early childhood: results from the prospective clinical trial HIT-2000 and an extended validation cohort. J Clin Oncol. 2020 Jun 20;38(18):2028–40. PMID:32330099
2187. Myung JK, Cho HJ, Park CK, et al. Clinicopathological and genetic characteristics of extraventricular neurocytomas. Neuropathology. 2013 Apr;33(2):111–21. PMID:22672632
2188. Nabavizadeh SA, Assadsangabi R, Hajmomenian M, et al. High accuracy of arterial spin labeling perfusion imaging in differentiation of pilomyxoid from pilocytic astrocytoma. Neuroradiology. 2015 May;57(5):527–33. PMID:25666232
2189. Nabbout R, Santos M, Rolland Y, et al. Early diagnosis of subependymal giant cell astrocytoma in children with tuberous sclerosis. J Neurol Neurosurg Psychiatry. 1999 Mar;66(3):370–5. PMID:10084537
2190. Nagaishi M, Kim YH, Mittelbronn M, et al. Amplification of the STOML3, FREM2, and LHFP genes is associated with mesenchymal differentiation in gliosarcoma. Am J Pathol. 2012 May;180(5):1816–23. PMID:22538188
2191. Nagaishi M, Paulus W, Brokinkel B, et al. Transcriptional factors for epithelial-mesenchymal transition are associated with mesenchymal differentiation in gliosarcoma. Brain Pathol. 2012 Sep;22(5):670–6. PMID:22288519
2192. Nagaishi M, Yokoo H, Nobusawa S, et al. Localized overexpression of alpha-internexin within nodules in multinodular and vacuolating neuronal tumors. Neuropathology. 2015 Dec;35(6):561–8. PMID:26073706
2193. Nagaraja S, Vitanza NA, Woo PJ, et al. Transcriptional dependencies in diffuse intrinsic pontine glioma. Cancer Cell. 2017 May 8;31(5):635–652.e6. PMID:28434841
2194. Nagashima T, Hoshino T, Cho KG. Proliferative potential of vascular components in human glioblastoma multiforme. Acta Neuropathol. 1987;73(3):301–5. PMID:3039783
2195. Naggara O, Varlet P, Page P, et al. Suprasellar paraganglioma: a case report and review of the literature. Neuroradiology. 2005 Oct;47(10):753–7. PMID:16047139
2196. Nair P, Das KK, Srivastava AK, et al. Primary intracranial rhabdomyosarcoma of the cerebellopontine angle mimicking a vestibular schwannoma in a child. Asian J Neurosurg. 2017 Jan-Mar;12(1):109–11. PMID:28413550
2197. Naitoh Y, Sasajima T, Kinouchi H, et al. Medulloblastoma with extensive nodularity: single photon emission CT study with iodine-123 metaiodobenzylguanidine. AJNR Am J Neuroradiol. 2002 Oct;23(9):1564–7. PMID:12372749
2198. Nakagawa Y, Perentes E, Rubinstein LJ. Immunohistochemical characterization of oligodendrogliomas: an analysis of multiple markers. Acta Neuropathol. 1986;72(1):15–22. PMID:2435103
2199. Nakagawa Y, Perentes E, Rubinstein LJ. Non-specificity of anti-carbonic anhydrase C antibody as a marker in human neurooncology. J Neuropathol Exp Neurol. 1987 Jul;46(4):451–60. PMID:3110380
2200. Nakajima N, Nobusawa S, Nakata S, et al. BRAF V600E, TERT promoter mutations and CDKN2A/B homozygous deletions are frequent in epithelioid glioblastomas: a histological and molecular analysis focusing on intratumoral heterogeneity. Brain Pathol. 2018 Sep;28(5):663–73. PMID:29105198
2201. Nakama S, Higashi T, Kimura A, et al. Double myxopapillary ependymoma of the cauda equina. J Orthop Sci. 2005 Sep;10(5):543–5. PMID:16193371
2202. Nakamura M, Chiba K, Matsumoto M, et al. Pleomorphic xanthoastrocytoma of the spinal cord. Case report. J Neurosurg Spine. 2006 Jul;5(1):72–5. PMID:16850961
2203. Nakamura M, Saeki N, Iwadate Y, et al. Neuroradiological characteristics of pineocytoma and pineoblastoma. Neuroradiology. 2000 Jul;42(7):509–14. PMID:10952183
2204. Nakamura M, Watanabe T, Yonekawa Y, et al. Promoter methylation of the DNA repair gene MGMT in astrocytomas is frequently associated with G:C -> A:T mutations of the TP53 tumor suppressor gene. Carcinogenesis. 2001 Oct;22(10):1715–9. PMID:11577014
2205. Nakamura T, Tateishi K, Niwa T, et al. Recurrent mutations of CD79B and MYD88 are the hallmark of primary central nervous system lymphomas. Neuropathol Appl Neurobiol. 2016 Apr;42(3):279–90. PMID:26111727
2206. Nakashima Y, Miyagi-Shiohira C, Kobayashi N, et al. Adhesion characteristics of porcine pancreatic islets and exocrine tissue to coating materials. Islets. 2018 May 4;10(3):e1460294. PMID:29757700
2207. Nambirajan A, Sharma MC, Rajeshwari M, et al. A comparative immunohistochemical study of epithelial membrane antigen and NHERF1/EBP50 in the diagnosis of ependymomas. Appl Immunohistochem Mol Morphol. 2018 Jan;26(1):71–8. PMID:27753657
2208. Nambirajan A, Suri V, Kedia S, et al. Paediatric diffuse leptomeningeal tumor with glial and neuronal differentiation harbouring chromosome 1p/19q co-deletion and H3.3 K27M mutation: unusual molecular profile and its therapeutic implications. Brain Tumor Pathol. 2018 Jul;35(3):186–91. PMID:30030640
2209. Nandu H, Wen PY, Huang RY. Imaging in neuro-oncology. Ther Adv Neurol Disord. 2018 Feb 28;11:1756286418759865. PMID:29511385
2210. Narayan V, Savardekar AR, Mahadevan A, et al. Unusual occurrence of multifocal desmoplastic infantile astrocytoma: a case report and review of the literature. Pediatr Neurosurg. 2017;52(3):173–80. PMID:28222441
2211. Narla S, Govindraj J, Chandrasekar K, et al. Craniopharyngioma with malignant transformation: review of literature. Neurol India. 2017 Mar-Apr;65(2):418–20. PMID:28290422
2212. Nascimento AF, Fletcher CD. The controversial nosology of benign nerve sheath tumors: neurofilament protein staining demonstrates intratumoral axons in many sporadic schwannomas. Am J Surg Pathol. 2007 Sep;31(9):1363–70. PMID:17721192
2213. Nasit J, Vaghsiya V, Hiryur S, et al. Intraoperative squash cytologic features of subependymal giant cell astrocytoma. J Lab Physicians. 2016 Jan-Jun;8(1):58–61. PMID:27013816
2214. Nassiri F, Mamatjan Y, Suppiah S, et al. DNA methylation profiling to predict recurrence risk in meningioma: development and validation of a nomogram to optimize clinical management. Neuro Oncol. 2019 Jul 11;21(7):901–10. PMID:31158293
2215. Nasu M, Emi M, Pastorino S, et al. High Incidence of Somatic BAP1 alterations in sporadic malignant mesothelioma. J Thorac Oncol. 2015 Apr;10(4):565–76. PMID:25658628
2216. National Comprehensive Cancer Network (NCCN). NCCN clinical practice guidelines in

oncology (NCCN guidelines): genetic/familial high-risk assessment: breast and ovarian cancer. Version 1.2010. Fort Washington (PA): NCCN; 2010. Available from: https://www.nccn.org/professionals/physician_gls/default.aspx.
2217. National Institutes of Health Consensus Development Conference. Neurofibromatosis. Conference statement. Arch Neurol. 1988 May;45(5):575–8. PMID:3128965
2218. Naudin ten Cate L, Vermeij-Keers C, Smit DA, et al. Intracranial teratoma with multiple fetuses: pre- and post-natal appearance. Hum Pathol. 1995 Jul;26(7):804–7. PMID:7628856
2219. Nayak L, Abrey LE, Iwamoto FM. Intracranial dural metastases. Cancer. 2009 May 1;115(9):1947–53. PMID:19241421
2220. Nayak L, Iwamoto FM, LaCasce A, et al. PD-1 blockade with nivolumab in relapsed/refractory primary central nervous system and testicular lymphoma. Blood. 2017 Jun 8;129(23):3071–3. PMID:28356247
2221. Naylor RM, Wohl A, Raghunathan A, et al. Novel suprasellar location of desmoplastic infantile astrocytoma and ganglioglioma: a single institution's experience. J Neurosurg Pediatr. 2018 Oct;22(4):397–403. PMID:29979130
2222. Nayyar M, Mayo MC, Shiroishi M, et al. Atypical central neurocytoma with metastatic craniospinal dissemination: a case report. Clin Imaging. 2016 Nov-Dec;40(6):1108–11. PMID:27450443
2223. Nayyar N, White MD, Gill CM, et al. MYD88 L265P mutation and CDKN2A loss are early mutational events in primary central nervous system diffuse large B-cell lymphomas. Blood Adv. 2019 Feb 12;3(3):375–83. PMID:30723112
2224. Neal MT, Ellis TL, Stanton CA. Pleomorphic xanthoastrocytoma in two siblings with neurofibromatosis type 1 (NF-1). Clin Neuropathol. 2012 Jan-Feb;31(1):54–6. PMID:22192706
2225. Nedialkova DD, Leidel SA. Optimization of codon translation rates via trna modifications maintains proteome integrity. Cell. 2015 Jun 18;161(7):1606–18. PMID:26052047
2226. Neftel C, Laffy J, Filbin MG, et al. An integrative model of cellular states, plasticity, and genetics for glioblastoma. Cell. 2019 Aug 8;178(4):835–849.e21. PMID:31327527
2227. Nelen MR, Kremer H, Konings IB, et al. Novel PTEN mutations in patients with Cowden disease: absence of clear genotype-phenotype correlations. Eur J Hum Genet. 1999 Apr;7(3):267–73. PMID:10234502
2228. Nelen MR, Padberg GW, Peeters EA, et al. Localization of the gene for Cowden disease to chromosome 10q22-23. Nat Genet. 1996 May;13(1):114–6. PMID:8673088
2229. Nelen MR, van Staveren WC, Peeters EA, et al. Germline mutations in the PTEN/MMAC1 gene in patients with Cowden disease. Hum Mol Genet. 1997 Aug;6(8):1383–7. PMID:9259288
2230. Nelson AJ, Zakaria R, Jenkinson MD, et al. Extent of resection predicts risk of progression in adult pilocytic astrocytoma. Br J Neurosurg. 2019 Jun;33(3):343–7. PMID:30653383
2231. Nelson DS, Quispel W, Badalian-Very G, et al. Somatic activating ARAF mutations in Langerhans cell histiocytosis. Blood. 2014 May 15;123(20):3152–5. PMID:24652991
2232. Neou M, Villa C, Armignacco R, et al. Pangenomic classification of pituitary neuroendocrine tumors. Cancer Cell. 2020 Jan 13;37(1):123–134.e5. PMID:31883967
2233. Neuhold JC, Friesenhahn J, Gerdes N, et al. Case reports of fatal or metastasizing melanoma in children and adolescents: a systematic analysis of the literature. Pediatr Dermatol. 2015 Jan-Feb;32(1):13–22. PMID:25487565
2234. Neumann HP, Bausch B, McWhinney SR, et al. Germ-line mutations in nonsyndromic pheochromocytoma. N Engl J Med. 2002 May 9;346(19):1459–66. PMID:12000816
2235. Neumann JE, Dorostkar MM, Korshunov A, et al. Distinct histomorphology in molecular subgroups of glioblastomas in young patients. J Neuropathol Exp Neurol. 2016 May;75(5):408–14. PMID:26975364
2236. Neumann JE, Spohn M, Obrecht D, et al. Molecular characterization of histopathological ependymoma variants. Acta Neuropathol. 2020 Feb;139(2):305–18. PMID:31679042
2237. Neves S, Mazal PR, Wanschitz J, et al. Pseudogliomatous growth pattern of anaplastic small cell carcinomas metastatic to the brain. Clin Neuropathol. 2001 Jan-Feb;20(1):38–42. PMID:11220694
2238. Ng A, Levy ML, Malicki DM, et al. Unusual high-grade and low-grade glioma in an infant with PPP1CB-ALK gene fusion. BMJ Case Rep. 2019 Feb 1;12(2):e228248. PMID:30709888
2239. Ng HK. Cytologic diagnosis of intracranial germinomas in smear preparations. Acta Cytol. 1995 Jul-Aug;39(4):693–7. PMID:7543235
2240. Ng HK, Poon WS. Gliosarcoma of the posterior fossa with features of a malignant fibrous histiocytoma. Cancer. 1990 Mar 1;65(5):1161–6. PMID:2154322
2241. Ng Wing Tin S, Martin-Duverneuil N, Idbaih A, et al. Efficacy of vinblastine in central nervous system Langerhans cell histiocytosis: a nationwide retrospective study. Orphanet J Rare Dis. 2011 Dec 12;6:83. PMID:22151964
2242. Nguyen HS, Doan N, Gelsomino M, et al. Dysembryoplastic neuroectodermal tumor: an analysis from the Surveillance, Epidemiology, and End Results Program, 2004-2013. World Neurosurg. 2017 Jul;103:380–5. PMID:28438654
2243. Nguyen HS, Doan N, Gelsomino M, et al. Intracranial subependymoma: a SEER analysis 2004-2013. World Neurosurg. 2017 May;101:599–605. PMID:28232153
2244. Nguyen HS, Doan NB, Gelsomino M, et al. Intracranial hemangioblastoma - A SEER-based analysis 2004-2013. Oncotarget. 2018 Jun 15;9(46):28009–15. PMID:29963258
2245. Nguyen HS, Doan NB, Gelsomino M, et al. Subependymal giant cell astrocytoma: a Surveillance, Epidemiology, and End Results Program-based analysis from 2004 to 2013. World Neurosurg. 2018 Oct;118:e263–8. PMID:29966782
2246. Nguyen-Them L, Costopoulos M, Tanguy ML, et al. The CSF IL-10 concentration is an effective diagnostic marker in immunocompetent primary CNS lymphoma and a potential prognostic biomarker in treatment-responsive patients. Eur J Cancer. 2016 Jul;61:69–76. PMID:27156226
2247. Ni HC, Chen SY, Chen L, et al. Angiocentric glioma: a report of nine new cases, including four with atypical histological features. Neuropathol Appl Neurobiol. 2015 Apr;41(3):333–46. PMID:24861831
2248. Ni Y, He X, Chen J, et al. Germline SDHx variants modify breast and thyroid cancer risks in Cowden and Cowden-like syndrome via FAD/NAD-dependant destabilization of p53. Hum Mol Genet. 2012 Jan 15;21(2):300–10. PMID:21979946
2249. Ni Y, Seballos S, Fletcher B, et al. Germline compound heterozygous poly-glutamine deletion in USF3 may be involved in predisposition to heritable and sporadic epithelial thyroid carcinoma. Hum Mol Genet. 2017 Jan 15;26(2):243–57. PMID:28011713
2250. Ni Y, Zbuk KM, Sadler T, et al. Germline mutations and variants in the succinate dehydrogenase genes in Cowden and Cowden-like syndromes. Am J Hum Genet. 2008 Aug;83(2):261–8. PMID:18678321
2251. Nichols KE, Malkin D, Garber JE, et al. Germ-line p53 mutations predispose to a wide spectrum of early-onset cancers. Cancer Epidemiol Biomarkers Prev. 2001 Feb;10(2):83–7. PMID:11219776
2252. Nieder C, Spanne O, Mehta MP, et al. Presentation, patterns of care, and survival in patients with brain metastases: what has changed in the last 20 years? Cancer. 2011 Jun 1;117(11):2505–12. PMID:24048799
2253. Nielsen EH, Feldt-Rasmussen U, Poulsgaard L, et al. Incidence of craniopharyngioma in Denmark (n = 189) and estimated world incidence of craniopharyngioma in children and adults. J Neurooncol. 2011 Sep;104(3):755–63. PMID:21336771
2254. Nielsen GP, Dickersin GR, Provenzal JM, et al. Lipomatous hemangiopericytoma. A histologic, ultrastructural and immunohistochemical study of a unique variant of hemangiopericytoma. Am J Surg Pathol. 1995 Jul;19(7):748–56. PMID:7793472
2255. Nieuwenhuis MH, Kets CM, Murphy-Ryan M, et al. Cancer risk and genotype-phenotype correlations in PTEN hamartoma tumor syndrome. Fam Cancer. 2014 Mar;13(1):57–63. PMID:23934601
2256. Niida Y, Stemmer-Rachamimov AO, Logrip M, et al. Survey of somatic mutations in tuberous sclerosis complex (TSC) hamartomas suggests different genetic mechanisms for pathogenesis of TSC lesions. Am J Hum Genet. 2001 Sep;69(3):493–503. PMID:11468687
2257. Niiro T, Tokimura H, Hanaya R, et al. MRI findings in patients with central neurocytomas with special reference to differential diagnosis from other ventricular tumours near the foramen of Monro. J Clin Neurosci. 2012 May;19(5):681–6. PMID:22410173
2258. Nikbakht H, Panditharatna E, Mikael LG, et al. Spatial and temporal homogeneity of driver mutations in diffuse intrinsic pontine glioma. Nat Commun. 2016 Apr 6;7:11185. PMID:27048880
2259. Nishikawa R, Furnari FB, Lin H, et al. Loss of P16INK4 expression is frequent in high grade gliomas. Cancer Res. 1995 May 1;55(9):1941–5. PMID:7728764
2260. Nishimoto T, Kaya B. Cerebellar liponeurocytoma. Arch Pathol Lab Med. 2012 Aug;136(8):965–9. PMID:22849747
2261. Nishimura H, Fukami S, Endo K, et al. A Case of rapidly-progressing cervical spine subependymoma with atypical features. Spine Surg Relat Res. 2018 May 29;3(1):91–4. PMID:31435558
2262. Nishioka H, Inoshita N, Mete O, et al. The complementary role of transcription factors in the accurate diagnosis of clinically nonfunctioning pituitary adenomas. Endocr Pathol. 2015 Dec;26(4):349–55. PMID:26481628
2263. Nitta H, Hayase H, Moriyama Y, et al. Gliosarcoma of the posterior cranial fossa: MRI findings. Neuroradiology. 1993;35(4):279–80. PMID:8492894
2264. Niu X, Wang T, Yang Y, et al. Prognostic factors for the survival outcome of bilateral thalamic glioma: an integrated survival analysis. World Neurosurg. 2018 Feb;110:e222–30. PMID:29102752
2265. Njauw CN, Kim I, Piris A, et al. Germline BAP1 inactivation is preferentially associated with metastatic ocular melanoma and cutaneous-ocular melanoma families. PLoS One. 2012;7(4):e35295. PMID:22545102
2266. Nobusawa S, Hirato J, Kurihara H, et al. Intratumoral heterogeneity of genomic imbalance in a case of epithelioid glioblastoma with BRAF V600E mutation. Brain Pathol. 2014 Apr;24(3):239–46. PMID:24354918
2267. Nobusawa S, Hirato J, Sugai T, et al. Atypical teratoid/rhabdoid tumor (AT/RT) arising from ependymoma: a type of AT/RT secondarily developing from other primary central nervous system tumors. J Neuropathol Exp Neurol. 2016 Feb;75(2):167–74. PMID:26769252
2268. Nobusawa S, Nakata S, Yoshida Y, et al. Secondary INI1-deficient rhabdoid tumors of the central nervous system: analysis of four cases and literature review. Virchows Arch. 2020 May;476(5):763–72. PMID:31707588
2269. Nobusawa S, Watanabe T, Kleihues P, et al. IDH1 mutations as molecular signature and predictive factor of secondary glioblastomas. Clin Cancer Res. 2009 Oct 1;15(19):6002–7. PMID:19755387
2270. Nobusawa S, Yokoo H, Hirato J, et al. Analysis of chromosome 19q13.42 amplification in embryonal brain tumors with ependymoblastic multilayered rosettes. Brain Pathol. 2012 Sep;22(5):689–97. PMID:22324795
2271. Noell S, Beschorner R, Bisdas S, et al. Simultaneous subependymomas in monozygotic female twins: further evidence for a common genetic or developmental disorder background. J Neurosurg. 2014 Sep;121(3):570–5. PMID:24655099
2272. Noell S, Fallier-Becker P, Mack AF, et al. Water channels aquaporin 4 and -1 expression in subependymoma depends on the localization of the tumors. PLoS One. 2015 Jun 26;10(6):e0131367. PMID:26115524
2273. Nolan MA, Sakuta R, Chuang N, et al. Dysembryoplastic neuroepithelial tumors in childhood: long-term outcome and prognostic features. Neurology. 2004 Jun 22;62(12):2270–6. PMID:15210893
2274. Nomani L, Cotta CV, Hsi ED, et al. Extranodal marginal zone lymphoma of the central nervous system includes parenchymal-based cases with characteristic features. Am J Clin Pathol. 2020 Jun 8;154(1):124–32. PMID:32318699
2275. Nomura M, Narita Y, Miyakita Y, et al. Clinical presentation of anaplastic large-cell lymphoma in the central nervous system. Mol Clin Oncol. 2013 Jul;1(4):655–60. PMID:24649224
2276. Nonaka D, Chiriboga L, Rubin BP. Sox10: a pan-schwannian and melanocytic marker. Am J Surg Pathol. 2008 Sep;32(9):1291–8. PMID:18636017
2277. Nonoguchi N, Ohta T, Oh JE, et al. TERT promoter mutations in primary and secondary glioblastomas. Acta Neuropathol. 2013 Dec;126(6):931–7. PMID:23955565
2278. Norman MG, Harrison KJ, Poskitt KJ, et al. Duplication of 9P and hyperplasia of the choroid plexus: a pathologic, radiologic, and molecular cytogenetics study. Pediatr Pathol Lab Med. 1995 Jan-Feb;15(1):109–20. PMID:8736601
2279. Northcott PA, Buchhalter I, Morrissy AS, et al. The whole-genome landscape of medulloblastoma subtypes. Nature. 2017 Jul 19;547(7663):311–7. PMID:28726821
2280. Northcott PA, Jones DT, Kool M, et al. Medulloblastomics: the end of the beginning. Nat Rev Cancer. 2012 Dec;12(12):818–34. PMID:23175120
2281. Northcott PA, Lee C, Zichner T, et al. Enhancer hijacking activates GFI1 family oncogenes in medulloblastoma. Nature. 2014 Jul 24;511(7510):428–34. PMID:25043047
2282. Northcott PA, Nakahara Y, Wu X, et al. Multiple recurrent genetic events converge on control of histone lysine methylation in medulloblastoma. Nat Genet. 2009 Apr;41(4):465–72. PMID:19270706
2283. Northcott PA, Robinson GW, Kratz CP, et al. Medulloblastoma. Nat Rev Dis Primers. 2019 Feb 14;5(1):11. PMID:30765705
2284. Northcott PA, Shih DJ, Peacock J, et al.

Subgroup-specific structural variation across 1,000 medulloblastoma genomes. Nature. 2012 Aug 2;488(7409):49–56. PMID:22832581
2285. Northrup H, Koenig MK, Pearson DA, et al. Tuberous sclerosis complex. In: Adam MP, Ardinger HH, Pagon RA, et al., editors. GeneReviews. Seattle (WA): University of Washington, Seattle; 1999 Jul 13 [updated 2020 Apr 16]. PMID:20301399
2286. Northrup H, Krueger DA, International Tuberous Sclerosis Complex Consensus Group. Tuberous sclerosis complex diagnostic criteria update: recommendations of the 2012 Iinternational Tuberous Sclerosis Complex Consensus Conference. Pediatr Neurol. 2013 Oct;49(4):243–54. PMID:24053982
2287. Noushmehr H, Weisenberger DJ, Diefes K, et al. Identification of a CpG island methylator phenotype that defines a distinct subgroup of glioma. Cancer Cell. 2010 May 18;17(5):510–22. PMID:20399149
2288. Nowak J, Jünger ST, Huflage H, et al. MRI Phenotype of RELA-fused Pediatric Supratentorial Ependymoma. Clin Neuroradiol. 2019 Dec;29(4):595–604. PMID:30027327
2289. Nowak J, Nemes K, Hohm A, et al. Magnetic resonance imaging surrogates of molecular subgroups in atypical teratoid/rhabdoid tumor. Neuro Oncol. 2018 Nov 12;20(12):1672–9. PMID:30010851
2290. Nowak J, Seidel C, Berg F, et al. MRI characteristics of ependymoblastoma: results from 22 centrally reviewed cases. AJNR Am J Neuroradiol. 2014 Oct;35(10):1996–2001. PMID:24948504
2291. Numoto RT. Pineal parenchymal tumors: cell differentiation and prognosis. J Cancer Res Clin Oncol. 1994;120(11):683–90. PMID:7525594
2292. Nunes RH, Hsu CC, da Rocha AJ, et al. Multinodular and vacuolating neuronal tumor of the cerebrum: a new "leave me alone" lesion with a characteristic imaging pattern. AJNR Am J Neuroradiol. 2017 Oct;38(10):1899–904. PMID:28705817
2293. Nutt CL, Mani DR, Betensky RA, et al. Gene expression-based classification of malignant gliomas correlates better with survival than histological classification. Cancer Res. 2003 Apr 1;63(7):1602–7. PMID:12670911
2294. Oakley GJ, Fuhrer K, Seethala RR. Brachyury, SOX-9, and podoplanin, new markers in the skull base chordoma vs chondrosarcoma differential: a tissue microarray-based comparative analysis. Mod Pathol. 2008 Dec;21(12):1461–9. PMID:18820665
2295. Obari A, Sano T, Ohyama K, et al. Clinicopathological features of growth hormone-producing pituitary adenomas: difference among various types defined by cytokeratin distribution pattern including a transitional form. Endocr Pathol. 2008 Summer;19(2):82–91. PMID:18629656
2296. Ochalski PG, Edinger JT, Horowitz MB, et al. Intracranial angiomatoid fibrous histiocytoma presenting as recurrent multifocal intraparenchymal hemorrhage. J Neurosurg. 2010 May;112(5):978–82. PMID:19731989
2297. Offit K, Levran O, Mullaney B, et al. Shared genetic susceptibility to breast cancer, brain tumors, and Fanconi anemia. J Natl Cancer Inst. 2003 Oct 15;95(20):1548–51. PMID:14559878
2298. Ogawa K, Kurose A, Kamataki A, et al. Giant cell glioblastoma is a distinctive subtype of glioma characterized by vulnerability to DNA damage. Brain Tumor Pathol. 2020 Jan;37(1):5–13. PMID:31655917
2299. Ogawa T, Kawai N, Miyake K, et al. Diagnostic value of PET/CT with 11C-methionine (MET) and 18F-fluorothymidine (FLT) in newly diagnosed glioma based on the 2016 WHO classification. EJNMMI Res. 2020 May 7;10(1):44. PMID:32382870
2300. Ogilvy KM, Jakubowski J, Shortland JR. Letter: Spinal subarachnoid spread of pituitary adenoma. J Neurol Neurosurg Psychiatry. 1974 Oct;37(10):1186. PMID:4443813
2301. Ogino H, Shibamoto Y, Takanaka T, et al. CNS germinoma with elevated serum human chorionic gonadotropin level: clinical characteristics and treatment outcome. Int J Radiat Oncol Biol Phys. 2005 Jul 1;62(3):803–8. PMID:15936563
2302. Ognjanovic S, Olivier M, Bergemann TL, et al. Sarcomas in TP53 germline mutation carriers: a review of the IARC TP53 Database. Cancer. 2012 Mar 1;118(5):1387–96. PMID:21837677
2303. Ogura R, Aoki H, Natsumeda M, et al. Epstein-Barr virus-associated primary central nervous system cytotoxic T-cell lymphoma. Neuropathology. 2013 Aug;33(4):436–41. PMID:23279449
2304. Oh JE, Ohta T, Nonoguchi N, et al. Genetic alterations in gliosarcoma and giant cell glioblastoma. Brain Pathol. 2016 Jul;26(4):517–22. PMID:26443480
2305. Oh JE, Ohta T, Satomi K, et al. Alterations in the NF2/LATS1/LATS2/YAP Pathway in Schwannomas. J Neuropathol Exp Neurol. 2015 Oct;74(10):952–9. PMID:26360373
2306. Oh MC, Tarapore PE, Kim JM, et al. Spinal ependymomas: benefits of extent of resection for different histological grades. J Clin Neurosci. 2013 Oct;20(10):1390–7. PMID:23768966
2307. Oh T, Rutkowski MJ, Safaee M, et al. Survival outcomes of giant cell glioblastoma: institutional experience in the management of 20 patients. J Clin Neurosci. 2014 Dec;21(12):2129–34. PMID:25037316
2308. Ohar JA, Cheung M, Talarchek J, et al. Germline BAP1 mutational landscape of asbestos-exposed malignant mesothelioma patients with family history of cancer. Cancer Res. 2016 Jan 15;76(2):206–15. PMID:26719535
2309. Ohgaki H, Dessen P, Jourde B, et al. Genetic pathways to glioblastoma: a population-based study. Cancer Res. 2004 Oct 1;64(19):6892–9. PMID:15466178
2310. Ohgaki H, Kleihues P. Epidemiology and etiology of gliomas. Acta Neuropathol. 2005 Jan;109(1):93–108. PMID:15685439
2311. Ohgaki H, Kleihues P. Genetic pathways to primary and secondary glioblastoma. Am J Pathol. 2007 May;170(5):1445–53. PMID:17456751
2312. Ohgaki H, Kleihues P. Population-based studies on incidence, survival rates, and genetic alterations in astrocytic and oligodendroglial gliomas. J Neuropathol Exp Neurol. 2005 Jun;64(6):479–89. PMID:15977639
2313. Ohgaki H, Kleihues P. The definition of primary and secondary glioblastoma. Clin Cancer Res. 2013 Feb 15;19(4):764–72. PMID:23209033
2314. Ojha BK, Sharma MC, Rastogi M, et al. Dumbbell-shaped paraganglioma of the cervical spine in a child. Pediatr Neurosurg. 2007;43(1):60–4. PMID:17190992
2315. Okada M, Yano H, Hirose Y, et al. Olig2 is useful in the differential diagnosis of oligodendrogliomas and extraventricular neurocytomas. Brain Tumor Pathol. 2011 Apr;28(2):157–61. PMID:21312066
2316. Okada Y, Nishikawa R, Matsutani M, et al. Hypomethylated X chromosome gain and rare isochromosome 12p in diverse intracranial germ cell tumors. J Neuropathol Exp Neurol. 2002 Jun;61(6):531–8. PMID:12071636
2317. Okimoto RA, Breitenbuecher F, Olivas VR, et al. Inactivation of Capicua drives cancer metastasis. Nat Genet. 2017 Jan;49(1):87–96. PMID:27869830
2318. Olar A, Wani KM, Alfaro-Munoz KD, et al. IDH mutation status and role of WHO grade and mitotic index in overall survival in grade II-III diffuse gliomas. Acta Neuropathol. 2015 Apr;129(4):585–96. PMID:25701198
2319. Olar A, Wani KM, Sulman EP, et al. Mitotic index is an independent predictor of recurrence-free survival in meningioma. Brain Pathol. 2015 May;25(3):266–75. PMID:25040885
2320. Olivier M, Goldgar DE, Sodha N, et al. Li-Fraumeni and related syndromes: correlation between tumor type, family structure, and TP53 genotype. Cancer Res. 2003 Oct 15;63(20):6643–50. PMID:14583457
2321. Olschwang S, Serova-Sinilnikova OM, Lenoir GM, et al. PTEN germ-line mutations in juvenile polyposis coli. Nat Genet. 1998 Jan;18(1):12–4. PMID:9425889
2322. Olsen TK, Panagopoulos I, Meling TR, et al. Fusion genes with ALK as recurrent partner in ependymoma-like gliomas: a new brain tumor entity? Neuro Oncol. 2015 Oct;17(10):1365–73. PMID:25795305
2323. Olsson DS, Andersson E, Bryngelsson IL, et al. Excess mortality and morbidity in patients with craniopharyngioma, especially in patients with childhood onset: a population-based study in Sweden. J Clin Endocrinol Metab. 2015 Feb;100(2):467–74. PMID:25375987
2324. O'Malley S, Weitman D, Olding M, et al. Multiple neoplasms following craniospinal irradiation for medulloblastoma in a patient with nevoid basal cell carcinoma syndrome. Case report. J Neurosurg. 1997 Feb;86(2):286–8. PMID:9010431
2325. O'Marcaigh AS, Ledger GA, Roche PC, et al. Aromatase expression in human germinomas with possible biological effects. J Clin Endocrinol Metab. 1995 Dec;80(12):3763–6. PMID:8530631
2326. Onishi S, Yamasaki F, Nakano Y, et al. RELA fusion-positive anaplastic ependymoma: molecular characterization and advanced MR imaging. Brain Tumor Pathol. 2018 Jan;35(1):41–5. PMID:29063976
2327. Oosterhuis JW, Stoop H, Honecker F, et al. Why human extragonadal germ cell tumours occur in the midline of the body: old concepts, new perspectives. Int J Androl. 2007 Aug;30(4):256–63. PMID:17705807
2328. Ordóñez-Rubiano EG, Forbes JA, Morgenstern PF, et al. Preserve or sacrifice the stalk? Endocrinological outcomes, extent of resection, and recurrence rates following endoscopic endonasal resection of craniopharyngiomas. J Neurosurg. 2018 Nov 1:1–9. PMID:30497145
2329. Orloff MS, Eng C. Genetic and phenotypic heterogeneity in the PTEN hamartoma tumour syndrome. Oncogene. 2008 Sep 18;27(41):5387–97. PMID:18794875
2330. Orloff MS, He X, Peterson C, et al. Germline PIK3CA and AKT1 mutations in Cowden and Cowden-like syndromes. Am J Hum Genet. 2013 Jan 10;92(1):76–80. PMID:23246288
2331. Orr BA, Clay MR, Pinto EM, et al. An update on the central nervous system manifestations of Li-Fraumeni syndrome. Acta Neuropathol. 2020 Apr;139(4):669–87. PMID:31468188
2332. Orrell JM, Hales SA. Paragangliomas of the cauda equina have a distinctive cytokeratin immunophenotype. Histopathology. 1992 Nov;21(5):479–81. PMID:1280616
2333. Ortega A, Nuño M, Walia S, et al. Treatment and survival of patients harboring histological variants of glioblastoma. J Clin Neurosci. 2014 Oct;21(10):1709–13. PMID:24980627
2334. Orton A, Frandsen J, Jensen R, et al. Anaplastic meningioma: an analysis of the National Cancer Database from 2004 to 2012. J Neurosurg. 2018 Jun;128(6):1684–9. PMID:28731397
2335. Ortonne N, Wolkenstein P, Blakeley JO, et al. Cutaneous neurofibromas: current clinical and pathologic issues. Neurology. 2018 Jul 10;91(2 Suppl 1):S5–13. PMID:29987130
2336. Osawa T, Tosaka M, Nagaishi M, et al. Factors affecting peritumoral brain edema in meningioma: special histological subtypes with prominently extensive edema. J Neurooncol. 2013 Jan;111(1):49–57. PMID:23104516
2337. Osborn AG, Blaser SI, Salzman KL, et al., editors. Diagnostic imaging: brain. 1st ed. Altona (MB): Amirsys; 2004.
2338. Osbun JW, Reynolds MR, Barrow DL. Arteriovenous malformations: epidemiology, clinical presentation, and diagnostic evaluation. Handb Clin Neurol. 2017;143:25–9. PMID:28552148
2339. Osorio JA, Hervey-Jumper SL, Walsh KM, et al. Familial gliomas: cases in two pairs of brothers. J Neurooncol. 2015 Jan;121(1):135–40. PMID:25208478
2340. Ostendorf AP, Gutmann DH, Weisenberg JL. Epilepsy in individuals with neurofibromatosis type 1. Epilepsia. 2013 Oct;54(10):1810–4. PMID:24032542
2341. Ostertun B, Wolf HK, Campos MG, et al. Dysembryoplastic neuroepithelial tumors: MR and CT evaluation. AJNR Am J Neuroradiol. 1996 Mar;17(3):419–30. PMID:8881234
2342. Ostrom QT, Bauchet L, Davis FG, et al. The epidemiology of glioma in adults: a "state of the science" review. Neuro Oncol. 2014 Jul;16(7):896–913. PMID:24842956
2343. Ostrom QT, Chen Y, M de Blank P, et al. The descriptive epidemiology of atypical teratoid/rhabdoid tumors in the United States, 2001-2010. Neuro Oncol. 2014 Oct;16(10):1392–9. PMID:24847086
2344. Ostrom QT, Cioffi G, Gittleman H, et al. CBTRUS statistical report: primary brain and other central nervous system tumors diagnosed in the United States in 2012-2016. Neuro Oncol. 2019 Nov 1;21(Suppl 5):v1–100. PMID:31675094
2345. Ostrom QT, Gittleman H, Liao P, et al. CBTRUS statistical report: primary brain and central nervous system tumors diagnosed in the United States in 2007-2011. Neuro Oncol. 2014 Oct;16(Suppl 4):iv1–63. PMID:25304271
2346. Ostrom QT, Gittleman H, Stetson L, et al. Epidemiology of gliomas. Cancer Treat Res. 2015;163:1–14. PMID:25468222
2347. Ostrom QT, Gittleman H, Truitt G, et al. CBTRUS statistical report: primary brain and other central nervous system tumors diagnosed in the United States in 2011-2015. Neuro Oncol. 2018 Oct 1;20(suppl_4):iv1–86. PMID:30445539
2348. Otero JJ, Rowitch D, Vandenberg S. OLIG2 is differentially expressed in pediatric astrocytic and in ependymal neoplasms. J Neurooncol. 2011 Sep;104(2):423–38. PMID:21193945
2349. Otvos B, Silver DJ, Mulkearns-Hubert EE, et al. Cancer stem cell-secreted macrophage migration inhibitory factor stimulates myeloid derived suppressor cell function and facilitates glioblastoma immune evasion. Stem Cells. 2016 Aug;34(8):2026–39. PMID:27145382
2350. Ou A, Sumrall A, Phuphanich S, et al. Primary CNS lymphoma commonly expresses immune response biomarkers. Neurooncol Adv. 2020 Jan-Dec;2(1):a018. PMID:32201861
2351. Ouladan S, Trautmann M, Orouji E, et al. Differential diagnosis of solitary fibrous tumors: a study of 454 soft tissue tumors indicating the diagnostic value of nuclear STAT6 relocation and ALDH1 expression combined

with in situ proximity ligation assay. Int J Oncol. 2015;46(6):2595–605. PMID:25901508
2352. Owler BK, Makeham JM, Shingde M, et al. Cerebellar liponeurocytoma. J Clin Neurosci. 2005 Apr;12(3):326–9. PMID:15851097
2353. Owonikoko TK, Arbiser J, Zelnak A, et al. Current approaches to the treatment of metastatic brain tumours. Nat Rev Clin Oncol. 2014 Apr;11(4):203–22. PMID:24569448
2354. Owosho AA, Chen S, Kashikar S, et al. Clinical and molecular heterogeneity of head and neck spindle cell and sclerosing rhabdomyosarcoma. Oral Oncol. 2016 Jul;58:e6–11. PMID:27261172
2355. Oya S, Saito A, Okano A, et al. The pathogenesis of intracranial growing teratoma syndrome: proliferation of tumor cells or formation of multiple expanding cysts? Two case reports and review of the literature. Childs Nerv Syst. 2014 Aug;30(8):1455–61. PMID:24633581
2356. Oyama T, Yamamoto K, Asano N, et al. Age-related EBV-associated B-cell lymphoproliferative disorders constitute a distinct clinicopathologic group: a study of 96 patients. Clin Cancer Res. 2007 Sep 1;13(17):5124–32. PMID:17785567
2357. Ozawa T, Arora S, Szulzewsky F, et al. A de novo mouse model of C11orf95-RELA fusion-driven ependymoma identifies driver functions in addition to NF-κB. Cell Rep. 2018 Jun 26;23(13):3787–97. PMID:29949764
2358. Ozawa T, Brennan CW, Wang L, et al. PDGFRA gene rearrangements are frequent genetic events in PDGFRA-amplified glioblastomas. Genes Dev. 2010 Oct 1;24(19):2205–18. PMID:20889717
2359. Ozek MM, Sav A, Pamir MN, et al. Pleomorphic xanthoastrocytoma associated with von Recklinghausen neurofibromatosis. Childs Nerv Syst. 1993 Feb;9(1):39–42. PMID:8481944
2360. Ozpinar A, Mendez G, Abla AA. Epidemiology, genetics, pathophysiology, and prognostic classifications of cerebral arteriovenous malformations. Handb Clin Neurol. 2017;143:5–13. PMID:28552158
2361. Ozpinar A, Weiner GM, Ducruet AF. Epidemiology, clinical presentation, diagnostic evaluation, and prognosis of spinal arteriovenous malformations. Handb Clin Neurol. 2017;143:145–52. PMID:28552136
2362. Özyörük D, Kocayozgat A, Yaman-Bajin İ, et al. A synchronous occurrence of bifocal intracranial germinoma and bilateral testicular epidermoid cyst in an adolescent patient with Klinefelter's syndrome. Turk J Pediatr. 2019;61(3):456–9. PMID:31916730
2363. Özyurt J, Müller HL, Thiel CM. A systematic review of cognitive performance in patients with childhood craniopharyngioma. J Neurooncol. 2015 Oct;125(1):9–21. PMID:26369768
2364. Packer RJ, Iavarone A, Jones DTW, et al. Implications of new understandings of gliomas in children and adults with NF1: report of a consensus conference. Neuro Oncol. 2020 Jun 9;22(6):773–84. PMID:32055852
2365. Paek SH, Shin HY, Kim JW, et al. Primary culture of central neurocytoma: a case report. J Korean Med Sci. 2010 May;25(5):798–803. PMID:20436722
2366. Paganini I, Chang VY, Capone GL, et al. Expanding the mutational spectrum of LZTR1 in schwannomatosis. Eur J Hum Genet. 2015 Jul;23(7):963–8. PMID:25335493
2367. Paganini I, Sestini R, Cacciatore M, et al. Broadening the spectrum of SMARCB1-associated malignant tumors: a case of uterine leiomyosarcoma in a patient with schwannomatosis. Hum Pathol. 2015 Aug;46(8):1226–31. PMID:26001331
2368. Pagès M, Beccaria K, Boddaert N, et al. Co-occurrence of histone H3 K27M and BRAF V600E mutations in paediatric midline grade I ganglioglioma. Brain Pathol. 2018 Jan;28(1):103–11. PMID:27984673
2369. Pages M, Lacroix L, Tauziede-Espariat A, et al. Papillary glioneuronal tumors: histological and molecular characteristics and diagnostic value of SLC44A1-PRKCA fusion. Acta Neuropathol Commun. 2015 Dec 15;3:85. PMID:26671581
2370. Pagès M, Pajtler KW, Puget S, et al. Diagnostics of pediatric supratentorial RELA ependymomas: integration of information from histopathology, genetics, DNA methylation and imaging. Brain Pathol. 2019 May;29(3):325–35. PMID:30325077
2371. Pagura L, de Prada I, López-Pino MA, et al. Isolated intracranial juvenile xanthogranuloma. A report of two cases and review of the literature. Childs Nerv Syst. 2015 Mar;31(3):493–8. PMID:25281434
2372. Pajtler KW, Wei Y, Okonechnikov K, et al. YAP1 subgroup supratentorial ependymoma requires TEAD and nuclear factor I-mediated transcriptional programmes for tumorigenesis. Nat Commun. 2019 Sep 2;10(1):3914. PMID:31477715
2373. Pajtler KW, Wen J, Sill M, et al. Molecular heterogeneity and CXorf67 alterations in posterior fossa group A (PFA) ependymomas. Acta Neuropathol. 2018 Aug;136(2):211–26. PMID:29909548
2374. Pajtler KW, Witt H, Sill M, et al. Molecular classification of ependymal tumors across all CNS compartments, histopathological grades, and age groups. Cancer Cell. 2015 May 11;27(5):728–43. PMID:25965575
2375. Pakos EE, Goussia AC, Zina VP, et al. Multi-focal gliosarcoma: a case report and review of the literature. J Neurooncol. 2005 Sep;74(3):301–4. PMID:16086111
2376. Pal P, Fernandes H, Ellison DW. Woman aged 24 years with fourth ventricular mass. Brain Pathol. 2005 Oct;15(4):367–8. PMID:16389948
2377. Palmer RD, Murray MJ, Saini HK, et al. Malignant germ cell tumors display common microRNA profiles resulting in global changes in expression of messenger RNA targets. Cancer Res. 2010 Apr 1;70(7):2911–23. PMID:20332240
2378. Palsgrove DN, Brosnan-Cashman JA, Giannini C, et al. Subependymal giant cell astrocytoma-like astrocytoma: a neoplasm with a distinct phenotype and frequent neurofibromatosis type-1-association. Mod Pathol. 2018 Dec;31(12):1787–800. PMID:29973652
2379. Palta M, Riedel RF, Vredenburgh JJ, et al. Primary meningeal rhabdomyosarcoma. Sarcoma. 2011;2011:312802. PMID:21772793
2380. Pan J, Qi S, Liu Y, et al. Growth patterns of craniopharyngiomas: clinical analysis of 226 patients. J Neurosurg Pediatr. 2016 Apr;17(4):418–33. PMID:26636252
2381. Pan Z, Kleinschmidt-DeMasters BK. CNS Erdheim-Chester disease: a challenge to diagnose. J Neuropathol Exp Neurol. 2017 Dec 1;76(12):986–96. PMID:29096034
2382. Pandey N, Singh PK, Mahapatra AK, et al. Pediatric bilateral large concurrent thalamic glioblastoma: an unusual case report. J Pediatr Neurosci. 2014 Jan;9(1):76–8. PMID:24891914
2383. Pantazis G, Harter PN, Capper D, et al. The embryonic stem cell factor UTF1 serves as a reliable diagnostic marker for germinomas. Pathology. 2014 Apr;46(3):225–9. PMID:24614704
2384. Panwalkar P, Clark J, Ramaswamy V, et al. Immunohistochemical analysis of H3K27me3 demonstrates global reduction in group-A childhood posterior fossa ependymoma and is a powerful predictor of outcome. Acta Neuropathol. 2017 Nov;134(5):705–14. PMID:28733933
2385. Panwalkar P, Pratt D, Chung C, et al. SWI/SNF complex heterogeneity is related to polyphenotypic differentiation, prognosis, and immune response in rhabdoid tumors. Neuro Oncol. 2020 Jun 9;22(6):785–96. PMID:31912158
2386. Papale M, Buccarelli M, Mollinari C, et al. Hypoxia, inflammation and necrosis as determinants of glioblastoma cancer stem cells progression. Int J Mol Sci. 2020 Apr 11;21(8):E2660. PMID:32290386
2387. Papanicolau-Sengos A, Wang-Rodriguez J, Wang HY, et al. Rare case of a primary non-dural central nervous system low grade B-cell lymphoma and literature review. Int J Clin Exp Pathol. 2012;5(1):89–95. PMID:22295152
2388. Papo M, Diamond EL, Cohen-Aubart F, et al. High prevalence of myeloid neoplasms in adults with non-Langerhans cell histiocytosis. Blood. 2017 Aug 24;130(8):1007–13. PMID:28679734
2389. Papo M, Emile JF, Maciel TT, et al. Erdheim-Chester disease: a concise review. Curr Rheumatol Rep. 2019 Dec 5;21(12):66. PMID:31807955
2390. Paramasivam N, Hübschmann D, Toprak UH, et al. Mutational patterns and regulatory networks in epigenetic subgroups of meningioma. Acta Neuropathol. 2019 Aug;138(2):295–308. PMID:31069492
2391. Paraskevopoulou C, Fairhurst SA, Lowe DJ, et al. The Elongator subunit Elp3 contains a Fe4S4 cluster and binds S-adenosylmethionine. Mol Microbiol. 2006 Feb;59(3):795–806. PMID:16420352
2392. Paret C, Theruvath J, Russo A, et al. Activation of the basal cell carcinoma pathway in a patient with CNS HGNET-BCOR diagnosis: consequences for personalized targeted therapy. Oncotarget. 2016 Dec 13;7(50):83378–91. PMID:27825128
2393. Parham DM, Barr FG. Classification of rhabdomyosarcoma and its molecular basis. Adv Anat Pathol. 2013 Nov;20(6):387–97. PMID:24113309
2394. Park CC, Hartmann C, Folkerth R, et al. Systemic metastasis in glioblastoma may represent the emergence of neoplastic subclones. J Neuropathol Exp Neurol. 2000 Dec;59(12):1044–50. PMID:11138924
2395. Park DH, Park YK, Oh JI, et al. Oncocytic paraganglioma of the cauda equina in a child. Case report and review of the literature. Pediatr Neurosurg. 2002 May;36(5):260–5. PMID:12053045
2396. Park HK, Yu DB, Sung M, et al. Molecular changes in solitary fibrous tumor progression. J Mol Med (Berl). 2019 Oct;97(10):1413–25. PMID:31321477
2397. Park JJ, Diefenbach RJ, Joshua AM, et al. Oncogenic signaling in uveal melanoma. Pigment Cell Melanoma Res. 2018 Nov;31(6):661–72. PMID:29738114
2398. Park JS, Park H, Park S, et al. Primary central nervous system ALK positive anaplastic large cell lymphoma with predominantly leptomeningeal involvement in an adult. Yonsei Med J. 2013 May 1;54(3):791–6. PMID:23549832
2399. Park JY, Kim E, Kim DW, et al. Cribriform neuroepithelial tumor in the third ventricle: a case report and literature review. Neuropathology. 2012 Oct;32(5):570–6. PMID:22239490
2400. Parker BC, Annala MJ, Cogdell DE, et al. The tumorigenic FGFR3-TACC3 gene fusion escapes miR-99a regulation in glioblastoma. J Clin Invest. 2013 Feb;123(2):855–65. PMID:23298836
2401. Parker M, Mohankumar KM, Punchihewa C, et al. C11orf95-RELA fusions drive oncogenic NF-κB signalling in ependymoma. Nature. 2014 Feb 27;506(7489):451–5. PMID:24553141
2402. Parks NE, Goyal G, Go RS, et al. Neuroradiologic manifestations of Erdheim-Chester disease. Neurol Clin Pract. 2018 Feb;8(1):15–20. PMID:29517068
2403. Parmar HA, Hawkins C, Ozelame R, et al. Fluid-attenuated inversion recovery ring sign as a marker of dysembryoplastic neuroepithelial tumors. J Comput Assist Tomogr. 2007 May-Jun;31(3):348–53. PMID:17538277
2404. Parry DM, Eldridge R, Kaiser-Kupfer MI, et al. Neurofibromatosis 2 (NF2): clinical characteristics of 63 affected individuals and clinical evidence for heterogeneity. Am J Med Genet. 1994 Oct 1;52(4):450–61. PMID:7747758
2405. Parsons DW, Jones S, Zhang X, et al. An integrated genomic analysis of human glioblastoma multiforme. Science. 2008 Sep 26;321(5897):1807–12. PMID:18772396
2406. Partap S, Curran EK, Propp JM, et al. Medulloblastoma incidence has not changed over time: a CBTRUS study. J Pediatr Hematol Oncol. 2009 Dec;31(12):970–1. PMID:19887963
2407. Pascual JM, Prieto R, Castro-Dufourny I, et al. Craniopharyngiomas primarily involving the hypothalamus: a model of neurosurgical lesions to elucidate the neurobiological basis of psychiatric disorders. World Neurosurg. 2018 Dec;120:e1245–78. PMID:30240857
2408. Pascual JM, Prieto R, Castro-Dufourny I, et al. Topographic diagnosis of papillary craniopharyngiomas: the need for an accurate MRI-surgical correlation. AJNR Am J Neuroradiol. 2015 Aug;36(8):E55–6. PMID:26113067
2409. Pasmant E, Parfait B, Luscan A, et al. Neurofibromatosis type 1 molecular diagnosis: what can NGS do for you when you have a large gene with loss of function mutations? Eur J Hum Genet. 2015 May;23(5):596–601. PMID:25074460
2410. Pasquier B, Gasnier F, Pasquier D, et al. Papillary meningioma. Clinicopathologic study of seven cases and review of the literature. Cancer. 1986 Jul 15;58(2):299–305. PMID:3719522
2411. Pasquier B, Péoc'H M, Fabre-Bocquentin B, et al. Surgical pathology of drug-resistant partial epilepsy. A 10-year-experience with a series of 327 consecutive resections. Epileptic Disord. 2002 Jun;4(2):99–119. PMID:12105073
2412. Pasquier B, Péoc'h M, Morrison AL, et al. Chordoid glioma of the third ventricle: a report of two new cases, with further evidence supporting an ependymal differentiation, and review of the literature. Am J Surg Pathol. 2002 Oct;26(10):1330–42. PMID:12360048
2413. Passos J, Quidet M, Brahimi A, et al. Familial adenomatous polyposis associated craniopharyngioma secondary to both germline and somatic mutations in the APC gene. Acta Neuropathol. 2020 Dec;140(6):967–9. PMID:33025138
2414. Pastorino S, Yoshikawa Y, Pass HI, et al. A subset of mesotheliomas with improved survival occurring in carriers of BAP1 and other germline mutations. J Clin Oncol. 2018 Oct 30;36(35):JCO2018790352. PMID:30376426
2415. Patay Z, DeSain LA, Hwang SN, et al. MR imaging characteristics of wingless-type-subgroup pediatric medulloblastoma. AJNR Am J Neuroradiol. 2015 Dec;36(12):2386–93. PMID:26338912
2416. Patel AP, Tirosh I, Trombetta JJ, et al. Single-cell RNA-seq highlights intratumoral heterogeneity in primary glioblastoma. Science. 2014 Jun 20;344(6190):1396–401. PMID:24925914
2417. Patel N, Fallah A, Provias J, et al. Cerebellar liponeurocytoma. Can J Surg. 2009 Aug;52(4):E117–9. PMID:19680499

2418. Patel SH, Bansal AG, Young EB, et al. Extent of surgical resection in lower-grade gliomas: differential impact based on molecular subtype. AJNR Am J Neuroradiol. 2019 Jul;40(7):1149–55. PMID:31248860
2419. Patel SH, Poisson LM, Brat DJ, et al. T2-FLAIR mismatch, an imaging biomarker for IDH and 1p/19q status in lower-grade gliomas: a TCGA/TCIA project. Clin Cancer Res. 2017 Oct 15;23(20):6078–85. PMID:28751449
2420. Patil CG, Yi A, Elramsisy A, et al. Prognosis of patients with multifocal glioblastoma: a case-control study. J Neurosurg. 2012 Oct;117(4):705–11. PMID:22920963
2421. Patil S, Perry A, Maccollin M, et al. Immunohistochemical analysis supports a role for INI1/SMARCB1 in hereditary forms of schwannomas, but not in solitary, sporadic schwannomas. Brain Pathol. 2008 Oct;18(4):517–9. PMID:18422762
2422. Patronas NJ, Courcoutsakis N, Bromley CM, et al. Intramedullary and spinal canal tumors in patients with neurofibromatosis 2: MR imaging findings and correlation with genotype. Radiology. 2001 Feb;218(2):434–42. PMID:11161159
2423. Patsalides AD, Atac G, Hedge U, et al. Lymphomatoid granulomatosis: abnormalities of the brain at MR imaging. Radiology. 2005 Oct;237(1):265–73. PMID:16100084
2424. Pattwell SS, Konnick EQ, Liu YJ, et al. Neurotrophic receptor tyrosine kinase 2 (NTRK2) alterations in low-grade gliomas: report of a novel gene fusion partner in a pilocytic astrocytoma and review of the literature. Case Rep Pathol. 2020 Jan 30;2020:5903863. PMID:32082673
2425. Paugh BS, Zhu X, Qu C, et al. Novel oncogenic PDGFRA mutations in pediatric high-grade gliomas. Cancer Res. 2013 Oct 15;73(20):6219–29. PMID:23970477
2426. Paulsson AK, Holmes JA, Peiffer AM, et al. Comparison of clinical outcomes and genomic characteristics of single focus and multifocal glioblastoma. J Neurooncol. 2014 Sep;119(2):429–35. PMID:24990827
2427. Paulus W, Honegger J, Keyvani K, et al. Xanthogranuloma of the sellar region: a clinicopathological entity different from adamantinomatous craniopharyngioma. Acta Neuropathol. 1999 Apr;97(4):377–82. PMID:10208277
2428. Paulus W, Jänisch W. Clinicopathologic correlations in epithelial choroid plexus neoplasms: a study of 52 cases. Acta Neuropathol. 1990;80(6):635–41. PMID:1703384
2429. Paulus W, Jellinger K, Hallas C, et al. Human herpesvirus-6 and Epstein-Barr virus genome in primary cerebral lymphomas. Neurology. 1993 Aug;43(8):1591–3. PMID:8394522
2430. Paulus W, Lisle DK, Tonn JC, et al. Molecular genetic alterations in pleomorphic xanthoastrocytoma. Acta Neuropathol. 1996;91(3):293–7. PMID:8834542
2431. Paulus W, Schlote W, Perentes E, et al. Desmoplastic supratentorial neuroepithelial tumours of infancy. Histopathology. 1992 Jul;21(1):43–9. PMID:1634201
2432. Paulus W, Slowik F, Jellinger K. Primary intracranial sarcomas: histopathological features of 19 cases. Histopathology. 1991 May;18(5):395–402. PMID:1715839
2433. Paulus W, Stöckel C, Krauss J, et al. Odontogenic classification of craniopharyngiomas: a clinicopathological study of 54 cases. Histopathology. 1997 Feb;30(2):172–6. PMID:9067743
2434. Pearce MS, Salotti JA, Little MP, et al. Radiation exposure from CT scans in childhood and subsequent risk of leukaemia and brain tumours: a retrospective cohort study. Lancet. 2012 Aug 4;380(9840):499–505. PMID:22681860
2435. Peckham-Gregory EC, Montenegro RE, Stevenson DA, et al. Racial/ethnic disparities and incidence of malignant peripheral nerve sheath tumors: results from the Surveillance, Epidemiology, and End Results Program, 2000-2014. J Neurooncol. 2018 Aug;139(1):69–75. PMID:29663170
2436. Pedersen M, Küsters-Vandevelde HVN, Viros A, et al. Primary melanoma of the CNS in children is driven by congenital expression of oncogenic NRAS in melanocytes. Cancer Discov. 2013 Apr;3(4):458–69. PMID:23303902
2437. Pei Y, Moore CE, Wang J, et al. An animal model of MYC-driven medulloblastoma. Cancer Cell. 2012 Feb 14;21(2):155–67. PMID:22340590
2438. Pekmezci M, Louie J, Gupta N, et al. Clinicopathological characteristics of adamantinomatous and papillary craniopharyngiomas: University of California, San Francisco experience 1985-2005. Neurosurgery. 2010 Nov;67(5):1341–9. PMID:20871436
2439. Pekmezci M, Perry A. Neuropathology of brain metastases. Surg Neurol Int. 2013 May 2;4(Suppl 4):S245–55. PMID:23717796
2440. Pekmezci M, Phillips JJ, Dirilenoglu F, et al. Loss of H3K27 trimethylation by immunohistochemistry is frequent in oligodendroglioma, IDH-mutant and 1p/19q-codeleted, but is neither a sensitive nor a specific marker. Acta Neuropathol. 2020 Mar;139(3):597–600. PMID:31912209
2441. Pekmezci M, Reuss DE, Hirbe AC, et al. Morphologic and immunohistochemical features of malignant peripheral nerve sheath tumors and cellular schwannomas. Mod Pathol. 2015 Feb;28(2):187–200. PMID:25189642
2442. Pekmezci M, Rice T, Molinaro AM, et al. Adult infiltrating gliomas with WHO 2016 integrated diagnosis: additional prognostic roles of ATRX and TERT. Acta Neuropathol. 2017 Jun;133(6):1001–16. PMID:28255664
2443. Pekmezci M, Stevers M, Phillips JJ, et al. Multinodular and vacuolating neuronal tumor of the cerebrum is a clonal neoplasm defined by genetic alterations that activate the MAP kinase signaling pathway. Acta Neuropathol. 2018 Mar;135(3):485–8. PMID:29428973
2444. Pekmezci M, Villanueva-Meyer JE, Goode B, et al. The genetic landscape of ganglioglioma. Acta Neuropathol Commun. 2018 Jun 7;6(1):47. PMID:29880043
2445. Pels H, Montesinos-Rongen M, Schaller C, et al. VH gene analysis of primary CNS lymphomas. J Neurol Sci. 2005 Feb 15;228(2):143–7. PMID:15694195
2446. Pels H, Schlegel U. Primary central nervous system lymphoma. Curr Treat Options Neurol. 2006 Jul;8(4):346–57. PMID:16942677
2447. Pelz D, Khezri N, Mainprize T, et al. Multifocal cerebellar liponeurocytoma. Can J Neurol Sci. 2013 Nov;40(6):870–2. PMID:24257232
2448. Pemberton LS, Dougal M, Magee B, et al. Experience of external beam radiotherapy given adjuvantly or at relapse following surgery for craniopharyngioma. Radiother Oncol. 2005 Oct;77(1):99–104. PMID:16216361
2449. Pemov A, Hansen NF, Sindiri S, et al. Low mutation burden and frequent loss of CDKN2A/B and SMARCA2, but not PRC2, define premalignant neurofibromatosis type 1-associated atypical neurofibromas. Neuro Oncol. 2019 Aug 5;21(8):981–92. PMID:30722027
2450. Pemov A, Li H, Patidar R, et al. The primacy of NF1 loss as the driver of tumorigenesis in neurofibromatosis type 1-associated plexiform neurofibromas. Oncogene. 2017 Jun 1;36(22):3168–77. PMID:28068329
2451. Pencalet P, Maixner W, Sainte-Rose C, et al. Benign cerebellar astrocytomas in children. J Neurosurg. 1999 Feb;90(2):265–73. PMID:9950497
2452. Pendleton C, Spinner RJ, Dyck PJB, et al. Association of intraneural perineurioma with neurofibromatosis type 2. Acta Neurochir (Wien). 2020 Aug;162(8):1891–7. PMID:32529330
2453. Per H, Kontaş O, Kumandaş S, et al. A report of a desmoplastic non-infantile ganglioglioma in a 6-year-old boy with review of the literature. Neurosurg Rev. 2009 Jul;32(3):369–74. PMID:19280238
2454. Peraud A, Watanabe K, Plate KH, et al. p53 mutations versus EGF receptor expression in giant cell glioblastomas. J Neuropathol Exp Neurol. 1997 Nov;56(11):1236–41. PMID:9370234
2455. Pereira AM, Schmid EM, Schutte PJ, et al. High prevalence of long-term cardiovascular, neurological and psychosocial morbidity after treatment for craniopharyngioma. Clin Endocrinol (Oxf). 2005 Feb;62(2):197–204. PMID:15670196
2456. Pereira BD, Raimundo L, Mete O, et al. Monomorphous plurihormonal pituitary adenoma of Pit-1 lineage in a giant adolescent with central hyperthyroidism. Endocr Pathol. 2016 Mar;27(1):25–33. PMID:26330191
2457. Perez-Rivas LG, Theodoropoulou M, Ferraù F, et al. The gene of the ubiquitin-specific protease 8 is frequently mutated in adenomas causing Cushing's disease. J Clin Endocrinol Metab. 2015 Jul;100(7):E997–1004. PMID:25942478
2458. Pérez-Rivas LG, Theodoropoulou M, Puar TH, et al. Somatic USP8 mutations are frequent events in corticotroph tumor progression causing Nelson's tumor. Eur J Endocrinol. 2018 Jan;178(1):57–63. PMID:28982703
2459. Perilongo G, Carollo C, Salviati L, et al. Diencephalic syndrome and disseminated juvenile pilocytic astrocytomas of the hypothalamic-optic chiasm region. Cancer. 1997 Jul 1;80(1):142–6. PMID:9210720
2460. Perkins SM, Mitra N, Fei W, et al. Patterns of care and outcomes of patients with pleomorphic xanthoastrocytoma: a SEER analysis. J Neurooncol. 2012 Oct;110(1):99–104. PMID:22843450
2461. Pernicone PJ, Scheithauer BW, Sebo TJ, et al. Pituitary carcinoma: a clinicopathologic study of 15 cases. Cancer. 1997 Feb 15;79(4):804–12. PMID:9024719
2462. Perreault S, Larouche V, Tabori U, et al. A phase 2 study of trametinib for patients with pediatric glioma or plexiform neurofibroma with refractory tumor and activation of the MAPK/ERK pathway: TRAM-01. BMC Cancer. 2019 Dec 27;19(1):1250. PMID:31881853
2463. Perreault S, Ramaswamy V, Achrol AS, et al. MRI surrogates for molecular subgroups of medulloblastoma. AJNR Am J Neuroradiol. 2014 Jul;35(7):1263–9. PMID:24831600
2464. Perry A, Aldape KD, George DH, et al. Small cell astrocytoma: an aggressive variant that is clinicopathologically and genetically distinct from anaplastic oligodendroglioma. Cancer. 2004 Nov 15;101(10):2318–26. PMID:15470710
2465. Perry A, Banerjee R, Lohse CM, et al. A role for chromosome 9p21 deletions in the malignant progression of meningiomas and the prognosis of anaplastic meningiomas. Brain Pathol. 2002 Apr;12(2):183–90. PMID:11958372
2466. Perry A, Burton SS, Fuller GN, et al. Oligodendroglial neoplasms with ganglioglioma-like maturation: a diagnostic pitfall. Acta Neuropathol. 2010 Aug;120(2):237–52. PMID:20464403
2467. Perry A, Giannini C, Raghavan R, et al. Aggressive phenotypic and genotypic features in pediatric and NF2-associated meningiomas: a clinicopathologic study of 53 cases. J Neuropathol Exp Neurol. 2001 Oct;60(10):994–1003. PMID:11589430
2468. Perry A, Giannini C, Scheithauer BW, et al. Composite pleomorphic xanthoastrocytoma and ganglioglioma: report of four cases and review of the literature. Am J Surg Pathol. 1997 Jul;21(7):763–71. PMID:9236832
2469. Perry A, Kurtkaya-Yapicier O, Scheithauer BW, et al. Insights into meningioangiomatosis with and without meningioma: a clinicopathologic and genetic series of 24 cases with review of the literature. Brain Pathol. 2005 Jan;15(1):55–65. PMID:15779237
2470. Perry A, Miller CR, Gujrati M, et al. Malignant gliomas with primitive neuroectodermal tumor-like components: a clinicopathologic and genetic study of 53 cases. Brain Pathol. 2009 Jan;19(1):81–90. PMID:18452568
2471. Perry A, Scheithauer BW, Macaulay RJ, et al. Oligodendrogliomas with neurocytic differentiation. A report of 4 cases with diagnostic and histogenetic implications. J Neuropathol Exp Neurol. 2002 Nov;61(11):947–55. PMID:12430711
2472. Perry A, Scheithauer BW, Nascimento AG. The immunophenotypic spectrum of meningeal hemangiopericytoma: a comparison with fibrous meningioma and solitary fibrous tumor of meninges. Am J Surg Pathol. 1997 Nov;21(11):1354–60. PMID:9351573
2473. Perry A, Scheithauer BW, Stafford SL, et al. "Malignancy" in meningiomas: a clinicopathologic study of 116 patients, with grading implications. Cancer. 1999 May 1;85(9):2046–56. PMID:10223247
2474. Perry A, Scheithauer BW, Stafford SL, et al. "Rhabdoid" meningioma: an aggressive variant. Am J Surg Pathol. 1998 Dec;22(12):1482–90. PMID:9850174
2475. Perry A, Stafford SL, Scheithauer BW, et al. Meningioma grading: an analysis of histologic parameters. Am J Surg Pathol. 1997 Dec;21(12):1455–65. PMID:9414189
2476. Perry JR, Laperriere N, O'Callaghan CJ, et al. Short-course radiation plus temozolomide in elderly patients with glioblastoma. N Engl J Med. 2017 Mar 16;376(11):1027–37. PMID:28296618
2477. Persson AI, Petritsch C, Swartling FJ, et al. Non-stem cell origin for oligodendroglioma. Cancer Cell. 2010 Dec 14;18(6):669–82. PMID:21156288
2478. Persu A, Hamoir M, Grégoire V, et al. High prevalence of SDHB mutations in head and neck paraganglioma in Belgium. J Hypertens. 2008 Jul;26(7):1395–401. PMID:18551016
2479. Peruzzi L, Iuvone L, Ruggiero A, et al. Neuropsychological deterioration predicts tumor progression in a young boy with bithalamic glioma. Appl Neuropsychol Child. 2016;5(1):76–81. PMID:25650783
2480. Pesatori AC, Baccarelli A, Consonni D, et al. Aryl hydrocarbon receptor-interacting protein and pituitary adenomas: a population-based study on subjects exposed to dioxin after the Seveso, Italy, accident. Eur J Endocrinol. 2008 Dec;159(6):699–703. PMID:18787049
2481. Pesce A, Palmieri M, Armocida D, et al. Spinal myxopapillary ependymoma: the Sapienza University experience and comprehensive literature review concerning the clinical course of 1602 patients. World Neurosurg. 2019 Sep;129:245–53. PMID:31152881
2482. Petitjean A, Mathe E, Kato S, et al. Impact of mutant p53 functional properties on TP53 mutation patterns and tumor phenotype: lessons from recent developments in the IARC TP53 Database. Hum Mutat. 2007 Jun;28(6):622–9. PMID:17311302
2483. Petrossians P, Daly AF, Natchev E, et al. Acromegaly at diagnosis in 3173 patients from

the Liège Acromegaly Survey (LAS) Database. Endocr Relat Cancer. 2017 Oct;24(10):505–18. PMID:28733467
2484. Petruzzellis G, Valentini D, Del Bufalo F, et al. Vemurafenib treatment of pleomorphic xanthoastrocytoma in a child with down syndrome. Front Oncol. 2019 Apr 12;9:277. PMID:31032231
2485. Peyrat JP, Révillion F, Bonneterre J. Plasma insulin-like growth factor in primary breast cancer patients treated with adjuvant chemotherapy. Br J Cancer. 1998 May;77(10):1669–71. PMID:9635846
2486. Peyre M, Bah A, Kalamarides M. Multifocal choroid plexus papillomas: case report. Acta Neurochir (Wien). 2012 Feb;154(2):295–9. PMID:21953479
2487. Peyre M, Gaillard S, de Marcellus C, et al. Progestin-associated shift of meningioma mutational landscape. Ann Oncol. 2018 Mar 1;29(3):681–6. PMID:29206892
2488. Peyre M, Gauchotte G, Giry M, et al. De novo and secondary anaplastic meningiomas: a study of clinical and histomolecular prognostic factors. Neuro Oncol. 2018 Jul 5;20(8):1113–21. PMID:29216385
2489. Peyre M, Stemmer-Rachamimov A, Clermont-Taranchon E, et al. Meningioma progression in mice triggered by Nf2 and Cdkn2ab inactivation. Oncogene. 2013 Sep 5;32(36):4264–72. PMID:23045274
2490. Pfaff E, Aichmüller C, Sill M, et al. Molecular subgrouping of primary pineal parenchymal tumors reveals distinct subtypes correlated with clinical parameters and genetic alterations. Acta Neuropathol. 2020 Feb;139(2):243–57. PMID:31768671
2491. Pfister S, Janzarik WG, Remke M, et al. BRAF gene duplication constitutes a mechanism of MAPK pathway activation in low-grade astrocytomas. J Clin Invest. 2008 May;118(5):1739–49. PMID:18398503
2492. Phi JH, Koh EJ, Kim SK, et al. Desmoplastic infantile astrocytoma: recurrence with malignant transformation into glioblastoma: a case report. Childs Nerv Syst. 2011 Dec;27(12):2177–81. PMID:21947035
2493. Phi JH, Park AK, Lee S, et al. Genomic analysis reveals secondary glioblastoma after radiotherapy in a subset of recurrent medulloblastomas. Acta Neuropathol. 2018 Jun;135(6):939–53. PMID:29644394
2494. Phi JH, Park SH, Chae JH, et al. Congenital subependymal giant cell astrocytoma: clinical considerations and expression of radial glial cell markers in giant cells. Childs Nerv Syst. 2008 Dec;24(12):1499–503. PMID:18629509
2495. Philips A, Henshaw DL, Lamburn G, et al. Authors' comment on "Brain tumours: rise in glioblastoma multiforme incidence in england 1995-2015 suggests an adverse environmental or lifestyle factor". J Environ Public Health. 2018 Jun 25;2018:2170208. PMID:30046315
2496. Philips A, Henshaw DL, Lamburn G, et al. Brain tumours: rise in glioblastoma multiforme incidence in England 1995-2015 suggests an adverse environmental or lifestyle factor. J Environ Public Health. 2018 Jun 24;2018:7910754. PMID:30034480
2497. Phillips CL, Miles L, Jones BV, et al. Medulloblastoma with melanotic differentiation: case report and review of the literature. J Neurooncol. 2011 Jul;103(3):759–64. PMID:20953660
2498. Phillips JJ, Aranda D, Ellison DW, et al. PDGFRA amplification is common in pediatric and adult high-grade astrocytomas and identifies a poor prognostic group in IDH1 mutant glioblastoma. Brain Pathol. 2013 Sep;23(5):565–73. PMID:23438035
2499. Phillips JJ, Gong H, Chen K, et al. The genetic landscape of anaplastic pleomorphic xanthoastrocytoma. Brain Pathol. 2019 Jan;29(1):85–96. PMID:30051528
2500. Phoenix TN, Patmore DM, Boop S, et al. Medulloblastoma genotype dictates blood brain barrier phenotype. Cancer Cell. 2016 Apr 11;29(4):508–22. PMID:27050100
2501. Picard C, Silvy M, Gerard C, et al. Gs alpha overexpression and loss of Gs alpha imprinting in human somatotroph adenomas: association with tumor size and response to pharmacologic treatment. Int J Cancer. 2007 Sep 15;121(6):1245–52. PMID:17514647
2502. Picard D, Miller S, Hawkins CE, et al. Markers of survival and metastatic potential in childhood CNS primitive neuro-ectodermal brain tumours: an integrative genomic analysis. Lancet Oncol. 2012 Aug;13(8):838–48. PMID:22691720
2503. Picarsic J, Pysher T, Zhou H, et al. BRAF V600E mutation in Juvenile Xanthogranuloma family neoplasms of the central nervous system (CNS-JXG): a revised diagnostic algorithm to include pediatric Erdheim-Chester disease. Acta Neuropathol Commun. 2019 Nov 4;7(1):168. PMID:31685033
2504. Piccirillo SG, Reynolds BA, Zanetti N, et al. Bone morphogenetic proteins inhibit the tumorigenic potential of human brain tumour-initiating cells. Nature. 2006 Dec 7;444(7120):761–5. PMID:17151667
2505. Pickles JC, Fairchild AR, Stone TJ, et al. DNA methylation-based profiling for paediatric CNS tumour diagnosis and treatment: a population-based study. Lancet Child Adolesc Health. 2020 Feb;4(2):121–30. PMID:31786093
2506. Pickles JC, Mankad K, Aizpurua M, et al. A case series of diffuse glioneuronal tumours with oligodendroglioma-like features and nuclear clusters (DGONC). Neuropathol Appl Neurobiol. 2021 Apr;47(3):464–7. PMID:33325069
2507. Pienkowska M, Choufani S, Turinsky AL, et al. DNA methylation signature is prognostic of choroid plexus tumor aggressiveness. Clin Epigenetics. 2019 Aug 13;11(1):117. PMID:31409384
2508. Pietsch T, Haberler C. Update on the integrated histopathological and genetic classification of medulloblastoma - a practical diagnostic guideline. Clin Neuropathol. 2016 Nov/Dec;35(6):344–52. PMID:27781424
2509. Pietsch T, Schmidt R, Remke M, et al. Prognostic significance of clinical, histopathological, and molecular characteristics of medulloblastomas in the prospective HIT2000 multicenter clinical trial cohort. Acta Neuropathol. 2014 Jul;128(1):137–49. PMID:24791927
2510. Pietsch T, Waha A, Koch A, et al. Medulloblastomas of the desmoplastic variant carry mutations of the human homologue of Drosophila patched. Cancer Res. 1997 Jun 1;57(11):2085–8. PMID:9187099
2511. Pietsch T, Wohlers I, Goschzik T, et al. Supratentorial ependymomas of childhood carry C11orf95-RELA fusions leading to pathological activation of the NF-κB signaling pathway. Acta Neuropathol. 2014 Apr;127(4):609–11. PMID:24562983
2513. Pikis S, Fellig Y, Margolin E. Cerebellar liponeurocytoma in two siblings suggests a possible familial predisposition. J Clin Neurosci. 2016 Oct;32:154–6. PMID:27349466
2514. Pilarski R, Cebulla CM, Massengill JB, et al. Expanding the clinical phenotype of hereditary BAP1 cancer predisposition syndrome, reporting three new cases. Genes Chromosomes Cancer. 2014 Feb;53(2):177–82. PMID:24243779
2515. Pinato DJ, Ramachandran R, Toussi ST, et al. Immunohistochemical markers of the hypoxic response can identify malignancy in phaeochromocytomas and paragangliomas and optimize the detection of tumours with VHL germline mutations. Br J Cancer. 2013 Feb 5;108(2):429–37. PMID:23257898
2516. Pinna V, Lanari V, Daniele P, et al. p.Arg1809Cys substitution in neurofibromin is associated with a distinctive NF1 phenotype without neurofibromas. Eur J Hum Genet. 2015 Aug;23(8):1068–71. PMID:25370043
2517. Pinto Gama HP, da Rocha AJ, Braga FT, et al. Comparative analysis of MR sequences to detect structural brain lesions in tuberous sclerosis. Pediatr Radiol. 2006 Feb;36(2):119–25. PMID:16283285
2518. Piotrowski A, Xie J, Liu YF, et al. Germline loss-of-function mutations in LZTR1 predispose to an inherited disorder of multiple schwannomas. Nat Genet. 2014 Feb;46(2):182–7. PMID:24362817
2519. Pirini MG, Mascalchi M, Salvi F, et al. Primary diffuse meningeal melanomatosis: radiologic-pathologic correlation. AJNR Am J Neuroradiol. 2003 Jan;24(1):115–8. PMID:12533338
2520. Piunti A, Smith ER, Morgan MAJ, et al. CATACOMB: an endogenous inducible gene that antagonizes H3K27 methylation activity of Polycomb repressive complex 2 via an H3K27M-like mechanism. Sci Adv. 2019 Jul 3;5(7):eaax2887. PMID:31281901
2521. Pivonello R, Matrone C, Filippella M, et al. Dopamine receptor expression and function in clinically nonfunctioning pituitary tumors: comparison with the effectiveness of cabergoline treatment. J Clin Endocrinol Metab. 2004 Apr;89(4):1674–83. PMID:15070930
2522. Plank TL, Logginidou H, Klein-Szanto A, et al. The expression of hamartin, the product of the TSC1 gene, in normal human tissues and in TSC1- and TSC2-linked angiomyolipomas. Mod Pathol. 1999 May;12(5):539–45. PMID:10349994
2523. Plank TL, Yeung RS, Henske EP. Hamartin, the product of the tuberous sclerosis 1 (TSC1) gene, interacts with tuberin and appears to be localized to cytoplasmic vesicles. Cancer Res. 1998 Nov 1;58(21):4766–70. PMID:9809973
2524. Plotkin SR, Blakeley JO, Evans DG, et al. Update from the 2011 International Schwannomatosis Workshop: from genetics to diagnostic criteria. Am J Med Genet A. 2013 Mar;161A(3):405–16. PMID:23401320
2525. Plotkin SR, O'Donnell CC, Curry WT, et al. Spinal ependymomas in neurofibromatosis Type 2: a retrospective analysis of 55 patients. J Neurosurg Spine. 2011 Apr;14(4):543–7. PMID:21294614
2526. Plotkin SR, Wick A. Neurofibromatosis and schwannomatosis. Semin Neurol. 2018 Feb;38(1):73–85. PMID:29548054
2527. Podsypanina K, Ellenson LH, Nemes A, et al. Mutation of Pten/Mmac1 in mice causes neoplasia in multiple organ systems. Proc Natl Acad Sci U S A. 1999 Feb 16;96(4):1563–8. PMID:9990064
2528. Poh B, Koso H, Momota H, et al. Foxr2 promotes formation of CNS-embryonal tumors in a Trp53-deficient background. Neuro Oncol. 2019 Aug 5;21(8):993–1004. PMID:30976792
2529. Polchi A, Magini A, Meo DD, et al. mTOR signaling and neural stem cells: the tuberous sclerosis complex model. Int J Mol Sci. 2018 May 16;19(5):E1474. PMID:29772672
2530. Policarpio-Nicolas ML, Le BH, Mandell JW, et al. Granular cell tumor of the neurohypophysis: report of a case with intraoperative cytologic diagnosis. Diagn Cytopathol. 2008 Jan;36(1):58–63. PMID:18064694
2531. Pollack IF, Hamilton RL, Sobol RW, et al. IDH1 mutations are common in malignant gliomas arising in adolescents: a report from the Children's Oncology Group. Childs Nerv Syst. 2011 Jan;27(1):87–94. PMID:20725730
2532. Pollack IF, Hurtt M, Pang D, et al. Dissemination of low grade intracranial astrocytomas in children. Cancer. 1994 Jun 1;73(11):2869–78. PMID:8194029
2533. Pomper MG, Passe TJ, Burger PC, et al. Chordoid glioma: a neoplasm unique to the hypothalamus and anterior third ventricle. AJNR Am J Neuroradiol. 2001 Mar;22(3):464–9. PMID:11237967
2534. Pompili A, Calvosa F, Caroli F, et al. The transdural extension of gliomas. J Neurooncol. 1993 Jan;15(1):67–74. PMID:8455064
2535. Ponzoni M, Arrigoni G, Gould VE, et al. Lack of CD 29 (beta1 integrin) and CD 54 (ICAM-1) adhesion molecules in intravascular lymphomatosis. Hum Pathol. 2000 Feb;31(2):220–6. PMID:10685637
2536. Ponzoni M, Berger F, Chassagne-Clement C, et al. Reactive perivascular T-cell infiltrate predicts survival in primary central nervous system B-cell lymphomas. Br J Haematol. 2007 Aug;138(3):316–23. PMID:17555470
2537. Ponzoni M, Bonetti F, Poliani PL, et al. Central nervous system marginal zone B-cell lymphoma associated with Chlamydophila psittaci infection. Hum Pathol. 2011 May;42(5):738–42. PMID:21239044
2538. Ponzoni M, Campo E, Nakamura S. Intravascular large B-cell lymphoma: a chameleon with multiple faces and many masks. Blood. 2018 Oct 11;132(15):1561–7. PMID:30111607
2539. Ponzoni M, Terreni MR, Ciceri F, et al. Primary brain CD30+ ALK1+ anaplastic large cell lymphoma ('ALKoma'): the first case with a combination of 'not common' variants. Ann Oncol. 2002 Nov;13(11):1827–32. PMID:12419758
2540. Popova T, Hebert L, Jacquemin V, et al. Germline BAP1 mutations predispose to renal cell carcinomas. Am J Hum Genet. 2013 Jun 6;92(6):974–80. PMID:23684012
2541. Poretti A, Meoded A, Huisman TA. Neuroimaging of pediatric posterior fossa tumors including review of the literature. J Magn Reson Imaging. 2012 Jan;35(1):32–47. PMID:21989968
2542. Portail Epidemiologie France: Health Databases [Internet]. Paris (France): Institut thématique Santé Publique - Inserm; 2020. POLA - National POLA Network for the Treatment of High-Grade Oligodendroglial Tumours; updated 2015 Jun 23. Available from: https://epidemiologie-france.aviesan.fr/fr/content/view/full/87575.
2543. Portela A, Esteller M. Epigenetic modifications and human disease. Nat Biotechnol. 2010 Oct;28(10):1057–68. PMID:20944598
2544. Portet S, Naoufal R, Tachon G, et al. Histomolecular characterization of intracranial meningiomas developed in patients exposed to high-dose cyproterone acetate: an antiandrogen treatment. Neurooncol Adv. 2019 May 28;1(1):vdz003. PMID:32642646
2545. Potorac I, Petrossians P, Daly AF, et al. T2-weighted MRI signal predicts hormone and tumor responses to somatostatin analogs in acromegaly. Endocr Relat Cancer. 2016 Nov;23(11):871–81. PMID:27649724
2546. Pouget C, Hergalant S, Lardenois E, et al. Ki-67 and MCM6 labeling indices are correlated with overall survival in anaplastic oligodendroglioma, IDH1-mutant and 1p/19q-codeleted: a multicenter study from the French POLA network. Brain Pathol. 2020 May;30(3):465–78. PMID:31561286
2547. Poulgrain K, Gurgo R, Winter C, et al. Papillary tumour of the pineal region. J Clin Neurosci. 2011 Aug;18(8):1007–17. PMID:21658955
2548. Powell SZ, Yachnis AT, Rorke LB, et al. Divergent differentiation in pleomorphic xanthoastrocytoma. Evidence for a neuronal

element and possible relationship to ganglion cell tumors. Am J Surg Pathol. 1996 Jan;20(1):80–5. PMID:8540612
2549. Powers J, Pinto EM, Barnoud T, et al. A rare TP53 mutation predominant in Ashkenazi Jews confers risk of multiple cancers. Cancer Res. 2020 Sep 1;80(17):3732–44. PMID:32675277
2550. Prabowo AS, Iyer AM, Veersema TJ, et al. BRAF V600E mutation is associated with mTOR signaling activation in glioneuronal tumors. Brain Pathol. 2014 Jan;24(1):52–66. PMID:23941441
2551. Prabowo AS, van Thuijl HF, Scheinin I, et al. Landscape of chromosomal copy number aberrations in gangliogliomas and dysembryoplastic neuroepithelial tumours. Neuropathol Appl Neurobiol. 2015 Oct;41(6):743–55. PMID:25764012
2552. Prada CE, Jousma E, Rizvi TA, et al. Neurofibroma-associated macrophages play roles in tumor growth and response to pharmacological inhibition. Acta Neuropathol. 2013 Jan;125(1):159–68. PMID:23099891
2553. Prajapati HJ, Vincentelli C, Hwang SN, et al. Primary CNS natural killer/T-cell lymphoma of the nasal type presenting in a woman: case report and review of the literature. J Clin Oncol. 2014 Mar 10;32(8):e26–9. PMID:24419127
2554. Prakash V, Batanian JR, Guzman MA, et al. Malignant transformation of a desmoplastic infantile ganglioglioma in an infant carrier of a nonsynonymous TP53 mutation. Pediatr Neurol. 2014 Jul;51(1):138–43. PMID:24768217
2555. Prasad G, Haas-Kogan DA. Radiation-induced gliomas. Expert Rev Neurother. 2009 Oct;9(10):1511–7. PMID:19831840
2556. Pratt D, Natarajan SK, Banda A, et al. Circumscribed/non-diffuse histology confers a better prognosis in H3K27M-mutant gliomas. Acta Neuropathol. 2018 Feb;135(2):299–301. PMID:29302777
2557. Prayer D, Grois N, Prosch H, et al. MR imaging presentation of intracranial disease associated with Langerhans cell histiocytosis. AJNR Am J Neuroradiol. 2004 May;25(5):880–91. PMID:15140741
2558. Prayson RA. Clinicopathologic study of 61 patients with ependymoma including MIB-1 immunohistochemistry. Ann Diagn Pathol. 1999 Feb;3(1):11–8. PMID:9990108
2559. Prayson RA. Myxopapillary ependymomas: a clinicopathologic study of 14 cases including MIB-1 and p53 immunoreactivity. Mod Pathol. 1997 Apr;10(4):304–10. PMID:9110291
2560. Prayson RA. Pleomorphic xanthoastrocytoma arising in neurofibromatosis type 1. Clin Neuropathol. 2012 May-Jun;31(3):152–4. PMID:22551920
2561. Prayson RA, Chahlavi A, Luciano M. Cerebellar paraganglioma. Ann Diagn Pathol. 2004 Aug;8(4):219–23. PMID:15290673
2562. Prayson RA, Khajavi K, Comair YG. Cortical architectural abnormalities and MIB1 immunoreactivity in gangliogliomas: a study of 60 patients with intracranial tumors. J Neuropathol Exp Neurol. 1995 Jul;54(4):513–20. PMID:7541447
2563. Prendergast N, Goldstein JD, Beier AD. Choroid plexus adenoma in a child: expanding the clinical and pathological spectrum. J Neurosurg Pediatr. 2018 Apr;21(4):428–33. PMID:29393815
2564. Pressey JG, Anderson JR, Crossman DK, et al. Hedgehog pathway activity in pediatric embryonal rhabdomyosarcoma and undifferentiated sarcoma: a report from the Children's Oncology Group. Pediatr Blood Cancer. 2011 Dec 1;57(6):930–8. PMID:21618411
2565. Preston DL, Ron E, Yonehara S, et al. Tumors of the nervous system and pituitary gland associated with atomic bomb radiation exposure. J Natl Cancer Inst. 2002 Oct 16;94(20):1555–63. PMID:12381708
2566. Preuss M, Christiansen H, Merkenschlager A, et al. Disseminated oligodendroglial-like leptomeningeal tumors: preliminary diagnostic and therapeutic results for a novel tumor entity [corrected]. J Neurooncol. 2015 Aug;124(1):65–74. PMID:25672644
2567. Preusser M, Budka H, Rössler K, et al. OLIG2 is a useful immunohistochemical marker in differential diagnosis of clear cell primary CNS neoplasms. Histopathology. 2007 Feb;50(3):365–70. PMID:17257132
2568. Preusser M, Capper D, Ilhan-Mutlu A, et al. Brain metastases: pathobiology and emerging targeted therapies. Acta Neuropathol. 2012 Feb;123(2):205–22. PMID:22212630
2569. Preusser M, Dietrich W, Czech T, et al. Rosette-forming glioneuronal tumor of the fourth ventricle. Acta Neuropathol. 2003 Nov;106(5):506–8. PMID:12915951
2570. Preusser M, Woehrer A, Koperek O, et al. Primary central nervous system lymphoma: a clinicopathological study of 75 cases. Pathology. 2010;42(6):547–52. PMID:20854073
2571. Priest JR, Magnuson J, Williams GM, et al. Cerebral metastasis and other central nervous system complications of pleuropulmonary blastoma. Pediatr Blood Cancer. 2007 Sep;49(3):266–73. PMID:16807914
2572. Priest JR, Watterson J, Strong L, et al. Pleuropulmonary blastoma: a marker for familial disease. J Pediatr. 1996 Feb;128(2):220–4. PMID:8636815
2573. Priesterbach-Ackley LP, Boldt HB, Petersen JK, et al. Brain tumour diagnostics using a DNA methylation-based classifier as a diagnostic support tool. Neuropathol Appl Neurobiol. 2020 Aug;46(5):478–92. PMID:32072658
2574. Prieto R, Pascual JM, Barrios L. Letter: A clinical rule for preoperative prediction of BRAF mutation status in craniopharyngiomas. Neurosurgery. 2019 Nov 1;85(5):E962–5. PMID:31435663
2575. Prieto R, Pascual JM, Barrios L. Optic chiasm distortions in craniopharyngiomas: a sign of hypothalamic involvement. Acta Neurochir (Wien). 2017 Aug;159(8):1533–5. PMID:28660394
2576. Prieto-Granada CN, Wiesner T, Messina JL, et al. Loss of H3K27me3 Expression Is a Highly Sensitive Marker for Sporadic and Radiation-induced MPNST. Am J Surg Pathol. 2016 Apr;40(4):479–89. PMID:26645727
2577. Proescholdt MA, Mayer C, Kubitza M, et al. Expression of hypoxia-inducible carbonic anhydrases in brain tumors. Neuro Oncol. 2005 Oct;7(4):465–75. PMID:16212811
2578. Prosniak M, Harshyne LA, Andrews DW, et al. Glioma grade is associated with the accumulation and activity of cells bearing M2 monocyte markers. Clin Cancer Res. 2013 Jul 15;19(14):3776–86. PMID:23741072
2579. Puchalski RB, Shah N, Miller J, et al. An anatomic transcriptional atlas of human glioblastoma. Science. 2018 May 11;360(6389):660–3. PMID:29748285
2580. Pugh TJ, Yu W, Yang J, et al. Exome sequencing of pleuropulmonary blastoma reveals frequent biallelic loss of TP53 and two hits in DICER1 resulting in retention of 5p-derived miRNA hairpin loop sequences. Oncogene. 2014 Nov 6;33(45):5295–302. PMID:24909177
2581. Pulido R, Baker SJ, Barata JT, et al. A unified nomenclature and amino acid numbering for human PTEN. Sci Signal. 2014 Jul 1;7(332):pe15. PMID:24985344
2582. Purav P, Ganapathy K, Mallikarjuna VS, et al. Rosai-Dorfman disease of the central nervous system. J Clin Neurosci. 2005 Aug;12(6):656–9. PMID:16099162
2583. Pytel P, Krausz T, Wollmann R, et al. Ganglioneuromatous paraganglioma of the cauda equina–a pathological case study. Hum Pathol. 2005 Apr;36(4):444–6. PMID:15892009
2584. Qaddoumi I, Orisme W, Wen J, et al. Genetic alterations in uncommon low-grade neuroepithelial tumors: BRAF, FGFR1, and MYB mutations occur at high frequency and align with morphology. Acta Neuropathol. 2016 Jun;131(6):833–45. PMID:26810070
2585. Qian H, Lin S, Zhang M, et al. Surgical management of intraventricular central neurocytoma: 92 cases. Acta Neurochir (Wien). 2012 Nov;154(11):1951–60. PMID:22941394
2586. Qin J, Wang Z, Hoogeveen-Westerveld M, et al. Structural basis of the interaction between tuberous sclerosis complex 1 (TSC1) and Tre2-Bub2-Cdc16 domain family member 7 (TBC1D7). J Biol Chem. 2016 Apr 15;291(16):8591–601. PMID:26893383
2587. Qu M, Olofsson T, Sigurdardottir S, et al. Genetically distinct astrocytic and oligodendroglial components in oligoastrocytomas. Acta Neuropathol. 2007 Feb;113(2):129–36. PMID:17031656
2588. Quillien V, Lavenu A, Karayan-Tapon L, et al. Comparative assessment of 5 methods (methylation-specific polymerase chain reaction, MethyLight, pyrosequencing, methylation-sensitive high-resolution melting, and immunohistochemistry) to analyze O6-methylguanine-DNA-methyltranferase in a series of 100 glioblastoma patients. Cancer. 2012 Sep 1;118(17):4201–11. PMID:22294349
2589. Rabenhorst U, Thalheimer FB, Gerlach K, et al. Single-stranded DNA-binding transcriptional regulator FUBP1 is essential for fetal and adult hematopoietic stem cell self-renewal. Cell Rep. 2015 Jun 30;11(12):1847–55. PMID:26095368
2590. Racher H, Soliman S, Argiropoulos B, et al. Molecular analysis distinguishes metastatic disease from second cancers in patients with retinoblastoma. Cancer Genet. 2016 Jul-Aug;209(7-8):359–63. PMID:27318443
2591. Rades D, Schild SE. Treatment recommendations for the various subgroups of neurocytomas. J Neurooncol. 2006 May;77(3):305–9. PMID:16575540
2592. Rades D, Schild SE, Fehlauer F. Prognostic value of the MIB-1 labeling index for central neurocytomas. Neurology. 2004 Mar 23;62(6):987–9. PMID:15037708
2593. Radhakrishnan VV, Saraswathy A, Rout D. Papillary meningioma–a clinicopathological study of six cases. Indian J Cancer. 1993 Dec;30(4):164–8. PMID:8206498
2594. Radke J, Gehlhaar C, Lenze D, et al. The evolution of the anaplastic cerebellar liponeurocytoma: case report and review of the literature. Clin Neuropathol. 2015 Jan-Feb;34(1):19–25. PMID:25250652
2595. Raffeld M, Abdullaev Z, Pack SD, et al. High level MYCN amplification and distinct methylation signature define an aggressive subtype of spinal cord ependymoma. Acta Neuropathol Commun. 2020 Jul 8;8(1):101. PMID:32641156
2596. Rafique MZ, Ahmad MN, Yaqoob N, et al. Diffuse bilateral thalamic astrocytoma. J Coll Physicians Surg Pak. 2007 Mar;17(3):170–2. PMID:17374306
2597. Ragazzini R, Pérez-Palacios R, Baymaz IH, et al. EZHIP constrains polycomb repressive complex 2 activity in germ cells. Nat Commun. 2019 Aug 26;10(1):3858. PMID:31451685
2598. Ragel BT, Couldwell WT. Pituitary carcinoma: a review of the literature. Neurosurg Focus. 2004 Apr 15;16(4):E7. PMID:15191336
2599. Raggi F, Russo D, Urbani C, et al. Divergent effects of dioxin- or non-dioxin-like polychlorinated biphenyls on the apoptosis of primary cell culture from the mouse pituitary gland. PLoS One. 2016 Jan 11;11(1):e0146729. PMID:26752525
2600. Raghavan R, Dickey WT Jr, Margraf LR, et al. Proliferative activity in craniopharyngiomas: clinicopathological correlations in adults and children. Surg Neurol. 2000 Sep;54(3):241–7. PMID:11118571
2601. Raghavan R, Steart PV, Weller RO. Cell proliferation patterns in the diagnosis of astrocytomas, anaplastic astrocytomas and glioblastoma multiforme: a Ki-67 study. Neuropathol Appl Neurobiol. 1990 Apr;16(2):123–33. PMID:2161084
2602. Raghavan SS, Mooney KL, Folpe AL, et al. OLIG2 is a marker of the fusion protein-driven neurodevelopmental transcriptional signature in alveolar rhabdomyosarcoma. Hum Pathol. 2019 Sep;91:77–85. PMID:31299267
2603. Raghunathan A, Olar A, Vogel H, et al. Isocitrate dehydrogenase 1 R132H mutation is not detected in angiocentric glioma. Ann Diagn Pathol. 2012 Aug;16(4):255–9. PMID:22445362
2604. Rai K, Pilarski R, Cebulla CM, et al. Comprehensive review of BAP1 tumor predisposition syndrome with report of two new cases. Clin Genet. 2016 Mar;89(3):285–94. PMID:26096145
2605. Raisanen J, Biegel JA, Hatanpaa KJ, et al. Chromosome 22q deletions in atypical teratoid/rhabdoid tumors in adults. Brain Pathol. 2005 Jan;15(1):23–8. PMID:15779233
2606. Rajaram V, Brat DJ, Perry A. Anaplastic meningioma versus meningeal hemangiopericytoma: immunohistochemical and genetic markers. Hum Pathol. 2004 Nov;35(11):1413–8. PMID:15668900
2607. Rajput DK, Mehrotra A, Srivastav AK, et al. Bilateral thalamic glioma in a 6-year-old child. J Pediatr Neurosci. 2010 Jan;5(1):45–8. PMID:21042509
2608. Raju GP, Urion DK, Sahin M. Neonatal subependymal giant cell astrocytoma: new case and review of literature. Pediatr Neurol. 2007 Feb;36(2):128–31. PMID:17275668
2609. Ralte AM, Rao S, Sharma MC, et al. Myxopapillary ependymoma of the temporal lobe-report of a rare case of temporal lobe epilepsy. Clin Neuropathol. 2004 Mar-Apr;23(2):53–8. PMID:15074578
2610. Ramani B, Gupta R, Wu J, et al. The immunohistochemical, DNA methylation, and chromosomal copy number profile of cauda equina paraganglioma is distinct from extra-spinal paraganglioma. Acta Neuropathol. 2020 Dec;140(6):907–17. PMID:32892244
2611. Ramaswamy V, Delaney H, Haque S, et al. Spectrum of central nervous system abnormalities in neurocutaneous melanocytosis. Dev Med Child Neurol. 2012 Jun;54(6):563–8. PMID:22469364
2612. Ramaswamy V, Hielscher T, Mack SC, et al. Therapeutic impact of cytoreductive surgery and irradiation of posterior fossa ependymoma in the molecular era: a retrospective multicohort analysis. J Clin Oncol. 2016 Jul 20;34(21):2468–77. PMID:27269943
2613. Ramaswamy V, Nör C, Taylor MD. p53 and Meduloblastoma. Cold Spring Harb Perspect Med. 2015 Dec 18;6(2):a026278. PMID:26684332
2614. Ramaswamy V, Remke M, Bouffet E, et al. Recurrence patterns across medulloblastoma subgroups: an integrated clinical and molecular analysis. Lancet Oncol. 2013 Nov;14(12):1200–7. PMID:24140199
2615. Ramaswamy V, Remke M, Bouffet E, et al. Risk stratification of childhood medulloblastoma in the molecular era: the current consensus. Acta Neuropathol. 2016 Jun;131(6):821–31. PMID:27040285

2616. Ramkissoon LA, Horowitz PM, Craig JM, et al. Genomic analysis of diffuse pediatric low-grade gliomas identifies recurrent oncogenic truncating rearrangements in the transcription factor MYBL1. Proc Natl Acad Sci U S A. 2013 May 14;110(20):8188–93. PMID:23633565
2617. Ramsay JA, Asa SL, van Nostrand AW, et al. Lipid degeneration in pheochromocytomas mimicking adrenal cortical tumors. Am J Surg Pathol. 1987 Jun;11(6):480–6. PMID:3592062
2618. Rankine AJ, Filion PR, Platten MA, et al. Perineurioma: a clinicopathological study of eight cases. Pathology. 2004 Aug;36(4):309–15. PMID:15370128
2619. Raoux D, Duband S, Forest F, et al. Primary central nervous system lymphoma: immunohistochemical profile and prognostic significance. Neuropathology. 2010 Jun;30(3):232–40. PMID:19925562
2620. Rasmussen SA, Yang Q, Friedman JM. Mortality in neurofibromatosis 1: an analysis using U.S. death certificates. Am J Hum Genet. 2001 May;68(5):1110–8. PMID:11283797
2621. Rasul FT, Jaunmuktane Z, Khan AA, et al. Plurihormonal pituitary adenoma with concomitant adrenocorticotropic hormone (ACTH) and growth hormone (GH) secretion: a report of two cases and review of the literature. Acta Neurochir (Wien). 2014 Jan;156(1):141–6. PMID:24081787
2622. Rausch T, Jones DT, Zapatka M, et al. Genome sequencing of pediatric medulloblastoma links catastrophic DNA rearrangements with TP53 mutations. Cell. 2012 Jan 20;148(1-2):59–71. PMID:22265402
2623. Raverot G, Burman P, McCormack A, et al. European Society of Endocrinology Clinical Practice Guidelines for the management of aggressive pituitary tumours and carcinomas. Eur J Endocrinol. 2018 Jan;178(1):G1–24. PMID:29046323
2624. Raverot G, Castinetti F, Jouanneau E, et al. Pituitary carcinomas and aggressive pituitary tumours: merits and pitfalls of temozolomide treatment. Clin Endocrinol (Oxf). 2012 Jun;76(6):769–75. PMID:22404748
2625. Raverot G, Wierinckx A, Jouanneau E, et al. Clinical, hormonal and molecular characterization of pituitary ACTH adenomas without (silent corticotroph adenomas) and with Cushing's disease. Eur J Endocrinol. 2010 Jul;163(1):35–43. PMID:20385723
2626. Ray A, Manjila S, Hdeib AM, et al. Extracranial metastasis of glioblastoma: three illustrative cases and current review of the molecular pathology and management strategies. Mol Clin Oncol. 2015 May;3(3):479–86. PMID:26137254
2627. Ray WZ, Blackburn SL, Casavilca-Zambrano S, et al. Clinicopathologic features of recurrent dysembryoplastic neuroepithelial tumor and rare malignant transformation: a report of 6 cases and review of the literature. J Neurooncol. 2009 Sep;94(2):283–92. PMID:19267228
2628. Raymond AA, Halpin SF, Alsanjari N, et al. Dysembryoplastic neuroepithelial tumor. Features in 16 patients. Brain. 1994 Jun;117(Pt 3):461–75. PMID:8032857
2629. Reardon W, Zhou XP, Eng C. A novel germline mutation of the PTEN gene in a patient with macrocephaly, ventricular dilatation, and features of VATER association. J Med Genet. 2001 Dec;38(12):820–3. PMID:11748304
2630. Reddy AT, Strother DR, Judkins AR, et al. Efficacy of high-dose chemotherapy and three-dimensional conformal radiation for atypical teratoid/rhabdoid tumor: a report from the Children's Oncology Group trial ACNS0333. J Clin Oncol. 2020 Apr 10;38(11):1175–85. PMID:32105509
2631. Rednam SP, Erez A, Druker H, et al. Von Hippel-Lindau and hereditary pheochromocytoma/paraganglioma syndromes: clinical features, genetics, and surveillance recommendations in childhood. Clin Cancer Res. 2017 Jun 15;23(12):e68–75. PMID:28620007
2632. Reese TS. The molecular basis of axonal transport in the squid giant axon. Res Publ Assoc Res Nerv Ment Dis. 1987;65:89–102. PMID:2455314
2633. Reid S, Schindler D, Hanenberg H, et al. Biallelic mutations in PALB2 cause Fanconi anemia subtype FA-N and predispose to childhood cancer. Nat Genet. 2007 Feb;39(2):162–4. PMID:17200671
2634. Reifenberger G, Hentschel B, Felsberg J, et al. Predictive impact of MGMT promoter methylation in glioblastoma of the elderly. Int J Cancer. 2012 Sep 15;131(6):1342–50. PMID:22139906
2635. Reifenberger G, Kaulich K, Wiestler OD, et al. Expression of the CD34 antigen in pleomorphic xanthoastrocytomas. Acta Neuropathol. 2003 Apr;105(4):358–64. PMID:12624789
2636. Reifenberger G, Reifenberger J, Ichimura K, et al. Amplification of multiple genes from chromosomal region 12q13-14 in human malignant gliomas: preliminary mapping of the amplicons shows preferential involvement of CDK4, SAS, and MDM2. Cancer Res. 1994 Aug 15;54(16):4299–303. PMID:8044775
2637. Reifenberger G, Szymas J, Wechsler W. Differential expression of glial- and neuronal-associated antigens in human tumors of the central and peripheral nervous system. Acta Neuropathol. 1987;74(2):105–23. PMID:3314309
2638. Reifenberger G, Weber RG, Riehmer V, et al. Molecular characterization of long-term survivors of glioblastoma using genome- and transcriptome-wide profiling. Int J Cancer. 2014 Oct 15;135(8):1822–31. PMID:24615357
2639. Reifenberger G, Weber T, Weber RG, et al. Chordoid glioma of the third ventricle: immunohistochemical and molecular genetic characterization of a novel tumor entity. Brain Pathol. 1999 Oct;9(4):617–26. PMID:10517500
2640. Reifenberger J, Reifenberger G, Liu L, et al. Molecular genetic analysis of oligodendroglial tumors shows preferential allelic deletions on 19q and 1p. Am J Pathol. 1994 Nov;145(5):1175–90. PMID:7977648
2641. Reilly KM, Kim A, Blakely J, et al. Neurofibromatosis type 1-associated MPNST state of the science: outlining a research agenda for the future. J Natl Cancer Inst. 2017 Aug 1;109(8):djx124. PMID:29117388
2642. Reincke M, Sbiera S, Hayakawa A, et al. Mutations in the deubiquitinase gene USP8 cause Cushing's disease. Nat Genet. 2015 Jan;47(1):31–8. PMID:25485838
2643. Reinhardt A, Stichel D, Schrimpf D, et al. Anaplastic astrocytoma with piloid features, a novel molecular class of IDH wildtype glioma with recurrent MAPK pathway, CDKN2A/B and ATRX alterations. Acta Neuropathol. 2018 Aug;136(2):273–91. PMID:29564591
2644. Reinhardt A, Stichel D, Schrimpf D, et al. Tumors diagnosed as cerebellar glioblastoma comprise distinct molecular entities. Acta Neuropathol Commun. 2019 Oct 28;7(1):163. PMID:31661039
2645. Reis F, Faria AV, Zanardi VA, et al. Neuroimaging in pineal tumors. J Neuroimaging. 2006 Jan;16(1):52–8. PMID:16483277
2646. Reis RM, Könü-Lebleblicioglu D, Lopes JM, et al. Genetic profile of gliosarcomas. Am J Pathol. 2000 Feb;156(2):425–32. PMID:10666371
2647. Reis-Filho JS, Faoro LN, Carrilho C, et al. Evaluation of cell proliferation, epidermal growth factor receptor, and bcl-2 immunoexpression as prognostic factors for patients with World Health Organization grade 2 oligodendroglioma. Cancer. 2000 Feb 15;88(4):862–9. PMID:10679656
2648. Reithmeier T, Gumprecht H, Stölzle A, et al. Intracerebral paraganglioma. Acta Neurochir (Wien). 2000;142(9):1063–6. PMID:11086818
2649. Remke M, Hielscher T, Northcott PA, et al. Adult medulloblastoma comprises three major molecular variants. J Clin Oncol. 2011 Jul 1;29(19):2717–23. PMID:21632505
2650. Remke M, Ramaswamy V, Peacock J, et al. TERT promoter mutations are highly recurrent in SHH subgroup medulloblastoma. Acta Neuropathol. 2013 Dec;126(6):917–29. PMID:24174164
2651. Rencic A, Gordon J, Otte J, et al. Detection of JC virus DNA sequence and expression of the viral oncoprotein, tumor antigen, in brain of immunocompetent patient with oligoastrocytoma. Proc Natl Acad Sci U S A. 1996 Jul 9;93(14):7352–7. PMID:8692997
2652. Reni M, Ferreri AJ, Zoldan MC, et al. Primary brain lymphomas in patients with a prior or concomitant malignancy. J Neurooncol. 1997 Apr;32(2):135–42. PMID:9120542
2653. Repo P, Järvinen RS, Jäntti JE, et al. Population-based analysis of BAP1 germline variations in patients with uveal melanoma. Hum Mol Genet. 2019 Jul 15;28(14):2415–26. PMID:31058963
2654. Reuss DE, Habel A, Hagenlocher C, et al. Neurofibromin specific antibody differentiates malignant peripheral nerve sheath tumors (MPNST) from other spindle cell neoplasms. Acta Neuropathol. 2014 Apr;127(4):565–72. PMID:24464231
2655. Reuss DE, Mamatjan Y, Schrimpf D, et al. IDH mutant diffuse and anaplastic astrocytomas have similar age at presentation and little difference in survival: a grading problem for WHO. Acta Neuropathol. 2015 Jun;129(6):867–73. PMID:25962792
2656. Reuss DE, Piro RM, Jones DT, et al. Secretory meningiomas are defined by combined KLF4 K409Q and TRAF7 mutations. Acta Neuropathol. 2013 Mar;125(3):351–8. PMID:23404370
2657. Reuss DE, Sahm F, Schrimpf D, et al. ATRX and IDH1-R132H immunohistochemistry with subsequent copy number analysis and IDH sequencing as a basis for an "integrated" diagnostic approach for adult astrocytoma, oligodendroglioma and glioblastoma. Acta Neuropathol. 2015 Jan;129(1):133–46. PMID:25427834
2658. Reyes-Botero G, Dehais C, Idbaih A, et al. Contrast enhancement in 1p/19q-codeleted anaplastic oligodendrogliomas is associated with 9p loss, genomic instability, and angiogenic gene expression. Neuro Oncol. 2014 May;16(5):662–70. PMID:24353325
2659. Rhiew RB, Manjila S, Lozen A, et al. Leptomeningeal dissemination of a pediatric neoplasm with 1p19q deletion showing mixed immunohistochemical features of an oligodendroglioma and neurocytoma. Acta Neurochir (Wien). 2010 Aug;152(8):1425–9. PMID:20446099
2660. Ribeiro S, Napoli I, White IJ, et al. Injury signals cooperate with Nf1 loss to relieve the tumor-suppressive environment of adult peripheral nerve. Cell Rep. 2013 Oct 17;5(1):126–36. PMID:24075988
2661. Ribi S, Baumhoer D, Lee K, et al. TP53 intron 1 hotspot rearrangements are specific to sporadic osteosarcoma and can cause Li-Fraumeni syndrome. Oncotarget. 2015 Apr 10;6(10):7727–40. PMID:25762628
2662. Richards S, Aziz N, Bale S, et al. Standards and guidelines for the interpretation of sequence variants: a joint consensus recommendation of the American College of Medical Genetics and Genomics and the Association for Molecular Pathology. Genet Med. 2015 May;17(5):405–24. PMID:25741868
2663. Richardson TE, Tang K, Vasudevaraja V, et al. GOPC-ROS1 fusion due to microdeletion at 6q22 is an oncogenic driver in a subset of pediatric gliomas and glioneuronal tumors. J Neuropathol Exp Neurol. 2019 Dec 1;78(12):1089–99. PMID:31626289
2664. Rickard KA, Parker JR, Vitaz TW, et al. Papillary tumor of the pineal region: two case studies and a review of the literature. Ann Clin Lab Sci. 2011 Spring;41(2):174–81. PMID:21844577
2665. Rickert CH, Paulus W. Lack of chromosomal imbalances in adamantinomatous and papillary craniopharyngiomas. J Neurol Neurosurg Psychiatry. 2003 Feb;74(2):260–1. PMID:12531965
2666. Rickert CH, Paulus W. No chromosomal imbalances detected by comparative genomic hybridisation in a case of fetal immature teratoma. Childs Nerv Syst. 2002 Nov;18(11):639–43. PMID:12420126
2667. Rickert CH, Paulus W. Tumors of the choroid plexus. Microsc Res Tech. 2001 Jan 1;52(1):104–11. PMID:11135453
2668. Rickert CH, Simon R, Bergmann M, et al. Comparative genomic hybridization in pineal parenchymal tumors. Genes Chromosomes Cancer. 2001 Jan;30(1):99–104. PMID:11107183
2669. Rickert CH, Wiestler OD, Paulus W. Chromosomal imbalances in choroid plexus tumors. Am J Pathol. 2002 Mar;160(3):1105–13. PMID:11891207
2670. Ricklefs FL, Fita KD, Rotermund R, et al. Genome-wide DNA methylation profiles distinguish silent from non-silent ACTH adenomas. Acta Neuropathol. 2020 Jul;140(1):95–7. PMID:32185515
2671. Rickman DS, Bobek MP, Misek DE, et al. Distinctive molecular profiles of high-grade and low-grade gliomas based on oligonucleotide microarray analysis. Cancer Res. 2001 Sep 15;61(18):6885–91. PMID:11559565
2672. Riegert-Johnson DL, Gleeson FC, Roberts M, et al. Cancer and Lhermitte-Duclos disease are common in Cowden syndrome patients. Hered Cancer Clin Pract. 2010 Jun 17;8(1):6. PMID:20565722
2673. Riemenschneider MJ, Reifenberger G. Molecular neuropathology of gliomas. Int J Mol Sci. 2009 Jan;10(1):184–212. PMID:19333441
2674. Riemersma SA, Jordanova ES, Schop RF, et al. Extensive genetic alterations of the HLA region, including homozygous deletions of HLA class II genes in B-cell lymphomas arising in immune-privileged sites. Blood. 2000 Nov 15;96(10):3569–77. PMID:11071656
2675. Riemersma SA, Oudejans JJ, Vonk MJ, et al. High numbers of tumour-infiltrating activated cytotoxic T lymphocytes, and frequent loss of HLA class I and II expression, are features of aggressive B cell lymphomas of the brain and testis. J Pathol. 2005 Jul;206(3):328–36. PMID:15887291
2676. Righi A, Sbaraglia M, Gambarotti M, et al. Extra-axial chordoma: a clinicopathologic analysis of six cases. Virchows Arch. 2018 Jun;472(6):1015–20. PMID:29560513
2677. Rimm DL, Han G, Taube JM, et al. A prospective, multi-institutional, pathologist-based assessment of 4 immunohistochemistry assays for pd-l1 expression in non-small cell lung cancer. JAMA Oncol. 2017 Aug 1;3(8):1051–8. PMID:28278348
2678. Rindi G, Klimstra DS, Abedi-Ardekani B, et al. A common classification framework for neuroendocrine neoplasms: an International Agency for Research on Cancer (IARC) and World Health Organization (WHO) expert

consensus proposal. Mod Pathol. 2018 Dec;31(12):1770–86. PMID:30140036
2679. Riva G, Cima L, Villanova M, et al. Low-grade neuroepithelial tumor: unusual presentation in an adult without history of seizures. Neuropathology. 2018 Oct;38(5):557–60. PMID:30051533
2680. Rivera B, Gayden T, Carrot-Zhang J, et al. Germline and somatic FGFR1 abnormalities in dysembryoplastic neuroepithelial tumors. Acta Neuropathol. 2016 Jun;131(6):847–63. PMID:26920151
2681. Rivera B, Nadaf J, Fahiminiya S, et al. DGCR8 microprocessor defect characterizes familial multinodular goiter with schwannomatosis. J Clin Invest. 2020 Mar 2;130(3):1479–90. PMID:31805011
2682. Rizk T, Taslakian B, Torbey PH, et al. Sequential development of Wilms tumor and medulloblastoma in a child: an unusual presentation of fanconi anemia. Pediatr Hematol Oncol. 2013 Aug;30(5):400–2. PMID:23698033
2683. Roach ES, Sparagana SP. Diagnostic criteria for tuberous sclerosis complex. In: Kwiatkowski DJ, Whittemore VH, Thiele EA, editors. Tuberous sclerosis complex: genes, clinical features, and therapeutics. Weinheim (Germany): Wiley-Blackwell; 2010. pp. 21–5.
2684. Robbins P, Segal A, Narula S, et al. Central neurocytoma. A clinicopathological, immunohistochemical and ultrastructural study of 7 cases. Pathol Res Pract. 1995 Mar;191(2):100–11. PMID:7567679
2685. Roberts CW, Biegel JA. The role of SMARCB1/INI1 in development of rhabdoid tumor. Cancer Biol Ther. 2009 Mar;8(5):412–6. PMID:19305156
2686. Roberts RO, Lynch CF, Jones MP, et al. Medulloblastoma: a population-based study of 532 cases. J Neuropathol Exp Neurol. 1991 Mar;50(2):134–44. PMID:2010773
2687. Robinson C, Kleinschmidt-DeMasters BK. IDH1-mutation in diffuse gliomas in persons age 55 years and over. J Neuropathol Exp Neurol. 2017 Feb 1;76(2):151–4. PMID:28110298
2688. Robinson DR, Wu YM, Kalyana-Sundaram S, et al. Identification of recurrent NAB2-STAT6 gene fusions in solitary fibrous tumor by integrative sequencing. Nat Genet. 2013 Feb;45(2):180–5. PMID:23313952
2689. Robinson G, Parker M, Kranenburg TA, et al. Novel mutations target distinct subgroups of medulloblastoma. Nature. 2012 Aug 2;488(7409):43–8. PMID:22722829
2690. Robinson GW, Gajjar A. Genomics paves the way for better infant medulloblastoma therapy. J Clin Oncol. 2020 Jun 20;38(18):2010–3. PMID:32352857
2691. Robinson GW, Rudneva VA, Buchhalter I, et al. Risk-adapted therapy for young children with medulloblastoma (SJYC07): therapeutic and molecular outcomes from a multicentre, phase 2 trial. Lancet Oncol. 2018 Jun;19(6):768–84. PMID:29778738
2692. Roche PH, Figarella-Branger D, Regis J, et al. Cauda equina paraganglioma with subsequent intracranial and intraspinal metastases. Acta Neurochir (Wien). 1996;138(4):475–9. PMID:8738400
2693. Rodriguez FJ, Brosnan-Cashman JA, Allen SJ, et al. Alternative lengthening of telomeres, ATRX loss and H3-K27M mutations in histologically defined pilocytic astrocytoma with anaplasia. Brain Pathol. 2019 Jan;29(1):126–40. PMID:30192422
2694. Rodriguez FJ, Graham MK, Brosnan-Cashman JA, et al. Telomere alterations in neurofibromatosis type 1-associated solid tumors. Acta Neuropathol Commun. 2019 Aug 28;7(1):139. PMID:31462295
2695. Rodriguez FJ, Perry A, Gutmann DH, et al. Gliomas in neurofibromatosis type 1: a clinicopathologic study of 100 patients. J Neuropathol Exp Neurol. 2008 Mar;67(3):240–9. PMID:18344915
2696. Rodriguez FJ, Perry A, Rosenblum MK, et al. Disseminated oligodendroglial-like leptomeningeal tumor of childhood: a distinctive clinicopathologic entity. Acta Neuropathol. 2012 Nov;124(5):627–41. PMID:22941225
2697. Rodriguez FJ, Scheithauer BW, Burger PC, et al. Anaplasia in pilocytic astrocytoma predicts aggressive behavior. Am J Surg Pathol. 2010 Feb;34(2):147–60. PMID:20061938
2698. Rodriguez FJ, Scheithauer BW, Giannini C, et al. Epithelial and pseudoepithelial differentiation in glioblastoma and gliosarcoma: a comparative morphologic and molecular genetic study. Cancer. 2008 Nov 15;113(10):2779–89. PMID:18816605
2699. Rodriguez FJ, Scheithauer BW, Jenkins R, et al. Gliosarcoma arising in oligodendroglial tumors ("oligosarcoma"): a clinicopathologic study. Am J Surg Pathol. 2007 Mar;31(3):351–62. PMID:17325476
2700. Rodriguez FJ, Scheithauer BW, Perry A, et al. Ependymal tumors with sarcomatous change ("ependymosarcoma"): a clinicopathologic and molecular cytogenetic study. Am J Surg Pathol. 2008 May;32(5):699–709. PMID:18347506
2701. Rodriguez FJ, Scheithauer BW, Tsunoda S, et al. The spectrum of malignancy in craniopharyngioma. Am J Surg Pathol. 2007 Jul;31(7):1020–8. PMID:17592268
2702. Rodriguez FJ, Schniederjan MJ, Nicolaides T, et al. High rate of concurrent BRAF-KIAA1549 gene fusion and 1p deletion in disseminated oligodendroglioma-like leptomeningeal neoplasms (DOLN). Acta Neuropathol. 2015 Apr;129(4):609–10. PMID:25720745
2703. Rodriguez FJ, Tihan T, Lin D, et al. Clinicopathologic features of pediatric oligodendrogliomas: a series of 50 patients. Am J Surg Pathol. 2014 Aug;38(8):1058–70. PMID:24805856
2704. Rodriguez FJ, Vizcaino MA, Blakeley J, et al. Frequent alternative lengthening of telomeres and ATRX loss in adult NF1-associated diffuse and high-grade astrocytomas. Acta Neuropathol. 2016 Nov;132(5):761–3. PMID:27650176
2705. Rodriguez HA, Berthrong M. Multiple primary intracranial tumors in von Recklinghausen's neurofibromatosis. Arch Neurol. 1966 May;14(5):467–75. PMID:4957904
2706. Rodriguez LA, Edwards MS, Levin VA. Management of hypothalamic gliomas in children: an analysis of 33 cases. Neurosurgery. 1990 Feb;26(2):242–6. PMID:2308672
2707. Rodriguez-Galindo C, Allen CE. Langerhans cell histiocytosis. Blood. 2020 Apr 16;135(16):1319–31. PMID:32106306
2708. Rogers S, Jones DTW, Ireland A, et al. Unusual paediatric spinal myxopapillary ependymomas: unique molecular entities or pathological variations on a theme? J Clin Neurosci. 2018 Apr;50:144–8. PMID:29402569
2709. Röhrich M, Koelsche C, Schrimpf D, et al. Methylation-based classification of benign and malignant peripheral nerve sheath tumors. Acta Neuropathol. 2016 Jun;131(6):877–87. PMID:26857854
2710. Rojnueangnit K, Xie J, Gomes A, et al. High incidence of Noonan syndrome features including short stature and pulmonic stenosis in patients carrying NF1 missense mutations affecting p.Arg1809: genotype-phenotype correlation. Hum Mutat. 2015 Nov;36(11):1052–63. PMID:26178382
2711. Rollins BJ. Genomic alterations in Langerhans cell histiocytosis. Hematol Oncol Clin North Am. 2015 Oct;29(5):839–51. PMID:26461146
2712. Rollison DE, Utaipat U, Ryschkewitsch C, et al. Investigation of human brain tumors for the presence of polyomavirus genome sequences by two independent laboratories. Int J Cancer. 2005 Feb 20;113(5):769–74. PMID:15499616
2713. Romano N, Federici M, Castaldi A. Imaging of extraventricular neurocytoma: a systematic literature review. Radiol Med. 2020 Oct;125(10):961–70. PMID:32335813
2714. Romero-Rojas AE, Diaz-Perez JA, Ariza-Serrano LM, et al. Primary gliosarcoma of the brain: radiologic and histopathologic features. Neuroradiol J. 2013 Dec;26(6):639–48. PMID:24355182
2715. Romero-Rojas AE, Melo-Uribe MA, Barajas-Solano PA, et al. Spindle cell oncocytoma of the adenohypophysis. Brain Tumor Pathol. 2011 Oct;28(4):359–64. PMID:21833579
2716. Ron E, Modan B, Boice JD Jr, et al. Tumors of the brain and nervous system after radiotherapy in childhood. N Engl J Med. 1988 Oct 20;319(16):1033–9. PMID:3173432
2717. Roncaroli F, Riccioni L, Cerati M, et al. Oncocytic meningioma. Am J Surg Pathol. 1997 Apr;21(4):375–82. PMID:9130983
2718. Roncaroli F, Scheithauer BW, Cenacchi G, et al. 'Spindle cell oncocytoma' of the adenohypophysis: a tumor of folliculostellate cells? Am J Surg Pathol. 2002 Aug;26(8):1048–55. PMID:12170092
2719. Ronellenfitsch MW, Harter PN, Kirchner M, et al. Targetable ERBB2 mutations identified in neurofibroma/schwannoma hybrid nerve sheath tumors. J Clin Invest. 2020 May 1;130(5):2488–95. PMID:32017710
2720. Rong Y, Durden DL, Van Meir EG, et al. 'Pseudopalisading' necrosis in glioblastoma: a familiar morphologic feature that links vascular pathology, hypoxia, and angiogenesis. J Neuropathol Exp Neurol. 2006 Jun;65(6):529–39. PMID:16783163
2721. Rorke LB, Packer RJ, Biegel JA. Central nervous system atypical teratoid/rhabdoid tumors of infancy and childhood: definition of an entity. J Neurosurg. 1996 Jul;85(1):56–65. PMID:8683283
2722. Rosemberg S, Fujiwara D. Epidemiology of pediatric tumors of the nervous system according to the WHO 2000 classification: a report of 1,195 cases from a single institution. Childs Nerv Syst. 2005 Nov;21(11):940–4. PMID:16044344
2723. Rosenbaum JN, Guo Z, Baus RM, et al. INSM1: a novel immunohistochemical and molecular marker for neuroendocrine and neuroepithelial neoplasms. Am J Clin Pathol. 2015 Oct;144(4):579–91. PMID:26386079
2724. Rosenberg AE, Nielsen GP, Keel SB, et al. Chondrosarcoma of the base of the skull: a clinicopathologic study of 200 cases with emphasis on its distinction from chordoma. Am J Surg Pathol. 1999 Nov;23(11):1370–8. PMID:10555005
2725. Rosenberg PS, Tamary H, Alter BP. How high are carrier frequencies of rare recessive syndromes? Contemporary estimates for Fanconi anemia in the United States and Israel. Am J Med Genet A. 2011 Aug;155A(8):1877–83. PMID:21739583
2726. Rosenberg S, Simeonova I, Bielle F, et al. A recurrent point mutation in PRKCA is a hallmark of chordoid gliomas. Nat Commun. 2018 Jun 18;9(1):2371. PMID:29915258
2727. Rosenblum MK, Erlandson RA, Aleksic SN, et al. Melanotic ependymoma and subependymoma. Am J Surg Pathol. 1990 Aug;14(8):729–36. PMID:2378394
2728. Rosenblum MK, Erlandson RA, Budzilovich GN. The lipid-rich epithelioid glioblastoma. Am J Surg Pathol. 1991 Oct;15(10):925–34. PMID:1718177
2729. Roser F, Nakamura M, Brandis A, et al. Transition from meningeal melanocytoma to primary cerebral melanoma. Case report. J Neurosurg. 2004 Sep;101(3):528–31. PMID:15352613
2730. Rossi S, Rodriguez FJ, Mota RA, et al. Primary leptomeningeal oligodendroglioma with documented progression to anaplasia and t(1;19)(q10;p10) in a child. Acta Neuropathol. 2009 Oct;118(4):575–7. PMID:19562354
2731. Roth J, Roach ES, Bartels U, et al. Subependymal giant cell astrocytoma: diagnosis, screening, and treatment. Recommendations from the International Tuberous Sclerosis Complex Consensus Conference 2012. Pediatr Neurol. 2013 Dec;49(6):439–44. PMID:24138953
2732. Rothová N, Houbová J. [Histiocytosis X]. Cesk Pediatr. 1968 Oct;23(10):890–3. Czech. PMID:5701259
2733. Rotman JA, Kucharczyk W, Zadeh G, et al. Spindle cell oncocytoma of the adenohypophysis: a case report illustrating its natural history with 8-year observation and a review of the literature. Clin Imaging. 2014 Jul-Aug;38(4):499–504. PMID:24721021
2734. Rouleau GA, Merel P, Lutchman M, et al. Alteration in a new gene encoding a putative membrane-organizing protein causes neuro-fibromatosis type 2. Nature. 1993 Jun 10;363(6429):515–21. PMID:8379998
2735. Rousseau G, Noguchi T, Bourdon V, et al. SMARCB1/INI1 germline mutations contribute to 10% of sporadic schwannomatosis. BMC Neurol. 2011 Jan 24;11:9. PMID:21255467
2736. Roussel-Gervais A, Couture C, Langlais D, et al. The cables1 gene in glucocorticoid regulation of pituitary corticotrope growth and Cushing disease. J Clin Endocrinol Metab. 2016 Feb;101(2):513–22. PMID:26695862
2737. Routman DM, Raghunathan A, Giannini C, et al. Anaplastic ependymoma and posterior fossa grouping in a patient with h3k27me3 loss of expression but chromosomal imbalance. Adv Radiat Oncol. 2019 Mar 14;4(3):466–72. PMID:31360801
2738. Roux A, Pallud J, Saffroy R, et al. High-grade gliomas in adolescents and young adults highlight histomolecular differences from their adult and pediatric counterparts. Neuro Oncol. 2020 Aug 17;22(8):1190–202. PMID:32025728
2739. Roux A, Tauziede-Espariat A, Zanello M, et al. Imaging growth as a predictor of grade of malignancy and aggressiveness of IDH-mutant and 1p/19q-codeleted oligodendrogliomas in adults. Neuro Oncol. 2020 Jul 7;22(7):993–1005. PMID:32025725
2740. Rowland BD, Bernards R, Peeper DS. The KLF4 tumour suppressor is a transcriptional repressor of p53 that acts as a context-dependent oncogene. Nat Cell Biol. 2005 Nov;7(11):1074–82. PMID:16244670
2741. Roy MS, Podgor MJ, Rick ME. Plasma fibrinopeptide A, beta-thromboglobulin, and platelet factor 4 in diabetic retinopathy. Invest Ophthalmol Vis Sci. 1988 Jun;29(6):856–60. PMID:2967258
2741A. Roy S, Chu A, Trojanowski JQ, et al. D2-40, a novel monoclonal antibody against the M2A antigen as a marker to distinguish hemangioblastomas from renal cell carcinomas. Acta Neuropathol. 2005 May;109(5):497–502. PMID:15864611
2742. Rubenstein JL, Wong VS, Kadoch C, et al. CXCL13 plus interleukin 10 is highly specific for the diagnosis of CNS lymphoma. Blood. 2013 Jun 6;121(23):4740–8. PMID:23570798
2743. Rubinstein LJ. The malformative central nervous system lesions in the central and peripheral forms of neurofibromatosis. A neuropathological study of 22 cases. Ann N Y Acad Sci. 1986;486:14–29. PMID:3105387
2744. Rudà R, Gilbert M, Soffietti R.

Ependymomas of the adult: molecular biology and treatment. Curr Opin Neurol. 2008 Dec;21(6):754–61. PMID:18989122

2745. Rudà R, Reifenberger G, Frappaz D, et al. EANO guidelines for the diagnosis and treatment of ependymal tumors. Neuro Oncol. 2018 Mar 27;20(4):445–56. PMID:29194500

2746 Rueda-Pedraza ME, Heifetz SA, Sesterhenn IA, et al. Primary intracranial germ cell tumors in the first two decades of life. A clinical, light-microscopic, and immunohistochemical analysis of 54 cases. Perspect Pediatr Pathol. 1987;10:160–207. PMID:3588245

2747. Ruiz VY, Praska CE, Armstrong G, et al. Molecular subtyping of tumors from patients with familial glioma. Neuro Oncol. 2018 May 18;20(6):810–7. PMID:29040662

2748. Ruland V, Hartung S, Kordes U, et al. Choroid plexus carcinomas are characterized by complex chromosomal alterations related to patient age and prognosis. Genes Chromosomes Cancer. 2014 May;53(5):373–80. PMID:24478045

2749. Rumeh ASAL, Bafaqeeh M, Khairan SJA, et al. Pituicytoma associated with Cushing's disease: a case report and literature review. J Surg Case Rep. 2020 Jun 15;2020(6):a104. PMID:32577204

2750. Runyan C, Schaible K, Molyneaux K, et al. Steel factor controls midline cell death of primordial germ cells and is essential for their normal proliferation and migration. Development. 2006 Dec;133(24):4861–9. PMID:17107997

2751. Rupani A, Modi C, Desai S, et al. Primary anaplastic large cell lymphoma of central nervous system-a case report. J Postgrad Med. 2005 Oct-Dec;51(4):326–7. PMID:16388180

2752. Rusch A, Ziltener G, Nackaerts K, et al. Prevalence of BRCA-1 associated protein 1 germline mutation in sporadic malignant pleural mesothelioma cases. Lung Cancer. 2015 Jan;87(1):77–9. PMID:25468148

2753. Rush S, Foreman N, Liu A. Brainstem ganglioglioma successfully treated with vemurafenib. J Clin Oncol. 2013 Apr 1;31(10):e159–60. PMID:23358987

2754. Rushing EJ, Armonda RA, Ansari Q, et al. Mesenchymal chondrosarcoma: a clinicopathologic and flow cytometric study of 13 cases presenting in the central nervous system. Cancer. 1996 May 1;77(9):1884–91. PMID:8646689

2755. Rushing EJ, Cooper PB, Quezado M, et al. Subependymoma revisited: clinicopathological evaluation of 83 cases. J Neurooncol. 2007 Dec;85(3):297–305. PMID:17569000

2756. Rushing EJ, Thompson LD, Mena H. Malignant transformation of a dysembryoplastic neuroepithelial tumor after radiation and chemotherapy. Ann Diagn Pathol. 2003 Aug;7(4):240–4. PMID:12913847

2757. Rushlow DE, Mol BM, Kennett JY, et al. Characterisation of retinoblastomas without RB1 mutations: genomic, gene expression, and clinical studies. Lancet Oncol. 2013 Apr;14(4):327–34. PMID:23498719

2758. Rusiecki D, Lach B. Lhermitte-Duclos disease with neurofibrillary tangles in heterotopic cerebral grey matter. Folia Neuropathol. 2016;54(2):190–6. PMID:27543776

2759. Russell DS, Rubinstein LJ. Pathology of tumours of the nervous system. 5th ed. London (UK): Edward Arnold; 1989.

2760. Russo C, Nastro A, Cicala D, et al. Neuroimaging in tuberous sclerosis complex. Childs Nerv Syst. 2020 Oct;36(10):2497–509. PMID:32519125

2761. Russo C, Pellarin M, Tingby O, et al. Comparative genomic hybridization in patients with supratentorial and infratentorial primitive neuroectodermal tumors. Cancer. 1999 Jul 15;86(2):331–9. PMID:10421270

2762. Rutenberg MS, Rotondo RL, Rao D, et al. Clinical outcomes following proton therapy for adult craniopharyngioma: a single-institution cohort study. J Neurooncol. 2020 Apr;147(2):387–95. PMID:32086697

2763. Rutkowski S, Bode U, Deinlein F, et al. Treatment of early childhood medulloblastoma by postoperative chemotherapy alone. N Engl J Med. 2005 Mar 10;352(10):978–86. PMID:15758008

2764. Rutkowski S, von Hoff K, Emser A, et al. Survival and prognostic factors of early childhood medulloblastoma: an international meta-analysis. J Clin Oncol. 2010 Nov 20;28(33):4961–8. PMID:20940197

2765. Ryall S, Guzman M, Elbabaa SK, et al. H3 K27M mutations are extremely rare in posterior fossa group A ependymoma. Childs Nerv Syst. 2017 Jul;33(7):1047–51. PMID:28623522

2766. Ryall S, Krishnatry R, Arnoldo A, et al. Targeted detection of genetic alterations reveal the prognostic impact of H3K27M and MAPK pathway aberrations in paediatric thalamic glioma. Acta Neuropathol Commun. 2016 Aug 31;4(1):93. PMID:27577993

2767. Ryall S, Tabori U, Hawkins C. Pediatric low-grade glioma in the era of molecular diagnostics. Acta Neuropathol Commun. 2020 Mar 12;8(1):30. PMID:32164789

2768. Ryall S, Zapotocky M, Fukuoka K, et al. Integrated molecular and clinical analysis of 1,000 pediatric low-grade gliomas. Cancer Cell. 2020 Apr 13;37(4):569–583.e5. PMID:32289278

2769. Sabbaghian N, Hamel N, Srivastava A, et al. Germline DICER1 mutation and associated loss of heterozygosity in a pineoblastoma. J Med Genet. 2012 Jul;49(7):417–9. PMID:22717647

2770. Sachdeva MU, Vankalakunti M, Rangan A, et al. The role of immunohistochemistry in medullomyoblastoma–a case series highlighting divergent differentiation. Diagn Pathol. 2008 Apr 25;3:18. PMID:18439235

2771. Sadashiva N, Sharma A, Shukla D, et al. Intracranial extraskeletal mesenchymal chondrosarcoma. World Neurosurg. 2016 Nov;95:618.e1–6. PMID:27565470

2772. Sadashivam S, Menon G, Abraham M, et al. Adult craniopharyngioma: the role of extent of resection in tumor recurrence and long-term functional outcome. Clin Neurol Neurosurg. 2020 May;192:105711. PMID:32036264

2773. Saeed Kamil Z, Sinson G, Gucer H, et al. TTF-1 expressing sellar neoplasm with ependymal rosettes and oncocytic change: mixed ependymal and oncocytic variant pituicytoma. Endocr Pathol. 2014 Dec;25(4):436–8. PMID:24242699

2774. Saeger W, Ebrahimi A, Beschorner R, et al. Teratoma of the sellar region: a case report. Endocr Pathol. 2017 Dec;28(4):315–9. PMID:28102527

2775. Saeger W, Lüdecke DK, Buchfelder M, et al. Pathohistological classification of pituitary tumors: 10 years of experience with the German Pituitary Tumor Registry. Eur J Endocrinol. 2007 Feb;156(2):203–16. PMID:17287410

2776. Sahakitrungruang T, Srichomthong C, Pornkunwilai S, et al. Germline and somatic DICER1 mutations in a pituitary blastoma causing infantile-onset Cushing's disease. J Clin Endocrinol Metab. 2014 Aug;99(8):E1487–92. PMID:24823459

2777. Sahm F, Bissel J, Koelsche C, et al. AKT1E17K mutations cluster with meningothelial and transitional meningiomas and can be detected by SFRP1 immunohistochemistry. Acta Neuropathol. 2013 Nov;126(5):757–62. PMID:24096618

2778. Sahm F, Capper D, Preusser M, et al. BRAFV600E mutant protein is expressed in cells of variable maturation in Langerhans cell histiocytosis. Blood. 2012 Sep 20;120(12):e28–34. PMID:22859608

2779. Sahm F, Koelsche C, Meyer J, et al. CIC and FUBP1 mutations in oligodendrogliomas, oligoastrocytomas and astrocytomas. Acta Neuropathol. 2012 Jun;123(6):853–60. PMID:22588899

2780. Sahm F, Korshunov A, Schrimpf D, et al. Gain of 12p encompassing CCND2 is associated with gemistocytic histology in IDH mutant astrocytomas. Acta Neuropathol. 2017 Feb;133(2):325–7. PMID:28000032

2781. Sahm F, Reuss D, Koelsche C, et al. Farewell to oligoastrocytoma: in situ molecular genetics favor classification as either oligodendroglioma or astrocytoma. Acta Neuropathol. 2014 Oct;128(4):551–9. PMID:25143301

2782. Sahm F, Schrimpf D, Olar A, et al. TERT promoter mutations and risk of recurrence in meningioma. J Natl Cancer Inst. 2015 Dec 13;108(5):djv377. PMID:26668184

2783. Sahm F, Schrimpf D, Stichel D, et al. DNA methylation-based classification and grading system for meningioma: a multicentre, retrospective analysis. Lancet Oncol. 2017 May;18(5):682–94. PMID:28314689

2784. Sainz J, Figueroa K, Baser ME, et al. High frequency of nonsense mutations in the NF2 gene caused by C to T transitions in five CGA codons. Hum Mol Genet. 1995 Jan;4(1):137–9. PMID:7711726

2785. Saito T, Sugiyama K, Yamasaki F, et al. Familial occurrence of dysembryoplastic neuroepithelial tumor-like neoplasm of the septum pellucidum: case report. Neurosurgery. 2008 Aug;63(2):E370–2. PMID:18797318

2786. Saitou M, Yamaji M. Primordial germ cells in mice. Cold Spring Harb Perspect Biol. 2012 Nov 1;4(11):a008375. PMID:23125014

2787. Sajjad EA, Sikora K, Paciejewski T, et al. Intraparenchymal mesenchymal chondrosarcoma of the frontal lobe–a case report and molecular detection of specific gene fusions from archival FFPE sample. Clin Neuropathol. 2015 Sep-Oct;34(5):288–93. PMID:25907264

2788. Sakaguchi M, Nakano Y, Honda-Kitahara M, et al. Two cases of primary supratentorial intracranial rhabdomyosarcoma with DICER1 mutation which may belong to a "spindle cell sarcoma with rhabdomyosarcoma-like feature, DICER1 mutant". Brain Tumor Pathol. 2019 Oct;36(4):174–82. PMID:31487013

2789. Sakuta R, Otsubo H, Nolan MA, et al. Recurrent intractable seizures in children with cortical dysplasia adjacent to dysembryoplastic neuroepithelial tumor. J Child Neurol. 2005 Apr;20(4):377–84. PMID:15921242

2790. Salgado CM, Basu D, Nikiforova M, et al. Amplification of mutated NRAS leading to congenital melanoma in neurocutaneous melanocytosis. Melanoma Res. 2015 Oct;25(5):453–60. PMID:26266759

2791. Salgado CM, Basu D, Nikiforova M, et al. BRAF mutations are also associated with neurocutaneous melanocytosis and large/giant congenital melanocytic nevi. Pediatr Dev Pathol. 2015 Jan-Feb;18(1):1–9. PMID:25490715

2792. Salge-Arrieta FJ, Carrasco-Moro R, Rodríguez-Berrocal V, et al. Clinical features, diagnosis and therapy of pituicytoma: an update. J Endocrinol Invest. 2019 Apr;42(4):371–84. PMID:30030746

2793. Salpea P, Horvath A, London E, et al. Deletions of the PRKAR1A locus at 17q24.2-q24.3 in Carney complex: genotype-phenotype correlations and implications for genetic testing. J Clin Endocrinol Metab. 2014 Jan;99(1):E183–8. PMID:24170103

2794. Salunke PS, Gupta K, Srinivasa R, et al. Functional? Paraganglioma of the cerebellum. Acta Neurochir (Wien). 2011 Jul;153(7):1527–8. PMID:21491190

2795. Salvati M, Frati A, Russo N, et al. Radiation-induced gliomas: report of 10 cases and review of the literature. Surg Neurol. 2003 Jul;60(1):60–7. PMID:12865017

2796. Sampson JR, Scahill SJ, Stephenson JD, et al. Genetic aspects of tuberous sclerosis in the west of Scotland. J Med Genet. 1989 Jan;26(1):28–31. PMID:2918523

2797. Samstein RM, Lee CH, Shoushtari AN, et al. Tumor mutational load predicts survival after immunotherapy across multiple cancer types. Nat Genet. 2019 Feb;51(2):202–6. PMID:30643254

2798. Sancak O, Nellist M, Goedbloed M, et al. Mutational analysis of the TSC1 and TSC2 genes in a diagnostic setting: genotype–phenotype correlations and comparison of diagnostic DNA techniques in Tuberous Sclerosis Complex. Eur J Hum Genet. 2005 Jun;13(6):731–41. PMID:15798777

2799. Sandoval-Sus JD, Sandoval-Leon AC, Chapman JR, et al. Rosai-Dorfman disease of the central nervous system: report of 6 cases and review of the literature. Medicine (Baltimore). 2014 May;93(3):165–75. PMID:24797172

2800. Sangoi AR, Dulai MS, Beck AH, et al. Distinguishing chordoid meningiomas from their histologic mimics: an immunohistochemical evaluation. Am J Surg Pathol. 2009 May;33(5):669–81. PMID:19194275

2801. Sankhla S, Khan GM. Cauda equina paraganglioma presenting with intracranial hypertension: case report and review of the literature. Neurol India. 2004 Jun;52(2):243–4. PMID:15269482

2802. Sano T, Kovacs K, Asa SL, et al. Immunoreactive luteinizing hormone in functioning corticotroph adenomas of the pituitary. Immunohistochemical and tissue culture studies of two cases. Virchows Arch A Pathol Anat Histopathol. 1990;417(4):361–7. PMID:2173251

2803. Sano T, Ohshima T, Yamada S. Expression of glycoprotein hormones and intracytoplasmic distribution of cytokeratin in growth hormone-producing pituitary adenomas. Pathol Res Pract. 1991 Jun;187(5):530–3. PMID:1717959

2804. Santagata S, Hornick JL, Ligon KL. Comparative analysis of germ cell transcription factors in CNS germinoma reveals diagnostic utility of NANOG. Am J Surg Pathol. 2006 Dec;30(12):1613–8. PMID:17122519

2805. Santagata S, Ligon KL, Hornick JL. Embryonic stem cell transcription factor signatures in the diagnosis of primary and metastatic germ cell tumors. Am J Surg Pathol. 2007 Jun;31(6):836–45. PMID:17527070

2806. Santagata S, Maire CL, Idbaih A, et al. CRX is a diagnostic marker of retinal and pineal lineage tumors. PLoS One. 2009 Nov 20;4(11):e7932. PMID:19936203

2807. Santiago T, Clay MR, Allen SJ, et al. Recurrent BCOR internal tandem duplication and BCOR or BCL6 expression distinguish primitive myxoid mesenchymal tumor of infancy from congenital infantile fibrosarcoma. Mod Pathol. 2017 Jun;30(6):884–91. PMID:28256570

2808. Santosh V, Sravya P, Gupta T, et al. ISNO consensus guidelines for practical adaptation of the WHO 2016 classification of adult diffuse gliomas. Neurol India. 2019 Jan-Feb;67(1):173–82. PMID:30860119

2809. Sargen MR, Merrill SL, Chu EY, et al. CDKN2A mutations with p14 loss predisposing to multiple nerve sheath tumours, melanoma, dysplastic naevi and internal malignancies: a case series and review of the literature. Br J Dermatol. 2016 Oct;175(4):785–9. PMID:26876133

2810. Sari N, Akyuz C, Aktas D, et al. Wilms tumor, AML and medulloblastoma in a child with cancer prone syndrome of total premature chromatid separation and Fanconi anemia. Pediatr Blood Cancer. 2009 Aug;53(2):208–10. PMID:19373780
2811. Sarkar H, K S, Ghosh S. Pure intraventricular origin of gliosarcoma - a rare entity. Turk Neurosurg. 2013;23(3):392–4. PMID:23756982
2812. Sartoretti-Schefer S, Wichmann W, Aguzzi A, et al. MR differentiation of adamantinous and squamous-papillary craniopharyngiomas. AJNR Am J Neuroradiol. 1997 Jan;18(1):77–87. PMID:9010523
2813. Sasayama T, Tanaka K, Mizowaki T, et al. Tumor-associated macrophages associate with cerebrospinal fluid interleukin-10 and survival in primary central nervous system lymphoma (PCNSL). Brain Pathol. 2016 Jul;26(4):479–87. PMID:26314692
2814. Sastre X, Chantada GL, Doz F, et al. Proceedings of the consensus meetings from the International Retinoblastoma Staging Working Group on the pathology guidelines for the examination of enucleated eyes and evaluation of prognostic risk factors in retinoblastoma. Arch Pathol Lab Med. 2009 Aug;133(8):1199–202. PMID:19653709
2815. Sato K, Oka H, Utsuki S, et al. Ciliated craniopharyngioma may arise from Rathke cleft cyst. Clin Neuropathol. 2006 Jan-Feb;25(1):25–8. PMID:16465771
2816. Sato TS, Kirby PA, Buatti JM, et al. Papillary tumor of the pineal region: report of a rapidly progressive tumor with possible multicentric origin. Pediatr Radiol. 2009 Feb;39(2):188–90. PMID:19037636
2817. Sawamura Y, Ikeda J, Shirato H, et al. Germ cell tumours of the central nervous system: treatment consideration based on 111 cases and their long-term clinical outcomes. Eur J Cancer. 1998 Jan;34(1):104–10. PMID:9624246
2818. Sayegh ET, Aranda D, Kim JM, et al. Prognosis by tumor location in adults with intracranial ependymomas. J Clin Neurosci. 2014 Dec;21(12):2096–101. PMID:25037313
2819. Sbiera S, Perez-Rivas LG, Taranets L, et al. Driver mutations in USP8 wild-type Cushing's disease. Neuro Oncol. 2019 Oct 9;21(10):1273–83. PMID:31222332
2820. Schaefer IM, Dong F, Garcia EP, et al. Recurrent SMARCB1 inactivation in epithelioid malignant peripheral nerve sheath tumors. Am J Surg Pathol. 2019 Jun;43(6):835–43. PMID:30864974
2821. Schaefer IM, Fletcher CD. Malignant peripheral nerve sheath tumor (MPNST) arising in diffuse-type neurofibroma: clinicopathologic characterization in a series of 9 cases. Am J Surg Pathol. 2015 Sep;39(9):1234–41. PMID:25929351
2822. Schaefer IM, Fletcher CD, Hornick JL. Loss of H3K27 trimethylation distinguishes malignant peripheral nerve sheath tumors from histologic mimics. Mod Pathol. 2016 Jan;29(1):4–13. PMID:26585554
2823. Schaefer IM, Ströbel P, Thiha A, et al. Soft tissue perineurioma and other unusual tumors in a patient with neurofibromatosis type 1. Int J Clin Exp Pathol. 2013 Nov 15;6(12):3003–8. PMID:24294391
2824. Schäfer S, Behling F, Skardelly M, et al. Low FoxG1 and high Olig-2 labelling indices define a prognostically favourable subset in isocitrate dehydrogenase (IDH)-mutant gliomas. Neuropathol Appl Neurobiol. 2018 Feb;44(2):207–23. PMID:29053887
2825. Scheil S, Brüderlein S, Eicker M, et al. Low frequency of chromosomal imbalances in anaplastic ependymomas as detected by comparative genomic hybridization. Brain Pathol. 2001 Apr;11(2):133–43. PMID:11303789
2826. Scheithauer BW. Pathobiology of the pineal gland with emphasis on parenchymal tumors. Brain Tumor Pathol. 1999;16(1):1–9. PMID:10532417
2827. Scheithauer BW. Symptomatic subependymoma. Report of 21 cases with review of the literature. J Neurosurg. 1978 Nov;49(5):689–96. PMID:712391
2828. Scheithauer BW, Horvath E, Abel TW, et al. Pituitary blastoma: a unique embryonal tumor. Pituitary. 2012 Sep;15(3):365–73. PMID:21805093
2829. Scheithauer BW, Kovacs K, Horvath E, et al. Pituitary blastoma. Acta Neuropathol. 2008 Dec;116(6):657–66. PMID:18551299
2830. Schernthaner-Reiter MH, Trivellin G, Stratakis CA. MEN1, MEN4, and Carney complex: pathology and molecular genetics. Neuroendocrinology. 2016;103(1):18–31. PMID:25592387
2831. Scheurer ME, Bondy ML, Aldape KD, et al. Detection of human cytomegalovirus in different histological types of gliomas. Acta Neuropathol. 2008 Jul;116(1):79–86. PMID:18351367
2832. Scheurlen WG, Schwabe GC, Joos S, et al. Molecular analysis of childhood primitive neuroectodermal tumors defines markers associated with poor outcome. J Clin Oncol. 1998 Jul;16(7):2478–85. PMID:9667267
2833. Schiariti M, Goetz P, El-Maghraby H, et al. Hemangiopericytoma: long-term outcome revisited. Clinical article. J Neurosurg. 2011 Mar;114(3):747–55. PMID:20672899
2834. Schiefer AI, Vastagh I, Molnar MJ, et al. Extranodal marginal zone lymphoma of the CNS arising after a long-standing history of atypical white matter disease. Leuk Res. 2012 Jul;36(7):e155–7. PMID:22520340
2835. Schiff D, O'Neill B, Wijdicks E, et al. Gliomas arising in organ transplant recipients: an unrecognized complication of transplantation? Neurology. 2001 Oct 23;57(8):1486–8. PMID:11673595
2836. Schiffer D, Cavalla P, Migheli A, et al. Apoptosis and cell proliferation in human neuroepithelial tumors. Neurosci Lett. 1995 Aug 4;195(2):81–4. PMID:7478273
2837. Schiffer D, Chiò A, Giordana MT, et al. Histologic prognostic factors in ependymoma. Childs Nerv Syst. 1991 Aug;7(4):177–82. PMID:1933913
2838. Schild SE, Scheithauer BW, Haddock MG, et al. Histologically confirmed pineal tumors and other germ cell tumors of the brain. Cancer. 1996 Dec 15;78(12):2564–71. PMID:8952565
2839. Schild SE, Scheithauer BW, Schomberg PJ, et al. Pineal parenchymal tumors. Clinical, pathologic, and therapeutic aspects. Cancer. 1993 Aug 1;72(3):870–80. PMID:8334641
2840. Schindeler A, Little DG. Recent insights into bone development, homeostasis, and repair in type 1 neurofibromatosis (NF1). Bone. 2008 Apr;42(4):616–22. PMID:18248783
2841. Schindler G, Capper D, Korshunov A, et al. Spinal metastasis of gliosarcoma: array-based comparative genomic hybridization for confirmation of metastatic spread. J Clin Neurosci. 2014 Nov;21(11):1945–50. PMID:25065849
2842. Schindler G, Capper D, Meyer J, et al. Analysis of BRAF V600E mutation in 1,320 nervous system tumors reveals high mutation frequencies in pleomorphic xanthoastrocytoma, ganglioglioma and extra-cerebellar pilocytic astrocytoma. Acta Neuropathol. 2011 Mar;121(3):397–405. PMID:21274720
2843. Schittenhelm J, Psaras T. Glioblastoma with granular cell astrocytoma features: a case report and literature review. Clin Neuropathol. 2010 Sep-Oct;29(5):323–9. PMID:20860896
2844. Schittenhelm J, Roser F, Tatagiba M, et al. Diagnostic value of EAAT-1 and Kir7.1 for distinguishing endolymphatic sac tumors from choroid plexus tumors. Am J Clin Pathol. 2012 Jul;138(1):85–9. PMID:22706862
2845. Schlaffer SM, Buchfelder M, Stoehr R, et al. Rathke's cleft cyst as origin of a pediatric papillary craniopharyngioma. Front Genet. 2018 Feb 22;9:49. PMID:29520296
2846. Schlamann A, von Bueren AO, Hagel C, et al. An individual patient data meta-analysis on characteristics and outcome of patients with papillary glioneuronal tumor, rosette glioneuronal tumor with neuropil-like islands and rosette forming glioneuronal tumor of the fourth ventricle. PLoS One. 2014 Jul 3;9(7):e101211. PMID:24991807
2847. Schlegel U. Primary CNS lymphoma. Ther Adv Neurol Disord. 2009 Mar;2(2):93–104. PMID:21180644
2848. Schmalisch K, Beschorner R, Psaras T, et al. Postoperative intracranial seeding of craniopharyngiomas–report of three cases and review of the literature. Acta Neurochir (Wien). 2010 Feb;152(2):313–9. PMID:19859655
2849. Schmidbauer M, Budka H, Pilz P. Neuroepithelial and ectomesenchymal differentiation in a primitive pineal tumor ("pineal anlage tumor"). Clin Neuropathol. 1989 Jan-Feb;8(1):7–10. PMID:2650944
2850. Schmidt MC, Antweiler S, Urban N, et al. Impact of genotype and morphology on the prognosis of glioblastoma. J Neuropathol Exp Neurol. 2002 Apr;61(4):321–8. PMID:11939587
2851. Schneider DT, Zahn S, Sievers S, et al. Molecular genetic analysis of central nervous system germ cell tumors with comparative genomic hybridization. Mod Pathol. 2006 Jun;19(6):864–73. PMID:16607373
2852. Schneider N, Hallin M, Thway K. STAT6 loss in dedifferentiated solitary fibrous tumor. Int J Surg Pathol. 2017 Feb;25(1):58–60. PMID:27189111
2853. Schneppenheim R, Frühwald MC, Gesk S, et al. Germline nonsense mutation and somatic inactivation of SMARCA4/BRG1 in a family with rhabdoid tumor predisposition syndrome. Am J Hum Genet. 2010 Feb 12;86(2):279–84. PMID:20137775
2854. Schniederjan MJ, Alghamdi S, Castellano-Sanchez A, et al. Diffuse leptomeningeal neuroepithelial tumor: 9 pediatric cases with chromosome 1p/19q deletion status and IDH1 (R132H) immunohistochemistry. Am J Surg Pathol. 2013 May;37(5):763–71. PMID:23588371
2855. Schofield D, West DC, Anthony DC, et al. Correlation of loss of heterozygosity at chromosome 9q with histological subtype in medulloblastomas. Am J Pathol. 1995 Feb;146(2):472–80. PMID:7856756
2856. Schrager CA, Schneider D, Gruener AC, et al. Clinical and pathological features of breast disease in Cowden's syndrome: an underrecognized syndrome with an increased risk of breast cancer. Hum Pathol. 1998 Jan;29(1):47–53. PMID:9445133
2857. Schramm J, Luyken C, Urbach H, et al. Evidence for a clinically distinct new subtype of grade II astrocytomas in patients with long-term epilepsy. Neurosurgery. 2004 Aug;55(2):340–7. PMID:15271240
2858. Schroers R, Baraniskin A, Heute C, et al. Diagnosis of leptomeningeal disease in diffuse large B-cell lymphomas of the central nervous system by flow cytometry and cytopathology. Eur J Haematol. 2010 Dec;85(6):520–8. PMID:20727005
2859. Schuettpelz LG, McDonald S, Whitesell K, et al. Pilocytic astrocytoma in a child with Noonan syndrome. Pediatr Blood Cancer. 2009 Dec;53(6):1147–9. PMID:19621452
2860. Schüller U, Heine VM, Mao J, et al. Acquisition of granule neuron precursor identity is a critical determinant of progenitor cell competence to form Shh-induced medulloblastoma. Cancer Cell. 2008 Aug 12;14(2):123–34. PMID:18691547
2861. Schulte SL, Waha A, Steiger B, et al. CNS germinomas are characterized by global demethylation, chromosomal instability and mutational activation of the Kit-, Ras/Raf/Erk- and Akt-pathways. Oncotarget. 2016 Aug 23;7(34):55026–42. PMID:27391150
2862. Schultz KAP, Williams GM, Kamihara J, et al. DICER1 and associated conditions: identification of at-risk individuals and recommended surveillance strategies. Clin Cancer Res. 2018 May 15;24(10):2251–61. PMID:29343557
2863. Schuss P, Ulrich CT, Harter PN, et al. Gliosarcoma with bone infiltration and extracranial growth: case report and review of literature. J Neurooncol. 2011 Jul;103(3):765–70. PMID:20957407
2864. Schwalbe EC, Hicks D, Rafiee G, et al. Minimal methylation classifier (MIMIC): a novel method for derivation and rapid diagnostic detection of disease-associated DNA methylation signatures. Sci Rep. 2017 Oct 18;7(1):13421. PMID:29044166
2865. Schwalbe EC, Lindsey JC, Nakjang S, et al. Novel molecular subgroups for clinical classification and outcome prediction in childhood medulloblastoma: a cohort study. Lancet Oncol. 2017 Jul;18(7):958–71. PMID:28545823
2866. Schwalbe EC, Williamson D, Lindsey JC, et al. DNA methylation profiling of medulloblastoma allows robust subclassification and improved outcome prediction using formalin-fixed biopsies. Acta Neuropathol. 2013 Mar;125(3):359–71. PMID:23291781
2867. Schwartzentruber J, Korshunov A, Liu XY, et al. Driver mutations in histone H3.3 and chromatin remodelling genes in paediatric glioblastoma. Nature. 2012 Jan 29;482(7384):226–31. PMID:22286061
2868. Schwechheimer K, Huang S, Cavenee WK. EGFR gene amplification–rearrangement in human glioblastomas. Int J Cancer. 1995 Jul 17;62(2):145–8. PMID:7622287
2869. Schweizer L, Capper D, Hölsken A, et al. BRAF V600E analysis for the differentiation of papillary craniopharyngiomas and Rathke's cleft cysts. Neuropathol Appl Neurobiol. 2015 Oct;41(6):733–42. PMID:25442675
2870. Schweizer L, Koelsche C, Sahm F, et al. Meningeal hemangiopericytoma and solitary fibrous tumors carry the NAB2-STAT6 fusion and can be diagnosed by nuclear expression of STAT6 protein. Acta Neuropathol. 2013 May;125(5):651–8. PMID:23575898
2871. Schweizer L, Thierfelder F, Thomas C, et al. Molecular characterization of CNS paragangliomas identifies cauda equina paragangliomas as a distinct tumor entity. Acta Neuropathol. 2020 Dec;140(6):893–906. PMID:32926213
2872. Schwindt H, Vater I, Kreuz M, et al. Chromosomal imbalances and partial uniparental disomies in primary central nervous system lymphoma. Leukemia. 2009 Oct;23(10):1875–84. PMID:19494841
2873. Sciot R, Jacobs S, Calenbergh FV, et al. Primary myxoid mesenchymal tumour with intracranial location: report of a case with a EWSR1-ATF1 fusion. Histopathology. 2018 Apr;72(5):880–3. PMID:29143432
2874. Scope A, Friedman E, Azizi E. A familial syndromic association between cutaneous malignant melanoma and neural system tumours. Br J Dermatol. 2004 Dec;151(6):1278–9. PMID:15606533
2875. Scoppetta TL, Brito MC, Prado JL, et al. Multifocal cerebellar liponeurocytoma.

Neurology. 2015 Nov 24;85(21):1912. PMID:26598433
2876. Sebro R, DeLaney T, Hornicek F, et al. Differences in sex distribution, anatomic location and MR imaging appearance of pediatric compared to adult chordomas. BMC Med Imaging. 2016 Sep 8;16(1):53. PMID:27609115
2877. Sekine S, Shibata T, Kokubu A, et al. Craniopharyngiomas of adamantinomatous type harbor beta-catenin gene mutations. Am J Pathol. 2002 Dec;161(6):1997–2001. PMID:12466115
2878. Selvadurai K, Wang P, Seimetz J, et al. Archaeal Elp3 catalyzes tRNA wobble uridine modification at C5 via a radical mechanism. Nat Chem Biol. 2014 Oct;10(10):810–2. PMID:25151136
2879. Semenza GL. The genomics and genetics of oxygen homeostasis. Annu Rev Genomics Hum Genet. 2020 Aug 31;21:183–204. PMID:32255719
2880. Seol HJ, Hwang SK, Choi YL, et al. A case of recurrent subependymoma with subependymal seeding: case report. J Neurooncol. 2003 May;62(3):315–20. PMID:12777084
2881. Seppälä MT, Sainio MA, Haltia MJ, et al. Multiple schwannomas: schwannomatosis or neurofibromatosis type 2? J Neurosurg. 1998 Jul;89(1):36–41. PMID:9647170
2882. Serracino HS, Kleinschmidt-Demasters BK. Skull invaders: when surgical pathology and neuropathology worlds collide. J Neuropathol Exp Neurol. 2013 Jul;72(7):600–13. PMID:23771219
2883. Sestini R, Bacci C, Provenzano A, et al. Evidence of a four-hit mechanism involving SMARCB1 and NF2 in schwannomatosis-associated schwannomas. Hum Mutat. 2008 Feb;29(2):227–31. PMID:18072270
2884. Seth R, Messersmith H, Kaur V, et al. Systemic therapy for melanoma: ASCO guideline. J Clin Oncol. 2020 Nov 20;38(33):3947–70. PMID:32228358
2885. Sévenet N, Sheridan E, Amram D, et al. Constitutional mutations of the hSNF5/INI1 gene predispose to a variety of cancers. Am J Hum Genet. 1999 Nov;65(5):1342–8. PMID:10521299
2886. Shah AH, Khatib Z, Niazi T. Extracranial extra-CNS spread of embryonal tumor with multilayered rosettes (ETMR): case series and systematic review. Childs Nerv Syst. 2018 Apr;34(4):649–54. PMID:29177676
2887. Shakur SF, McGirt MJ, Johnson MW, et al. Angiocentric glioma: a case series. J Neurosurg Pediatr. 2009 Mar;3(3):197–202. PMID:19338465
2888. Shankar GM, Abedalthagafi M, Vaubel RA, et al. Germline and somatic BAP1 mutations in high-grade rhabdoid meningiomas. Neuro Oncol. 2017 Apr 1;19(4):535–45. PMID:28170043
2889. Shankar GM, Chen L, Kim AH, et al. Composite ganglioneuroma-paraganglioma of the filum terminale. J Neurosurg Spine. 2010 Jun;12(6):709–13. PMID:20515359
2890. Shankar GM, Santagata S. BAP1 mutations in high-grade meningioma: implications for patient care. Neuro Oncol. 2017 Oct 19;19(11):1447–56. PMID:28482042
2890A. Shankar GM, Taylor-Weiner A, Lelic N, et al. Sporadic hemangioblastomas are characterized by cryptic VHL inactivation. Acta Neuropathol Commun. 2014 Dec 24;2:167. PMID:25589003
2891. Shanley S, Ratcliffe J, Hockey A, et al. Nevoid basal cell carcinoma syndrome: review of 118 affected individuals. Am J Med Genet. 1994 Apr 15;50(3):282–90. PMID:8042673
2892. Shanmugam V, Griffin GK, Jacobsen ED, et al. Identification of diverse activating mutations of the RAS-MAPK pathway in histiocytic sarcoma. Mod Pathol. 2019 Jun;32(6):830–43. PMID:30626916
2893. Shapiro S, Mealey J Jr. Late anaplastic gliomas in children previously treated for acute lymphoblastic leukemia. Pediatr Neurosci. 1989;15(4):176–80. PMID:2485912
2894. Sharaf AF, Hamouda FS, Teo JG. Bilateral thalamic and right fronto-temporo-parietal gliomas in a 4 years old child diagnosed by magnetic resonance imaging. J Radiol Case Rep. 2016 Jan 31;10(1):1–13. PMID:27200150
2895. Sharma M, Ralte A, Arora R, et al. Subependymal giant cell astrocytoma: a clinicopathological study of 23 cases with special emphasis on proliferative markers and expression of p53 and retinoblastoma gene proteins. Pathology. 2004 Apr;36(2):139–44. PMID:15203749
2896. Sharma MC, Ralte AM, Gaekwad S, et al. Subependymal giant cell astrocytoma–a clinicopathological study of 23 cases with special emphasis on histogenesis. Pathol Oncol Res. 2004;10(4):219–24. PMID:15619643
2897. Sharma MK, Mansur DB, Reifenberger G, et al. Distinct genetic signatures among pilocytic astrocytomas relate to their brain region origin. Cancer Res. 2007 Feb 1;67(3):890–900. PMID:17283119
2898. Sharma MK, Zehnbauer BA, Watson MA, et al. RAS pathway activation and an oncogenic RAS mutation in sporadic pilocytic astrocytoma. Neurology. 2005 Oct 25;65(8):1335–6. PMID:16247081
2899. Sharma S, Deb P. Intraoperative neurocytology of primary central nervous system neoplasia: a simplified and practical diagnostic approach. J Cytol. 2011 Oct;28(4):147–58. PMID:22090687
2900. Sharma T, Schwalbe EC, Williamson D, et al. Second-generation molecular subgrouping of medulloblastoma: an international meta-analysis of Group 3 and Group 4 subtypes. Acta Neuropathol. 2019 Aug;138(2):309–26. PMID:31076851
2901. Shen WH, Balajee AS, Wang J, et al. Essential role for nuclear PTEN in maintaining chromosomal integrity. Cell. 2007 Jan 12;128(1):157–70. PMID:17218262
2902. Shenkier TN, Blay JY, O'Neill BP, et al. Primary CNS lymphoma of T-cell origin: a descriptive analysis from the international primary CNS lymphoma collaborative group. J Clin Oncol. 2005 Apr 1;23(10):2233–9. PMID:15800313
2903. Shepherd CW, Gomez MR, Lie JT, et al. Causes of death in patients with tuberous sclerosis. Mayo Clin Proc. 1991 Aug;66(8):792–6. PMID:1861550
2904. Shepherd CW, Houser OW, Gomez MR. MR findings in tuberous sclerosis complex and correlation with seizure development and mental impairment. AJNR Am J Neuroradiol. 1995 Jan;16(1):149–55. PMID:7900584
2905. Shern JF, Chen L, Chmielecki J, et al. Comprehensive genomic analysis of rhabdomyosarcoma reveals a landscape of alterations affecting a common genetic axis in fusion-positive and fusion-negative tumors. Cancer Discov. 2014 Feb;4(2):216–31. PMID:24436047
2906. Shern JF, Yohe ME, Khan J. Pediatric rhabdomyosarcoma. Crit Rev Oncog. 2015;20(3-4):227–43. PMID:26349418
2907. Shete S, Hosking FJ, Robertson LB, et al. Genome-wide association study identifies five susceptibility loci for glioma. Nat Genet. 2009 Aug;41(8):899–904. PMID:19578367
2908. Shi ZF, Li KK, Kwan JSH, et al. Whole-exome sequencing revealed mutational profiles of giant cell glioblastomas. Brain Pathol. 2019 Nov;29(6):782–92. PMID:30861589
2909. Shibahara J, Todo T, Morita A, et al. Papillary neuroepithelial tumor of the pineal region. A case report. Acta Neuropathol. 2004 Oct;108(4):337–40. PMID:15221340
2910. Shibamoto Y, Takahashi M, Sasai K. Prognosis of intracranial germinoma with syncytiotrophoblastic giant cells treated by radiation therapy. Int J Radiat Oncol Biol Phys. 1997 Feb 1;37(3):505–10. PMID:9112445
2911. Shibuya M. Welcoming the new WHO classification of pituitary tumors 2017: revolution in TTF-1-positive posterior pituitary tumors. Brain Tumor Pathol. 2018 Apr;35(2):62–70. PMID:29500747
2912. Shih AR, Cote GM, Chebib I, et al. Clinicopathologic characteristics of poorly differentiated chordoma. Mod Pathol. 2018 Aug;31(8):1237–45. PMID:29483606
2913. Shih DJ, Northcott PA, Remke M, et al. Cytogenetic prognostication within medulloblastoma subgroups. J Clin Oncol. 2014 Mar 20;32(9):886–96. PMID:24493713
2914. Shin SA, Ahn B, Kim SK, et al. Brainstem astroblastoma with MN1 translocation. Neuropathology. 2018 Dec;38(6):631–7. PMID:30238518
2915. Shinojima N, Kochi M, Hamada J, et al. The influence of sex and the presence of giant cells on postoperative long-term survival in adult patients with supratentorial glioblastoma multiforme. J Neurosurg. 2004 Aug;101(2):219–26. PMID:15309911
2916. Shirahata M, Ono T, Stichel D, et al. Novel, improved grading system(s) for IDH-mutant astrocytic gliomas. Acta Neuropathol. 2018 Jul;136(1):153–66. PMID:29687258
2917. Shiran SI, Ben-Sira L, Elhasid R, et al. Multiple brain developmental venous anomalies as a marker for constitutional mismatch repair deficiency syndrome. AJNR Am J Neuroradiol. 2018 Oct;39(10):1943–6. PMID:30166433
2918. Shitara S, Tokime T, Akiyama Y. Multinodular and vacuolating neuronal tumor: a case report and literature review. Surg Neurol Int. 2018 Mar 19;9:63. PMID:29629230
2919. Shiurba RA, Buffinger NS, Spencer EM, et al. Basic fibroblast growth factor and somatomedin C in human medulloepithelioma. Cancer. 1991 Aug 15;68(4):798–808. PMID:1855180
2920. Shlien A, Campbell BB, de Borja R, et al. Combined hereditary and somatic mutations of replication error repair genes result in rapid onset of ultra-hypermutated cancers. Nat Genet. 2015 Mar;47(3):257–62. PMID:25642631
2921. Short MP, Richardson EP Jr, Haines JL, et al. Clinical, neuropathological and genetic aspects of the tuberous sclerosis complex. Brain Pathol. 1995 Apr;5(2):173–9. PMID:7670658
2922. Showalter TN, Andrel J, Andrews DW, et al. Multifocal glioblastoma multiforme: prognostic factors and patterns of progression. Int J Radiat Oncol Biol Phys. 2007 Nov 1;69(3):820–4. PMID:17499453
2923. Shuch B, Ricketts CJ, Metwalli AR, et al. The genetic basis of pheochromocytoma and paraganglioma: implications for management. Urology. 2014 Jun;83(6):1225–32. PMID:24642075
2924. Shupnik MA, Pitt LK, Soh AY, et al. Selective expression of estrogen receptor alpha and beta isoforms in human pituitary tumors. J Clin Endocrinol Metab. 1998 Nov;83(11):3965–72. PMID:9814476
2925. Sieg EP, Payne R, Langan S, et al. Case report: a rosette-forming glioneuronal tumor in the tectal plate in a patient with neurofibromatosis type I. Cureus. 2016 Nov 1;8(11):e857. PMID:27917325
2926. Siegfried A, Cances C, Denuelle M, et al. Noonan syndrome, PTPN11 mutations, and brain tumors. A clinical report and review of the literature. Am J Med Genet A. 2017 Apr;173(4):1061–5. PMID:28328117
2927. Siegfried A, Morin S, Munzer C, et al. A French retrospective study on clinical outcome in 102 choroid plexus tumors in children. J Neurooncol. 2017 Oct;135(1):151–60. PMID:28677107
2928. Siegfried A, Rousseau A, Maurage CA, et al. EWSR1-PATZ1 gene fusion may define a new glioneuronal tumor entity. Brain Pathol. 2019 Jan;29(1):53–62. PMID:29679497
2929. Sievers P, Appay R, Schrimpf D, et al. Rosette-forming glioneuronal tumors share a distinct DNA methylation profile and mutations in FGFR1, with recurrent co-mutation of PIK3CA and NF1. Acta Neuropathol. 2019 Sep;138(3):497–504. PMID:31250151
2930. Sievers P, Chiang J, Schrimpf D, et al. YAP1-fusions in pediatric NF2-wild-type meningioma. Acta Neuropathol. 2020 Jan;139(1):215–8. PMID:31734728
2931. Sievers P, Hielscher T, Schrimpf D, et al. CDKN2A/B homozygous deletion is associated with early recurrence in meningiomas. Acta Neuropathol. 2020 Sep;140(3):409–13. PMID:32642869
2932. Sievers P, Schrimpf D, Stichel D, et al. Posterior fossa pilocytic astrocytomas with oligodendroglial features show frequent FGFR1 activation via fusion or mutation. Acta Neuropathol. 2020 Feb;139(2):403–6. PMID:31729570
2933. Sievers P, Sill M, Schrimpf D, et al. A subset of pediatric-type thalamic gliomas share a distinct DNA methylation profile, H3K27me3 loss and frequent alteration of EGFR. Neuro Oncol. 2021 Jan 30;23(1):34–43. PMID:33130881
2934. Sievers P, Stichel D, Hielscher T, et al. Chordoid meningiomas can be sub-stratified into prognostically distinct DNA methylation classes and are enriched for heterozygous deletions of chromosomal arm 2p. Acta Neuropathol. 2018 Dec;136(6):975–8. PMID:30382370
2935. Sievers P, Stichel D, Schrimpf D, et al. FGFR1:TACC1 fusion is a frequent event in molecularly defined extraventricular neurocytoma. Acta Neuropathol. 2018 Aug;136(2):293–302. PMID:29978331
2936. Sievert AJ, Jackson EM, Gai X, et al. Duplication of 7q34 in pediatric low-grade astrocytomas detected by high-density single-nucleotide polymorphism-based genotype arrays results in a novel BRAF fusion gene. Brain Pathol. 2009 Jul;19(3):449–58. PMID:19016743
2937. Silveira AB, Kasper LH, Fan Y, et al. H3.3 K27M depletion increases differentiation and extends latency of diffuse intrinsic pontine glioma growth in vivo. Acta Neuropathol. 2019 Apr;137(4):637–55. PMID:30770999
2938. Simanshu DK, Nissley DV, McCormick F. RAS Proteins and Their Regulators in Human Disease. Cell. 2017 Jun 29;170(1):17–33. PMID:28666118
2939. Simon M, Park TW, Köster G, et al. Alterations of INK4a(p16-p14ARF)/INK4b(p15) expression and telomerase activation in meningioma progression. J Neurooncol. 2001 Dec;55(3):149–58. PMID:11859969
2940. Simón-Carrasco L, Graña O, Salmón M, et al. Inactivation of Capicua in adult mice causes T-cell lymphoblastic lymphoma. Genes Dev. 2017 Jul 15;31(14):1456–68. PMID:28827401
2941. Simpson LN, Hughes BD, Karikari IO, et al. Catecholamine-secreting paraganglioma of the thoracic spinal column: report of an unusual case and review of the literature. Neurosurgery. 2012 Apr;70(4):E1049–52. PMID:21788916
2942. Singh D, Chan JM, Zoppoli P, et al. Transforming fusions of FGFR and TACC genes in human glioblastoma. Science. 2012

Sep 7;337(6099):1231–5. PMID:22837387
2943. Singh SK, Hawkins C, Clarke ID, et al. Identification of human brain tumour initiating cells. Nature. 2004 Nov 18;432(7015):396–401. PMID:15549107
2944. Singh U, Kalavakonda C, Venkitachalam S, et al. Intraosseous hemangioma of sella: case report and review of literature. World Neurosurg X. 2019 Mar 9;3:100030. PMID:31225522
2945. Singh VK, Singh S, Bhupalam L. Anaplastic oligodendroglioma metastasizing to the bone marrow: a unique case report and literature review. Int J Neurosci. 2019 Jul;129(7):722–8. PMID:30526175
2946. Sinicrope FA, Sargent DJ. Molecular pathways: microsatellite instability in colorectal cancer: prognostic, predictive, and therapeutic implications. Clin Cancer Res. 2012 Mar 15;18(6):1506–12. PMID:22302899
2947. Sivaraju L, Aryan S, Ghosal N, et al. Cerebellar liponeurocytoma presenting as multifocal bilateral cerebellar hemispheric mass lesions. Neurol India. 2017 Mar-Apr;65(2):422–4. PMID:28290424
2948. Sjöblom T, Jones S, Wood LD, et al. The consensus coding sequences of human breast and colorectal cancers. Science. 2006 Oct 13;314(5797):268–74. PMID:16959974
2949. Skapek SX, Ferrari A, Gupta AA, et al. Rhabdomyosarcoma. Nat Rev Dis Primers. 2019 Jan 7;5(1):1. PMID:30617281
2950. Skardelly M, Pantazis G, Bisdas S, et al. Primary cerebral low-grade B-cell lymphoma, monoclonal immunoglobulin deposition disease, cerebral light chain deposition disease and "aggregoma": an update on classification and diagnosis. BMC Neurol. 2013 Aug 15;13:107. PMID:23947787
2951. Skullerud K, Stenwig AE, Brandtzaeg P, et al. Intracranial primary leiomyosarcoma arising in a teratoma of the pineal area. Clin Neuropathol. 1995 Jul-Aug;14(4):245–8. PMID:8521631
2952. Slade I, Bacchelli C, Davies H, et al. DICER1 syndrome: clarifying the diagnosis, clinical features and management implications of a pleiotropic tumour predisposition syndrome. J Med Genet. 2011 Apr;48(4):273–8. PMID:21266384
2953. Slegers RJ, Blumcke I. Low-grade developmental and epilepsy associated brain tumors: a critical update 2020. Acta Neuropathol Commun. 2020 Mar 9;8(1):27. PMID:32151273
2954. Sloan EA, Chiang J, Villanueva-Meyer JE, et al. Intracranial mesenchymal tumor with FET-CREB fusion-a unifying diagnosis for the spectrum of intracranial myxoid mesenchymal tumors and angiomatoid fibrous histiocytoma-like neoplasms. Brain Pathol. 2020 Nov 3;e12918. PMID:33141488
2955. Sloan EA, Hilz S, Gupta R, et al. Gliomas arising in the setting of Li-Fraumeni syndrome stratify into two molecular subgroups with divergent clinicopathologic features. Acta Neuropathol. 2020 May;139(5):953–7. PMID:32157385
2956. Smedby KE, Brandt L, Bäcklund ML, et al. Brain metastases admissions in Sweden between 1987 and 2006. Br J Cancer. 2009 Dec 1;101(11):1919–24. PMID:19826419
2957. Smith AB, Horkanyne-Szakaly I, Schroeder JW, et al. From the radiologic pathology archives: mass lesions of the dura: beyond meningioma-radiologic-pathologic correlation. Radiographics. 2014 Mar-Apr;34(2):295–312. PMID:24617680
2958. Smith AB, Rushing EJ, Smirniotopoulos JG. From the archives of the AFIP: lesions of the pineal region: radiologic-pathologic correlation. Radiographics. 2010 Nov;30(7):2001–20. PMID:21057132
2959. Smith AB, Rushing EJ, Smirniotopoulos JG. Pigmented lesions of the central nervous system: radiologic-pathologic correlation. Radiographics. 2009 Sep-Oct;29(5):1503–24. PMID:19755608
2960. Smith DR, Wu CC, Saadatmand HJ, et al. Clinical and molecular characteristics of gliosarcoma and modern prognostic significance relative to conventional glioblastoma. J Neurooncol. 2018 Apr;137(2):303–11. PMID:29264835
2961. Smith JS, Tachibana I, Passe SM, et al. PTEN mutation, EGFR amplification, and outcome in patients with anaplastic astrocytoma and glioblastoma multiforme. J Natl Cancer Inst. 2001 Aug 15;93(16):1246–56. PMID:11504770
2962. Smith MJ. Germline and somatic mutations in meningiomas. Cancer Genet. 2015 Apr;208(4):107–14. PMID:25857641
2963. Smith MJ, Beetz C, Williams SG, et al. Germline mutations in SUFU cause Gorlin syndrome-associated childhood medulloblastoma and redefine the risk associated with PTCH1 mutations. J Clin Oncol. 2014 Dec 20;32(36):4155–61. PMID:25403219
2964. Smith MJ, Bowers NL, Bulman M, et al. Revisiting neurofibromatosis type 2 diagnostic criteria to exclude LZTR1-related schwannomatosis. Neurology. 2017 Jan 3;88(1):87–92. PMID:27856782
2965. Smith MJ, Higgs JE, Bowers NL, et al. Cranial meningiomas in 411 neurofibromatosis type 2 (NF2) patients with proven gene mutations: clear positional effect of mutations, but absence of female severity effect on age at onset. J Med Genet. 2011 Apr;48(4):261–5. PMID:21278391
2966. Smith MJ, Isidor B, Beetz C, et al. Mutations in LZTR1 add to the complex heterogeneity of schwannomatosis. Neurology. 2015 Jan 13;84(2):141–7. PMID:25480913
2967. Smith MJ, Kulkarni A, Rustad C, et al. Vestibular schwannomas occur in schwannomatosis and should not be considered an exclusion criterion for clinical diagnosis. Am J Med Genet A. 2012 Jan;158A(1):215–9. PMID:22105938
2968. Smith MJ, O'Sullivan J, Bhaskar SS, et al. Loss-of-function mutations in SMARCE1 cause an inherited disorder of multiple spinal meningiomas. Nat Genet. 2013 Mar;45(3):295–8. PMID:23377182
2969. Smith MJ, Wallace AJ, Bowers NL, et al. SMARCB1 mutations in schwannomatosis and genotype correlations with rhabdoid tumors. Cancer Genet. 2014 Sep;207(9):373–8. PMID:24933152
2970. Smits M. Imaging of oligodendroglioma. Br J Radiol. 2016;89(1060):20150857. PMID:26849038
2971. Smits M, van den Bent MJ. Imaging correlates of adult glioma genotypes. Radiology. 2017 Aug;284(2):316–31. PMID:28723281
2972. Smoll NR, Drummond KJ. The incidence of medulloblastomas and primitive neurectodermal tumours in adults and children. J Clin Neurosci. 2012 Nov;19(11):1541–4. PMID:22981874
2973. Smolle E, Al-Qubati S, Stefanits H, et al. Medullomyoblastoma: a case report and literature review of a rare tumor entity. Anticancer Res. 2012 Nov;32(11):4939–44. PMID:23155263
2974. Snuderl M, Eichler AF, Ligon KL, et al. Polysomy for chromosomes 1 and 19 predicts earlier recurrence in anaplastic oligodendrogliomas with concurrent 1p/19q loss. Clin Cancer Res. 2009 Oct 15;15(20):6430–7. PMID:19808867
2975. Snuderl M, Fazlollahi L, Le LP, et al. Mosaic amplification of multiple receptor tyrosine kinase genes in glioblastoma. Cancer Cell. 2011 Dec 13;20(6):810–7. PMID:22137795
2976. Snuderl M, Kannan K, Pfaff E, et al. Recurrent homozygous deletion of DROSHA and microduplication of PDE4DIP in pineoblastoma. Nat Commun. 2018 Jul 20;9(1):2868. PMID:30030436
2977. Snyder LA, Wolf AB, Oppenlander ME, et al. The impact of extent of resection on malignant transformation of pure oligodendrogliomas. J Neurosurg. 2014 Feb;120(2):309–14. PMID:24313617
2978. So JS, Epstein JI. GATA3 expression in paragangliomas: a pitfall potentially leading to misdiagnosis of urothelial carcinoma. Mod Pathol. 2013 Oct;26(10):1365–70. PMID:23599157
2979. Sobel RA. Vestibular (acoustic) schwannomas: histologic features in neurofibromatosis 2 and in unilateral cases. J Neuropathol Exp Neurol. 1993 Mar;52(2):106–13. PMID:8440992
2980. Sofela AA, Hettige S, Curran O, et al. Malignant transformation in craniopharyngiomas. Neurosurgery. 2014 Sep;75(3):306–14. PMID:24978859
2981. Soffer D, Pittaluga S, Caine Y, et al. Paraganglioma of cauda equina. A report of a case and review of the literature. Cancer. 1983 May 15;51(10):1907–10. PMID:6831356
2982. Soffietti R, Abacioglu U, Baumert B, et al. Diagnosis and treatment of brain metastases from solid tumors: guidelines from the European Association of Neuro-Oncology (EANO). Neuro Oncol. 2017 Feb 1;19(2):162–74. PMID:28391295
2983. Sohda T, Yun K. Insulin-like growth factor II expression in primary meningeal hemangiopericytoma and its metastasis to the liver accompanied by hypoglycemia. Hum Pathol. 1996 Aug;27(8):858–61. PMID:8760024
2984. Sohier P, Luscan A, Lloyd A, et al. Confirmation of mutation landscape of NF1-associated malignant peripheral nerve sheath tumors. Genes Chromosomes Cancer. 2017 May;56(5):421–6. PMID:28124441
2985. Soliman SE, Racher H, Zhang C, et al. Genetics and molecular diagnostics in retinoblastoma–an update. Asia Pac J Ophthalmol (Phila). 2017 Mar-Apr;6(2):197–207. PMID:28399338
2986. Sollfrank L, Lettmaier S, Erdmann M, et al. Panniculitis under successful targeted inhibition of the MAPK/ERK signaling pathway in a patient with BRAF V600E-mutated spindle cell oncocytoma of the pituitary gland. Anticancer Res. 2019 Jul;39(7):3955–9. PMID:31262927
2987. Solomon DA, Korshunov A, Sill M, et al. Myxoid glioneuronal tumor of the septum pellucidum and lateral ventricle is defined by a recurrent PDGFRA p.K385 mutation and DNT-like methylation profile. Acta Neuropathol. 2018 Aug;136(2):339–43. PMID:30006677
2988. Solomon DA, Wood MD, Tihan T, et al. Diffuse midline gliomas with histone H3-K27M mutation: a series of 47 cases assessing the spectrum of morphologic variation and associated genetic alterations. Brain Pathol. 2016 Sep;26(5):569–80. PMID:26517431
2989. Solomon JP, Benayed R, Hechtman JF, et al. Identifying patients with NTRK fusion cancer. Ann Oncol. 2019 Nov;30 Suppl 8:viii16–22. PMID:32223934
2990. Song MK, Chung JS, Joo YD, et al. Clinical importance of Bcl-6-positive non-deep-site involvement in non-HIV-related primary central nervous system diffuse large B-cell lymphoma. J Neurooncol. 2011 Sep;104(3):825–31. PMID:21380743
2991. Song X, Andrew Allen R, Terence Dunn S, et al. Glioblastoma with PNET-like components has a higher frequency of isocitrate dehydrogenase 1 (IDH1) mutation and likely a better prognosis than primary glioblastoma. Int J Clin Exp Pathol. 2011;4(7):651–60. PMID:22076165
2992. Sonneland PR, Scheithauer BW, LeChago J, et al. Paraganglioma of the cauda equina region. Clinicopathologic study of 31 cases with special reference to immunocytology and ultrastructure. Cancer. 1986 Oct 15;58(8):1720–35. PMID:2875784
2993. Sonneland PR, Scheithauer BW, Onofrio BM. Myxopapillary ependymoma. A clinicopathologic and immunocytochemical study of 77 cases. Cancer. 1985 Aug 15;56(4):883–93. PMID:4016681
2994. Sonoda Y, Yokoo H, Tanaka S, et al. Practical procedures for the integrated diagnosis of astrocytic and oligodendroglial tumors. Brain Tumor Pathol. 2019 Apr;36(2):56–62. PMID:30847711
2995. Soukup J, Kasparova P, Kohout A, et al. Evaluation of expression of somatostatin receptor 1, 2, 3, 5 and dopamine D2 receptor in spindle cell oncocytomas of posterior pituitary. Pituitary. 2019 Feb;22(1):70–8. PMID:30607746
2996. Sousa J, O'Brien D, Crooks D. Paraganglioma of the filum terminale. J Clin Neurosci. 2005 Jun;12(5):584–5. PMID:15921911
2997. Soylemezoglu F, Onder S, Tezel GG, et al. Neuronal nuclear antigen (NeuN): a new tool in the diagnosis of central neurocytoma. Pathol Res Pract. 2003;199(7):463–8. PMID:14521262
2998. Söylemezoglu F, Scheithauer BW, Esteve J, et al. Atypical central neurocytoma. J Neuropathol Exp Neurol. 1997 May;56(5):551–6. PMID:9143268
2999. Soylemezoglu F, Soffer D, Onol B, et al. Lipomatous medulloblastoma in adults. A distinct clinicopathological entity. Am J Surg Pathol. 1996 Apr;20(4):413–8. PMID:8604807
3000. Spada A, Arosio M, Bochicchio D, et al. Clinical, biochemical, and morphological correlates in patients bearing growth hormone-secreting pituitary tumors with or without constitutively active adenylyl cyclase. J Clin Endocrinol Metab. 1990 Dec;71(6):1421–6. PMID:1977758
3001. Spanberger T, Berghoff AS, Dinhof C, et al. Extent of peritumoral brain edema correlates with prognosis, tumoral growth pattern, HIF1a expression and angiogenic activity in patients with single brain metastases. Clin Exp Metastasis. 2013 Apr;30(4):357–68. PMID:23076770
3002. Spatz M, Nussbaum ES, Lyons L, et al. Primary intracranial angiomatoid fibrous histiocytoma: a case report and literature review. Br J Neurosurg. 2021 Apr;35(2):233–5. PMID:29540076
3003. Specht K, Sung YS, Zhang L, et al. Distinct transcriptional signature and immunoprofile of CIC-DUX4 fusion-positive round cell tumors compared to EWSR1-rearranged Ewing sarcomas: further evidence toward distinct pathologic entities. Genes Chromosomes Cancer. 2014 Jul;53(7):622–33. PMID:24723486
3004. Spence T, Perotti C, Sin-Chan P, et al. A novel C19MC amplified cell line links Lin28/let-7 to mTOR signaling in embryonal tumor with multilayered rosettes. Neuro Oncol. 2014 Jan;16(1):62–71. PMID:24311633
3005. Spence T, Sin-Chan P, Picard D, et al. CNS-PNETs with C19MC amplification and/or LIN28 expression comprise a distinct histogenetic diagnostic and therapeutic entity. Acta Neuropathol. 2014 Aug;128(2):291–303. PMID:24839957
3006. Sperduto PW, Chao ST, Sneed PK, et al. Diagnosis-specific prognostic factors, indexes, and treatment outcomes for patients with newly diagnosed brain metastases: a multi-institutional analysis of 4,259 patients. Int J Radiat Oncol Biol Phys. 2010 Jul 1;77(3):655–61. PMID:19942357

3007. Sperduto PW, Jiang W, Brown PD, et al. Estimating survival in melanoma patients with brain metastases: an update of the graded prognostic assessment for melanoma using molecular markers (Melanoma-molGPA). Int J Radiat Oncol Biol Phys. 2017 Nov 15;99(4):812–6. PMID:29063850
3008. Sperduto PW, Mesko S, Li J, et al. Beyond an updated graded prognostic assessment (Breast GPA): a prognostic index and trends in treatment and survival in breast cancer brain metastases from 1985 to today. Int J Radiat Oncol Biol Phys. 2020 Jun 1;107(2):334–43. PMID:32084525
3009. Sperduto PW, Mesko S, Li J, et al. Estrogen/progesterone receptor and HER2 discordance between primary tumor and brain metastases in breast cancer and its effect on treatment and survival. Neuro Oncol. 2020 Sep 29;22(9):1359–67. PMID:32034917
3010. Sperduto PW, Yang TJ, Beal K, et al. Estimating survival in patients with lung cancer and brain metastases: an update of the graded prognostic assessment for lung cancer using molecular markers (Lung-molGPA). JAMA Oncol. 2017 Jun 1;3(6):827–31. PMID:27892978
3011. Sperfeld AD, Hein C, Schröder JM, et al. Occurrence and characterization of peripheral nerve involvement in neurofibromatosis type 2. Brain. 2002 May;125(Pt 5):996–1004. PMID:11960890
3012. Spiegel E. Hyperplasie des Kleinhirns. Beitr Pathol Anat. 1920;67:539–48. German.
3013. Srirangam Nadhamuni V, Korbonits M. Novel insights into pituitary tumorigenesis: genetic and epigenetic mechanisms. Endocr Rev. 2020 Dec 1;41(6):bnaa006. PMID:32201880
3014. Stafford JM, Lee CH, Voigt P, et al. Multiple modes of PRC2 inhibition elicit global chromatin alterations in H3K27M pediatric glioma. Sci Adv. 2018 Oct 31;4(10):eaau5935. PMID:30402543
3015. Stambolic V, Suzuki A, de la Pompa JL, et al. Negative regulation of PKB/Akt-dependent cell survival by the tumor suppressor PTEN. Cell. 1998 Oct 2;95(1):29–39. PMID:9778245
3016. Stanescu Cosson R, Varlet P, Beuvon F, et al. Dysembryoplastic neuroepithelial tumors: CT, MR findings and imaging follow-up: a study of 53 cases. J Neuroradiol. 2001 Dec;28(4):230–40. PMID:11924137
3017. Stapleton CJ, Walcott BP, Kahle KT, et al. Diffuse central neurocytoma with craniospinal dissemination. J Clin Neurosci. 2012 Jan;19(1):163–6. PMID:22088950
3018. Star P, Goodwin A, Kapoor R, et al. Germline BAP1-positive patients: the dilemmas of cancer surveillance and a proposed interdisciplinary consensus monitoring strategy. Eur J Cancer. 2018 Mar;92:48–53. PMID:29413689
3019. Starink TM, van der Veen JP, Arwert F, et al. The Cowden syndrome: a clinical and genetic study in 21 patients. Clin Genet. 1986 Mar;29(3):222–33. PMID:3698331
3020. Starzyk J, Starzyk B, Bartnik-Mikuta A, et al. Gonadotropin releasing hormone-independent precocious puberty in a 5 year-old girl with suprasellar germ cell tumor secreting beta-hCG and alpha-fetoprotein. J Pediatr Endocrinol Metab. 2001 Jun;14(6):789–96. PMID:11453531
3021. Stavrou T, Bromley CM, Nicholson HS, et al. Prognostic factors and secondary malignancies in childhood medulloblastoma. J Pediatr Hematol Oncol. 2001 Oct;23(7):431–6. PMID:11878577
3022. Stead LF, Verhaak RGW. Doomed from the TERT? A two-stage model of tumorigenesis in IDH-wild-type glioblastoma. Cancer Cell. 2019 Apr 15;35(4):542–4. PMID:30991024
3023. Steck PA, Pershouse MA, Jasser SA, et al. Identification of a candidate tumour suppressor gene, MMAC1, at chromosome 10q23.3 that is mutated in multiple advanced cancers. Nat Genet. 1997 Apr;15(4):356–62. PMID:9090379
3024. Steffen-Smith EA, Baker EH, Venzon D, et al. Measurements of the pons as a biomarker of progression for pediatric DIPG. J Neurooncol. 2014 Jan;116(1):127–33. PMID:24113877
3025. Stein TD, Chae YS, Won N, et al. A 34-year-old man with bitemporal hemianopsia. Brain Pathol. 2014 Jan;24(1):107–10. PMID:24345226
3026. Steinbok P, Gopalakrishnan CV, Hengel AR, et al. Pediatric thalamic tumors in the MRI era: a Canadian perspective. Childs Nerv Syst. 2016 Feb;32(2):269–80. PMID:26597682
3027. Steklov M, Pandolfi S, Baietti MF, et al. Mutations in LZTR1 drive human disease by dysregulating RAS ubiquitination. Science. 2018 Dec 7;362(6419):1177–82. PMID:30442762
3028. Stemmer-Rachamimov AO, Gonzalez-Agosti C, Xu L, et al. Expression of NF2-encoded merlin and related ERM family proteins in the human central nervous system. J Neuropathol Exp Neurol. 1997 Jun;56(6):735–42. PMID:9184664
3029. Stemmer-Rachamimov AO, Horgan MA, Taratuto AL, et al. Meningioangiomatosis is associated with neurofibromatosis 2 but not with somatic alterations of the NF2 gene. J Neuropathol Exp Neurol. 1997 May;56(5):485–9. PMID:9143261
3030. Stemmer-Rachamimov AO, Ino Y, Lim ZY, et al. Loss of the NF2 gene and merlin occur by the tumorlet stage of schwannoma development in neurofibromatosis 2. J Neuropathol Exp Neurol. 1998 Dec;57(12):1164–7. PMID:9862639
3031. Stemmer-Rachamimov AO, Xu L, Gonzalez-Agosti C, et al. Universal absence of merlin, but not other ERM family members, in schwannomas. Am J Pathol. 1997 Dec;151(6):1649–54. PMID:9403715
3032. Stenzel W, Pels H, Staib P, et al. Concomitant manifestation of primary CNS lymphoma and Toxoplasma encephalitis in a patient with AIDS. J Neurol. 2004 Jun;251(6):764–6. PMID:15311360
3033. Sterkenburg AS, Hoffmann A, Gebhardt U, et al. Survival, hypothalamic obesity, and neuropsychological/psychosocial status after childhood-onset craniopharyngioma: newly reported long-term outcomes. Neuro Oncol. 2015 Jul;17(7):1029–38. PMID:25838139
3034. Stewart DR, Korf BR, Nathanson KL, et al. Care of adults with neurofibromatosis type 1: a clinical practice resource of the American College of Medical Genetics and Genomics (ACMG). Genet Med. 2018 Jul;20(7):671–82. PMID:30006586
3035. Stewart DR, Messinger Y, Williams GM, et al. Nasal chondromesenchymal hamartomas arise secondary to germline and somatic mutations of DICER1 in the pleuropulmonary blastoma tumor predisposition disorder. Hum Genet. 2014 Nov;133(11):1443–50. PMID:25118636
3036. Stichel D, Ebrahimi A, Reuss D, et al. Distribution of EGFR amplification, combined chromosome 7 gain and chromosome 10 loss, and TERT promoter mutation in brain tumors and their potential for the reclassification of IDHwt astrocytoma to glioblastoma. Acta Neuropathol. 2018 Nov;136(5):793–803. PMID:30187121
3037. Stichel D, Schrimpf D, Casalini B, et al. Routine RNA sequencing of formalin-fixed paraffin-embedded specimens in neuropathology diagnostics identifies diagnostically and therapeutically relevant gene fusions. Acta Neuropathol. 2019 Nov;138(5):827–35. PMID:31278449
3038. Stiles CE, Korbonits M. Familial isolated pituitary adenoma. In: Feingold KR, Anawalt B, Boyce A, et al., editors. Endotext. South Dartmouth (MA): MDText.com, Inc.; 2000 [updated 2020 May 28]. PMID:25905184
3039. Stivaros SM, Stemmer-Rachamimov AO, Alston R, et al. Multiple synchronous sites of origin of vestibular schwannomas in neurofibromatosis Type 2. J Med Genet. 2015 Aug;52(8):557–62. PMID:26104281
3040. Stockhammer F, Misch M, Helms HJ, et al. IDH1/2 mutations in WHO grade II astrocytomas associated with localization and seizure as the initial symptom. Seizure. 2012 Apr;21(3):194–7. PMID:22217666
3041. Stödberg T, Deniz Y, Esteitie N, et al. A case of diffuse leptomeningeal oligodendrogliomatosis associated with HHV-6 variant A. Neuropediatrics. 2002 Oct;33(5):266–70. PMID:12536370
3042. Stojanova A, Penn LZ. The role of INI1/hSNF5 in gene regulation and cancer. Biochem Cell Biol. 2009 Feb;87(1):163–77. PMID:19234532
3043. Stone DM, Hynes M, Armanini M, et al. The tumour-suppressor gene patched encodes a candidate receptor for Sonic hedgehog. Nature. 1996 Nov 14;384(6605):129–34. PMID:8906787
3044. Stone DM, Murone M, Luoh S, et al. Characterization of the human suppressor of fused, a negative regulator of the zinc-finger transcription factor Gli. J Cell Sci. 1999 Dec;112(Pt 23):4437–48. PMID:10564661
3045. Stone TJ, Keeley A, Virasami A, et al. Comprehensive molecular characterisation of epilepsy-associated glioneuronal tumours. Acta Neuropathol. 2018 Jan;135(1):115–29. PMID:29058119
3046. Stone TJ, Rowell R, Jayasekera BAP, et al. Review: Molecular characteristics of long-term epilepsy-associated tumours (LEATs) and mechanisms for tumour-related epilepsy (TRE). Neuropathol Appl Neurobiol. 2018 Feb;44(1):56–69. PMID:29315734
3047. Stowe IB, Mercado EL, Stowe TR, et al. A shared molecular mechanism underlies the human rasopathies Legius syndrome and Neurofibromatosis-1. Genes Dev. 2012 Jul 1;26(13):1421–6. PMID:22751498
3048. Stratakis CA, Carney JA, Lin JP, et al. Carney complex, a familial multiple neoplasia and lentiginosis syndrome. Analysis of 11 kindreds and linkage to the short arm of chromosome 2. J Clin Invest. 1996 Feb 1;97(3):699–705. PMID:8609225
3049. Stratakis CA, Kirschner LS, Carney JA. Clinical and molecular features of the Carney complex: diagnostic criteria and recommendations for patient evaluation. J Clin Endocrinol Metab. 2001 Sep;86(9):4041–6. PMID:11549623
3050. Stratakis CA, Raygada M. Carney complex. In: Adam MP, Ardinger HH, Pagon RA, et al., editors. GeneReviews. Seattle (WA): University of Washington, Seattle; 2003 Feb 5 [updated 2018 Aug 16]. PMID:20301463
3051. Stratmann R, Krieg M, Haas R, et al. Putative control of angiogenesis in hemangioblastomas by the von Hippel-Lindau tumor suppressor gene. J Neuropathol Exp Neurol. 1997 Nov;56(11):1242–52. PMID:9370235
3052. Strickland MR, Gill CM, Nayyar N, et al. Targeted sequencing of SMO and AKT1 in anterior skull base meningiomas. J Neurosurg. 2017 Aug;127(2):438–44. PMID:27885953
3053. Strommer KN, Brandner S, Sarioglu AC, et al. Symptomatic cerebellar metastasis and late local recurrence of a cauda equina paraganglioma. Case report. J Neurosurg. 1995 Jul;83(1):166–9. PMID:7782837
3054. Strong MJ, Blanchard E 4th, Lin Z, et al. A comprehensive next generation sequencing-based virome assessment in brain tissue suggests no major virus - tumor association. Acta Neuropathol Commun. 2016 Jul 11;4(1):71. PMID:27402152
3055. Stuivenvolt M, Mandl E, Verheul J, et al. Atypical transformation in sacral drop metastasis from posterior fossa choroid plexus papilloma. BMJ Case Rep. 2012 Aug 24;2012:bcr0120125681. PMID:22922909
3056. Stupp R, Hegi ME, Gorlia T, et al. Cilengitide combined with standard treatment for patients with newly diagnosed glioblastoma with methylated MGMT promoter (CENTRIC EORTC 26071-22072 study): a multicentre, randomised, open-label, phase 3 trial. Lancet Oncol. 2014 Sep;15(10):1100–8. PMID:25163906
3057. Stupp R, Hegi ME, Mason WP, et al. Effects of radiotherapy with concomitant and adjuvant temozolomide versus radiotherapy alone on survival in glioblastoma in a randomised phase III study: 5-year analysis of the EORTC-NCIC trial. Lancet Oncol. 2009 May;10(5):459–66. PMID:19269895
3058. Sturm D, Bender S, Jones DT, et al. Paediatric and adult glioblastoma: multiform (epi)genomic culprits emerge. Nat Rev Cancer. 2014 Feb;14(2):92–107. PMID:24457416
3059. Sturm D, Orr BA, Toprak UH, et al. New brain tumor entities emerge from molecular classification of CNS-PNETs. Cell. 2016 Feb 25;164(5):1060–72. PMID:26919435
3060. Sturm D, Witt H, Hovestadt V, et al. Hotspot mutations in H3F3A and IDH1 define distinct epigenetic and biological subgroups of glioblastoma. Cancer Cell. 2012 Oct 16;22(4):425–37. PMID:23079654
3061. Suchorska B, Schüller U, Biczok A, et al. Contrast enhancement is a prognostic factor in IDH1/2 mutant, but not in wild-type WHO grade II/III glioma as confirmed by machine learning. Eur J Cancer. 2019 Jan;107:15–27. PMID:30529899
3062. Suerink M, Ripperger T, Messiaen L, et al. Constitutional mismatch repair deficiency as a differential diagnosis of neurofibromatosis type 1: consensus guidelines for testing a child without malignancy. J Med Genet. 2019 Feb;56(2):53–62. PMID:30415209
3063. Sugawa N, Ekstrand AJ, James CD, et al. Identical splicing of aberrant epidermal growth factor receptor transcripts from amplified rearranged genes in human glioblastomas. Proc Natl Acad Sci U S A. 1990 Nov;87(21):8602–6. PMID:2236070
3064. Sughrue ME, Sanai N, Shangari G, et al. Outcome and survival following primary and repeat surgery for World Health Organization Grade III meningiomas. J Neurosurg. 2010 Aug;113(2):202–9. PMID:20225922
3065. Sugiarto S, Persson AI, Munoz EG, et al. Asymmetry-defective oligodendrocyte progenitors are glioma precursors. Cancer Cell. 2011 Sep 13;20(3):328–40. PMID:21907924
3066. Sugita S, Arai Y, Aoyama T, et al. NUTM2A-CIC fusion small round cell sarcoma: a genetically distinct variant of CIC-rearranged sarcoma. Hum Pathol. 2017 Jul;65:225–30. PMID:28188754
3067. Sugita S, Arai Y, Tonooka A, et al. A novel CIC-FOXO4 gene fusion in undifferentiated small round cell sarcoma: a genetically distinct variant of Ewing-like sarcoma. Am J Surg Pathol. 2014 Nov;38(11):1571–6. PMID:25007147
3068. Sukov WR, Cheville JC, Giannini C, et al. Isochromosome 12p and polysomy 12 in primary central nervous system germ cell tumors: frequency and association with

clinicopathologic features. Hum Pathol. 2010 Feb;41(2):232–8. PMID:19801160

3069. Sullivan JP, Nahed BV, Madden MW, et al. Brain tumor cells in circulation are enriched for mesenchymal gene expression. Cancer Discov. 2014 Nov;4(11):1299–309. PMID:25139148

3070. Sumerauer D, Krskova L, Vicha A, et al. Rare IDH1 variants are common in pediatric hemispheric diffuse astrocytomas and frequently associated with Li-Fraumeni syndrome. Acta Neuropathol. 2020 Apr;139(4):795–7. PMID:31897644

3071. Sunderland AJ, Steiner RE, Al Zahrani M, et al. An international multicenter retrospective analysis of patients with extranodal marginal zone lymphoma and histologically confirmed central nervous system and dural involvement. Cancer Med. 2020 Jan;9(2):663–70. PMID:31808316

3072. Sundgren P, Annertz M, Englund E, et al. Paragangliomas of the spinal canal. Neuroradiology. 1999 Oct;41(10):788–94. PMID:10552032

3073. Sung CC, Collins R, Li J, et al. Glycolipids and myelin proteins in human oligodendrogliomas. Glycoconj J. 1996 Jun;13(3):433–43. PMID:8781974

3074. Surawicz TS, McCarthy BJ, Kupelian V, et al. Descriptive epidemiology of primary brain and CNS tumors: results from the Central Brain Tumor Registry of the United States, 1990-1994. Neuro Oncol. 1999 Jan;1(1):14–25. PMID:11554386

3075. Surrey LF, Jain P, Zhang B, et al. Genomic analysis of dysembryoplastic neuroepithelial tumor spectrum reveals a diversity of molecular alterations dysregulating the MAPK and PI3K/mTOR pathways. J Neuropathol Exp Neurol. 2019 Dec 1;78(12):1100–11. PMID:31617914

3076. Surun A, Varlet P, Brugières L, et al. Medulloblastomas associated with an APC germline pathogenic variant share the good prognosis of CTNNB1-mutated medulloblastomas. Neuro Oncol. 2020 Jan 11;22(1):128–38. PMID:31504825

3077. Süß P, Volz F, Lang C, et al. A case of large meningeal epithelioid hemangioendothelioma with WWTR1-CAMTA1 gene rearrangement and slow growth over 15 Years. J Neuropathol Exp Neurol. 2018 Oct 1;77(10):871–6. PMID:30085199

3078. Suvà ML, Rheinbay E, Gillespie SM, et al. Reconstructing and reprogramming the tumor-propagating potential of glioblastoma stem-like cells. Cell. 2014 Apr 24;157(3):580–94. PMID:24726434

3079. Suvà ML, Riggi N, Bernstein BE. Epigenetic reprogramming in cancer. Science. 2013 Mar 29;339(6127):1567–70. PMID:23539597

3080. Suvà ML, Tirosh I. The glioma stem cell model in the era of single-cell genomics. Cancer Cell. 2020 May 11;37(5):630–6. PMID:32396858

3081. Suzuki A, de la Pompa JL, Stambolic V, et al. High cancer susceptibility and embryonic lethality associated with mutation of the PTEN tumor suppressor gene in mice. Curr Biol. 1998 Oct 22;8(21):1169–78. PMID:9799734

3082. Suzuki H, Aoki K, Chiba K, et al. Mutational landscape and clonal architecture in grade II and III gliomas. Nat Genet. 2015 May;47(5):458–68. PMID:25848751

3083. Suzuki H, Kumar SA, Shuai S, et al. Recurrent noncoding U1 snRNA mutations drive cryptic splicing in SHH medulloblastoma. Nature. 2019 Oct;574(7780):707–11. PMID:31664194

3084. Svajdler M Jr, Rychlý B, Gajdoš M, et al. Gliosarcoma with alveolar rhabdomyosarcoma-like component: report of a case with a hitherto undescribed sarcomatous component. Cesk Patol. 2012 Oct;48(4):210–4. PMID:23121030

3085. Svojgr K, Sumerauer D, Puchmajerova A, et al. Fanconi anemia with biallelic FANCD1/BRCA2 mutations - Case report of a family with three affected children. Eur J Med Genet. 2016 Mar;59(3):152–7. PMID:26657402

3086. Swaidan MY, Hussaini M, Sultan I, et al. Radiological findings in gliosarcoma. A single institution experience. Neuroradiol J. 2012 May;25(2):173–80. PMID:24028910

3087. Swanson AA, Raghunathan A, Jenkins RB, et al. Spinal cord ependymomas with MYCN amplification show aggressive clinical behavior. J Neuropathol Exp Neurol. 2019 Sep 1;78(9):791–7. PMID:31373367

3088. Swanson KR, Bridge C, Murray JD, et al. Virtual and real brain tumors: using mathematical modeling to quantify glioma growth and invasion. J Neurol Sci. 2003 Dec 15;216(1):1–10. PMID:14607296

3089. Swartling FJ, Savov V, Persson AI, et al. Distinct neural stem cell populations give rise to disparate brain tumors in response to N-MYC. Cancer Cell. 2012 May 15;21(5):601–13. PMID:22624711

3090. Sweet K, Willis J, Zhou XP, et al. Molecular classification of patients with unexplained hamartomatous and hyperplastic polyposis. JAMA. 2005 Nov 16;294(19):2465–73. PMID:16287957

3091. Sweiss FB, Lee M, Sherman JH. Extraventricular neurocytomas. Neurosurg Clin N Am. 2015 Jan;26(1):99–104. PMID:25432188

3092. Swensen JJ, Keyser J, Coffin CM, et al. Familial occurrence of schwannomas and malignant rhabdoid tumour associated with a duplication in SMARCB1. J Med Genet. 2009 Jan;46(1):68–72. PMID:19124645

3093. Szeifert GT, Pásztor E. Could craniopharyngiomas produce pituitary hormones? Neurol Res. 1993 Feb;15(1):68–9. PMID:8098858

3094. Taal W, Oosterkamp HM, Walenkamp AM, et al. Single-agent bevacizumab or lomustine versus a combination of bevacizumab plus lomustine in patients with recurrent glioblastoma (BELOB trial): a randomised controlled phase 2 trial. Lancet Oncol. 2014 Aug;15(9):943–53. PMID:25035291

3095. Taal W, van der Rijt CC, Dinjens WN, et al. Treatment of large low-grade oligodendroglial tumors with upfront procarbazine, lomustine, and vincristine chemotherapy with long follow-up: a retrospective cohort study with growth kinetics. J Neurooncol. 2015 Jan;121(2):365–72. PMID:25344884

3096. Tabori U, Baskin B, Shago M, et al. Universal poor survival in children with medulloblastoma harboring somatic TP53 mutations. J Clin Oncol. 2010 Mar 10;28(8):1345–50. PMID:20142599

3097. Tabori U, Shlien A, Baskin B, et al. TP53 alterations determine clinical subgroups and survival of patients with choroid plexus tumors. J Clin Oncol. 2010 Apr 20;28(12):1995–2001. PMID:20308654

3098. Tabouret E, Bequet C, Denicolaï E, et al. BRAF mutation and anaplasia may be predictive factors of progression-free survival in adult pleomorphic xanthoastrocytoma. Eur J Surg Oncol. 2015 Dec;41(12):1685–90. PMID:26454767

3099. Tabouret E, Chinot O, Metellus P, et al. Recent trends in epidemiology of brain metastases: an overview. Anticancer Res. 2012 Nov;32(11):4655–62. PMID:23155227

3100. Tabouret E, Nguyen AT, Dehais C, et al. Prognostic impact of the 2016 WHO classification of diffuse gliomas in the French POLA cohort. Acta Neuropathol. 2016 Oct;132(4):625–34. PMID:27573687

3101. Tachibana O, Yamashima T, Yamashita J, et al. Immunohistochemical expression of human chorionic gonadotropin and P-glycoprotein in human pituitary glands and craniopharyngiomas. J Neurosurg. 1994 Jan;80(1):79–84. PMID:7903692

3102. Tada T, Katsuyama T, Aoki T, et al. Mixed glioblastoma and sarcoma with osteoid-chondral tissue. Clin Neuropathol. 1987 Jul-Aug;6(4):160–3. PMID:3115659

3103. Taggard DA, Menezes AH. Three choroid plexus papillomas in a patient with Aicardi syndrome. A case report. Pediatr Neurosurg. 2000 Oct;33(4):219–23. PMID:11124640

3104. Tai HC, Chuang IC, Chen TC, et al. NAB2-STAT6 fusion types account for clinicopathological variations in solitary fibrous tumors. Mod Pathol. 2015 Oct;28(10):1324–35. PMID:26226844

3105. Taillibert S, Laigle-Donadey F, Chodkiewicz C, et al. Leptomeningeal metastases from solid malignancy: a review. J Neurooncol. 2005 Oct;75(1):85–99. PMID:16215819

3106. Tajima S, Koda K. Germinoma with an extensive rhabdoid cell component centered at the corpus callosum. Med Mol Morphol. 2017 Mar;50(1):52–8. PMID:26012485

3107. Takahashi M, Yamamoto J, Aoyama Y, et al. Efficacy of multi-staged surgery and adjuvant chemotherapy for successful treatment of atypical choroid plexus papilloma in an infant: case report. Neurol Med Chir (Tokyo). 2009 Oct;49(10):484–7. PMID:19855149

3108. Takami H, Fukuoka K, Fukushima S, et al. Integrated clinical, histopathological, and molecular data analysis of 190 central nervous system germ cell tumors from the iGCT Consortium. Neuro Oncol. 2019 Dec 17;21(12):1565–77. PMID:31420671

3109. Takami H, Fukushima S, Aoki K, et al. Intratumoural immune cell landscape in germinoma reveals multipotent lineages and exhibits prognostic significance. Neuropathol Appl Neurobiol. 2020 Feb;46(2):111–24. PMID:31179566

3110. Takami H, Graffeo CS, Perry A, et al. Epidemiology, natural history, and optimal management of neurohypophyseal germ cell tumors. J Neurosurg. 2020 Feb 7:1–9. PMID:32032947

3111. Takami H, Perry A, Graffeo CS, et al. Comparison on epidemiology, tumor location, histology, and prognosis of intracranial germ cell tumors between Mayo Clinic and Japanese consortium cohorts. J Neurosurg. 2020 Jan 31:1–11. PMID:32005022

3112. Takami H, Yoshida A, Fukushima S, et al. Revisiting TP53 Mutations and Immunohistochemistry–A Comparative Study in 157 Diffuse Gliomas. Brain Pathol. 2015 May;25(3):256–65. PMID:25040820

3113. Takei H, Dauser RC, Adesina AM. Cytomorphologic characteristics, differential diagnosis and utility during intraoperative consultation for medulloblastoma. Acta Cytol. 2007 Mar-Apr;51(2):183–92. PMID:17425200

3114. Takei Y, Mirra SS, Miles ML. Eosinophilic granular ceels in oligodendrogliomas. An ultrastructural study. Cancer. 1976 Nov;38(5):1968–76. PMID:991110

3115. Takei Y, Seyama S, Pearl GS, et al. Ultrastructural study of the human neurohypophysis. II. Cellular elements of neural parenchyma, the pituicytes. Cell Tissue Res. 1980;205(2):273–87. PMID:7188885

3116. Takeshima H, Kawahara Y, Hirano H, et al. Postoperative regression of desmoplastic infantile gangliogliomas: report of two cases. Neurosurgery. 2003 Oct;53(4):979–83. PMID:14519230

3117. Takeuchi H, Kitai R, Hosoda T, et al. Clinicopathologic features of small cell glioblastomas. J Neurooncol. 2016 Apr;127(2):337–44. PMID:26725094

3118. Tallegas M, Miquelestorena-Standley É, Labit-Bouvier C, et al. IDH mutation status in a series of 88 head and neck chondrosarcomas: different profile between tumors of the skull base and tumors involving the facial skeleton and the laryngotracheal tract. Hum Pathol. 2019 Feb;84:183–91. PMID:30296521

3119. Tamai S, Kinoshita M, Sabit H, et al. Case of metastatic glioblastoma with primitive neuronal component to the lung. Neuropathology. 2019 Jun;39(3):218–23. PMID:31025405

3120. Tampourlou M, Ntali G, Ahmed S, et al. Outcome of nonfunctioning pituitary adenomas that regrow after primary treatment: a study from two large UK centers. J Clin Endocrinol Metab. 2017 Jun 1;102(6):1889–97. PMID:28323946

3121. Tamura M, Gu J, Matsumoto K, et al. Inhibition of cell migration, spreading, and focal adhesions by tumor suppressor PTEN. Science. 1998 Jun 5;280(5369):1614–7. PMID:9616126

3122. Tan C, Scotting PJ. Stem cell research points the way to the cell of origin for intracranial germ cell tumours. J Pathol. 2013 Jan;229(1):4–11. PMID:22926997

3123. Tan CL, Vellayappan B, Wu B, et al. Molecular profiling of different glioma specimens from an Ollier disease patient suggests a multifocal disease process in the setting of IDH mosaicism. Brain Tumor Pathol. 2018 Oct;35(4):202–8. PMID:30159860

3124. Tan MH, Mester J, Peterson C, et al. A clinical scoring system for selection of patients for PTEN mutation testing is proposed on the basis of a prospective study of 3042 probands. Am J Hum Genet. 2011 Jan 7;88(1):42–56. PMID:21194675

3125. Tan MH, Mester JL, Ngeow J, et al. Lifetime cancer risks in individuals with germline PTEN mutations. Clin Cancer Res. 2012 Jan 15;18(2):400–7. PMID:22252256

3126. Tan TSE, Patel L, Gopal-Kothandapani JS, et al. The neuroendocrine sequelae of paediatric craniopharyngioma: a 40-year meta-data analysis of 185 cases from three UK centres. Eur J Endocrinol. 2017 Mar;176(3):359–69. PMID:28073908

3127. Tan W, Huang W, Xiong J, et al. Neuroradiological features of papillary glioneuronal tumor: a study of 8 cases. J Comput Assist Tomogr. 2014 Sep-Oct;38(5):634–8. PMID:24879457

3128. Tanaka F, Matsukawa M, Kogue R, et al. A case of a rosette-forming glioneuronal tumor arising from the pons with disappearance of contrast enhancement. Radiol Case Rep. 2019 May 22;14(8):899–902. PMID:31193570

3129. Tanaka K, Waga S, Itho H, et al. Superficial location of malignant glioma with heavily lipidized (foamy) tumor cells: a case report. J Neurooncol. 1989 Sep;7(3):293–7. PMID:2795123

3130. Tanaka Y, Yokoo H, Komori T, et al. A distinct pattern of Olig2-positive cellular distribution in papillary glioneuronal tumors: a manifestation of the oligodendroglial phenotype? Acta Neuropathol. 2005 Jul;110(1):39–47. PMID:15906048

3131. Tanboon J, Williams EA, Louis DN. The diagnostic use of immunohistochemical surrogates for signature molecular genetic alterations in gliomas. J Neuropathol Exp Neurol. 2016 Jan;75(1):4–18. PMID:26671986

3132. Tang H, Zhu H, Wang X, et al. KLF4 is a tumor suppressor in anaplastic meningioma stem-like cells and human meningiomas. J Mol Cell Biol. 2017 Aug 1;9(4):315–24. PMID:28651379

3133. Tanizaki Y, Jin L, Scheithauer BW, et al. P53 gene mutations in pituitary carcinomas. Endocr Pathol. 2007 Winter;18(4):217–22. PMID:18026859

3134. Tao R, Murad N, Xu Z, et al. MYC drives group 3 medulloblastoma through transformation of Sox2+ astrocyte progenitor cells. Cancer Res. 2019 Apr 15;79(8):1967–80. PMID:30862721
3135. Tapella L, Sesta A, Cassarino MF, et al. Benzene and 2-ethyl-phthalate induce proliferation in normal rat pituitary cells. Pituitary. 2017 Jun;20(3):311–8. PMID:27853917
3136. Taratuto AL, Monges J, Lylyk P, et al. Superficial cerebral astrocytoma attached to dura. Report of six cases in infants. Cancer. 1984 Dec 1;54(11):2505–12. PMID:6498740
3137. Tarpey PS, Behjati S, Young MD, et al. The driver landscape of sporadic chordoma. Nat Commun. 2017 Oct 12;8(1):890. PMID:29026114
3138. Tashjian VS, Khanlou N, Vinters HV, et al. Hemangiopericytoma of the cerebellopontine angle: a case report and review of the literature. Surg Neurol. 2009 Sep;72(3):290–5. PMID:18786704
3139. Tate M, Sughrue ME, Rutkowski MJ, et al. The long-term postsurgical prognosis of patients with pineoblastoma. Cancer. 2012 Jan 1;118(1):173–9. PMID:21717450
3140. Tateishi K, Nakamura T, Juratli TA, et al. PI3K/AKT/mTOR pathway alterations promote malignant progression and xenograft formation in oligodendroglial tumors. Clin Cancer Res. 2019 Jul 15;25(14):4375–87. PMID:30975663
3141. Tateno T, Zhu X, Asa SL, et al. Chromatin remodeling and histone modifications in pituitary tumors. Mol Cell Endocrinol. 2010 Sep 15;326(1-2):66–70. PMID:20060434
3142. Tatevossian RG, Tang B, Dalton J, et al. MYB upregulation and genetic aberrations in a subset of pediatric low-grade gliomas. Acta Neuropathol. 2010 Dec;120(6):731–43. PMID:21046410
3143. Tateyama H, Tada T, Okabe M, et al. Different keratin profiles in craniopharyngioma subtypes and ameloblastomas. Pathol Res Pract. 2001;197(11):735–42. PMID:11770017
3144. Tauziéde-Espariat A, Bresson D, Polivka M, et al. Prognostic and therapeutic markers in chordomas: a study of 287 tumors. J Neuropathol Exp Neurol. 2016 Feb;75(2):111–20. PMID:26733585
3145. Tauziède-Espariat A, Debily MA, Castel D, et al. An integrative radiological, histopathological and molecular analysis of pediatric pontine histone-wildtype glioma with MYCN amplification (HGG-MYCN). Acta Neuropathol Commun. 2019 Jun 10;7(1):87. PMID:31177990
3146. Tauziède-Espariat A, Debily MA, Castel D, et al. The pediatric supratentorial MYCN-amplified high-grade gliomas methylation class presents the same radiological, histopathological and molecular features as their pontine counterparts. Acta Neuropathol Commun. 2020 Jul 9;8(1):104. PMID:32646492
3147. Tauziède-Espariat A, Pagès M, Roux A, et al. Pediatric methylation class HGNET-MN1: unresolved issues with terminology and grading. Acta Neuropathol Commun. 2019 Nov 10;7(1):176. PMID:31707996
3148. Tauziede-Espariat A, Parfait B, Besnard A, et al. Loss of SMARCE1 expression is a specific diagnostic marker of clear cell meningioma: a comprehensive immunophenotypical and molecular analysis. Brain Pathol. 2018 Jul;28(4):466–74. PMID:28474749
3149. Tavangar SM, Larijani B, Mahta A, et al. Craniopharyngioma: a clinicopathological study of 141 cases. Endocr Pathol. 2004 Winter;15(4):339–44. PMID:15681858
3150. Taylor KR, Mackay A, Truffaux N, et al. Recurrent activating ACVR1 mutations in diffuse intrinsic pontine glioma. Nat Genet. 2014 May;46(5):457–61. PMID:24705252
3151. Taylor MD, Gokgoz N, Andrulis IL, et al. Familial posterior fossa brain tumors of infancy secondary to germline mutation of the hSNF5 gene. Am J Hum Genet. 2000 Apr;66(4):1403–6. PMID:10739763
3152. Taylor MD, Liu L, Raffel C, et al. Mutations in SUFU predispose to medulloblastoma. Nat Genet. 2002 Jul;31(3):306–10. PMID:12068298
3153. Taylor MD, Northcott PA, Korshunov A, et al. Molecular subgroups of medulloblastoma: the current consensus. Acta Neuropathol. 2012 Apr;123(4):465–72. PMID:22134537
3154. Taylor MD, Perry J, Zlatescu MC, et al. The hPMS2 exon 5 mutation and malignant glioma. Case report. J Neurosurg. 1999 May;90(5):946–50. PMID:10223463
3155. Taylor MD, Poppleton H, Fuller C, et al. Radial glia cells are candidate stem cells of ependymoma. Cancer Cell. 2005 Oct;8(4):323–35. PMID:16226707
3156. Taylor SS, Ilouz R, Zhang P, et al. Assembly of allosteric macromolecular switches: lessons from PKA. Nat Rev Mol Cell Biol. 2012 Oct;13(10):646–58. PMID:22992589
3157. Tchoghandjian A, Fernandez C, Colin C, et al. Pilocytic astrocytoma of the optic pathway: a tumour deriving from radial glia cells with a specific gene signature. Brain. 2009 Jun;132(Pt 6):1523–35. PMID:19336457
3158. Tee AR, Fingar DC, Manning BD, et al. Tuberous sclerosis complex-1 and -2 gene products function together to inhibit mammalian target of rapamycin (mTOR)-mediated downstream signaling. Proc Natl Acad Sci U S A. 2002 Oct 15;99(21):13571–6. PMID:12271141
3159. Teferi N, Abukhiran I, Noeller J, et al. Vertebral hemangiomas: diagnosis and management. A single center experience. Clin Neurol Neurosurg. 2020 Mar;190:105745. PMID:32097829
3160. Tehrani M, Friedman TM, Olson JJ, et al. Intravascular thrombosis in central nervous system malignancies: a potential role in astrocytoma progression to glioblastoma. Brain Pathol. 2008 Apr;18(2):164–71. PMID:18093251
3161. Telera S, Carosi M, Cerasoli V, et al. Hemothorax presenting as a primitive thoracic paraganglioma. Case illustration. J Neurosurg Spine. 2006 Jun;4(6):515. PMID:16776367
3162. Telfeian AE, Judkins A, Younkin D, et al. Subependymal giant cell astrocytoma with cranial and spinal metastases in a patient with tuberous sclerosis. Case report. J Neurosurg. 2004 May;100(5 Suppl Pediatrics):498–500. PMID:15287462
3163. Temming P, Arendt M, Viehmann A, et al. How eye-preserving therapy affects long-term overall survival in heritable retinoblastoma survivors. J Clin Oncol. 2016 Sep 10;34(26):3183–8. PMID:27382102
3164. Teo WY, Shen J, Su JM, et al. Implications of tumor location on subtypes of medulloblastoma. Pediatr Blood Cancer. 2013 Sep;60(9):1408–10. PMID:23512859
3165. Terada T. Expression of cytokeratins in glioblastoma multiforme. Pathol Oncol Res. 2015 Jul;21(3):817–9. PMID:25633990
3166. Terashima K, Yu A, Chow WY, et al. Genome-wide analysis of DNA copy number alterations and loss of heterozygosity in intracranial germ cell tumors. Pediatr Blood Cancer. 2014 Apr;61(4):593–600. PMID:24249158
3167. Terrier LM, Bauchet L, Rigau V, et al. Natural course and prognosis of anaplastic gangliogliomas: a multicenter retrospective study of 43 cases from the French Brain Tumor Database. Neuro Oncol. 2017 May 1;19(5):678–88. PMID:28453747
3168. Tesileanu CMS, Dirven L, Wijnenga MMJ, et al. Survival of diffuse astrocytic glioma, IDH1/2 wildtype, with molecular features of glioblastoma, WHO grade IV: a confirmation of the cIMPACT-NOW criteria. Neuro Oncol. 2020 Apr 15;22(4):515–23. PMID:31637414
3169. Testa JR, Cheung M, Pei J, et al. Germline BAP1 mutations predispose to malignant mesothelioma. Nat Genet. 2011 Aug 28;43(10):1022–5. PMID:21874000
3170. Thakkar JP, Kumthekar P, Dixit KS, et al. Leptomeningeal metastasis from solid tumors. J Neurol Sci. 2020 Apr 15;411:116706. PMID:32007755
3171. Thieblemont C, Bertoni F, Copie-Bergman C, et al. Chronic inflammation and extra-nodal marginal-zone lymphomas of MALT-type. Semin Cancer Biol. 2014 Feb;24:33–42. PMID:24333758
3172. Thiel E, Korfel A, Martus P, et al. High-dose methotrexate with or without whole brain radiotherapy for primary CNS lymphoma (G-PCNSL-SG-1): a phase 3, randomised, non-inferiority trial. Lancet Oncol. 2010 Nov;11(11):1036–47. PMID:20970380
3173. Thiele EA. Managing and understanding epilepsy in tuberous sclerosis complex. Epilepsia. 2010 Feb;51 Suppl 1:90–1. PMID:20331728
3174. Thiessen B, Finlay J, Kulkarni R, et al. Astroblastoma: does histology predict biologic behavior? J Neurooncol. 1998 Oct;40(1):59–65. PMID:9874187
3175. Thimsen V, John N, Buchfelder M, et al. Expression of SRY-related HMG box transcription factors (Sox) 2 and 9 in craniopharyngioma subtypes and surrounding brain tissue. Sci Rep. 2017 Nov 20;7(1):15856. PMID:29158570
3176. Thines L, Lejeune JP, Ruchoux MM, et al. Management of delayed intracranial and intraspinal metastases of intradural spinal paragangliomas. Acta Neurochir (Wien). 2006 Jan;148(1):63–6. PMID:16283104
3177. Thom M, Blümcke I, Aronica E. Long-term epilepsy-associated tumors. Brain Pathol. 2012 May;22(3):350–79. PMID:22497610
3178. Thom M, Gomez-Anson B, Revesz T, et al. Spontaneous intralesional haemorrhage in dysembryoplastic neuroepithelial tumours: a series of five cases. J Neurol Neurosurg Psychiatry. 1999 Jul;67(1):97–101. PMID:10369831
3179. Thom M, Liu J, Bongaarts A, et al. Multinodular and vacuolating neuronal tumors in epilepsy: dysplasia or neoplasia? Brain Pathol. 2018 Mar;28(2):155–71. PMID:28833756
3180. Thom M, Toma A, An S, et al. One hundred and one dysembryoplastic neuroepithelial tumors: an adult epilepsy series with immunohistochemical, molecular genetic, and clinical correlations and a review of the literature. J Neuropathol Exp Neurol. 2011 Oct;70(10):859–78. PMID:21937911
3181. Thomas AA, Fisher JL, Rahme GJ, et al. Regulatory T cells are not a strong predictor of survival for patients with glioblastoma. Neuro Oncol. 2015 Jun;17(6):801–9. PMID:25618892
3182. Thomas C, Metrock K, Kordes U, et al. Epigenetics impacts upon prognosis and clinical management of choroid plexus tumors. J Neurooncol. 2020 May;148(1):39–45. PMID:32342334
3183. Thomas C, Ruland V, Kordes U, et al. Pediatric atypical choroid plexus papilloma reconsidered: increased mitotic activity is prognostic only in older children. Acta Neuropathol. 2015 Jun;129(6):925–7. PMID:25935663
3184. Thomas C, Sill M, Ruland V, et al. Methylation profiling of choroid plexus tumors reveals 3 clinically distinct subgroups. Neuro Oncol. 2016 Jun;18(6):790–6. PMID:26826203
3185. Thomas C, Wefers A, Bens S, et al. Desmoplastic myxoid tumor, SMARCB1-mutant: clinical, histopathological and molecular characterization of a pineal region tumor encountered in adolescents and adults. Acta Neuropathol. 2020 Feb;139(2):277–86. PMID:31732806
3186. Thomas PK, King RH, Chiang TR, et al. Neurofibromatous neuropathy. Muscle Nerve. 1990 Feb;13(2):93–101. PMID:2156160
3187. Thomas RP, Recht L, Nagpal S. Advances in the management of glioblastoma: the role of temozolomide and MGMT testing. Clin Pharmacol. 2013;5:1–9. PMID:23293540
3188. Thommen F, Hewer E, Schäfer SC, et al. Rosette-forming glioneuronal tumor of the cerebellum in statu nascendi: an incidentally detected diminutive example indicates derivation from the internal granule cell layer. Clin Neuropathol. 2013 Sep-Oct;32(5):370–6. PMID:23547894
3189. Thompsett AR, Ellison DW, Stevenson FK, et al. V(H) gene sequences from primary central nervous system lymphomas indicate derivation from highly mutated germinal center B cells with ongoing mutational activity. Blood. 1999 Sep 1;94(5):1738–46. PMID:10477699
3190. Thomson N, Pacak K, Schmidt MH, et al. Leptomeningeal dissemination of a low-grade lumbar paraganglioma: case report. J Neurosurg Spine. 2017 Apr;26(4):501–6. PMID:28128698
3191. Thurston B, Gunny R, Anderson G, et al. Fourth ventricle rosette-forming glioneuronal tumour in children: an unusual presentation in an 8-year-old patient, discussion and review of the literature. Childs Nerv Syst. 2013 May;29(5):839–47. PMID:23239254
3192. Tian L, Li Y, Edmonson MN, et al. CICERO: a versatile method for detecting complex and diverse driver fusions using cancer RNA sequencing data. Genome Biol. 2020 May 28;21(1):126. PMID:32466770
3193. Tian R, Hao S, Hou Z, et al. Clinical characteristics and prognostic analysis of recurrent hemangiopericytoma in the central nervous system: a review of 46 cases. J Neurooncol. 2013 Oct;115(1):53–9. PMID:23824534
3194. Tian Y, Wang J, Ge Jz, et al. Intracranial Rosai-Dorfman disease mimicking multiple meningiomas in a child: a case report and review of the literature. Childs Nerv Syst. 2015 Feb;31(2):317–23. PMID:25183389
3195. Tien RD, Barkovich AJ, Edwards MS. MR imaging of pineal tumors. AJR Am J Roentgenol. 1990 Jul;155(1):143–51. PMID:2162137
3196. Tihan T, Ersen A, Qaddoumi I, et al. Pathologic characteristics of pediatric intracranial pilocytic astrocytomas and their impact on outcome in 3 countries: a multi-institutional study. Am J Surg Pathol. 2012 Jan;36(1):43–55. PMID:21989351
3197. Tihan T, Fisher PG, Kepner JL, et al. Pediatric astrocytomas with monomorphous pilomyxoid features and a less favorable outcome. J Neuropathol Exp Neurol. 1999 Oct;58(10):1061–8. PMID:10515229
3198. Tihan T, Vohra P, Berger MS, et al. Definition and diagnostic implications of gemistocytic astrocytomas: a pathological perspective. J Neurooncol. 2006 Jan;76(2):175–83. PMID:16132490
3199. Tinat J, Bougeard G, Baert-Desurmont S, et al. 2009 version of the Chompret criteria for Li Fraumeni syndrome. J Clin Oncol. 2009 Sep 10;27(26):e108–9. PMID:19652052
3200. Tirabosco R, Mangham DC, Rosenberg AE, et al. Brachyury expression in extra-axial skeletal and soft tissue chordomas: a marker that distinguishes chordoma from mixed tumor/myoepithelioma/parachordoma in soft tissue. Am J Surg Pathol. 2008 Apr;32(4):572–80. PMID:18301055
3201. Tirode F, Surdez D, Ma X, et al. Genomic landscape of Ewing sarcoma defines an aggressive subtype with co-association of STAG2 and TP53 mutations. Cancer Discov.

2014 Nov;4(11):1342–53. PMID:25223734
3202. Tirosh I, Venteicher AS, Hebert C, et al. Single-cell RNA-seq supports a developmental hierarchy in human oligodendroglioma. Nature. 2016 Nov 10;539(7628):309–13. PMID:27806376
3203. Tischkowitz M, Huang S, Banerjee S, et al. Small-cell carcinoma of the ovary, hypercalcemic type-genetics, new treatment targets, and current management guidelines. Clin Cancer Res. 2020 Aug 1;26(15):3908–17. PMID:32156746
3204. Tischkowitz MD, Chisholm J, Gaze M, et al. Medulloblastoma as a first presentation of fanconi anemia. J Pediatr Hematol Oncol. 2004 Jan;26(1):52–5. PMID:14707715
3205. Tish S, Habboub G, Jones J, et al. The epidemiology of central and extraventricular neurocytoma in the United States between 2006 and 2014. J Neurooncol. 2019 May;143(1):123–7. PMID:30859483
3206. Tiwari N, Powell SZ, Takei H. Recurrent subependymoma of fourth ventricle with unusual atypical histological features: a case report. Pathol Int. 2015 Aug;65(8):438–42. PMID:26059172
3207. Tjörnstrand A, Gunnarsson K, Evert M, et al. The incidence rate of pituitary adenomas in western Sweden for the period 2001-2011. Eur J Endocrinol. 2014 Oct;171(4):519–26. PMID:25084775
3208. Toki S, Wakai S, Sekimizu M, et al. PAX7 immunohistochemical evaluation of Ewing sarcoma and other small round cell tumours. Histopathology. 2018 Oct;73(4):645–52. PMID:29920735
3209. Tokumitsu T, Sato Y, Fukushima T, et al. Squash cytology findings of subependymomas: a report of three cases and differential diagnosis. Diagn Cytopathol. 2018 Mar;46(3):258–62. PMID:29024543
3210. Toledano H, Orenstein N, Sofrin E, et al. Paediatric systemic lupus erythematosus as a manifestation of constitutional mismatch repair deficiency. J Med Genet. 2020 Jul;57(7):505–8. PMID:31501241
3211. Tomić TT, Olausson J, Wilzén A, et al. A new GTF2I-BRAF fusion mediating MAPK pathway activation in pilocytic astrocytoma. PLoS One. 2017 Apr 27;12(4):e0175638. PMID:28448514
3212. Tomlinson FH, Scheithauer BW, Kelly PJ, et al. Subependymoma with rhabdomyosarcomatous differentiation: report of a case and literature review. Neurosurgery. 1991 May;28(5):761–8. PMID:1876259
3213. Tomura N, Hirano H, Watanabe O, et al. Central neurocytoma with clinically malignant behavior. AJNR Am J Neuroradiol. 1997 Jun-Jul;18(6):1175–8. PMID:9194446
3214. Tong Y, Merino D, Nimmervoll B, et al. Cross-species genomics identifies TAF12, NFYC, and RAD54L as choroid plexus carcinoma oncogenes. Cancer Cell. 2015 May 11;27(5):712–27. PMID:25965574
3215. Torchia J, Golbourn B, Feng S, et al. Integrated (epi)-genomic analyses identify subgroup-specific therapeutic targets in CNS rhabdoid tumors. Cancer Cell. 2016 Dec 12;30(6):891–908. PMID:27960086
3216. Torchia J, Picard D, Lafay-Cousin L, et al. Molecular subgroups of atypical teratoid rhabdoid tumours in children: an integrated genomic and clinicopathological analysis. Lancet Oncol. 2015 May;16(5):569–82. PMID:25882982
3217. Tordjman KM, Greenman Y, Ram Z, et al. Plurihormonal pituitary tumor of Pit-1 and SF-1 lineages, with synchronous collision corticotroph tumor: a possible stem cell phenomenon. Endocr Pathol. 2019 Mar;30(1):74–80. PMID:30610567
3218. Torre M, Meredith DM, Dubuc A, et al. Recurrent EP300-BCOR fusions in pediatric gliomas with distinct clinicopathologic features. J Neuropathol Exp Neurol. 2019 Apr 1;78(4):305–14. PMID:30816933
3219. Torres-Mora J, Dry S, Li X, et al. Malignant melanotic schwannian tumor: a clinicopathologic, immunohistochemical, and gene expression profiling study of 40 cases, with a proposal for the reclassification of "melanotic schwannoma". Am J Surg Pathol. 2014 Jan;38(1):94–105. PMID:24145644
3220. Tortosa F, Webb SM. Atypical pituitary adenomas: 10 years of experience in a reference centre in Portugal. Neurologia. 2016 Mar;31(2):97–105. PMID:26300499
3221. Touat M, Gratieux J, Condette Auliac S, et al. Vemurafenib and cobimetinib overcome resistance to vemurafenib in BRAF-mutant ganglioglioma. Neurology. 2018 Sep 11;91(11):523–5. PMID:30120137
3222. Touat M, Li YY, Boynton AN, et al. Mechanisms and therapeutic implications of hypermutation in gliomas. Nature. 2020 Apr;580(7804):517–23. PMID:32322066
3223. Trassard M, Le Doussal V, Bui BN, et al. Angiosarcoma arising in a solitary schwannoma (neurilemoma) of the sciatic nerve. Am J Surg Pathol. 1996 Nov;20(11):1412–7. PMID:8898847
3224. Trehan G, Bruge H, Vinchon M, et al. MR imaging in the diagnosis of desmoplastic infantile tumor: retrospective study of six cases. AJNR Am J Neuroradiol. 2004 Jun-Jul;25(6):1028–33. PMID:15205142
3225. Trépant AL, Bouchart C, Rorive S, et al. Identification of OLIG2 as the most specific glioblastoma stem cell marker starting from comparative analysis of data from similar DNA chip microarray platforms. Tumour Biol. 2015 Mar;36(3):1943–53. PMID:25384509
3226. Trisolini E, Wardighi DE, Giry M, et al. Actionable FGFR1 and BRAF mutations in adult circumscribed gliomas. J Neurooncol. 2019 Nov;145(2):241–5. PMID:31673897
3227. Trofatter JA, MacCollin MM, Rutter JL, et al. A novel moesin-, ezrin-, radixin-like gene is a candidate for the neurofibromatosis 2 tumor suppressor. Cell. 1993 Mar 12;72(5):791–800. PMID:8453669
3228. Trouillas J, Jaffrain-Rea ML, Vasiljevic A, et al. Are aggressive pituitary tumors and carcinomas two sides of the same coin? Pathologists reply to clinician's questions. Rev Endocr Metab Disord. 2020 Jun;21(2):243–51. PMID:32504268
3229. Trouillas J, Roy P, Sturm N, et al. A new prognostic clinicopathological classification of pituitary adenomas: a multicentric case-control study of 410 patients with 8 years post-operative follow-up. Acta Neuropathol. 2013 Jul;126(1):123–35. PMID:23400299
3230. Trouillas J, Vasiljevic A, Lapoirie M, et al. Pathological markers of somatotroph pituitary neuroendocrine tumors predicting the response to medical treatment. Minerva Endocrinol. 2019 Jun;44(2):129–36. PMID:30531694
3231. Ts'o MO, Fine BS, Zimmerman LE. The Flexner-Wintersteiner rosettes in retinoblastoma. Arch Pathol. 1969 Dec;88(6):664–71. PMID:5357720
3232. Tsou HC, Teng DH, Ping XL, et al. The role of MMAC1 mutations in early-onset breast cancer: causative in association with Cowden syndrome and excluded in BRCA1-negative cases. Am J Hum Genet. 1997 Nov;61(5):1036–43. PMID:9345101
3233. Tsuchida T, Matsumoto M, Shirayama Y, et al. Neuronal and glial characteristics of central neurocytoma: electron microscopical analysis of two cases. Acta Neuropathol. 1996;91(6):573–7. PMID:8781655
3234. Tsukamoto K, Murakami M, Seo Y, et al. Energetic recovery from hypothermic preservation in the rat liver. J Surg Res. 1990 Jan;48(1):46–50. PMID:2296180
3235. Tsumanuma I, Tanaka R, Washiyama K. Clinicopathological study of pineal parenchymal tumors: correlation between histopathological features, proliferative potential, and prognosis. Brain Tumor Pathol. 1999;16(2):61–8. PMID:10746962
3236. Tsuyuguchi S, Sugiyama K, Kinoshita Y, et al. Primary and recurrent growing teratoma syndrome in central nervous system nongerminomatous germ cell tumors: case series and review of the literature. World Neurosurg. 2020 Feb;134:e360–71. PMID:31751614
3237. Tu PH, Giannini C, Judkins AR, et al. Clinicopathologic and genetic profile of intracranial marginal zone lymphoma: a primary low-grade CNS lymphoma that mimics meningioma. J Clin Oncol. 2005 Aug 20;23(24):5718–27. PMID:16009945
3238. Tumaitis TD, Lane BG. Differential labelling of the carboxymethyl and methyl substituents of 5-carboxymethyluridine methyl ester, a trace nucleoside constituent of yeast transfer RNA. Biochim Biophys Acta. 1970 Dec 14;224(2):391–403. PMID:5498072
3239. Turcan S, Makarov V, Taranda J, et al. Mutant-IDH1-dependent chromatin state reprogramming, reversibility, and persistence. Nat Genet. 2018 Jan;50(1):62–72. PMID:29180699
3240. Turcan S, Rohle D, Goenka A, et al. IDH1 mutation is sufficient to establish the glioma hypermethylator phenotype. Nature. 2012 Feb 15;483(7390):479–83. PMID:22343889
3241. Turchini J, Cheung VKY, Tischler AS, et al. Pathology and genetics of phaeochromocytoma and paraganglioma. Histopathology. 2018 Jan;72(1):97–105. PMID:29239044
3242. Turchini J, Gill AJ. Morphologic clues to succinate dehydrogenase (SDH) deficiency in pheochromocytomas and paragangliomas. Am J Surg Pathol. 2020 Mar;44(3):422–4. PMID:31789631
3243. Turchini J, Sioson L, Clarkson A, et al. Utility of GATA-3 expression in the analysis of Pituitary Neuroendocrine Tumour (PitNET) transcription factors. Endocr Pathol. 2020 Jun;31(2):150–5. PMID:32193825
3244. Turkoglu E, Kertmen H, Sanli AM, et al. Clinical outcome of adult choroid plexus tumors: retrospective analysis of a single institute. Acta Neurochir (Wien). 2014 Aug;156(8):1461–8. PMID:24866474
3245. Turner AL, D'Souza P, Belirgen M, et al. Atypical presentation of multinodular and vacuolating neuronal tumor of the cerebrum in a boy. J Neurosci Rural Pract. 2020 Jan;11(1):214–5. PMID:32140033
3246. Tyburczy ME, Dies KA, Glass J, et al. Mosaic and intronic mutations in TSC1/TSC2 explain the majority of TSC patients with no mutation identified by conventional testing. PLoS Genet. 2015 Nov 5;11(11):e1005637. PMID:26540169
3247. Ud Din N, Memon A, Aftab K, et al. Oligodendroglioma arising in the glial component of ovarian teratomas: a series of six cases and review of literature. J Clin Pathol. 2012 Jul;65(7):631–4. PMID:22496515
3248. Ueba T, Okawa M, Abe H, et al. Central nervous system marginal zone B-cell lymphoma of mucosa-associated lymphoid tissue type involving the brain and spinal cord parenchyma. Neuropathology. 2013 Jun;33(3):306–11. PMID:22994302
3249. Ueki K, Ono Y, Henson JW, et al. CDKN2/p16 or RB alterations occur in the majority of glioblastomas and are inversely correlated. Cancer Res. 1996 Jan 1;56(1):150–3. PMID:8548755
3250. Ueno-Yokohata H, Okita H, Nakasato K, et al. Consistent in-frame internal tandem duplications of BCOR characterize clear cell sarcoma of the kidney. Nat Genet. 2015 Aug;47(8):861–3. PMID:26098867
3251. UICC [Internet]. Geneva (Switzerland): Union for International Cancer Control; 2020. TNM Publications and Resources – Errata; updated 2020 Oct 6. Available from: https://www.uicc.org/resources/tnm/publications-resources.
3252. Ulbright TM, Hattab EM, Zhang S, et al. Primitive neuroectodermal tumors in patients with testicular germ cell tumors usually resemble pediatric-type central nervous system embryonal neoplasms and lack chromosome 22 rearrangements. Mod Pathol. 2010 Jul;23(7):972–80. PMID:20348883
3253. Umphlett M, Shea S, Tome-Garcia J, et al. Widely metastatic glioblastoma with BRCA1 and ARID1A mutations: a case report. BMC Cancer. 2020 Jan 20;20(1):47. PMID:31959133
3254. Uneda A, Kurozumi K, Fujimura A, et al. Intracranial mesenchymal chondrosarcoma lacking the typical histopathological features diagnosed by HEY1-NCOA2 gene fusion. NMC Case Rep J. 2020 Mar 24;7(2):47–52. PMID:32322450
3255. Uno K, Takita J, Yokomori K, et al. Aberrations of the hSNF5/INI1 gene are restricted to malignant rhabdoid tumors or atypical teratoid/rhabdoid tumors in pediatric solid tumors. Genes Chromosomes Cancer. 2002 May;34(1):33–41. PMID:11921280
3256. Unruh D, Schwarze SR, Khoury L, et al. Mutant IDH1 and thrombosis in gliomas. Acta Neuropathol. 2016 Dec;132(6):917–30. PMID:27664011
3257. Upadhyaya M, Huson SM, Davies M, et al. An absence of cutaneous neurofibromas associated with a 3-bp inframe deletion in exon 17 of the NF1 gene (c.2970-2972 delAAT): evidence of a clinically significant NF1 genotype-phenotype correlation. Am J Hum Genet. 2007 Jan;80(1):140–51. PMID:17160901
3258. Upadhyaya SA, Robinson GW, Onar-Thomas A, et al. Molecular grouping and outcomes of young children with newly diagnosed ependymoma treated on the multi-institutional SJYC07 trial. Neuro Oncol. 2019 Oct 9;21(10):1319–30. PMID:30976811
3259. Uro-Coste E, Masliah-Planchon J, Siegfried A, et al. ETMR-like infantile cerebellar embryonal tumors in the extended morphologic spectrum of DICER1-related tumors. Acta Neuropathol. 2019 Jan;137(1):175–7. PMID:30446821
3260. Uusitalo E, Leppävirta J, Koffert A, et al. Incidence and mortality of neurofibromatosis: a total population study in Finland. J Invest Dermatol. 2015 Mar;135(3):904–6. PMID:25354145
3261. Vajtai I, Beck J, Kappeler A, et al. Spindle cell oncocytoma of the pituitary gland with follicle-like component: organotypic differentiation to support its origin from folliculo-stellate cells. Acta Neuropathol. 2011 Aug;122(2):253–8. PMID:21590491
3262. Valdez R, McKeever P, Finn WG, et al. Composite germ cell tumor and B-cell non-Hodgkin's lymphoma arising in the sella turcica. Hum Pathol. 2002 Oct;33(10):1044–7. PMID:12395379
3263. Valera ET, McConechy MK, Gayden T, et al. Methylome analysis and whole-exome sequencing reveal that brain tumors associated with encephalocraniocutaneous lipomatosis are midline pilocytic astrocytomas. Acta Neuropathol. 2018 Oct;136(4):657–60. PMID:30143858
3264. Valera ET, Neder L, Queiroz RG, et al. Perinatal complex low- and high-grade glial tumor harboring a novel GIGYF2-ALK fusion. Pediatr Blood Cancer. 2020 Jan;67(1):e28015.

PMID:31556208
3265. Valiente M, Ahluwalia MS, Boire A, et al. The evolving landscape of brain metastasis. Trends Cancer. 2018 Mar;4(3):176–96. PMID:29506669
3266. Vallat-Decouvelaere AV, Wassef M, Lot G, et al. Spinal melanotic schwannoma: a tumour with poor prognosis. Histopathology. 1999 Dec;35(6):558–66. PMID:10583580
3267. Valle L, Hernández-Illán E, Bellido F, et al. New insights into POLE and POLD1 germline mutations in familial colorectal cancer and polyposis. Hum Mol Genet. 2014 Jul 1;23(13):3506–12. PMID:24501277
3268. van de Nes J, Gessi M, Sucker A, et al. Targeted next generation sequencing reveals unique mutation profile of primary melanocytic tumors of the central nervous system. J Neurooncol. 2016 May;127(3):435–44. PMID:26744134
3269. van de Nes J, Wrede K, Ringelstein A, et al. Diagnosing a primary leptomeningeal melanoma by gene mutation signature. J Invest Dermatol. 2016 Jul;136(7):1526–8. PMID:27060446
3270. van de Nes JA, Nelles J, Kreis S, et al. Comparing the prognostic value of BAP1 mutation pattern, chromosome 3 status, and BAP1 immunohistochemistry in uveal melanoma. Am J Surg Pathol. 2016 Jun;40(6):796–805. PMID:27015033
3271. van de Nes JAP, Koelsche C, Gessi M, et al. Activating CYSLTR2 and PLCB4 mutations in primary leptomeningeal melanocytic tumors. J Invest Dermatol. 2017 Sep;137(9):2033–5. PMID:28499758
3272. van den Bent MJ, Afra D, de Witte O, et al. Long-term efficacy of early versus delayed radiotherapy for low-grade astrocytoma and oligodendroglioma in adults: the EORTC 22845 randomised trial. Lancet. 2005 Sep 17-23;366(9490):985–90. PMID:16168780
3273. van den Bent MJ, Brandes AA, Taphoorn MJ, et al. Adjuvant procarbazine, lomustine, and vincristine chemotherapy in newly diagnosed anaplastic oligodendroglioma: long-term follow-up of EORTC brain tumor group study 26951. J Clin Oncol. 2013 Jan 20;31(3):344–50. PMID:23071237
3274. van den Bent MJ, Carpentier AF, Brandes AA, et al. Adjuvant procarbazine, lomustine, and vincristine improves progression-free survival but not overall survival in newly diagnosed anaplastic oligodendrogliomas and oligoastrocytomas: a randomized European Organisation for Research and Treatment of Cancer phase III trial. J Clin Oncol. 2006 Jun 20;24(18):2715–22. PMID:16782911
3275. Van den Bent MJ, Reni M, Gatta G, et al. Oligodendroglioma. Crit Rev Oncol Hematol. 2008 Jun;66(3):262–72. PMID:18272388
3276. van den Bent MJ, Smits M, Kros JM, et al. Diffuse infiltrating oligodendroglioma and astrocytoma. J Clin Oncol. 2017 Jul 20;35(21):2394–401. PMID:28640702
3277. van den Bent MJ, Wefel JS, Schiff D, et al. Response assessment in neuro-oncology (a report of the RANO group): assessment of outcome in trials of diffuse low-grade gliomas. Lancet Oncol. 2011 Jun;12(6):583–93. PMID:21474379
3278. van den Munckhof P, Christiaans I, Kenter SB, et al. Germline SMARCB1 mutation predisposes to multiple meningiomas and schwannomas with preferential location of cranial meningiomas at the falx cerebri. Neurogenetics. 2012 Feb;13(1):1–7. PMID:22038540
3279. van der Voort SR, Incekara F, Wijnenga MMJ, et al. Predicting the 1p/19q codeletion status of presumed low-grade glioma with an externally validated machine learning algorithm. Clin Cancer Res. 2019 Dec 15;25(24):7455–62. PMID:31548344
3280. van Engelen K, Villani A, Wasserman JD, et al. DICER1 syndrome: approach to testing and management at a large pediatric tertiary care center. Pediatr Blood Cancer. 2018 Jan;65(1). PMID:28960912
3281. van Engen-van Grunsven AC, Rabold K, Küsters-Vandevelde HV, et al. Copy number variations as potential diagnostic and prognostic markers for CNS melanocytic neoplasms in neurocutaneous melanosis. Acta Neuropathol. 2017 Feb;133(2):333–5. PMID:27988846
3282. van Iersel L, Brokke KE, Adan RAH, et al. Pathophysiology and individualized treatment of hypothalamic obesity following craniopharyngioma and other suprasellar tumors: a systematic review. Endocr Rev. 2019 Feb 1;40(1):193–235. PMID:30247642
3283. van Nederveen FH, Gaal J, Favier J, et al. An immunohistochemical procedure to detect patients with paraganglioma and phaeochromocytoma with germline SDHB, SDHC, or SDHD gene mutations: a retrospective and prospective analysis. Lancet Oncol. 2009 Aug;10(8):764–71. PMID:19576851
3284. van Schaijik B, Wickremesekera AC, Mantamadiotis T, et al. Circulating tumor stem cells and glioblastoma: a review. J Clin Neurosci. 2019 Mar;61:5–9. PMID:30622004
3285. van Slegtenhorst M, de Hoogt R, Hermans C, et al. Identification of the tuberous sclerosis gene TSC1 on chromosome 9q34. Science. 1997 Aug 8;277(5327):805–8. PMID:9242607
3286. van Slegtenhorst M, Verhoef S, Tempelaars A, et al. Mutational spectrum of the TSC1 gene in a cohort of 225 tuberous sclerosis complex patients: no evidence for genotype-phenotype correlation. J Med Genet. 1999 Apr;36(4):285–9. PMID:10227394
3287. VandenBerg SR. Desmoplastic infantile ganglioglioma and desmoplastic cerebral astrocytoma of infancy. Brain Pathol. 1993 Jul;3(3):275–81. PMID:8293187
3288. VandenBerg SR, May EE, Rubinstein LJ, et al. Desmoplastic supratentorial neuroepithelial tumors of infancy with divergent differentiation potential ("desmoplastic infantile gangliogliomas"). Report on 11 cases of a distinctive embryonal tumor with favorable prognosis. J Neurosurg. 1987 Jan;66(1):58–71. PMID:3097276
3289. Vandeva S, Daly AF, Petrossians P, et al. Somatic and germline mutations in the pathogenesis of pituitary adenomas. Eur J Endocrinol. 2019 Dec;181(6):R235–54. PMID:31658440
3290. Van Effenterre R, Boch AL. Craniopharyngioma in adults and children: a study of 122 surgical cases. J Neurosurg. 2002 Jul;97(1):3–11. PMID:12134929
3291. Vanneste R, Smith E, Graham G. Multiple neurofibromas as the presenting feature of familial atypical multiple malignant melanoma (FAMMM) syndrome. Am J Med Genet A. 2013 Jun;161A(6):1425–31. PMID:23613284
3292. Varlet P, Le Teuff G, Le Deley MC, et al. WHO grade has no prognostic value in the pediatric high-grade glioma included in the HERBY trial. Neuro Oncol. 2020 Jan 11;22(1):116–27. PMID:31419298
3293. Varma A, Giraldi D, Mills S, et al. Surgical management and long-term outcome of intracranial subependymoma. Acta Neurochir (Wien). 2018 Sep;160(9):1793–9. PMID:29915887
3294. Vasen HF, Ghorbanoghli Z, Bourdeaut F, et al. Guidelines for surveillance of individuals with constitutional mismatch repair-deficiency proposed by the European Consortium "Care for CMMR-D" (C4CMMR-D). J Med Genet. 2014 May;51(5):283–93. PMID:24556086
3295. Vasiljevic A, Champier J, Figarella-Branger D, et al. Molecular characterization of central neurocytomas: potential markers for tumor typing and progression. Neuropathology. 2013 Apr;33(2):149–61. PMID:22816789
3296. Vasiljevic A, François P, Loundou A, et al. Prognostic factors in central neurocytomas: a multicenter study of 71 cases. Am J Surg Pathol. 2012 Feb;36(2):220–7. PMID:22251941
3297. Vasovčák P, Senkeříková M, Hatlová J, et al. Multiple primary malignancies and subtle mucocutaneous lesions associated with a novel PTEN gene mutation in a patient with Cowden syndrome: case report. BMC Med Genet. 2011 Mar 15;12:38. PMID:21406108
3298. Vater I, Montesinos-Rongen M, Schlesner M, et al. The mutational pattern of primary lymphoma of the central nervous system determined by whole-exome sequencing. Leukemia. 2015 Mar;29(3):677–85. PMID:25189415
3299. Vaubel R, Zschernack V, Tran QT, et al. Biology and grading of pleomorphic xanthoastrocytoma-what have we learned about it? Brain Pathol. 2021 Jan;31(1):20–32. PMID:32619305
3300. Vaubel RA, Caron AA, Yamada S, et al. Recurrent copy number alterations in low-grade and anaplastic pleomorphic xanthoastrocytoma with and without BRAF V600E mutation. Brain Pathol. 2018 Mar;28(2):172–82. PMID:28181325
3301. Vaubel RA, Chen SG, Raleigh DR, et al. Meningiomas with rhabdoid features lacking other histologic features of malignancy: a study of 44 cases and review of the literature. J Neuropathol Exp Neurol. 2016 Jan;75(1):44–52. PMID:26705409
3302. Vege KD, Giannini C, Scheithauer BW. The immunophenotype of ependymomas. Appl Immunohistochem Mol Morphol. 2000 Mar;8(1):25–31. PMID:10937045
3303. Velázquez Vega JE, Brat DJ. Incorporating advances in molecular pathology into brain tumor diagnostics. Adv Anat Pathol. 2018 May;25(3):143–71. PMID:29521646
3304. Velz J, Agaimy A, Frontzek K, et al. Molecular and clinicopathologic heterogeneity of intracranial tumors mimicking extraskeletal myxoid chondrosarcoma. J Neuropathol Exp Neurol. 2018 Aug 1;77(8):727–35. PMID:29924341
3305. Venencie PY, Boffa GA, Delmas PD, et al. Pachydermoperiostosis with gastric hypertrophy, anemia, and increased serum bone Gla-protein levels. Arch Dermatol. 1988 Dec;124(12):1831–4. PMID:3263841
3306. Venkataraman G, Rizzo KA, Chavez JJ, et al. Marginal zone lymphomas involving meningeal dura: possible link to IgG4-related diseases. Mod Pathol. 2011 Mar;24(3):355–66. PMID:21102421
3307. Venkatesh HS, Morishita W, Geraghty AC, et al. Electrical and synaptic integration of glioma into neural circuits. Nature. 2019 Sep;573(7775):539–45. PMID:31534222
3308. Venneti S, Santi M, Felicella MM, et al. A sensitive and specific histopathologic prognostic marker for H3F3A K27M mutant pediatric glioblastomas. Acta Neuropathol. 2014 Nov;128(5):743–53. PMID:25200322
3309. Venteicher AS, Tirosh I, Hebert C, et al. Decoupling genetics, lineages, and microenvironment in IDH-mutant gliomas by single-cell RNA-seq. Science. 2017 Mar 31;355(6332):eaai8478. PMID:28360267
3310. Ventii KH, Devi NS, Friedrich KL, et al. BRCA1-associated protein-1 is a tumor suppressor that requires deubiquitinating activity and nuclear localization. Cancer Res. 2008 Sep 1;68(17):6953–62. PMID:18757409
3311. Vera-Bolanos E, Aldape K, Yuan Y, et al. Clinical course and progression-free survival of adult intracranial and spinal ependymoma patients. Neuro Oncol. 2015 Mar;17(3):440–7. PMID:25121770
3312. Veraldi N, Parra A, Urso E, et al. Structural features of heparan sulfate from multiple osteochondromas and chondrosarcomas. Molecules. 2018 Dec 11;23(12):E3277. PMID:30544937
3313. Verdijk RM, den Bakker MA, Dubbink HJ, et al. TP53 mutation analysis of malignant peripheral nerve sheath tumors. J Neuropathol Exp Neurol. 2010 Jan;69(1):16–26. PMID:20010306
3314. Vergeer RA, Vink R, Avenarius JK, et al. A 71-year-old woman with an intracranial dural-based mesenchymal chondrosarcoma. J Clin Neurosci. 2012 Aug;19(8):1170–1. PMID:22658242
3315. Verhaak RG, Hoadley KA, Purdom E, et al. Integrated genomic analysis identifies clinically relevant subtypes of glioblastoma characterized by abnormalities in PDGFRA, IDH1, EGFR, and NF1. Cancer Cell. 2010 Jan 19;17(1):98–110. PMID:20129251
3316. Vernooij MW, Ikram MA, Tanghe HL, et al. Incidental findings on brain MRI in the general population. N Engl J Med. 2007 Nov 1;357(18):1821–8. PMID:17978290
3317. Veronese F, Miglino B, Boggio P, et al. Gorlin-Goltz syndrome: a case series from north Italy. Eur J Dermatol. 2018 Oct 1;28(5):687–8. PMID:30129523
3318. Versteege I, Sévenet N, Lange J, et al. Truncating mutations of hSNF5/INI1 in aggressive paediatric cancer. Nature. 1998 Jul 9;394(6689):203–6. PMID:9671307
3319. Verstegen MJ, van den Munckhof P, Troost D, et al. Multiple meningiomas in a patient with Rubinstein-Taybi syndrome. Case report. J Neurosurg. 2005 Jan;102(1):167–8. PMID:15658110
3320. Vettermann FJ, Felsberg J, Reifenberger G, et al. Characterization of diffuse gliomas with histone H3-G34 mutation by MRI and dynamic 18F-FET PET. Clin Nucl Med. 2018 Dec;43(12):895–8. PMID:30358620
3321. Veugelers M, Wilkes D, Burton K, et al. Comparative PRKAR1A genotype-phenotype analyses in humans with Carney complex and prkar1a haploinsufficient mice. Proc Natl Acad Sci U S A. 2004 Sep 28;101(39):14222–7. PMID:15371594
3322. Viaene AN, Lee EB, Nasrallah MP. Intraoperative cytology of pituicytomas. Diagn Cytopathol. 2020 Apr;48(4):342–9. PMID:31883319
3323. Viaene AN, Lee EB, Rosenbaum JN, et al. Histologic, immunohistochemical, and molecular features of pituicytomas and atypical pituicytomas. Acta Neuropathol Commun. 2019 May 2;7(1):69. PMID:31046843
3324. Vij M, Krishnani N, Agrawal V, et al. Cytomorphology of intraparenchymal mesenchymal chondrosarcoma in frontal lobe: report of a case. Diagn Cytopathol. 2011 Nov;39(11):837–42. PMID:21994195
3325. Villà S, Miller RC, Krengli M, et al. Primary pineal tumors: outcome and prognostic factors–a study from the Rare Cancer Network (RCN). Clin Transl Oncol. 2012 Nov;14(11):827–34. PMID:22914906
3326. Villani A, Shore A, Wasserman JD, et al. Biochemical and imaging surveillance in germline TP53 mutation carriers with Li-Fraumeni syndrome: 11 year follow-up of a prospective observational study. Lancet Oncol. 2016 Sep;17(9):1295–305. PMID:27501770
3327. Villano JL, Koshy M, Shaikh H, et al. Age, gender, and racial differences in incidence and survival in primary CNS lymphoma. Br J Cancer. 2011 Oct 25;105(9):1414–8. PMID:21915121
3328. Villaume MT, Patel D, Lopez C, et al. Dural marginal zone lymphoma in a patient with a hepatitis C virus infection. World J Oncol.

2020 Jun;11(3):122–5. PMID:32494320
3329. Villegas VM, Hess DJ, Wildner A, et al. Retinoblastoma. Curr Opin Ophthalmol. 2013 Nov;24(6):581–8. PMID:24100372
3330. Villeneuve PJ, Agnew DA, Johnson KC, et al. Brain cancer and occupational exposure to magnetic fields among men: results from a Canadian population-based case-control study. Int J Epidemiol. 2002 Feb;31(1):210–7. PMID:11914323
3331. Vinchon M, Blond S, Lejeune JP, et al. Association of Lhermitte-Duclos and Cowden disease: report of a new case and review of the literature. J Neurol Neurosurg Psychiatry. 1994 Jun;57(6):699–704. PMID:8006650
3332. Vinci M, Burford A, Molinari V, et al. Functional diversity and cooperativity between subclonal populations of pediatric glioblastoma and diffuse intrinsic pontine glioma cells. Nat Med. 2018 Aug;24(8):1204–15. PMID:29967352
3333. Vinters HV, Park SH, Johnson MW, et al. Cortical dysplasia, genetic abnormalities and neurocutaneous syndromes. Dev Neurosci. 1999 Nov;21(3-5):248–59. PMID:10575248
3334. Viskochil D, Buchberg AM, Xu G, et al. Deletions and a translocation interrupt a cloned gene at the neurofibromatosis type 1 locus. Cell. 1990 Jul 13;62(1):187–92. PMID:1694727
3335. Visser J, Hukin J, Sargent M, et al. Late mortality in pediatric patients with craniopharyngioma. J Neurooncol. 2010 Oct;100(1):105–11. PMID:20204458
3336. Vivekanandan S, Dickinson P, Bessell E, et al. An unusual case of primary anaplastic large cell central nervous system lymphoma: an 8-year success story. BMJ Case Rep. 2011 Feb 24;2011:bcr1120103550. PMID:22707580
3337. Vizcaino MA, Palsgrove DN, Yuan M, et al. Granular cell astrocytoma: an aggressive IDH-wildtype diffuse glioma with molecular genetic features of primary glioblastoma. Brain Pathol. 2019 Mar;29(2):193–204. PMID:30222900
3338. Vladoiu MC, El-Hamamy I, Donovan LK, et al. Childhood cerebellar tumours mirror conserved fetal transcriptional programs. Nature. 2019 Aug;572(7767):67–73. PMID:31043743
3339. Vogazianou AP, Chan R, Bäcklund LM, et al. Distinct patterns of 1p and 19q alterations identify subtypes of human gliomas that have different prognoses. Neuro Oncol. 2010 Jul;12(7):664–78. PMID:20164239
3340. Vogels R, Macagno N, Griewank K, et al. Prognostic significance of NAB2-STAT6 fusion variants and TERT promotor mutations in solitary fibrous tumors/hemangiopericytomas of the CNS: not (yet) clear. Acta Neuropathol. 2019 Apr;137(4):679–82. PMID:30761420
3341. Vogt J, Wagener R, Montesinos-Rongen M, et al. Array-based profiling of the lymphoma cell DNA methylome does not unequivocally distinguish primary lymphomas of the central nervous system from non-CNS diffuse large B-cell lymphomas. Genes Chromosomes Cancer. 2019 Jan;58(1):66–9. PMID:30284345
3342. Volkow ND, Tomasi D, Wang GJ, et al. Effects of cell phone radiofrequency signal exposure on brain glucose metabolism. JAMA. 2011 Feb 23;305(8):808–13. PMID:21343580
3343. Voltaggio L, Murray R, Lasota J, et al. Gastric schwannoma: a clinicopathologic study of 51 cases and critical review of the literature. Hum Pathol. 2012 May;43(5):650–9. PMID:22137423
3344. von Deimling A, Janzer R, Kleihues P, et al. Patterns of differentiation in central neurocytoma. An immunohistochemical study of eleven biopsies. Acta Neuropathol. 1990;79(5):473–9. PMID:2109481
3345. von Deimling A, Kleihues P, Saremaslani P, et al. Histogenesis and differentiation potential of central neurocytomas. Lab Invest. 1991 Apr;64(4):585–91. PMID:1901927
3346. von Deimling A, Ono T, Shirahata M, et al. Grading of diffuse astrocytic gliomas: a review of studies before and after the advent of IDH testing. Semin Neurol. 2018 Feb;38(1):19–23. PMID:29548048
3347. von Hoff K, Hinkes B, Dannenmann-Stern E, et al. Frequency, risk-factors and survival of children with atypical teratoid rhabdoid tumors (AT/RT) of the CNS diagnosed between 1988 and 2004, and registered to the German HIT database. Pediatr Blood Cancer. 2011 Dec 1;57(6):978–85. PMID:21796761
3348. von Spreckelsen N, Waldt N, Poetschke R, et al. KLF4K409Q-mutated meningiomas show enhanced hypoxia signaling and respond to mTORC1 inhibitor treatment. Acta Neuropathol Commun. 2020 Apr 3;8(1):41. PMID:32245394
3349. von Witzleben A, Goerttler LT, Lennerz J, et al. In chordoma, metastasis, recurrences, Ki-67 index, and a matrix-poor phenotype are associated with patients' shorter overall survival. Eur Spine J. 2016 Dec;25(12):4016–24. PMID:26399506
3349A. Vortmeyer AO, Falke EA, Gläsker S, et al. Nervous system involvement in von Hippel-Lindau disease: pathology and mechanisms. Acta Neuropathol. 2013 Mar;125(3):333–50. PMID:23400300
3350. Vortmeyer AO, Frank S, Jeong SY, et al. Developmental arrest of angioblastic lineage initiates tumorigenesis in von Hippel-Lindau disease. Cancer Res. 2003 Nov 1;63(21):7051–5. PMID:14612494
3351. Vortmeyer AO, Tran MG, Zeng W, et al. Evolution of VHL tumourigenesis in nerve root tissue. J Pathol. 2006 Nov;210(3):374–82. PMID:16981244
3352. Vortmeyer AO, Yuan Q, Lee YS, et al. Developmental effects of von Hippel-Lindau gene deficiency. Ann Neurol. 2004 May;55(5):721–8. PMID:15122713
3353. Wadt KA, Aoude LG, Johansson P, et al. A recurrent germline BAP1 mutation and extension of the BAP1 tumor predisposition spectrum to include basal cell carcinoma. Clin Genet. 2015 Sep;88(3):267–72. PMID:25225168
3354. Waitkus MS, Pirozzi CJ, Moure CJ, et al. Adaptive evolution of the GDH2 allosteric domain promotes gliomagenesis by resolving IDH1R132H-induced metabolic liabilities. Cancer Res. 2018 Jan 1;78(1):36–50. PMID:29097607
3355. Wakamatsu T, Matsuo T, Kawano S, et al. Glioblastoma with extracranial metastasis through ventriculopleural shunt. Case report. J Neurosurg. 1971 May;34(5):697–701. PMID:4326303
3356. Walker C, Baborie A, Crooks D, et al. Biology, genetics and imaging of glial cell tumours. Br J Radiol. 2011 Dec;84 Spec No 2(Spec Iss 2):S90–106. PMID:22433833
3357. Walker C, Joyce KA, Thompson-Hehir J, et al. Characterisation of molecular alterations in microdissected archival gliomas. Acta Neuropathol. 2001 Apr;101(4):321–33. PMID:11355303
3358. Walker EV, Davis FG, CBTR founding affiliates. Malignant primary brain and other central nervous system tumors diagnosed in Canada from 2009 to 2013. Neuro Oncol. 2019 Feb 19;21(3):360–9. PMID:30649461
3359. Wallace AJ, Watson CJ, Oward E, et al. Mutation scanning of the NF2 gene: an improved service based on meta-PCR/sequencing, dosage analysis, and loss of heterozygosity analysis. Genet Test. 2004 Winter;8(4):368–80. PMID:15684865
3360. Wallace MR, Marchuk DA, Andersen LB, et al. Type 1 neurofibromatosis gene: identification of a large transcript disrupted in three NF1 patients. Science. 1990 Jul 13;249(4965):181–6. PMID:2134734
3361. Walpole S, Pritchard AL, Cebulla CM, et al. Comprehensive study of the clinical phenotype of germline BAP1 variant-carrying families worldwide. J Natl Cancer Inst. 2018 Dec 1;110(12):1328–41. PMID:30517737
3362. Wan YCE, Liu J, Chan KM. Histone H3 Mutations in Cancer. Curr Pharmacol Rep. 2018;4(4):292–300. PMID:30101054
3363. Wanebo JE, Lonser RR, Glenn GM, et al. The natural history of hemangioblastomas of the central nervous system in patients with von Hippel-Lindau disease. J Neurosurg. 2003 Jan;98(1):82–94. PMID:12546356
3364. Wang AC, Jones DTW, Abecassis IJ, et al. Desmoplastic infantile ganglioglioma/astrocytoma (DIG/DIA) are distinct entities with frequent BRAFV600 mutations. Mol Cancer Res. 2018 Oct;16(10):1491–8. PMID:30006355
3365. Wang B, Jin H, Zhao Y, et al. The clinical diagnosis and management options for intracranial juvenile xanthogranuloma in children: based on four cases and another 39 patients in the literature. Acta Neurochir (Wien). 2016 Jul;158(7):1289–97. PMID:27173098
3366. Wang B, Krall EB, Aguirre AJ, et al. ATXN1L, CIC, and ETS transcription factors modulate sensitivity to MAPK pathway inhibition. Cell Rep. 2017 Feb 7;18(6):1543–57. PMID:28178529
3367. Wang F, He Y, Li C, et al. Malignant craniopharyngioma: a report of seven cases and review of the literature. World Neurosurg. 2020 Mar;135:e194–201. PMID:31785438
3368. Wang G, Zhang X, Feng M, et al. Comparing survival outcomes of gross total resection and subtotal resection with radiotherapy for craniopharyngioma: a meta-analysis. J Surg Res. 2018 Jun;226:131–9. PMID:29661278
3369. Wang GX, Mu YD, Che JY, et al. Compressive myelopathy and compression fracture of aggressive vertebral hemangioma after parturition: a case report and review of literature. Medicine (Baltimore). 2019 Dec;98(50):e18285. PMID:31852104
3370. Wang H, Zhang S, Wu C, et al. Melanocytomas of the central nervous system: a clinicopathological and molecular study. Eur J Clin Invest. 2013 Aug;43(8):809–15. PMID:23683178
3371. Wang HW, Wu YH, Hsieh JY, et al. Pediatric primary central nervous system germ cell tumors of different prognosis groups show characteristic miRNome traits and chromosome copy number variations. BMC Genomics. 2010 Feb 24;11:132. PMID:20178649
3372. Wang J, Cazzato E, Ladewig E, et al. Clonal evolution of glioblastoma under therapy. Nat Genet. 2016 Jul;48(7):768–76. PMID:27270107
3373. Wang J, Liu Z, Fang J, et al. Atypical teratoid/rhabdoid tumors with multilayered rosettes in the pineal region. Brain Tumor Pathol. 2016 Oct;33(4):261–6. PMID:27307151
3374. Wang L, Yamaguchi S, Burstein MD, et al. Novel somatic and germline mutations in intracranial germ cell tumours. Nature. 2014 Jul 10;511(7508):241–5. PMID:24896186
3375. Wang L, Zehir A, Sadowska J, et al. Consistent copy number changes and recurrent PRKAR1A mutations distinguish melanotic schwannomas from melanomas: SNP-array and next generation sequencing analysis. Genes Chromosomes Cancer. 2015 Aug;54(8):463–71. PMID:26031761
3376. Wang M, Jia D, Shen J, et al. Clinical and imaging features of central neurocytomas. J Clin Neurosci. 2013 May;20(5):679–85. PMID:23522930
3377. Wang M, Tihan T, Rojiani AM, et al. Monomorphous angiocentric glioma: a distinctive epileptogenic neoplasm with features of infiltrating astrocytoma and ependymoma. J Neuropathol Exp Neurol. 2005 Oct;64(10):875–81. PMID:16215459
3378. Wang M, Zhang R, Liu X, et al. Supratentorial extraventricular ependymomas: a retrospective study focused on long-term outcomes and prognostic factors. Clin Neurol Neurosurg. 2018 Feb;165:1–6. PMID:29253745
3379. Wang M, Zhou P, Zhang S, et al. Clinical features, treatment, and long-term outcomes of central neurocytoma: a 20-year experience at a single center. World Neurosurg. 2018 Jan;109:e59–66. PMID:28958923
3380. Wang PF, Ji WJ, Zhang XH, et al. Allergy reduces the risk of meningioma: a meta-analysis. Sci Rep. 2017 Jan 10;7:40333. PMID:28071746
3381. Wang Q, Hu B, Hu X, et al. Tumor evolution of glioma-intrinsic gene expression subtypes associates with immunological changes in the microenvironment. Cancer Cell. 2017 Jul 10;32(1):42–56.e6. PMID:28697342
3382. Wang X, Dubuc AM, Ramaswamy V, et al. Medulloblastoma subgroups remain stable across primary and metastatic compartments. Acta Neuropathol. 2015 Mar;129(3):449–57. PMID:25689980
3383. Wang X, Lee RS, Alver BH, et al. SMARCB1-mediated SWI/SNF complex function is essential for enhancer regulation. Nat Genet. 2017 Feb;49(2):289–95. PMID:27941797
3384. Wang XQ, Zhou Q, Li ST, et al. Solitary fibrous tumors of the central nervous system: clinical features and imaging findings in 22 patients. J Comput Assist Tomogr. 2013 Sep-Oct;37(5):658–65. PMID:24045237
3385. Wang Y, Li M, Deng H, et al. The systems of metastatic potential prediction in pheochromocytoma and paraganglioma. Am J Cancer Res. 2020 Mar 1;10(3):769–80. PMID:32266090
3386. Wang Y, Xiong J, Chu SG, et al. Rosette-forming glioneuronal tumor: report of an unusual case with intraventricular dissemination. Acta Neuropathol. 2009 Dec;118(6):813–9. PMID:19585134
3387. Wang Y, Yang J, Wild AT, et al. G-quadruplex DNA drives genomic instability and represents a targetable molecular abnormality in ATRX-deficient malignant glioma. Nat Commun. 2019 Feb 26;10(1):943. PMID:30808951
3388. Wanggou S, Jiang X, Li Q, et al. HESRG: a novel biomarker for intracranial germinoma and embryonal carcinoma. J Neurooncol. 2012 Jan;106(2):251–9. PMID:21861197
3389. Warmuth-Metz M, Gnekow AK, Müller H, et al. Differential diagnosis of suprasellar tumors in children. Klin Padiatr. 2004 Nov-Dec;216(6):323–30. PMID:15565547
3390. Warnick RE, Raisanen J, Adornato BT, et al. Intracranial myxopapillary ependymoma: case report. J Neurooncol. 1993 Mar;15(3):251–6. PMID:8360710
3391. Warren M, Hiemenz MC, Schmidt R, et al. Expanding the spectrum of dicer1-associated sarcomas. Mod Pathol. 2020 Jan;33(1):164–74. PMID:31537896
3392. Waszak SM, Northcott PA, Buchhalter I, et al. Spectrum and prevalence of genetic predisposition in medulloblastoma: a retrospective genetic study and prospective validation in a clinical trial cohort. Lancet Oncol. 2018 Jun;19(6):785–98. PMID:29753700
3393. Waszak SM, Robinson GW, Gudenas BL, et al. Germline elongator mutations in sonic hedgehog medulloblastoma. Nature. 2020 Apr;580(7803):396–401. PMID:32296180
3394. Watanabe K, Peraud A, Gratas C, et al. p53 and PTEN gene mutations in gemistocytic astrocytomas. Acta Neuropathol. 1998

Jun;95(6):559–64. PMID:9650746

3395. Watanabe K, Tachibana O, Yonekawa Y, et al. Role of gemistocytes in astrocytoma progression. Lab Invest. 1997 Feb;76(2):277–84. PMID:9042164

3396. Watanabe T, Mizowaki T, Arakawa Y, et al. Pineal parenchymal tumor of intermediate differentiation: treatment outcomes of five cases. Mol Clin Oncol. 2014 Mar;2(2):197–202. PMID:24649332

3397. Watanabe T, Nobusawa S, Kleihues P, et al. IDH1 mutations are early events in the development of astrocytomas and oligodendrogliomas. Am J Pathol. 2009 Apr;174(4):1149–53. PMID:19246647

3398. Watanabe T, Vital A, Nobusawa S, et al. Selective acquisition of IDH1 R132C mutations in astrocytomas associated with Li-Fraumeni syndrome. Acta Neuropathol. 2009 Jun;117(6):653–6. PMID:19340432

3399. Weaver KJ, Crawford LM, Bennett JA, et al. Brainstem angiocentric glioma: report of 2 cases. J Neurosurg Pediatr. 2017 Oct;20(4):347–51. PMID:28753090

3400. Weber DC, Wang Y, Miller R, et al. Long-term outcome of patients with spinal myxopapillary ependymoma: treatment results from the MD Anderson Cancer Center and institutions from the Rare Cancer Network. Neuro Oncol. 2015 Apr;17(4):588–95. PMID:25301811

3401. Weber HC, Marsh D, Lubensky I, et al. Germline PTEN/MMAC1/TEP1 mutations and association with gastrointestinal manifestations in Cowden disease. Gastroenterology. 1998;114(Suppl 1):A702. doi:10.1016/S0016-5085(98)82880-1.

3402. Wechsler-Reya RJ, Scott MP. Control of neuronal precursor proliferation in the cerebellum by Sonic Hedgehog. Neuron. 1999 Jan;22(1):103–14. PMID:10027293

3403. Wefel JS, Noll KR, Rao G, et al. Neurocognitive function varies by IDH1 genetic mutation status in patients with malignant glioma prior to surgical resection. Neuro Oncol. 2016 Dec;18(12):1656–63. PMID:27576872

3404. Wefers AK, Stichel D, Schrimpf D, et al. Isomorphic diffuse glioma is a morphologically and molecularly distinct tumour entity with recurrent gene fusions of MYBL1 or MYB and a benign disease course. Acta Neuropathol. 2020 Jan;139(1):193–209. PMID:31563982

3405. Wefers AK, Warmuth-Metz M, Pöschl J, et al. Subgroup-specific localization of human medulloblastoma based on pre-operative MRI. Acta Neuropathol. 2014;127(6):931–3. PMID:24699697

3406. Wehrli BM, Huang W, De Crombrugghe B, et al. Sox9, a master regulator of chondrogenesis, distinguishes mesenchymal chondrosarcoma from other small blue round cell tumors. Hum Pathol. 2003 Mar;34(3):263–9. PMID:12673561

3407. Wei D, Rich P, Bridges L, et al. Rare case of cerebral MALToma presenting with stroke-like symptoms and seizures. BMJ Case Rep. 2013 Apr 22;2013:bcr2012008494. PMID:23608841

3408. Wei G, Zhang W, Li Q, et al. Magnetic resonance characteristics of adult-onset Lhermitte-Duclos disease: an indicator for active cancer surveillance? Mol Clin Oncol. 2014 May;2(3):415–20. PMID:24772310

3409. Weil S, Osswald M, Solecki G, et al. Tumor microtubes convey resistance to surgical lesions and chemotherapy in gliomas. Neuro Oncol. 2017 Oct 1;19(10):1316–26. PMID:28419303

3410. Weiner HL, Wisoff JH, Rosenberg ME, et al. Craniopharyngiomas: a clinicopathological analysis of factors predictive of recurrence and functional outcome. Neurosurgery. 1994 Dec;35(6):1001–10. PMID:7885544

3411. Weingart MF, Roth JJ, Hutt-Cabezas M, et al. Disrupting LIN28 in atypical teratoid rhabdoid tumors reveals the importance of the mitogen activated protein kinase pathway as a therapeutic target. Oncotarget. 2015 Feb 20;6(5):3165–77. PMID:25638158

3412. Weiss WA, Burns MJ, Hackett C, et al. Genetic determinants of malignancy in a mouse model for oligodendroglioma. Cancer Res. 2003 Apr 1;63(7):1589–95. PMID:12670909

3413. Weissferdt A, Kalhor N, Moran CA. Ewing sarcoma with extensive neural differentiation: a clinicopathologic, immunohistochemical, and molecular analysis of three cases. Am J Clin Pathol. 2015 May;143(5):659–64. PMID:25873499

3414. Weller M, Butowski N, Tran DD, et al. Rindopepimut with temozolomide for patients with newly diagnosed, EGFRvIII-expressing glioblastoma (ACT IV): a randomised, double-blind, international phase 3 trial. Lancet Oncol. 2017 Oct;18(10):1373–85. PMID:28844499

3415. Weller M, Felsberg J, Hartmann C, et al. Molecular predictors of progression-free and overall survival in patients with newly diagnosed glioblastoma: a prospective translational study of the German Glioma Network. J Clin Oncol. 2009 Dec 1;27(34):5743–50. PMID:19805672

3416. Weller M, Tabatabai G, Kästner B, et al. MGMT promoter methylation is a strong prognostic biomarker for benefit from dose-intensified temozolomide rechallenge in progressive glioblastoma: the DIRECTOR trial. Clin Cancer Res. 2015 May 1;21(9):2057–64. PMID:25655102

3417. Weller M, van den Bent M, Tonn JC, et al. European Association for Neuro-Oncology (EANO) guideline on the diagnosis and treatment of adult astrocytic and oligodendroglial gliomas. Lancet Oncol. 2017 Jun;18(6):e315–29. PMID:28483413

3418. Weller M, Weber RG, Willscher E, et al. Molecular classification of diffuse cerebral WHO grade II/III gliomas using genome- and transcriptome-wide profiling improves stratification of prognostically distinct patient groups. Acta Neuropathol. 2015 May;129(5):679–93. PMID:25783747

3419. Werbrouck C, Evangelista CCS, Lobón-Iglesias MJ, et al. TP53 pathway alterations drive radioresistance in diffuse intrinsic pontine gliomas (DIPG). Clin Cancer Res. 2019 Nov 15;25(22):6788–800. PMID:31481512

3420. Werner MT, Zhao C, Zhang Q, et al. Nucleophosmin-anaplastic lymphoma kinase: the ultimate oncogene and therapeutic target. Blood. 2017 Feb 16;129(7):823–31. PMID:27879258

3421. Wesseling P, Schlingemann RO, Rietveld FJ, et al. Early and extensive contribution of pericytes/vascular smooth muscle cells to microvascular proliferation in glioblastoma multiforme: an immuno-light and immuno-electron microscopic study. J Neuropathol Exp Neurol. 1995 May;54(3):304–10. PMID:7745429

3422. Wharton SB, Chan KK, Anderson JR, et al. Replicative Mcm2 protein as a novel proliferation marker in oligodendrogliomas and its relationship to Ki67 labelling index, histological grade and prognosis. Neuropathol Appl Neurobiol. 2001 Aug;27(4):305–13. PMID:11532161

3423. White B, Belzberg A, Ahlawat S, et al. Intraneural perineurioma in neurofibromatosis type 2 with molecular analysis. Clin Neuropathol. 2020 Jul/Aug;39(4):167–71. PMID:32271143

3424. White FV, Dehner LP, Belchis DA, et al. Congenital disseminated malignant rhabdoid tumor: a distinct clinicopathologic entity demonstrating abnormalities of chromosome 22q11. Am J Surg Pathol. 1999 Mar;23(3):249–56. PMID:10078913

3425. White W, Shiu MH, Rosenblum MK, et al. Cellular schwannoma. A clinicopathologic study of 57 patients and 58 tumors. Cancer. 1990 Sep 15;66(6):1266–75. PMID:2400975

3425A. WHO Classification of Tumours Editorial Board. Endocrine and neuroendocrine tumours. Lyon (France): International Agency for Research on Cancer; forthcoming. (WHO classification of tumours series, 5th ed.). https://publications.iarc.fr/.

3426. WHO Classification of Tumours Editorial Board. Soft tissue and bone tumours. Lyon (France): International Agency for Research on Cancer; 2020. (WHO classification of tumours series, 5th ed.; vol. 3). https://publications.iarc.fr/588.

3427. Wick A, Kessler T, Platten M, et al. Superiority of temozolomide over radiotherapy for elderly patients with RTK II methylation class, MGMT promoter methylated malignant astrocytoma. Neuro Oncol. 2020 Aug 17;22(8):1162–72. PMID:32064499

3428. Wick W, Dettmer S, Berberich A, et al. N2M2 (NOA-20) phase I/II trial of molecularly matched targeted therapies plus radiotherapy in patients with newly diagnosed non-MGMT hypermethylated glioblastoma. Neuro Oncol. 2019 Jan 1;21(1):95–105. PMID:30277538

3429. Wick W, Meisner C, Hentschel B, et al. Prognostic or predictive value of MGMT promoter methylation in gliomas depends on IDH1 mutation. Neurology. 2013 Oct 22;81(17):1515–22. PMID:24068788

3430. Wick W, Platten M, Meisner C, et al. Temozolomide chemotherapy alone versus radiotherapy alone for malignant astrocytoma in the elderly: the NOA-08 randomised, phase 3 trial. Lancet Oncol. 2012 Jul;13(7):707–15. PMID:22578793

3431. Wick W, Weller M, van den Bent M, et al. MGMT testing–the challenges for biomarker-based glioma treatment. Nat Rev Neurol. 2014 Jul;10(7):372–85. PMID:24912512

3432. Wicking C, Gillies S, Smyth I, et al. De novo mutations of the Patched gene in nevoid basal cell carcinoma syndrome help to define the clinical phenotype. Am J Med Genet. 1997 Dec 19;73(3):304–7. PMID:9415689

3433. Wicking C, Shanley S, Smyth I, et al. Most germ-line mutations in the nevoid basal cell carcinoma syndrome lead to a premature termination of the PATCHED protein, and no genotype-phenotype correlations are evident. Am J Hum Genet. 1997 Jan;60(1):21–6. PMID:8981943

3434. Widemann BC. Current status of sporadic and neurofibromatosis type 1-associated malignant peripheral nerve sheath tumors. Curr Oncol Rep. 2009 Jul;11(4):322–8. PMID:19508838

3435. Wiemels J, Wrensch M, Claus EB. Epidemiology and etiology of meningioma. J Neurooncol. 2010 Sep;99(3):307–14. PMID:20821343

3436. Wiens AL, Cheng L, Bertsch EC, et al. Polysomy of chromosomes 1 and/or 19 is common and associated with less favorable clinical outcome in oligodendrogliomas: fluorescent in situ hybridization analysis of 84 consecutive cases. J Neuropathol Exp Neurol. 2012 Jul;71(7):618–24. PMID:22710961

3437. Wiens AL, Hattab EM. The pathological spectrum of solid CNS metastases in the pediatric population. J Neurosurg Pediatr. 2014 Aug;14(2):129–35. PMID:24926970

3438. Wiesner T, Obenauf AC, Murali R, et al. Germline mutations in BAP1 predispose to melanocytic tumors. Nat Genet. 2011 Aug 28;43(10):1018–21. PMID:21874003

3439. Wiestler B, Claus R, Hartlieb SA, et al. Malignant astrocytomas of elderly patients lack favorable molecular markers: an analysis of the NOA-08 study collective. Neuro Oncol. 2013 Aug;15(8):1017–26. PMID:23595628

3440. Wiestler OD, von Siebenthal K, Schmitt HP, et al. Distribution and immunoreactivity of cerebral micro-hamartomas in bilateral acoustic neurofibromatosis (neurofibromatosis 2). Acta Neuropathol. 1989;79(2):137–43. PMID:2596263

3441. Wijnenga MMJ, French PJ, Dubbink HJ, et al. Prognostic relevance of mutations and copy number alterations assessed with targeted next generation sequencing in IDH mutant grade II glioma. J Neurooncol. 2018 Sep;139(2):349–57. PMID:29663171

3442. Wijnenga MMJ, French PJ, Dubbink HJ, et al. The impact of surgery in molecularly defined low-grade glioma: an integrated clinical, radiological, and molecular analysis. Neuro Oncol. 2018 Jan 10;20(1):103–12. PMID:29016833

3443. Wijnenga MMJ, van der Voort SR, French PJ, et al. Differences in spatial distribution between WHO 2016 low-grade glioma molecular subgroups. Neurooncol Adv. 2019 May 31;1(1):vdz001. PMID:33889844

3444. Wilcox P, Li CC, Lee M, et al. Oligoastrocytomas: throwing the baby out with the bathwater? Acta Neuropathol. 2015 Jan;129(1):147–9. PMID:25304041

3445. Wildeman ME, Shepard MJ, Oldfield EH, et al. Central nervous system germinomas express programmed death ligand 1. J Neuropathol Exp Neurol. 2018 Apr 1;77(4):312–6. PMID:29415126

3446. Wilding A, Ingham SL, Lalloo F, et al. Life expectancy in hereditary cancer predisposing diseases: an observational study. J Med Genet. 2012 Apr;49(4):264–9. PMID:22362873

3447. Williams D, Mori T, Reiter A, et al. Central nervous system involvement in anaplastic large cell lymphoma in childhood: results from a multicentre European and Japanese study. Pediatr Blood Cancer. 2013 Oct;60(10):E118–21. PMID:23720354

3448. Williams EA, Miller JJ, Tummala SS, et al. TERT promoter wild-type glioblastomas show distinct clinical features and frequent PI3K pathway mutations. Acta Neuropathol Commun. 2018 Oct 17;6(1):106. PMID:30333046

3449. Williams EA, Wakimoto H, Shankar GM, et al. Frequent inactivating mutations of the PBAF complex gene PBRM1 in meningioma with papillary features. Acta Neuropathol. 2020 Jul;140(1):89–93. PMID:32405805

3450. Williams LA, Pankratz N, Lane J, et al. Klinefelter syndrome in males with germ cell tumors: a report from the Children's Oncology Group. Cancer. 2018 Oct 1;124(19):3900–8. PMID:30291793

3451. Williams SR, Juratli TA, Castro BA, et al. Genomic analysis of posterior fossa meningioma demonstrates frequent AKT1 E17K mutations in foramen magnum meningiomas. J Neurol Surg B Skull Base. 2019 Dec;80(6):562–7. PMID:31750041

3452. Willis SN, Mallozzi SS, Rodig SJ, et al. The microenvironment of germ cell tumors harbors a prominent antigen-driven humoral response. J Immunol. 2009 Mar 1;182(5):3310–7. PMID:19234230

3453. Wilson BG, Roberts CW. SWI/SNF nucleosome remodellers and cancer. Nat Rev Cancer. 2011 Jun 9;11(7):481–92. PMID:21654818

3454. Wilson BG, Wang X, Shen X, et al. Epigenetic antagonism between polycomb and SWI/SNF complexes during oncogenic transformation. Cancer Cell. 2010 Oct 19;18(4):316–28. PMID:20951942

3455. Wilson C, Bonnet C, Guy C, et al. Tsc1 haploinsufficiency without mammalian target of rapamycin activation is sufficient for renal cyst formation in Tsc1+/- mice. Cancer Res. 2006

Aug 15;66(16):7934–8. PMID:16912167
3456. Wilson TJ, Amrami KK, Howe BM, et al. Clinical and radiological follow-up of intraneural perineuriomas. Neurosurgery. 2019 Dec 1;85(6):786–92. PMID:30481319
3457. Wimmer K, Kratz CP, Vasen HF, et al. Diagnostic criteria for constitutional mismatch repair deficiency syndrome: suggestions of the European consortium 'care for CMMRD' (C4CMMRD). J Med Genet. 2014 Jun;51(6):355–65. PMID:24737826
3458. Winek RR, Scheithauer BW, Wick MR. Meningioma, meningeal hemangiopericytoma (angioblastic meningioma), peripheral hemangiopericytoma, and acoustic schwannoma. A comparative immunohistochemical study. Am J Surg Pathol. 1989 Apr;13(4):251–61. PMID:2648875
3459. Winkler F, Wick W. Harmful networks in the brain and beyond. Science. 2018 Mar 9;359(6380):1100–1. PMID:29590028
3460. Wippold FJ 2nd, Smirniotopoulos JG, Pilgram TK. Lesions of the cauda equina: a clinical and pathology review from the Armed Forces Institute of Pathology. Clin Neurol Neurosurg. 1997 Dec;99(4):229–34. PMID:9491294
3461. Witkowski L, Lalonde E, Zhang J, et al. Familial rhabdoid tumour 'avant la lettre'–from pathology review to exome sequencing and back again. J Pathol. 2013 Sep;231(1):35–43. PMID:23775540
3462. Witt H, Gramatzki D, Hentschel B, et al. DNA methylation-based classification of ependymomas in adulthood: implications for diagnosis and treatment. Neuro Oncol. 2018 Nov 12;20(12):1616–24. PMID:30053291
3463. Witt H, Mack SC, Ryzhova M, et al. Delineation of two clinically and molecularly distinct subgroups of posterior fossa ependymoma. Cancer Cell. 2011 Aug 16;20(2):143–57. PMID:21840481
3464. Wizigmann-Voos S, Breier G, Risau W, et al. Up-regulation of vascular endothelial growth factor and its receptors in von Hippel-Lindau disease-associated and sporadic hemangioblastomas. Cancer Res. 1995 Mar 15;55(6):1358–64. PMID:7533661
3464A. Wizigmann-Voos S, Plate KH. Pathology, genetics and cell biology of hemangioblastomas. Histol Histopathol. 1996 Oct;11(4):1049–61. PMID:8930647
3465. Woehrer A, Slavc I, Peyrl A, et al. Embryonal tumor with abundant neuropil and true rosettes (ETANTR) with loss of morphological but retained genetic key features during progression. Acta Neuropathol. 2011 Dec;122(6):787–90. PMID:22057788
3466. Wolf A, Alghefari H, Krivosheya D, et al. Cerebellar liponeurocytoma: a rare intracranial tumor with possible familial predisposition. Case report. J Neurosurg. 2016 Jul;125(1):57–61. PMID:26613167
3467. Wolf HK, Müller MB, Spänle M, et al. Ganglioglioma: a detailed histopathological and immunohistochemical analysis of 61 cases. Acta Neuropathol. 1994;88(2):166–73. PMID:7985497
3468. Wolff JE, Sajedi M, Brant R, et al. Choroid plexus tumours. Br J Cancer. 2002 Nov 4;87(10):1086–91. PMID:12402146
3469. Wong D, Lounsbury K, Lum A, et al. Transcriptomic analysis of CIC and ATXN1L reveal a functional relationship exploited by cancer. Oncogene. 2019 Jan;38(2):273–90. PMID:30093628
3470. Wong D, Shen Y, Levine AB, et al. The pivotal role of sampling recurrent tumors in the precision care of patients with tumors of the central nervous system. Cold Spring Harb Mol Case Stud. 2019 Aug 1;5(4):a004143. PMID:31371350
3471. Wong D, Yip S. Making heads or tails - the emergence of capicua (CIC) as an important multifunctional tumour suppressor. J Pathol. 2020 Apr;250(5):532–40. PMID:32073140
3472. Wong GC, Li KK, Wang WW, et al. Clinical and mutational profiles of adult medulloblastoma groups. Acta Neuropathol Commun. 2020 Nov 10;8(1):191. PMID:33172502
3473. Woo PYM, Lam TC, Pu JKS, et al. Regression of BRAFV600E mutant adult glioblastoma after primary combined BRAF-MEK inhibitor targeted therapy: a report of two cases. Oncotarget. 2019 Jun 4;10(38):3818–26. PMID:31217909
3474. Wood MD, Tihan T, Perry A, et al. Multimodal molecular analysis of astroblastoma enables reclassification of most cases into more specific molecular entities. Brain Pathol. 2018 Mar;28(2):192–202. PMID:28960623
3475. Woodruff JM, Godwin TA, Erlandson RA, et al. Cellular schwannoma: a variety of schwannoma sometimes mistaken for a malignant tumor. Am J Surg Pathol. 1981 Dec;5(8):733–44. PMID:7337161
3476. Woodruff JM, Scheithauer BW, Kurtkaya-Yapicier O, et al. Congenital and childhood plexiform (multinodular) cellular schwannoma: a troublesome mimic of malignant peripheral nerve sheath tumor. Am J Surg Pathol. 2003 Oct;27(10):1321–9. PMID:14508393
3477. Woodruff JM, Selig AM, Crowley K, et al. Schwannoma (neurilemoma) with malignant transformation. A rare, distinctive peripheral nerve tumor. Am J Surg Pathol. 1994 Sep;18(9):882–95. PMID:8067509
3478. Woroniecka K, Chongsathidkiet P, Rhodin K, et al. T-Cell exhaustion signatures vary with tumor type and are severe in glioblastoma. Clin Cancer Res. 2018 Sep 1;24(17):4175–86. PMID:29437767
3479. Wrede B, Hasselblatt M, Peters O, et al. Atypical choroid plexus papilloma: clinical experience in the CPT-SIOP-2000 study. J Neurooncol. 2009 Dec;95(3):383–92. PMID:19543851
3480. Wrensch M, Minn Y, Chew T, et al. Epidemiology of primary brain tumors: current concepts and review of the literature. Neuro Oncol. 2002 Oct;4(4):278–99. PMID:12356358
3481. Wu G, Broniscer A, McEachron TA, et al. Somatic histone H3 alterations in pediatric diffuse intrinsic pontine gliomas and non-brainstem glioblastomas. Nat Genet. 2012 Jan 29;44(3):251–3. PMID:22286216
3482. Wu G, Diaz AK, Paugh BS, et al. The genomic landscape of diffuse intrinsic pontine glioma and pediatric non-brainstem high-grade glioma. Nat Genet. 2014 May;46(5):444–50. PMID:24705251
3483. Wu MK, Vujanic GM, Fahiminiya S, et al. Anaplastic sarcomas of the kidney are characterized by DICER1 mutations. Mod Pathol. 2018 Jan;31(1):169–78. PMID:28862265
3484. Wu W, Tanrivermis Sayit A, Vinters HV, et al. Primary central nervous system histiocytic sarcoma presenting as a postradiation sarcoma: case report and literature review. Hum Pathol. 2013 Jun;44(6):1177–83. PMID:23356953
3485. Wu YT, Ho JT, Lin YJ, et al. Rhabdoid papillary meningioma: a clinicopathologic case series study. Neuropathology. 2011 Dec;31(6):599–605. PMID:21382093
3486. Wysozan TR, Khelifa S, Turchan K, et al. The morphologic spectrum of germline-mutated BAP1-inactivated melanocytic tumors includes lesions with conventional nevic melanocytes: a case report and review of literature. J Cutan Pathol. 2019 Nov;46(11):852–7. PMID:31206729
3487. Xi S, Sai K, Hu W, et al. Clinical significance of the histological and molecular characteristics of ependymal tumors: a single institution case series from China. BMC Cancer. 2019 Jul 19;19(1):717. PMID:31324163
3488. Xiao GH, Jin F, Yeung RS. Identification of tuberous sclerosis 2 messenger RNA splice variants that are conserved and differentially expressed in rat and human tissues. Cell Growth Differ. 1995 Sep;6(9):1185–91. PMID:8519695
3489. Xiao X, Zhou J, Wang J, et al. Clinical, radiological, pathological and prognostic aspects of intraventricular oligodendroglioma: comparison with central neurocytoma. J Neurooncol. 2017 Oct;135(1):57–65. PMID:28900829
3490. Xie J, Murone M, Luoh SM, et al. Activating smoothened mutations in sporadic basal-cell carcinoma. Nature. 1998 Jan 1;391(6662):90–2. PMID:9422511
3491. Xin W, Rubin MA, McKeever PE. Differential expression of cytokeratins 8 and 20 distinguishes craniopharyngioma from rathke cleft cyst. Arch Pathol Lab Med. 2002 Oct;126(10):1174–8. PMID:12296753
3492. Xiong J, Liu Y, Chu SG, et al. Dysembryoplastic neuroepithelial tumor-like neoplasm of the septum pellucidum: review of 2 cases with chromosome 1p/19q and IDH1 analysis. Clin Neuropathol. 2012 Jan-Feb;31(1):31–8. PMID:22192702
3493. Xiong J, Liu Y, Chu SG, et al. Rosette-forming glioneuronal tumor of the septum pellucidum with extension to the supratentorial ventricles: rare case with genetic analysis. Neuropathology. 2012 Jun;32(3):301–5. PMID:22017246
3494. Xu F, De Las Casas LE, Dobbs LJ Jr. Primary meningeal rhabdomyosarcoma in a child with hypomelanosis of Ito. Arch Pathol Lab Med. 2000 May;124(5):762–5. PMID:10782165
3495. Xu G, Zheng H, Li JY. Next-generation whole exome sequencing of glioblastoma with a primitive neuronal component. Brain Tumor Pathol. 2019 Jul;36(3):129–34. PMID:30715630
3496. Xu HM, Gutmann DH. Merlin differentially associates with the microtubule and actin cytoskeleton. J Neurosci Res. 1998 Feb 1;51(3):403–15. PMID:9486775
3497. Xu J, Yang Y, Liu Y, et al. Rosette-forming glioneuronal tumor in the pineal gland and the third ventricle: a case with radiological and clinical implications. Quant Imaging Med Surg. 2012 Sep;2(3):227–31. PMID:23256084
3498. Xu L, Du J, Wang J, et al. The clinicopathological features of liponeurocytoma. Brain Tumor Pathol. 2017 Jan;34(1):28–35. PMID:28236115
3499. Xu L, Ouyang Z, Wang J, et al. A clinicopathologic study of extraventricular neurocytoma. J Neurooncol. 2017 Mar;132(1):75–82. PMID:27864704
3500. Xu N, Cai J, Du J, et al. Clinical features and prognosis for intraventricular liponeurocytoma. Oncotarget. 2017 Mar 8;8(37):62641–7. PMID:28977976
3501. Xu W, Yang H, Liu Y, et al. Oncometabolite 2-hydroxyglutarate is a competitive inhibitor of α-ketoglutarate-dependent dioxygenases. Cancer Cell. 2011 Jan 18;19(1):17–30. PMID:21251613
3502. Xu X, Zhao J, Xu Z, et al. Structures of human cytosolic NADP-dependent isocitrate dehydrogenase reveal a novel self-regulatory mechanism of activity. J Biol Chem. 2004 Aug 6;279(32):33946–57. PMID:15173171
3503. Yakubov E, Ghoochani A, Buslei R, et al. Hidden association of Cowden syndrome, PTEN mutation and meningioma frequency. Oncoscience. 2016 Jun 30;3(5-6):149–55. PMID:27489861
3504. Yamada H, Haratake J, Narasaki T, et al. Embryonal craniopharyngioma. Case report of the morphogenesis of a craniopharyngioma. Cancer. 1995 Jun 15;75(12):2971–7. PMID:7773950
3505. Yamada S, Aiba T, Sano T, et al. Growth hormone-producing pituitary adenomas: correlations between clinical characteristics and morphology. Neurosurgery. 1993 Jul;33(1):20–7. PMID:7689191
3506. Yamada S, Fukuhara N, Horiguchi K, et al. Clinicopathological characteristics and therapeutic outcomes in thyrotropin-secreting pituitary adenomas: a single-center study of 90 cases. J Neurosurg. 2014 Dec;121(6):1462–73. PMID:25237847
3507. Yamada S, Muto J, De Leon JCA, et al. Primary spinal intramedullary Ewing-like sarcoma harboring CIC-DUX4 translocation: a similar cytological appearance as its soft tissue counterpart but no lobulation in association with desmoplastic stroma. Brain Tumor Pathol. 2020 Jul;37(3):111–7. PMID:32449046
3508. Yamaguchi U, Hasegawa T, Hirose T, et al. Sclerosing perineurioma: a clinicopathological study of five cases and diagnostic utility of immunohistochemical staining for GLUT1. Virchows Arch. 2003 Aug;443(2):159–63. PMID:12836021
3509. Yamamoto K, Yamada K, Nakahara T, et al. Rapid regrowth of solitary subependymal giant cell astrocytoma–case report. Neurol Med Chir (Tokyo). 2002 May;42(5):224–7. PMID:12064158
3510. Yamane Y, Mena H, Nakazato Y. Immunohistochemical characterization of pineal parenchymal tumors using novel monoclonal antibodies to the pineal body. Neuropathology. 2002 Jun;22(2):66–76. PMID:12075938
3511. Yamanouchi H, Ho M, Jay V, et al. Giant cells in cortical tubers in tuberous sclerosis showing synaptophysin-immunoreactive halos. Brain Dev. 1997 Jan;19(1):21–4. PMID:9071486
3512. Yamasaki K, Nakano Y, Nobusawa S, et al. Spinal cord astroblastoma with an EWSR1-BEND2 fusion classified as a high-grade neuroepithelial tumour with MN1 alteration. Neuropathol Appl Neurobiol. 2020 Feb;46(2):190–3. PMID:31863478
3513. Yamasaki T, Sakai N, Shinmura K, et al. Anaplastic changes of diffuse leptomeningeal glioneuronal tumor with polar spongioblastoma pattern. Brain Tumor Pathol. 2018 Oct;35(4):209–16. PMID:30051174
3514. Yan H, Parsons DW, Jin G, et al. IDH1 and IDH2 mutations in gliomas. N Engl J Med. 2009 Feb 19;360(8):765–73. PMID:19228619
3515. Yan J, Liu W, Wang X, et al. Primary central nervous system extranodal natural killer/T-cell lymphoma, nasal type colliding with meningioma. World Neurosurg. 2018 Dec;120:17–26. PMID:30144614
3516. Yang C, Fang J, Li G, et al. Spinal meningeal melanocytomas: clinical manifestations, radiological and pathological characteristics, and surgical outcomes. J Neurooncol. 2016 Apr;127(2):279–86. PMID:26940907
3517. Yang C, Li G, Fang J, et al. Clinical characteristics and surgical outcomes of primary spinal paragangliomas. J Neurooncol. 2015 May;122(3):539–47. PMID:25720695
3518. Yang FC, Ingram DA, Chen S, et al. Nf1-dependent tumors require a microenvironment containing Nf1+/– and c-kit-dependent bone marrow. Cell. 2008 Oct 31;135(3):437–48. PMID:18984156
3519. Yang I, Tihan T, Han SJ, et al. CD8+ T-cell infiltrate in newly diagnosed glioblastoma is associated with long-term survival. J Clin Neurosci. 2010 Nov;17(11):1381–5. PMID:20727764
3520. Yang JC, Wexler LH, Meyers PA, et al. Parameningeal rhabdomyosarcoma: outcomes and opportunities. Int J Radiat Oncol Biol Phys.

2013 Jan 1;85(1):e61–6. PMID:23021437
3521. Yang P, Kollmeyer TM, Buckner K, et al. Polymorphisms in GLTSCR1 and ERCC2 are associated with the development of oligodendrogliomas. Cancer. 2005 Jun 1;103(11):2363–72. PMID:15834925
3522. Yang RR, Shi ZF, Zhang ZY, et al. IDH mutant lower grade (WHO Grades II/III) astrocytomas can be stratified for risk by CDKN2A, CDK4 and PDGFRA copy number alterations. Brain Pathol. 2020 May;30(3):541–53. PMID:31733156
3523. Yang S, Zheng X, Lu C, et al. Molecular basis for oncohistone H3 recognition by SETD2 methyltransferase. Genes Dev. 2016 Jul 15;30(14):1611–6. PMID:27474439
3524. Yang SY, Jin YJ, Park SH, et al. Paragangliomas in the cauda equina region: clinicopathoradiologic findings in four cases. J Neurooncol. 2005 Mar;72(1):49–55. PMID:15803375
3525. Yang Y, Shrestha D, Shi XE, et al. Ectopic recurrence of craniopharyngioma: reporting three new cases. Br J Neurosurg. 2015 Apr;29(2):295–7. PMID:25311042
3526. Yang ZJ, Ellis T, Markant SL, et al. Medulloblastoma can be initiated by deletion of Patched in lineage-restricted progenitors or stem cells. Cancer Cell. 2008 Aug 12;14(2):135–45. PMID:18691548
3527. Yao H, Price TT, Cantelli G, et al. Leukaemia hijacks a neural mechanism to invade the central nervous system. Nature. 2018 Aug;560(7716):55–60. PMID:30022166
3528. Yao K, Duan Z, Wang Y, et al. Detection of H3K27M mutation in cases of brain stem subependymoma. Hum Pathol. 2019 Feb;84:262–9. PMID:30389438
3529. Yao K, Qi XL, Mei X, et al. Gliosarcoma with primitive neuroectodermal, osseous, cartilage and adipocyte differentiation: a case report. Int J Clin Exp Pathol. 2015 Feb 1;8(2):2079–84. PMID:25973108
3530. Yao ZG, Wu HB, Hao YH, et al. Papillary solitary fibrous tumor/hemangiopericytoma: an uncommon morphological form with NAB2-STAT6 gene fusion. J Neuropathol Exp Neurol. 2019 Jul 4;nlz053. PMID:31271432
3531. Yasargil MG, von Ammon K, von Deimling A, et al. Central neurocytoma: histopathological variants and therapeutic approaches. J Neurosurg. 1992 Jan;76(1):32–7. PMID:1727166
3532. Yde CW, Sehested A, Mateu-Regué À, et al. A new NFIA:RAF1 fusion activating the MAPK pathway in pilocytic astrocytoma. Cancer Genet. 2016 Oct;209(10):440–4. PMID:27810072
3533. Yehia L, Eng C. PTEN hamartoma tumour syndrome: what happens when there is no PTEN germline mutation? Hum Mol Genet. 2020 Oct 20;29 R2:R150–7. PMID:32568377
3534. Yehia L, Niazi F, Ni Y, et al. Germline heterozygous variants in SEC23B are associated with Cowden syndrome and enriched in apparently sporadic thyroid cancer. Am J Hum Genet. 2015 Nov 5;97(5):661–76. PMID:26522472
3535. Yi KS, Sohn CH, Yun TJ, et al. MR imaging findings of extraventricular neurocytoma: a series of ten patients confirmed by immunohistochemistry of IDH1 gene mutation. Acta Neurochir (Wien). 2012 Nov;154(11):1973–9. PMID:22945896
3536. Yi X, Cao H, Tang H, et al. Gliosarcoma: a clinical and radiological analysis of 48 cases. Eur Radiol. 2019 Jan;29(1):429–38. PMID:29948068
3537. Yip S, Butterfield YS, Morozova O, et al. Concurrent CIC mutations, IDH mutations, and 1p/19q loss distinguish oligodendrogliomas from other cancers. J Pathol. 2012 Jan;226(1):7–16. PMID:22072542
3538. Yip S, Miao J, Cahill DP, et al. MSH6 mutations arise in glioblastomas during temozolomide therapy and mediate temozolomide resistance. Clin Cancer Res. 2009 Jul 15;15(14):4622–9. PMID:19584161
3539. Yoda RA, Marxen T, Longo L, et al. Mitotic index thresholds do not predict clinical outcome for IDH-mutant astrocytoma. J Neuropathol Exp Neurol. 2019 Nov 1;78(11):1002–10. PMID:31529048
3540. Yokota T, Tachizawa T, Fukino K, et al. A family with spinal anaplastic ependymoma: evidence of loss of chromosome 22q in tumor. J Hum Genet. 2003;48(11):598–602. PMID:14566482
3541. Yoo JH, Rivera A, Naeini RM, et al. Melanotic paraganglioma arising in the temporal horn following Langerhans cell histiocytosis. Pediatr Radiol. 2008 May;38(5):571–4. PMID:18196230
3542. Yoshida A, Arai Y, Kobayashi E, et al. CIC break-apart fluorescence in-situ hybridization misses a subset of CIC-DUX4 sarcomas: a clinicopathological and molecular study. Histopathology. 2017 Sep;71(3):461–9. PMID:28493604
3543. Yoshida A, Goto K, Kodaira M, et al. CIC-rearranged sarcomas: a study of 20 cases and comparisons with Ewing sarcomas. Am J Surg Pathol. 2016 Mar;40(3):313–23. PMID:26685084
3544. Yoshida K, Miwa T, Akiyama T, et al. Primary intracranial rhabdomyosarcoma in the cerebellopontine angle resected after preoperative embolization. World Neurosurg. 2018 Aug;116:110–5. PMID:29777888
3545. Yoshida KI, Machado I, Motoi T, et al. NKX3-1 is a useful immunohistochemical marker of EWSR1-NFATC2 sarcoma and mesenchymal chondrosarcoma. Am J Surg Pathol. 2020 Jun;44(6):719–28. PMID:31972596
3546. Yoshida M, Fushiki S, Takeuchi Y, et al. Diffuse bilateral thalamic astrocytomas as examined serially by MRI. Childs Nerv Syst. 1998 Aug;14(8):384–8. PMID:9753406
3547. Yoshida Y, Nobusawa S, Nakata S, et al. CNS high-grade neuroepithelial tumor with BCOR internal tandem duplication: a comparison with its counterparts in the kidney and soft tissue. Brain Pathol. 2018 Sep;28(5):710–20. PMID:29226988
3548. Yoshimoto T, Takahashi-Fujigasaki J, Inoshita N, et al. TTF-1-positive oncocytic sellar tumor with follicle formation/ependymal differentiation: non-adenomatous tumor capable of two different interpretations as a pituicytoma or a spindle cell oncocytoma. Brain Tumor Pathol. 2015 Jul;32(3):221–7. PMID:25893822
3549. Yoshimoto T, Tanaka M, Homme M, et al. CIC-DUX4 induces small round cell sarcomas distinct from Ewing sarcoma. Cancer Res. 2017 Jun 1;77(11):2927–37. PMID:28404587
3550. You H, Kim YI, Im SY, et al. Immunohistochemical study of central neurocytoma, subependymoma, and subependymal giant cell astrocytoma. J Neurooncol. 2005 Aug;74(1):1–8. PMID:16078101
3551. Young RJ, Sills AK, Brem S, et al. Neuroimaging of metastatic brain disease. Neurosurgery. 2005 Nov;57(5 Suppl):S10–23. PMID:16237282
3552. Youngblood MW, Duran D, Montejo JD, et al. Correlations between genomic subgroup and clinical features in a cohort of more than 3000 meningiomas. J Neurosurg. 2019 Oct 25:1–10. PMID:31653806
3553. Yu KK, Zanation AM, Moss JR, et al. Familial head and neck cancer: molecular analysis of a new clinical entity. Laryngoscope. 2002 Sep;112(9):1587–93. PMID:12352668
3554. Yu T, Sun X, Wang J, et al. Twenty-seven cases of pineal parenchymal tumours of intermediate differentiation: mitotic count, Ki-67 labelling index and extent of resection predict prognosis. J Neurol Neurosurg Psychiatry. 2016 Apr;87(4):386–95. PMID:25911570
3555. Yu XR, Jun-Zhang, Zhang BY, et al. Magnetic resonance imaging findings of intracranial papillary meningioma: a study on eight cases. Clin Imaging. 2014 Sep-Oct;38(5):611–5. PMID:24993640
3556. Yue Q, Yu Y, Shi Z, et al. Prediction of BRAF mutation status of craniopharyngioma using magnetic resonance imaging features. J Neurosurg. 2018 Jul;129(1):27–34. PMID:28984520
3557. Yuh WT, Chung CK, Park SH, et al. Spinal cord subependymoma surgery: a multi-institutional experience. J Korean Neurosurg Soc. 2018 Mar;61(2):233–42. PMID:29526067
3558. Yun J, Park JE, Lee H, et al. Radiomic features and multilayer perceptron network classifier: a robust MRI classification strategy for distinguishing glioblastoma from primary central nervous system lymphoma. Sci Rep. 2019 Apr 5;9(1):5746. PMID:30952930
3559. Yust Katz S, Cachia D, Kamiya-Matsuoka C, et al. Ependymomas arising outside of the central nervous system: a case series and literature review. J Clin Neurosci. 2018 Jan;47:202–7. PMID:29054328
3560. Yust-Katz S, Anderson MD, Liu D, et al. Clinical and prognostic features of adult patients with gangliogliomas. Neuro Oncol. 2014 Mar;16(3):409–13. PMID:24305706
3561. Yuzawa S, Nishihara H, Wang L, et al. Analysis of NAB2-STAT6 gene fusion in 17 cases of meningeal solitary fibrous tumor/hemangiopericytoma: review of the literature. Am J Surg Pathol. 2016 Aug;40(8):1031–40. PMID:26927892
3562. Zacharia BE, Bruce SS, Goldstein H, et al. Incidence, treatment and survival of patients with craniopharyngioma in the surveillance, epidemiology and end results program. Neuro Oncol. 2012 Aug;14(8):1070–8. PMID:22735773
3563. Zacharoulis S, Morales La Madrid A, Bandopadhayay P, et al. Central versus extraventricular neurocytoma in children: a clinicopathologic comparison and review of the literature. J Pediatr Hematol Oncol. 2016 Aug;38(6):479–85. PMID:27438020
3564. Zacher A, Kaulich K, Stepanow S, et al. Molecular diagnostics of gliomas using next generation sequencing of a glioma-tailored gene panel. Brain Pathol. 2017 Mar;27(2):146–59. PMID:26919320
3565. Zada G, Woodmansee WW, Ramkissoon S, et al. Atypical pituitary adenomas: incidence, clinical characteristics, and implications. J Neurosurg. 2011 Feb;114(2):336–44. PMID:20868211
3566. Zafar A, Fiani B, Hadi H, et al. Cerebral vascular malformations and their imaging modalities. Neurol Sci. 2020 Sep;41(9):2407–21. PMID:32335778
3567. Zafar A, Quadri SA, Farooqui M, et al. Familial cerebral cavernous malformations. Stroke. 2019 May;50(5):1294–301. PMID:30909834
3568. Zafar M, Ezzat S, Ramyar L, et al. Cell-specific expression of estrogen receptor in the human pituitary and its adenomas. J Clin Endocrinol Metab. 1995 Dec;80(12):3621–7. PMID:8530610
3569. Zagzag D, Esencay M, Mendez O, et al. Hypoxia- and vascular endothelial growth factor-induced stromal cell-derived factor-1alpha/CXCR4 expression in glioblastomas: one plausible explanation of Scherer's structures. Am J Pathol. 2008 Aug;173(2):545–60. PMID:18599607
3570. Zagzag D, Krishnamachary B, Yee H, et al. Stromal cell-derived factor-1alpha and CXCR4 expression in hemangioblastoma and clear cell-renal cell carcinoma: von Hippel-Lindau loss-of-function induces expression of a ligand and its receptor. Cancer Res. 2005 Jul 15;65(14):6178–88. PMID:16024619
3571. Zagzag D, Lukyanov Y, Lan L, et al. Hypoxia-inducible factor 1 and VEGF upregulate CXCR4 in glioblastoma: implications for angiogenesis and glioma cell invasion. Lab Invest. 2006 Dec;86(12):1221–32. PMID:17075581
3572. Zagzag D, Zhong H, Scalzitti JM, et al. Expression of hypoxia-inducible factor 1alpha in brain tumors: association with angiogenesis, invasion, and progression. Cancer. 2000 Jun 1;88(11):2606–18. PMID:10861440
3573. Zaidi HA, Cote DJ, Dunn IF, et al. Predictors of aggressive clinical phenotype among immunohistochemically confirmed atypical adenomas. J Clin Neurosci. 2016 Dec;34:246–51. PMID:27765563
3574. Zajac V, Kirchhoff T, Levy ER, et al. Characterisation of X;17(q12;p13) translocation breakpoints in a female patient with hypomelanosis of Ito and choroid plexus papilloma. Eur J Hum Genet. 1997 Mar-Apr;5(2):61–8. PMID:9195154
3575. Zakrzewska M, Wojcik I, Zakrzewski K, et al. Mutational analysis of hSNF5/INI1 and TP53 genes in choroid plexus carcinomas. Cancer Genet Cytogenet. 2005 Jan 15;156(2):179–82. PMID:15642401
3576. Zaky W, Dhall G, Khatua S, et al. Choroid plexus carcinoma in children: the Head Start experience. Pediatr Blood Cancer. 2015 May;62(5):784–9. PMID:25662896
3577. Zaky W, Patil SS, Park M, et al. Ganglioglioma in children and young adults: single institution experience and review of the literature. J Neurooncol. 2018 Sep;139(3):739–47. PMID:29882043
3578. Zanello M, Pages M, Tauziède-Espariat A, et al. Clinical, imaging, histopathological and molecular characterization of anaplastic ganglioglioma. J Neuropathol Exp Neurol. 2016 Oct;75(10):971–80. PMID:27539475
3579. Zapka P, Dörner E, Dreschmann V, et al. Type, frequency, and spatial distribution of immune cell infiltrates in CNS germinomas: evidence for inflammatory and immunosuppressive mechanisms. J Neuropathol Exp Neurol. 2018 Feb 1;77(2):119–27. PMID:29237087
3580. Zapotocky M, Beera K, Adamski J, et al. Survival and functional outcomes of molecularly defined childhood posterior fossa ependymoma: cure at a cost. Cancer. 2019 Jun 1;125(11):1867–76. PMID:30768777
3581. Zapotocky M, Mata-Mbemba D, Sumerauer D, et al. Differential patterns of metastatic dissemination across medulloblastoma subgroups. J Neurosurg Pediatr. 2018 Feb;21(2):145–52. PMID:29219788
3582. Zarate JO, Sampaolesi R. Pleomorphic xanthoastrocytoma of the retina. Am J Surg Pathol. 1999 Jan;23(1):79–81. PMID:9888706
3583. Zatelli MC, Piccin D, Tagliati F, et al. Dopamine receptor subtype 2 and somatostatin receptor subtype 5 expression influences somatostatin analogs effects on human somatotroph pituitary adenomas in vitro. J Mol Endocrinol. 2005 Oct;35(2):333–41. PMID:16216913
3584. Zbuk KM, Eng C. Cancer phenomics: RET and PTEN as illustrative models. Nat Rev Cancer. 2007 Jan;7(1):35–45. PMID:17167516
3585. Zec N, De Girolami U, Schofield DE, et al. Giant cell ependymoma of the filum terminale. A report of two cases. Am J Surg Pathol. 1996 Sep;20(9):1091–101. PMID:8764746
3585A. Zeltser L, Desplan C, Heintz N. Hoxb-13: a new Hox gene in a distant region of the HOXB cluster maintains colinearity. Development. 1996 Aug;122(8):2475–84.

PMID:8756292

3586. Zeng Q, Michael IP, Zhang P, et al. Synaptic proximity enables NMDAR signalling to promote brain metastasis. Nature. 2019 Sep;573(7775):526–31. PMID:31534217

3587. Zeng Y, Zhu X, Wang Y, et al. Clinicopathological, immunohistochemical and molecular genetic study on epithelioid glioblastoma: a series of fifteen cases with literature review. Onco Targets Ther. 2020 May 8;13:3943–52. PMID:32440157

3588. Zepeda-Mendoza CJ, Vaubel RA, Zarei S, et al. Concomitant 1p/19q co-deletion and IDH1/2, ATRX, and TP53 mutations within a single clone of "dual-genotype" IDH-mutant infiltrating gliomas. Acta Neuropathol. 2020 Jun;139(6):1105–7. PMID:32170402

3589. Zetterling M, Berhane L, Alafuzoff I, et al. Prognostic markers for survival in patients with oligodendroglial tumors; a single-institution review of 214 cases. PLoS One. 2017 Nov 29;12(11):e0188419. PMID:29186201

3590. Zhang A, Brown DF, Colpan EM. Mesial temporal extraventricular neurocytoma (mtEVN): a case report and literature review. Epilepsy Behav Case Rep. 2018 Oct 23;11:26–30. PMID:30603610

3591. Zhang C, Ostrom QT, Hansen HM, et al. European genetic ancestry associated with risk of childhood ependymoma. Neuro Oncol. 2020 Nov 26;22(11):1637–46. PMID:32607579

3592. Zhang GJ, Zhang GB, Zhang YS, et al. World Health Organization grade III (nonanaplastic) meningioma: experience in a series of 23 cases. World Neurosurg. 2018 Apr;112:e754–62. PMID:29382616

3593. Zhang H, Ma L, Shu C, et al. Spinal clear cell meningioma: clinical features and factors predicting recurrence. World Neurosurg. 2020 Feb;134:e1062–76. PMID:31765868

3594. Zhang HY, Yang GH, Chen HJ, et al. Clinicopathological, immunohistochemical, and ultrastructural study of 13 cases of melanotic schwannoma. Chin Med J (Engl). 2005 Sep 5;118(17):1451–61. PMID:16157048

3595. Zhang J, Cheng H, Qiao Q, et al. Malignant solitary fibrous tumor arising from the pineal region: case study and literature review. Neuropathology. 2010 Jun;30(3):294–8. PMID:19845865

3596. Zhang J, Walsh MF, Wu G, et al. Germline mutations in predisposition genes in pediatric cancer. N Engl J Med. 2015 Dec 10;373(24):2336–46. PMID:26580448

3597. Zhang J, Wu G, Miller CP, et al. Whole-genome sequencing identifies genetic alterations in pediatric low-grade gliomas. Nat Genet. 2013 Jun;45(6):602–12. PMID:23583981

3598. Zhang M, Wang Y, Jones S, et al. Somatic mutations of SUZ12 in malignant peripheral nerve sheath tumors. Nat Genet. 2014 Nov;46(11):1170–2. PMID:25305755

3599. Zhang Y, Shan CM, Wang J, et al. Molecular basis for the role of oncogenic histone mutations in modulating H3K36 methylation. Sci Rep. 2017 Mar 3;7:43906. PMID:28256625

3600. Zhang Y, Teng Y, Zhu H, et al. Granular cell tumor of the neurohypophysis: 3 cases and a systematic literature review of 98 cases. World Neurosurg. 2018 Oct;118:e621–30. PMID:30017767

3601. Zhao F, Li C, Zhou Q, et al. Distinctive localization and MRI features correlate of molecular subgroups in adult medulloblastoma. J Neurooncol. 2017 Nov;135(2):353–60. PMID:28808827

3602. Zhao K, Sun G, Wang Q, et al. The diagnostic value of conventional MRI and CT features in the identification of the IDH1-mutant and 1p/19q co-deletion in WHO Grade II gliomas. Acad Radiol. 2020 Apr 28;S1076-6332(20)30149-5. PMID:32359929

3603. Zheng JJ, Zhang GJ, Huo XL, et al. Treatment strategy and long-term outcomes of primary intracranial rhabdomyosarcoma: a single-institution experience and systematic review. J Neurosurg. 2019 Sep 13:1–11. PMID:31518985

3604. Zheng W, Huang Y, Guan T, et al. Application of nomograms to predict overall and cancer-specific survival in patients with chordoma. J Bone Oncol. 2019 Jun 24;18:100247. PMID:31528536

3605. Zheng Z, Liebers M, Zhelyazkova B, et al. Anchored multiplex PCR for targeted next-generation sequencing. Nat Med. 2014 Dec;20(12):1479–84. PMID:25384085

3606. Zhou J, Shrikhande G, Xu J, et al. Tsc1 mutant neural stem/progenitor cells exhibit migration deficits and give rise to subependymal lesions in the lateral ventricle. Genes Dev. 2011 Aug 1;25(15):1595–600. PMID:21828270

3607. Zhou R, Xu A, Gingold J, et al. Li-Fraumeni syndrome disease model: a platform to develop precision cancer therapy targeting oncogenic p53. Trends Pharmacol Sci. 2017 Oct;38(10):908–27. PMID:28818333

3608. Zhou X, Hampel H, Thiele H, et al. Association of germline mutation in the PTEN tumour suppressor gene and Proteus and Proteus-like syndromes. Lancet. 2001 Jul 21;358(9277):210–1. PMID:11476841

3609. Zhou XP, Marsh DJ, Morrison CD, et al. Germline inactivation of PTEN and dysregulation of the phosphoinositol-3-kinase/Akt pathway cause human Lhermitte-Duclos disease in adults. Am J Hum Genet. 2003 Nov;73(5):1191–8. PMID:14566704

3610. Zhou XP, Waite KA, Pilarski R, et al. Germline PTEN promoter mutations and deletions in Cowden/Bannayan-Riley-Ruvalcaba syndrome result in aberrant PTEN protein and dysregulation of the phosphoinositol-3-kinase/Akt pathway. Am J Hum Genet. 2003 Aug;73(2):404–11. PMID:12844284

3611. Zhou YX, Flint NC, Murtie JC, et al. Retroviral lineage analysis of fibroblast growth factor receptor signaling in FGF2 inhibition of oligodendrocyte progenitor differentiation. Glia. 2006 Nov 1;54(6):578–90. PMID:16921523

3612. Zhu L, Ren G, Li K, et al. Pineal parenchymal tumours: minimum apparent diffusion coefficient in prediction of tumour grading. J Int Med Res. 2011;39(4):1456–63. PMID:21986148

3613. Zhu X, Mao X, Hurren R, et al. Deoxyribonucleic acid methyltransferase 3B promotes epigenetic silencing through histone 3 chromatin modifications in pituitary cells. J Clin Endocrinol Metab. 2008 Sep;93(9):3610–7. PMID:18544619

3614. Zhukova N, Ramaswamy V, Remke M, et al. Subgroup-specific prognostic implications of TP53 mutation in medulloblastoma. J Clin Oncol. 2013 Aug 10;31(23):2927–35. PMID:23835706

3615. Ziegler DS, Wong M, Mayoh C, et al. Brief Report: Potent clinical and radiological response to larotrectinib in TRK fusion-driven high-grade glioma. Br J Cancer. 2018 Sep;119(6):693–6. PMID:30220707

3616. Zimmerman LE, Burns RP, Wankum G, et al. Trilateral retinoblastoma: ectopic intracranial retinoblastoma associated with bilateral retinoblastoma. J Pediatr Ophthalmol Strabismus. 1982 Nov-Dec;19(6):320–5. PMID:7153826

3617. Zlatescu MC, TehraniYazdi A, Sasaki H, et al. Tumor location and growth pattern correlate with genetic signature in oligodendroglial neoplasms. Cancer Res. 2001 Sep 15;61(18):6713–5. PMID:11559541

3618. Zoli M, Sambati L, Milanese L, et al. Postoperative outcome of body core temperature rhythm and sleep-wake cycle in third ventricle craniopharyngiomas. Neurosurg Focus. 2016 Dec;41(6):E12. PMID:27903128

3619. Zong H, Parada LF, Baker SJ. Cell of origin for malignant gliomas and its implication in therapeutic development. Cold Spring Harb Perspect Biol. 2015 Jan 29;7(5):a020610. PMID:25635044

3620. Zorludemir S, Scheithauer BW, Hirose T, et al. Clear cell meningioma. A clinicopathologic study of a potentially aggressive variant of meningioma. Am J Surg Pathol. 1995 May;19(5):493–505. PMID:7726360

3621. Zou H, Duan Y, Wei D, et al. Molecular features of pleomorphic xanthoastrocytoma. Hum Pathol. 2019 Apr;86:38–48. PMID:30496796

3622. Zuccaro G, Taratuto AL, Monges J. Intracranial neoplasms during the first year of life. Surg Neurol. 1986 Jul;26(1):29–36. PMID:3715697

3623. Zumel-Marne A, Castano-Vinyals G, Kundi M, et al. Environmental factors and the risk of brain tumours in young people: a systematic review. Neuroepidemiology. 2019;53(3-4):121–41. PMID:31167200

3624. Zunino V, Catalano MG, Zenga F, et al. Benzene affects the response to octreotide treatment of growth hormone secreting pituitary adenoma cells. Environ Res. 2019 Jun;173:489–96. PMID:30986651

Subject index

Bold page numbers indicate the main discussion(s) of the topic.

medulloblastoma with extensive nodularity 201–202, 213–214, 217, 219, 459

medulloblastoma, WNT-activated 10, 199, 203–204

medulloepithelioma 228, 230–231, 464–465, 474

MEK 68, 89, 115, 266, 342, 346, 371, 400, 427–428

melan-A 50, 274, 319, 347, 420

melanin 230, 251, 267, 274, 341–347, 419

melanocytoma 339–340, 343–348

melanocytosis 339–343

melanoma 46, 49–50, 274, 294–295, 328, **339–348**, 418–421, 449, 471, 474–476

melanoma-astrocytoma syndrome 20, 96, 423, 425, **471–472**

melanomatosis 339–343, 347

MEN1 402, 409, 468

meningioangiomatosis 295, 430, 432

meningioma 8, 10–11, 13, 35, 45, 47–48, 106, **283–297**, 301–303, 317, 319, 324–325, 331, 347, 350–352, 363, 369, 372, 402, 424, 430, 432, 434, 436, 458, 475–476

meningothelial meningioma 284, 288

merlin (NF2) 262, 431–432

mesenchymal chondrosarcoma 14, 299, 303, 328, 330–331

mesothelioma 294, 475–477

MET 23, 27, 43–44, 54, 67, 79, 81, 84, 121–122, 276, 287, 420, 450

metabolic syndrome 396

metaplastic meningioma 284, 291

metastasis 40–41, 45–46, 48, 182–183, 185, 193, 197, 204–206, 208, 210–212, 219, 225, 231–232, 234, 237, 239, 252, 255, 282, 293, 304–305, 316, 320, 325, 335, 337, 340, 343–344, 347–348, 418–419, 421–422, 457, 464, 467, 470, 477, 482

met-enkephalin 281

methylome 9–10, 12–13, 16, 26–27, 37, 86, 99, 103, 197, 238, 297, 322, 352

MGMT 22, 33, 44, 54–55, 72, 75–76, 93, 154, 352, 355, 414

MIB1 13, 33–35, 52, 82, 102, 151–152, 157–158, 216–217, 227, 257, 309, 414

microcalcification 33, 36, 50, 116–117, 128, 131, 134, 137, 145, 153–154, 244

microcystic meningioma 284, 290

microcystic/reticular schwannoma 261, 264

microRNA 9–10, 229, 231, 251, 280, 324, 402, 415, 465

microvascular proliferation 18, 21, 24–27, 29, 31–35, 37–39, 42, 45–49, 51, 53–54,

58, 60, 63, 66–68, 71, 75, 80, 82, 87, 96, 101, 107, 113, 120, 131, 141–142, 151, 154, 157, 162, 170, 173, 176, 180–181, 184, 237

miR-17-92 229

miR-19 354

miR-21 354

miR-30 354

miR-92a 354

miR-302 384

miR-335 384

miR-371-3 384

miR-654-3p 384

MIRLET7BHG 229

mismatch repair 20, 23–24, 30, 40, 44, 46–47, 70, 78, 80, 203, 216, 297, 420, 423–424, 428, 452–455

missense 27, 30–31, 37, 44, 73–75, 97, 104, 106, 125–126, 157, 269, 308, 324–325, 352, 355, 416, 428, 433, 438, 442, 448, 450, 458, 463–466, 475–477, 482

MITF 319, 347

MLH1 23–24, 44, 409, 420, 452–454

MLL 44

MLLT10 286

MMP2 49, 360

MMP9 49, 360

MMP16 58

MN1 9, 107–110, 128, 237

MNF116 281

moesin 431

monosomy 42, 109, 127–129, 176, 200, 203–204, 286, 297, 340, 345, 347–348, 461

mosaic neurofibromatosis type 1 426

MSA 316, 319

MSH 416

MSH2 44, 78, 409, 414, 420, 452–454

MSH6 44, 78, 409, 414, 420, 452–454

mTOR, MTOR 41, 43, 100–103, 114, 147, 266, 342, 380, 384, 427, 432, 442–443, 445

MTR 352

MU213-UC 404

MUC4 319

MUC5AC 320

mucin 33, 184

multinodular and vacuolating neuronal tumour 9, 13, 15–16, 114, 116, 118, **143–145**

multiple endocrine neoplasia type 2 468

MYB 9, 35, 37, 56–61, 67, 114–115, 125, 128

MYBL1 9, 35, 37, 56–58, 67, 114–115

MYC 23, 32, 38, 52, 54–55, 76, 181, 200, 202, 211–212, 219, 223, 242, 249–251,

352–353, 355

MYCL 206

MYCN 9, 23, 27, 52, 54–55, 71, 75–80, 150, 159, 177, 179–182, 200, 206–211, 448, 473

MYD88 250, 252, 254, 264

myelin-associated glycoprotein (MAG) 35

myelin basic protein (MBP) 35

myelin proteolipid protein (PLP) 35

myelodysplastic syndrome 478

MYO5A 239

MYO9B 229

MYOD1 316, 319, 330

myogenin 315–316, 319, 324, 330

myoglobin 319

myxoid glioneuronal tumour 9, 13, 15–16, 125, 136–138

myxoma 462–463

myxopapillary ependymoma 15, 159–160, 177, 179, **183–185**, 281

N

NAB2 10, 301–305, 324, 331

NADP+ 22

naevoid basal cell carcinoma syndrome (Gorlin syndrome) 200, 202, 205, 215, 285, 315, 423, **458–459**

naevus of Ota 344

NANOG 386

napsin A 420

National Comprehensive Cancer Network (NCCN) 449, 451

NBN 200

NBS1 See NBN

NCOA2 316, 328, 330–331

nestin 53, 102, 230, 405, 444

NeuN 35, 63, 85, 102–103, 113–114, 116–117, 120, 124–125, 128, 131, 134, 141, 145, 147, 151, 154, 157–158, 217–218, 230, 236–237, 247, 327, 443

neuroblastoma 10, 13, 114, 128, 182, 199, 213, 220, 232–234, 239, 328, 414, 419, 468

neuroblastoma, FOXR2-activated 10, 13, 199, 232–234

neurocutaneous melanosis 341–343, 346

NeuroD1 407

neurofibroma 259, **265–268**, 271–272, 277–278, 288, 424, 426–428, 431–432, 435–436, 468, 471–472

neurofibroma/perineurioma 271, 272

neurofibroma/schwannoma 271, 272, 424, 436

neurofibromatosis-Noonan syndrome 426

neurofibromatosis type 1 20, 40, 59, 65, 83–84, 90, 96, 101, 111, 123, 133, 260,

thyrotroph adenoma/PitNET 407, 411
TIA1 369
Tinea capitis 285
tissue factor (TF) 42
TLE1 303, 324
TMEM127 468
TNF-α 286
TNFAIP3 363–364
TNFRSF16 See p75-NGFR
toll-like receptor 350, 352
TOP2A 33
TOP2B 187
toxoplasmosis 356
TP53 10, 19–23, 26–27, 35–36, 40, 42–43,
    47–49, 54, 61, 64, 70–71, 73, 75, 78–79,
    96, 106, 122, 157, 191, 195, 197, 200–210,
    218–219, 230, 276, 302, 324, 326–327,
    407, 427, 446–448, 453, 465, 479, 481
TPIT 407–410, 412
TRAF7 10, 269, 284, 286, 288, 290,
    296–297, 324
transitional meningioma 284, 289
transthyretin 191–192, 194, 196–197, 254
TRH 463
trichorhinophalangeal syndrome type 1 186
trilateral retinoblastoma syndrome 252
trisomy 42, 176, 191, 384
triton tumour 277
TRPM3 190
TRPS1 186–187
truncating 31–32, 44, 325, 433, 435, 448,
    458, 461, 464, 475
TSC 100–101, 443, 445

TSH 393, 411–412
TSH-β 407
TTR 253
TTYH1 229, 231
tuberin 101–103, 442–444
tuberous sclerosis 100, 103, 336, 409,
    423–425, **441–445**
TUJ1 102
tumour-associated macrophage 41–42
Turcot syndrome 425, 452, 456
TWIST 49
tyrosinase 222, 224, 227, 274
tyrosine hydroxylase 414, 469

U

ubiquitin ligase 311, 432, 435, 439
ultrahypermutation 452–453, 455
unclassified plurihormonal tumour 407
USF3 147, 451
USP8 407, 410
USP8-related syndrome 409
USP48 407
UTF1 386, 388

V

vascular malformation 430
VATER/VACTERL association 450
VE1 97, 113, 115, 121
VEGF 42, 106, 311
VEGF-A, VEGFA 439
vemurafenib 112
Verocay body 261, 263–264, 272, 431
VGLL2 316

VHL 285, 310–313, 437–440, 468, 470
vimentin 25, 53, 105, 117, 152, 178, 192,
    224, 227, 230, 233, 237, 239, 254, 287,
    319, 347, 402–404, 444
Virchow–Robin space 120, 140, 255, 325,
    341, 343, 363, 431
von Hippel–Lindau syndrome 310, 313,
    423–424, **437–440**, 468, 470
von Willebrand factor 313

W

Warburg metabolic phenotype 183
Wishart phenotype 429, 433
Wiskott–Aldrich syndrome 356
WNT 10, 150, 200–204, 211–212, 236, 251,
    273, 394, 432, 456
WT1 321–322, 420
WWP1 147, 450–451

Y

YAP1 9, 13, 15, 17, 159, 161–163, 167–168,
    206, 209, 212, 218, 237, 286, 296, 346,
    461
yolk sac tumour 382–383, 386, 388–390
YY1 477

Z

ZFHX4 253
ZFTA 9, 14–15, 35, 109, 159, 161–166, 237
ZIC1 211
ZMYM3 200, 211

The World Health Organization Classification of Tumours

Urinary system and male genital organs
Moch H, Humphrey PA, Ulbright TM, et al., editors. WHO classification of tumours of the urinary system and male genital organs. Lyon (France): International Agency for Research on Cancer; 2016. (WHO classification of tumours series, 4th ed.; vol. 8). https://publications.iarc.fr/540.

Head and neck
El-Naggar AK, Chan JKC, Grandis JR, et al., editors. WHO classification of head and neck tumours. Lyon (France): International Agency for Research on Cancer; 2017. (WHO classification of tumours series, 4th ed.; vol. 9). https://publications.iarc.fr/548.

Endocrine organs
Lloyd RV, Osamura RY, Klöppel G, et al., editors. WHO classification of tumours of endocrine organs. Lyon (France): International Agency for Research on Cancer; 2017. (WHO classification of tumours series, 4th ed.; vol. 10). https://publications.iarc.fr/554.

Haematopoietic and lymphoid tissues
Swerdlow SH, Campo E, Harris NL, et al., editors. WHO classification of tumours of haematopoietic and lymphoid tissues. Lyon (France): International Agency for Research on Cancer; 2017. (WHO classification of tumours series, 4th rev. ed.; vol. 2). https://publications.iarc.fr/556.

Skin
Elder DE, Massi D, Scolyer RA, et al., editors. WHO classification of skin tumours. Lyon (France): International Agency for Research on Cancer; 2018. (WHO classification of tumours series, 4th ed.; vol. 11). https://publications.iarc.fr/560.

Eye
Grossniklaus HE, Eberhart CG, Kivelä TT, editors. WHO classification of tumours of the eye. Lyon (France): International Agency for Research on Cancer; 2018. (WHO classification of tumours series, 4th ed.; vol. 12). https://publications.iarc.fr/561.

Digestive system
WHO Classification of Tumours Editorial Board. Digestive system tumours. Lyon (France): International Agency for Research on Cancer; 2019. (WHO classification of tumours series, 5th ed.; vol. 1). https://publications.iarc.fr/579.

Breast
WHO Classification of Tumours Editorial Board. Breast tumours. Lyon (France): International Agency for Research on Cancer; 2019. (WHO classification of tumours series, 5th ed.; vol. 2). https://publications.iarc.fr/581.

Soft tissue and bone
WHO Classification of Tumours Editorial Board. Soft tissue and bone tumours. Lyon (France): International Agency for Research on Cancer; 2020. (WHO classification of tumours series, 5th ed.; vol. 3). https://publications.iarc.fr/588.

Female genital tract
WHO Classification of Tumours Editorial Board. Female genital tumours. Lyon (France): International Agency for Research on Cancer; 2020. (WHO classification of tumours series, 5th ed.; vol. 4). https://publications.iarc.fr/592.

Thorax
WHO Classification of Tumours Editorial Board. Thoracic tumours. Lyon (France): International Agency for Research on Cancer; 2021. (WHO classification of tumours series, 5th ed.; vol. 5). https://publications.iarc.fr/595.

Central nervous system
WHO Classification of Tumours Editorial Board. Central nervous system tumours. Lyon (France): International Agency for Research on Cancer; 2021. (WHO classification of tumours series, 5th ed.; vol. 6). https://publications.iarc.fr/601.

WHO Classification of Tumours Online
The content of this renowned classification series is now also available in a convenient digital format:
https://tumourclassification.iarc.who.int